SAUNDERS

COMPREHENSIVE REVIEW FOR THE

NCLEX-PN®

EXAMINATION

SAUNDERS

COMPREHENSIVE REVIEW FOR THE

NCLEX-PN®

EXAMINATION

8 EDITION

AUTHORS

LINDA ANNE SILVESTRI, PHD, RN, FAAN

Nursing Instructor, School of Nursing
University of Nevada, Las Vegas
Las Vegas, Nevada

President
Nursing Reviews, Inc. and Professional Nursing Seminars, Inc.
Henderson, Nevada

Elsevier
Next Generation NCLEX® (NGN) Thought Leader

ANGELA ELIZABETH SILVESTRI, PHD, APRN, FNP-BC, CNE

Assistant Professor **and BSN Program Director**
University of Nevada, Las Vegas
Las Vegas, Nevada

President
Nurse Prep, LLC
Henderson, Nevada

ASSOCIATE EDITORS

ALENA GREWAL, MSN, APRN, FNP-BC

Nursing Instructor, School of Nursing
University of Nevada, Las Vegas
Las Vegas, Nevada

EILEEN H. GRAY, DNP, RN, CPNP

Nursing Instructor, School of Nursing
University of Nevada, Las Vegas
Las Vegas, Nevada

Consultant and Reviewer
Nursing Reviews, Inc.
Henderson, Nevada

ELSEVIER

Elsevier
3251 Riverport Lane
St. Louis, Missouri 63043

SAUNDERS COMPREHENSIVE REVIEW FOR THE NCLEX-PN®
EXAMINATION, EIGHTH EDITION

ISBN: 978-0-323-73305-2

Notice

Practitioners and researchers must always rely on their own experience and knowledge in evaluating
and using any information, methods, compounds or experiments described herein. Because of rapid
advances in the medical sciences, in particular, independent verification of diagnoses and drug dosages
should be made. To the fullest extent of the law, no responsibility is assumed by Elsevier, authors, editors
or contributors for any injury and/or damage to persons or property as a matter of products liability,
negligence or otherwise, or from any use or operation of any methods, products, instructions, or ideas
contained in the material herein.

Previous editions copyrighted 2019, 2016, 2013, 2010, 2008, 2005, 2002, and 1999.

NCLEX®, NCLEX-RN®, and NCLEX-PN® are registered trademarks of the National Council of State Boards of
Nursing, Inc.

Library of Congress Control Number: 2020944772

Content Strategist: Heather Bays-Petrovic
Senior Content Development Specialist: Melissa Rawe
Publishing Services Manager: Julie Eddy
Senior Project Manager: Cindy Thoms
Design Direction: Amy Buxton

Printed in India

Last digit is the print number: 9 8 7 6 5 4 3 2 1

Working together
to grow libraries in
developing countries

www.elsevier.com • www.bookaid.org

To All Future Licensed Practical Nurses,

Congratulations to you!

You should be very proud of yourself for your most recent, well-deserved accomplishment of completing your nursing program to become a licensed practical nurse. We know that you have worked very hard to become successful and that you have proven to yourself that indeed you can achieve your goals.

In our opinion, you are about to enter the most wonderful and rewarding profession that exists. Your willingness, desire, and ability to assist those who need nursing care will bring great satisfaction to your life. In the profession of nursing, your learning will be a lifelong process. This aspect of the profession makes it stimulating and dynamic. Your learning process will continue to expand and grow as the profession continues to evolve. Your next very important endeavor will be the learning process involved to achieve success on your examination to become a licensed practical nurse.

We are excited and pleased to be able to provide you with the Saunders Pyramid to Success products, which will help you prepare for this important professional goal. We want to thank all of our former nursing students whom we have assisted in their studies for the NCLEX-PN® exam for their willingness to offer ideas regarding their needs in preparing for licensure. Student ideas have certainly added a special uniqueness to all of the products available in the Saunders Pyramid to Success.

Saunders Pyramid to Success products provide you with everything you need to prepare yourself for the NCLEX-PN exam. These products include material that is required for the NCLEX-PN exam for all nursing students regardless of educational background, specific strengths, areas in need of improvement, or clinical experience during the nursing program.

So let's get started and begin our journey through the Saunders Pyramid to Success! Welcome to the wonderful profession of nursing!

Sincerely,
Linda Anne Silvestri, PhD, RN, FAAN
Angela Elizabeth Silvestri, PhD, APRN, FNP-BC CNE

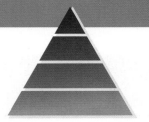

About the Authors

Linda Anne Silvestri

(Photo by Laurent W. Valliere.)

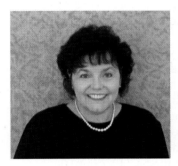

As a child, I always dreamed of becoming either a nurse or a teacher. Initially, I chose to become a nurse because I really wanted to help others, especially those who were ill. Then I realized that both of my dreams could come true: I could be both a nurse and a teacher. So I pursued my dreams.

I received my diploma in nursing at Cooley Dickinson Hospital School of Nursing in Northampton, Massachusetts. Afterward, I worked at Baystate Medical Center in Springfield, Massachusetts, where I cared for clients in acute medical-surgical units, the intensive care unit, the emergency department, pediatric units, and other acute care units. Later, I received an associate degree from Holyoke Community College in Holyoke, Massachusetts, my BSN from American International College in Springfield, Massachusetts, and my MSN from Anna Maria College in Paxton, Massachusetts, with a dual major in Nursing Management and Patient Education. I received my PhD in Nursing from the University of Nevada, Las Vegas (UNLV), and conducted and published research on self-efficacy and the predictors of NCLEX success. In 2012, I received the UNLV School of Nursing, Alumna of the Year Award. I am a member of the Honor Society of Nursing, Sigma Theta Tau International, Phi Kappa Phi, the Western Institute of Nursing, the Eastern Nursing Research Society, the Golden Key International Honour Society, the National League for Nursing, and the American Nurses Association. Additionally, I am a Fellow in the American Academy of Nursing.

As a native of Springfield, Massachusetts, I began my teaching career as an instructor of medical-surgical nursing and leadership-management nursing in 1981 at Baystate Medical Center School of Nursing. In 1989, I relocated to Rhode Island and began teaching advanced medical-surgical nursing and psychiatric nursing to RN and LPN students at the Community College of Rhode Island. While teaching there, a group of students approached me for assistance in preparing for the NCLEX examination. I have always had a very special interest in test success for nursing students because of my own personal experiences with testing. Taking tests was never easy for me, and as a student I needed to find methods and strategies that would bring success. My own difficult experiences, desire, and dedication to assist nursing students to overcome the obstacles associated with testing inspired me to develop and write the many products that would foster success with testing. My experiences as a student, nursing educator, and item writer for the NCLEX exams aided me as I developed a comprehensive review course to prepare nursing graduates for the NCLEX examination.

Later, in 1994, I began teaching medical-surgical nursing at Salve Regina University in Newport, Rhode Island. I also prepared nursing students at Salve Regina University for the NCLEX examination. Currently, I am a part-time nursing instructor at the University of Nevada, Las Vegas—Las Vegas, Nevada. I am the President of Nursing Reviews, Inc. established in 2000, and Professional Nursing Seminars, Inc. established in 1991. Both companies are located in Henderson, Nevada and are dedicated to helping nursing graduates achieve their goals of becoming registered nurses, licensed practical/vocational nurses, or both.

Today, I am the successful author of numerous NCLEX review products published by Elsevier and I am passionate about assisting nursing students with achieving success. Also, I work with Elsevier as a Thought Leader for the Next Generation NCLEX® (NGN). I am so pleased that you have decided to join us on your journey to success in testing for nursing examinations and for the NCLEX examination!

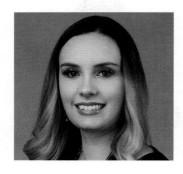

Angela Elizabeth Silvestri

When asked what I wanted to do with my life and as a career, I always answered that I wanted to work in the medical field. At first my ambition was to become a physician; however, learning that nurses interact with their patients more often than physicians do swayed me to pursue nursing. While in nursing school, I worked as a tutor for my peers. I realized how much I enjoyed doing this and how much of a difference my help made in these students' college careers and ultimately their lives.

I received my baccalaureate degree in Nursing and Sociology at Salve Regina University in Newport, Rhode Island. After earning my degree, I worked in long-term care, rehabilitation, and acute care settings. I then went on to earn my master's degree and PhD in nursing, and published the findings related to cultural competence in the curriculum. I completed my family nurse practitioner post-master's graduate certificate program and am practicing as a family nurse practitioner on a college campus. I am a member of the Nevada Nurses Association, Sigma Theta Tau International, and Golden Key International Honour Society. I am an assistant professor and the BSN Program Director at the University of Nevada, Las Vegas, and teach the transition to practice and leadership in nursing course, focusing on preparation for NCLEX. My short-term goals include conducting research focused on nursing education and nursing student success to help students transition to successful nurses in practice.

Working with students while having been a student for quite some time helped me understand and realize the individual needs of each student. This experience, in addition to my experience in item writing and other contributions to nursing textbooks, has helped me co-author this text. I am very excited to be a part of this opportunity to further assist nursing students in their ultimate goal: passing nursing school and the NCLEX exam!

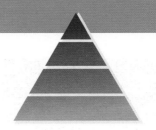

Contributors and Reviewers

Associate Editors

Alena Grewal, MSN, APRN, FNP-BC
Nursing Instructor, School of Nursing
University of Nevada, Las Vegas
Las Vegas, Nevada

Eileen H. Gray, DNP, RN, CPNP
Nursing Instructor, School of Nursing
University of Nevada, Las Vegas
Las Vegas, Nevada;
Consultant and Reviewer
Nursing Reviews, Inc.
Henderson, Nevada

Consultants

Dianne E. Fiorentino
Research Coordinator
Nursing Reviews, Inc.
Henderson, Nevada

James Guilbault, BS, PharmD Jr.
Rite Aid Pharmacy
Greenfield, Massachusetts;
Mercy Medical Center
Springfield, Massachusetts

Contributors

Alena Grewal, MSN, APRN, FNP-BC
Nursing Instructor, School of Nursing
University of Nevada, Las Vegas
Las Vegas, Nevada

Eileen H. Gray, DNP, RN, CPNP
Nursing Instructor, School of Nursing
University of Nevada, Las Vegas

Las Vegas, Nevada;
Consultant and Reviewer
Nursing Reviews, Inc.
Henderson, Nevada

Kristen Hickey, RN, BSN
Graduate, Salve Regina University
Newport, Rhode Island

Karen Machnacz, LPN
Greenfield Community College
Greenfield, Massachusetts

Gabrielle Machnacz, LPN
Greenfield Community College
Greenfield, Massachusetts

Katherine M. Silvestri, BSN, RN
Editorial and Reviewer Consultant
Nursing Reviews, Inc.
Henderson, Nevada

Bethany Sykes, EdD, RN, CEN, CCRN
Adjunct Faculty
Department of Nursing
Salve Regina University
Newport, Rhode Island

Laurent W. Valliere, BS, DD
Vice President
Nursing Reviews, Inc.
Henderson, Nevada;
Eastern New Mexico University
Alumni
Portales, New Mexico

The authors would like to acknowledge the following individuals who contributed to previous editions of this resource.

Barbara Callahan, MEd, BSN, RN, NCC, CHSE
Retired ADN Faculty
ADN Program
Health Sciences Department
Lenoir Community College
Kinston, North Carolina

Margie Francisco, EdD, MSN, RN
Nursing Professor, Health Division
Illinois Valley Community College
Oglesby, Illinois

Louise S. Frantz, MHA, Ed, BSN, RN
Program Coordinator, Practical
Nursing
Penn State Berks
Reading, Pennsylvania

Eileen H. Gray, DNP, RN, CPNP
Nursing Instructor, School of Nursing
University of Nevada, Las Vegas
Las Vegas, Nevada;
Consultant and Reviewer
Nursing Reviews, Inc.
Henderson, Nevada

Joyce Hammer, RN, MSN
Adjunct Faculty, Nursing
Monroe County Community College
Monroe, Michigan

David Petersen, BSN, RN
Adjunct Faculty, Department of
Nursing
Estrella Mountain Community College
Avondale, Arizona;
Visiting Professor
Chamberlain College of Nursing
Phoenix, Arizona

Karen Petersen, BSN, RN
Clinical Faculty, Nursing
Maricopa Community College District
Phoenix, Arizona

Jennifer Ponto, RN, BSN
Faculty, Vocational Nursing
South Plains College
Levelland, Texas

Russlyn Ann St. John, MSN, RN
Professor, Nursing & Allied Health
St. Charles Community College
Cottleville, Missouri

Bethany Sykes, EdD, RN, CEN, CCRN
Adjunct Faculty, Department of
Nursing
Salve Regina University
Newport, Rhode Island

Laurent W. Valliere, BS, DD
Vice President
Nursing Reviews, Inc.
Henderson, Nevada;
Eastern New Mexico University
Alumni
Portales, New Mexico

Michelle Willihnganz, MS, RN, CNE
Nursing Instructor
Rochester Community and Technical
College
Rochester, Minnesota

Donna Elise Wilsker, MSN, BSN
Assistant Professor
Dishman Department of Nursing
Lamar University
Beaumont, Texas

Reviewers

Linda F. Gambill, RN, MSN/Ed, ENPC
Instructor/Clinical Coordinator,
Nursing
Southwest Virginia Community
College
Cedar Bluff, Virginia

Melanie Gray, MSN, BSN, RN
Faculty
Milwaukee Area Technical College
School of Nursing
Associate Degree Program
Milwaukee, Wisconsin

Alice M. Hupp, BS, RN
Vocational Nursing Instructor
Vocational Nursing
North Central Texas College
Gainesville, Texas

David Petersen, BSN, RN
Adjunct Faculty, Department of
Nursing
Estrella Mountain Community College
Avondale, Arizona;
Visiting Professor
Chamberlain College of Nursing
Phoenix, Arizona

Karen Petersen, BSN, RN
Clinical Faculty, Nursing
Maricopa Community College District
Phoenix, Arizona

Claudia Stoffel, MSN, RN, CNE
Professor and Practical Nursing
Program Coordinator, Nursing
West Kentucky Community and
Technical College
Paducah, Kentucky

Elaine Kay Strouss, MSN, RN, CNE
Professor–Coordinator for the PN
Program and First Year of the ADN
Program
Nursing
Community College of Beaver County
Monaca, Pennsylvania

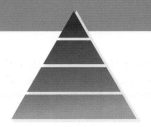

Preface

To laugh often and much, to appreciate beauty, to find the best in others, to leave the world a bit better, to know that even one life has breathed easier because you have lived, this is to have succeeded.

Ralph Waldo Emerson

Welcome to Saunders *Pyramid to Success!*

An Essential Resource for Test Success

Saunders Comprehensive Review for the NCLEX-PN® Examination is one in a series of products designed to assist you in achieving your goal of becoming a licensed practical nurse. This text provides you with a comprehensive review of all of the nursing content areas specifically related to the new 2020 test plan for the NCLEX-PN examination, which is implemented by the National Council of State Boards of Nursing. This resource will help you achieve success on your nursing examinations during nursing school and on the NCLEX-PN examination.

Organization

This book contains 19 units and 65 chapters. The chapters are designed to identify specific components of nursing content, and they contain practice questions, including multiple-choice and alternate item formats that reflect the chapter content and the 2020 test plan for the NCLEX-PN exam.

The test plan identifies a framework based on *Client Needs*. These Client Needs categories include Safe and Effective Care Environment, Health Promotion and Maintenance, Psychosocial Integrity, and Physiological Integrity. *Integrated Processes* are also identified as a component of the test plan. These include Caring, Communication and Documentation, Culture and Spirituality, Nursing Process (Clinical Problem-Solving Process), and Teaching and Learning. All chapters address the components of the test plan framework.

Special Features of the Book

Pyramid Terms

Pyramid Terms are important to the discussion of the content in the chapters of the unit. Therefore they are in bold green type throughout the content section of each chapter. In addition, these *Pyramid Terms* are defined and located in the Glossary in the backmatter of this book.

Pyramid to Success

The *Pyramid to Success*, a feature part of the unit introduction, provides you with an overview, guidance, and direction regarding the focus of review in the particular content area, as well as the content areas of relative importance to the 2020 test plan for the NCLEX-PN exam. The *Pyramid to Success* reviews the Client Needs as they pertain to the content in that unit or chapter; in addition Learning Objectives are provided. These points identify the specific test plan components to keep in mind as you review the chapter.

Priority Concepts

Each chapter identifies two *Priority Concepts* reflective of its content. These *Priority Concepts* will assist you to focus on the important aspects of the content and associated nursing interventions.

Pyramid Points

Pyramid Points are the little icons that are placed next to specific content throughout the chapters. The *Pyramid Points* highlight content that is important for preparing for the NCLEX-PN examination and identify content that typically appears on the NCLEX-PN examination.

Pyramid Alerts

Pyramid Alerts are the red text found throughout the chapters that alert you to important nursing information. These alerts identify content that typically appears on the NCLEX-PN examination.

Priority Nursing Actions

Numerous *Priority Nursing Actions* boxes have been placed throughout the chapters. These boxes present a clinical nursing situation and the priority actions to take in the event of its occurrence.

"What Would You Do?" Questions

Each chapter begins with a "What Would You Do?" Question. These questions provide a brief clinical scenario related to the content of the chapter and ask you what you would do about the client situation presented. A narrative answer and its location is provided.

Special Features Found on Evolve

Pretest, Post-Test, and Study Calendar

The accompanying Evolve site contains a 75-question pretest and post-test that provide you with feedback on your strengths and weaknesses. The results of your pretest will generate an individualized study calendar to guide you in your preparation for the NCLEX-PN examination.

Heart and Lung Sound Questions

The accompanying Evolve site contains *Audio Questions* representative of content addressed in the 2020 test plan for the NCLEX-PN exam. These questions are in NCLEX-style format, and each question presents an audio sound as a component of the question.

Audio Review Summaries

The companion Evolve site includes three Audio Review Summaries that cover challenging subject areas under the 2020 NCLEX-PN test plan, including Pharmacology, Acid-Base Balance, and Fluids and Electrolytes.

Next Generation NCLEX® (NGN) Case Studies and NGN Test Questions

The accompanying Evolve site contains single-episode case studies and unfolding case studies. These case studies are accompanied by NGN test questions representative of the NGN testing format. The single episode case studies are accompanied by one NGN test question that measures one of the cognitive skills of the NCSBN Clinical Judgment Measurement Model (NCJMM). The unfolding case studies are accompanied by 6 NGN test questions and the questions measure all six cognitive skills of the NCJMM. These cognitive skills include Recognize Cue, Analyze Cues, Prioritize Hypotheses, Generate Solutions, Take Action, and Evaluate Outcomes.

Practice Questions

While preparing for the NCLEX-PN examination, it is crucial for students to practice answering test questions. This book contains 730 NCLEX-style multiple-choice and alternate item format questions. The accompanying software includes all the questions from the book, plus additional new Evolve questions for a total of more than 4600 questions. Both multiple choice and alternate item formats are included. The alternate item format questions in the book and on the accompanying Evolve site may be presented as one of the following:

Fill-in-the-blank question
Multiple response (select all that apply) question
Priority Order (ordered response) question, also known as a drag-and-drop question
Figure/chart question
Graphic options question, in which each option contains a figure or illustration
Hot spot question
Audio question that includes a heart or lung sound
NGN® Case Studies and NGN test questions

These questions provide you with practice in prioritizing, decision-making and critical thinking, and strengthen your clinical judgment skills. In addition, each practice question provides a review button that links you to common laboratory values for your reference while studying on the Evolve site.

Multiple-Choice and Alternate Item Format Questions

Starting with Unit II, each chapter is followed by a practice test. Each practice test contains several questions reflective of the content of the chapter and those presented on the NCLEX-PN examination.

These questions provide you with practice in prioritizing, decision-making, and clinical judgment skills. Chapter 1 of this book provides a description of each question type and the answer section for the Evolve questions. The answer section includes the correct answer, rationale, test-taking strategy, and question categories. The question categories identified with each practice question include Level of Cognitive Ability, Client Needs, Integrated Process, Clinical Judgment/Cognitive Skill, the specific nursing Content Area, Health Problem, and Priority Concepts. Every question on the accompanying Evolve site is organized by these question codes, so you can customize your study session to be as specific or as generic as you need.

Following each practice question, a rationale for both the correct and incorrect options is provided. Additionally, a specific test-taking strategy is provided that will assist in answering the question correctly. The specific test-taking strategy is highlighted in bold blue type. The specific test-taking strategy and the Content Area and Health Problem categories will provide you with guidance on what topics to review for further remediation in *Saunders Strategies for Test Success: Passing Nursing School and the NCLEX® Exam, Saunders Comprehensive Review for the NCLEX-PN® Exam*, and *Saunders Q&A Review for the NCLEX-PN® Exam*.

Pharmacology and Medication Calculations Review

Students consistently state that pharmacology is an area with which they need assistance. The 2020 NCLEX-PN test plan continues to incorporate pharmacology in the examination, but only generic drug names will be included. Therefore pharmacology chapters have been included for your review and practice. This book includes 13 pharmacology chapters, a medication and intravenous calculation chapter, and a pediatric medication calculation chapter. Each of these chapters is followed by a practice test that uses the same question format described earlier. This book contains numerous pharmacology questions. Additionally, more than 675 pharmacology questions can be found on the accompanying Evolve site.

Next Generation NCLEX® (NGN) Questions

The NCSBN is currently piloting research questions for a project known as the "Next Generation NCLEX." An NCLEX candidate may encounter these questions once they complete their examination, and they will have the option to answer these questions as part of NCSBN's research on these new item types. The NCSBN is currently aiming to launch the NGN questions on the examination in 2023, and these item types are designed to test the candidate's ability to make safe and competent clinical judgments. This resource includes NGN item types, and although these item types are not live on the NCLEX now, practicing these questions will assist the current candidate in preparing for the NCLEX examination. The NGN questions are located on the Evolve site.

How to Use This Book

Saunders Comprehensive Review for the NCLEX-PN® Examination is especially designed to help you with your successful journey to the peak of the Saunders *Pyramid to Success:* becoming a licensed practical nurse. As you begin your journey through this book, you will be introduced to all the important points regarding the 2020 NCLEX-PN examination, the process of testing, and unique and special tips regarding how to prepare yourself for this very important examination.

You should begin your process through the Saunders *Pyramid to Success* by reading Chapter 1 and becoming familiar with the central points regarding the NCLEX-PN examination. Chapter 1 is titled "Clinical Judgment and the NCLEX-PN® Examination". It addresses information about clinical judgment and the related cognitive skills as defined by the National Council of State Boards of Nursing (NCSBN) and all of the information related to the NCLEX-PN test plan and the examination testing procedures. This chapter answers all of the questions that you may have regarding this information. Chapter 2 is an important chapter that presents nonacademic test preparation such as techniques to control anxiety and other strategies. Read Chapter 3, which was written by nursing graduates who recently passed the examination, and note what they have to say about the testing experience. Chapter 4, "Clinical Judgment and Test-Taking Strategies", includes information about using clinical judgment and the six cognitive skills to answer questions and all of the strategies that will assist in teaching you how to read a question, how not to read into a question, and how to use the process of elimination and various other strategies to select the correct response from the options presented. Continue on your journey by studying the specific content areas addressed in Units II through XIX. Review the definitions of the *Pyramid Terms* located in the Glossary and the *Pyramid to Success* notes, and identify the Client Needs and Learning Objectives specific to the test plan in each area. Read through the chapters, and focus on the *Pyramid Points* and *Pyramid Alerts* that identify the areas most likely to be tested on the NCLEX-PN examination. Pay particular attention to the *Priority Nursing Actions* boxes because they provide information about the steps that you will take in clinical situations requiring prioritization.

As you read each chapter, identify your areas of strength and those in need of further review. Highlight these areas, and test your abilities by taking all the practice tests provided at the end of the chapters. Be sure to review all the rationales and the test-taking strategies.

In preparation for the NCLEX, be sure to take the pretest on the Evolve site and generate your study calendar. Follow the calendar for your review because the calendar represents your pretest results and the best study path to follow based on your strong and weak content areas. Then, when you feel ready, take the posttest on the Evolve site. Also, be sure to access the Audio Review Summaries as part of your preparation for the NCLEX.

Climbing the Pyramid to Success

The purpose of this book is to provide a **comprehensive review** of the nursing content you will be tested on during the NCLEX-PN examination. However, *Saunders Comprehensive Review for the NCLEX-PN® Examination* is intended to do more than simply prepare you for the rigors of the NCLEX-PN. This book is also meant to serve as a valuable study tool that you can refer to throughout your nursing program, with customizable Evolve site selections to help identify and reinforce key content areas and prepare you for your nursing exams.

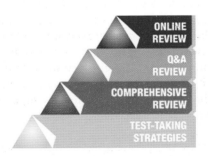

At the base of the *Pyramid to Success* is our **test-taking strategies** book, which provide a foundation for understanding and unpacking the complexities of NCLEX-PN exam questions, including alternate item formats. *Saunders Strategies for Test Success: Passing Nursing School and the NCLEX® Exam* takes a detailed look at all the test-taking strategies you will need to know to pass any nursing examination, including the NCLEX-PN. Special tips are integrated for nursing students, and there are more than 1200 practice questions included so you can apply the testing strategies.

The next important step in the Pyramid to Success is to get additional practice with a Q&A review product. *Saunders Q&A Review for the NCLEX-PN® Examination* offers more than 5700 unique practice questions in the book and on the companion Evolve site. The questions are focused on the Client Needs and Integrated Processes of the NCLEX test plan, making it easy to access your study area of choice.

For on-the-go Q&A review, you can pick up *Saunders Q&A Review Cards for the NCLEX-PN® Examination*, which features 1200 practice NCLEX-type questions spanning all content areas.

Your final step on the *Pyramid to Success* is to master the online review. *Saunders Online Review for the NCLEX-PN® Examination* provides an interactive and individualized platform to get you ready for your final licensure exam. This online course provides 10 high-level content modules, supplemented with instructional videos, animations, audio, illustrations, case studies, and several subject matter exams. End of module practice tests are provided along with several Crossing the Finish Line: Practice Tests, and two Test Yourself Quizzes. In addition, you can assess your progress with a pre-test and comprehensive exam in a computerized environment that prepares you for the actual NCLEX-PN exam.

To obtain any of these resources that will prepare you for your nursing exams and the NCLEX-PN exam, visit the Elsevier Health Sciences website at elsevierhealth.com.

Good luck with your journey through the Saunders *Pyramid to Success*. We wish you continued success throughout your new career as a licensed practical nurse!

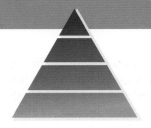

Acknowledgments

Sincere appreciation and warmest thanks are extended to the many individuals who in their own ways have contributed to the publication of this book.

First, we want to thank all of our nursing students who we have assisted to prepare to take the NCLEX examination. Their enthusiasm and inspiration led to the commencement of our professional endeavors in conducting review courses for the NCLEX exam for nursing students. We also thank the numerous nursing students who have attended our review courses for their willingness to share their needs and ideas. Their input has certainly added a special uniqueness to this publication.

We wish to acknowledge all the nursing faculty who taught in our NCLEX review courses. Their commitment, dedication, and expertise have certainly helped nursing students achieve success with the NCLEX exam. Additionally, we want to acknowledge and sincerely thank our husbands: Laurent (Larry) and Brent. We thank Laurent W. Valliere, or Larry, for his contribution to this publication, for teaching in our NCLEX review courses, and for his commitment and dedication in helping our nursing students prepare for the NCLEX from a nonacademic point of view.

From Linda: Larry has supported my many professional endeavors and was so loyal and loving to me each and every moment as I worked to achieve my professional goals. Larry, thank you so much - I love you!

From Angela: Brent has always been there to support me through anything and everything. He is generous and caring and knows how to make me laugh when I need it most. Brent, thank you and I love you!

A very special thank you also goes to Karen Machnacz, LPN and Gabrielle Machnacz, LPN, for writing a chapter for this book about their experiences preparing for and taking the NCLEX-PN examination. Thank you, Karen and Gabby!

We sincerely acknowledge and thank many very important individuals from Elsevier who are so dedicated to our work in creating NCLEX products for nursing students. We thank our former Senior Content Strategist, Jamie Blum, and our former Senior Content Development Specialist, Laura Goodrich, for their continuous assistance, enthusiasm, support, and expert professional guidance as we prepared our NCLEX-PN products over the past several years. We also thank Laurie Gower, Director, Content Development, for her expert ideas as we planned the project and for her continuous support through its production process.

And a very special and sincere thank you to Melissa Rawe, Senior Content Development Specialist. This was the first time Melissa worked with us on a project and we thank her for all of her hard work and willingness to learn about all of the complexities associated with the book and its production. Thank you, Melissa!!!

A very special thank you to Alena Grewal and Eileen Gray, our associate editors, who so expertly managed the editing of the entire book and Evolve site. We also want to acknowledge Bethany Sykes who reviewed all the chapters completed by Alena and Eileen and prepared them for the final production process. And, a special thank you to Lisa Nicolas who wrote many of the new practice questions added to this book. We especially want to thank Elodia Dianne Fiorentino for researching content for each practice question and for electronically adding our new practice questions; and James Guilbault for researching and updating medications. We thank Kristen Hickey for her initial work in coding the practice questions and Katie Silvestri for editing, formatting, and organizing manuscript files for us and coding practice questions. A very special thank you to all of you for providing continuous support and dedication to our work in preparing this publication and maintaining its excellent quality.

We also thank our team of helpers who assisted us with the many tasks needed to bring this project to fruition. We thank Gabby Machnacz, Brianna Machnacz, Karen Machnacz, Mary Silvestri, and Larry Silvestri. Their assistance and willingness to complete so many tasks for us and their loyalty and dedication to our success will never be forgotten. A big thank you to all of you.

We want to acknowledge all of the staff at Elsevier for their tremendous assistance throughout the preparation and production of this publication and all of the Elsevier staff involved in the publication of previous editions of this outstanding NCLEX review product. A special thank you to all of them. We thank all the important people in the Production department, including Cindy Thoms, Senior Project Manager; Julie Eddy, Publishing Services Manager; Bergen Farthing, Marketing Manager; and Amy Buxton, Designer, who all played such significant roles in finalizing this publication. We sincerely thank those in the marketing department who helped with the promotion of this book. And a special thank you to Kristin Green, Loren Wilson, Shelly Hayden, and Nancy O'Brien for their past years of expert guidance and continuous support for all the products in the *Pyramid to Success*. A sincere and very special thank you goes to Cindy Thoms, Senior Project Manager. Cindy has been fantastic. Her patience and complete support and her expertise has been greatly appreciated. We could not have done this without you Cindy! So a big thank you from both of us!

From Linda: I want to acknowledge my parents, who opened my door of opportunity in education. I thank my mother, Frances Mary, for all of her love, support, and assistance as I continuously worked to achieve my professional goals. I thank my father, Arnold Lawrence, who always provided insightful words of encouragement. My memories of their love and support will always remain in my heart. I am certain that they are very proud of my professional accomplishments. I also want to acknowledge my husband, Larry, for being there each and every moment supporting and encouraging me as I faced the many challenges in life that came my way. And, I thank my brother Lawrence Peter and my sister Dianne Elodia for their never-ending caring support they give me.

From Angela: I want to acknowledge my parents, Mary Elizabeth and Lawrence Peter, for their advice and support throughout the years. I would also like to acknowledge my husband and children, and my brother, Nicholas Lawrence, and sister, Katherine Silvestri. Their support has been monumental in my success.

We also thank all our family for being continuously supportive, giving, and helpful during our research and preparation of this publication.

We want to especially acknowledge each and every individual who contributed to this publication—our associate editors Alena and Eileen, our contributors, item writers, and updaters—for their expert input and ideas. We also thank the many faculty and student reviewers of the manuscript for their thoughts and ideas. A very special thank you to all of you!

Finally, we extend a very special thank you to all our nursing students, past, present, and future. All of you light up our lives! Your love and dedication to the profession of nursing and your commitment to provide health care will bring never-ending rewards!

Linda Anne Silvestri
Angela E. Silvestri

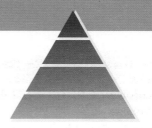

Contents

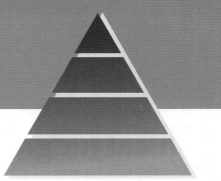

NCLEX-PN® Exam Preparation

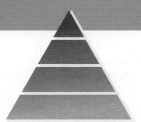

CHAPTER 1

NCLEX Preparation

Clinical Judgment and the NCLEX-PN® Examination

 The Pyramid to Success

Welcome to the Pyramid to Success

Saunders Comprehensive Review for the NCLEX-PN® Examination

Saunders Comprehensive Review for the NCLEX-PN® Examination is specially designed to help you begin your successful journey to the peak of the pyramid, becoming a licensed practical/vocational nurse. As you begin your journey, you will be introduced to all of the important points regarding the NCLEX-PN examination and the process of testing, and to the unique and special tips regarding how to prepare yourself for this important examination. You will read what two nursing graduates, a mother and daughter team who recently passed the NCLEX-PN examination, have to say about their tests. Important test-taking strategies are detailed. These details will guide you in selecting the correct option or assist you in selecting an answer to a question at which you must guess.

Each unit in this book begins with the Pyramid to Success. The Pyramid to Success addresses specific points related to the NCLEX-PN examination. Client Needs as identified in the test plan framework for the examination are listed, as well as learning objectives for the unit. Pyramid Terms are key words that are defined in the glossary at the end of the book and set in color throughout each chapter to direct your attention to significant points for the examination.

Throughout each chapter, you will find Pyramid Point bullets that identify areas most likely to be tested on the NCLEX-PN examination. Read each chapter, and identify your strengths and areas that are in need of further review. Test your strengths and abilities by answering all of the practice questions provided in this book and on the accompanying Evolve site. Be sure to read all of the rationales and test-taking strategies. The rationale provides you with significant information regarding the correct and incorrect options. The test-taking strategy provides you with the logical path to selecting the correct option. Each question on Evolve is coded on the basis of the Level of Cognitive Ability, the Client Needs category, Clinical Judgment/Cognitive skills code if applicable, the Integrated Process, Content Area, the Health Problem if applicable, and Priority Concepts.

Other Resources

Additional products in Saunders Pyramid to Success include *Saunders Q&A Review for the NCLEX-PN Examination, Saunders Strategies for Test Success: Passing Nursing School and the NCLEX Examination, Saunders Q&A Review Cards for the NCLEX-PN Examination*, and the *HESI/Saunders Online Review for the NCLEX-PN Examination*. Specific information about these ideal NCLEX preparation tools can be found in the preface of this book. You can visit the App Store and Google Play to locate the App for both this resource and the *Saunders Q&A Review for the NCLEX-PN® Examination*. Additionally, products in the Saunders Pyramid to Success can be obtained online by visiting http://elsevierhealth.com or by calling 1-800-545-2522.

Let's begin our journey through the Pyramid to Success.

Clinical Judgment and Next Generation NCLEX Items

Clinical judgment is the observed outcome of critical thinking and decision-making (Dickison, Haerling, & Lasater, 2019). There is heightened attention being paid to clinical judgment as a means of teaching, learning, assessment, and testing. The NCLEX-PN examination requires candidates to demonstrate the ability to use clinical judgment in the delivery of client care. Clinical judgment can also be used as a test-taking strategy to

TABLE 1.1   Cognitive Skills/Processes and Descriptions

Cognitive Skill/Process	Description
Recognize cues	Identifying significant data; data can be from many sources (assessment)
Analyze cues	Connecting data to the client's clinical presentation—determining if the data is expected? Unexpected? (analysis)
Prioritize hypotheses	Ranking hypotheses; what are the concerns or client needs/problems and their priority? (analysis)
Generate solutions	Using hypotheses to determine interventions for an expected outcome (planning)
Take action	Implementing the generated solutions addressing the highest priorities or hypotheses (implementation)
Evaluate outcomes	Comparing observed outcomes with expected ones (evaluation)

From Dickison, P., Haerling, K. A., & Lasater, K. (2019). Integrating the National Council of State Boards of Nursing Clinical Judgment Model into Nursing Educational Frameworks. *Journal of Nursing Education*, 58(2), 72–78.

TABLE 1.2   Next Generation NCLEX (NGN) Item Types and Descriptions

NGN Item Type	Description
Extended multiple response	Items allow candidates to select one or more answer options at a time. This item type is similar to the current NCLEX multiple response items but with more options, from 7 up to 10 options.
Extended drag and drop	Items allow candidates to move or place response options into answer spaces. This item type is like the current NCLEX ordered response items but it is possible that not all of the response options may be required to answer the item.
Cloze	Items allow candidates to select an option from a drop-down list. There can be more than 1 drop-down list in a cloze item. These drop-down lists can be used as words or phrases within a sentence, within tables, and/or charts.
Highlight	Items allow candidates to select their answer by highlighting predefined words or phrases. Candidates can select and deselect the highlighted parts by clicking on the words or phrases. These types of items allow an individual to read a portion of a client medical record, such as a nursing note, medical history, lab values, medication record, etc. and then select the words or phrases that answer the item.
Matrix	Items allow the candidate to select 1 answer option for each row and/or column. This item type can be useful in measuring multiple aspects of the clinical scenario with a single item.

From NCSBN. (Fall 2019). Next Generation NCLEX News: Approved NGN Item Types. Chicago: NCSBN.

answer test questions (refer to Chapter 4). The National Council of State Boards of Nursing (NCSBN) has created the NCSBN Clinical Judgment Measurement Model (NCJMM) that consists of applying 6 cognitive skills or processes. These include: (1) recognizing cues; (2) analyzing cues; (3) prioritizing hypotheses; (4) generating solutions; (5) taking action; and (6) evaluating outcomes (Dickison et al., 2019). Table 1.1 provides a description of these six cognitive skills/processes identified in the NCJMM. This model also serves as a guide for the NCSBN to create Next Generation NCLEX (NGN) questions. The NCJMM continues to evolve, as may the NGN item types that will be presented in the exam. Currently, the test items that will be used are extended multiple response, extended drag and drop, cloze, highlight, and matrix (Table 1.2). It is expected that the NGN test items will be scored items in the new test plan implemented in 2023. Some of these NGN item types can be found on the Evolve site accompanying this book. We highly encourage you to frequently access the NCSBN website at www.ncsbn.org for updates.

Examination Process

An important step in the Pyramid to Success is to become as familiar as possible with the examination process. Candidates facing the challenge of this examination can experience significant anxiety. Knowing what the examination is all about and knowing what you will encounter during the process of testing will assist in alleviating fear and anxiety. The information contained in this chapter was obtained from the NCSBN website

(http://www.ncsbn.org) and from the NCSBN 2020 test plan for the NCLEX-PN and includes some procedures related to registering for the examination, testing procedures, and the answers to the questions most commonly asked by nursing students and graduates preparing to take the NCLEX. You can obtain additional information regarding the test and its development by accessing the NCSBN website and clicking on the NCLEX and Other Exams tab or by writing to the National Council of State Boards of Nursing, 111 East Wacker Drive, Suite 2900, Chicago, IL 60601. You are encouraged to access the NCSBN website because this site provides you with valuable information about the NCLEX and other resources available to an NCLEX candidate.

Computer Adaptive Testing

The acronym *CAT* stands for computer adaptive test, which means that the examination is created as the test-taker answers each question. Test questions are categorized on the basis of the test plan structure and the level of difficulty of the question. As you answer a question, the computer determines your competency based on the answer you selected. If you selected a correct answer, the computer scans the question bank and selects a more difficult question. If you selected an incorrect answer, the computer scans the question bank and selects an easier question. This process continues until all test plan requirements are met and a reliable pass-or-fail decision is made.

When taking a CAT, once an answer is recorded, all subsequent questions administered depend, to an extent, on the answer selected for that question. Skipping and/or returning to earlier questions is not compatible with the logical methodology of a CAT. The inability to skip questions and/or go back to change previous answers will not be a disadvantage to you; you will not fall into that "trap" of changing a correct answer to an incorrect one with the CAT system.

If you are faced with a question that contains unfamiliar content, you may need to guess at the answer because the test will not move on until you answer the question on the computer screen. Although guessing is discouraged for any examination that you take, there is no penalty for guessing on this examination. With most of the questions, the answer will be right there in front of you. If you need to guess, use your nursing knowledge and clinical experiences and clinical judgment skills to their fullest extent and all of the test-taking strategies you have practiced in this review program.

You do not need any computer experience to take this examination. A keyboard tutorial is provided. The tutorial will instruct you on the use of the on-screen optional calculator, the use of the mouse, and how to record an answer. The tutorial provides instructions on how to respond to all question types on this examination and is provided on the NCSBN website; you are encouraged to view the tutorial when you are preparing for the NCLEX examination. In addition, at the testing site, a test administrator is present to assist in explaining the use of the computer to ensure your full understanding of how to proceed.

Development of the Test Plan

The test plan for the NCLEX-PN examination is developed by the NCSBN. It is a national examination; the NCSBN considers the legal scope of nursing practice as governed by state laws and regulations, including the Nurse Practice Act, and uses these laws to define the areas on the examination that will assess the competence of the test-taker for licensure.

The NCSBN also conducts an important study every 3 years, known as a practice analysis study, to determine the framework for the test plan for the examination. The participants in this study include newly licensed practical or vocational nurses. From a list of nursing care activities provided, the participants are asked about the frequency and importance of performing them in relation to client safety and the setting in which they are performed. A panel of content experts at the NCSBN analyzes the results of the study and makes decisions regarding the test plan framework. The results of this recently conducted study provided the structure for the test plan implemented in April 2020.

Test Plan

The content of the NCLEX-PN examination reflects the activities identified in the practice analysis study conducted by the NCSBN. The questions are written to address Level of Cognitive Ability, Client Needs, and Integrated Processes as identified in the test plan developed by the NCSBN.

Level of Cognitive Ability

Levels of cognitive ability include remembering, understanding, applying, analyzing, evaluating, and synthesizing/creating. The practice of nursing requires critical thinking in decision-making and making clinical judgments. Therefore, you will not encounter any remembering or understanding questions on the NCLEX. Questions on this examination are written at the applying level or at higher Levels of Cognitive Ability. Table 1.3 provides descriptions and examples of each level of cognitive ability. Box 1.1 presents an example of a question that requires you to apply data.

Client Needs

The NCSBN identifies a test plan framework based on Client Needs, which includes four major categories. Some of these categories are divided further into subcategories. The Client Needs categories are Safe and Effective Care Environment, Health Promotion and Maintenance, Psychosocial Integrity, and Physiological Integrity. For further information, go to: http://www.ncsbn.org/2020_NCLEXPN_TestPlan-English.pdf

Safe and Effective Care Environment

The Safe and Effective Care Environment category includes two subcategories: Coordinated Care and Safety and Infection Control. According to the NCSBN, Coordinated Care (18%–24%) addresses content that tests the nurse's knowledge, skills, and ability required to collaborate with the interprofessional health care team to facilitate effective client care. The NCSBN indicates that Safety and Infection Control (10%–16%) addresses content that tests the nurse's knowledge, skills, and ability required to protect clients, families, significant others, visitors, and health care personnel from health and environmental hazards. Box 1.2 presents examples of questions that address these two subcategories.

Health Promotion and Maintenance

The Health Promotion and Maintenance category (6%–12% of questions) addresses the principles related to

TABLE 1.3   Levels of Cognitive Ability: Descriptions and Examples

Level	Description and Example
Remembering	Recalling information from memorizing. Example: A normal blood glucose level is 70–99 mg/dL.
Understanding	Recognizing the meaning of information. Example: A blood glucose level of 60 mg/dL is less than the normal reference range.
Applying	Carrying out an appropriate action based on information. Example: Administering 10–15 g of carbohydrate such as a ½ glass of fruit juice to treat mild hypoglycemia.
Analyzing	Examining a broad concept and breaking it down into smaller parts. Example: The broad concept is mild hypoglycemia and the smaller concepts are the signs and symptoms of mild hypoglycemia, such as hunger, irritability, weakness, headache, blood glucose level less than 70 mg/dL.*
Evaluating	Making judgments, conclusion, or validations based on evidence; determining outcomes. Example: Determining that treatment for mild hypoglycemia was effective if the blood glucose level returned to a normal level between 70 and 99 mg/dL.
Synthesizing/Creating	Examining smaller parts of information, determining the broad concept, and creating a plan of care. Example: The smaller concepts are manifestations such as polyuria, polydipsia, polyphagia, vomiting, abdominal pain, weakness, confusion, and Kussmaul respirations. The broad concept is diabetic ketoacidosis (DKA). Creating a safe and individualized plan of care with the interprofessional health care team to treat DKA.

*The blood glucose level at which hypoglycemic symptoms begin to be experienced are individualized.

Reference: Ignatavicius, Workman (2016), pp. 1331–1333.

Adapted from Understanding Bloom's (and Anderson and Krathwohl's) Taxonomy, 2015, ProEdit, Inc. http://www.proedit.com/understanding-blooms-and-anderson-and-krathwohls-taxonomy/

BOX 1.1   Level of Cognitive Ability: Applying

The nurse notes blanching, coolness, and edema at the peripheral intravenous (IV) site. On the basis of these findings, the nurse would implement which action?

1. Remove the IV.
2. Apply a warm compress.
3. Check for a blood return.
4. Measure the area of infiltration.

Answer: 1

This question requires that you focus on the data in the question and determine that the client is experiencing an infiltration. Next, you need to consider the harmful effects of infiltration and determine the action to take. Because infiltration can be damaging to the surrounding tissue, the appropriate action is to remove the IV to prevent any further damage. Applying a warm compress, checking for a blood return, or measuring the area of infiltration would not be appropriate actions when the IV has infiltrated.

growth and development. According to the NCSBN, the Client Needs category also addresses content required to assist clients, family members, and significant others to prevent health problems; to recognize alterations in health; and to develop health practices that promote and support wellness. See Box 1.3 for an example of a question in the Client Needs category.

Psychosocial Integrity

The Psychosocial Integrity category (9%–15% of questions) addresses content required to promote and support the ability of the client, client's family, and client's significant other to cope, adapt, and problem-solve during stressful events. The NCSBN also indicates that the Client Needs category addresses the emotional, mental, and social well-being of the client, family, or significant other, and care for the client with an acute or chronic mental health problem. See Box 1.4 for an example of a question in the Client Needs category.

Physiological Integrity

The Physiological Integrity category includes four subcategories: Basic Care and Comfort, Pharmacological Therapies, Reduction of Risk Potential, and Physiological Adaptation. The NCSBN describes these subcategories as follows. Basic Care and Comfort (7%–13% of questions) addresses content for providing comfort and assistance to the client in the performance of activities of daily living. Pharmacological Therapies (10%–16% of questions) addresses content for administering medications and parenteral therapies, including dosage calculations and pharmacological pain management. Reduction of Risk Potential (9%–15% of questions) addresses content for preventing complications or health problems related to the client's condition or any prescribed treatments or procedures. Physiological Adaptation (7%–13% of questions) addresses content for providing care to clients with acute, chronic, or life-threatening conditions. See Box 1.5 for examples of questions in the Client Needs category.

Integrated Processes

The NCSBN identifies five processes in the test plan that are fundamental to the practice of nursing. These processes are incorporated throughout the major categories of Client Needs. The Integrated Process subcategories are Caring, Communication and Documentation, Culture and Spirituality, Clinical Problem-Solving Process (Nursing Process), and Teaching and Learning. See Box 1.6 for an example of a question that incorporates the Integrated Process of Caring.

BOX 1.2   Safe and Effective Care Environment

Coordinated Care

The nurse has received the client assignment for the day. Which client would the nurse attend to **first**?

1. The client who has a nasogastric tube attached to intermittent suction
2. The client who needs to receive subcutaneous insulin before breakfast
3. The client who is 2 days postoperative and is complaining of incisional pain
4. The client who has a blood glucose level of 50 mg/dL and complains of blurred vision

Answer: 4

This question addresses the subcategory, Coordinated Care, in the Client Needs category, Safe and Effective Care Environment. Note the strategic word, *first*. It requires you to establish priorities by comparing the needs of each client and deciding which need is urgent. The client described in option 4 has a low blood glucose level and symptoms reflective of hypoglycemia. This client would be attended to first so that treatment can be implemented. Although the clients in options 1, 2, and 3 have needs that require attention, they are not the priority and can wait until the client in option 4 is stabilized.

Safety and Infection Control

The nurse prepares to care for a client on contact precautions who has a hospital-acquired infection caused by methicillin-resistant *Staphylococcus aureus* (MRSA). The client has an abdominal wound that requires irrigation and has a tracheostomy attached to a mechanical ventilator, which requires frequent suctioning. The nurse would assemble which necessary protective items before entering the client's room?

1. Gloves and a gown
2. Gloves, mask, and goggles
3. Gloves, mask, gown, and goggles
4. Gloves, gown, and shoe protectors

Answer: 3

This question addresses the subcategory, Safety and Infection Control, in the Client Needs category, Safe and Effective Care Environment. It addresses content related to protecting oneself from contracting an infection and requires that you consider the methods of possible transmission of infection, based on the client's condition. Note the data in the question. Because splashes of infective material can occur during wound irrigation or suctioning of the tracheostomy, option 3 is correct.

BOX 1.3   Health Promotion and Maintenance

The nurse is choosing age-appropriate toys for a toddler. Which toy is the **best** choice for this age?

1. A puzzle
2. Toy soldiers
3. Large stacking blocks
4. A card game with large pictures

Answer: 3

This question addresses the Client Needs category Health Promotion and Maintenance and specifically relates to the principles of growth and development of a toddler. Note the strategic word, *best*. Toddlers like to master activities independently, such as stacking blocks. Because toddlers do not have the developmental ability to determine what could be harmful, toys that are safe need to be provided. A puzzle and toy soldiers provide objects that can be placed in the mouth and may be harmful for a toddler. A card game with large pictures may require cooperative play, which is more appropriate for a school-age child.

BOX 1.4   Psychosocial Integrity

A client with coronary artery disease has selected guided imagery to help cope with psychological stress. Which client statement indicates an understanding of this stress reduction measure?

1. "This will help only if I play music at the same time."
2. "This will work for me only if I am alone in a quiet area."
3. "I need to do this only when I lie down in case I fall asleep."
4. "The best thing about this is that I can use it anywhere, anytime."

Answer: 4

This question addresses the Client Needs category Psychosocial Integrity and the content addresses coping mechanisms. Focus on the subject, client understanding of guided imagery. Guided imagery involves the client creating an image in the mind, concentrating on the image, and gradually becoming less aware of the offending stimulus. It can be done anytime and anywhere; some clients may use other relaxation techniques or play music with it.

Types of Questions on the Examination

The types of questions that may be administered on the examination include multiple-choice; fill-in-the-blank; multiple-response; ordered-response (also known as drag and drop); questions that contain a figure, chart/exhibit, or graphic option item; case studies and accompanying items, and audio formats. Some questions may require you to use the mouse and cursor on the computer. For example, you may be presented with a visual that displays the heart of an adult client. In this visual, you may be asked to "point and click" (using the mouse) on the area where you would place the stethoscope to obtain the apical heart rate. In all types of questions the answer is scored as either right or wrong. Credit is not given for a partially correct answer. In addition, all question types may include pictures, graphics, tables, charts, or sound. The NCSBN provides specific directions for you to follow with all question types to guide you through the testing process. Be sure to read these directions as they appear on the computer screen. Examples of some of these types of questions are noted in this chapter. Most question types are placed in this book, and all types, including the new NGN, are on the accompanying Evolve site.

BOX 1.5 Physiological Integrity

Basic Care and Comfort

A client with Parkinson's disease develops akinesia while ambulating, increasing the risk for falls. Which suggestion would the nurse provide to the client to alleviate this problem?

1. Use a wheelchair to move around.
2. Stand erect and use a cane to ambulate.
3. Keep the feet close together while ambulating, and use a walker.
4. Consciously think about walking over imaginary lines on the floor.

Answer: 4

This question addresses the subcategory Basic Care and Comfort in the Client Needs category Physiological Integrity and addresses client mobility and promoting assistance in an activity of daily living to maintain safety. Focus on the subject, a suggestion that will ensure client safety. Clients with Parkinson's disease can develop bradykinesia (slow movement) or akinesia (freezing or no movement). Having these clients imagine lines on the floor to walk over can keep them moving forward while remaining safe.

Pharmacological Therapies

The nurse monitors a client receiving digoxin for which **early** manifestation of digoxin toxicity?

1. Anorexia
2. Facial pain
3. Photophobia
4. Yellow color perception

Answer: 1

This question addresses the subcategory Pharmacological Therapies in the Client Needs category Physiological Integrity. Note the strategic word, *early*. Digoxin is a cardiac glycoside that is used to manage and treat heart failure and to control ventricular rates in clients with atrial fibrillation. The most common early manifestations of toxicity include gastrointestinal disturbances such as anorexia, nausea, and vomiting. Neurological abnormalities can also occur early and include fatigue, headache, depression, weakness, drowsiness, confusion, and nightmares. Facial pain, personality changes, and ocular disturbances (photophobia, diplopia, light flashes, halos around bright objects, yellow or green color perception) are also signs of toxicity, but are not early signs.

Reduction of Risk Potential

A magnetic resonance imaging (MRI) study is prescribed for a client with a suspected brain tumor. The nurse would implement which action to prepare the client for this test?

1. Shave the groin for insertion of a femoral catheter.
2. Remove all metal-containing objects from the client.
3. Keep the client NPO (*nil per os*; nothing by mouth) for 6 hours before the test.
4. Instruct the client in inhalation techniques for the administration of the radioisotope.

Answer: 2

This question addresses the subcategory, Reduction of Risk Potential, in the Client Needs category Physiological Integrity, and the nurse's responsibilities in preparing the client for the diagnostic test. Focus on the subject, preparation for an MRI. In an MRI study, radiofrequency pulses in a magnetic field are converted into pictures. All metal objects, such as rings, bracelets, hairpins, and watches, would be removed. In addition, a history would be taken to ascertain whether the client has any internal metallic devices, such as orthopedic hardware, pacemakers, or shrapnel. NPO status is not necessary for an MRI study of the head. The groin may be shaved for an angiogram, and inhalation of the radioisotope may be prescribed with other types of scans but is not a part of the procedures for an MRI.

Physiological Adaptation

A client with renal insufficiency has a magnesium level of 3.5 mEq/L. On the basis of this laboratory result, the nurse interprets which sign as significant?

1. Hyperpnea
2. Drowsiness
3. Hypertension
4. Physical hyperactivity

Answer: 2

This question addresses the subcategory, Physiological Adaptation, in the Client Needs category Physiological Integrity. Determine whether an abnormality exists. The laboratory value noted in the question addresses an alteration in body systems. The normal magnesium level is 1.8 to 2.6 mEq/L. A magnesium level of 3.5 mEq/L indicates hypermagnesemia. Neurological manifestations occur when magnesium levels are elevated and are noted as symptoms of neurological depression such as drowsiness, sedation, lethargy, respiratory depression, muscle weakness, and areflexia. Bradycardia and hypotension also occur.

BOX 1.6 Integrated Processes

A client is scheduled for angioplasty. The client says to the nurse, "I'm so afraid that it will hurt and make me worse off than I am." Which response by the nurse is therapeutic?

1. "Can you tell me what you understand about the procedure?"
2. "Your fears are a sign that you really should have this procedure."
3. "Try not to worry. This is a well-known and easy procedure for your doctor."
4. "Those are very normal fears, but please be assured that everything will be okay."

Answer: 1

This question addresses the subcategory, Caring, in the category Integrated Processes. The correct option is a therapeutic communication technique that explores the client's feelings, determines the level of client understanding about the procedure, and displays caring. Option 2 demeans the client and does not encourage further sharing by the client. Option 3 diminishes the client's feelings by directing attention away from the client and toward the doctor's importance. Option 4 does not address the client's fears, provides false reassurance, and puts the client's feelings on hold.

BOX 1.7 **Fill-in-the-Blank Question**

A prescription reads: acetaminophen liquid, 650 mg orally every 4 hours PRN for pain. The medication label reads: 500 mg/15 mL. The nurse prepares how many milliliters to administer one dose? **Fill in the blank. Record your answer using one decimal place.**

Answer: *19.5 mL*

Formula:

$$\frac{Desired}{Available} \times Volume = mL$$

$$\frac{650 \text{ mg}}{500 \text{ mg}} \times 15 \text{ mL} = 19.5 \text{ mL}$$

Note the data in the question, then use the formula for calculating a medication dose. Once the dose is determined, you will need to type your numeric answer in the answer box. Always follow the specific directions noted on the computer screen. Also, remember that there will be an on-screen calculator available for your use.

Multiple-Choice Questions

Many of the questions that you will be asked to answer will be in the multiple-choice format. These questions provide you with data about a client situation and four answer options.

Fill-in-the-Blank Questions

Fill-in-the-blank questions may ask you to perform a medication calculation, determine an intravenous flow rate, or calculate an intake or output record on a client. You will need to type only a number (your answer) in the answer box. If the question requires rounding the answer, this needs to be performed at the end of the calculation. The rules for rounding an answer are described in the tutorial provided by the NCSBN and are also provided in the specific question on the computer screen. In addition, you must type in a decimal point if necessary. See Box 1.7 for an example.

Multiple-Response Questions

For a multiple-response question, you will be asked to select or check all of the options, such as nursing interventions, that relate to the information in the question. In these question types, there may be one or more correct answers. No partial credit is given for correct selections. You need to do exactly as the question asks, which will be to select all of the options that apply. See Box 1.8 for an example.

Ordered-Response (Prioritizing) Questions

In this type of question, you will be asked to use the computer mouse to drag and drop your nursing actions in order of priority. Information will be presented in a question, and, based on the data, you need to determine what you will do first, second, third, and so forth. The unordered options will be located in boxes on the left side of the screen, and you need to move all options in order of priority to ordered-response boxes on the right side of the screen. Specific directions for moving the options are provided with the question. See Fig 1.1 for an example. Examples of this question type are located on the accompanying Evolve site.

Figure Questions

A question with a picture or graphic will ask you to answer the question based on the picture or graphic. The question could contain a chart, table, figure, or illustration. You also may be asked to use the computer mouse to point and click on a specific area in the visual. A figure or illustration may appear in any type of question, including a multiple-choice question. See Box 1.9 for an example.

Chart/Exhibit Questions

In this type of question, you will be presented with a client situation and a chart or exhibit. You will be provided with tabs or buttons that you need to click to obtain the information needed to answer the question. A prompt or message will appear that will indicate the need to click on a tab or button. See Box 1.10 for an example.

Graphic Option Questions

In this type of question, the option selections will be pictures rather than text. Each option will be preceded by a circle, and you will need to use the computer mouse to click in the circle that represents your answer choice. See Box 1.11 for an example.

Audio Questions

Audio questions will require listening to a sound to answer the question. These questions will prompt you to use the headset provided and to click on the sound icon. You will be able to click on the volume button to adjust the volume to your comfort level, and you will be able to listen to the sound as many times as necessary. Content examples include, but are not limited to, various lung sounds, heart sounds, or bowel sounds. Examples of this question type are located on the accompanying Evolve site (Fig. 1.2).

Refer to the COVID-19 Modifications section at the end of this chapter.

Registering to Take the Examination

It is important to obtain an NCLEX Examination Candidate Bulletin from the NCSBN website at www.ncsbn.org because this bulletin provides all of the information you need to register for and schedule your examination. It also provides you with website and telephone information for NCLEX examination contacts. The initial step in the registration process is to submit an application to the state board of nursing in the state in which you intend to

BOX 1.8	Multiple-Response Question

The emergency department nurse is caring for a child suspected of acute epiglottitis. Which interventions apply in the care of the child? **Select all that apply.**

- ☐ 1. Obtain a throat culture.
- ☑ 2. Ensure a patent airway.
- ☑ 3. Prepare the child for a chest x-ray.
- ☐ 4. Maintain the child in a supine position.
- ☑ 5. Obtain a pediatric-size tracheostomy tray.
- ☑ 6. Place the child on an oxygen saturation monitor.

Answer: 2, 3, 5, 6

In a multiple-response question, you will be asked to select or check all of the options, such as interventions that relate to the data in the question. To answer this question, recall that acute epiglottitis is a serious obstructive inflammatory process that requires immediate intervention and that airway patency is a priority. Examination of the throat with a tongue depressor or attempting to obtain a throat culture is contraindicated because the examination can precipitate further obstruction. A lateral neck and chest x-ray is obtained to determine the degree of obstruction, if present. To reduce respiratory distress, the child would sit upright. The child is placed on an oxygen saturation monitor to monitor oxygenation status. Tracheostomy and intubation may be necessary if respiratory distress is severe. Remember to follow the specific directions given on the computer screen and for this question, select all that apply.

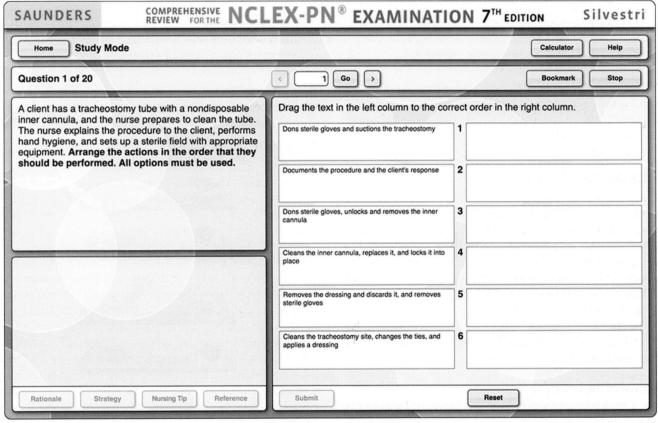

FIGURE 1.1 Sample of an ordered-response question.

obtain licensure. You need to obtain information from the board of nursing regarding the specific registration process because the process may vary from state to state. Then, use the NCLEX Examination Candidate Bulletin as your guide to complete the registration process.

Following the registration instructions and completing the registration forms precisely and accurately are important. Registration forms not properly completed or not accompanied by the proper fees in the required method of payment will be returned to you and will delay testing. You must pay a fee for taking the examination; you also may have to pay additional fees to the board of nursing in the state in which you are applying.

Authorization to Test Form and Scheduling an Appointment

Once you are eligible to test, you will receive an Authorization to Test (ATT) form. You cannot make an appointment until you receive an ATT form. Note the validity dates on the ATT form, and schedule a

BOX 1.9   Figure Question

A client who experienced a myocardial infarction is being monitored via cardiac telemetry. The nurse notes the sudden onset of this cardiac rhythm on the monitor **(refer to figure)** and would plan to take which **immediate** action?

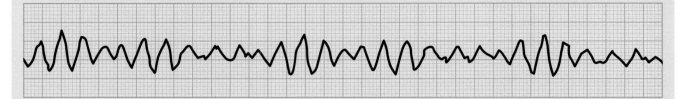

1. Take the client's blood pressure.
2. Initiate cardiopulmonary resuscitation (CPR).
3. Place a nitroglycerin tablet under the client's tongue.
4. Continue to monitor the client and then contact the primary health care provider (PHCP).

Answer: 2

This question requires you to identify the cardiac rhythm and then determine the priority nursing action. Note the strategic word, *immediate*. This cardiac rhythm identifies a coarse ventricular fibrillation (VF). The goals of treatment are to terminate VF promptly and to convert it to an organized rhythm. The PHCP or an Advanced Cardiac Life Support (ACLS)–qualified nurse must immediately defibrillate the client. If a defibrillator is not readily available, CPR is initiated until the defibrillator arrives. Options 1, 3, and 4 are incorrect actions and delay life-saving treatment.

BOX 1.10   Chart/Exhibit Question

The nurse reviews the history and physical examination documented in the medical record of a client requesting a prescription for oral contraceptives. The nurse determines that oral contraceptives are contraindicated because of which documented item? **Refer to chart.**

Client's Chart		
History and Physical	**Medications**	**Diagnostic Results**
Item 1: Has renal calculi Item 2: Had thrombophlebitis 1 year ago	Item 3: Daily multivitamin taken orally	Item 4: Electrocardiogram normal

Answer: 2

This chart/exhibit question provides you with data from the client's medical record and asks you to identify the item that is a contraindication to the use of oral contraceptives. Therefore, note the data in the question. Oral contraceptives are contraindicated in women with a history of any of the following: thrombophlebitis and thromboembolic disorders, cardiovascular or cerebrovascular diseases (including stroke), any estrogen-dependent cancer or breast cancer, benign or malignant liver tumors, impaired liver function, hypertension, and diabetes mellitus with vascular involvement. Adverse effects of oral contraceptives include increased risk of superficial and deep venous thrombosis, pulmonary embolism, thrombotic stroke (or other types of strokes), myocardial infarction, and accelerations of preexisting breast tumors.

BOX 1.11   Graphic Options Question

The nurse would place the client in which position to administer an enema? **(Refer to the figures in 1-4).**

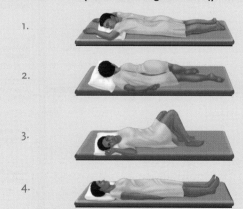

Answer: 2

This question requires you to select the picture that represents your answer choice. Focus on the subject, administering an enema. To administer an enema, the nurse assists the client into the left side-lying (Sims') position with the right knee flexed. This position allows the enema solution to flow downward by gravity along the natural curve of the sigmoid colon and rectum, improving the retention of solution. Option 1 is a prone position. Option 3 is a dorsal recumbent position used for performing a vaginal examination. Option 4 is a supine position.

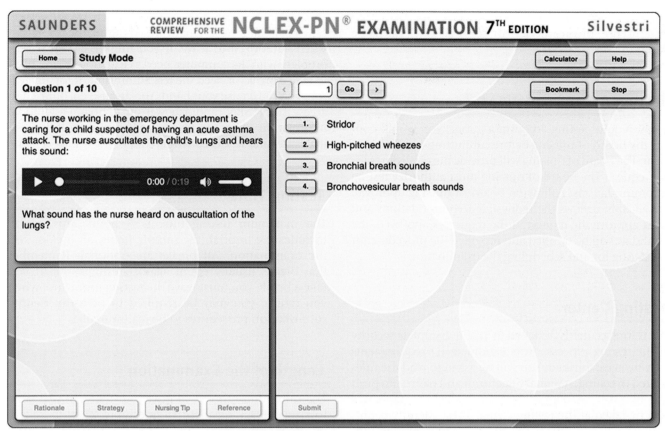

FIGURE 1.2 Sample of an audio question.

testing date and time before the expiration date on the ATT form. The NCLEX Examination Candidate Bulletin provides you with the directions for scheduling an appointment, and you do not have to take the examination in the same state in which you are seeking licensure.

The ATT form contains important information, including your test authorization number, candidate identification (ID) number, and validity date. You need to take your ATT form to the testing center on the day of your examination. You will not be admitted to the examination if you do not have it.

Changing Your Appointment

If for any reason you need to change your appointment to test, you can make the change on the candidate website or by calling candidate services. Refer to the NCLEX Examination Candidate Bulletin for this contact information and other important procedures for canceling and changing an appointment. If you fail to arrive for the examination or fail to cancel your appointment to test without providing appropriate notice, you will forfeit your examination fee and your ATT form will be invalidated. This information will be reported to the

board of nursing in the state in which you have applied for licensure, and you will be required to register and pay the testing fees again.

Day of the Examination

It is important that you arrive at the testing center at least 30 minutes before the test is scheduled. If you arrive late for the scheduled testing appointment, you may be required to forfeit your examination appointment. If it is necessary to forfeit your appointment, you will need to reregister for the examination and pay an additional fee. The board of nursing will be notified that you did not take the test. A few days before your scheduled date of testing, take the time to drive to the testing center to determine its exact location, the length of time required to arrive at that destination, and any potential obstacles that might delay you, such as road construction, traffic, or parking sites.

In addition to the ATT form, you must have proper ID such as a US driver's license, passport, US state ID, or US military ID to be admitted to take the examination. All acceptable ID must be valid, not expired, and contain a photograph and signature (in English). In addition, the first and last names on the ID must match the ATT form. According to the NCSBN guidelines, any name discrepancies require legal documentation, such as a marriage license, divorce decree, or court action legal name change.

Testing Accommodations

If you require testing accommodations, you would contact the board of nursing before submitting a registration form. The board of nursing will provide the procedures for the request. The board of nursing must authorize testing accommodations. Following board of nursing approval, the NCSBN reviews the requested accommodations and must approve the request. If the request is approved, the candidate will be notified and provided the procedure for registering for and scheduling the examination.

Testing Center

The testing center is designed to ensure complete security of the testing process. Strict candidate ID requirements have been established. You will be asked to read the rules related to testing. A digital fingerprint and palm vein print will be taken. A digital signature and photograph will also be taken at the testing center. These identity confirmations will accompany the NCLEX examination results. In addition, if you leave the testing room for any reason, you may be required to perform these identity confirmation procedures again to be readmitted to the room.

Personal belongings are not allowed in the testing room; all electronic devices must be placed in a sealable bag provided by the test administrator and kept in a locker. Any evidence of tampering with the bag could result in an incident and a result cancellation. A locker and locker key will be provided for you; however, storage space is limited, so you must plan accordingly. In addition, the testing center will not assume responsibility for your personal belongings. The testing waiting areas are generally small; friends or family members who accompany you are not permitted to wait in the testing center during the time of your examination.

Once you have completed the admission process, the test administrator will escort you to the assigned computer. You will be seated at an individual workspace that includes computer equipment, appropriate lighting, an erasable note board, and a marker. No items, including unauthorized scratch paper, are allowed into the testing room. Eating, drinking, or the use of tobacco is not allowed in the testing room. You will be observed at all times by the test administrator while taking the examination. In addition, video and audio recordings of all test sessions are made. The testing center has no control over the sounds made by typing on the computer by others. If these sounds are distracting, raise your hand to summon the test administrator. Earplugs are available on request.

You must follow the directions given by the testing center staff and must remain seated during the test except when authorized to leave. If you think that you have a problem with the computer, need a clean note board, need to take a break, or need the test administrator for any reason, you must raise your hand. You are also encouraged to access the NCSBN candidate website to obtain additional information about the physical environment of the testing center and to view a virtual tour of the testing center.

Testing Time

The maximum testing time is 5 hours; this period includes the tutorial, the sample items, all breaks, and the examination. All breaks are optional. Remember that breaks usually count against testing time. If you take a break, you must leave the testing room and, when you return, you may be required to perform identity confirmation procedures to be readmitted.

Length of the Examination

The minimum number of questions that you will need to answer is 85. Of these 85 questions, 25 of these will be pretest (unscored) questions. The maximum number of questions in the test is 205. The pretest questions are questions that may be presented as scored questions on future examinations. These pretest questions are not identified as such. In other words, you do not know which questions are the pretest (unscored) questions; however, these pretest (unscored) questions will be administered among the first 85 questions of the test.

Pass-or-Fail Decisions

All examination questions are categorized by test plan area and level of difficulty. This is an important point to keep in mind when you consider how the computer makes a pass-or-fail decision, because a pass-or-fail decision is not based on a percentage of correctly answered questions.

The NCSBN indicates that a pass-or-fail decision is governed by three different scenarios. The first scenario is the 95% Confidence Interval Rule, in which the computer stops administering test questions when it is 95% certain that the test-taker's ability is clearly above the passing standard or clearly below the passing standard. The second scenario is known as the Maximum-Length Examination, in which the final ability estimate of the test-taker is considered. If the final ability estimate is above the passing standard, the test-taker passes; if it is below the passing standard, the test-taker fails.

The third scenario is the Run-Out-Of-Time (ROOT) Rule. If the examination ends because the test-taker ran out of time, the computer may not have enough information with 95% certainty to make a clear pass-or-fail decision. If this is the case, the computer will review the test-taker's performance during testing. If the test-taker has not answered the minimum number of required questions, the test-taker fails. If the test-taker's ability estimate was consistently above the passing standard on the last 60 questions, the test-taker passes. If the test-taker's ability estimate falls to or is below the passing standard, even once, the test-taker fails. Additional information about pass-or-fail decisions can be found in the NCLEX Examination Candidate Bulletin located at www.ncsbn.org.

Completing the Examination

When the examination has ended, you may be asked to participate in an NCSBN research project in which you will be provided a case study and accompanying test questions and asked to answer the test questions. Participation is optional and whether or not you decide to participate has no effect at all on your NCLEX score. Likewise, if you do participate, your responses to the case study test questions do not affect your score on NCLEX.

You will also be asked to complete a brief computer-delivered questionnaire about your testing experience. After you complete this questionnaire, you need to raise your hand to summon the test administrator. The test administrator will collect and inventory all note boards and then permit you to leave.

Processing Results

Every computerized examination is scored twice, once by the computer at the testing center and again after the examination is transmitted to the test scoring center. No results are released at the testing center; testing center staff do not have access to examination results. The board of nursing receives your result, and your result will be mailed to you approximately one month after you take the examination. In some states, an unofficial result can be obtained via the Quick Results Service two business days after taking the examination. There is a fee for this service, and information about obtaining your NCLEX result by this method can be obtained on the NCSBN website under candidate services.

Candidate Performance Report

A candidate performance report is provided to a test-taker who failed the examination. This report provides the test-taker with information about her or his strengths and weaknesses in relation to the test plan framework and provides a guide for studying and retaking the examination. If a retake is necessary, the candidate must wait 45 to 90 days between examination administration, depending on state procedures.

Interstate Endorsement

Because the NCLEX-PN examination is a national examination, you can apply to take it in any state. When licensure is received you can apply for interstate endorsement, which allows you to obtain another nursing license in another state. The procedures and requirements for interstate endorsement may vary from state to state, and these procedures can be obtained from the state board of nursing in the state in which endorsement is sought.

Nurse Licensure Compact

It may be possible to practice nursing in another state under the mutual recognition model of nursing licensure if the state has enacted a Nurse Licensure Compact. To obtain information about the Nurse Licensure Compact and the states that are part of this interstate compact, access the NCSBN website at http://www.ncsbn.org.

The Internationally-Educated Nurse

An important first step in the process of obtaining information about becoming a licensed nurse in the United States is to access the NCSBN website at http://www.ncsbn.org and obtain information provided for international nurses in the NCLEX website link. The NCSBN provides information about some of the documents you need to obtain as an international nurse seeking licensure in the United States and about credentialing agencies. Refer to Box 1.12 for a listing of some of these documents. The NCSBN also provides information regarding the requirements for education and English proficiency, and immigration requirements such as visas and VisaScreen. You are encouraged to access the NCSBN website to obtain the most current information about seeking licensure as a nurse in the United States.

An important factor to consider as you pursue this process is that some requirements may vary from state to state. You need to contact the board of nursing in the state in which you are planning to obtain licensure to determine the specific requirements and documents that you need to submit.

Boards of nursing can decide either to use a credentialing agency to evaluate your documents or to

BOX 1.12	Internationally-Educated Nurse: Some Documents Needed to Obtain Licensure

1. Proof of citizenship or lawful alien status
2. Work visa
3. VisaScreen certificate
4. Commission on Graduates of Foreign Nursing Schools (CGFNS) certificate
5. Criminal background check documents
6. Official transcripts of educational credentials sent directly to credentialing agency or board of nursing from home country school of nursing
7. Validation of a comparable nursing education as that provided in US nursing programs; this may include theoretical instruction and clinical practice in a variety of nursing areas, including, but not limited to, medical nursing, surgical nursing, pediatric nursing, maternity and newborn nursing, community and public health nursing, and mental health nursing
8. Validation of safe professional nursing practice in home country
9. Copy of nursing license or diploma or both
10. Proof of proficiency in the English language
11. Photograph(s)
12. Social Security number
13. Application and fees

review your documents at the specific state board, known as in-house evaluation. When you contact the board of nursing in the state in which you intend to work as a nurse, inform them that you were educated outside of the United States and ask that they send you an application to apply for licensure by examination. Be sure to specify that you are applying for PN licensure. You would also ask about the specific documents needed to become eligible to take the NCLEX examination. You can obtain contact information for each state board of nursing through the NCSBN website at http://www.ncsbn.org. In addition, you can write to the NCSBN regarding the NCLEX examination. The address is 111 East Wacker Drive, Suite 2900, Chicago, IL 60601. The telephone number for the NCSBN is 1-866-293-9600; international telephone is 011 1 312 525 3600; the fax number is 1-312-279-1032.

COVID-19 Test Modifications

The testing procedures described in this chapter are the standard and normal procedures developed by the NCSBN. However, in response to the COVID-19 pandemic, modifications to testing have been implemented. These modifications affect such procedures as testing time, the length of the examination, pass and fail decisions, among other procedures. According to the NCSBN, these modifications will remain in effect until further notice. Additionally, all Centers for Disease Control and Prevention guidelines are being followed in all test centers including social distancing and enhanced cleaning between each test-taker. All personnel and test-takers are required to wear a mask. You are encouraged to frequently access the NCSBN web site for updated information on these COVID-19 modifications at https://www.ncsbn.org/SummaryofModificationstoNCLEX.pdf.

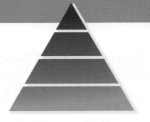

CHAPTER **2**

Pathways to Success

Laurent W. Valliere, BS, DD

Pyramid to Success

Preparing to take the NCLEX-PN® examination can produce a great deal of anxiety. You may be thinking that it is the most important examination that you will ever have to take and that it reflects the culmination of everything for which you have worked so hard. The NCLEX-PN is important because receiving that nursing license means that you can begin your career as a licensed practical/vocational nurse. Your success on the NCLEX-PN involves expelling all thoughts from your mind that allow this examination to appear overwhelming and intimidating; such thoughts will take complete control over your destiny. A positive attitude, a structured plan for preparation, and maintaining control of your pathway to success will ensure your achievement of reaching the peak of the Pyramid to Success (Fig. 2.1).

Pathways to Success (Box 2.1)

The Foundation

The foundation of the Pathways to Success begins with a positive attitude, the belief that you will achieve success, and the development of control. It also includes the creation of a list of your personal short- and long-term goals and a plan for preparation. A positive attitude, belief in yourself, control, and a list of personal goals will lead you to becoming a licensed practical/vocational nurse. Without these components, your Pathway to Success leads to nowhere and has no end point. You will expend energy and valuable time in your journey, but you will lack control over where you are heading, and you will experience exhaustion without any accomplishment. Therefore, it is imperative that you take the time to develop that positive attitude and to establish your short- and long-term goals.

Where do you start? To begin this process, find a location that offers solitude. Sit or lie in a comfortable position, close your eyes, relax, inhale deeply, hold your breath to a count of 4, exhale slowly, and again relax. Repeat this breathing exercise several times until you begin to feel relaxed, free from anxiety, and in control of your destiny. Allow your mind to become void of all of the mind chatter; you are now in control, and your mind can see for miles. Your highway of life has a multitude of destinations to which you may travel. Next, reflect on all that you have accomplished and the path that brought you to where you are today. Keep a journal of your reflections as you plan the order of your journey to the Pyramid to Success.

The List

It is time to create "The List." "The List" is your set of short- and long-term goals. Begin by developing the goals you wish to accomplish today, tomorrow, over the next month, and into the future. Allow yourself the opportunity to list all that is flowing from your mind. Write your goals in your personal journal. When "the list" is complete, put it away for 2 or 3 days. After that time, retrieve and review it, and begin the process of planning for preparing for the NCLEX-PN examination.

The Plan for Preparation

Now that you have "The List" in order, look at the goals that relate to studying for the licensing examination. The first task is to decide what study pattern works best for you. Think about what has worked most successfully for you in the past. There are questions that must be addressed to develop your plan for study. These questions are identified in Box 2.2.

The plan must include a schedule. Use a calendar to plan and document the times and nursing content areas for your study sessions. Establish a realistic schedule that includes your daily, weekly, and future goals, and

15

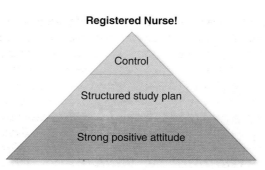

FIGURE 2.1 The Pyramid to Success.

Registered Nurse!

Control

Structured study plan

Strong positive attitude

BOX 2.1   Pathways to Success

The Foundation
- Maintaining a positive attitude
- Thinking about realistic short- and long-term goals
- Preparing a plan for studying for the NCLEX
- Maintaining control

The List
- Journaling realistic short- and long-term goals

The Plan for Preparation
- Developing a study plan and schedule
- Deciding on the place to study
- Balancing personal and work obligations with the study schedule
- Sharing the study schedule and personal needs with others
- Implementing the study plan

Positive Pampering
- Planning time for exercise and fun activities
- Establishing healthy eating habits
- Including activities in the schedule that provide positive mental stimulation

Final Preparation
- Reviewing and identifying goals that have been achieved
- Remaining focused on completing the plan of study
- Writing down the date and time of the examination and posting it next to your name with the letters "LPN" or "LVN" after it, along with the word "YES!"
- Taking a test drive to the testing center
- Enjoying relaxing activities on the day before the examination

The Day of the Examination
- Grooming yourself for success
- Eating a healthy and nutritious breakfast
- Maintaining a confident and positive attitude
- Maintaining control
- Meeting the challenges of the day
- Reaching the peak of the Pyramid to Success

BOX 2.2   Developing a Plan of Study

- Do I work better alone or in a group study environment?
- If I work best in a group, does the group consist of one, two, or more study partners?
- Who are these study partners?
- How long should my study sessions last?
- Does the time of day that I study make a difference for me?
- Do I retain more if I study in the morning?
- How does my work schedule affect my study pattern?
- How do I balance my family obligations with my need to study?
- Do I have a comfortable study area at home, or do I need to find another environment that is more conducive to my study needs?

---

adhere to it. This consistency will provide advantages to you and those supporting you. A daily schedule allows you to plan your content areas for study more carefully. Stick to your plan of study. Adherence to the plan helps you develop a rhythm that can only enhance your retention and positive momentum. The people who are supporting you will share this rhythm, and they will be able to schedule their activities and life better because you are consistent with your study schedule. You are moving forward, and you are in control!

The length of the study session will depend on you and your ability to focus and concentrate. What you need to think about is *quality* rather than *quantity* when you are determining a realistic amount of time for each session. Plan to schedule at least 2 hours of daily quality study time. If you can spend more than 2 hours studying, then by all means do so.

You may be asking yourself, "What do you mean by quality time?" Quality time means spending uninterrupted quiet time focusing on your study session. This may mean that you will have to isolate yourself for these study sessions. Think again about what has worked for you during nursing school when you studied for examinations and select a study place that has also worked for you in the past. If you have a special study room at home that you have always used, then plan your study sessions in that special room. If you have always studied at a library, then plan your study sessions for the library. If you plan to study at home, make the time spent studying uninterrupted and quiet. Sometimes it is difficult to balance your study time with your family obligations and possibly a work schedule, but if you can, plan your study time for when you know that you will be at home alone. Try to eliminate anything that may be distracting during your study time. Shut off your cell phone so that you will not be disturbed. If you have small children, plan your study time during their nap time or school hours.

Your plan must include the ways in which you will manage your study needs and the demands of your work, family, and friends. Take time to think about how you will balance your everyday commitments with your plan for study. Your family and friends are key players in your life, and they will become a part of your Pyramid to Success. After you have established your study needs, communicate your needs and the importance of your study plan to your family and friends. Help them to understand that you must follow this plan in order to achieve your goal of becoming a licensed practical/vocational nurse.

A difficult part of the plan may be finding ways to deal with those family members and friends who choose not to participate in your Pathways to Success. What if an individual or individuals choose not to be part of your plan? For example, what would you do if a friend asked you to go to a movie during your scheduled study time? Your friend might say, "Come on. Take some time off. You have plenty of time to study. Study later when we get back!" Then you will be faced with a decision. You must weigh all the factors carefully. You must keep your goals in mind and remember that it is critical to maintain a positive momentum. Your decision may not be an easy one, but it must be one that will help you to meet your goal of becoming a licensed practical/vocational nurse. Remember, positive momentum and meeting your goal are the most important considerations.

Positive Pampering

Positive pampering means that you must continue to care for yourself holistically. Positive momentum can be maintained only if you are properly balanced. Proper exercise, diet, and positive mental stimulation are critical to achieving your goal of becoming a licensed practical/vocational nurse. Just as you have developed a schedule for study, you should have a schedule that includes some fun and some form of physical activity. It is your choice—aerobics, running, walking, weightlifting, bowling, or whatever makes you feel good about yourself. Time spent away from the hard study schedule and devoted to some form of fun and physical exercise pays its rewards 100-fold. You will feel alive and more energetic with a schedule that includes these activities.

Establish healthy eating habits. Stay away from fatty foods, because they will slow you down. Eat lighter meals and eat more frequently. Include complex carbohydrates in your diet for energy, and be careful not to include too much caffeine in your daily diet. Drink plenty of water to stay hydrated. Continue to feel good about yourself because you are in control.

Take the time to pamper yourself with activities that make you feel even better about who you are. Make dinner reservations at your favorite restaurant with someone who is special and who is supporting your goal of becoming a licensed practical/vocational nurse. Take walks in a place that has a particular tranquility that enables you to reflect on the positive momentum that you have achieved and maintained. Whatever it is and wherever it takes you, allow yourself the time to do some positive pampering.

Final Preparation

You have established the foundation of your Pyramid to Success. You have developed your list of goals and

your study plan, and you have maintained your positive momentum. You are moving forward, and you are in control. When you receive your date and time for the NCLEX-PN examination you may immediately think, "I'm not ready!" Stop! Reflect on all that you have achieved. Think about your goal, your accomplishment, and the organization of the positive life momentum with which you have surrounded yourself. Think about all those individuals who love and support your effort to become a licensed practical/vocational nurse. Believe that the challenge that awaits you is one that you have successfully prepared for and that will lead you to your goal of becoming a licensed practical/vocational nurse!

Take a deep breath and organize the remaining days so that they support your educational and personal needs. Support your positive momentum with a visual technique. Write your name in large letters and write the letters "LPN" or "LVN" after it. Post one or more of these visual reinforcements in areas that you frequent. This form of visual motivational technique works for many individuals preparing for this examination.

Through all that you have accomplished to this point, it is imperative that you not fall into the trap of expecting too much of yourself. The idea of perfection must not drive you to a point that causes your positive momentum to hesitate. You must believe in who you are as you are, and you need to stay focused on your goal. Allow yourself the opportunity to continue to carry out your plan in a manner that is the most conducive to who you are. The date and time are in hand. Write down the date and time, and underneath write the word "YES!" Post this next to your note with your name plus "LPN" or "LVN."

You must ensure that you know how to get to the testing center. A test run is a must. Time the drive and allow for road construction or other problems that may slow down traffic. During the test run, when you arrive at the testing facility, you may want to walk into it. Walk in and become familiar with the lobby and the surroundings. This may help to alleviate some of the peripheral nervousness associated with entering an unknown building. Remember, you must do whatever it takes to keep yourself in control. If familiarizing yourself with the facility will help you to maintain positive momentum, then by all means be sure to do so. Who is in control? *You* are!

It is time to check your study plan and make the necessary adjustments now that a firm date and time are set. Adjust your review so that it flows to your needs and so that your study plan ends 2 days before the examination. Remember that the mind is like a muscle. If it is overworked, it has no strength or stamina. Your strategy is to rest the body and mind on the day before the examination. Your strategy is to stay in control and allow yourself the opportunity to be absolutely fresh and attentive on the day of the examination. This will help you to control the nervousness that is natural, achieve the clear thought processes required, and feel confident that you have done all that is necessary to prepare for and conquer this challenge. The day before the examination is to be one of pleasure. Treat yourself to what you enjoy the most.

Relax! Take a deep breath, hold it to a count of 4, and exhale slowly. You have prepared yourself well for the challenge of tomorrow. Allow yourself a good night's sleep and wake up on the day of the examination knowing that you are absolutely ready to succeed. Look at your name with "LPN" or "LVN" after it and write the word "YES!"

The Day of the Examination (Box 2.3)

Wake up believing in yourself and knowing that all you have accomplished is about to propel you to the professional level of becoming a licensed practical/vocational nurse. Allow yourself plenty of time, eat a nutritious breakfast, and groom yourself for success. You are ready to meet the challenges of the day and overcome any obstacle that may face you. Your test day will soon be history and then you will receive your test result, which will have your name with the letters "LPN" or "LVN" after it.

Be proud and confident of your achievements. You have worked hard to achieve your goal of becoming a licensed practical/vocational nurse. If you believe in yourself and your goals, no one person or obstacle can move you off the pathway that leads to success and to the peak of the Pyramid!

Congratulations! I wish you the very best in your career as a licensed practical/vocational nurse!

This Is Not a Test

1. What are the factors needed to ensure a productive study environment? **Select all that apply.**
   1. Secure a location that offers solitude
   2. Plan breaks during your study session
   3. Establish a realistic study schedule that includes your goals
   4. Continue with the study pattern that has worked best for you
   Answer: 1, 2, 3, 4

> **BOX 2.3** **The Day of the Examination**
>
> *Breathe*—Inhale deeply, hold your breath to a count of 4, and exhale slowly.
> *Believe*—Have positive thoughts today and keep those thoughts focused on your achievements.
> *Control*—You are in command!
> *Believe*—This is your day!
> *Visualize*—The letters "LPN" or "LVN" next to your name!

Rationale: A location of solitude helps to ensure concentration. Taking breaks during your study session helps to clear your mind and increase your ability to concentrate and focus. Establishing a realistic study pattern will keep you in control. Do not vary your study pattern. It has been successful for you until now, so why change it?

2. What are the key factors in your final preparation? **Select all that apply.**
   1. Remain focused on the study plan
   2. Visualize the letters "LPN/LVN" after your name
   3. Stop studying the day before the examination and relax
   4. Know where the testing facility is and how long it takes to get there
   Answer: 1, 2, 3, 4
   Rationale: Focus on your plan of study and success will follow. Positive reinforcement: write your name in large letters on a piece of paper with "LPN/LVN" after your name and post it where you see it often. Allow yourself a day of pampering before the test. Wake up on the day of the test refreshed and ready to succeed. Ensure that you know where the testing facility is; map out your route and the average time it takes to arrive.

3. What key points do the Pathways to Success emphasize to help ensure your success? **Select all that apply.**
   1. A strong positive attitude
   2. Believing in your ability to succeed
   3. Being proud and confident of your achievements
   4. Maintaining control of your mind, the surrounding environment, and your physical being
   Answer: 1, 2, 3, 4
   Rationale: A strong, positive attitude leads to success. Believe in who you are and the goals that you have set for yourself. Be "proud and confident." If you believe in yourself, you will achieve success. Maintain control and all your goals will be attainable.

Final Result

Your grade: A+
Continue to *"Believe"* and you will *succeed.*
LPN/LVN belongs to you!

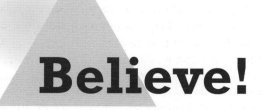

Believe!

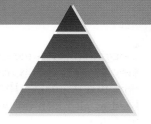

CHAPTER 3

The NCLEX-PN® Examination: From a Graduate's Perspective

Karen Machnacz, LPN and Gabrielle (Gabby) Machnacz, LPN

Nursing Students and Graduates

We want to thank two very special recent graduates, now licensed practical nurses (LPNs), for writing letters to you in this chapter. We are pleased to introduce you to Karen Machnacz, LPN, and Gabrielle (Gabby) Machnacz, LPN, a mother (Karen) and daughter (Gabby) team, who attended nursing school together. Listen to what they have to say to you—their information, tips, and suggestions will be very helpful!

A Letter From Karen

Congratulations to all of you!

The moment I entered nursing school my life changed. Everything was overwhelming; in fact, "overwhelming" was an understatement, let alone thinking about taking the NCLEX exam. We all know that the stress of going through nursing school can be high. I would sometimes feel exhausted and nauseous when I thought about test questions.

During nursing school, I was one of those students who had anxiety about studying and doing well on tests. I quickly learned that the verbiage and question structures are much different than any other college course tests that I took before. Nursing tests were all critical thinking! Each question challenges you to think: What would you as a nurse do in a real-world scenario? Feeling overwhelmed, I started to research different supplemental books that might help me during nursing school to get a better handle on how to break down each question and provide tips that will assist me throughout the program. That is when I discovered *Saunders Strategies for Test Success: Passing Nursing School and the NCLEX® Exam.* The book is outstanding with breaking down the questions by question types such as multiple choice, select

all that apply (SATA), prioritization, and pharmacology, to name a few. The book also provides additional free resources and practice questions. It helped me so much while I was in nursing school and with preparing for the NCLEX. The other book that helped me both while I was in nursing school and preparing for the NCLEX was *Saunders Comprehensive Review for the NCLEX-PN® Examination.* This book has thousands of practice questions, and the great thing is that you could use the Evolve site and select specific content areas for practice questions. So, when I had a test on, for example, endocrine, I would go to Evolve for this book and select Endocrine and be provided with hundreds of practice questions on this area. This was perfect for exam preparation and helped me pass my nursing tests.

Before I knew it, 10 months had flown by and I was graduating from nursing school and had one more challenging thing to accomplish—to pass that dreaded NCLEX. I definitely suggest doing practice questions in preparation for NCLEX, as many as you can, and I would say that you need to practice at least 3000 to 4000; through repetition you'll start to identify the format and structure of each question and the different strategic words that help direct you to the correct answer.

After graduation, I would do practice questions for about 2 to 3 hours a day. My daughter and I were in the LPN nursing program together, and it was great to do study sessions with her during the program and especially when studying for the NCLEX. I had about 3 weeks after graduation for final preparation for NCLEX and of course similar to other nursing graduates, had several other life stressors simultaneously going on. There were some days that I didn't think I could accomplish this last feat and felt defeated about studying. I would reach out to my family and friends to seek support. This is just so important and I want to tell you never to be ashamed or disappointed in yourself if you to reach out to others for support. Sometimes as nurses we feel like we are the ones that everyone needs to lean on; well I realized we need to also lean on others sometimes to get through the tough times. My uncle gave me great advice; he told me to take small breaks when studying and when stressed to close my eyes and sit back and take some deep breaths. This really helped. I was also worried about getting through the test and not running out of time. My uncle advised me to take the total number of questions on NCLEX, which is 205, divide it by the hours allotted (5 hours) and you will know approximately how many minutes you have for each question. That turns out to be 1.46 minutes and if you closed your eyes and relaxed for that time period it feels like a long time. However, it is important to remember that the question does not disappear from the screen after this time period—you can spend as much time as you need on a question and the question does not leave the screen until you answer it and click "submit."

The night before the NCLEX my stomach felt like it was in knots. I studied as much as my mental capacity allowed and I needed to clear my mind. I decided to watch some of my favorite movies until my body would relax and I would fall asleep. When morning came after a restless night, I made breakfast and went to the testing site, which was about 2 hours away. I left my house 5 hours before my scheduled time of my exam because I wanted to make sure I arrived with plenty of time to focus and clear my mind.

When the time finally came, I walked into the testing center and was greeted by a very firm receptionist. She verified my license, took my photo, and then my fingerprints. I was provided a locker for personal belongings. The receptionist spoke to me about the guidelines of the exam and what you could have with you during the exam, which was your license, erase board, erase marker for math, one tissue, earplugs, and noise-blocking headphones and that is it! The erase board, marker, earplugs, and headphones are provided to you. My heart started to race and just when I was about to walk in, the receptionist stopped me. I had completely forgotten you could not bring in any jewelry. I pleaded with her explaining that it was my grandma's and provided me comfort and less anxiety, but she told me it was against the guidelines. I ended up placing the jewelry in my locker. I took a few minutes to collect myself again, closed my eyes, took a deep breath to clear my mind, and I went in to take the test.

The receptionist walked me to the computer desk, and I placed the noise-blocking headphones on and began the NCLEX exam. There were a few example questions that showed the format of what the exam was going to look like, then the actual exam began. There were a good majority of SATA questions, pharmacology, pediatrics, and prioritizing and delegation questions that I had on my exam. Slowly, I crept up to question 85,

the minimum number of questions. Once I had submitted question 85 and my computer did not shut down, my anxiety and panic came over me once again. I wasn't sure when the exam would end, so I was starting to lose focus. After question 95, I had to refocus my thinking and took lots of deep breaths to relax. Then, after question 98, my computer shut off. My anxiety was not really relieved and I still thought the worst possible scenario, which is that I failed the NCLEX. Many other nursing students I talked with felt the same way when their computer shut off. Now I had to wait for results. I knew that these next few days were going to go by so slowly. Luckily, I had a lot planned to help keep my mind occupied.

Finally, these post-test days passed and when I checked the results site, the screen read that I had passed! I cried… I couldn't believe that all the stress and hard work had paid off. Thank you to my mom and grandma, forever in my heart; and to my daughters and sons and my entire family, and my nursing professors for their support and constantly telling me that if I believed in myself, I COULD do this!

Preparing for the NCLEX is hard but worth it. So definitely hang in there. I am proud to say I passed NCLEX, you can do it too! Trust yourself, be positive, believe in yourself, and NEVER give up… you WILL pass the NCLEX exam.
I wish you the best of luck!
Karen

A Letter From Gabby

Congratulations to all of you!

If you are a student, it's great that you are using this book while you are in nursing school. It will help you with preparing for your nursing exams and will help you prepare for NCLEX at the same time. Hang in there – soon you will be graduating and taking the NCLEX. If you have officially completed nursing school, your final step is that you need to pass the NCLEX to become an LPN/LVN.

The NCLEX is a giant comprehensive test of everything you learn in nursing school. The test can ask questions you learned in fundamentals, medical-surgical, mental health, and pediatrics and maternity. It's the final test that determines the competency of your nursing skills and knowledge. Thinking of it can be an emotional roller coaster filled with stress, anxiety, and determination. Even after taking the NCLEX, not everyone feels 100% on how they did until they get the Quick Results that Pearson VUE offers post-test. Here is my personal story on what helped me prepare and pass the NCLEX.

Halfway through my nursing program I wanted to find supplemental material that would not only help me prepare for my medical-surgical nursing course, but the NCLEX as well. Through researching and watching

YouTube reviews on what helped previous PN students, I discovered Saunders products. I purchased *Saunders Comprehensive Review for the NCLEX-PN*, the book you are now reading, and was beyond impressed. The book breaks down topics and explains material clearly that the NCLEX may test on; it also provides test-taking strategies and tips on how to break down each question to figure out what the question is asking. What I really feel that prepared me was the library of practice questions this book has on Evolve, which is included with the purchase of the book. There are well over 5,000 questions and you can focus on a specific content area like cardiovascular, respiratory, etc. Another book that I would highly recommend is *Saunders' Strategies for Test Success—Passing Nursing School and the NCLEX*. The book has multiple strategies on how to combat test anxiety, break down critical thinking questions, and pick out strategic words to identify what the question is asking you.

I prepared for the NCLEX while I was in school. Then, I really focused and studied for the NCLEX starting the day after I graduated from nursing school. I graduated in June and took my exam in July, which gave me 1 month to do final preparation. I attempted looking at other review material but found that each different company had different verbiage associated with their practice questions. This became a little overwhelmed, so I decided to use only the Saunders products and I am so happy that I made this decision. I also would look up videos on the internet for mnemonics on the many drugs and lab values that are needed to know for the NCLEX. Each day I would spend 2 hours reviewing material I was not confident with and practicing at least 200 practice questions a day. From the strategies I used—reading material, going over various different visual videos, and doing practice questions—doing the practice questions consistently is what truly prepared me for the NCLEX.

The night before the NCLEX, my body and mind were at its limits, so I decided to close all my books and laptop computer and I tried to get some sleep. Before I knew it, it was 5:00 a.m. and exactly 4 hours away from taking my NCLEX. The butterflies and anxiety were starting to bubble up inside of me. I ate a good breakfast and headed to the Pearson testing center a little over an hour before my test time. Once at the testing center, the receptionist checked me in with my identification. They have very strict guidelines at the testing center that must be followed before you can step foot in front of a testing screen. Any personal items get placed in a locker. If you bring any electronic device, it must be fully shut off, sealed in a bag, and placed in your locker. You cannot wear any jewelry; you will be asked to remove it. You are not allowed to bring in writing utensils; they will be provided. They will provide tissues if needed and hand sanitizer; you cannot bring your own. They also provide noise-blocking headphones; I would highly recommend using these especially for when getting distracted easily from background noise. Lastly, no food or beverages are allowed either. Then, after locking up all personal items, the test proctor nicely instructs that you are allotted 5 hours to complete the exam and may get anywhere between 85 and 205 to determine your competency. You are allowed two breaks at different intervals during testing.

You are provided with practice time to get accustomed to how to navigate the exam software. But shortly after that trial, the test begins. The questions differ for each person who takes the exam. I remember having a lot of questions pertaining to pharmacology, diabetes, prioritization, medical-surgical, and fundamentals. Roughly, every 1 out of 3 questions I had were SATA type questions. It's important to remember that on NCLEX, SATA questions may have just one correct answer out of the multiple options or all the options could be the correct answer. So, when in doubt, trust your gut. I would try to read the question twice and think about what the question is asking and look for any strategic words that might clue me into what is the most correct answer they are looking for. When the test got closer to question 80, the nerves came back and I became self-conscious on whether or not I was spending too much time on certain questions. After I answered question 85, my test was over. Again, nerves and anxiety overwhelmed me and I knew that the next few days would drag on until I was able to view my Quick Results. I heard stories of people still failing their exam even after shutting off after the minimum of questions. So, my anxiety wasn't really relieved knowing that I had shut off after 85 questions.

While awaiting the results, trying to keep busy is a must. In the meantime, I cleaned and reorganized my kitchen, deep cleaned the basement, and took a trip to the beach just to preoccupy my mind from thinking of my NCLEX results. Finally, at 8:00 a.m., 2 days and 1 hour after I took my exam, I knew my results would be posted. I quickly paid the fee to see it early and when the page finally loaded I took a big sigh of relief. I HAD PASSED MY NCLEX! I was officially a licensed practical nurse! It felt like a weight lifted off my chest. I'm proud to say that I have been a practicing nurse now for about 5 months and I wanted to give a quick and sincere thank you to my mom (who was my rock, support, and classmate), my boyfriend Eddie, my family, and aunts that have inspired me to become a nurse, my school professors, and a big thank you to Elsevier and the Saunders products. These products guided me to understanding the rationale behind the critical thinking that goes into the nursing process and I couldn't have passed the NCLEX without using this material. Thank you! And to the future PN students—you got this! And, you too will pass the NCLEX!

I wish you the very best!
Gabby

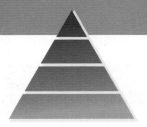

CHAPTER 4

Clinical Judgment and Test-Taking Strategies

If you would like to read more about test-taking strategies after completing this chapter, *Saunders Strategies for Test Success: Passing Nursing School and the NCLEX® Exam* focuses on the test-taking strategies that will help you to pass your nursing examinations while in nursing school and will prepare you for the NCLEX-PN® examination.

I. Clinical Judgment

Clinical judgment is the observed outcome of critical thinking and decision-making (Dickison et al., 2019). The NCLEX-PN examination requires candidates to demonstrate the ability to use clinical judgment in client care. Thus, clinical judgment skills along with other traditional test-taking strategies should be used to answer test questions. The National Council of State Boards of Nursing (NCSBN) has created the NCSBN Clinical Judgment Measurement Model (NCJMM) that consists of applying 6 cognitive skills or processes: (1) recognizing cues; (2) analyzing cues; (3) prioritizing hypotheses; (4) generating solutions; (5) taking action; and (6) evaluating outcomes. See Chapter 1, Table 1.1 for a description of these six cognitive skills/processes. Also see Box 4.18 for an example of how to apply the six cognitive skills/ processes when answering test questions. From Dickison P, Haerling KA, Lasater K: Integrating the NCSBN Clinical Judgment Model into Nursing Educational Frameworks. *J Nurs Educ* 58(2):72–78, 2019.

II. Key Test-Taking Strategies (Box 4.1)

III. How to Avoid Reading Into the Question (Box 4.2)

A. Pyramid Points
1. Avoid asking yourself the forbidden words, "Well, what if …?" because this will lead you to the "forbidden" area: Reading into the question.
2. Focus only on the data in the question, read every word, and make a decision about what the question is asking. Recognize cues presented in the question. Reread the question more than one time; ask yourself, "What is this question asking?" and "What content is this question testing?" (see Box 4.2).
3. Determine whether an abnormality exists. Look at data or information in the question and in the responses and decide what is significant. What is abnormal data? Analyze the cues. Pay close attention to this information as you read the question and as you answer the question.
4. Focus on the client in the question. At times, there are other people discussed in the question who also impact how the question should be answered. Remember the concepts of client-centered and family-centered care.
5. Look for the strategic words in the question, such as *immediate, initial, first, priority, initial, best, need for follow-up,* and *need for further teaching;* strategic words make a difference regarding what the question is asking and will assist in prioritizing hypotheses (Box 4.3).
6. Consider available resources as you generate solutions and answer the question. Remember that you will have all resources you need at the client's bedside to provide quality client care.
7. In multiple-choice questions, multiple-response questions, extended multiple response questions, matrix-type questions, cloze questions, or questions that require you to arrange nursing interventions or other data in order of priority (drag and drop or extended drag and drop), read every choice or option presented before answering.
8. *Always* use the process of elimination when choices or options are presented; after you have eliminated options, reread the question before selecting your final choice or choices. Focus on the data in both the question and the options to assist in the process of elimination and directing you to the correct answer. In taking action questions, think about the client's presentation and needs to answer correctly. In evaluating outcomes questions, read carefully especially if the question is asking which option indicates the need for further teaching or follow-up.
9. With questions that require you to fill in the blank or complete a sentence (cloze questions), focus on the information in the question and determine what the question is asking; if the question requires you to calculate a medication dose, an intravenous flow rate, or intake and output amounts, recheck your work in calculating and always use the on-screen calculator to verify the answer.

BOX 4.1 Key Test-Taking Strategies

The Question

- Focus on the data or information, read every word, recognize cues, and make a decision about what the question is asking.
- Note the subject and determine what content is being tested.
- Visualize the event; analyze cues and note if an abnormality exists in the data provided.
- Determine who "the client of the question" is.
- Look for the strategic words; strategic words make a difference regarding what the question is asking about and prioritizing hypotheses.
- Think about the client's presenting situation and needs to generate solutions and determine which actions to take.
- Determine whether the question presents a positive or negative event query; negative event queries are usually most associated with the skill of evaluating outcomes.
- Avoid asking yourself, "Well, what if …?" because this will lead you to reading into the question.
- Apply the NCSBN Clinical Judgment Measurement Model (NCJMM) and the 6 cognitive skills/processes alongside other test-taking strategies.

The Options

- Always use the process of elimination when choices or options are presented, and always read each option carefully; once you have eliminated options, reread the question before selecting your final choice or choices.
- Look for comparable or alike options and eliminate these.
- Determine whether there is an umbrella option or comprehensive option; if so, this could be the correct option.
- Identify any closed-ended words; if present, the option is likely incorrect.
- Use the ABCs, Maslow's Hierarchy of Needs (remembering that physiological needs are a priority), and the steps of the nursing process to answer questions that require prioritizing; use CAB for cardiopulmonary resuscitation (CPR).
- Use therapeutic communication techniques to answer communication questions, and remember to focus on the client's thoughts, feelings, concerns, anxieties, and fears.
- Use delegating and assignment-making guidelines to match the client's needs with the scope of practice of the health care provider.
- Use pharmacology guidelines to select the correct option if the question addresses a medication.

BOX 4.2 Practice Question: Avoiding the "What If …?" Syndrome and Reading Into the Question

The nurse is changing the tapes on a tracheostomy tube. The client coughs, and the tube is dislodged. What is the **initial** nursing action?

1. Call the surgeon to reinsert the tube.
2. Ventilate the client using a manual resuscitation bag and face mask.
3. Cover the tracheostomy site with a sterile dressing to prevent infection.
4. Call the respiratory therapy department to reinsert the tracheostomy tube.

Answer: 2

Test-Taking Strategy

You may immediately think, "The tube is dislodged, and I need the surgeon!" Read the question carefully, and note the strategic word, *initial*. You need to quickly prioritize and take action. Focus on the data in the question—the tube is dislodged—and determine that an abnormality exists. Apply the cognitive skill, *take action*. The question is asking you to analyze cues and determine a nursing action, so that is what you need to look for as you eliminate the incorrect options. Eliminate options 1 and 4 because they are comparable or alike and delay the *initial* intervention needed. Eliminate option 3 because this action will block the airway. If the tube is dislodged, the *initial* nursing action is to ventilate the client using a manual resuscitation bag and face mask. Additionally, use of the ABCs—airway, breathing, and circulation—will direct you to the correct option. Remember: Avoid the "What if …?" syndrome and reading into the question!

B. Ingredients of a question (Box 4.4)
  1. The ingredients of a question include the event, which is a client or clinical scenario; the event query; and the options or answers.
  2. The event provides you with the content about the client or clinical case situation that you need to think about when answering the question.
  3. The event query asks something specific about the content of the event.
  4. The options are all of the answers provided with the question.

5. Traditional NCLEX® test questions
  a. In a multiple-choice question, there will be four options and you must select one; read every option carefully and think about the event and the event query as you use the process of elimination.
  b. In a multiple-response question, there will be several options (up to six) and you must select all options that apply to the event in the question. The correct answer could be *only* one of the options, *all* of the options, *or* any number of the total options provided. Visualize the event, and use your nursing knowledge and clinical experiences to answer the question.
  c. In an ordered-response (prioritizing)/drag-and-drop question, you will be required to arrange in order of priority nursing actions or other data; visualize the event and use your nursing knowledge and clinical experiences to answer the question. These questions are usually related to nursing procedures.
  d. A fill-in-the-blank question does not contain options, and some figure/illustration questions and audio item formats may or may not con-

BOX 4.3 Common Strategic Words

Words That Indicate the Need to Prioritize
Best
Early or late
Essential
First
Highest priority
Immediate
Initial
Most
Most appropriate
Most important
Most likely
Next
Priority
Primary
Vital

Words That Reflect Assessment
Ascertain
Assess
Check
Collect
Determine
Find out
Gather
Identify
Monitor
Observe
Obtain information
Recognize

Additional Strategic Words
Need for further teaching or education
Need for follow-up
On the day of
After several days

BOX 4.4 Ingredients of a Question: Event, Event Query, and Options

Event
The nurse instructs an adolescent with iron deficiency anemia about the administration of oral iron preparations.

Event Query
The nurse would tell the adolescent that it is **best** to take the iron with which item?

Options
1. Cola
2. Soda
3. Water
4. Tomato juice

Answer: 4
Test-Taking Strategy
Note the strategic word, *best*. Apply the cognitive skill, *generate solutions*. Use knowledge about the administration of iron to determine the action you will take and what instruction you will provide to the adolescent. Remember that vitamin C enhances the absorption of the iron preparation. Tomato juice has a high ascorbic acid (vitamin C) content, whereas cola, soda, and water do not contain vitamin C. Note that options 1 and 2 are comparable or alike, so eliminate these options. Next, recalling that vitamin C increases the absorption of iron will direct you to option 4, tomato juice. As you read a question, remember to note its ingredients: the event, event query, and options!

tain options. A graphic option item will contain options in the form of a picture or graphic.
  e. A chart/exhibit question will most likely contain options; read the question carefully and all of the information in the chart or exhibit before selecting an answer. In this question type, there will be information in the chart/exhibit that is pertinent to how the question is answered, and there may also be information that is not pertinent. Read all of the information in the chart before answering. It is necessary to discern what information is important and what the "distractors" are.

6. Next Generation NCLEX® (NGN) Item Types
  a. The NGN item types will use a case study approach and accompanying test questions will be designed to assess the six cognitive skills identified in the NCJMM developed by the NCSBN.
  b. There will be single episode case studies and unfolding case studies.

  c. Single episode case studies will be accompanied by a test question that will most likely assess one of the cognitive skills. However, note that there may be some single episode case studies that will be accompanied by a test question that assesses more than one cognitive skill.
  d. Unfolding case studies will be accompanied by six test questions in which all six cognitive skills are assessed.
  e. It is important to read all of the data in the case study and look for abnormalities in the information presented before answering the accompanying questions.
  f. Use nursing knowledge and clinical experiences to assist in answering the questions.
  g. Currently, the NGN item types include highlight, extended multiple response, extended drag and drop, matrix, and cloze. Examples of these NGN item types can be located on the Evolve site accompanying this book.

IV. Strategic Words (See Box 4.3 and Box 4.5)
A. Strategic words focus your attention on a critical point to consider when answering the question and will assist you in eliminating the incorrect options. These words can be located in either the event or the query of the question.

BOX 4.5	Practice Question: Strategic Words

The nurse visits a client with chronic obstructive pulmonary disease (COPD) who is on home oxygen at 2 L/minute. The client's respiratory rate is 22 breaths/minute, and the client is complaining of increased dyspnea. The nurse would take which **initial** action?

1. Determine the need to increase the oxygen.
2. Call emergency services to come to the home.
3. Reassure the client that there is no need to worry.
4. Collect more information about the client's respiratory status.

Answer: 4
Test-Taking Strategy
Note the strategic word, *initial*. Recognize and analyze cues in order to determine the action to take. Completing the assessment and collecting additional information regarding the client's respiratory status is the *initial* nursing action. The oxygen is not increased without validation of the need for further oxygen and the approval of the primary health care provider. Calling emergency services is a premature action. Reassuring the client is appropriate, but it is inappropriate to tell the client not to worry. Using the steps of the nursing process will assist in remembering that assessment (data collection) is the first step. Also, use the ABCs—airway, breathing, and circulation—to direct you to option 4. Remember to look for strategic words!

B. With certain item types, some strategic words may indicate that all options are correct and that it will be necessary to prioritize to select the correct option; words that reflect the process of assessment or recognizing cues are also important to note (see Box 4.3). Words that reflect assessment usually indicate the need to look for an option that is a first step, because assessment (data collection) is the first step in the nursing process.

C. As you read the question, look for the strategic words; strategic words make a difference regarding the focus of the question. Throughout this book, *strategic words* presented in the question, such as those that indicate the need to prioritize, are **bolded.** If the test-taking strategy is to focus on *strategic words,* then the term *strategic words* is highlighted in blue where it appears in the test-taking strategy.

V. Subject of the Question (Box 4.6)

A. The subject of the question is the specific topic that the question is asking about.

B. Identifying the subject of the question will assist you in eliminating the incorrect options and direct you in selecting the correct option. Throughout this book, if the *subject* of the question is a specific strategy to use in answering the question correctly, it is highlighted in blue in the test-taking strategy.

C. The highlighting of the strategy will provide you with guidance on what strategies to review in *Saunders Strategies for Test Success: Passing Nursing School and the NCLEX Exam* and the content areas and Health Problem in need of further remediation in *Saunders Comprehensive Review for the NCLEX-PN® Examination.*

BOX 4.6	Practice Question: Subject of the Question

The nurse would implement which measures to prevent infection in a hospitalized immunocompromised client? **Select all that apply.**

1. Use strict aseptic technique for all invasive procedures.
2. Use good hand-washing technique before touching the client.
3. Insert a urinary catheter to eliminate the need to use a bedpan.
4. Keep fresh flowers and potted plants out of the client's room.
5. Place the client in a semiprivate room with another client who is immunocompromised.
6. Keep frequently used equipment such as a blood pressure cuff in the client's room for use by the client.

Answer: 1, 2, 4, 6
Test-Taking Strategy
Focus on the subject, measures to prevent infection. The nurse needs to use knowledge to generate solutions and the actions to take to prevent infection. An immunocompromised client is at high risk for infection, and specific measures are taken to prevent infection. Strict aseptic technique is necessary for all invasive procedures; however, invasive procedures are avoided as much as possible. Urinary catheters are avoided because of the risk of infection associated with their use. Good hand-washing technique is used before touching the client. Fresh fruits, fresh flowers, and potted plants are kept out of the client's room because they harbor organisms, placing the client at risk for infection. The client is placed in a private room. Frequently used equipment such as a blood pressure cuff, stethoscope, or thermometer is kept in the client's room for use by the client only. The client is also monitored daily for any signs of infection. Remember to focus on the subject of the question!

VI. Positive and Negative Event Queries (Boxes 4.7 and 4.8)

A. A positive event query uses strategic words that ask you to select an option that is correct; for example, the event query may read, "Which statement by a client *indicates an understanding* of the side effects of the prescribed medication?"

B. A negative event query uses strategic words that ask you to select an option that is an incorrect item or statement; for example, the event query may read, "Which statement by a client *indicates a need for further teaching* about the side effects of the prescribed medication?"

VII. Questions That Require Prioritizing

A. Many questions in the examination will require you to use the skill of prioritizing hypotheses or nursing actions.

B. Look for the strategic words in the question that indicate the need to prioritize (see Box 4.3).

C. Remember that when a question requires prioritization, all options may be correct and you need to determine the correct order.

BOX 4.7	Practice Question: Positive Event Query

The nurse is teaching a postpartum woman how to bathe her newborn. The nurse would provide which instructions to the mother? **Select all that apply.**

1. Support the newborn's body during the bath.
2. Clean any eye discharge using a wet cotton ball.
3. Fill the bathtub with no more than 10 inches of water.
4. Clean the eyes, moving from the outer canthus to the inner canthus.
5. Cover the newborn's body except for the part being washed or rinsed.
6. Begin the bath with the face, and clean the newborn's diaper area next.

Answer: 1, 2, 5
Test-Taking Strategy
Focus on the subject, instructions for bathing the newborn, and apply the cogntive skill, *generate solutions*. Note that the question identifies a positive event query, and you need to select the correct instructions for bathing a newborn. The nurse needs to use knowledge when teaching the mother to ensure actions that will provide a safe environment. Visualize each option carefully, keeping the principles of safety and infection control in mind. During bathing, the newborn's body is supported at all times by placing a hand under the newborn's head and neck. If the newborn is bathed in a bathtub, the tub should be lined with a towel to provide comfort and traction to prevent slipping, and it is filled with no more than 3 inches of water. The newborn's body is covered except for the part being washed or rinsed. Any eye discharge is cleaned using a wet cotton ball moving from the inner canthus to the outer canthus. The bath is started with the face, then other body areas are washed, and the diaper area is cleaned last. Remember to read the event query and note if it is a positive event type.

BOX 4.8	Practice Question: Negative Event Query

The nurse provides home care instructions to a client who is taking lithium carbonate. Which statement by the client indicates a **need for further instructions**?

1. "I need to take the medication with meals."
2. "My blood levels must be monitored very closely."
3. "I need to decrease my salt and fluid intake while taking the medication."
4. "I need to call my doctor if I have excessive diarrhea, vomiting, or sweating."

Answer: 3
Test-Taking Strategy
This question identifies an example of a negative event query question. Note the strategic words, *need for further instructions*. These strategic words indicate that you need to select an option that identifies an incorrect client statement. The nurse needs to use knowledge about lithium carbonate to evaluate the outcomes of teaching and to determine what the client needs regarding further instructions. Lithium is irritating to the gastric mucosa; therefore, lithium should be taken with meals. Because therapeutic and toxic dosage ranges are so close, lithium blood levels must be monitored very closely, more frequently at first and then once every several months after that per health care provider's prescription. The client should be instructed to withhold the medication if excessive diarrhea, vomiting, or diaphoresis occurs, and to inform the primary health care provider if any of these problems occur. A normal diet with daily recommended sodium (1500 mg) and fluid (3000 mL) intake should be maintained because lithium decreases sodium reabsorption by the renal tubules, which could cause sodium depletion. A low-sodium intake causes a relative increase in lithium retention and could lead to toxicity. Remember that negative event queries ask you to select an option that is an *incorrect* item or statement! Watch for negative event queries!

D. Strategies to use to prioritize include the ABCs—airway, breathing, and circulation, Maslow's Hierarchy of Needs theory (recalling that physiological needs are a priority), steps of the nursing process recalling that data collection (assessment) is the first step, and the cognitive skills in the NCJMM focusing on what the question is asking.

E. The ABCs (Box 4.9)
1. Use the ABCs—airway, breathing, and circulation—when selecting an answer or determining the order of priority.
2. Remember the order of priority: airway, breathing, and circulation.
3. Airway is always the first priority. Note that an exception occurs when cardiopulmonary resuscitation (CPR) is performed; in this situation, the nurse follows the CAB (compressions, airway, breathing) guidelines.

F. Maslow's Hierarchy of Needs theory (Box 4.10 and Fig. 4.1)
1. According to Maslow's Hierarchy of Needs theory, physiological needs are the priority, followed by safety and security needs, love and belonging needs, self-esteem needs, and, finally, self-actualization needs; select the option or determine the order of priority by addressing physiological needs first.
2. When a physiological need is not addressed in the question or noted in one of the options, continue to use Maslow's Hierarchy of Needs theory sequentially as a guide and look for the option that addresses safety.

G. Steps of the nursing process and NCJMM and Cognitive Skills
1. Data Collection (Assessment)/Recognize Cues
   a. The nurse recognizes cues by identifying significant data from many sources,
   b. These questions address the process of gathering subjective and objective data and cues relative to the client and the client's problem, confirming the data, and communicating and documenting the data.

| BOX 4.9 | Practice Question: Use of the ABCs |

A client is admitted to the emergency department with complaints of severe chest pain. The client is extremely restless, frightened, and dyspneic. Immediate admission prescriptions include oxygen by nasal cannula at 4 L per minute, troponin level, creatinine phosphokinase and isoenzymes blood levels, a chest x-ray, and a 12-lead electrocardiogram (ECG). Which action would the nurse take **first?**

1. Obtain the 12-lead ECG.
2. Draw the blood specimens.
3. Apply the oxygen to the client.
4. Call radiology to obtain the chest x-ray study.

Answer: *3*
Test-Taking Strategy
Note the strategic word, *first*. The nurse needs to recognize the cues and analyze them to determine that the priority hypothesis is oxygenation. The nurse would then generate solutions and take action by applying the oxygen to the client first. Also, use the ABCs—airway, breathing, and circulation. The *first* action would be to apply the oxygen because the client can be experiencing myocardial ischemia. The ECG can provide evidence of cardiac damage and the location of myocardial ischemia. However, oxygen is the priority to prevent further cardiac damage. Drawing the blood specimens would be done after oxygen administration and just before or after the ECG, depending on the situation. Although the chest x-ray can show cardiac enlargement, having the chest x-ray would not influence immediate treatment. Remember to use the ABCs—airway, breathing, and circulation—to help prioritize actions you will take!

| BOX 4.10 | Practice Question: Maslow's Hierarchy of Needs Theory |

A female client arrives at the emergency department and states that she was just raped. In preparing a plan of care, which is the **priority** intervention?

1. Providing instructions for medical follow-up
2. Obtaining appropriate counseling for the victim
3. Providing anticipatory guidance for police investigations, medical questions, and court proceedings
4. Exploring safety concerns by obtaining permission to notify significant others who can provide shelter

Answer: *4*
Test-Taking Strategy
Note the strategic word, *priority*. The nurse needs to have knowledge of the client's priority needs and generate solutions. Use Maslow's Hierarchy of Needs theory. After the provision of medical treatment, the nurse's next *priority* would be obtaining support and planning for safety. Option 1 is concerned with ensuring that the victim understands the importance of and commits to the need for medical follow-up. Options 2 and 3 seek to meet the emotional needs related to the rape and emotional readiness for the process of discovery and legal action. These are not *priority* interventions. Remember that physiological needs are the *priority*, followed by safety needs. Therefore, select option 4 because it addresses the client's safety needs. Remember to use Maslow's Hierarchy of Needs theory to help prioritize and generate solutions!

---

c. Remember that data collection (assessment)/recognizing cues is a first step.

d. When you are asked to select your first, immediate, or initial nursing action, collect data (assess) and recognize cues *first* to prioritize when selecting the correct option.

e. Look for strategic words in the options that reflect data collection (assessment)/recognizing cues (see Boxes 4.3 and 4.5).

f. If an option contains the concept of collection of client data, the best choice is to select that option (Box 4.11).

g. Possible exception to the guideline—if the question presents an emergency situation, read carefully; in an emergency situation, an action may be the priority rather than taking the time to collect further data.

2. Analysis/Analyze Cues and Prioritize Hypotheses (Box 4.12)

a. The nurse analyzes cues by connecting significant data to the client's clinical presentation and determining: is the data expected? Unexpected? What are the concerns?

b. Although *Analysis* is not a part of the Clinical Problem-Solving Process, the licensed practical nurse is expected to analyze some of the data and collaborate with the registered nurse to confirm the analysis.

c. These questions are the most difficult questions because they require understanding of the principles of physiological responses and require interpretation of the data collected.

d. They require critical thinking and decision-making and determining the rationale for therapeutic prescriptions or actions that may be addressed in the question.

e. These questions may address the formulation and prioritization of a hypothesis that identifies a client need or problem and may also include the communication and documentation of the results from the process of analyzing cues.

3. Planning/Generating Solutions (Box 4.13)

a. These questions require the nurse to develop a plan of care based on the ranking of the hypotheses from highest to lowest priority.

b. These questions also require determining goals and outcome criteria for goals of care when developing the plan of care, and communicating and documenting the plan of care.

c. The nurse generates solutions by using hypotheses to determine interventions for an expected outcome.

d. Remember that actual client problems rather than potential client problems will be the priority in most client situations.

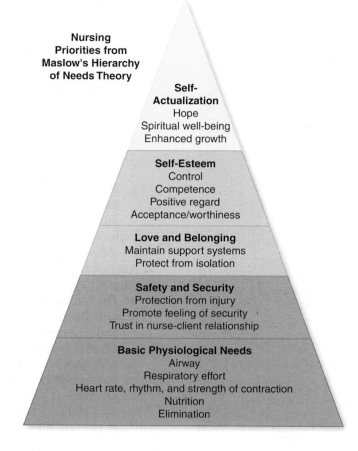

FIGURE 4.1 Use Maslow's Hierarchy of Needs theory to establish priorities.

BOX 4.11	Practice Question: Assessment (Data Collection)/Recognize Cues

The nurse assists in developing a diabetic teaching program. To meet the clients' needs, the nurse would suggest to take which action **first**?
1. Assess the clients' functional abilities.
2. Ensure that insurance will pay for participation in the program.
3. Discuss the focus of the program with the interprofessional team.
4. Include everyone who comes into the clinic in the teaching sessions.

Answer: 1
Test-Taking Strategy
Note the strategic word, *first*, which indicates the need to prioritize. The nurse needs to have knowledge of the teaching/learning process to recognize cues that affect preparation of an individualized teaching program for the clients. Use the steps of the nursing process to answer the question, remembering that assessment (data collection) is the first step. The only option that addresses data collection is option 1. The nurse should focus on individualized disease prevention and health promotion and maintenance. Therefore, the nurse must *first* assess and recognize cues so as to effectively plan the program. Options 2, 3, and 4 do not directly address the clients' needs.

BOX 4.12	Practice Question: Analysis/Analyze Cues/Prioritize Hypotheses

The nurse reviews the arterial blood gas results of a client and notes the following: pH of 7.30, $Paco_2$ of 50 mm Hg, and bicarbonate (HCO_3) of 22 mEq/L. The nurse analyzes these results as indicating which condition?
1. Metabolic acidosis
2. Respiratory alkalosis
3. Metabolic alkalosis
4. Respiratory acidosis

Answer: 4
Test-Taking Strategy
Focus on the data in the question and the subject, interpreting arterial blood gas results. The nurse needs to analyze the cues provided in the question and have knowledge of normal arterial blood gas results and acid-base disorders to determine the condition the client is experiencing. The normal pH is 7.35–7.45. In a respiratory condition, an opposite effect will be seen between the pH and the $Paco_2$. In this situation, the pH is lower than the normal value, and the $Paco_2$ is elevated. Therefore, you can eliminate options 1 and 3. In an acidotic condition, the pH is low. Therefore, the values identified in the question indicate respiratory acidosis. Remember the nurse needs to analyze cues, connect data to the client's presentation, identify client needs, and prioritize hypotheses.

BOX 4.13 Practice Question: Planning/ Generating Solutions

A client with active tuberculosis (TB) is to be admitted to a medical-surgical unit. Which action would the nurse take when assisting with planning a bed assignment?

1. Tell the admitting office to send the client to the intensive care unit.
2. Place the client in a private, airborne infection isolation room (AIIR).
3. Assign the client to a room with another client because intravenous antibiotics will be administered.
4. Assign the client to a room with another client and place a "strict hand washing" sign outside the door.

Answer: 2
Test-Taking Strategy
Focus on the subject, planning nursing care and identifying the safe bed assignment. The nurse needs to have knowledge of the transmission methods of TB in order to generate solutions for planning a bed assignment. Note that the question states "active tuberculosis." TB is spread via the airborne route. Preventing the spread of infection requires the use of special air handling and ventilation in an AIIR. Therefore, option 2 is the only correct option when planning a bed assignment for this client. Remember the nurse needs to plan and generate solutions to determine interventions for an expected outcome.

4. Implementation/Taking Action (Box 4.14)
   a. The nurse implements the generated solutions addressing the highest priorities or hypotheses.
   b. These questions address the process of organizing and managing care, counseling and teaching, providing care to achieve established goals, supervising and coordinating care, and communicating and documenting nursing interventions.
   c. Focus on a nursing action rather than on a medical action when you are answering a question, unless the question is asking you what prescribed medical action is anticipated.
   d. On the NCLEX-PN examination, the only client whom you need to be concerned about is the client in the question that you are answering; avoid the "What if ...?" syndrome and remember that the client in the question on the computer screen is your only assigned client.
   e. Answer the question from a textbook and ideal point of view; remember that the nurse has all of the time and all of the equipment needed to care for the client readily available at the bedside; remember that you do not need to run to the supply room to obtain, for example, sterile gloves because the sterile gloves will be at the client's bedside.

BOX 4.14 Practice Question: Implementation/ Taking Actions

The nurse is performing range-of-motion (ROM) exercises on a client when the client unexpectedly develops spastic muscle contractions. The nurse would implement which interventions? **Select all that apply.**

1. Stop movement of affected part.
2. Massage the affected part vigorously.
3. Force movement of the joint supporting the muscle.
4. Notify the primary health care provider immediately.
5. Ask the client to stand and walk rapidly around the room.
6. Place continuous gentle pressure on the muscle group until it relaxes.

Answer: 1, 6
Test-Taking Strategy
Implementation questions address the process of organizing and managing care. Focus on the subject, interventions to relieve spastic muscle contractions. In this question, the hypothesis is spastic muscle contractions. The nurse would use knowledge about the interventions to relieve spasticity, generate solutions, and take actions. ROM exercises should put each joint through as full a range of motion as possible without causing discomfort. The development of spastic muscle contraction is an unexpected outcome during ROM exercises. If this occurs, the nurse should stop movement of the affected part and place continuous gentle pressure on the muscle group until it relaxes. Once the contraction subsides, the exercises are resumed using slower, steady movement. Massaging the affected part vigorously may worsen the contraction. There is no need to notify the primary health care provider unless intervention is ineffective. The nurse should never force movement of a joint. Asking the client to stand and walk rapidly around the room is an inappropriate measure. Additionally, if the client is able to walk, ROM exercises are probably unnecessary. Remember the nurse needs to plan generated solutions and then take actions.

5. Evaluation/Evaluate Outcomes (Box 4.15)
   a. The nurse compares observed outcomes with expected ones.
   b. These questions focus on comparing the actual outcomes of care with the expected outcomes and on communicating and documenting findings.
   c. They also focus on assisting in determining the client's response to care and identifying factors that may interfere with achieving expected outcomes.
   d. In these question types, watch for negative event queries because they are frequently used.
H. Determine if an abnormality exists (Box 4.16)
   1. In the question, the client scenario will be described. Use your nursing knowledge and recognize cues that determine whether any of the information presented is indicating an abnormality.

BOX 4.15	Practice Question: Evaluation/ Evaluating Outcomes

The nurse instructs a client receiving external radiation therapy about skin care. Which statements by the client indicate an understanding of the instructions? **Select all that apply.**

1. "I can lie in the sun as long as I limit the time to 2 hours daily."
2. "I should wear snug clothing to support the irradiated skin area."
3. "I should wash the irradiated area gently each day with a mild soap and water."
4. "After bathing I should dry the area with a patting motion using a clean soft towel."
5. "I should avoid the use of powders, lotions, or creams on the skin area being irradiated."
6. "I should avoid removing the markings on the skin when bathing until my course of radiation is complete."

Answer: *3, 4, 5, 6*
Test-Taking Strategy
Focus on the subject, client's understanding of the instructions. The subject specifies that this is an evaluation-type question. The nurse needs to use knowledge about radiation therapy to evaluate the outcomes of teaching. Recall that external radiation therapy can cause altered skin integrity and special measures need to be taken to protect the skin. These measures include washing the irradiated area gently (using the hand rather than a wash cloth) each day with either water alone or water and a mild soap (rinse soap thoroughly); drying the area with a patting motion (not a rubbing motion) with a clean soft towel; avoiding removing the markings on the skin when bathing until the entire course of radiation is complete because these markings indicate exactly where the beam of radiation is to be focused; avoiding the use of powders, lotions, or creams on the skin area being irradiated unless prescribed by the radiologist; avoiding wearing clothing or items that bind or rub the irradiated skin area; and avoiding heat exposure or sun exposure to the irradiated area. Remember the nurse needs to evaluate outcomes by comparing observed outcomes with expected ones.

2. Look at the options. If an abnormality exists, either further nursing assessment and analysis or further nursing intervention will be required. Therefore, continuing to monitor or documenting will not likely be a correct answer; do not select these options if they are presented!

I. Focus on the data or information in the question and recognize cues (Box 4.17)
   1. With this strategy, data are provided in either the question or the answers (or both) that are important in answering the question correctly.
   2. Data needed to answer the question will be obviously abnormal, and will not likely be borderline data. If it is borderline, there will be another event in the question that could cause the data to become abnormal.

J. Choose options that ensure client safety (see Box 4.17)
   1. When choosing an option, think about whether the option could cause a compromise in client safety.

BOX 4.16	Practice Question: Determine If an Abnormality Exists

The nurse is caring for a client who is taking digoxin and is complaining of nausea. The nurse gathers additional data and checks the most recent laboratory results. Which laboratory value requires the **need for follow-up** by the nurse?

1. Sodium 138 mEq/L
2. Potassium 3.3 mEq/L
3. Phosphorus 3.1 mg/dL
4. Magnesium 1.8 mg/dL

Answer: *2*
Test-Taking Strategy
Note the strategic words, *need for follow-up*. The first step in approaching the answer to this question is to determine whether an abnormality exists. Recognize cues in the question that are significant and analyze the cues by connecting the data. The client is taking digoxin and is complaining of nausea and the nurse should suspect toxicity. The normal reference range for sodium is 135–145 mEq/L; potassium, 3.5–5.0 mEq/L; phosphorus, 3.0–4.5 mg/dL; and magnesium, 1.8–2.6 mEq/L. The laboratory values noted in the options are all within normal range except for the potassium level. Recall that the potassium level must stay consistent while the client is taking digoxin to prevent adverse effects such as toxicity from occurring. Remember to recognize cues, analyze them, and determine whether an abnormality exists before choosing the correct option.

2. If an option could potentially result in an adverse effect or increase the client's risk for injury, eliminate that option.

VIII. Using the NCJMM and the 6 Cognitive Skills to Answer a Test Question (Box 4.18)

IX. Client Needs
A. Physiological Integrity
   1. According to the NCSBN, these questions test the concepts that the nurse provides care as it relates to comfort and assistance in the performance of activities of daily living as well as care related to the administration of medications and parenteral therapies.
   2. These questions also address the nurse's ability to reduce the client's potential for developing complications or health problems related to treatments, procedures, or existing conditions and to provide care to clients with acute, chronic, or life-threatening physical health conditions.
   3. Focus on Maslow's Hierarchy of Needs theory in these types of questions and remember that physiological needs are a priority and are addressed first.
   4. Use the ABCs—airway, breathing, and circulation. Note that when CPR is necessary, follow the CAB guidelines rather than the ABCs.
   5. Use the nursing process and NCJMM when selecting an option addressing Physiological Integrity.

BOX 4.17 **Practice Question: Focus on the Data in the Question and Ensure Client Safety**

The nurse is providing discharge instructions to a client with diabetes mellitus. The client's glycosylated hemoglobin (HbA1c) level is 10%. What information would the nurse provide to the client?

1. "Increase the amount of vegetables and water intake in your diet regimen."
2. "Change the time of day you exercise because it may cause hypoglycemia."
3. "Continue with the same diet and exercise regimen you are currently using."
4. "Utilize a high-intensity exercise regimen and decrease carbohydrate consumption."

Answer: 1

Test-Taking Strategy

Focus on the **data in the question**, an HbA1c level of 10%. The nurse needs to recognize cues and analyze the cues to determine that the HbA1c level is greater than the recommended range for a client with diabetes mellitus, and indicates poor glycemic control. Therefore, an **abnormality exists**. Choose the option that addresses this abnormality and **ensures client safety**. Option 1 is a safe recommendation to make to a diabetic client and will help to reduce the HbA1c level. Changing the time of day for exercise and continuing with the same diet and exercise regimen will not address the client's problem. Note the words *high intensity* in option 4. Utilizing a high-intensity exercise regimen and decreasing carbohydrate consumption could potentially result in a hypoglycemic reaction and does not ensure client safety. Remember to focus on the data in the question and recognize and analyze cues to determine if an abnormality is present.

B. Safe and Effective Care Environment
   1. The NCSBN indicates that these questions test the concepts of providing safe nursing care and collaborating with interprofessional team members to facilitate effective client care; these questions also focus on the protection of clients, significant others, and health care personnel from environmental hazards.
   2. Focus on safety with these types of questions, and remember the importance of hand washing, call lights or bells, bed positioning, appropriate use of side rails, asepsis, use of standard and other precautions, triage, and emergency response planning.
C. Health Promotion and Maintenance
   1. According to the NCSBN, these questions test the concepts that the nurse provides and assists in directing nursing care to promote and maintain health.
   2. Content addressed in these questions relates to assisting the client and significant others during the normal expected stages of growth and development, and providing client care related to the prevention and early detection of health problems.
   3. Use the teaching and learning theory if the question addresses client teaching, remembering that the client's willingness, desire, and readiness to learn is the first priority.
   4. Watch for negative event queries because they are frequently used in questions that address Health Promotion and Maintenance and client education.
D. Psychosocial Integrity
   1. The NCSBN notes that these questions test the concepts of nursing care that promote and support the emotional, mental, and social well-being of the client and significant others.
   2. Content addressed in these questions relates to supporting and promoting the client's or significant others' ability to cope, adapt, or problem-solve in situations such as illnesses; disabilities; or stressful events, including abuse, neglect, or violence.
   3. In this Client Needs category, you may be asked communication-type questions that relate to how you would respond to a client, a client's family member or significant other, or other health care team members.
   4. Use therapeutic communication techniques to answer communication questions because of their effectiveness in the communication process (Box 4.19).
   5. Remember to identify the client of the question and select the option that focuses on the thoughts, feelings, concerns, anxieties, or fears of the client, client's family member, or significant other (see Box 4.19).
E. For additional information about Client Needs, refer to the NCLEX-PN test plan at the NCSBN web site (http://www.ncsbn.org).

X. **Eliminate Comparable or Alike Options (Box 4.20)**
A. When reading the options in multiple-choice or multiple-response questions, look for options that are comparable or alike.
B. Comparable or alike options can be eliminated as possible answers because it is unlikely that both options will be correct.

XI. **Eliminate Options Containing Closed-Ended Words (Box 4.21)**
A. Some closed-ended words are all, always, every, must, none, never, and only and there may be options accompanying a question that contain these words.
B. Eliminate options that contain closed-ended words because these words imply a fixed or extreme meaning; these types of options are usually incorrect.
C. Options that contain open-ended words, such as may, usually, normally, commonly, or generally, should be considered as possible correct options.

BOX 4.18 **Using the NCSBN Clinical Judgment Measurement Model and Cognitive Skills to Answer Test Questions**

Case Study

A client in the emergency department has anorexia, nausea, vomiting, and visual problems. The nurse asks about medications the client takes at home and the client provides a list.

Medication List:

- Amiodarone 400 mg orally daily
- Digoxin 0.25 mg orally daily
- Lisinopril 20 mg orally daily
- Furosemide 40 mg orally daily
- Metformin 1000 mg orally twice daily

Cognitive Skill: Recognize Cues

Question types that may be presented to measure your ability to recognize cues that are significant include highlight, cloze, extended multiple response, and extended drag and drop. Ask yourself: "What data matters the most?" Focus on the following to answer the question.

- Client observation cues: Anorexia, nausea, and vomiting, visual problems
- Environmental: Emergency department
- Medical record: Each medication taken by the client
- In this case, the client observation cues and medications are significant.

Cognitive Skill: Analyze Cues

Question types that may be presented to measure your ability to analyze cues include cloze, extended multiple response, matrix, and extended drag and drop. Ask yourself: "What does the significant assessment data mean?" Focus on the following to answer the question.

- Linking recognized cues with client data.
- What client conditions are consistent with the cues?
- Using knowledge of the medications and their adverse effects.
- In this case, make a determination that the client exhibits signs of digoxin toxicity.

Cognitive Skill: Prioritize Hypotheses

Question types that may be presented to measure your ability to prioritize hypotheses include cloze, extended multiple response, and extended drag and drop. Ask yourself: "What is happening to the client and what are the client needs?" Focus on the following to answer the question.

- Interpreting relevant data
- Considering all possibilities about what is happening and client needs

- Ranking the urgency of client needs with regard to planning care
- In this case, client needs can be ranked as 1) checking the digoxin level; 2) treating toxicity; 3) treating nausea and vomiting.

Cognitive Skill: Generate Solutions

Question types that may be presented to measure your ability to generate solutions include matrix, extended multiple response, and extended drag and drop. Ask yourself: "What must I do, what can I do, and what would I not do?" Focus on the following to answer the question.

- Identifying client goals and potential interventions
- Acceptable actual or potential evidence-based actions
- Actions that need to be avoided or are contraindicated
- In this case, goals are to 1) reduce the digoxin level—potential intervention is consider an antidote; 2) eliminate nausea and vomiting—potential intervention is consider an antiemetic.

Cognitive Skill: Take Action

Question types that may be presented to measure your ability to take action include cloze, extended multiple response, matrix, and extended drag and drop. Ask yourself: "What will I do?" Focus on the following to answer the question.

- Actions to take
- Actions that address the highest priorities of care
- In this case, actions are to 1) withhold the digoxin; 2) monitor vital signs (VS) and the apical heart rate; 3) notify the RN and the PHCP for prescriptions to treat digoxin toxicity and the nausea and vomiting; 4) administer antidote and antiemetics.

Cognitive Skill: Evaluate Outcomes

Question types that may be presented to measure your ability to evaluate outcomes include highlight, extended multiple response, matrix, and extended drag and drop. Ask yourself: "Did the action help?" Focus on the following to answer the question.

- Actions that resulted in improvement, a decline, or no change in the client's condition, or actions that were effective, ineffective, or were unrelated actions.
- In this case, to evaluate outcomes and determine effectiveness of actions the nurse would note that 1) the digoxin level is in the therapeutic range; 2) clinical symptoms are resolved; 3) vital signs and heart rate are stable.

XII. Look for the Umbrella Option (Box 4.22)

A. When answering a question, look for the umbrella option.

B. The umbrella option is one that is a broad, comprehensive, or universal statement and that usually contains the concepts of the other options within it.

C. The umbrella option is usually the correct answer.

XIII. Use the Guidelines for Delegating and Assignment-Making (Box 4.23)

A. You may be asked a question that will require you to decide how you will delegate a task or assign clients to other health care providers (HCPs).

B. Focus on the information in the question and what task or assignment is to be delegated and the available HCPs.

C. When you have determined what task or assignment is to be delegated and the available HCPs, consider the client's needs and match the client's needs with the scope of practice of the HCPs identified.

D. The Nurse Practice Act and any practice limitations define which aspects of care can be delegated and which must be performed by a licensed nurse. Use nursing scope of practice as a guide to assist in answering questions. Remember that the NCLEX is a national examination and national standards rather

BOX 4.19 Practice Questions: Communication and the Client of the Question

A client with a diagnosis of depression says to the nurse, "I should have died. I've always been a failure." The nurse would make which therapeutic response to the client?

1. "I see a lot of positive things in you."
2. "You still have a great deal to live for."
3. "Feeling like a failure is part of your illness."
4. "You've been feeling like a failure for some time now?"

Answer: 4
Test-Taking Strategy

Use therapeutic communication techniques to answer this question. Recognize cues in the question and analyze them to determine the significance of the client's statement. Remember to address the client's feelings and concerns. Option 4 is the only option that is stated in the form of a question and is open-ended, thus encouraging the verbalization of feelings. Remember to recognize and analyze cues, use therapeutic communication techniques, and focus on the client.

The nurse is caring for a terminally ill client. The client's wife, who has served as the caregiver, is at the bedside. She states, "I really hope my husband can just get better so we can go home." What statement would the nurse make to the client's wife?

1. "Has the doctor spoken with you about your husband's plan of care?"
2. "It sounds like this is difficult for you. What do you know about your husband's condition?"
3. "I hope your husband gets better too. It would be wonderful for you to be able to take him home."
4. "I know this is a difficult situation. I've seen this many times before. The spouse always has a hard time."

Answer: 2
Test-Taking Strategy

Focus on the client of the question, which in this case is the client's spouse. Recognize cues in the question and analyze them to determine the significance of the client's statement. Also, use therapeutic communication techniques. The correct option acknowledges the spouse's feelings and also asks for further information to determine her understanding of the situation. Option 1 does not acknowledge her feelings. Option 3 may offer false reassurance and false hope. Option 4 does not address the spouse's feelings and may cause further emotional distress. Remember to recognize and analyze cues, use therapeutic communication techniques, and focus on the client.

BOX 4.20 Practice Question: Eliminate Comparable or Alike Options

The nurse is assessing the leg pain of a client who has just undergone right femoral-popliteal artery bypass grafting. Which question would be **most** useful in determining whether the client is experiencing graft occlusion?

1. "Can you describe what the pain feels like?"
2. "Can you rate the pain on a scale of 1–10?"
3. "Did you get any relief from the last dose of pain medication?"
4. "Can you compare this pain to the pain you felt before surgery?"

Answer: 4
Test-Taking Strategy

Note the strategic word, *most*, and focus on recognizing cues related to differentiating expected postoperative pain from pain that indicates graft occlusion. The most frequent indication that a graft is occluding is the return of pain that is similar to that experienced preoperatively. Eliminate options 1, 2, and 3 because they are comparable or alike and are standard pain assessment questions. Remember to eliminate comparable or alike options.

BOX 4.21 Practice Question: Eliminate Options That Contain Closed-Ended Words

A client is to undergo a barium swallow test, and the nurse provides preprocedure instructions. The nurse would instruct the client to take which action in the preprocedure period?

1. Avoid eating or drinking after midnight before the test.
2. Limit self to only two cigarettes on the morning of the test.
3. Have a clear liquid breakfast only on the morning of the test.
4. Take all routine medications with a glass of water on the morning of the test.

Answer: 1
Test-Taking Strategy

The nurse needs to use knowledge about the preparation for a barium swallow test in order to take action with regard to preprocedure instructions. Note the closed-ended words "only" in options 2 and 3 and "all" in option 4. Eliminate options that contain closed-ended words because these options are usually incorrect. Also, note that options 2, 3, and 4 are comparable or alike options in that they all involve taking in something on the morning of the test. Remember to eliminate options that contain closed-ended words.

than agency-specific standards must be followed when delegating.

E. In general, noninvasive interventions, such as skin care, range-of-motion (ROM) exercises, ambulation, grooming, and hygiene measures, can be assigned to an assistive personnel (AP), also known as a nursing assistant or certified nursing assistant.

F. A licensed practical nurse (LPN) can perform the tasks that an AP can perform and can usually perform certain invasive tasks, such as dressings, suctioning, urinary catheterization, and administering medications orally or by the subcutaneous or intramuscular route; some selected piggyback intravenous medications may also be administered.

G. A registered nurse can perform the tasks that an LPN can perform and is responsible for assessment and planning care, analyzing client data, implementing and evaluating client care, supervising care, initiating teaching, and administering medications intravenously.

BOX 4.22 Practice Question: Look for the Umbrella Option

The nurse is caring for a client at home who has just been discharged from the hospital after implantation of a permanent pacemaker. The nurse would assess the client's home for the presence of which **priority** item?

1. Hair dryer
2. Electric blanket
3. Electric toothbrush with holder
4. Electrical items with strong magnetic fields

Answer: 4
Test-Taking Strategy
The nurse needs to use knowledge about safety measures for a client with a permanent pacemaker to recognize cues indicating risks. Note the strategic word, *priority*, and note the umbrella option. A pacemaker is shielded from interference from most electrical devices. Radios, televisions, electric blankets, toasters, microwave ovens, heating pads, and hair dryers are considered to be safe. Devices to be forewarned about include those with a strong electric current or magnetic field, such as antitheft devices in stores, metal detectors used in airports, and radiation therapy (if applicable and which might require relocation of the pacemaker). Note that option 4 uses the word "strong" and is the umbrella option addressing items with strong electric currents or magnetic fields. Remember that the umbrella option is a broad or universal option that includes the concepts of the other options in it.

XIV. Available Resources and Ideal Situations (Box 4.24)

A. When providing care to a client, particularly in emergency situations, keep in mind that all of the resources needed (i.e., blood pressure cuff, dressing supplies, gloves, masks) to provide client care will be readily available. Remember, you have everything you need wherever and whenever you need it!

B. Answer the question as if it were an ideal situation. Remember that NCLEX requires that you will answer questions based on textbook information.

XV. Answering Pharmacology Questions (Box 4.25)

A. If you are familiar with the medication, use nursing knowledge to answer the question.

B. Remember that the question will identify the generic name of the medication only.

C. If the question identifies a medical diagnosis, try to form a relationship between the medication and the diagnosis; for example, you can determine that cyclophosphamide is an antineoplastic medication if the question refers to a client with breast cancer who is taking this medication. Remember though that on the NCLEX a diagnosis may or may not be presented in a question.

D. Try to determine the classification of the medication being addressed to assist in answering the question. Identifying the classification will assist in determining a medication's action or side/adverse effects or both.

BOX 4.23 Practice Question: Use Guidelines for Delegating and Assignment Making

The licensed practical nurse (LPN) employed in a long-term care and rehabilitation agency is planning the client assignments for the day and has another licensed practical nurse (LPN) and an assistive personnel (AP) on the nursing team. Which client would the nurse **most appropriately** assign to the LPN?

1. A client with stable heart failure who has early stage Alzheimer's disease
2. A client who is scheduled for a physical therapy and an occupational therapy session
3. A client who was treated for dehydration and is weak and needs assistance with bathing
4. A client with emphysema who is receiving oxygen at 2 L by nasal cannula and becomes dyspneic on exertion

Answer: 4
Test-Taking Strategy
The nurse needs to have knowledge of the job descriptions and roles of the LPN and AP in order to generate solutions for planning safe client assignments. Note the strategic words, *most appropriately*, and focus on the subject, the assignment to be delegated to the LPN. When asked questions related to delegation, think about the role description of the employee and the needs of the client. The nurse would most appropriately assign the client with emphysema to the LPN. This client has an airway problem and has the highest priority needs of the clients presented in the options. The clients described in options 1, 2, and 3 can be cared for appropriately by the AP. Remember the nurse needs to match the client's needs with the scope of practice of the health care provider to plan and generate solutions for a safe client assignment!

BOX 4.24 Available Resources

The nurse is called to a client's room to assist the client who has a chest tube. The client states that it felt like the tube pulled out. The nurse assesses the client and finds that the tube has dislodged from the chest and is lying on the floor. What action would the nurse take **next**?

1. Obtain a pair of sterile gloves.
2. Contact the registered nurse for help.
3. Cover the insertion site with a sterile dressing.
4. Submerge the dislodged tube into sterile water.

Answer: 3
Test-Taking Strategy
Note the strategic word, *next*. Recognize cues in the question and analyze the cues for their significance to identify the action that needs to be taken. When providing care to a client, particularly in emergency situations, keep in mind that all of the resources needed to provide client care will be readily available at the client's bedside. Most students would eliminate option 4 first, knowing that this action is not necessary in this scenario since the tube has dislodged from the chest. From the remaining options, you may think, "I don't have sterile gloves or a sterile dressing with me, so let me call for help first." Remember, you have everything you need wherever and whenever you need it!

BOX 4.25 **Practice Question: Answering Pharmacology Questions**

The nurse is preparing to administer atenolol to a client. The nurse would check which **priority** item before administering the medication?

1. Temperature
2. Blood pressure
3. Potassium level
4. Blood glucose level

Answer: 2

Test-Taking Strategy

Note the strategic word, *priority*. The nurse needs to use knowledge about the medication in order to know the action that would be taken. Focus on the name of the medication. Recall that most beta-blocker medication names end with the letters *-lol* and that these medications are used to treat hypertension. This will direct you to option 2. Remember to use knowledge of medications and pharmacology guidelines to assist you in answering questions about medications!

E. Recognize the common side effects and adverse effects associated with each medication classification and relate the appropriate nursing interventions to each effect; for example, if a side effect is hypertension, the associated nursing intervention would be to monitor the blood pressure.

F. Focus on what the question is asking or the subject of the question; for example, intended effect, side effect, adverse effect, or toxic effect.

G. Learn medications that belong to a classification by commonalities in their medication names; for example, medications that act as beta blockers end with "*-lol*" (e.g., ateno*lol*).

H. If the question requires a medication calculation, remember that a calculator is available on the computer; talk yourself through each step to be sure that the answer makes sense, and recheck the calculation before answering the question, particularly if the answer seems like an unusual dosage.

I. Pharmacology: Pyramid Points to remember

   1. In general, the client should not take an antacid with medication because the antacid will affect the absorption of the medication.

   2. Enteric-coated and sustained-release tablets should not be crushed; also, capsules should not be opened unless specifically prescribed to do so.

   3. The client should never adjust or change a medication dose or abruptly stop taking a medication.

   4. The nurse never adjusts or changes the client's medication dosage and never discontinues a medication.

   5. The client needs to avoid taking any over-the-counter medications or any other medications, such as herbal preparations, unless they are approved for use by the primary health care provider (PHCP).

   6. The client needs to avoid consuming alcohol.

   7. Medications are never administered if the prescription is difficult to read, is unclear, or identifies a medication dose that is not a normal one.

   8. Additional strategies for answering pharmacology questions are presented in *Saunders Strategies for Test Success: Passing Nursing School and the NCLEX® Exam.*

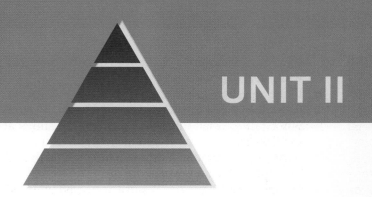

UNIT II

Professional Standards in Nursing

 Pyramid to Success

Nurses often care for clients who come from ethnic, cultural, or religious backgrounds that are different from their own. Awareness of, and sensitivity to, the unique health and illness beliefs and practices of people of different backgrounds is essential for the delivery of safe and effective care. Acknowledgment and acceptance of cultural differences with a nonjudgmental attitude are essential to providing culturally sensitive care. The NCLEX-PN® examination test plan is unique and individualized to the client's culture and beliefs. The nurse needs to avoid stereotyping and needs to be aware that there are several subcultures within cultures and there are several dialects within languages. In nursing practice, the nurse should assess the client's perceived needs before planning and implementing a plan of care.

Across all settings in the practice of nursing, nurses frequently are confronted with ethical and legal issues related to client care. The professional nurse has the responsibility to be aware of the ethical principles, laws, and guidelines related to providing safe and quality care to clients. In the Pyramid to Success, focus on ethical practices; the Nurse Practice Act and clients' rights, particularly confidentiality, information security and confidentiality, and informed consent; advocacy, documentation, and advance directives; and cultural, religious, and spiritual issues. Knowledgeable use of information technology, such as an electronic health record, is also an important role of the nurse.

The National Council of State Boards of Nursing (NCSBN) describes coordinated care as a process in which the practical nurse collaborates with health care team members to facilitate effective client care. A primary Pyramid Point focuses on the skills required to organize and prioritize client care activities. Pyramid Points also focus on participating as a member of the interprofessional health care team.

Client Needs: Learning Objectives

- **Safe and Effective Care Environment**
  Acting as a client advocate
  Assisting with triaging clients as appropriate
  Becoming familiar with the emergency response plan
  Collaborating with interprofessional teams
  Ensuring that ethical practices are implemented
  Ensuring that informed consent has been obtained
  Ensuring that legal rights and responsibilities are maintained
  Instituting quality improvement procedures
  Integrating advance directives into the plan of care
  Integrating case management concepts
  Maintaining confidentiality and information security issues related to the client's health care
  Organizing and prioritizing client care activities as appropriate and providing continuity of care
  Supervising the delivery of client care as appropriate
  Upholding client rights
  Using information technology in a confidential manner
- **Health Promotion and Maintenance**
  Considering cultural issues related to family systems and family planning
  Identifying changes related to the aging process
  Identifying high-risk behaviors of the client
  Performing physical assessment data collection techniques
  Promoting health and preventing disease

Promoting the client's ability to perform self-care

Providing health screening and health promotion programs

Respecting cultural preferences and lifestyle choices

- **Psychosocial Integrity**

Addressing end-of-life care based on the client's preferences and beliefs

Becoming aware of culture preferences and incorporating these preferences when planning and implementing care

Determining the client's use of effective coping mechanisms

Identifying abuse and neglect issues

Identifying clients who do not speak or understand English and determining how language needs will be met by the use of agency-approved interpreters

Identifying family dynamics as they relate to the client's culture

Identifying support systems for the client

Providing a therapeutic environment and building a relationship based on trust

Client Needs lists modified from: National Council of State Boards of Nursing, Inc. (NCSBN). *NCLEX-PN Examination: Test Plan for the National Council Licensure Examination for Practical Nurses,* effective April 2020. Chicago: NCSBN.

Respecting religious and spiritual influences on health

- **Physiological Integrity**

Assisting with emergency procedures

Identifying cultural differences for providing holistic client care

Identifying cultural issues related to alternative and complementary therapies

Identifying cultural issues related to receiving blood and blood products

Implementing therapeutic procedures considering cultural preferences

Providing nonpharmacological comfort interventions

Providing nutrition and oral hydration, considering cultural preferences

Ensuring that palliative and comfort care is provided to the client

Monitoring for alterations in body systems or unexpected responses to therapy

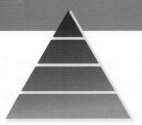

CHAPTER **5**

Care of Special Populations

Professional Standards

PRIORITY CONCEPTS **Caregiving, Health Disparities**

WHAT WOULD YOU DO?

The nurse is preparing to gather assessment data from a client who does not speak the same language as the nurse. What would the nurse do to gather accurate assessment data from the client?
Answer is located on p. 47.

I. Special Population Groups

A. Special population is a term that is generally used to refer to a disadvantaged group, meaning those who are vulnerable to health care disparities.
US Legal. https://definitions.uslegal.com/s/special-population/

B. The literature identifies numerous groups that may be designated as a special population group.

C. For this chapter, based on the literature, the authors have identified certain special groups most commonly cared for in the health care environment that require nursing's special attention, care, and sensitivity regarding their health care needs to ensure that their needs are met.

II. Health Care Disparities

A. Health disparities are differences in health care offered to different groups of people.

B. Some of the vulnerable groups that are at risk for health disparities include minority groups, those who are uninsured, those living in poverty or are homeless, those with chronic health problems and disabilities, immigrants, refugees, those with limited English proficiency, those who are incarcerated, and members of the lesbian, gay, bisexual, transgender, queer or questioning (LGBTQ) community.

C. Vulnerable groups experience greater risk factors, lack of necessary access to care, and increased morbidity and mortality as compared with the general population.
Joszt, L. (2018). 5 Vulnerable populations in health care. *The American Journal of Managed* Care (AJM). Retrieved from https://www.ajmc.com/view/5-vulnerable-populations-in-healthcare.

D. Nurses often care for clients who are vulnerable and are at risk for health disparities; nurses need to be aware that health care disparities exist and plan and provide care to prevent a disparity.

E. Nurses also need to be aware of the most prevalent chronic health problems and infectious diseases in the United States and their associated risk factors. This is important because on assessment, the nurse needs to screen for these health problems and infections, the associated risk factors, and determine necessary support services for the individual or family. Then, the nurse needs to plan appropriate educational strategies and teach about the measures that will either prevent or treat these health problems and infectious diseases and connect the client or family with identified support services. Box 5.1 identifies chronic health problems in the United States and associated risk factors. Box 5.2 identifies common infectious diseases.

III. Nursing Assessment

A. See Box 5.3 for a comprehensive nursing assessment tool written by the authors of this chapter, titled *Special Populations: Needs Assessment Tool*, that can be used to obtain information from the client about his or her special needs in order to plan care. This tool can be adapted, based on the individual or family group being cared for.

B. Nurses' self-awareness of their own culture, values, beliefs, ethics, personality, and communication style helps to promote optimal health outcomes for clients of diverse populations. Recognizing one's own biases and being respectful to all people despite differences can influence satisfaction of care.

⚠️ An encounter with a client needs to elicit the client's unique perspectives based on their own preferences. This will allow the nurse to understand what health care treatments will be realistic and acceptable.

BOX 5.1	Chronic Health Problems in the United States and Risk Factors

Chronic Health Problems

Heart disease
Cancer
Chronic lung disease
Stroke
Alzheimer's disease
Diabetes
Chronic kidney disease

Risk Factors

Tobacco use
Poor nutrition
Obesity
Lack of physical activity
Excessive alcohol use

Centers for Disease Control and Prevention. (2019). *Chronic diseases in America.* Retrieved from https://www.cdc.gov/chronicdisease/resources/infographic/chronic-diseases.htm.

BOX 5.2	Common Infectious Diseases in the United States

COVID* -19 (Coronavirus)
Sexually transmitted infections (chlamydia, syphilis, gonorrhea)
Human immunodeficiency virus and acquired immunodeficiency syndrome
Influenza
Staphylococcus aureus
Escherichia coli
Herpes simplex 1, herpes simplex 2
Shigellosis
Norovirus
Salmonella
Pneumonia
Hepatitis C

*Corona Virus Disease
Data in part from John Hopkins Medicine. (2020). *Infectious diseases.* Retrieved from https://www.hopkinsmedicine.org/health/infectious-diseases.

C. It is imperative for nurses to understand that special population groups may share dominant characteristics; however, all clients are individuals and stereotyping must be avoided.

D. It is also very important for nurses to be aware of the health problems that are common in a population group so that specific and special attention can be made when performing a comprehensive assessment.

IV. COVID-19—Coronavirus

A. The COVID-19 pandemic is a serious global health threat and has caused severe illness and even death in some individuals.

B. It is considered a respiratory illness that is caused by a virus called SARS-CoV. Although the illness is a respiratory one, the virus also attacks and affects many different body systems.

C. Symptoms of the illness include but are not limited to cough, shortness of breath, fever, muscle pain, sore throat, and loss of taste and/or smell.

D. COVID-19 is a highly contagious illness and controlling its spread is a primary goal.

E. There are special population groups that are at higher risk of contracting the infection and also at higher risk for dying because of the virus. Those at high risk include the elderly, those with a chronic health condition such as diabetes or respiratory disease, those who have cancer, those who are immunocompromised from chemotherapy or a disease, and minority groups. For additional information refer to: https://www.hopkinsmedicine.org/health/conditions-and-diseases/coronavirus/covid19-racial-disparities.

F. Other special population groups at risk are those that are living in crowded conditions or are institutionalized, such as those in a nursing home or prison.

G. Working in essential fields such as health care environments, inconsistent access to health care, stress, and a low immune response also play a role in increasing the risk for this infection.

H. When performing an assessment on a client, the nurse must assess for any risk factors for COVID-19 and must institute safety measures for protecting and preventing that client from contracting the illness.

I. The nurse must be aware of the critical measures needed to protect oneself from contracting the virus and must be an advocate in educating the public about the measures to prevent spread. These primary measures are handwashing, wearing a mask and eye protection, social distancing (at least 6 feet apart), avoiding crowded situations, avoiding close contact with people who are sick, covering your nose and mouth when coughing or sneezing, keeping the hands away from the eyes and face, and self-quarantine.

V. Minority Groups

A. Minority groups are more often affected by health care disparities than nonminority groups.

B. Some individuals in these groups may be less likely to have health insurance coverage or a regular source of health care. Center for American Progress. (2010). *Fact sheet: Health disparities by race and ethnicity.* https://cdn.americanprogress.org/wp-content/uploads/issues/2010/12/pdf/disparities_factsheet.pdf.

C. Obesity, diabetes mellitus, end-stage renal disease secondary to diabetes, and cervical cancer are more common among the Hispanic/Latino population.

D. The Native Hawaiians and other Pacific Islanders population is noted to have higher rates of smoking, alcohol consumption, obesity, and diabetes mellitus.

BOX 5.3 Special Populations: Needs Assessment Tool

Not all questions listed in this assessment tool will need to be used for the assessment. The nurse needs to make a judgment on appropriate questions for each population and needs to ask questions within that list, if appropriate for the client, based on the *General Background Questions*. Use the *General Background Questions* as a guide to determine additional questions that should be included in the assessment.

Initial
- Introduce yourself and describe your role.
- Example: "I would like to ask you some questions so that we have information about your individualized needs. Do I have your permission to ask you some questions?"

General Background Questions
- Are you comfortable talking to me?
- What name would you like us to use to address you?
- What is your primary language spoken?
- Do you speak and understand English?
- In which language do you wish to communicate?
- Do you need an interpreter?
- Do you feel you are able to adequately answer questions regarding your health?
- What is your age?
- Is there a specific gender which you identify with?
- What is your ethnicity?
- Do you have any cultural, religious, or spiritual preferences you would like us to consider in your plan of care?
- Do you have any dietary preferences that you would like us to include in your plan of care? Describe your eating patterns in a 24-hour period.
- Do you exercise? What do you do and how often?
- Do you use any remedies when you are sick?
- What do you do when you are sick?
- What is your living situation? Where do you live? Who do you live with? Do you have children?
- Do you have a support system?
- Would you like to name a support person or emergency contact person?
- Do you have access to financial resources needed to live?
- Do you have health insurance?
- Do you feel safe at home or where you live? Have you been abused within the last 12 months? Do you encounter crime or violence in your life? Is anyone hurting you, physically or emotionally or in any other way? Have you ever been or are you now being bullied?
- Do you smoke, drink alcohol, or use any type of drug?
- Do you have or need a health care proxy?
- Do you have an advance directive? If not, would you like more information about this?
- When was the last time you sought health care? For what reason?
- Do you have any fears about seeing your provider?
- Do you currently or have you ever had a communicable disease?
- Have you been exposed to anyone with a communicable disease? If so, how was this exposure treated?
- Have you ever been tested for COVID-19? Or tested for immunity?
- Have you traveled outside of the country recently?
- Are you up-to-date on immunizations?
- When was your last influenza vaccine?
- Have you ever been vaccinated for pneumonia? If so, when?
- Do you have a history of a mental health problem?
- Have you ever had feelings of committing suicide? If so, do you have these feelings now? Do you have a plan?
- Are you a veteran or member of the military?
- Do you have any chronic illness, disability, or other past medical history?
- Have you ever been incarcerated?
- Are you an immigrant or refugee?

Further Questions Based on Living Situation
- Do you have a home? Do you live alone? Who do you live with at home?
- Do you drink alcohol? Any other type of drug use?
- Have you been exposed to environmental irritants?
- Have you had problems with asthma, anemia, lead exposure, ear infections, gastrointestinal illness, or a mental health problem?
- Are you willing to follow up on your health care recommendations if given the necessary resources?

Further Questions Based on Health Insurance Coverage
- What health insurance do you have?
- Do you have the financial means to pay for your health care?
- Are you willing to work with a social worker to seek health coverage?

Further Questions Based on Financial Status and Access to Resources
- What is your education level?
- What is your income?
- Do you have family you are in contact with?
- Is anyone in your immediate family disabled?
- Do you have a support system?
- Do you live in a safe community?
- Do you seek health care on a routine basis?
- Are you willing to work with a social worker to increase your access to community resources?

Further Questions Related to Abuse
- Do you have or have you had any bruises, sprains, broken bones, fatigue, shortness of breath, muscle tension, involuntary shaking, changes in eating or sleeping, sexual dysfunction, or fertility problems?
- Do you experience nightmares, anxiety, uncontrollable thoughts, depression, or low self-esteem?
- Do you have anxiety or depression? Have you felt suicidal? If so, do you have a plan?
- Do you ever feel hopeless, worthless, apprehensive, discouraged? Do you lack motivation or faith? Have you questioned your trust in others?
- For a child: do you have any problems at school? Are you bullied?

Further Questions Based on Racial/Ethnic Background
- Are there any resources you need to ensure your ability to follow up on your health care recommendations?
- Do you have any past medical history or family history of chronic diseases, such as diabetes mellitus, hypertension, heart disease, stroke, cancer, renal disease, injuries or accidents, depression, or anxiety?

BOX 5.3   **Special Populations: Needs Assessment Tool -** *Continued*

Further Questions Based on Gender and Sexual Orientation
- Can you describe your sexual orientation preferences?
- Which pronoun would you like to be referred to by (he, she, other)?
- Do you seek regular and routine health care? When were you last seen?
- When was your last breast exam, mammogram, Pap smear, testicular exam, prostate exam?
- Do you do a breast self-examination or a testicular self-examination?
- Do you have any past medical history?
- Are you sexually active? If so, how many partners do you have? Do you use safe sex practices?
- Do you smoke, drink alcohol, or use any other type of drug?
- Do you have any problems with depression or anxiety? Have you ever felt suicidal? If so, do you have a plan?
- Do you take hormone therapy?
- Are you up to date on your immunizations?
- Do you have children? If not, do you wish to or plan on having children?
- Do you feel you have access to necessary resources such as health care or other benefits?

Further Questions Related to Mental Health
- Do you seek routine health care?
- Describe your eating habits in a 24-hour period.
- Describe your activity level.
- Do you have any past medical history?
- Do you take any medications? If so, what are they and do you experience any side effects?
- Do you smoke, drink, or use any other type of drug?
- Do you experience depression or anxiety? Have you ever had thoughts of suicide? If so, do you have a plan?

- Are you sexually active? If so, do you employ safe sex practices? How many partners do you have?

Further Questions Related to Veteran/Military Status
- Do you have any problems with a mental health problem, such as posttraumatic stress disorder, moral injury?
- Have you had any traumatic brain injuries?
- Have you had any other injuries?
- Describe your living situation.
- Are you interested in any community support groups?

Further Questions Related to Incarceration
- Have you ever been a victim of abuse or rape?
- Do you have any past medical history, particularly asthma, diabetes mellitus, hypertension, heart disease, mental health problem, or communicable diseases?

Further Questions Related to Immigration
- Do you have problems with mental health?
- Are you able to speak and understand English?
- Do you have access to resources such as housing, transportation, health care, and education services?
- Do you have any past medical history, such as accidents, injuries, hypothermia, gastrointestinal illness, heart problems, pregnancy complications, diabetes, hypertension, malnutrition, or infectious or communicable disease?

Further Questions Related to Chronic Illness
- Do you have access to a primary health care provider?
- Do you see a specialist on a regular basis?
- Are you able to follow up on the recommendations made by your primary health care provider and/or specialist?

Summary
- Is there anything else you would like to share regarding your ability to maintain your health or any other issue or concern?

Authors of the *Special Populations: Needs Assessment Tool.* Linda A. Silvestri, Angela E. Silvestri, and Paula Richards.

Hepatitis B, human immunodeficiency virus (HIV) and acquired immunodeficiency syndrome (AIDS), and tuberculosis are more frequent diseases. Noted is that there is a high incidence of infant mortality and sudden infant death syndrome (SIDS) in this population.

E. In the Native American and Alaska Native populations, geographic isolation and income may be factors with regard to receiving health care. Inadequate water supply and sewage disposal can be a factor with infectious diseases. Smoking and alcohol use are more common, and diabetes mellitus, cancer, stroke, heart disease, and accidents are a concern. Additional concerns include mental health alterations, suicide, infant mortality, SIDS, teenage pregnancy, liver disease, and hepatitis.

F. Obesity, diabetes mellitus, hypertension, heart disease, asthma, and cancer occur more commonly among the black population with leading causes of death being heart disease, cancer, and stroke.

G. Cancer, tuberculosis, and hepatitis are more common health problems of Asian Americans with leading causes of death being cancer, heart disease, and stroke.

⚠ Some people in minority groups report hesitancy in seeking health care due to a language barrier. Ineffective communication between the nurse or other health care provider and the client can affect the client's health care and the client's ability to comply with follow-up care.

H. Health care considerations for minority groups
   1. Cultural competence is critical in the effort to reduce health care disparity and is a necessary ability for health care professionals to acquire to provide care for a diverse population. This can help to improve health outcomes and quality of care.
   2. The nurse and other health care professionals need to be aware of health care variations and risk factors for various populations to facilitate appropriate care and access to needed health care services.

3. It is important for the nurse to examine his or her own values to competently care for someone of a differing population group; awareness is a useful tool in caring for these special populations.

4. Language barriers influence access to health care. It is important to remember that family members and friends must not be asked to be an interpreter for the client because of confidentiality, the potential for conflict of interest, and the risk associated with relaying inaccurate information; only specified individuals as designated by the health care agency need to be asked to interpret for a client.

5. Lack of access to preventative care needs to be addressed; lack of routine health care and delay in seeking health care for illness are common.

6. Some important education health topics include diet and meal planning, exercise, and other healthy lifestyle practices to prevent disease, including infectious and communicable diseases.

7. Return explanation and demonstration (teach-back) are of particular importance to ensure safety and mutual understanding.

VI. Lesbian, gay, bisexual, transgender and queer or questioning individuals

A. Commonly referred to as the "LGBTQ" community, this group is represented by a wide range of varying characteristics in terms of race, ethnicity, age, socioeconomic status (SES), and identity.

B. There is often a lack of awareness and understanding among health care professionals in managing the health care needs of this population—providing access to health care to meet their needs is critical.

C. When performing an assessment, the nurse needs to individualize and take into account the characteristics in terms of race, ethnicity, age, and SES; the assessment needs to focus on health concerns unique to each characteristic.

D. Some LGBTQ persons may be less likely to access health care than other population groups due to fear of stigmatization and being viewed as different.

E. Transgender individuals require special attention and care. They may be less likely than other groups to have certain screenings completed, such as mammograms, breast exams, cervical cancer screening, testicular cancer exams, and prostate screening. For additional information, refer to the GLAAD (Gay & Lesbian Alliance Against Defamation) Media Reference Guide: Transgender at https://www.glaad.org/reference/transgender.

F. Sexually transmitted infections (STIs) are of concern in this population.

G. Breast cancer and cervical cancer are a concern, likely a result of decreased screening and nulliparity.

H. Depression and suicide is a concern.

I. Rejection from friends, family members, and social support systems may be a stressor. Teenage members of the LGBTQ population are more likely to be threatened, bullied, injured, raped, and victimized. For these reasons, school absenteeism can be a problem. LGBTQ youth are at risk for abuse by family members due to their sexual orientation.

J. Many same-sex couples desire children; there may be some barriers to child-rearing for this population, such as the expenses associated with adoption, artificial insemination, and surrogacy.

 Members of the LGBTQ population are less likely to have family members who can assist them with elder or disability care. In addition, certain benefits may not be available to them, such as spousal death benefits, which could impact their ability to manage finances and expenses associated with health.

K. Health care considerations for the LGBTQ population

1. Health care professionals need to create a welcoming, nonjudgmental environment when caring for this population.

2. Using the preferred pronoun when addressing these clients is important in developing and maintaining a rapport.

3. Measures such as altering signage on paperwork and documents asking for gender identification will better serve the health needs of this population. In addition, the health care facility must develop institutional polices inclusive of all gender identities and preferences. Such measures will allow the primary health care provider to treat the client according to their preferences while also maintaining an understanding of their risk factors based on biological drivers of health.

4. Health promotion measures need to focus on screening for health concerns such as cancer, STIs, depression, and suicide and on educating on safe sex practices.

5. A careful sexual history and appropriate counseling is important for all members of the LGBTQ population.

6. Nonoccupational postexposure prophylaxis (nPEP), or the use of prophylactic antiretrovirals before and after potential HIV exposure, needs to be considered.

7. Transgender persons taking hormone therapy need to be monitored at regular intervals; associated complications, such as polycythemia occurring with exogenous testosterone use, need to be detected and treated early.

8. Transgendered persons who have undergone sexual reassignment surgery must have the respective preventive screenings. For example, male-to-female need to have breast cancer screening by way of mammography if they are older than 50 years. In addition, female-to-male would

still have mammography routinely as indicated due to the risk for residual breast tissue to develop cancerous growth.

VII. Homeless

A. Affects men, women, children, and persons of all backgrounds, and family units can be affected as a whole.

B. There is a risk for early death related to health problems (Box 5.4).

C. Disability often results from illness and becomes a barrier to employment, which further augments the problem of homelessness.

D. Infants affected by homelessness often have low birth weights and are more likely to die within the first 12 months of life than in other population groups.

E. Children affected by homelessness are sick more often with illnesses such as asthma, iron deficiency, lead poisoning, ear infections, gastrointestinal illness, and behavioral and mental health problems.

F. Children may begin to act out or become less attentive in the classroom when basic needs are not met.

G. Youth experience health problems related to risk-taking behaviors such as alcohol and drug abuse, and depression and suicide are concerns. Unintended pregnancy and STIs are a concern; physical and sexual abuse is also a concern.

H. Health care considerations for the homeless
   1. Identification of those who are homeless needs to be accomplished through avenues such as outreach programs.

BOX 5.4 Determinants of Health and Common Problems in the Homeless

Determinants of Health
Limited access to health care
Problems getting enough food
Difficulty staying safe
Violence
Stress
Unsanitary living conditions
Exposure to extremes in weather

Common Health Problems
Dental problems
Malnutrition
Sexually transmitted infections including HIV and AIDS
Lung diseases including bronchitis, tuberculosis, and pneumonia
Infectious and communicable diseases
Mental health problems
Substance abuse problems
Wounds and skin infections

MedlinePlus. (2020). *Homeless health concerns.* Retrieved from https://medlineplus.gov/homelesshealthconcerns.html.

---

2. The initial health care visit and every visit thereafter needs to be done with a nonjudgmental, nonthreatening approach.

3. The nurse needs to focus on reported symptoms first—this will encourage adherence and follow-up.

4. Subsequent care would include health maintenance, attention to common problems and concerns, and establishing an emergency contact person if available.

5. Members of the homeless population may not adhere to medical treatment recommendations and therefore require close follow-up as much as possible.

6. This population tends to have longer hospital stays, and have poorer health outcomes.

7. Certain medications must be avoided in the homeless population due to the potential for abuse and contraindications in chronic conditions; the nurse needs to ensure that any medication prescribed is safe for the person.

8. Multiple resources are available to increase access to health care for the homeless population and the nurse needs to establish connections for the client as appropriate.

9. See https://www.aafp.org/afp/2014/0415/p634.html for more information about the homeless population.

VIII. Socioeconomically Disadvantaged Individuals and Families

A. Disadvantage in the socioeconomic sense can correlate with poor health outcomes.

B. Education level, income, family, social support, and community safety are social determinants that can influence health and health outcomes.

C. In addition to healthy lifestyle and access to routine, quality care, the social determinants of health are equally as important in promoting positive health outcomes.

D. Individuals of low SES are more likely to engage in risky health behaviors.

E. Due to limited financial resources, these individuals are at a higher risk for chronic disease and any diseases associated with primary prevention.

F. The health of children can be affected later in life due to risk factors.

G. Health care considerations for socioeconomically disadvantaged individuals and families
   1. Social work services are helpful in connecting this population to needed health care services and resources to assist in paying for health care.
   2. The nurse needs to carefully assess the client for at-risk behaviors and intervene appropriately, including providing education.
   3. The nurse also needs to initiate social service contacts to ensure adequate health care.

IX. Uninsured and Underinsured Individuals

A. Individuals with low incomes are most at risk for being uninsured or underinsured.

B. Those who are uninsured or underinsured are at increased risk for health complications due to lack of access to care and the likelihood that preventive care services and chronic disease management will not be sought.

C. Most individuals receive health insurance coverage through an employer. If the employer does not offer this coverage, the employee is at risk for being uninsured or underinsured.

D. Medicaid is an option for some low-income families who meet eligibility criteria. Commercial insurance is another option but may still be cost prohibitive depending on the individual circumstance. The client would be referred to social services or financial services to apply for Medicaid.

E. Risk factors: Refer to risk factors for socioeconomically disadvantaged individuals and families.

F. Health care considerations for uninsured and underinsured individuals: Refer to health care considerations for socioeconomically disadvantaged individuals and families.

X. Intellectually Disabled Individuals

A. Intellectually disabled individuals are at high risk for certain health disorders.

B. Often, these health disorders go untreated due to atypical symptom presentation, which leads to additional problems later in life.

C. Communication barriers between health care professionals and those with an intellectual disability presents a unique challenge in identifying and managing health care needs in this population.

D. These clients may have difficulty recalling their personal medical history, so it may be necessary to take more time to ask questions in a variety of different ways.

E. More common health conditions include motor deficits, epilepsy, allergies, otitis media, gastroesophageal reflux disease (GERD), dysmenorrhea, sleep problems, mental health problems, vision and hearing impairments, constipation, and oral health problems.

BOX 5.5 **Some Mental Health Concerns for Foster Children**

Anxiety disorder
Attention-deficit/hyperactivity disorder
Bipolar disorder
Depression
Post-traumatic stress disorder

From Turney, K., & Wildeman, C. (2016). Mental and physical health of children in foster care. *Pediatrics*, 138(5), e20161118.

F. These clients may tend to eat quickly and so should be assessed for risk of choking and aspiration.

G. Certain conditions can cause changes in behavior; for example, there may be eating disturbances due to GERD or self-injury due to the presence of an ear infection.

H. Health care considerations for intellectually disabled individuals

   1. Safety is a priority; ensure a safe environment.

   2. Functional behavioral assessment is important in identifying existing health problems.

   3. Awareness of altered behavior as a manifestation of an illness is important in early identification and prevention of secondary problems.

   4. Health interventions must be focused on treating a medical condition, followed by behavioral interventions to prevent continued behavioral response to an illness.

XI. Battered Individuals and Victims of Abuse or Neglect

⚠ Health care professionals are often the first point of contact for victims of abuse or neglect.

A. Abuse of the older client (refer to Chapters 21 and 64).

B. Child abuse: Consequences are long lasting, both impacting initial development and influencing adult health (refer to Chapter 64).

C. Women are affected more than men.

D. Some of the outcomes of abuse or neglect may include physical, somatic, psychological, behavioral, sexual, and pregnancy-related effects.

E. Children from birth to 1 year of age are at risk of maltreatment—the majority are victims of neglect; maternal SES and parental behavioral issues impact a child's risk.

F. Victims are prone to certain health effects as a result of the abuse or neglect; these effects can include bruises, sprains or broken bones, chronic fatigue, shortness of breath, muscle tension, involuntary shaking, changes in eating and sleeping patterns, sexual dysfunction, and fertility issues.

G. Mental health problems can arise, including post-traumatic stress disorder (PTSD), nightmares, anxiety, uncontrollable thoughts, depression, low self-esteem, and alcohol and drug abuse.

H. Feelings of hopelessness, lack of worth, apprehension, discouragement, inability to trust others, and lack of motivation are common.

I. Children who witness violence are prone to fearfulness, anxiety, depression, and problems in school.

J. Health care considerations for battered individuals and victims of abuse or neglect

   1. Safety is a priority; provide a safe environment and ensure that the victim has a safe environment to live and has contact information for seeking a safe haven if necessary.

2. Treat victims with compassion and respect.
3. Acknowledge and respect the dignity of each person.
4. Nurses are mandated reporters of domestic violence and abuse incidents; it may be necessary to take photographs of injuries for legal reasons.
5. Cleaning and dressing wounds, administering pain medications, use of assistive devices such as for sprains or fractures, education for self-management and seeking safety, and emotional support may be needed in the care of these victims.
6. Provide parental education and support programs; increase awareness of potential battering and abuse or neglect.

XII. Single Parents

A. The nurse should establish a therapeutic relationship with the client and encourage the single parent to express any concerns and needs about single-parenting; this information will assist the nurse in identifying appropriate resources for the client.
B. Initiating access to community organizations can assist in alleviating some burden and provide needed services such as child care, food security, health care including immunizations, and employment.
C. The nurse may need to assist single parents to address the child's sexual development, especially those with a child of the opposite sex.
D. Preventive screenings are important in this population due to risk factors and the negative effects of stress from single parenting.

XIII. Foster Children

A. Needs that often go unmet for children in foster care include physical, mental, behavioral, and dental health; this increases the risk for health problems later in life (Box 5.5).
B. Some children in foster care may have complex and chronic health conditions.
C. Health care considerations for foster children
1. Community resources are important for this population to facilitate the provision of health, safety, stability, and permanence.
2. Social workers must be included in the care of a foster child to facilitate access to community resources.
3. Medically equipped homes may be needed, as well as in-home nursing care services for those children with complex or chronic health conditions.
4. Frequent health visits may be needed for children transitioning to and from foster care.

XIV. Individuals With a Mental Health Problem

A. Lifestyle choices, chronic health problems, psychotropic medications, limitation in access to health care, and lack of preventive screening are concerns.

B. Side effects of psychotropic medications may contribute to an altered health state. Certain psychotropic medications can contribute to weight gain.
C. Lack of exercise and poor diet, as well as features of an illness, such as depression or disorganized thought processes, may contribute to health problem development.
D. Side effects from psychotropic medications, such as sedation, weight gain, and increased appetite contribute to the incidence of diabetes mellitus and metabolic syndrome in this population.
E. Due to the higher frequency of substance abuse, risky sexual behaviors, and lack of knowledge regarding risks, individuals with a mental health problem are at increased risk for STIs.
F. Sexual dysfunction can result from a mental health problem as well as the medication used to treat it.
G. Xerostomia from reduction in salivary gland flow due to medications can result in difficulty maintaining oral hygiene and overall health.
H. Health care considerations for individuals with a mental health problem
1. Individuals with a mental health problem have a difficult time accessing needed and available health care services.
2. Family and social service support are important for these individuals.
3. Governmental insurance has expanded to cover individuals in need of mental health care.
4. Mental health screenings must be completed regularly for all individuals, which allows for prompt and accurate treatment strategies to prevent further health complications.
5. Refer to the mental health chapters for additional information about this special population.

XV. Older Adults

A. Elder abuse is a concern for this population; health care providers are mandated to report if there is suspicion of elder abuse. The most common type of abuse is neglect.
B. There are many health problems that can occur in the older client (Box 5.6 lists some of these health problems).
C. See Chapter 21 for more information on common health conditions experienced by older adults and care of the older adult.

XVI. Military Veterans

A. This population is at increased risk for injury-related and stress-related health illnesses.
B. Mental health or behavioral adjustment disorders are common.
C. Substance use disorders with tobacco, alcohol, or other drugs and suicide are more common.
D. PTSD and moral injury is common among this population.

BOX 5.6 Some Health Problems That Occur in Older Adults

Alzheimer's disease
Arthritis
Dementia
Depression
Falls
Heart disease
Influenza
Obesity
Oral/dental health problems
Osteoporosis
Pneumonia
Respiratory diseases
Shingles
Substance abuse

Healthy People 2020. (2020). *Older adults.* Retrieved from
https://www.healthypeople.gov/2020/topics-objectives/topic/older-adults;
Healthy West Orange. (n.d.). *15 common health concerns for seniors.* Retrieved
from https://healthywestorange.org/15-senior-concerns/.

E. Traumatic brain injury can occur as a result of external force injuries.

F. Limb amputations and disfigurement are more common.

G. Long-term health problems may result from exposure to chemicals and environmental irritants.

H. Military veterans can experience issues leading to homelessness.

I. Health care considerations for military veterans
1. Identifying and treating mental health problems assists in mitigating suicide risk.
2. Treatment of comorbid conditions such as PTSD or moral injury may help to address substance use disorders.
3. Use of screening tools in identifying substance use disorder will help to plan appropriate care.
4. Veterans Affairs Services can assist in managing some of the health issues experienced by these individuals.

XVII. Prisoners

⚠ The environment of a prison can predispose a person to different health conditions, such as tuberculosis, sexually transmitted infections, or other infectious or communicable diseases.

A. Social determinants of poor health are often present in prisoners.

B. Health concerns are asthma, diabetes, hypertension, heart disease, and mental health problems.

C. Infectious and communicable diseases are also a concern for this population.

D. Health care considerations for prisoners
1. The correctional facility is usually the sole provider of health care for this population.

2. Screening protocols and procedures for individuals in this setting need to be thorough, consistent, and performed regularly.
3. Educational and vocational programs may help to mitigate the health problems associated with living in a prison.
4. History of incarceration increases the risk of poor health due to limited opportunities to reform; inadequate housing, employment, and education; and lack of family stability.
5. Failure to address mental health problems among this population may contribute to repeated crimes when released from prison; those who are in prison for life need adequate screening and health care as well.

XVIII. Immigrants and Refugees

A. Challenges include learning to speak English (or the adopted language of their new country), citizenship, raising children, employment, housing, accessing health care, transportation, and overcoming cultural barriers.

B. Acculturation to the United States increases the risk for poor health. Poor health can be the result of eating a less healthy diet, increased risk-taking behaviors, and separation from family support networks.

C. There are many health concerns for this population. Many result from the process of migration and include infectious diseases such as tuberculosis, hepatitis, vector-borne disease, influenza, coronavirus, sexually transmitted infections, childhood diseases such as measles, mumps, rubella, and polio; antimicrobial resistance is a concern.

D. For refugees, mental health problems due to war, violence, and rape occurring in camps is a concern.

E. Health care considerations for immigrants and refugees
1. A process for offering services and treating immigrants and refugees must be available regardless of insurance status.
2. Refugees may be eligible for short-term medical assistance in the United States but then may lack health care coverage due to ineligibility for state medical assistance or inability to afford private health insurance.
3. Nurses need to be aware of the limited access to health care resources and explore possible health care services for this population.
4. Vaccinations must be provided to prevent communicable diseases.

XIX. Individuals With Chronic Illness

A. Individuals with multiple chronic illnesses need special attention.

B. Chronic illness is the leading cause of death and disability in the United States; the prevalence increases with age and is a major cause of disability.

C. Chronic illnesses include cardiovascular disease, cancer, respiratory disease, diabetes, mental health problems, vision and hearing impairment, oral diseases, bone and joint disorders, and genetic disorders.

D. Poor health outcomes and high health care costs are associated with chronic illness.

E. Optimal care for individuals with multiple chronic illnesses may be limited because of multiple health needs present.

F. Many health professionals do not feel adequately prepared to manage individuals with multiple chronic illnesses.

G. Individuals with one chronic illness are at risk for developing multiple chronic illnesses.

H. Modifiable factors include an unhealthy diet, physical inactivity, and tobacco use; nonmodifiable factors include age and genetics.

I. Health care considerations for individuals with chronic illness

1. Follow-up care is important in promoting health for individuals with chronic illness.

2. Focusing on a single illness does not effectively manage an individual with multiple chronic diseases—rather, the "big picture" needs to be understood in managing these clients.

3. Interprofessional collaboration is important in safely managing individuals with chronic diseases.

4. Nurses play a key role in facilitating interprofessional communication between providers and specialists.

5. Inclusion of the client and support person(s) in health care decisions helps to increase adherence to a complex health care regimen.

WHAT WOULD YOU DO?

Answer: If the nurse needs to care for a client who speaks a different language, the nurse would need to seek an interpreter. The nurse needs to seek an agency approved interpreter to assist because this will ensure the collection of accurate data. The nurse would not ask a family member or anyone else, except the agency approved interpreter, to assist with communicating with the client. This could lead to the collection of inaccurate data and also can violate confidentiality.

PRACTICE QUESTIONS

1. Which teaching method is **most effective** when providing instruction to members of special populations?
   1. Teach-back
   2. Video instruction
   3. Written materials
   4. Verbal explanation

2. Which is **most appropriate** when communicating with a transgender person?
   1. Using preferred pronouns
   2. Using their first name to address them
   3. Using pronouns associated with birth sex
   4. Anticipating the client's needs and making suggestions

3. The nurse is volunteering with an outreach program to provide basic health care for homeless people. Which finding, if noted, must be addressed **first**?
   1. Blood pressure 154/72 mm Hg
   2. Visual acuity of 20/200 in both eyes
   3. Random blood glucose level of 206 mg/dL
   4. Complaints of pain associated with numbness and tingling in both feet

4. The nurse is completing the admission assessment of a client who is intellectually disabled. Which part of the client encounter may require more time to complete?
   1. The history
   2. The physical assessment
   3. The nursing plan of care
   4. The readmission risk assessment

5. The nurse working in a correctional facility is caring for a new prisoner. The client asks about health risks associated with living in a prison. How would the nurse respond?
   1. "Health care is very limited in the prison setting."
   2. "Living in a prison isn't different than living at home."
   3. "Living in a prison can predispose a person to different health conditions."
   4. "Living in a prison is similar to living in a condominium complex or dormitory."

6. The nurse is caring for a female client in the emergency department who presents with a complaint of fatigue and shortness of breath. Which physical assessment findings, if noted by the nurse, warrant a **need for follow-up**?
   1. Reddened sclera of the eyes
   2. Dry flaking noted on the scalp
   3. A reddish-purple mark on the neck
   4. A scaly rash noted on the elbows and knees

7. The nurse working in a community outreach program for foster children plans care knowing that which health conditions are common in this population? **Select all that apply.**
   ❑ 1. Asthma
   ❑ 2. Claustrophobia
   ❑ 3. Sleep problems
   ❑ 4. Bipolar disorder
   ❑ 5. Aggressive behavior
   ❑ 6. Attention-deficit/hyperactivity disorder (ADHD)

8. The nurse assisting in planning care for a military veteran must **prioritize** nursing interventions targeted at managing which condition, if present, that commonly occurs in this population?
1. Hypertension
2. Hyperlipidemia
3. Substance abuse disorder
4. Post-traumatic stress disorder

9. The nurse caring for a refugee considers which health care need a **priority** for this client?
1. Access to housing
2. Access to clean water
3. Access to transportation
4. Access to mental health care services

10. Which action by the nurse will **best** facilitate adherence to the treatment regimen for a client with a chronic illness?
1. Arranging for home health care
2. Focusing on managing a single illness at a time
3. Communicating with one provider only to avoid confusion for the client
4. Allowing the client to teach a support person about their treatment regimen

ANSWERS

1. 1
Rationale: When providing education to members of special populations, return explanation and demonstration (teach-back) are of particular importance to ensure safety and mutual understanding. This method is the most reliable in confirming client understanding of the instructions. Video instruction, written materials, and verbal explanation are helpful and may be incorporated with the teach-back method.
Test-Taking Strategy: Note the strategic words, *most effective.* Note that the correct option—the teach-back method—is the umbrella option, which encompasses all other options. Recall that asking the client to perform a return demonstration is the best way to confirm his or her understanding.

2. 1
Rationale: The nurse needs to address the client with the name and pronouns that the client prefers, and the first name may not necessarily be preferred. For the transgender person, it is likely that they would like to be addressed using pronouns associated with the sex they identify with now, which typically is not their birth sex. Anticipating the client's needs and making suggestions may be seen as passing judgment, so the nurse should refrain from doing this.
Test-Taking Strategy: Note the strategic words, *most appropriate.* Recalling that clarification regarding name preference for any client is important will assist you in eliminating option 2. Recalling that use of pronouns associated with birth sex is inappropriate will assist you in eliminating option 3. Noting the word *making suggestions* in option 4 will assist you in eliminating this option.

3. 4
Rationale: The nurse needs to address the complaints of pain and numbness and tingling in both feet first with this population. If the client perceives value to the service provided and his or her complaint is addressed, they will be more likely to return for follow-up care. Although the blood pressure, blood glucose, and vision results are concerning, the client's stated concern must be addressed first.
Test-Taking Strategy: Note the subject, the finding to be addressed, and focus on the strategic word, *first.* Recalling that adherence is a problem for this population will direct you to the correct option. Also note that the correct option is the only subjective finding.

4. 1
Rationale: Intellectually disabled clients tend to have difficulty trying to remember their medical history. It may be necessary for the nurse to take more time to ask questions in a variety of different ways when collecting the history data. The physical assessment, nursing plan of care, and readmission risk assessment portions, although they rely on the history, take less time because they require less client questioning.
Test-Taking Strategy: Note the subject, conducting an admission assessment for an intellectually disabled client and the part that may take more time to complete. Recall that individuals in this special population group tend to have difficulty remembering their medical history. The use of questioning in a variety of ways may be necessary to obtain the necessary assessment data.

5. 3
Rationale: The environment of a prison can predispose a person to different health conditions, such as tuberculosis, sexually transmitted infections, or other infectious diseases. Option 1 does not address the client's question. Options 2 and 4 convey incorrect information.
Test-Taking Strategy: Note the subject, health conditions associated with living in a prison. Remember that the prison is a confined environment, and a variety of health problems including infectious diseases are prevalent.

6. 3
Rationale: The client in this question must be screened for abuse. Battered women experience bruises, particularly around the eyes, red or purple marks on the neck, sprained or broken wrists, chronic fatigue, shortness of breath, muscle tension, involuntary shaking, changes in eating and sleeping, sexual dysfunction, and fertility issues. Mental health problems can also arise, including posttraumatic stress disorder, nightmares, anxiety, uncontrollable thoughts, depression, low self-esteem, and alcohol and drug abuse. Reddened sclera, a dry rash on the elbows, and flaking of the scalp do not pose an indication of abuse.
Test-Taking Strategy: Note the strategic words, *need for follow-up.* Also focus on the data in the question, and select the option that indicates the most concern and is indicative of abuse. Remember that battered women often present with bruising around the eyes or on the neck.

7. 3, 4, 5, 6
Rationale: Foster children are at risk for a variety of health conditions, including attention-deficit/hyperactivity disorder,

aggressive behavior, anxiety disorder, bipolar disorder, depression, mood disorder, post-traumatic stress disorder (PTSD), reactive detachment disorder, sleep problems, and personality disorder. Claustrophobia and asthma are not specifically associated with foster children.

Test-Taking Strategy: Note the subject, health concerns for foster children. Specific knowledge of the health concerns associated with these children is needed to answer correctly.

8. 4

Rationale: PTSD is extremely common in this population. Identifying and treating mental health problems assists in mitigating suicide risk. Treatment of comorbid conditions such as PTSD may also help to address any substance use disorder. Use of screening tools in identifying substance use disorder is helpful. Treatment of PTSD includes exposure therapy, psychotherapy, and family/group therapy. Hypertension and hyperlipidemia are important but are not the priority; the risk of suicide and other safety concerns associated with PTSD are the priority for this population.

Test-Taking Strategy: Note the strategic word, *prioritize*. This word indicates that although all options may be important, one option is a priority due to safety considerations. Also note that options 1 and 2 are comparable or alike and therefore can be eliminated. Although substance abuse may be a concern, PTSD is the priority.

9. 4

Rationale: Mental health problems are the primary issue for this population as a result of difficult events. Although all other options are important for all clients, they do not address the specific needs of this special population.

Test-Taking Strategy: Note the strategic word, *priority*. This indicates that all options are important and are most likely correct. It is necessary to recall that due to the potential trauma experienced by refugees, mental health is a priority.

10. 1

Rationale: Nursing follow-up visits are important in promoting health for individuals with chronic illness; therefore, arranging for home health care is an important strategy. Focusing on a single illness does not effectively manage an individual with multiple chronic diseases—rather, the "big picture" needs to be understood in managing these clients. Interprofessional collaboration is important in safely managing individuals with chronic diseases and often involves consulting with specialist providers. Nurses play a key role in facilitating communication between providers and specialists. Inclusion of the client and support persons in health care decisions helps to increase adherence to a complex health care regimen. The nurse would be the facilitator of this communication.

Test-Taking Strategy: Note the strategic word, *best*. Recalling that these clients often have complex histories and health care needs will assist you in choosing the option that relates to nursing support services.

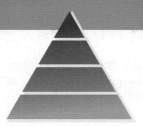

Professional Standards

CHAPTER 6

Ethical and Legal Issues

PRIORITY CONCEPTS Ethics; Health Care Law

WHAT WOULD YOU DO?

While preparing a client for surgery scheduled in 1 hour, the client states to the nurse, "I have changed my mind. I don't want this surgery." What would the nurse do?
Answer is located on p. 60.

I. Ethics
A. Description: The branch of philosophy concerned with the distinction between right and wrong on the basis of a body of knowledge, not based only on opinions
B. Morals: Behavior in accordance with customs or traditions, usually reflecting personal or religious beliefs
C. Ethical principles: Codes that direct or govern nursing actions (Box 6.1)
D. Values: Beliefs and attitudes that may influence behavior and the process of decision making
E. Values clarification: Process of analyzing one's own values to understand oneself more completely regarding what is truly important
F. Ethical codes
   1. Ethical codes provide broad principles for determining and evaluating client care.
   2. These codes are not legally binding, but the board of nursing has authority in most states to reprimand nurses for unprofessional conduct that results from violation of the ethical codes.
   3. Specific ethical codes are as follows:
      a. The Code of Ethics for Nurses was developed by the International Council of Nurses. The code can be found at: https://www.icn.ch/sites/default/files/inline-files/2012_ICN_Codeofethicsfornurses_%20eng.pdf
      b. The American Nurses Association Code of Ethics can be viewed on the American Nurses As-

sociation website: https://www.nursingworld.org/practice-policy/nursing-excellence/ethics/
G. Ethical dilemma
   1. An ethical dilemma occurs when there is a conflict between two or more ethical principles.
   2. No correct decision exists, and the nurse must make a choice between two alternatives that are equally unsatisfactory.
   3. Such dilemmas may occur as a result of differences in cultural or religious beliefs.
   4. Ethical reasoning is the process of thinking through what one would do in an orderly and systematic manner to provide justification for actions based on principles. The nurse would gather all information to determine whether an ethical dilemma exists, examine his or her own values, verbalize the problem, consider possible courses of action, negotiate the outcome, and evaluate the action taken.
H. Advocate
   1. An advocate is a person who speaks up for, or acts on the behalf of the client, protects the client's right to make his or her own decisions, and upholds the principle of fidelity.
   2. An advocate represents the client's viewpoint to others.
   3. An advocate avoids letting personal values influence advocacy for the client and supports the client's decision, vveven when it conflicts with the advocate's own preferences or choices.
I. Ethics committees
   1. Ethics committees take an interprofessional approach to facilitate dialogue regarding ethical dilemmas.
   2. These committees develop and establish policies and procedures to facilitate the prevention and resolution of dilemmas.

   ⚠ An important nursing responsibility is to act as a client advocate and protect the client's rights.

BOX 6.1 Ethical Principles

Autonomy	Respect for an individual's right to self-determination.
Nonmaleficence	The obligation to do or cause no harm to another.
Beneficence	The duty to do good to others and maintain a balance between benefit and harm. Paternalism is an undesirable outcome of beneficence, in which the primary health care provider decides what is best for the client and encourages the client to act against his or her own choices.
Justice	The equitable distribution of potential benefits and tasks determining the order in which clients would be cared for.
Veracity	The obligation to tell the truth.
Fidelity	The duty to do what one has promised.

II. Regulation of Nursing Practice

A. Nurse Practice Act

1. A nurse practice act is a series of statutes that have been enacted by each state legislature to regulate the practice of nursing in that state. The nurse practice act is designed to protect the public.

2. Nurse practice acts set educational requirements for the nurse, distinguish between nursing practice and medical practice, and define the scope of nursing practice.

3. Additional issues covered by nurse practice acts include licensure requirements for the protection of the public, grounds for disciplinary action, rights of the nurse licensee if a disciplinary action is taken, and related topics.

4. All nurses are responsible for knowing the provisions of the act of the state or province in which they work.

B. Standards of care

1. Standards of care are guidelines that identify what the client can expect to receive in terms of nursing care.

2. The guidelines determine whether nurses have performed duties in an appropriate manner.

3. If the nurse does not perform duties within accepted standards of care, the nurse could harm the client and place himself or herself in jeopardy of legal action.

4. If the nurse is named as a defendant in a malpractice lawsuit and proceedings show that the nurse followed neither the accepted standards of care outlined by the state or province nurse practice act nor the policies of the employing institution, the nurse's legal liability is clear; he or she is liable.

C. Employee guidelines

1. Respondent superior: The employer is held liable for any negligent acts of an employee if the alleged negligent act occurred during the employment relationship and was within the scope of the employee's responsibilities.

2. Contracts

   a. Nurses are responsible for carrying out the terms of a contractual agreement with the employing agency and the client.

   b. The nurse–employee relationship is governed by established employee handbooks and client care policies and procedures that create obligations, rights, and duties between those parties.

3. Institutional policies

   a. Written policies and procedures of the employing institution detail how nurses are to perform their duties.

   b. Policies and procedures are usually specific and describe the expected behavior on the part of the nurse.

   c. Although policies are not laws, courts generally rule against nurses who violate policies.

   d. If the nurse practices nursing according to client care policies and procedures established by the employer, functions within the job responsibility, and provides care consistently in a nonnegligent manner, the nurse minimizes the potential for liability.

⚠ The nurse must protect the client from harm and follow the guidelines identified in the nurse practice act and agency policies and procedures when delivering client care.

D. Hospital staffing

1. Charges of abandonment may be made against nurses who "walk out" when staffing is inadequate.

2. Nurses in short-staffing situations are obligated to make a report to the nursing administration.

E. Floating

1. Floating is an acceptable, legal practice used by health care facilities to alleviate understaffing and overstaffing.

2. Legally, the nurse cannot refuse to float unless a written contract guarantees that nurses can work only in a specified area or the nurse can prove lack of competence in the area.

3. Nurses in a floating situation must not assume responsibility beyond their level of experience or qualification.

4. Nurses who float would inform the supervisor of any lack of experience in caring for the type of clients on the new nursing unit.

5. A resource nurse who is skilled in the care of clients on the unit would also be assigned to the float nurse; in addition, the float nurse would be given an orientation of the unit, and the standards of care for the unit would be reviewed (the float nurse would care for clients whose acuity

level is more matched with the nurse's experience).

F. Disciplinary action

1. Boards of nursing may restrict, revoke, or suspend any license to practice as a nurse, according to their statutory authority.
2. Some causes for disciplinary action are as follows:
   a. Unprofessional conduct
   b. Conduct that could affect the health and welfare of the client or public adversely
   c. Breach of client confidentiality
   d. Failure to use sufficient knowledge, skills, or nursing judgment
   e. Physically or verbally abusing a client
   f. Assuming duties without sufficient preparation
   g. Knowingly delegating to unlicensed personnel nursing care that places the client at risk for injury
   h. Failure to maintain an accurate record for each client
   i. Falsifying a client's record
   j. Leaving a nursing assignment without properly notifying appropriate personnel

III. Legal Liability

A. Laws

1. Nurses are governed by civil and criminal law in roles as providers of services, employees of institutions, and private citizens.
2. The nurse has a personal and legal obligation to provide a standard of client care expected of a reasonably competent professional nurse.
3. Professional nurses are held responsible (liable) for harm resulting from their negligent acts or their failure to act.

B. Types of law (Box 6.2)

C. Negligence and malpractice (Box 6.3)

1. Negligence is conduct that falls below the standard of care.
2. Negligence can include acts of commission and acts of omission.
3. The nurse who does not meet appropriate standards of care may be held liable.
4. Malpractice is negligence on the part of the nurse.
5. Malpractice is determined by assessing if the nurse owed a duty to the client and did not carry out that duty, causing the client harm or injury.
6. Proof of liability
   a. Duty: At the time of injury, a duty existed between the plaintiff and the defendant.
   b. Breach of duty: The defendant breached duty of care to the plaintiff.
   c. Proximate cause: The breach of the duty was the legal cause of injury to the client.
   d. Damage or injury: The plaintiff experienced injury or damages, or both, and can be compensated by law.

BOX 6.2 **Types of Law**

Contract Law
Contract law is concerned with enforcement of agreements among private individuals.

Civil Law
Civil law is concerned with relationships among persons and the protection of a person's rights. Violation may cause harm to an individual or property, but no grave threat to society exists.

Criminal Law
Criminal law is concerned with relationships between individuals and governments, and with acts that threaten society and its order; a crime is an offense against society that violates a law and is defined as a misdemeanor (less serious nature) or felony (serious nature).

Tort Law
A tort is a civil wrong, other than a breach in contract, in which the law allows an injured person to seek damages from the party that caused the injury.

BOX 6.3 **Examples of Negligent Acts**

- Failure to assess and/or monitor, including recognizing significant cues
- Failure to notify the registered nurse of significant changes in a client's status
- Failure to use, calibrate, or replace equipment required to safely care for the client
- Failure to document care and evaluate care provided to the client in a timely manner
- Failure to respond to or correctly implement new and existing prescriptions
- Failure to follow the rights of medication administration and causing medication errors that result in injury to the client
- Failure to monitor an intravenous flow rate that results in injury to the client, infiltration, or phlebitis
- Failure to convey discharge instructions to the client, his or her family, or providers who are assuming responsibility for the client
- Failure to ensure client safety, especially clients who have a history of falling, are sedated or confused, are frail, are mentally impaired, get up in the night, or are uncooperative
- Failure to follow policies and procedures
- Failure to properly delegate and supervise other licensed practical nurses or nursing assistive personnel

Adapted from Potter et al. (2017), p. 309, St. Louis: Mosby.

⚠ The nurse must meet appropriate standards of care when delivering care to the client; otherwise the nurse would be held liable if the client is harmed.

D. Professional liability insurance

1. Nurses need their own liability insurance for protection against malpractice lawsuits.
2. Having their own insurance provides nurses protection as individuals. This allows the nurse to

have an attorney, who has only the nurse's interests in mind, present if necessary.

E. Good Samaritan laws

  1. State legislatures pass Good Samaritan laws, which may vary from state to state.

  2. These laws encourage health care professionals to assist in emergency situations, limit liability, and offer legal immunity for persons helping in an emergency, provided that they give reasonable care.

  3. Immunity from suit applies only when all conditions of the state law are met, such as the care giver receives no compensation for the care provided and the care given is not intentionally negligent.

F. Controlled substances

  1. The nurse would adhere to facility policies and procedures concerning administration of controlled substances, which are governed by federal and state laws.

  2. Controlled substances must be kept locked securely, and only authorized personnel would have access to them.

  3. Controlled substances must be properly signed out for administration and a correct inventory must be maintained.

IV. Collective Bargaining

A. Collective bargaining is a formalized decision-making process between representatives of management and representatives of labor to negotiate wages and conditions of employment.

B. When collective bargaining breaks down because the parties cannot reach an agreement, the employees may call a strike or take other work actions.

C. Striking presents a moral dilemma to many nurses because nursing practice is a service to people.

V. Legal Risk Areas

A. Assault

  1. Assault occurs when a person puts another person in fear of a harmful or offensive contact.

  2. The victim fears and believes that harm will result because of the threat.

B. Battery is an intentional touching of another's body without the other's consent.

C. Invasion of privacy includes violating confidentiality, intruding on private client or family matters, and sharing client information with unauthorized persons.

D. False imprisonment

  1. False imprisonment occurs when a client is not allowed to leave a health care facility when there is no legal justification to detain the client.

  2. False imprisonment occurs when restraining devices are used without an appropriate clinical need.

  3. A client can sign an Against Medical Advice form when the client refuses care and is competent to make such decisions.

BOX 6.4	**Client's Rights When Hospitalized**

- Right to considerate and respectful care
- Right to be informed about diagnosis, possible treatments, likely outcomes, and to discuss this information with the primary health care provider
- Right to know the names and roles of the persons who are involved in care
- Right to consent to or refuse a treatment
- Right to have an advance directive
- Right to privacy
- Right to expect that medical records are confidential
- Right to review the medical record and to have information explained
- Right to expect that the hospital will provide necessary health services
- Right to know if the hospital has relationships with outside parties that may influence treatment or care
- Right to consent or refuse to take part in research
- Right to be told of realistic care alternatives when hospital care is no longer appropriate
- Right to know about hospital rules that affect treatment, and about charges and payment methods

Adapted from Linton (2012). St. Louis: Saunders and adapted from American Hospital Association: The patient care partnership: Understanding expectations, rights and responsibilities. Available at http://www.aha.org/content/00-10/pcp_english_030730.pdf.

  4. The nurse would document circumstances in the medical record to avoid allegations by the client that cannot be defended.

E. Defamation is a false communication that causes damage to someone's reputation, either written (libel) or verbal (slander).

F. Fraud results from a deliberate deception intended to produce unlawful gains.

G. There may be exceptions to certain legal risk areas, such as assault, battery, and false imprisonment, when caring for a client with an alteration in normal mental status experiencing acute distress who poses a risk to himself, herself, or others. In this situation, the nurse must assess the client to determine loss of control and intervene accordingly; the nurse would use the least restrictive methods initially, but then use interventions such as restraint if the client's behavior indicates the need for this intervention.

VI. Client's Rights

A. Description

  1. The client's rights document, also called the Client's (Patient's) Bill of Rights, reflects acknowledgment of a client's right to participate in her or his health care with an emphasis on client autonomy.

  2. The document provides a list of the rights of the client and responsibilities that the hospital cannot violate (Box 6.4).

  3. The client's rights protect the client's ability to determine the level and type of care received. All

---

> ### BOX 6.5 Laws and Standards
>
> ***American Hospital Association:*** Issued Patient's Bill of Rights
>
> ***American Nurses Association:*** Developed the Code for Nurses, which defines the nurse's responsibility for upholding the client's rights
>
> ***Mental Health Systems Act:*** Developed rights for clients with a mental health problem
>
> ***The Joint Commission:*** Developed policy statements on the rights of individuals, including those with a mental health problem
>
> ***Americans With Disabilities Act:*** Prohibits discrimination against an individual with disabilities in all areas of public life

---

> ### BOX 6.6 Rights for the Mentally Ill
>
> - Right to be treated with dignity and respect
> - Right to communicate with persons outside the hospital
> - Right to keep clothing and personal effects with them
> - Right to religious freedom
> - Right to be employed
> - Right to manage property
> - Right to execute wills
> - Right to enter into contractual agreements
> - Right to make purchases
> - Right to education
> - Right to habeas corpus (written request for release from the hospital)
> - Right to an independent psychiatric examination
> - Right to civil service status, including the right to vote
> - Right to retain licenses, privileges, or permits
> - Right to sue or be sued
> - Right to marry or divorce
> - Right to treatment in the least restrictive setting
> - Right not to be subject to unnecessary restraints
> - Right to privacy and confidentiality
> - Right to informed consent
> - Right to treatment and to refuse treatment
> - Right to refuse participation in experimental treatments or research
>
> Adapted from deWit, Kumagai (2013), St. Louis: Saunders.

health care agencies are required to have a Client's Bill of Rights posted in a visible area.

    4. Several laws and standards pertain to clients' rights (Box 6.5).

B. Rights for the mentally ill (Box 6.6)

    1. The Mental Health Systems Act created rights for mentally ill people.

    2. The Joint Commission has developed policy statements on the rights of mentally ill people.

    3. Psychiatric facilities are required to have a Client's Bill of Rights posted in a visible area.

C. Organ donation and transplantation

    1. A client has the right to decide to become an organ donor and a right to refuse organ transplantation as a treatment option.

    2. An individual who is at least 18 years old may indicate a wish to become a donor on his or her driver's license (state-specific) or in an advance directive.

    3. The Uniform Anatomical Gift Act provides a list of individuals who can provide informed consent for the donation of a deceased individual's organs.

    4. The United Network for Organ Sharing sets the criteria for organ donations.

    5. Some organs, such as the heart, lungs, and liver, can be obtained only from a person who is dependent on mechanical ventilation and has suffered brain death, whereas other organs or tissues can be removed several hours after death.

    6. A donor must be free of infectious disease and cancer.

    7. Requests to the deceased's family for organ donation usually are done by the PHCP or nurse specially trained for making such requests.

    8. Donation of organs does not delay funeral arrangements, no obvious evidence that the organs were removed from the body shows when the body is dressed, and the family incurs no cost for removal of the organs donated.

D. Religious beliefs: Organ donation and transplantation:

    1. Catholic Church: Organ donation and transplants are acceptable

    2. Orthodox Church: Church usually discourages organ donation

    3. Islam (Muslim) beliefs: Body parts should not be removed or donated for transplantation.

    4. Jehovah's Witness: An organ transplant may be accepted, but the organ must be cleansed with a nonblood solution before transplantation.

    5. Orthodox Judaism:

        a. All body parts removed during autopsy must be buried with the body because it is believed that the entire body must be returned to the earth; organ donation may not be considered by family members.

        b. Organ transplantation may be allowed with the rabbi's approval.

    6. Refer to Chapter 20 for information on end-of-life care.

VII. Consents

A. Description

    1. Consents, or releases, are legal documents that indicate the client's permission to perform surgery, perform a treatment or procedure, or give information to a third party.

    2. There are different types of consents (Box 6.7).

    3. Informed consent indicates the client's participation in the decision regarding health care.

BOX 6.7 Types of Consents

Admission Agreement

Admission agreements are obtained at the time of admission and identify the health care agency's responsibility to the client.

Immunization Consent

An immunization consent may be required before the administration of certain immunizations. The consent indicates that the client was informed of the benefits and risks of the immunization.

Blood Transfusion Consent

A blood transfusion consent indicates that the client was informed of the benefits and risks of the transfusion. Some clients hold religious beliefs that would prohibit them from receiving a blood transfusion, even in a life-threatening situation.

Surgical Consent

Surgical consent is obtained for all surgical or invasive procedures or diagnostic tests that are invasive. The primary health care provider, surgeon, or anesthesiologist who performs the operative or other procedure is responsible for explaining the procedure, its risks and benefits, and possible alternative options.

Research Consent

The research consent obtains permission from the client regarding participation in a research study. The consent informs the client about the possible risks, consequences, and benefits of the research.

Special Consents

Special consents are required for the use of restraints, photographing the client, disposal of body parts during surgery, donating organs after death, or performing an autopsy.

BOX 6.8 Mentally or Emotionally Incompetent Clients

- Declared incompetent
- Unconscious
- Under the influence of chemical agents such as alcohol or drugs
- Chronic dementia or other mental deficiency that impairs thought processes and the ability to make decisions

4. The client must be informed, in understandable terms, of the risks and benefits of the surgery or treatment, what the consequences are for not having the surgery or procedure performed, treatment options, and the name of the PHCP performing the surgery or procedure.
5. A client's questions about the surgery or procedure must be answered by the person performing the procedure before signing the consent.
6. A consent must be signed freely by the client without threat or pressure and must be witnessed (witness must be an adult).
7. A client who has been medicated with sedating medications or any other medications that can affect the client's cognitive abilities must not be asked to sign a consent form.
8. Legally, the client must be mentally and emotionally competent to give consent.
9. If a client is declared mentally or emotionally incompetent, the next of kin, appointed guardian (appointed by the court), or durable power of attorney for health care has legal authority to give consent (Box 6.8).

10. A competent client older than 18 years of age must sign the consent.
11. In most states, when the nurse is involved in the informed consent process, the nurse is witnessing only the signature of the client on the informed consent form.
12. An informed consent can be waived for urgent medical or surgical intervention as long as institutional policy so indicates.
13. A client has the right to refuse information and waive the informed consent and undergo treatment, but this decision must be documented in the medical record.
14. A client may withdraw consent at any time.

⚠ An informed consent is a legal document and the client must be informed by the PHCP (i.e., physician, surgeon), in understandable terms, of the risks and benefits of surgery, treatments, procedures, and plan of care. The client needs to be a participant in decisions regarding health care.

B. Minors
1. A minor is a client under legal age as defined by state statute (usually younger than 18 years).
2. A minor may not give legal consent, and consent must be obtained from a parent or the legal guardian.
3. Parental or guardian consent would be obtained before treatment is initiated for a minor, except in the following cases: an emergency; situations in which the consent of the minor is sufficient, including treatment related to substance abuse, treatment of a sexually transmitted infection, human immunodeficiency virus (HIV) testing and acquired immunodeficiency syndrome (AIDS) treatment, birth control services, pregnancy or psychiatric services; the minor is an emancipated minor; or a court order or other legal authorization has been obtained. Refer to the Guttmacher Report on Public Policy for additional information: https://www.guttmacher.org/sites/default/files/article_files/gr030404.pdf

C. Emancipated minor
1. An emancipated minor has established independence from his or her (client) parents through marriage, pregnancy, service in the armed forces, or by a court order.
2. An emancipated minor is considered legally capable of signing an informed consent.

VIII. Health Insurance Portability and Accountability Act

A. Description

1. The Health Insurance Portability and Accountability Act (HIPAA) describes how personal health information (PHI) may be used and how the client can obtain access to the information.

2. PHI includes individually identifiable information that relates to the client's past, present, or future health; treatment; and payment for health care services.

3. The act requires health care agencies to keep PHI private, provides information to the client about the legal responsibilities regarding privacy, and explains the client's rights with respect to PHI.

4. The client has various rights as a consumer of health care under HIPAA, and any client requests may need to be placed in writing. A fee may be attached to certain client requests.

5. The client may file a complaint if the client believes that privacy rights have been violated.

6. For 2019 HIPAA regulations visit this website: https://www.hipaaguide.net/new-hipaa-regulations/

B. Client's rights include the right to:

1. Inspect a copy of PHI.

2. Ask the health care agency to amend the PHI that is contained in a record if the PHI is inaccurate.

3. Request a list of disclosures made regarding the PHI as specified by HIPAA.

4. Request to restrict how the health care agency uses or discloses PHI regarding treatment, payment, or health care services, unless information is needed to provide emergency treatment.

5. Request that the health care agency communicate with the client in a certain way or at a certain location. The request must specify how or where the client wishes to be contacted.

6. Request a paper copy of the HIPAA notice.

C. Health care agency use and disclosure of PHI

1. The health care agency obtains PHI in the course of providing or administering health insurance benefits.

2. Use or disclosure of PHI may be done for the following:
   a. Health care payment purposes
   b. Health care operations purposes
   c. Treatment purposes
   d. Providing information about health care services
   e. Data aggregation purposes to make health care benefit decisions
   f. Administering health care benefits

3. There are additional uses or disclosures of PHI (Box 6.9).

BOX 6.9 Uses or Disclosures of Personal Health Information

- Compliance with legal proceedings or for limited law enforcement purposes
- To a family member or significant other in a medical emergency
- To a personal representative appointed by the client or designated by law
- For research purposes in limited circumstances
- To a coroner, medical examiner, or funeral director about a deceased person
- To an organ procurement organization in limited circumstances
- To avert a serious threat to the client's health or safety or the health or safety of others
- To a governmental agency authorized to oversee the health care system or government programs
- To the Department of Health and Human Services for the investigation of compliance with the Health Insurance Portability and Accountability Act or to fulfill another lawful request
- To federal officials for lawful intelligence or national security purposes
- To protect health authorities for public health purposes
- To appropriate military authorities if a client is a member of the armed forces
- In accordance with a valid authorization signed by the client

Adapted from U.S. Department of Health and Human Services Office for Civil Rights: Health information privacy. Available at http://www.hhs.gov/ocr/privacy/.

IX. Confidentiality/Information Security

A. Description

1. In the health care system, confidentiality/information security refers to the protection of privacy of the client's PHI.

2. Clients have a right to privacy in the health care system.

3. A special relationship exists between the client and the nurse, in which information discussed is not shared with a third party who is not directly involved in the client's care.

4. Violations of privacy occur in various ways (Box 6.10).

B. Nurse's responsibility

1. Nurses are bound to protect client confidentiality by most nurse practice acts, by ethical principles and standards, and by institutional and agency policies and procedures.

2. Disclosure of confidential information exposes the nurse to liability for invasion of the client's privacy.

3. The nurse needs to protect the client from indiscriminate disclosure of health care information that may cause harm (Box 6.11).

C. Social networks and health care (Box 6.12)

D. Medical records

1. Medical records are confidential.

BOX 6.10 Violations and Invasion of Client Privacy

- Taking photographs of the client
- Release of medical information to an unauthorized person, such as a member of the press, family, friend, or neighbor of the client, without the client's permission
- Use of the client's name or picture for the health care agency's sole advantage
- Intrusion by the health care agency regarding the client's affairs
- Publication of information about the client or photographs of the client, including on a social networking site
- Publication of embarrassing facts
- Public disclosure of private information
- Leaving the curtains or room door open during a treatment or procedure
- Allowing individuals to observe a treatment or procedure without the client's consent
- Leaving a confused or agitated client sitting in the nursing unit hallway
- Interviewing a client in a room with only a curtain between clients, or where conversation can be overheard
- Accessing medical records when unauthorized to do so

BOX 6.11 Maintenance of Confidentiality

- Not discussing client issues with other clients or staff uninvolved in the client's care
- Not sharing health care information with others without the client's consent (includes family members or friends of the client)
- Keeping all information about a client private, and not revealing it to someone not directly involved in care
- Discussing client information only in private and secluded areas
- Protecting the medical record from all unauthorized readers

BOX 6.12 Social Networking and Health Care

- Specific social networking sites can be beneficial to health care providers and clients. Misuse of social networking sites by health care providers can lead to Health Insurance Portability and Accountability Act violations and subsequent termination of the employee.
- Nurses need to adhere to the code of ethics, confidentiality rules, and social media rules. Additional information about these code and rules can be located at the American Nurses Association Social Media Principles website at https://www.nursingworld.org/social/
- Standards of professionalism need to be maintained, and any information obtained through any nurse–client relationship cannot be shared.
- The nurse is responsible for reporting any breach of privacy or confidentiality.

2. The client has the right to read the medical record and have copies of it.

3. Only staff members directly involved in care have legitimate access to a client's records. These may include PHCPs and nurses caring for the client, technicians, therapists, social workers, unit secretaries, client advocates, and administrators (e.g., for statistical analysis, staffing, quality care review). Others must ask permission from the client.

4. Per health care facilities policies, the medical record is sent to the records or the health information department after discharge of the client from the facility.

E. Information technology/computerized medical records

1. Health care employees would have access only to the client's records in the nursing unit or work area.

2. Confidentiality/information security can be protected by the use of special computer access codes to limit what employees have access to in computer systems.

3. The use of a password or an identification code is needed to enter and sign off a computer system.

4. A password or an identification code would never be shared with another person.

5. Personal passwords would be changed periodically to prevent unauthorized computer access.

F. When conducting research, any information provided by the client is not to be reported in any manner that identifies the client and is not to be made accessible to anyone outside the research team.

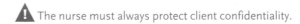 The nurse must always protect client confidentiality.

X. Legal Safeguards

A. Risk management

1. Risk management is a planned method to identify, analyze, and evaluate risks, followed by a plan for reducing the frequency of accidents and injuries.

2. Programs are based on a systematic reporting system for incidents or unusual occurrences.

B. Occurrence reports (Box 6.13)

1. The occurrence report is used as a means of identifying risk situations and improving client care.

2. Follow specific documentation guidelines.

3. Fill out the report completely, accurately, and factually.

4. The report form would not be copied or placed in the client's record.

5. Make no reference to the occurrence report form in the client's record.

6. The report is not a substitute for a complete entry in the client's record regarding the occurrence.

7. If a client injury or error in care occurred, assess the client frequently.

BOX 6.13 Examples of Occurrences That Need to Be Reported

- Accidental omission of prescribed therapies
- Circumstances that led to injury or a risk for client injury (i.e. safety hazards)
- Client falls
- Medication or intravenous administration errors
- Needle-stick injuries
- Procedure or equipment-related accidents
- A visitor injury that occurred on the health care agency's premises
- A visitor who exhibits symptoms of a communicable disease

BOX 6.14 Telephone Prescriptions

- Date and time the entry.
- Repeat the prescription to the primary health care provider (PHCP) and record the prescription.
- Sign the prescription; begin with "to." (telephone order), write the PHCP's name, and sign the prescription.
- If another nurse witnessed the prescription, that nurse's signature follows.
- The PHCP needs to countersign the prescription within a time frame according to agency policy.

---

8. The PHCP must be notified of the occurrence and the client's condition.

C. Safeguarding valuables

1. Client's valuables would be given to a family member or secured for safekeeping in a stored and locked designated location, such as the agency's safe if this is a part of the agency's procedures. The location of the client's valuables would be documented per agency policy.
2. Many health care agencies require a client to sign a release to free the agency of the responsibility for lost valuables.
3. A client's wedding band can be taped in place unless a risk exists for swelling of the hands or fingers.
4. Religious items, such as medals, may be pinned to the client's gown if allowed by agency policy.

D. PHCP's prescriptions

1. The nurse is obligated to carry out a PHCP's prescription, except when the nurse believes a prescription to be inappropriate or inaccurate.
2. The nurse carrying out an inaccurate prescription may be legally responsible for any harm suffered by the client.
3. If no resolution occurs regarding the prescription in question, the nurse would contact the nurse manager or supervisor.
4. The nurse would follow specific agency guidelines for telephone prescriptions (Box 6.14).

BOX 6.15 Components of a Medication Prescription

- Date and time the prescription was written
- Medication name
- Medication dosage
- Route of administration
- Frequency of administration
- Prescriber's signature

BOX 6.16 Dos and Don'ts Documentation Guidelines: Narrative and Information Technology

- Date and time entries.
- Provide objective, factual, and complete documentation.
- Document care, medications, treatments, and procedures as soon as possible after completion.
- Document client responses to interventions.
- Document consent for, or refusal of, treatments.
- Document calls made to other primary health care providers.
- Use quotes as appropriate for subjective data.
- Use correct spelling, grammar, and punctuation.
- Sign and title each entry.
- Follow agency policies when an error is made.
- Follow agency guidelines regarding late entries.
- Use only the user identification code, name, or password for computerized documentation.
- Maintain privacy and confidentiality of documented information printed from the computer.
- Do not document for others or change documentation for other individuals.
- Do not use unacceptable abbreviations.
- Do not use judgmental or evaluative statements, such as "uncooperative client."
- Do not leave blank spaces on documentation forms.
- Do not lend access identification computer codes to another person; change password at regular intervals.

---

5. The nurse would ensure that all components of a medication prescription are documented (Box 6.15).

⚠ The nurse would never carry out a prescription if it is unclear or inappropriate. The PHCP would be contacted immediately.

E. Documentation

1. Documentation is legally required by accrediting agencies, state licensing laws, and state nurse and medical practice acts.
2. The nurse would follow agency guidelines and procedures (Box 6.16).
3. Refer to the Joint Commission website for acceptable abbreviations and documentation guidelines: http://www.jointcommission.org/standards_information/npsgs.aspx.

F. Client and family teaching

1. Provide complete instructions in a language that the client or family can understand; consult agency

medical interpreter and/or follow agency protocol. A family member or other individual should not be asked to act as an interpreter for the client.

2. Document client and family teaching, what was taught, evaluation of understanding, and who was present during the teaching.

3. Inform the client of what could happen if information shared during teaching is not followed.

 XI. Advance Directives

A. Patient Self-Determination Act

1. The Patient Self-Determination Act is a law that indicates clients must be provided with information about their rights to identify written directions about the care they wish to receive in the event that they become incapacitated and are unable to make health care decisions.

2. During admission to a health care facility, the client is asked about the existence of an advance directive, and if one exists. It must be documented and included as a part of the medical record; if the client signs an advance directive at the time of admission, it must be documented in the client's medical record.

3. The two basic types of advance directives include instructional directives and durable powers of attorney for health care.

   a. Instructional directive: Lists the medical treatment that a client chooses to omit or refuse if the client becomes unable to make decisions and is terminally ill.

   b. Durable powers of attorney for health care: Appoints a person (health care proxy) chosen by the client to make health care decisions on the client's behalf when the client can no longer make decisions.

B. Do not resuscitate (DNR) prescriptions

1. A DNR prescription would be written if the client and PHCP have made the decision that the client's health is deteriorating and the client chooses not to undergo cardiopulmonary resuscitation (CPR) if needed.

2. The client or his or her legal representative must provide informed consent for the DNR status.

3. The DNR prescription must be defined clearly so that other treatment, not refused by the client, will be continued.

4. Some states offer DNR Comfort Care and DNR Comfort Care Arrest protocols; these protocols list specific actions that PHCPs will take when providing CPR.

5. All health care personnel must know whether a client has a DNR prescription; if a client does not have a DNR prescription, health care personnel need to make every effort to revive the client.

6. A DNR prescription needs to be reviewed regularly according to agency policy and may need to be changed if the client's status changes.

7. DNR protocols may vary from state to state, and it is important for the nurse to know his or her state's protocols.

C. The nurse's role

1. Discussing advance directives with the client opens the communication channel to establish what is important to the client and what the client may view as promoting life versus prolonging dying.

2. The nurse needs to ensure that the client has been provided with information about the right to identify written directions about the care that the client wishes to receive.

3. During admission to a health care facility, the nurse determines whether an advance directive exists and ensures that it is part of the medical record.

4. The nurse ensures that the PHCP is aware of the presence of an advance directive.

5. All health care workers need to follow the directions of an advance directive to be safe from liability.

6. Some agencies have specific policies that prohibit the nurse from signing as a witness to a legal document, such as an instructional directive.

7. If allowed by the agency, when the nurse acts as a witness to a legal document, the nurse must document the event and the factual circumstances surrounding the signing in the medical record. Documentation as a witness would include who was present, any significant comments made by the client, and the nurse's observations of the client's conduct during this process.

XII. Reporting Responsibilities

A. Nurses are required to report certain communicable diseases or criminal activities, such as child or elder abuse or domestic violence; dog bite or other animal bite; gunshot or stab wounds, assaults, and homicides; and suicides, to the appropriate authorities.

B. Impaired nurse

1. If the nurse suspects that a coworker is abusing chemicals and potentially jeopardizing a client's safety, the nurse must report the individual to the nursing administration in a confidential manner. (Client safety is always the first priority.)

2. Nursing administration notifies the board of nursing regarding the nurse's behavior.

3. Many institutions have policies that allow for drug testing if impairment is suspected.

C. Occupational Safety and Health Administration (OSHA)

1. OSHA requires that an employer provide a safe workplace for employees according to regulations.

2. Employees can confidentially report working conditions that violate regulations.

3. An employee who reports unsafe working conditions cannot be retaliated against by the employer.

D. Sexual harassment

1. Sexual harassment is prohibited by state and federal laws.

2. Sexual harassment includes unwelcome conduct of a sexual nature.

3. Follow agency policies and procedures to handle reporting a concern or complaint.

WHAT WOULD YOU DO?

Answer: If the client indicates that he or she does not want a prescribed therapy, treatment, or procedure such as surgery, then the nurse would further investigate the client's request. If the client indicates that he or she has changed his/her mind about surgery, the nurse would assess the client and explore with the client his or her concerns about not wanting the surgery. The nurse would then withhold further surgical preparation and contact the surgeon to report the client's request so that the surgeon can discuss the consequences of not having the surgery with the client. The nurse would also document the client's request and that the surgeon was notified. Under no circumstances would the nurse continue with surgical preparation if the client has indicated that he or she does not want the surgery. Further assessment and follow-up related to the client's request need to be done. In addition, it is the client's right to refuse treatment.

PRACTICE QUESTIONS

❖ **1.** Which identifies accurate nursing documentation notations? *Select all that apply.*

   1. The client slept through the night.

   2. Abdominal wound dressing is dry and intact without drainage.

   3. The client seemed angry when awakened for vital sign measurement.

   4. The client appears to become anxious when it is time for respiratory treatments.

   5. The client's left lower medial leg wound is 3 cm in length without redness, drainage, or edema.

2. The licensed practical nurse (LPN) enters a client's room and finds the client lying on the bathroom floor. The LPN calls the registered nurse, who checks the client thoroughly and then assists the client back into bed. The LPN completes an incident report, and the nursing supervisor and primary health care provider (PHCP) are notified of the incident. Which is the *next* nursing action regarding the incident?

   1. Place the incident report in the client's chart.

   2. Make a copy of the incident report for the PHCP.

   3. Document a complete entry in the client's record concerning the incident.

   4. Document in the client's record that an incident report has been completed.

3. An unconscious client, bleeding profusely, is brought to the emergency department after a serious accident. Surgery is required immediately to save the client's life. With regard to informed consent for the surgical procedure, which is the *best* action?

   1. Call the nursing supervisor to initiate a court order for the surgical procedure.

   2. Try calling the client's spouse to obtain telephone consent before the surgical procedure.

   3. Ask the friend who accompanied the client to the emergency department to sign the consent form.

   4. Transport the client to the operating department immediately without obtaining an informed consent.

4. The nurse arrives at work and is told to report (float) to the pediatric unit for the day because the unit is understaffed and needs additional nurses to care for the clients. The nurse has never worked in the pediatric unit. Which is the appropriate nursing action?

   1. Call the hospital lawyer.

   2. Call the nursing supervisor.

   3. Refuse to float to the pediatric unit.

   4. Report to the pediatric unit and identify tasks that can be safely performed.

5. The nurse enters a client's room and notes that the client's lawyer is present and that the client is preparing a living will. The living will requires that the client's signature be witnessed, and the client asks the nurse to witness the signature. Which is the appropriate nursing action?

   1. Decline to sign the will.

   2. Sign the will as a witness to the signature only.

   3. Call the hospital lawyer before signing the will.

   4. Sign the will, clearly identifying credentials and employment agency.

6. The nurse finds the client lying on the floor. The nurse calls the registered nurse, who checks the client and then calls the nursing supervisor and the primary health care provider (PHCP) to inform them of the occurrence. The nurse completes the incident report for which purpose?

   1. Providing clients with necessary stabilizing treatments

   2. A method of promoting quality care and risk management

   3. Determining the effectiveness of interventions in relation to outcomes

   4. The appropriate method of reporting to local, state, and federal agencies

7. The nurse observes that a client received pain medication 1 hour ago from another nurse, but the client still has severe pain. The nurse has previously observed this same occurrence several times. Based on the nurse practice act, the observing nurse would plan to take which action?
   1. Report the information to the police.
   2. Call the impaired nurse organization.
   3. Talk with the nurse who gave the medication.
   4. Report the information to a nursing supervisor.

8. A client has died, and the nurse asks a family member about the funeral arrangements. The family member refuses to discuss the issue. Which is the appropriate nursing action at this time?
   1. Show acceptance of feelings.
   2. Provide information needed for decision making.
   3. Suggest a referral to a mental health professional.
   4. Remain with the family member without discussing funeral arrangements.

9. A nurse lawyer provides an education session to the nursing staff regarding client rights with an emphasis on invasion of these rights. The nurse lawyer asks a staff nurse to identify a situation that represents an example of invasion of client privacy. Which situation, if identified by a staff nurse, indicates an understanding of a violation of this client right?
   1. Threatening to place a client in restraints
   2. Performing a surgical procedure without consent
   3. Taking photographs of the client without consent
   4. Telling the client that he or she cannot leave the hospital

10. An older woman is brought to the emergency department. When caring for the client, the nurse notes old and new ecchymotic areas on both of the client's arms and buttocks. The nurse asks the client how the bruises were sustained. The client, although reluctant, tells the nurse in confidence that her daughter frequently hits her if she gets in the way. Which is the appropriate nursing response?
    1. "I have a legal obligation to report this type of abuse."
    2. "I promise I won't tell anyone, but let's see what we can do about this."
    3. "Let's talk about ways that will prevent your daughter from hitting you."
    4. "This should not be happening. If it happens again, you must call the emergency department."

ANSWERS

❖ **1.   1, 2, 5**
Rationale: Factual documentation contains descriptive and objective information about what the nurse sees, hears, feels, or smells. The use of inferences without supporting factual data is not acceptable because it can be misunderstood. The use of vague terms, such as *seems* or *appears*, is not acceptable because these words suggest the nurse is stating an opinion.
Test-Taking Strategy: Focus on the subject, accurate documentation notations. Eliminate options 3 and 4 because they are comparable or alike and include vague terms (*seemed*, *appears*).

2.   3
Rationale: The incident report is confidential and privileged information, and it would not be copied, placed in the chart, or have any reference made to it in the client's record. The incident report is not a substitute for a complete entry in the client's record concerning the incident.
Test-Taking Strategy: Note the strategic word, *next*. Eliminate options 1 and 4 first because they are comparable or alike. Recalling that incident reports would not be copied will direct you to the correct option.

3.   4
Rationale: Generally, there are only two instances in which the informed consent of an adult client is not needed. One instance is when an emergency is present and delaying treatment for the purpose of obtaining informed consent would result in injury or death to the client. The second instance is when the client waives the right to give informed consent. Options 1, 2, and 3 are inappropriate.
Test-Taking Strategy: Note the strategic word, *best*. Option 3 can easily be eliminated first: a friend would not be asked to sign a consent. Note the subject, surgery is required immediately. Options 1 and 2 would delay treatment and would be eliminated.

4.   4
Rationale: Floating is an acceptable legal practice used by hospitals to solve their understaffing problems. Legally the nurse cannot refuse to float unless a union contract guarantees that the nurse can only work in a specified area or the nurse can prove a lack of knowledge for the performance of assigned tasks. When faced with this situation, the nurse would identify potential areas of harm to the client and only perform tasks that he or she is trained and experienced in.
Test-Taking Strategy: Options 1 and 2 can be eliminated first because they are comparable or alike. From the remaining options, eliminate option 3, because refusal is unacceptable behavior for a professional.

5.   1
Rationale: Living wills are required to be in writing and signed by the client. The client's signature either must be witnessed by specified individuals or notarized. Many states prohibit any employee from being a witness, including the nurse in a facility in which the client is receiving care.
Test-Taking Strategy: Options 2 and 4 are comparable or alike and would be eliminated first. From the remaining options, option 1 is the appropriate action.

6. 2

Rationale: Proper documentation of unusual occurrences, incidents, accidents, and the nursing actions taken as a result of the occurrence are internal to the institution or agency. Documentation on the incident report allows the nurse and administration to review the quality of care and determine any potential risks present. Options 1, 3, and 4 are incorrect.

Test-Taking Strategy: Focus on the subject, the purpose of completing incident reports. Eliminate options 1 and 3, because incident reports are not routinely filled out for interventions or treatment measures. Eliminate option 4, because incident reports are not used to report occurrences to other agencies; medical records are used for this purpose.

7. 4

Rationale: Nurse practice acts require reporting the suspicion of impaired nurses. The state board of nursing has jurisdiction over the practice of nursing and may develop plans for treatment and supervision. This suspicion needs to be reported to the nursing supervisor, who will then report to the board of nursing. Options 1 and 2 are inappropriate. Option 3 may cause a conflict.

Test-Taking Strategy: Focus on the subject, following the channels of communication in a health care agency. By reporting the information, the nurse alerts the institution to the potential problem and sets the stage for further investigation and appropriate action.

8. 4

Rationale: The family member is exhibiting the first stage of grief (denial), and the nurse would remain with the family member. Option 1 is an appropriate intervention for the acceptance or reorganization and restitution stage. Option 2 may be an appropriate intervention for the bargaining stage. Option 3 may be an appropriate intervention for depression.

Test-Taking Strategy: Note the words, *at this time*. Use therapeutic communication techniques to direct you to option 4. Note that the family member is exhibiting denial and remember to address client and family feelings and be supportive.

9. 3

Rationale: Invasion of privacy takes place when an individual's private affairs are intruded on unreasonably. Threatening to place a client in restraints constitutes assault. Performing a surgical procedure without consent is an example of battery. Not allowing a client to leave the hospital constitutes false imprisonment.

Test-Taking Strategy: Note the subject, invasion of client privacy. These words would direct you to the correct option. Also reading each option carefully will assist in answering correctly.

10. 1

Rationale: Confidential issues are not to be discussed with nonmedical personnel or with the client's family or friends without the client's permission. Clients would be assured that information is kept confidential unless it places the nurse under a legal obligation. The nurse must report situations related to child, older adult abuse, and other types of abuse, depending on state laws; gunshot wounds; stabbings; and certain infectious diseases.

Test-Taking Strategy: Focus on the subject, elderly abuse. Option 4 can be eliminated first because this action does not protect the client from injury. Options 2 and 3 are comparable or alike and would be eliminated next.

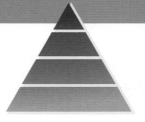

CHAPTER **7**

Prioritizing Client Care: Leadership, Delegation, and Emergency Response Planning

---

PRIORITY CONCEPTS Leadership; Health Care Organizations

WHAT WOULD YOU DO?

The nurse notes that there has been an increase in the number of intravenous (IV) site infections that developed in the clients being cared for on the nursing unit. How would the nurse proceed to implement a quality improvement program?
Answer is located on p. 74.

 I. Health Care Delivery Systems

A. Managed care
1. *Managed care* is a broad term used to describe strategies used in the health care delivery system that reduce the costs of health care.
2. Client care is outcome driven and is managed by a case management process.
3. Managed care emphasizes the promotion of health, client education and responsible self-care, early identification of disease, and the use of health care resources.

B. Case management
1. Case management is a health care delivery strategy that supports managed care. It uses an interprofessional approach that provides comprehensive client care throughout their illness and uses available resources to promote high-quality and cost-effective care.
2. Case management includes data collection and development of a plan of care, coordination of all services, referral, and follow-up.
3. Critical pathways are used, and variation analysis is conducted.
4. The core functions of case management are assessment, treatment planning, linking, advocacy, and monitoring.

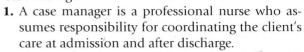 Case management involves collaboration with an interprofessional health care team.

C. Case manager
1. A case manager is a professional nurse who assumes responsibility for coordinating the client's care at admission and after discharge.
2. The case manager establishes a plan of care with the client, coordinates any interprofessional consultations and referrals, and facilitates discharge.
3. A case manager is knowledgeable in various types of health insurance, which allows them to assist clients in navigating health care options covered by insurance.

D. Health Insurance
1. There are state and federal insurance plans.
2. An aim of the Affordable Care Act (ACA) is to reduce the amount of uncompensated care the average U.S. family pays for by requiring everyone to have health insurance or pay a tax penalty. Its goals are to expand access to health insurance, to reduce cost, and to protect clients against arbitrary actions by insurance companies.
3. There are many insurance companies that provide state marketplace insurance; some include Aetna, Blue Cross Blue Shield, Cigna, Humana, Kaiser, United, and TriCare/Humana.
4. Types of insurance plans include health maintenance organizations (HMOs), preferred provider organizations (PPOs), exclusive provider organizations (EPOs), point-of-service (POS) plans, high-deductible health plans (HDHPs), and health saving accounts (HSAs); these offer varying options in terms of insurance coverage and out-of-pocket costs and premiums.
5. Medicare is a federal health insurance program for persons aged 65 or older, and may be for

certain younger people with disabilities, and people with end stage renal disease (ESRD) requiring dialysis or renal transplant; certain premiums are attached to each part.

  a. Part A: Covers hospital stays, skilled nursing facility stays, hospice care, and some home health care

  b. Part B: Helps pay for some services not covered by Part A. Medicare usually covers 80% for approved services; the remaining 20% is the client's responsibility and a supplemental insurance needs to be obtained.

  c. Part C: A health plan offered by a private insurance agency that contracts with Medicare to supplement coverage

  d. Part D: Covers prescription and medication needs

  6. Medicaid is a joint federal and state program that provides health benefits to eligible low-income adults, children, pregnant women, elderly individuals, and people with disabilities. A concern associated with these programs is fraud and abuse; a case manager needs to know how to complete insurance, state, and federal applications and be astute enough to know if an individual is reporting incorrect information.

E. Critical pathway

  1. A critical pathway is a clinical management care plan for providing client-centered care and for planning and monitoring the client's progress within an established time frame; interprofessional collaboration and teamwork ensure shared decision making and quality client care.

  2. Critical pathways are based on evidence-based practice and include evidence-based medical practice, budgetary, organizational, and systems-wide information.

  3. Variation analysis is a continuous process that the case manager and other caregivers conduct by comparing the specific client outcomes with the expected outcomes described on the critical pathway.

  4. The goal of a critical pathway is to anticipate and recognize negative client problems early so that appropriate action can be taken and positive client outcomes can result.

  5. Critical pathways are used to ensure medical care is consistent within budget constraints and to allow primary health care providers (PHCPs) to care for more complex clients. For example, some ambulatory practices have critical pathways for certain conditions such as blood pressure monitoring or urinary tract infections.

 F. Care Planning and Clinical Judgment Processes

  1. Nursing care plan

    a. A written guideline and communication tool that identifies the client's pertinent assessment data (data collection and recognize cues), client problems (analyze cues and prioritize hypotheses), goals (generate solutions, planning), interventions (implementation, take action), and provides a framework for evaluation of the client's response to nursing actions (evaluation, evaluate outcomes)

    b. The plan enhances continuity of care by identifying specific nursing actions necessary to achieve the goals of care.

    c. The client and family are involved in developing the plan of care, and the plan identifies short- and long-term goals.

    d. Client problems, goals, interventions, and expected outcomes are documented in the care plan, which provides a framework for evaluation of the client's response to nursing actions. The care plan is modified as the client condition changes.

  2. Assessment, Diagnosis, Planning, Implementation, Evaluation (ADPIE); note that nurses do not diagnose, rather the nurse identifies client problems.

  3. Data Collection, Planning, Implementation, Evaluation (Clinical Problem-Solving Process/Nursing Process)

  4. National Council of State Board of Nursing (NCSBN) Clinical Judgment Skills: Recognize cues, Analyze Cues, Prioritize hypotheses, Generate solutions, Take action, Evaluate outcomes

II. **Nursing Delivery Systems**

A. Functional nursing:

  1. Functional nursing involves a task approach to client care, with tasks being delegated by the charge nurse to individual members of the team.

  2. This type of system is task-oriented, and the team member focuses on the delegated task rather than the total client. This results in fragmentation of care and lack of accountability by the team member.

B. Team nursing

  1. The team is led by a team leader (generally a registered nurse [RN]) who determines the work assignment. Each staff member works fully within the realm of his or her educational and clinical expertise and job description.

  2. The team leader determines the work assignment.

  3. Each staff member is accountable for client care and outcomes of care delivered in accordance with the licensing and practice scope as determined by health care agency policy and state law.

  4. Modular nursing is similar to team nursing, but it takes into account the structure of the unit. The unit is divided into modules, allowing nurses to care for a group of clients who are geographically close by.

C. Relationship-based practice (primary nursing)
1. Relationship-based practice is concerned with keeping the nurse at the bedside, actively involved in client care, while planning goal-directed, individualized care.
2. One primary nurse is responsible for managing and coordinating the client's care while in the hospital and for discharge, and an associate nurse cares for the client when the primary nurse is off duty.

D. Client-focused care
1. This is also known as the total care or case method; the nurse assumes total responsibility for planning and delivering care to a client.
2. The client may have different nurses assigned during a 24-hour period; the nurse provides all necessary care needed for the assigned time period.

III. Professional Responsibilities

A. Accountability
1. The process in which individuals have an obligation (or duty) to act and are answerable for their choices, decisions, and actions
2. Involves assuming only the responsibilities that are within one's scope of practice and not assuming responsibility for activities in which competence has not been achieved
3. Involves admitting mistakes rather than blaming others and evaluating the outcomes of one's own actions
4. Includes a responsibility to the client to be competent, providing nursing care in accordance with standards of nursing practice, and adhering to the professional codes of ethics

⚠ Accountability is accepting responsibility for one's choices, decisions and actions. The nurse is always responsible for his or her actions when providing care to a client.

B. Leadership and management
1. Leadership is the interpersonal process that involves influencing others (followers) to achieve goals.
2. Management is the accomplishment of tasks or goals by oneself or by directing others.

C. Leader and manager approaches
1. Autocratic
   a. The authoritarian leader or manager is focused and maintains strong control, makes decisions, and addresses all problems.
   b. The leader or manager dominates the group and commands rather than seeks suggestions or input.
2. Democratic
   a. This is also called participative management.
   b. It is based on the belief that every group member needs to have input into the development of goals and problem solving; leader obtains participation/input from the group and then makes the best decision for the organization.
   c. The democratic style is a more "talk with the members" style and much less authoritarian than the autocratic style.
3. Laissez-faire
   a. A laissez-faire leader or manager assumes a passive, nondirective, and inactive approach and relinquishes part or all of the responsibilities to the members of the group.
   b. Decision making is left to the group with the laissez-faire leader or manager providing little, if any, guidance, support, or feedback.
4. Situational
   a. Situational style uses a combination of styles based on the current circumstances and events.
   b. Situational styles are assumed according to the needs of the group and the tasks to be achieved.
5. Bureaucratic
   a. The leader or manager believes that individuals are motivated by external forces.
   b. The leader/manager relies on organizational policies and procedures for decision making.
6. Transformational Leadership
   a. Focused on building relationships
   b. Motivates staff members through a shared vision and mission
   c. Encourages and praises staff members and inspires them to improve performance levels while earning staff respect and loyalty
7. Servant Leadership
   a. Servant leaders influence and motivate others by building relationships and developing the skills of individual team members.
   b. Servant leaders make sure to meet the needs of the individual team members and to give each person input in decisions.

D. Effective leader and manager behaviors and qualities (Box 7.1)

E. Problem-solving process and decision making
1. Problem solving involves obtaining information and using it to reach an acceptable solution to a problem.
2. Decision making involves identifying a problem and deciding which alternatives can best achieve objectives.
3. Steps of the problem-solving process are similar to the steps of the nursing process and the cognitive skills of the NCSBN Clinical Judgment Measurement Model (Table 7.1).

IV. Empowerment

A. Empowerment is an interpersonal process of enabling others to do for themselves.

BOX 7.1 **Effective Leader and Manager Behaviors and Qualities**

Behaviors

Treats followers as unique individuals

Inspires followers and stimulates critical thinking

Shows followers how to think about old problems in new ways

Is visible to followers; is flexible; and provides guidance, assistance, and feedback

Communicates a vision, establishes trust, and empowers employees

Motivates employees to achieve goals

Qualities

Effective communicator; promotes interprofessional collaboration

Credible

Critical thinker

Initiator of action

Risk taker

Is persuasive and influences employees

Adapted from Potter P, Perry AG, Stockert PA, Hall AM: *Fundamentals of nursing*, ed 8, St. Louis, 2013, Mosby; and Huber D: *Leadership and nursing care management*, ed 4, Philadelphia, 2010, Saunders.

TABLE 7.1 **Similarities of the Problem-Solving Process, Nursing Process, and National Council of State Board of Nursing Cognitive Processes/Skills**

Problem-Solving Process	Nursing Process	Cognitive Processes/ Skills
Identifying a problem and collecting data about the problem	Data collection/ assessment	Recognize cues
Determining the exact nature of the problem	Analysis	Analyze cues Prioritize hypotheses
Deciding on a plan of action	Planning	Generate solutions
Carrying out the plan	Implementation	Take action
Evaluating the plan	Evaluation	Evaluate outcomes

B. Empowerment occurs when individuals are able to influence what happens to them more effectively.

C. Empowerment involves open communication, mutual goal setting, and shared decision making.

D. Nurses can empower clients through teaching and advocacy.

V. Formal Organizations

A. An organization's mission statement communicates in broad terms its reason for existence; the geographical area that the organization serves; and the attitudes, beliefs, and values from which the organization functions.

B. Goals and objectives are measurable activities specific to the development of designated services and programs of an organization.

C. The organizational chart depicts and communicates how activities are arranged, how authority relationships are defined, and how communication channels are established.

D. Policies, procedures, and protocols

  1. Policies are guidelines that define the organization's standpoint on courses of action.

  2. Procedures are based on policy and define methods for tasks.

  3. Protocols prescribe a specific course of action for a specific type of client or problem.

    a. Centralization is the making of decisions by a few individuals at the top of the organization or by managers of a department or unit, and decisions are communicated thereafter to the employees.

    b. Decentralization is the distribution of authority throughout the organization to allow for increased responsibility and delegation in decision making; decentralization tries to move the decision making as close to the client as possible.

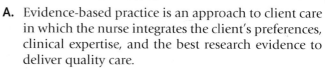
The nurse must follow policies, procedures, and protocols of the health care agency in which he or she is employed.

VI. Evidence-Based Practice

A. Evidence-based practice is an approach to client care in which the nurse integrates the client's preferences, clinical expertise, and the best research evidence to deliver quality care.

B. Determining the client's personal, social, cultural, and religious preferences ensures individualization and is a component of implementing evidence-based practice.

C. The nurse needs to be an observer and identify and question situations that require change or result in a less than desirable outcome.

D. Use of information technology such as online resources, including research publications, provides current research findings related to areas of practice.

E. The nurse needs to follow evidence-based practice protocols developed by the institution and question the rationale for nursing approaches identified in the protocols as necessary.

Evidence-based practice requires that the nurse base nursing practice on evidence from clinical research studies. The nurse would also be alert to clinical issues that warrant investigation and report these issues to the RN.

Professional Standards

VII. Quality Improvement

A. Also known as *performance improvement*, quality improvement focuses on processes or systems that significantly contribute to client safety and effective client care outcomes without attaching or looking for blame. Criteria are used to monitor outcomes of care and to determine the need for change to improve the quality of care.

B. Quality improvement processes or systems may be named *quality assurance, continuous quality management,* or *continuous quality improvement.*

C. When quality improvement is part of the philosophy of a health care agency, every staff member becomes involved in ways to improve client care and outcomes.

D. A retrospective ("looking back") audit is an evaluation method used to inspect the medical record after the client's discharge for documentation of compliance with the standards.

E. A concurrent ("at the same time") audit is an evaluation method used to inspect compliance of nurses with predetermined standards and criteria during the time that the nurses are providing care for the client.

F. Peer review is a process in which nurses employed in an organization, or consultants from outside of the organization, evaluate the quality of nursing care delivered to the client.

G. The quality improvement process is similar to the nursing process and involves a systematic interprofessional approach.

H. An outcome describes the most positive response to care; comparison of client responses to the expected outcomes indicates whether the interventions are effective, whether the client has progressed, how well standards are met, and whether changes are necessary.

I. The nurse is responsible for recognizing trends in nursing practice, identifying recurrent problems, reporting these problems, and initiating opportunities to improve the quality of care.

⚠ Quality improvement processes improve the quality of care delivery to clients and the safety of health care agencies.

VIII. Conflict

A. Conflict is an internal or external friction that arises from a perception of incompatibility or difference in beliefs, attitudes, values, goals, priorities, or decisions.

B. Types of conflict
   1. Intrapersonal: Occurs within a person
   2. Interpersonal: Occurs between and among clients, nurses, or other staff members
   3. Organizational: Occurs when an employee confronts the policies and procedures of the organization

C. Modes of conflict resolution
   1. Avoidance
      a. Avoiders are unassertive and uncooperative.
      b. Avoiders do not pursue their own needs, goals, or concerns, and they do not assist others to pursue theirs.
      c. Avoiders postpone dealing with the issue.
   2. Accommodation
      a. Accommodators neglect their own needs, goals, or concerns (unassertive) and try to satisfy those of others.
      b. Accommodators obey and serve others and often feel resentment and disappointment because they "get nothing in return."
   3. Competition
      a. Competitors pursue their own needs and goals at the expense of others.
      b. Competitors also may stand up for rights and defend important principles.
   4. Compromise
      a. Compromisers are assertive and cooperative.
      b. Compromisers work creatively and openly to find the solution that most fully satisfies all important goals and concerns to be achieved.

IX. Roles of Health Care Team Members

A. Nurse roles are as follows:
   1. Promote health and prevent disease
   2. Provide comfort and care to clients
   3. Assist to make decisions
   4. Act as a client advocate
   5. Manage client care
   6. Communicate effectively
   7. Reinforce teaching to clients and families
   8. Act as a resource person
   9. Use resources in a cost-effective manner

B. PHCP: A PHCP diagnoses and treats disease.

C. Nurse practitioner: An advanced practice RN who is educated to diagnose and treat acute illness and chronic conditions; health promotion and maintenance is a focus.

D. PHCP assistant (physician's assistant)
   1. The PHCP assistant acts to a limited extent in the role of the PHCP during the PHCP's absence.
   2. The PHCP assistant conducts physical examinations, performs diagnostic procedures, assists in the operating room and emergency department, and performs treatments.
   3. Certified and licensed PHCP assistants in some states have prescriptive powers.

E. Physical therapist: Assists in examining, testing, and treating physically disabled clients to determine functional ability and safety needs.

F. Occupational therapist: Develops adaptive devices that help chronically ill or handicapped clients perform activities of daily living.

G. Respiratory therapist: Delivers treatments designed to improve the client's ventilation and oxygenation status.

H. Speech therapist: Evaluates a client's ability to swallow safely and effectively and communicates a plan to improve a client's swallowing ability.

I. Nutritionist: Assists in planning dietary measures to improve or maintain a client's nutritional status.

J. Continuing care nurse: Coordinates discharge plans for the client.

K. Assistive personnel: Help the nurse with specified tasks and functions; also known as nursing assistant or unlicensed assistive personnel.

L. Pharmacist: Formulates and dispenses medications.

M. Social worker: Counsels clients and families about home care services and assists the continuing care nurse with planning discharge.

N. Chaplain: Offers spiritual support and guidance to clients and families.

O. Administrative staff: Support staff members organize and schedule diagnostic tests and procedures and arrange for services needed by the client and family.

X. Interprofessional Collaboration

A. Client care planning can be accomplished through referrals to, or consultations with, or interprofessional collaborations with other health care specialists and through client care conferences, which involve members from all health care disciplines. This approach helps ensure continuity of care.

B. Reports

    1. Reports need to be factual, accurate, current, complete, and organized.

    2. Reports need to include essential background information, subjective data, objective data, any changes in the client's status, client problems, treatments and procedures, medication administration, client teaching, discharge planning, family information, the client's response to treatments and procedures, and the client's priority needs.

    3. Change of shift report

      a. The report facilitates continuity of care among nurses who are responsible for a client.

      b. The report may be written, oral, audiotaped, or provided during walking rounds at the client's bedside.

      c. The report describes the client's health status and informs the nurse on the next shift about the client's needs and priorities for care.

      d. The report may be done at the client's bedside to allow the client to participate in care planning, as well as to establish the stability of the client before the oncoming nurse assumes care.

    4. Telephone reports

      a. Purposes include informing a PHCP of a client's change in status, communicating information about a client's transfer to or from

another unit or facility, and obtaining results of laboratory or diagnostic tests.

      b. The telephone report needs to be documented and needs to include when the call was made, who made the call, who was called, to whom information was given, what information was given, and what information was received.

    5. Transfer reports

      a. Transferring nurse reports provide continuity of care and may be given by telephone or in person (Box 7.2).

      b. Receiving nurse needs to repeat transfer information to ensure client safety and asks questions to clarify information about the client's status.

      c. The key to success is clear, concise, and thorough communication.

      d. Situation, background, assessment, recommendation (SBAR); (Table 7.2) is a systematic communication process that facilitates the exchange of important information regarding client care.

XI. Interprofessional Consultation

A. Consultation is a process in which a specialist is sought to identify methods of care or treatment plans to meet the needs of a client.

BOX 7.2	**Transfer Reports**

Client's name, age, primary health care provider, and diagnoses
Current health status and plan of care
Client's needs and priorities for care
Any interventions that need to be performed after transfer, such as laboratory tests, medication administration, or dressing changes
Need for any special equipment
Additional considerations such as allergies, resuscitation status, precautionary considerations, or family issues

---

TABLE 7.2   **Situation, Background, Assessment, Recommendation**

Process Step	Action
Situation	Identify self, client, location, diagnosis, and specific current situation
Background	Explain significant medical history and overview of current treatment
Assessment	Provide current vital signs and critical current assessment data, clinical impression, and any concerns
Recommendation	Make suggestions; clarify expectations; make recommendations as appropriate to ensure client safety and satisfaction, care continuity, and best outcomes

Adapted from Linton A: *Introduction to medical-surgical nursing*, ed 6, St. Louis, 2016, Saunders.

BOX 7.3   Process for Medication Reconciliation

1. Obtain a list of current medications from the client.
2. Develop an accurate list of newly prescribed medications.
3. Compare new medications to the list of current medications.
4. Identify and investigate any discrepancies and collaborate with the primary health care provider (PHCP) as necessary.
5. Communicate the finalized list with the client, caregivers, PHCP, and other team members.

BOX 7.4   Discharge Teaching

How to administer prescribed medications and the reason the medication is prescribed
Side effects of medications that need to be reported to the primary health care provider (PHCP)
Prescribed dietary and activity measures
Complications of the medical condition that need to be reported to the PHCP
How to perform prescribed treatments
How to use special equipment prescribed for the client
Schedule for home care services that are planned
How to access available community resources
When to obtain follow-up care
Note: The licensed practical nurse/licensed vocational nurse reinforces instructions prepared and initially taught by the registered nurse.

B. Consultation is needed when the nurse encounters a problem that cannot be solved using nursing knowledge, skills, and available resources.

C. Consultation is also needed when the exact problem remains unclear; a consultant can objectively and more clearly assess and identify the exact nature of the problem.

D. A rapid response team is a medical emergency team that responds to treat hospitalized clients on nonintensive care units exhibiting early signs of deterioration and life-threatening conditions to prevent respiratory or cardiac arrest.

E. Other types of "codes," such as a Code Blue or Code White, are developed within hospitals to alert expert clinicians and technicians or specific situations, such as cardiac arrest or brain attack (stroke), allowing for the mobilization of appropriate resources.

F. Medication reconciliation includes collaboration among the client, PHCPs, nurses, and pharmacists to ensure medication accuracy when clients experience changes in health care settings, or levels of care, or are transferred from one care unit to another, and upon discharge (Box 7.3).

XII. Discharge Planning

A. Discharge planning begins when the client is admitted to the hospital or health care facility.

B. Discharge planning is an interprofessional process that ensures that the client has a plan for continuing care after leaving the health care facility and assists in the client's transition from one environment to another.

C. All caregivers need to be involved in discharge planning, and referrals to other health care professionals or agencies may be needed. A PHCP's prescription may be needed for the referral, and the referral needs to be approved by the client's health care insurer.

D. The nurse needs to anticipate the client's discharge needs and report these to the RN so that referrals can be made as soon as possible (involving the client and family in the referral process).

E. The nurse needs to assist with teaching the client and family regarding care at home by reinforcing instructions prepared by the RN (Box 7.4).

XIII. Delegation and Assignments

A. Delegation

1. Delegation is a process of transferring performance of a selected nursing task in a situation to an individual who is competent to perform that specific task.
2. Delegation involves achieving outcomes and sharing activities with other individuals who have the authority to accomplish the task.
3. Nurse practice acts and any practice limitations define which aspects of care can be delegated.
4. Only the task, not the ultimate accountability, may be delegated to another.
5. The five rights of delegation are the right task, right circumstances, right person, right direction/communication, and right supervision/evaluation.

 The nurse delegates only tasks for which he or she is responsible. The nurse who delegates is accountable for the task; the person who assumes responsibility for the task is also accountable.

B. Principles and guidelines of delegating (Box 7.5)

C. Assignments

1. Assignment is the transfer of performance of client care activities to specific staff members.
2. Guidelines for client care assignments
   a. Always ensure client safety.
   b. Be aware of individual variations in work abilities.
   c. Determine which tasks can be delegated and to whom.
   d. Match the task to the delegate on the basis of the nurse practice act and any practice limitations (institutional policies and procedures and job descriptions of personnel provided by the institution).

BOX 7.5 Principles and Guidelines of Delegating

- Delegate the right task to the right delegate. Be familiar with the experience of the delegates, their scopes of practice, their job descriptions, agency policy and procedures, and the state nurse practice act.
- Provide clear directions about the task and ensure that the delegate understands the expectations.
- Determine the degree of supervision that may be required.
- Provide the delegate with the authority to complete the task. Provide a deadline for completion of the task.
- Evaluate the outcome of care that has been delegated.
- Provide feedback to the delegate regarding his or her performance.
- In general, noninvasive interventions, such as skin care, range-of-motion exercises, ambulation, grooming, and hygiene measures, can be assigned to assistive personnel (AP).
- In general, a licensed practical nurse (LPN) or licensed vocational nurse (LVN) can perform not only the tasks that a nursing assistant (assistive personnel [AP]) can perform but also certain invasive tasks, such as dressing changes, suctioning, urinary catheterization, and medication administration (oral, subcutaneous, intramuscular, and selected piggyback medications), according to the education and job description of the LPN or LVN. The LPN or LVN can also review teaching plans with the client that were initiated by the registered nurse (RN).
- An RN can perform the tasks that an LPN or LVN can perform and is responsible for assessment and planning care, initiating teaching, and administering medications intravenously.
- An RN can care for stable and unstable clients.
- An AP provides basic care that does not require any type of assessment; they can perform routine tasks in client care.

---

    e. Provide directions that are clear, concise, accurate, and complete.
    f. Validate the delegate's understanding of the directions.
    g. Communicate a feeling of confidence to the delegate and provide feedback promptly after the task is performed.
    h. Maintain continuity of care as much as possible when assigning client care.

▲ XIV. Time Management

A. Description
  1. Time management is a technique designed to assist in completing tasks within a definite time period.
  2. Learning how, when, and where to use one's time and establishing personal goals and time frames are part of time management.
  3. Time management requires an ability to anticipate the day's activities, to combine activities when possible, and not to be interrupted by nonessential activities.
  4. Time management involves efficiency in completing tasks as quickly as possible and effectiveness in deciding on the most important task to do (i.e., *prioritizing*) and doing it correctly.

B. Principles and guidelines
  1. Identify tasks, obligations, and activities and write them down.
  2. Organize the work day; identify which tasks must be completed in specified time frames.
  3. Prioritize client needs according to importance.
  4. Anticipate the needs of the day and provide time for unexpected and unplanned tasks that may arise.
  5. Focus on beginning the daily tasks, working on the most important first but also keeping the goals in mind. Look at the final goal for the day, which helps in the breakdown of tasks into manageable parts.
  6. Begin client rounds at the beginning of the shift, collecting data on each assigned client.
  7. Delegate tasks when appropriate.
  8. Keep a daily hour-by-hour log to assist in providing structure to the tasks that must be accomplished. Cross tasks off the list as they are accomplished.
  9. Use health care agency resources wisely, anticipate resource needs, and gather the necessary supplies before beginning the task.
  10. Organize paperwork and continuously document task completion and necessary client data throughout the day (i.e., documentation needs to be concurrent with the completion of a task or observation of pertinent client data).
  11. At the end of the day, evaluate the effectiveness of time management.

XV. Prioritizing Care

A. Prioritizing is deciding which needs or problems require immediate action and which ones could tolerate a delay in response because they are not urgent.
B. Guidelines for prioritizing (Box 7.6) ▲
C. Setting priorities for client teaching
  1. Determine the client's immediate learning needs.
  2. Identify types of learning needs for the individual; for example, consider the clients age, cognitive age, language needs, and generational concerns.
  3. Review the learning objectives established for the client.
  4. Determine what the client perceives as important.
  5. Determine the client's anxiety level and the time available to teach.

D. Prioritizing when caring for a group of clients (see Priority Nursing Actions)
  1. Review the problems of each client.
  2. Determine which client problems are most urgent based on their basic needs, changing or unstable status, and complexity of problems.
  3. Anticipate the time that it may take to care for the priority needs of each client.
  4. Combine activities, if possible, to resolve more than one problem at a time.
  5. Involve the client in his or her care as much as possible.

⚡ PRIORITY NURSING ACTIONS

Assessing a Group of Clients in Order of Priority

The nurse is assigned to the following clients. The order of priority for their assessment is as follows:

1. A client with heart failure who has a 4-pound weight gain since yesterday and is experiencing shortness of breath
2. A 24-hour postoperative client who had a wedge resection of the lung and has a closed chest tube drainage system
3. A client admitted to the hospital for observation who has absent bowel sounds
4. A client who is undergoing surgery for a hysterectomy on the following day

BOX 7.6 Guidelines for Prioritizing

- The nurse and the client mutually rank the client's needs in order of importance based on the client's preferences and expectations, safety, and physical and psychological needs. What the client sees as his or her priority needs may be different from what the nurse sees as the priority needs.
- Priorities are classified as high, intermediate, or low.
- Client needs that are life threatening or that could result in harm to the client if they are left untreated are high priorities.
- Nonemergency, non–life-threatening and nonurgent client needs are intermediate priorities.
- Client needs that are not related directly to the client's illness or prognosis are low priorities.
- When providing care, the nurse needs to decide which needs or problems require immediate action and which ones could be delayed until a later time because they are not urgent.
- The nurse considers client problems that involve actual or life-threatening concerns before potential health-threatening concerns.
- When prioritizing care, the nurse must consider time constraints and available resources.
- Problems identified as important by the client must be given high priority.
- The nurse can use the ABCs—airway, breathing, and circulation—as a guide when determining priorities; client needs related to maintaining a patent airway are always the priority.
- If the nurse determines that cardiopulmonary resuscitation is necessary, then the nurse uses CAB—compressions, airway, and breathing—as a guide to prioritize actions.
- The nurse can use Maslow's Hierarchy of Needs theory as a guide to determine priorities and identify the levels of physiological needs, safety, love and belonging, self-esteem, and self-actualization. (Basic needs are met before moving to other needs in the hierarchy.)
- The nurse can use the steps of the nursing process as a guide to determine priorities, remembering that data collection is the first step of the nursing process.
- Prioritization may be different in a disaster or emergency situation, where an action would be taken before gathering further information.

BOX 7.7 Types of Disasters

Human-Made Disasters
Accidents involving release of radioactive material
Dam failures resulting in flooding
Hazardous substance accidents such as pollution, chemical spills, or toxic gas leaks
Mass transportation accidents
Resource shortages such as food, water, and electricity
Structural collapse, fire, or explosions
Terrorist attacks such as bombing, riots, and bioterrorism

Natural Disasters
Avalanches
Blizzards
Communicable disease epidemics and pandemics
Cyclones
Droughts
Earthquakes
Floods
Forest fires
Hailstorms
Hurricanes
Landslides
Mudslides
Tidal waves (tsunami)
Tornadoes
Volcanic eruptions

⚠️ Use the ABCs—airway, breathing, and circulation—Maslow's Hierarchy of Needs theory, and the steps of the nursing process (assessment is first) to prioritize. If cardiopulmonary resuscitation (CPR) needs to be initiated, use CAB—compressions, airway, and breathing—as the priority guideline.

XVI. Disasters and Emergency Response Plan

A. Description

1. A disaster is any human-made or natural event that causes destruction and devastation that cannot be alleviated without assistance (Box 7.7).
2. Internal disasters are disasters that occur within a health care agency (e.g., health care agency fire, structural collapse, radiation spill), whereas external disasters are disasters that occur outside the health care agency.
3. A multicausality event can usually be managed by the hospital with the assistance of local resources; a mass casualty event requires multiple agencies and health care facilities, including state, regional, and national resources, to manage the event because the event is too overwhelming for local resources to manage.
4. An emergency response plan is a formal plan of action for coordinating the response of the health care agency staff in the event of a disaster in the health care agency or surrounding community.

B. American Red Cross (ARC)
1. The ARC has been given authority by the federal government to provide disaster relief.
2. All ARC disaster relief assistance is free and local offices are located across the United States.
3. The ARC participates with the government in developing and testing community disaster plans.
4. The ARC identifies and trains personnel for emergency response.
5. The ARC works with businesses and labor organizations to identify resources and individuals for disaster work.
6. The ARC educates the public about ways to prepare for a disaster.
7. The ARC operates shelters, provides assistance to meet immediate emergency needs, and provides disaster health services, including crisis counseling.
8. The ARC handles inquiries from family members.
9. The ARC coordinates relief activities with other agencies.
10. Nurses are involved directly with the ARC and assume functions such as managers, supervisors, and educators of first aid; they also participate in emergency response plans and disaster relief programs, and provide services, such as blood collection drives and immunization programs.

C. HAZMAT (Hazardous Materials) Team
1. HAZMAT teams are typically composed of emergency department health care providers and nursing staff because they will be the first individuals to encounter the potential exposure.
2. Members of HAZMAT teams have been educated on how to recognize patterns of illness that may be indicative of nuclear, biological, and chemical exposure; protocols for pharmacological treatment of infectious disease agents; availability of decontamination facilities and personal protective gear; safety measures; and the methods of responding to an exposure.

D. Phases of disaster management
1. The Federal Emergency Management Agency (FEMA) identifies four disaster management phases: mitigation, preparedness, response, and recovery.
2. Mitigation encompasses the following:
   a. Actions or measures that can prevent the occurrence of a disaster or reduce the damaging effects of a disaster
   b. Determination of community hazards and risks (actual and potential threats) before a disaster occurs
   c. Awareness of available community resources and health personnel to facilitate mobilization of activities and minimize chaos and confusion if a disaster occurs
   d. Determination of the resources available for care to infants, older adults, disabled individuals, and individuals with chronic health problems

3. Preparedness encompasses the following:
   a. Plans for rescue, evacuation, and caring for disaster victims
   b. Plans for training disaster personnel and gathering resources, equipment, and other materials needed for dealing with the disaster
   c. Identification of specific responsibilities for various emergency response personnel
   d. Establishment of a community emergency response plan and an effective public communication system
   e. Development of an emergency medical system and a plan for activation
   f. Verification of proper functioning of emergency equipment
   g. Collection of anticipatory provisions and creation of a location for providing food, water, clothing, shelter, other supplies, and needed medicine
   h. Inventory of supplies on a regular basis and replenishment of outdated supplies
   i. Practice of community emergency response plans (mock disaster drills)
4. Response encompasses the following:
   a. Putting disaster planning services into action and the actions taken to save lives and prevent further damage
   b. Primary concerns include safety of the victims and members of the disaster response team, physical health, and mental health of victims and members of the disaster response team
5. Recovery encompasses the following:
   a. Actions taken to return to a normal situation after the disaster
   b. Preventing debilitating effects and restoring personal, economic, and environmental health and stability to the community

E. Levels of disaster
1. Federal Emergency Management Agency (FEMA) identifies three levels of disaster with FEMA response (Box 7.8).

BOX 7.8   Federal Emergency Management Agency Levels of Disaster

Level III Disaster
A minor disaster that involves a minimal level of damage but could result in a presidential declaration of an emergency.

Level II Disaster
A moderate disaster that likely will result in a presidential declaration of an emergency, with moderate federal assistance.

Level I Disaster
A massive disaster that involves significant damage and results in a presidential disaster declaration, with major federal involvement and full engagement of federal, regional, and national resources.

2. When a federal emergency has been declared, the federal response plan may take effect and activate emergency support functions.

3. The emergency support functions of the ARC include performing emergency first aid, sheltering, feeding, providing a disaster welfare information system, and coordinating bulk distribution of emergency relief supplies.

4. Disaster medical assistant teams (teams of specially trained personnel) can be activated and sent to a disaster site to provide triage and medical care to victims until they can be transported to a hospital.

F. Nurse's role in disaster planning
   1. Personal and professional preparedness (Box 7.9)
      a. Make personal and family preparations.

BOX 7.9 **Emergency Plans and Supplies**

Plan a meeting place for family members.
Identify where to go if an evacuation is necessary.
Determine when and how to turn off water, gas, and electricity at main switches.
Locate the safe spots in the home for each type of disaster.
Replace stored water supply every 3 months and stored food supply every 6 months.
Include the following supplies:
- Backpack, clean clothing, sturdy footwear
- Pocket-knife or multitool
- A 3-day supply of water (1 gallon per person per day)
- A 3-day supply of nonperishable food
- Blankets/sleeping bags/pillows
- First-aid kit and over-the-counter medications and vitamins
- Adequate supply of prescription medication
- Battery-operated radio
- Flashlight and batteries
- Credit card, cash, or traveler's checks
- Personal ID card, list of emergency contacts, allergies, medication information, list of credit card numbers and bank accounts (all sealed in a water-tight package)
- Extra set of car keys and a full tank of gas in the car
- Sanitation supplies for washing, toileting, and disposing of trash; hand sanitizer
- Extra pair of eyeglasses/sunglasses
- Special items for infants, older adults, or disabled individuals
- Items needed for pets such as food, water, and leashes
- Paper, pens, pencils, maps
- Cell phone and charger
- Work gloves
- Rain gear
- Roll of duct tape and plastic sheeting
- Toiletries (basic daily needs, sunscreen, insect repellent, toilet paper)
- Household bleach for disinfection
- Whistle
- Matches in a waterproof container

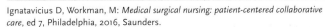
Ignatavicius D, Workman, M: *Medical surgical nursing: patient-centered collaborative care*, ed 7, Philadelphia, 2016, Saunders.

---

b. Be aware of the disaster plan at the place of employment and in the community.

c. Maintain certification in disaster training and in cardiopulmonary resuscitation.

d. Participate in mock disaster drills, including a bomb threat drill.

e. Prepare professional emergency response items, such as a copy of nursing license, personal health care equipment such as a stethoscope, cash, warm clothing, record-keeping materials, and other nursing care supplies.

2. Disaster response
   a. In the health care agency setting, if a disaster occurs, the agency disaster preparedness plan (emergency response plan) is activated immediately, and the nurse responds by following the directions identified in the plan.
   b. In the community setting, if the nurse is the first responder to a disaster, the nurse cares for the victims by attending to the victims with life-threatening problems first. When rescue workers arrive at the scene, immediate plans for triage would begin. (See Priority Nursing Actions.)

⚡ PRIORITY NURSING ACTIONS

Triaging Clients at the Site of an Accident

The nurse is the first responder at the scene of a school bus accident. The nurse triages the victims from highest to lowest priority as follows:
1. Confused child with bright red blood pulsating from a leg wound
2. Child with a closed head wound and multiple compound fractures of the arms and legs
3. Child with a simple fracture of the arm
4. Sobbing child with several minor lacerations on the face, arms, and legs

⚠ In the event of a disaster, activate the emergency response plan immediately.

G. Triage
   1. In a disaster or war, triage consists of brief assessment of victims that allows the nurse to classify victims according to the severity of the injury, urgency of treatment, and place for treatment.
   2. Simple Triage and Rapid Treatment (START) is a strategy used to evaluate the severity of injury of each victim as quickly as possible and tag the victims in about 30 to 60 seconds.
   3. In an emergency department, triage consists of brief assessment of clients, which allows the nurse to classify clients according to their need for care and establish priorities of care; the type of illness or injury, the severity of the problem, and the resources available govern the process.

BOX 7.10   Emergency Department Triage

Emergent (Red): Priority 1 (Highest)
This classification is assigned to clients who have life-threatening injuries and need immediate attention and continuous evaluation but have a high probability for survival when stabilized.

Such clients include trauma victims, clients with chest pain, clients with severe respiratory distress or cardiac arrest, clients with limb amputation, clients with acute neurological deficits, and clients who have sustained chemical splashes to the eyes.

Urgent (Yellow): Priority 2
This classification is assigned to clients who require treatment and whose injuries have complications that are not life-threatening, provided that they are treated within 30 minutes to 2 hours. These clients require continuous evaluation every 30–60 minutes thereafter.

Such clients include those with an open fracture with a distal pulse and large wounds.

Nonurgent (Green): Priority 3
This classification is assigned to clients with local injuries who do not have immediate complications and who can wait at least 2 hours for medical treatment. These clients require evaluation every 1–2 hours thereafter. Such clients include those with conditions such as a minor laceration, closed fracture, sprain, strains, or contusions.

Note: Some triage systems include tagging a client "black" if the victim is dead or soon will be deceased because of severe injuries; these are victims who would not benefit from any care because of the severity of their injuries.

H. Emergency department triage system
  1. A commonly used rating system in an emergency department is a three-tier system that uses the categories of emergent, urgent, and nonurgent; these categories may be identified by color codes or numbers (Box 7.10).
  2. The nurse needs to be familiar with the triage system of the health care agency.
  3. When caring for a client who has died, the nurse needs to recognize the importance of family and cultural and religious rituals and provide support to loved ones.
  4. Organ donation procedures of the health care agency need to be addressed if appropriate.

⚠ Think survivability. If you are the first responder to a scene of a disaster, such as a train crash, the priority victim is the one whose life can be saved.

I. Client assessment in the emergency department
  1. Primary assessment
    a. The purpose of primary assessment is to identify any client problem that poses an immediate or potential threat to life.
    b. The nurse gathers information primarily through objective data and, on finding any abnormalities, immediately initiates interventions.
    c. The nurse uses the ABCs—airway, breathing, and circulation—as a guide for assessing a client's needs and assesses a client who has sustained a traumatic injury for signs of a head injury or cervical spine injury; if CPR needs to be initiated, use CAB—compressions, airway, and breathing—as the priority guideline.
    d. Only central pulses, such as the carotid or femoral pulses would be used to assess circulation; they would be checked for at least 5 seconds but no longer than 10 seconds so as to not delay chest compressions.
  2. Secondary assessment
    a. The nurse performs secondary assessment after the primary assessment and after treatment for any primary problems identified.
    b. Secondary assessment identifies any other life-threatening problems that a client might be experiencing.
    c. The nurse obtains subjective and objective data, including a history, general overview, vital sign measurement, neurological assessment, pain assessment, and complete or focused physical assessment.

WHAT WOULD YOU DO?

Answer: Quality improvement, also known as performance improvement, focuses on processes or systems that significantly contribute to client safety and effective client care outcomes; criteria are used to monitor outcomes of care and to determine the need for change to improve the quality of care. If the nurse notes a particular problem, such as an increase in the number of intravenous (IV) site infections, the nurse would collaborate with the RN and assist to collect data about the problem. These data would include information, such as the primary and secondary diagnoses of the clients developing the infection, the type of IV catheters being used, the site of the catheter, IV site dressings being used, frequency of assessment and methods of care for the IV site, and length of time that the IV catheter has been inserted. Once these data are collected and analyzed by the RN, the nurse will assist to examine evidence-based practice protocols to identify the best practices for the care of IV sites to prevent infection. These practices can then be implemented and would be followed by an evaluation of the results of the protocols used.

PRACTICE QUESTIONS

1. The nurse is recording a nursing hands-off (end-of-shift) report for a client. Which information needs to be included?
   1. As-needed medications given that shift
   2. Normal vital signs that have been the same since admission

3. All of the tests and treatments the client has had since admission

4. Total number of scheduled medications that the client received on that shift

2. The nurse is planning the client assignments for the day. Which is the **most appropriate** assignment for the assistive personnel (AP)?
   1. A client who requires wound irrigation
   2. A client who requires frequent ambulation
   3. A client who is receiving continuous tube feedings
   4. A client who requires frequent vital signs after a cardiac catheterization

3. The nurse employed in a long-term care facility is planning the client assignments for the shift. Which client would the nurse assign to the assistive personnel (AP)?
   1. A client who requires a 24-hour urine collection
   2. A client who requires twice-daily dressing changes
   3. A client with diabetes mellitus who requires daily insulin and the reinforcement of dietary measures
   4. A client who has been placed on a bowel management program and requires rectal suppositories and a daily enema

4. The nurse is assigned to care for four clients. When planning client rounds, which client would the nurse check **first**?
   1. A client in skeletal traction
   2. A client who is dependent on a ventilator
   3. A postoperative client preparing for discharge
   4. A client admitted during the previous shift with a diagnosis of gastroenteritis

5. The nurse employed in an emergency department (ED) is assigned to assist with the triage of clients arriving at the ED. The nurse would assign **priority** to which client?
   1. A client complaining of muscle ache, headache, and malaise
   2. A client who twisted their ankle when they fell in-line skating
   3. A client with a minor laceration on the index finger sustained while cutting an eggplant
   4. A client with chest pain who states that they just ate pizza that was made with a very spicy sauce

❖ 6. The nurse is educating a new nurse about mass casualty events (disasters). Which statement by the new nurse indicates a **need for further teaching**? **Select all that apply.**
   ❏ 1. "An event is termed a mass casualty when it overwhelms local medical capabilities."
   ❏ 2. "Mass casualty events do not require an increase in the number of staff that are needed."
   ❏ 3. "A mass casualty event occurs only within the health care facility and could endanger staff."
   ❏ 4. "Mass casualty events may require the collaboration of many local agencies to handle the situation."
   ❏ 5. "A mass casualty event occurs if a fight between visitors occurs in the emergency department."

7. The nurse is attending an agency orientation meeting about the nursing model of practice implemented in the facility. The nurse is told that the nursing model is a team nursing approach. Which of the following describes the team-based model of nursing practice?
   1. A task approach method is used to provide care to clients.
   2. Managed care concepts and tools are used when providing client care.
   3. Nursing staff are led by the nurse when providing care to a group of clients.
   4. A single registered nurse is responsible for providing nursing care to a group of clients.

8. A client experiences cardiac arrest. The nurse leader quickly responds to the emergency and assigns clearly defined tasks to the work group. In this situation, the nurse is implementing which leadership style?
   1. Autocratic
   2. Situational
   3. Democratic
   4. Laissez-faire

9. The nurse has delegated several nursing tasks to staff members. Which is the nurse's **primary** responsibility after the delegation of tasks?
   1. Document that the task was completed.
   2. Assign the tasks that were not completed to the next nursing shift.
   3. Allow each staff member to make judgments when performing the tasks.
   4. Perform follow-up with each staff member regarding the performance and outcome of the task.

10. The nurse is assigned to care for four clients. When planning client rounds, which client would the nurse collect data from **first**?
   1. A client scheduled for a chest x-ray
   2. A client requiring daily dressing changes
   3. A postoperative client preparing for discharge
   4. A client receiving oxygen who is having difficulty breathing

ANSWERS

1. 1
Rationale: The nursing hands-off (end-of-shift) report needs to be an efficient and accurate account of the client's condition during the last shift. It needs to include pertinent information about the client, such as tests and treatments; as-needed medications given or therapies performed during the past 24 hours, including the client's response to them; changes in the client's condition; scheduled tests and treatments; current problems; and any other special concerns. It is not necessary to include the total number of medications given or a list of all the tests and treatments that the client has had since admission. Only significant vital signs need to be included.
Test-Taking Strategy: Focus on the subject of the question, the end-of-shift report. The purpose of this report is to communicate accurate and significant information about the client. Think about the word "significant." Eliminate option 2 because of the word *normal*. Eliminate option 3 because of the closed-ended word, *all*. Eliminate option 4 because of the words *total* and *scheduled medications*.

2. 2
Rationale: The nurse must determine the most appropriate assignment on the basis of the skills of the staff member and the needs of the client. In this case the best assignment for the AP would be to care for the client who requires frequent ambulation. The AP is skilled in this task. The client who had a cardiac catheterization will require specific monitoring in addition to that of the vital signs. Wound irrigations and tube feedings are not performed by unlicensed personnel.
Test-Taking Strategy: Note the strategic words, *most appropriate*, and focus on the subject, an assignment to the AP. Answer this question by recalling the principles of delegation and the supervision of work of others. Remember that work delegated to others must be done in a way that is consistent with the individual's level of expertise and that individual's licensure or lack of licensure.

3. 1
Rationale: The nurse must determine the appropriate assignment on the basis of the skills of the staff member and the needs of the client. The assignment of tasks needs to be implemented on the basis of the job description of the individual, the individual's level of clinical competence, and state law. Options 2, 3, and 4 involve care that requires the skill of a licensed nurse. An AP is not licensed.
Test-Taking Strategy: Focus on the subject of the question, safe delegation of tasks to an AP. Think about what an unlicensed person can perform for tasks. Eliminate options 2, 3, and 4, because these clients require care that needs to be provided by a licensed nurse.

4. 2
Rationale: The airway is always a priority, and the nurse first checks the client on a ventilator. The clients described in options 1, 3, and 4 have needs that would be identified as intermediate priorities.
Test-Taking Strategy: Note the strategic word, *first*. Use ABCs—airway, breathing, and circulation—to answer the question. Remember that the airway is always the first priority.

5. 4
Rationale: In an emergency department, triage involves classifying clients according to their need for care, and it includes establishing priorities of care, the type of illness, the severity of the problem, and the resources available to govern the process. Clients with trauma, chest pain, severe respiratory distress, cardiac arrest, limb amputation, or acute neurological deficits, and those who sustained a chemical splash to the eyes are classified as emergent, and these clients are the number 1 priority. Clients with conditions such as simple fractures, asthma without respiratory distress, fever, hypertension, abdominal pain, or renal stones have urgent needs, and these clients are classified as the number 2 priority. Clients with conditions such as minor lacerations, sprains, or cold symptoms are classified as nonurgent, and they are the number 3 priority.
Test-Taking Strategy: Note the strategic word, *priority*. Use the ABCs—airway, breathing, and circulation—to direct you to the correct option. A client who is experiencing chest pain is always classified as priority number 1 until a myocardial infarction has been ruled out.

❖ 6. 2, 3, 5
Rationale: Mass casualty events, also known as disasters, overwhelm local medical capabilities and may require the collaboration of multiple agencies and health care facilities to handle the crises. This type of event can occur in the health care facility or outside of it. Fights in the emergency department are not termed mass casualty events but are agency security and local enforcement issues. Mass casualty events almost always require an increase in staffing to ensure safe client care.
Test-Taking Strategy: Note the strategic words, *need for further teaching*. These words indicate a negative event query and the need to select the incorrect statements. Think about what a mass casualty event or disaster is to assist in answering. Eliminate options 1 and 4 because they are correct statements and therefore do not indicate a need for further teaching.

7. 3
Rationale: In team nursing, nursing personnel are led by the nurse when providing care to a group of clients. Option 1 identifies functional nursing. Option 2 identifies a component of case management. Option 4 identifies primary nursing.
Test-Taking Strategy: Note that the subject relates to team nursing. Think about the meaning of the word *team*. Option 3 is the only option that identifies the concept of a team approach.

8. 1
Rationale: Autocratic leadership is an approach in which the leader retains all authority and is primarily concerned with task accomplishment. It is an effective leadership style to implement in an emergency or crisis situation. The leader assigns clearly defined tasks and establishes one-way communication with the work group, and he or she makes all decisions independently. Situational leadership uses a combination of styles based on the current circumstances and events; this style is assumed according to the needs of the group and the tasks to be achieved. Democratic leadership is a people-centered approach that is primarily concerned with human relations and teamwork. This leadership style facilitates goal accomplishment and contributes to the growth and development of the

staff. Laissez-faire leadership is a permissive style in which the leader gives up control and delegates all decision making to the work group.

Test-Taking Strategy: Focus on the subject, identifying the type of leadership. Reviewing the nurse leader's actions described in the question and noting the words, *assigns clearly defined tasks* will assist you in choosing the correct option.

9. 4

Rationale: The ultimate responsibility for a task lies with the person who delegated it. Therefore, it is the nurse's primary responsibility to follow up with each staff member regarding the performance of the task and the outcomes related to implementing the task. Not all staff members have the education, knowledge, and ability to make judgments about tasks being performed. The nurse documents that the task has been completed, but this would not be done until follow-up was

implemented and outcomes were identified. It is not appropriate to assign the tasks that were not completed to the next nursing shift.

Test-Taking Strategy: Note the strategic word, *primary*. Recalling that the ultimate responsibility for a task lies with the person who delegated it will direct you to the correct option.

10. 4

Rationale: The airway is always a priority, and the nurse would attend to the client who has been experiencing an airway problem first. The clients described in options 1, 2, and 3 would have intermediate priority.

Test-Taking Strategy: Note the strategic word, *first*. Use the ABCs—airway, breathing, and circulation—to answer the question. Remember that the airway is always the first priority.

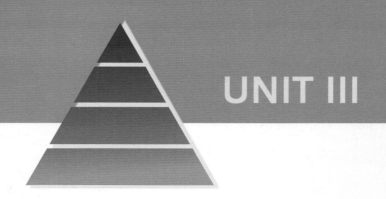

UNIT III

Nursing Sciences

Pyramid to Success

Pyramid Points focus on fluids and electrolytes, acid-base balance, laboratory reference intervals, nutrition, intravenous (IV) therapy, and blood administration. Fluids and electrolytes and acid–base balance constitute a content area that is sometimes complex and difficult to understand. For a client who is experiencing these imbalances, it is important to remember that maintenance of a patent airway is a priority and the nurse needs to monitor vital signs, physiological status, intake and output, laboratory reference intervals, and arterial blood gas values. It is also important to remember that normal laboratory reference levels may vary slightly, depending on the laboratory setting and equipment used in testing. If you are familiar with the normal reference intervals, you will be able to determine whether an abnormality exists when a laboratory value is presented in a question. The specific laboratory reference levels identified in the NCLEX® test plan that you need to know include arterial blood gases known as ABGs (pH, Po_2, Pco_2, Sao_2, HCO_3), blood urea nitrogen (BUN), cholesterol (total), glucose, hematocrit, hemoglobin, glycosylated hemoglobin (HgbA1C), platelets, potassium, sodium, white blood cell (WBC) count, creatinine, prothrombin time (PT), activated partial thromboplastin time (aPTT), and international normalized ratio (INR).

For some questions on the NCLEX-PN examination related to laboratory reference intervals, the normal reference ranges will be provided. Whereas, other questions will require you to identify whether the laboratory value is normal or abnormal, and then you will be required to think critically about the effects of the laboratory value in terms of the client. Note the health problem presented in the question and the associated body organ affected as a result of the health problem. This process will assist you in determining the correct answer.

Nutrition is a basic need that must be met for all clients. The NCLEX-PN examination addresses the dietary measures required for basic needs. When presented with a question related to nutrition, consider the client's health problem and the particular requirement or restriction necessary for treatment of the problem. With regard to IV therapy, checking the client for allergies, including latex sensitivity, and monitoring for complications are critical nursing responsibilities. Likewise, monitoring a client receiving blood components, the signs and symptoms of transfusion reaction, and the immediate interventions if a transfusion reaction occurs are a focus.

Client Needs: Learning Objectives

- **Safe and Effective Care Environment**
  Applying principles of infection control
  Collaborating with members of the health care team
  Ensuring that informed consent has been obtained for invasive procedures and for the administration of blood products and following agency procedures for blood administration
  Establishing priorities for care
  Handling hazardous and infectious materials to prevent injury to health care personnel and others
  Identifying the need for home health care referrals
  Maintaining asepsis and preventing infection in the client
  Maintaining standard, transmission-based, and other precautions to prevent transmission of infection to self and others
  Preventing accidents and ensuring safety of the client when a fluid or electrolyte imbalance exists, particularly when changes in cardiovascular, respiratory, gastrointestinal, neuromuscular, renal, or central nervous systems occur, or when the client is at risk for complications such as seizures, respiratory depression, or dysrhythmias

Providing safety for the client during implementation of treatments

Upholding client rights

- **Health Promotion and Maintenance**

Considering lifestyle choices related to home care needs

Determining the client's ability to perform self-care

Evaluating the client's home environment for self-care modifications

Identifying clients at risk for an acid-base imbalance

Identifying community resources available for follow-up

Identifying lifestyle choices related to receiving a blood transfusion

Implementing health screening and monitoring for the potential risk for a fluid or electrolyte imbalance

Performing physical data collection techniques

Providing information to the client about community classes for nutrition education

Reinforcing teaching points related to medication and diet management

Reinforcing teaching points about prevention, early detection, and treatment measures for health problems

Reinforcing teaching points about monitoring for signs and symptoms that indicate the need to notify the health care provider

- **Psychosocial Integrity**

Considering cultural and religious preferences related to nutritional patterns and lifestyle choices

Determining the client's emotional response to treatment

Discussing role changes and alterations in lifestyle related to the client's need to receive parenteral nutrition

Ensuring therapeutic interactions with the client regarding the procedure for blood administration

Identifying coping mechanisms

Identifying religious, spiritual, and cultural considerations related to blood administration

Providing emotional support to the client during testing

Providing reassurance to the client who is experiencing a fluid or electrolyte imbalance

Providing support and continuously informing the client of the purposes for prescribed interventions

- **Physiological Integrity**

Assisting and monitoring medications, IV fluids, and other therapeutic interventions

Assisting with obtaining an ABG specimen and analyzing the results

Checking for expected and unexpected responses to therapeutic interventions and reporting findings to the RN

Identifying clients who are at risk for a fluid or electrolyte imbalance

Managing medical emergencies as appropriate if a transfusion reaction or other complication occurs

Monitoring for changes in status and for complications; reporting changes and taking actions if a complication arises

Monitoring for clinical manifestations associated with an abnormal laboratory value

Monitoring for complications related to blood administration

Monitoring for expected effects of pharmacological and parenteral therapies

Monitoring laboratory reference intervals; determining the significance of an abnormal laboratory value and the need to report results

Monitoring of enteral feedings and the client's ability to tolerate feedings

Monitoring of nutritional intake and oral hydration

Client Needs lists modified from: National Council of State Boards of Nursing, Inc. (NCSBN). *NCLEX-PN Examination: Test Plan for the National Council Licensure Examination for Practical Nurses,* effective April 2020. Chicago: NCSBN.

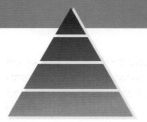

CHAPTER 8

Fluids and Electrolytes

PRIORITY CONCEPTS Cellular Regulation; Fluids and Electrolytes

WHAT WOULD YOU DO?

The licensed practical nurse (LPN) is observing the client's cardiac rhythm on the monitor screen and notes that there is an additional prominent wave following each T wave and suspects the presence of U waves. What actions would the LPN take?
Answer is located on p. 88.

I. Concepts of Fluid and Electrolyte Balance

A. Electrolytes
 1. An electrolyte is a substance that, once dissolved in solution, ionizes; that is, some of its molecules split or dissociate into electrically charged atoms or ions.
 2. Measurement
  a. The metric system is used to measure volumes of fluids: liters (L) or milliliters (mL).
  b. The unit of measure that expresses the combining activity of an electrolyte is the milliequivalent (mEq).
  c. Milliequivalents provide information about the number of anions or cations available to combine with other anions or cations.

B. Body fluid compartments (Fig. 8.1)
 1. Fluid in each of the body compartments contains electrolytes.
 2. Each compartment has a particular composition of electrolytes that differs from that of other compartments.
 3. To function normally, body cells must have fluids and electrolytes in the right compartments and in the right amounts.
 4. Whenever an electrolyte moves out of a cell, another electrolyte moves in to take its place.
 5. The numbers of cations and anions must be the same for **homeostasis** to exist.
 6. Compartments are separated by semipermeable membranes.

 7. Intravascular compartment: refers to fluid inside a **blood** vessel.
 8. Intracellular compartment: refers to all fluid inside of cells; most body fluids are inside the cells.
 9. Extracellular compartment
  a. Refers to all fluid outside of the cells
  b. Includes interstitial fluids, which is the fluid between cells (sometimes called *third space*), blood, lymph, bone, connective tissue, water, and transcellular fluid

C. Third-spacing
 1. The accumulation and sequestration of trapped extracellular fluid in an actual or potential body space as a result of disease or injury
 2. The trapped fluid represents a volume loss and is unavailable for normal physiological processes.
 3. Fluid may be trapped in body spaces such as the pericardial, pleural, peritoneal, or joint cavities; the bowel; the abdomen; or within soft tissues after trauma or burns.
 4. Gathering data about intravascular fluid loss is difficult. It may not be reflected in weight change or intake and output (I&O) records, and it may not become apparent until after organ malfunction occurs.

D. Edema
 1. An excess accumulation of fluid in the interstitial space; it occurs as a result of alterations in oncotic pressure, hydrostatic pressure, capillary permeability, and lymphatic obstruction.
 2. Localized edema occurs as a result of traumatic injury from accidents or surgery, local inflammatory processes, or burns.
 3. Generalized edema, also called *anasarca*, is an excessive accumulation of fluid in the interstitial space throughout the body as a result of a condition such as cardiac, renal, or liver failure.

E. Body fluid
 1. Description
  a. Body fluids transport **nutrients** to the cells and carry waste products from the cells.

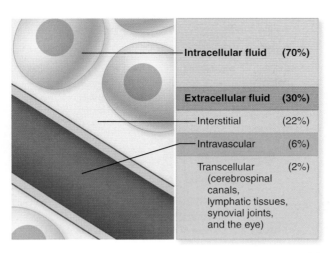

Intracellular fluid	**(70%)**
Extracellular fluid	**(30%)**
Interstitial	(22%)
Intravascular	(6%)
Transcellular (cerebrospinal canals, lymphatic tissues, synovial joints, and the eye)	(2%)

FIGURE. 8.1 Distribution of fluid by compartments in the average adult.

   b. Total body fluid (intracellular and extracellular) amounts to about 60% of body weight in the adult, 55% in the older adult, and 80% in the infant.

   c. Thus, infants and older adults are at higher risk for fluid-related problems than younger adults; children have a greater proportion of body water than adults; and the older adult has the least proportion of body water.

 2. Constituents of body fluids

   a. Body fluids consist of water and dissolved substances.

   b. The largest single fluid constituent of the body is water.

⚠ Infants and older adults need to be monitored closely for fluid imbalance.

F. Body fluid transport

 1. Diffusion

   a. Diffusion is the process whereby a solute (substance that is dissolved) may spread through a solution or solvent (solution in which the solute is dissolved).

   b. Diffusion of a solute spreads the molecules from an area of higher concentration to an area of lower concentration.

   c. Diffusion occurs within fluid compartments and from one compartment to another if the barrier between the compartments is permeable to the diffusing substances.

 2. Osmosis

   a. Osmosis is the movement of solvent molecules across a membrane in response to a concentration gradient, usually from a solution of lower to one of higher solute concentration.

   b. If a membrane is permeable to water but not to all solutes present, the membrane is a selective or semipermeable membrane.

   c. When a more concentrated solution is on one side of a selectively permeable membrane and a less concentrated solution is on the other side, a pull called *osmotic pressure* draws the water through the membrane to the more concentrated side, or the side with more solute.

 3. Filtration

   a. Filtration is the movement of solutes and solvents by hydrostatic pressure.

   b. The movement is from an area of higher pressure to an area of lower pressure.

 4. Hydrostatic pressure

   a. The force exerted by the weight of a solution

   b. When a difference exists in the hydrostatic pressure on two sides of a membrane, water and diffusible solutes move out of the solution that has the higher hydrostatic pressure by the process of filtration.

 5. Osmolality

   a. Refers to the number of osmotically active particles per kilogram of water; it is the concentration of a solution.

   b. In the body, osmotic pressure is measured in milliosmols (mOsm).

   c. The normal osmolality of **plasma** is 275 mOsm/kg to 295 mOsm/kg water.

G. Movement of body fluid

 1. Description

   a. Cell membranes and capillary walls separate body compartments.

   b. Cell membranes are selectively permeable; that is, the cell membrane and the capillary wall allow water and some solutes free passage through them.

   c. Several forces affect the movement of water and solutes through the walls of cells and capillaries; for example, the greater the number of particles within the cell, the more pressure that exists to force water through the cell membrane and out of the cell.

   d. If the body loses more electrolytes than fluids, as can happen with diarrhea, then the extracellular fluid will contain fewer electrolytes or less solute than the intracellular fluid.

   e. Fluids and electrolytes must be kept in balance for health; when they remain out of balance, death can occur.

 2. Isotonic solutions (Table 8.1)

   a. When the solutions on both sides of a selectively permeable membrane have established equilibrium or are equal in concentration, they are isotonic.

   b. Isotonic solutions are isotonic to human cells, and thus very little osmosis occurs; isotonic solutions have the same osmolality as body fluids.

Nursing Sciences

TABLE 8.1   Tonicity of Intravenous Fluids

Solution	Tonicity
0.45% saline (½ normal saline [NS])	Hypotonic
0.9% saline (NS)	Isotonic
5% dextrose in water (D₅W)	Isotonic
5% dextrose in 0.225% saline (D₅/¼ NS)	Isotonic
Lactated Ringer's solution	Isotonic
5% dextrose in lactated Ringer's solution	Hypertonic
5% dextrose in 0.45% saline (D₅/½ NS)	Hypertonic
5% dextrose in 0.9% saline (D₅/NS)	Hypertonic
10% dextrose in water (D₁₀W)	Hypertonic

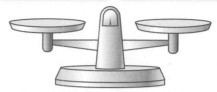

Fluid intake		Fluid output	
Ingested water	1200–1500 mL	Kidneys	1500 mL
Ingested food	800–1100 mL	Insensible loss through skin	600–800 mL
Metabolic oxidation	300 mL	Insensible loss through lungs	400–600 mL
		Gastrointestinal tract	100 mL
TOTAL	**2300–2900 mL**	**TOTAL**	**2600–3000 mL**

FIGURE 8.2 Sources of fluid intake and fluid output.

   3. Hypotonic solutions (see Table 8.1)
      a. When a solution contains a lower concentration of salt or solute than another more concentrated solution, it is considered hypotonic.
      b. A hypotonic solution has less salt or more water than an isotonic solution. These solutions have lower osmolality than body fluids.
      c. Hypotonic solutions are hypotonic to the cells; therefore, osmosis would continue in an attempt to bring about balance or equality.
   4. Hypertonic solutions: A solution that has a higher concentration of solutes than another less concentrated solution is hypertonic. These solutions have a higher osmolality than body fluids (see Table 8.1).
H. Body fluid intake and output (Fig. 8.2)
   1. Body fluid intake
      a. Water enters the body through three sources—orally ingested liquids, water in foods, and water formed by the oxidation of foods.
      b. About 10 mL of water is released by the metabolism of each 100 calories of fat, carbohydrates, or proteins.
   2. Body fluid output
      a. Water lost through the skin is called *insensible loss* (the individual is unaware of losing that water).
      b. The amount of water lost by perspiration varies according to the temperature of the environment and of the body, but the average amount of loss by perspiration alone is 100 mL/day.
      c. Water lost from the lungs is called *insensible loss* and is lost through expired air that is saturated with water vapor.
      d. The amount of water lost from the lungs varies with the rate and the depth of respiration.
      e. Large quantities of water are secreted into the gastrointestinal (GI) tract, but almost all this fluid is reabsorbed.
      f. A large volume of electrolyte-containing liquids moves into the GI tract and then returns again into the extracellular fluid.

      g. Severe diarrhea results in the loss of large quantities of fluids and electrolytes.
      h. The kidneys play a major role in regulating fluid and electrolyte balance and excrete the largest quantity of fluid.
      i. Normal kidneys can adjust the amount of water and electrolytes leaving the body.
      j. The quantity of fluid excreted by the kidneys is determined by the amount of water ingested and the amount of waste and solutes excreted.
      k. As long as all organs are functioning normally, the body is able to maintain balance in its fluid content.

   ⚠ The client with diarrhea is at high risk for a fluid and electrolyte imbalance.

II. Maintaining fluid and electrolyte balance
A. Description
   1. Homeostasis is a term that indicates the relative stability of the internal environment.
   2. Concentration and composition of body fluids must be nearly constant.
   3. When one of the substances in a client is deficient—either fluid or electrolytes—the substance must be replaced normally by the intake of food and water or by therapy, such as intravenous (IV) solutions and medications.
   4. When the client has an excess of fluid or electrolytes, therapy is directed toward assisting the body with eliminating the excess.
B. The kidneys play a major role in controlling the balance of fluid and electrolytes.
C. The adrenal glands, through the secretion of aldosterone, also aid with controlling the extracellular fluid volume by regulating the amount of sodium reabsorbed by the kidneys.
D. Antidiuretic hormone from the pituitary gland regulates the osmotic pressure of extracellular fluid by regulating the amount of water reabsorbed by the kidney.

III. Fluid Volume Deficit

A. Description
   1. Dehydration occurs when the body's fluid intake is not sufficient to meet the body's fluid needs.
   2. The goal of treatment is to restore fluid volume, replace electrolytes as needed, and eliminate the cause of the fluid volume deficit.

 B. Causes
   1. Vomiting and/or diarrhea
   2. Continuous GI irrigation
   3. GI suctioning
   4. Ileostomy or colostomy drainage
   5. Draining wounds, burns, or fistulas
   6. Increased urine output from the use of diuretics

C. Data collection
   1. Thirst
   2. Poor skin turgor and dry mucous membranes
   3. Increased heart rate, thready pulse, dyspnea, and postural hypotension
   4. Weight loss
   5. Flat neck or hand veins
   6. Dizziness or weakness
   7. Decrease in urine volume and dark, concentrated urine
   8. Increased specific gravity of the urine
   9. Confusion
   10. Increased hematocrit level

D. Interventions
   1. The cause of the fluid volume deficit is treated (e.g., antidiarrheal, antiemetic, antipyretic, and antimicrobial medications may be prescribed), and fluids are replaced through administration of IV solutions as prescribed and oral rehydration.
   2. Monitor vital signs and respiratory and neurological status closely.
   3. Administer oxygen as prescribed.
   4. Check mucous membranes and skin turgor.
   5. Monitor weight daily.
   6. Monitor I&O.
   7. Test urine for specific gravity.
   8. Monitor hematocrit and electrolyte levels; prepare to correct electrolyte imbalance if needed.

IV. Fluid Volume Excess

A. Description
   1. Fluid intake or retention exceeds the body's fluid needs.
   2. Also called *overhydration, fluid overload,* or circulatory overload
   3. The goals of treatment are to restore fluid balance; correct electrolyte imbalance, if present; and eliminate or control the underlying cause of the overload (impaired cardiac or renal function can lead to fluid volume excess).

B. Causes
   1. Overhydration with IV fluids
   2. Kidney damage
   3. Heart failure
   4. Long-term use of corticosteroids
   5. Excessive sodium ingestion

6. Syndrome of inappropriate antidiuretic hormone secretion
   7. Irrigation of wounds or body cavities with hypotonic fluids

C. Data collection
   1. Cough and dyspnea
   2. Lung crackles
   3. Increased respirations and heart rate
   4. Increased blood pressure and bounding pulse
   5. Pitting edema
   6. Weight gain
   7. Neck and hand vein distention
   8. Increased urine output if kidneys can compensate; decreased if kidney damage is the cause
   9. Confusion
   10. Decreased hematocrit level

D. Interventions
   1. Monitor vital signs and respiratory and neurological status closely.
   2. Position the client in semi-Fowler's position.
   3. Administer oxygen as prescribed.
   4. Check for edema.
   5. Monitor I&O.
   6. Monitor daily weight.
   7. Administer diuretics as prescribed.
   8. Monitor hematocrit and electrolyte levels.
   9. Restrict fluids as prescribed.
   10. Provide a low-sodium diet as prescribed.

 A client with kidney damage or failure is at high risk for fluid volume excess.

V. Hypokalemia

A. Description (Box 8.1)
   1. Hypokalemia is a serum potassium level lower than 3.5 mEq/L.
   2. Potassium deficit is potentially life-threatening because every body system is affected.

B. Causes and signs/symptoms (Table 8.2)

C. Interventions
   1. Assist to monitor cardiovascular, respiratory, neuromuscular, GI, and renal status; client is placed on a cardiac monitor; anticipate a prescription for an electrocardiogram (ECG).
   2. Monitor vital signs closely.
   3. Monitor I&O.
   4. Monitor electrolyte values.
   5. Check for adequate renal function before administering prescribed potassium; monitor I&O during administration.
   6. Administer potassium supplements as prescribed (orally or monitor by IV).
   7. Oral potassium supplements
      a. Oral potassium supplements may cause nausea and vomiting, and they would not be taken on an empty stomach; if the client complains of abdominal pain, distention, nausea, vomiting, diarrhea, or GI bleeding, the supplement may need to be discontinued.

BOX 8.1 **Potassium**

Normal Value
3.5 mEq/L–5.0 mEq/L

Common Food Sources
Avocados, bananas, cantaloupe, oranges, strawberries
Tomatoes
Carrots, mushrooms, spinach
Fish, pork, beef, veal
Potatoes
Raisins

TABLE 8.2 **Potassium Imbalances**

Hypokalemia	Hyperkalemia
Causes	
Use of potassium-losing diuretics	Kidney failure
Diarrhea	Intestinal obstruction
Vomiting	Cell damage
Inadequate intake of potassium	Excessive oral or parenteral
Excessive gastric suction	administration of potas-
Excessive fistula drainage	sium; potassium-retaining
Cushing's syndrome (increased	(sparing) diuretics
secretion of aldosterone)	Addison's disease
Chronic use of corticosteroids or	Excessive use of
laxatives	potassium-based salt
Kidney disease	substitutes
Parenteral nutrition	Transfusion of stored blood
Uncontrolled diabetes	(the breakdown of older red
Alkalosis	blood cells releases potas-
	sium) Acidosis
Signs and Symptoms	
Leg and abdominal cramps	Muscle weakness
Lethargy and weakness	Paresthesia
Shallow respirations and thready pulse	Hypotension
Confusion	Diarrhea
Decreased or absent reflexes	Hyperactive bowel sounds
Hypoactive bowel sounds and ileus	Flat P waves; widened QRS
Orthostatic hypotension	complex; prolonged PR
Shallow, flat or inverted T waves;	interval; and tall, peaked T
depressed ST segment and	waves
prominent U waves	

    b. Liquid potassium chloride has an unpleasant taste and would be taken with juice or another liquid.

  8. IV administered potassium

    a. The client receiving potassium by the IV route needs to be placed on a cardiac monitor and monitored closely, and the nurse needs to follow the registered nurse's (RN's) instructions regarding care.

    b. Monitor the IV site closely; if phlebitis or infiltration occurs, the IV must be stopped immediately, and the RN must be notified; the IV will be restarted at another site.

  9. Institute safety measures for the client experiencing muscle weakness.

  10. If the client is taking a potassium-excreting diuretic, it may be discontinued; a potassium-retaining (sparing) diuretic may be prescribed.

  11. Instruct the client about foods that are high in potassium content (see Box 8.1).

  12. Reinforce instructions to the client not to use salt substitutes containing potassium unless prescribed by the primary health care provider (PHCP).

⚠ Potassium is never administered by IV push, intramuscular, or subcutaneous routes. IV potassium is always diluted and administered using an infusion device.

VI. Hyperkalemia

A. Description

  1. Hyperkalemia is a serum potassium level that exceeds 5.0 mEq/L (see Box 8.1).

  2. Pseudohyperkalemia: a condition that can occur as a result of methods of blood specimen collection and cell lysis; if an increased serum value is obtained in the absence of clinical symptoms, the specimen needs to be redrawn and evaluated.

B. Causes and signs/symptoms (see Table 8.2)

C. Interventions

  1. Monitor cardiovascular, respiratory, neuromuscular, renal, and GI status; the client is placed on a cardiac monitor.

  2. If IV potassium is being administered, it is stopped immediately (however, the IV catheter is not removed and is kept patent); in addition, oral potassium supplements are withheld.

  3. Assist to initiate a potassium-restricted diet.

  4. Prepare to administer potassium-excreting diuretics as prescribed if renal function is not impaired.

  5. If renal function is impaired, prepare to administer sodium polystyrene sulfonate as prescribed, a cation-exchange resin that promotes GI sodium absorption and potassium excretion.

  6. Prepare the client for dialysis if potassium levels are critically high.

  7. IV calcium may be prescribed if the hyperkalemia is severe to avert myocardial excitability.

  8. IV hypertonic glucose followed by regular insulin may be prescribed to move excess potassium into the cells.

  9. When blood transfusions are prescribed for a client with a potassium imbalance, the client would receive fresh blood, if possible; transfusions of stored blood may elevate the potassium level because the breakdown of older blood cells releases potassium.

  10. Reinforce instructions to avoid foods high in potassium (see Box 8.1).

  11. Reinforce instructions to avoid the use of salt substitutes or other potassium-containing substances.

⚠ Monitor the serum potassium level closely when a client is receiving a potassium-sparing diuretic!

BOX 8.2   Sodium

Normal Value
135 mEq/L–145 mEq/L

Common Food Sources
  Bacon, hot dogs, lunch meats
  Butter, cheese
  Canned foods
  Ketchup, mustard
  Milk
  Processed foods
  Snack foods
  Soy sauce
  Table salt

TABLE 8.3   Sodium Imbalances

Hyponatremia	Hypernatremia
Causes	
Inadequate sodium intake (nothing by mouth)	Decreased water intake
	Fever
Gastrointestinal suction	Excessive perspiration
Excessive intake of water	Dehydration
Irrigation of gastrointestinal tubes with plain water	Hyperventilation
	Watery diarrhea
Diuretics	Enteral nutrition and parenteral nutrition deplete the cells of water
Increased perspiration	
Draining skin lesion(s)	
Burn(s)	Diabetes insipidus
Nausea and vomiting	Cushing's syndrome
Diabetic ketoacidosis	Impaired kidney function
Syndrome of inappropriate antidiuretic hormone secretion	Use of corticosteroids
	Excessive administration of sodium bicarbonate
Retention of fluid, such as with kidney or heart failure	
Signs and Symptoms	
Rapid, thready pulse	Dry mucous membranes
Postural blood pressure change	Loss of skin turgor
Weakness	Thirst
Abdominal cramping	Flushed skin
Poor skin turgor	Elevated temperature
Muscle twitching and seizure	Oliguria
Apprehension	Muscle twitching
Confusion	Fatigue
	Confusion
	Seizure

 VII. Hyponatremia

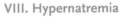 Hyponatremia precipitates lithium toxicity in a client taking lithium.

A. Description
  1. Hyponatremia is a serum **sodium** level less than 135 mEq/L (Box 8.2).
  2. Sodium imbalances are usually associated with fluid imbalances.
B. Causes and signs/symptoms (Table 8.3)
C. Interventions
  1. Monitor cardiovascular, respiratory, neuromuscular, cerebral, renal, and GI status.

2. If hyponatremia is accompanied by a fluid volume deficit (hypovolemia), IV sodium chloride infusions may be prescribed to restore sodium content and fluid volume.
3. If hyponatremia is accompanied by fluid volume excess (hypervolemia), osmotic diuretics may be prescribed to promote the excretion of water rather than sodium.
4. If hyponatremia is caused by inappropriate or excessive secretion of antidiuretic hormone, medications that antagonize antidiuretic hormone may be prescribed.
5. Reinforce instructions about the need to increase oral sodium intake and inform the client about what foods to include in his/her diet (see Box 8.2).
6. If the client is taking lithium, monitor the lithium level because hyponatremia can cause diminished lithium excretion, resulting in toxicity.

VIII. Hypernatremia

A. Description: Hypernatremia is a serum sodium level that exceeds 145 mEq/L (see Box 8.2).
B. Causes and signs/symptoms (see Table 8.3)
C. Interventions
  1. Monitor cardiovascular, respiratory, neuromuscular, cerebral, renal, and integumentary status.
  2. If the cause is fluid loss, IV fluids may be prescribed.
  3. If the cause is inadequate renal excretion of sodium, diuretics that promote sodium loss may be prescribed.
  4. Restrict sodium and fluid intake as prescribed (see Box 8.2).

IX. Hypocalcemia

A. Description: Hypocalcemia is a serum **calcium** level less than 9.0 mg/dL (Box 8.3).
B. Causes and signs/symptoms (Table 8.4 and Fig. 8.3)
C. Interventions
  1. Monitor cardiovascular, respiratory, neuromuscular, and GI status; the client is placed on a cardiac monitor.
  2. Assist to administer calcium supplements orally; calcium may be prescribed IV.
  3. Assist to monitor the client receiving IV calcium; monitor for electrocardiographic changes, observe for infiltration, and monitor for hypercalcemia.
  4. Medications that increase calcium absorption may be prescribed.
    a. Aluminum hydroxide reduces phosphorus levels, causing the counter effect of increasing calcium levels.
    b. Vitamin D aids in the absorption of calcium from the intestinal tract.
  5. Provide a quiet environment to reduce environmental stimuli.
  6. Initiate seizure precautions.

BOX 8.3 Calcium

Normal Value
9 mg/dL–10.5 mg/dL

Common Food Sources
Cheese
Collard greens
Kale
Milk and soy milk
Rhubarb
Sardines
Tofu
Yogurt

TABLE 8.4 Calcium Imbalances

Hypocalcemia	Hypercalcemia
Causes	
Inadequate dietary intake of calcium	Excessive intake of calcium supplements, milk, and antacid products that contain calcium
Inhibited absorption of calcium from the intestinal tract	Excessive intake of vitamin D
Inadequate vitamin D consumption	Increased bone resorption or destruction from conditions such as bone tumors, fractures, osteoporosis, and immobility
Diarrhea	
Excessive gastrointestinal losses from diarrhea or wound draining	Decreased excretion of calcium
End-stage kidney disease	Kidney disease
Calcium-excreting medications such as diuretics, caffeine, anticonvulsants, heparin, laxatives, and nicotine	Use of thiazide diuretics
	Hyperparathyroidism
	Use of lithium
Decreased secretion of parathyroid hormone	Adrenal insufficiency
Acute pancreatitis	
Crohn's disease	
Excessive administration of blood	
Signs and Symptoms	
Tachycardia	Increased heart rate and blood pressure
Hypotension	
Paresthesia	Bounding pulse
Twitching	Bradycardia (late stage)
Cramps	Muscle weakness (hypotonicity)
Tetany	Diminished deep tendon reflexes
Positive Chvostek's or Trousseau's sign	Nausea and vomiting
	Constipation
Diarrhea	Abdominal distention
Hyperactive bowel sounds	Confusion, lethargy, and coma
Prolonged QT interval; prolonged ST segment	Shortened QT interval and widened T wave

7. Calcium gluconate 10% needs to be readily available for treatment of acute calcium deficit.
8. Reinforce instructions regarding consuming foods high in calcium (see Box 8.3).

X. Hypercalcemia

A. Description: Hypercalcemia is a serum calcium level that exceeds 10.5 mg/dL (see Box 8.3).

B. Causes and signs/symptoms (see Table 8.4)
C. Interventions
1. Monitor cardiovascular, respiratory, neuromuscular, renal, and GI status; the client is placed on a cardiac monitor.
2. IV infusions of solutions containing calcium and oral medications containing calcium or vitamin D will be discontinued.
3. Thiazide diuretics may be discontinued and replaced with diuretics that enhance the excretion of calcium.
4. Assist to administer medications as prescribed that inhibit calcium resorption from the bone, such as phosphorus, calcitonin, bisphosphonates, and prostaglandin synthesis inhibitors (aspirin, nonsteroidal anti-inflammatory drugs).
5. Assist to prepare the client with severe hypercalcemia for dialysis if medications fail to reduce the serum calcium level.
6. Monitor for flank or abdominal pain and strain the urine to check for the presence of urinary stones.
7. Reinforce instructions about what foods to avoid that are high in calcium (see Box 8.3).

 A client with a calcium imbalance is at risk for a pathological fracture. Move the client carefully and slowly; assist the client with ambulation.

XI. Hypomagnesemia

A. Description: Hypomagnesemia is a serum magnesium level less than 1.8 mEq/L (Box 8.4).
B. Causes and signs/symptoms (Table 8.5)
C. Interventions
1. Monitor cardiovascular, respiratory, GI, neuromuscular, and central nervous system status; the client is placed on a cardiac monitor.
2. Because hypocalcemia frequently accompanies hypomagnesemia, interventions also aim to restore normal serum calcium levels.
3. Oral preparations of magnesium may cause diarrhea and increase magnesium loss.
4. Magnesium sulfate by the IV route may be prescribed in severe cases (intramuscular injections cause pain and tissue damage); assist to monitor the client closely during administration; seizure precautions are initiated, serum magnesium levels are monitored frequently, and the client is monitored for diminished deep tendon reflexes that suggest hypermagnesemia.
5. Reinforce instructions to the client to eat food that is high in magnesium (see Box 8.4).

XII. Hypermagnesemia

A. Description: Hypermagnesemia is a serum magnesium level that exceeds 2.6 mEq/L (Box 8.5).
B. Causes and signs/symptoms (see Table 8.5)
C. Interventions

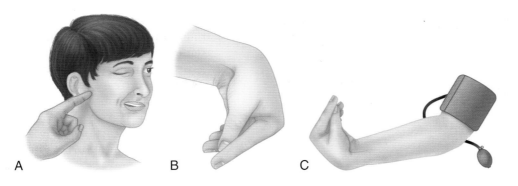

FIGURE 8.3 Tests for hypocalcemia. (A) Chvostek's sign is a contraction of facial muscles in response to a light tap over the facial nerve in front of the ear. (B) Trousseau's sign is a carpal spasm induced by inflating a blood pressure cuff (C) above the systolic pressure for a few minutes.

BOX 8.4   Magnesium

Normal Value
1.8 mEq/L–2.6 mEq/L

Common Food Sources
Avocados
Canned white tuna fish
Cauliflower
Oatmeal
Green leafy vegetables, such as spinach and broccoli
Milk
Wheat bran
Peanut butter, almonds
Peas
Pork, beef, chicken, soybeans
Potatoes
Raisins
Yogurt

TABLE 8.5   Magnesium Imbalances

Hypomagnesemia	Hypermagnesemia
Causes	
Malnutrition	Overuse of antacids or
Diarrhea	laxatives that contain
Celiac disease	magnesium
Crohn's disease	Renal insufficiency and
Alcoholism	kidney failure
Prolonged gastric suctioning	Treatment of preeclampsia with magnesium
Ileostomy, colostomy, or intestinal fistula(s)	
Acute pancreatitis	
Diabetic ketoacidosis	
Eclampsia	
Chemotherapy	
Sepsis	
Signs and Symptoms	
Twitching	Hypotension
Paresthesia	Bradycardia
Hyperactive reflexes	Weak pulse
Irritability	Sweating and flushing
Confusion	Respiratory depression
Positive Chvostek's or Trousseau's sign	Loss of deep tendon reflexes
Shallow respiration	Prolonged PR interval and widened QRS complexes
Tetany	
Seizure	
Tachycardia	
Tall T waves and depressed ST segment	

1. Monitor cardiovascular, respiratory, neuromuscular, and central nervous system status; the client is placed on a cardiac monitor.
2. Diuretics are prescribed to increase renal excretion of magnesium.
3. IV administered calcium chloride or calcium gluconate may be prescribed to reverse the effects of magnesium on cardiac muscle.
4. Reinforce instructions to restrict dietary intake of magnesium-containing foods (see Box 8.4).
5. Reinforce instructions to the client to avoid the use of laxatives and antacids that contain magnesium.

 Calcium gluconate is the antidote for magnesium overdose!

XIII. Hypophosphatemia

A. Description
1. Hypophosphatemia is a serum phosphorus level lower than 3.0 mg/dL (Box 8.5).
2. A decrease in the serum phosphorus level is accompanied by an increase in the serum calcium level.

B. Causes and signs/symptoms (Table 8.6)

C. Interventions
1. Monitor cardiovascular, respiratory, neuromuscular, central nervous system, and hematological status.
2. Medications that contribute to hypophosphatemia will be discontinued.
3. Prepare to administer phosphorus orally along with a vitamin D supplement.
4. IV phosphorus may be prescribed when serum phosphorus levels fall below 1 mg/dL and when the client experiences critical clinical manifestations; assist with monitoring the client closely if IV phosphorus is prescribed.
5. Check for adequate renal function before administering phosphorus.
6. Move the client carefully, and monitor for signs of a pathological fracture.
7. Reinforce instructions to increase the intake of phosphorus-containing foods while decreasing the intake of calcium-containing foods (see Boxes 8.3 and 8.5).

Nursing Sciences

BOX 8.5 Phosphorus

Normal Value
3.0 mg/dL–4.5 mg/dL

Common Food Sources
Dairy products
Fish
Organ meats
Nuts
Pork, beef, chicken
Whole-grain breads and cereal

TABLE 8.6 Phosphorus Imbalances

Hypophosphatemia	Hyperphosphatemia
Causes	
Decreased nutritional intake of phosphorus and malnutrition	Excessive dietary intake of phosphorus
Use of magnesium-based or aluminum hydroxide-based antacids	Overuse of phosphate-containing laxatives or enemas
Kidney failure	Vitamin D intoxication
Hyperparathyroidism	Hypoparathyroidism
Malignancy	Renal insufficiency
Hypercalcemia	Chemotherapy
Alcohol withdrawal	
Diabetic ketoacidosis	
Respiratory alkalosis	
Signs and Symptoms	
Confusion	Neuromuscular irritability
Seizure	Muscle weakness
Weakness	Hyperactive reflexes
Decreased deep tendon reflexes	Tetany
Shallow respiration	Positive Chvostek's or Trousseau's sign
Increased bleeding tendency	
Immunosuppression	
Bone pain	

 A decrease in the serum phosphorus level is accompanied by an increase in the serum calcium level, and an increase in the serum phosphorus level is accompanied by a decrease in the serum calcium level. This is called reciprocal relationship.

XIV. Hyperphosphatemia

A. Description
1. Hyperphosphatemia is a serum phosphorus level that exceeds 4.5 mg/dL (see Box 8.5).
2. Most body systems tolerate elevated serum phosphorus levels well.
3. An increase in the serum phosphorus level is accompanied by a decrease in the serum calcium level.
4. The problems that occur in hyperphosphatemia center on the hypocalcemia that results when serum phosphorus levels increase.

B. Causes and signs/symptoms (see Table 8.6)

C. Interventions
1. Interventions entail the management of hypocalcemia.
2. Assist to administer phosphate-binding medications that increase fecal excretion of phosphorus by binding phosphorus from food in the GI tract.
3. Reinforce instructions to avoid phosphate-containing medications, including laxatives and enemas.
4. Reinforce instructions to decrease the intake of food that is high in phosphorus (see Box 8.5).
5. Reinforce instructions in medication administration: take phosphate-binding medications, emphasizing that they must be taken with meals or immediately after meals.

WHAT WOULD YOU DO?

Answer: Cardiac changes in hypokalemia include impaired repolarization, resulting in the emergence of prominent U waves. Therefore, hypokalemia is suspected. The incidence of potentially lethal ventricular dysrhythmias is increased in hypokalemia. The nurse must immediately notify the RN and check the client's vital signs, cardiac status, and signs of hypokalemia. The nurse needs to stay with the client while the RN checks the client's most recent serum potassium level, contacts the PHCP to report the findings, and obtains prescriptions to treat the hypokalemic state.

PRACTICE QUESTIONS

1. The nurse who is caring for a client with renal failure notes that the client is dyspneic and crackles are heard when listening to breath sounds in the lungs. Which additional sign/symptom would the nurse expect to note in this client?
   1. Rapid weight loss
   2. Flat hand and neck veins
   3. A weak and thready pulse
   4. An increase in blood pressure
2. The nurse is reviewing the health records of assigned clients. The nurse would plan care knowing that which client is at risk for a potassium deficit?
   1. The client with Addison's disease
   2. The client with metabolic acidosis
   3. The client with intestinal obstruction
   4. The client receiving nasogastric suction
3. The nurse reviews a client's electrolyte results and notes a potassium level of 5.5 mEq/L. The nurse understands that a potassium value at this level would be noted with which condition?
   1. Diarrhea
   2. Traumatic burn
   3. Cushing's syndrome
   4. Overuse of laxatives

4. The nurse reviews a client's electrolyte results and notes that the potassium level is 5.4 mEq/L. What would the nurse look for on the cardiac monitor as a result of this laboratory value?
   1. ST elevation
   2. Peaked P waves
   3. Prominent U waves
   4. Narrow, peaked T waves

5. The nurse is reading the primary health care provider's (PHCP's) progress notes in the client's record and sees that the PHCP has documented "insensible fluid loss of approximately 800 mL daily." Which client is at risk for this loss?
   1. The client with a draining wound
   2. The client with a urinary catheter
   3. The client with a fast respiratory rate
   4. The client with a nasogastric tube to low suction

6. The nurse is reviewing the health records of assigned clients. The nurse would plan care knowing that which client is at the **least likely** risk for the development of third-spacing?
   1. The client with sepsis
   2. The client with cirrhosis
   3. The client with kidney failure
   4. The client with diabetes mellitus

7. The nurse is reviewing the health records of assigned clients. The nurse would plan care knowing that which client is at risk for fluid volume deficit?
   1. The client with cirrhosis
   2. The client with ileostomy
   3. The client with heart failure
   4. The client with decreased renal function

8. The nurse is caring for a client who has been taking diuretics on a long-term basis. Which finding would the nurse expect to note as a result of this long-term use?
   1. Gurgling respirations
   2. Increased blood pressure
   3. Decreased hematocrit level
   4. Increased specific gravity of the urine

9. The nurse reviews electrolyte values and notes a sodium level of 130 mEq/L. The nurse expects that this sodium level would be noted in a client with which condition?
   1. The client with watery diarrhea
   2. The client with diabetes insipidus
   3. The client with an inadequate daily water intake
   4. The client with the syndrome of inappropriate secretion of antidiuretic hormone

10. The nurse is caring for a client with leukemia and notes that the client has poor skin turgor and flat neck and hand veins. The nurse suspects hyponatremia. Which sign/symptom would the nurse expect to note in this client if hyponatremia is present?
    1. Intense thirst
    2. Slow bounding pulse
    3. Dry mucous membranes
    4. Postural blood pressure changes

11. The nurse is caring for a client with a diagnosis of hyperparathyroidism. Laboratory studies are performed and the serum calcium level is 12.0 mg/dL. Based on this laboratory value, the nurse would take which action?
    1. Document the value in the client's record.
    2. Inform the registered nurse of the laboratory value.
    3. Place the laboratory result form in the client's record.
    4. Reassure the client that the laboratory result is normal.

12. The nurse reviews the client's serum calcium level and notes that the level is 8.0 mg/dL. The nurse understands that which condition would cause this serum calcium level?
    1. Prolonged bed rest
    2. Adrenal insufficiency
    3. Hyperparathyroidism
    4. Excessive ingestion of vitamin D

13. The nurse is caring for a client with a suspected diagnosis of hypercalcemia. Which sign/symptom would be an indication of this electrolyte imbalance?
    1. Twitching
    2. Positive Trousseau's sign
    3. Hyperactive bowel sounds
    4. Generalized muscle weakness

14. The nurse is instructing a client on how to decrease the intake of calcium in the diet. The nurse would tell the client that which food item is **least likely** to contain calcium?
    1. Milk
    2. Butter
    3. Spinach
    4. Collard greens

15. The nurse is caring for a client with hyperparathyroidism and notes that the client's serum calcium level is 13 mg/dL. Which prescribed medication would the nurse plan to assist in administering to the client?
    1. Calcitonin
    2. Calcium chloride
    3. Calcium gluconate
    4. Large doses of vitamin D

Nursing Sciences

ANSWERS

1. 4

Rationale: Impaired cardiac or renal function can result in fluid volume excess. Findings associated with fluid volume excess include cough, dyspnea, crackles, tachypnea, tachycardia, an elevated blood pressure, a bounding pulse, an elevated central venous pressure, weight gain, edema, neck and hand vein distention, an altered level of consciousness, and a decreased hematocrit level.

Test-Taking Strategy: Note that rapid weight loss; flat hand and neck veins; and weak, thready pulse are comparable or alike in that they all relate to a decrease in fluid volume. The correct option is the only option that reflects an increase in fluid volume.

2. 4

Rationale: Potassium-rich gastrointestinal (GI) fluids are lost through GI suction, which places the client at risk for hypokalemia. The client with intestinal obstruction, Addison's disease, and metabolic acidosis is at risk for hyperkalemia.

Test-Taking Strategy: Focus on the subject, potassium deficit (hypokalemia). Read the question carefully and note that it asks for the client who is at risk for hypokalemia. Read each option and think about the electrolyte loss that can occur with each condition. Nasogastric suction not only results in a loss of body fluid, but also of electrolytes.

3. 2

Rationale: A serum potassium level that exceeds 5.0 mEq/L is indicative of hyperkalemia. Clients who experience the cellular shifting of potassium, as in the early stages of massive cell destruction (i.e., with trauma, burns, sepsis, or metabolic or respiratory acidosis), are at risk for hyperkalemia. The client with Cushing's syndrome or diarrhea and the client who has been overusing laxatives are at risk for hypokalemia.

Test-Taking Strategy: Eliminate diarrhea and overuse of laxatives first, because they are comparable or alike and reflect a gastrointestinal loss. From the remaining options, recalling that cell destruction, occurring with traumatic burns, causes potassium shifts will direct you to the correct option. Remember that Cushing's syndrome presents a risk for hypokalemia.

4. 4

Rationale: A serum potassium level of 5.4 mEq/L is indicative of hyperkalemia. Cardiac changes include a wide, flat P wave; a prolonged PR interval; a widened QRS complex; and narrow, peaked T waves.

Test-Taking Strategy: Focus on the subject, potassium level of 5.4 mEq/L. Determine next that this condition is a hyperkalemic one. From this point, it is necessary to know the cardiac changes that are expected when hyperkalemia exists.

5. 3

Rationale: Sensible losses are those that the person is aware of, such as those that occur through wound drainage, gastrointestinal (GI) tract losses, and urination. Insensible losses may occur without the person's awareness. Insensible losses occur daily through the skin and the lungs.

Test-Taking Strategy: Focus on the subject, insensible fluid loss. Note that wound drainage, urinary output, and gastric secretions are comparable or alike in that they represent vis-

ible losses. These types of losses can be measured for accurate output. Fluid loss through a fast respiratory rate cannot be accurately measured, only approximated.

6. 4

Rationale: Fluid that shifts into the interstitial space and remains there is referred to as *third-space fluid*. Common sites for third-spacing include the abdomen, pleural cavity, peritoneal cavity, and pericardial sac. Third-space fluid is physiologically useless because it does not circulate to provide nutrients for the cells. Risk factors include liver or kidney disease, major trauma, burns, sepsis, wound healing, major surgery, malignancy, malabsorption syndrome, malnutrition, alcoholism, and older age.

Test-Taking Strategy: Note the subject, the client least likely to develop third-spacing. Eliminate cirrhosis and kidney failure first, because it is likely that fluid balance disturbances will occur with these conditions. From the remaining options, sepsis is the option that is the most acute and therefore the most similar to cirrhosis and kidney failure.

7. 2

Rationale: Causes of a fluid volume deficit include vomiting, diarrhea, conditions that cause increased respirations or increased urinary output, insufficient IV fluid replacement, draining fistulas, ileostomy, and ileostomy. A client with cirrhosis, heart failure (HF), or decreased kidney function is at risk for fluid volume excess.

Test-Taking Strategy: Focus on the subject, fluid volume deficit. Read the question carefully and note that it asks for the client who is at risk for a deficit. Read each option and think about the fluid imbalance that can occur in each client. Clients with cirrhosis, HF, and decreased kidney function all retain fluid. The only condition that can cause a fluid volume deficit is the condition noted in the correct option.

8. 4

Rationale: Clients taking diuretics on a long-term basis are at risk for fluid volume deficit. Findings of fluid volume deficit include increased respiration and heart rate, decreased central venous pressure, weight loss, poor skin turgor, dry mucous membranes, decreased urine volume, increased specific gravity of the urine, dark-colored and odorous urine, an increased hematocrit level, and an altered level of consciousness. Gurgling respirations, increased blood pressure, and decreased hematocrit as a result of hemodilution are seen in a client with fluid volume excess.

Test-Taking Strategy: Focus on the subject, long-term use of diuretics, and realize that this can lead to a fluid volume deficit. Eliminate gurgling respiration and increased blood pressure first because they would be noted in clients with fluid volume excess. Next, remember that the specific gravity of urine is increased in a client with a fluid volume deficit.

9. 4

Rationale: Hyponatremia is a serum sodium level less than 135 mEq/L. Hyponatremia can occur secondary to syndrome of inappropriate secretion of antidiuretic hormone (SIADH). The client with an inadequate daily water intake, watery diarrhea, or diabetes insipidus is at risk for hypernatremia.

Test-Taking Strategy: Focus on the subject, sodium level of

130 mEq/L, and determine that this represents hyponatremia. Knowledge regarding the normal sodium level and the causes of hyponatremia is required to answer the question. Remember that hyponatremia can occur secondary to SIADH.

10. 4
Rationale: Postural blood pressure changes occur in the client with hyponatremia. Intense thirst and dry mucous membranes are seen in clients with hypernatremia. A slow, bounding pulse is not indicative of hyponatremia. In a client with hyponatremia, a rapid, thready pulse is noted.
Test-Taking Strategy: Focus on the subject, hyponatremia, and note the information in the question. Eliminate intense thirst and dry mucous membranes first because they are comparable or alike (a client with dry mucous membranes is likely to have intense thirst). From the remaining options, it is necessary to recall the signs of hyponatremia.

11. 2
Rationale: The normal serum calcium level ranges from 9 to 10.5 mg/dL. The client is experiencing hypercalcemia and the nurse would inform the registered nurse of the laboratory value. Because the client is experiencing hypercalcemia, the remaining options are incorrect actions.
Test-Taking Strategy: Focus on the laboratory value in the question to determine that the client is experiencing hypercalcemia. Note that options 1 and 3 are comparable or alike and indicate that no action would be taken to report the abnormal value. From the remaining options, eliminate option 4 because the value is elevated.

12. 1
Rationale: The normal serum calcium level is 9 to 10.5 mg/dL. A client with a serum calcium level of 8.0 mg/dL is experiencing hypocalcemia. The excessive ingestion of vitamin D, adrenal insufficiency, and hyperparathyroidism are causative factors associated with hypercalcemia. Although immobilization can initially cause hypercalcemia, the long-term effect of prolonged bed rest is hypocalcemia.
Test-Taking Strategy: Focus on the subject, serum calcium level of 8.0 mg/dL. Knowledge regarding the normal serum calcium level will assist you with determining that the client is experiencing hypocalcemia. This will help you to eliminate

excessive ingestion of vitamin D. Recalling the causative factors associated with hypocalcemia is necessary to select the correct option from those remaining. Remember that the long-term effect of prolonged bed rest is hypocalcemia.

13. 4
Rationale: Generalized muscle weakness is seen in clients with hypercalcemia. Twitching, positive Trousseau's sign, and hyperactive bowel sounds are signs of hypocalcemia.
Test-Taking Strategy: Recall the signs/symptoms of hypocalcemia and hypercalcemia. Note that twitching, positive Trousseau's sign, and hyperactive bowel sounds are comparable or alike, because they all reflect a hyperactivity of body systems. The option that is different is muscle weakness.

14. 2
Rationale: Butter comes from milk fat and does not contain significant amounts of calcium. Milk, spinach, and collard greens are calcium-containing foods and must be avoided by the client on a calcium-restricted diet.
Test-Taking Strategy: Note the subject, the item that is lowest in calcium. Milk can be easily eliminated first. Eliminate spinach and collard greens next because they are comparable or alike.

15. 1
Rationale: The normal serum calcium level is 9 to 10.5 mg/dL. This client is experiencing hypercalcemia. Calcium gluconate and calcium chloride are medications used for the treatment of tetany, which occurs as a result of acute hypocalcemia. In hypercalcemia, large doses of vitamin D need to be avoided. Calcitonin, a thyroid hormone, decreases the plasma calcium level by inhibiting bone resorption and lowering the serum calcium concentration.
Test-Taking Strategy: Focus on the subject, serum calcium level of 13 mg/dL. Recalling the normal serum calcium level will assist you with determining that the client is experiencing hypercalcemia. With this knowledge, you can easily eliminate calcium chloride and calcium gluconate, because you would not administer medication that adds calcium to the body. Remembering that excessive vitamin D is a causative factor of hypercalcemia will assist you with eliminating that option.

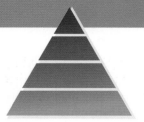
CHAPTER 9

Acid–Base Balance

PRIORITY CONCEPTS Acid–Base Balance; Oxygenation

WHAT WOULD YOU DO?

The nurse assists to perform an Allen's test on a client scheduled for an arterial blood gas (ABG) draw from the radial artery. During release of pressure from the ulnar artery, color in the hand returns after 20 seconds. The nurse would take which actions?
Answer is located on p. 97.

I. Hydrogen Ions, Acids, and Bases

A. Hydrogen (H^+) ions
1. Vital to life, because H^+ ions determine the pH of the body, which must be maintained in a narrow range
2. Expressed as pH; the pH scale is determined by the number of H^+ ions and goes from 1 to 14; 7 is considered neutral.
3. The number of H^+ ions in the body fluid determines whether it is acid (acidosis), alkaline (alkalosis), or neutral.

B. Acids
1. Produced as end products of metabolism
2. Contain H^+ ions
3. Are H^+ ion donors; they give up H^+ ions to neutralize or decrease the strength of an acid or to form a weaker base.

C. Bases
1. Contain no H^+ ions
2. Are H^+ ion acceptors; they accept H^+ ions from acids to neutralize or decrease the strength of a base or to form a weaker acid.
3. Normal serum levels of bicarbonate (HCO_3^-) are 21 to 28 mEq/L (21–28 mmol/L)

II. Regulatory Systems for Hydrogen Concentration in the Blood

A. Buffers
1. The fastest-acting regulatory system
2. Provide immediate protection against changes in H^+ ion concentration in the extracellular fluid (i.e., absorb or release H^+ ions as needed)

3. Serve as a transport mechanism that carries excess H^+ ions to the lungs
4. Once the primary buffer systems react, they are consumed, leaving the body less able to withstand further stress until the buffers are replaced.

B. Primary buffer systems in extracellular fluid
1. Hemoglobin system
   a. Red blood cells contain hemoglobin.
   b. System maintains the acid–base balance by a process called *chloride shift*.
   c. Chloride shifts in and out of the red blood cells in response to the levels of oxygen (O_2) in the blood.
   d. For each chloride ion that leaves a red blood cell, a bicarbonate ion enters.
   e. For each chloride ion that enters a red blood cell, a bicarbonate ion leaves.
2. Plasma proteins system
   a. Functions along with the liver to vary the amount of H^+ ions in the chemical structure of plasma proteins
   b. Plasma proteins have the ability to attract or release H^+ ions as the body needs them.
3. Carbonic acid–bicarbonate (HCO_3^-) system
   a. Primary buffer system in the body
   b. Maintains a pH of 7.4, with a ratio of 20 parts HCO_3^- to 1-part carbonic acid (H_2CO_3) (Fig. 9.1)
   c. This ratio (20:1) determines the concentration of H^+ ions in body fluid.
   d. The carbonic acid concentration is controlled by the excretion of carbon dioxide (CO_2) by the lungs. The rate and depth of respiration changes in response to CO_2 levels.
   e. The kidneys control the bicarbonate (HCO_3^-) concentration and selectively retain or excrete HCO_3^- in response to bodily needs.
4. Phosphate buffer system
   a. Present in cells and body fluids and is especially active in the kidneys
   b. Acts like HCO_3^- and neutralizes excess hydrogen (H^+) ions

C. Lungs

1. The body's second defense; interact with the buffer system to maintain the acid–base balance
2. During acidosis, the pH decreases and the respiratory rate and depth increase in an attempt to exhale acids. The carbonic acid created by the neutralizing action of HCO_3^- can be carried to the lungs, where it is reduced to CO_2 and water and is exhaled. Thus H⁺ ions are inactivated and exhaled.
3. During alkalosis, the pH increases, and the respiratory rate and depth decrease. CO_2 is retained, and carbonic acid increases to neutralize and decrease the strength of excess HCO_3.
4. The action of the lungs is reversible for controlling an excess or deficit.
5. The lungs can hold H⁺ ions until the deficit is corrected or can inactivate H⁺ ions, changing the ions to water molecules to be exhaled along with CO_2, thus correcting the excess.

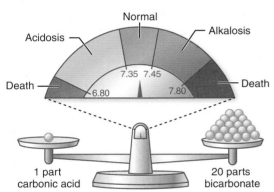

FIGURE. 9.1 Acid–base balance. In the healthy state, a ratio of 1 part carbonic acid to 20 parts bicarbonate provides a normal serum pH between 7.35 and 7.45. Any deviation to the left of 7.35 results in an acidotic state. Any deviation to the right of 7.45 results in an alkalotic state.

6. The lungs can inactivate only H⁺ ions carried by carbonic acid. Excess H⁺ ions created by other problems must be excreted by the kidneys.

⚠ Monitor the client's respiratory status closely. During acidosis, the respiratory rate and depth increase in an attempt to exhale acids. During alkalosis, the respiratory rate and depth decrease. CO_2 is retained to neutralize and decrease the strength of excess bicarbonate.

D. Kidneys

1. The kidneys provide a more inclusive corrective response to acid–base disturbances than other corrective mechanisms, even though the renal excretion of acids and alkalis occurs more slowly.
2. Compensation requires a few hours to several days; however, it is a more thorough and selective process than that of other regulators, such as the buffer systems and the lungs.
3. During acidosis, the pH decreases, and excess H⁺ ions are secreted into the tubules and combine with buffers for excretion in the urine.
4. During alkalosis, the pH increases, and excess HCO_3^- ions move into the tubules, combine with sodium, and are excreted in the urine.
5. Selective regulation of HCO_3^- in the kidneys
   a. The kidneys restore HCO_3^- by excreting H+ ions and retaining HCO_3^- ions.
   b. Excess H⁺ ions are excreted in the urine in the form of phosphoric acid.
   c. The alteration of certain amino acids in the renal tubules results in the diffusion of ammonia into the kidneys. The ammonia combines with excess H⁺ ions and is excreted into the urine.

E. Potassium (Fig. 9.2)

1. Plays an exchange role in maintaining the acid–base balance

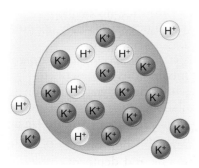

Under normal conditions, the intracellular potassium content is much greater than that of the extracellular fluid. The concentration of hydrogen ions is low in both compartments.

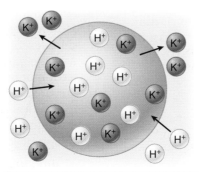

In acidosis, the extracellular hydrogen ion content increases, and the hydrogen ions move into the intracellular fluid. To keep the intracellular fluid electrically neutral, an equal number of potassium ions leave the cell, creating a relative hyperkalemia.

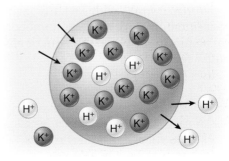

In alkalosis, more hydrogen ions are present in the intracellular fluid than in the extracellular fluid. Hydrogen ions move from the intracellular fluid into the extracellular fluid. To keep the intracellular fluid electrically neutral, potassium ions move from the extracellular fluid into the intracellular fluid, creating a relative hypokalemia.

FIGURE. 9.2 Movement of potassium in response to changes in the extracellular fluid hydrogen ion concentration.

BOX 9.1   Causes of Respiratory Acidosis

- Asthma
- Atelectasis
- Brain trauma
- Bronchiectasis
- Bronchitis
- Central nervous system depressants
- Emphysema
- Hypoventilation
- Pneumonia
- Pulmonary edema
- Pulmonary emboli

2. The body changes the potassium (K) level by drawing H⁺ ions into the cell or by pushing them out of the cells (potassium movement across cell membranes is facilitated by transcellular shifting in response to acid–base patterns).
3. During acidosis, the body protects itself from the acidic state by moving H⁺ ions into the cell. Therefore, K moves out to make room for H⁺ ions; the serum potassium level increases.
4. During alkalosis, the cells release H⁺ ions into the blood in an attempt to increase the acidity of the blood; this forces the serum potassium into the cell, and the serum potassium level decreases.

⚠️ When the client experiences an acid–base imbalance, monitor the potassium level closely because the potassium moves in or out of the cells in an attempt to maintain acid–base balance. The resulting hypokalemia or hyperkalemia predisposes the client to associated complications.

III. Respiratory Acidosis

A. Description: The total concentration of buffer base is lower than normal, with a relative increase in H⁺ ion concentration; thus, a greater number of H⁺ ions are circulating in the blood than can be absorbed by the buffer system.

B. Causes (Box 9.1)

⚠️ If the client has a condition that causes an obstruction of the airway or depresses the respiratory system, monitor the client for respiratory acidosis.

C. Data collection: In an attempt to compensate, the respiratory rate and depth increase (Table 9.1).

D. Interventions
1. Monitor for signs of respiratory distress.
2. Administer oxygen as prescribed.
3. Place the client in a semi-Fowler's position.
4. Encourage and assist the client to turn, cough, and deep-breathe.
5. Encourage hydration to thin secretions.

TABLE 9.1   Clinical Manifestations of Acidosis

Respiratory (↑ Pco_2)	Metabolic (↓ HCO_3^-)
Neurological	
Drowsiness	Drowsiness
Disorientation	Confusion
Dizziness	Headache
Headache	Coma
Coma	
Cardiovascular	
Decreased blood pressure	Decreased blood pressure
Dysrhythmia (related to hyperkalemia from compensation)	Dysrhythmia (related to hyperkalemia from compensation)
Warm, flushed skin (related to peripheral vasodilation)	Warm, flushed skin (related to peripheral vasodilation)
Gastrointestinal	
No significant findings	Nausea, vomiting, diarrhea, abdominal pain
Neuromuscular	
Seizure	No significant findings
Respiratory	
Hypoventilation with hypoxia (lungs are unable to compensate when there is a respiratory problem)	Deep, rapid respiration (compensatory action by the lungs)

From Lewis S, Dirksen S, Heitkemper M, Bucher L, Camera I: *Medical-surgical nursing: assessment and management of clinical problems*, ed 9, St. Louis, 2014, Mosby.

6. Reduce restlessness by improving ventilation rather than by administering tranquilizers, sedatives, or opioids because these medications further depress respirations.
7. Prepare to assist to administer respiratory treatments as prescribed.
8. Suction the client's airway, if necessary.
9. Monitor electrolyte values, particularly the potassium level.
10. Assist to administer antibiotics for respiratory infection or other medications as prescribed.
11. Prepare to assist with endotracheal intubation and mechanical ventilation (these measures may be instituted if CO_2 levels rise above 50 mm Hg and if signs of acute respiratory distress are present).

IV. Respiratory Alkalosis

A. Description: A deficit of carbonic acid and a decrease in H⁺ ion concentration that results from the accumulation of base or the loss of acid without a comparable loss of base in the body fluids

B. Causes (Box 9.2)

⚠️ If the client has a condition that causes overstimulation of the respiratory system, monitor the client for respiratory alkalosis.

BOX 9.2 Causes of Respiratory Alkalosis

- Fever
- Hyperventilation
- Hypoxia
- Hysteria
- Overventilation by mechanical ventilators
- Pain

BOX 9.3 Causes of Metabolic Acidosis

- Diabetes mellitus or diabetic ketoacidosis
- Excessive ingestion of acetylsalicylic acid (aspirin)
- High-fat diet
- Insufficient metabolism of carbohydrates
- Malnutrition
- Renal insufficiency or failure
- Severe diarrhea

TABLE 9.2   Clinical Manifestations of Alkalosis

Respiratory ($\downarrow$ Pco$_2$)	Metabolic ($\uparrow$ HCO$_3^-$)
Neurological	
Lethargy	Drowsiness
Lightheadedness	Dizziness
Confusion	Nervousness
	Confusion
Cardiovascular	
Tachycardia	Tachycardia
Dysrhythmia (related to hypokalemia from compensation)	Dysrhythmia (related to hypokalemia from compensation)
Gastrointestinal	
Nausea	Anorexia
Vomiting	Nausea
Epigastric pain	Vomiting
Neuromuscular	
Tetany	Tremors
Numbness	Hypertonic muscles
Tingling of extremities	Muscle cramps
Hyperreflexia	Tetany
Seizure	Tingling of extremities
	Seizure
Respiratory	
Hyperventilation (lungs are unable to compensate when there is a respiratory problem)	Hypoventilation (compensatory action by the lungs)

From Lewis S, Dirksen S, Heitkemper M, Bucher L, Camera I: *Medical-surgical nursing: assessment and management of clinical problems*, ed 9, St. Louis, 2014, Mosby.

 C. Data collection: In an attempt to compensate, the kidneys retain bicarbonate and excrete excess hydrogen ions into the urine (Table 9.2).

D. Interventions

1. Monitor for signs of respiratory distress.
2. Provide emotional support and reassurance to the client.
3. Assist with breathing techniques and breathing aids as prescribed.
   a. Voluntary holding of the breath if appropriate
   b. Use of a rebreathing mask as prescribed
   c. Carbon dioxide breaths as prescribed (rebreathing into a paper bag)

4. Monitor ventilator clients to be sure that they are not forced to take breaths too deeply or rapidly.
5. Monitor electrolyte values, particularly potassium and calcium levels.
6. Calcium gluconate may be prescribed for tetany; assist with administration.

V. Metabolic Acidosis

A. Description: A total concentration of buffer base that is lower than normal, with a relative increase in the H$^+$ ion concentration resulting from loss of too much base and/or retention of too much acid

B. Causes (Box 9.3)

⚠ An insufficient supply of insulin in a client with diabetes mellitus can result in metabolic acidosis, known as diabetic ketoacidosis.

C. Data collection: To compensate for the acidosis, hyperpnea with Kussmaul's respiration occurs as the lungs attempt to exhale the excess CO$_2$ (see Table 9.1).

D. Interventions

1. Monitor for signs of respiratory distress.
2. Check level of consciousness for central nervous system depression.
3. Monitor intake and output and assist with fluid and electrolyte replacement as prescribed.
4. Initiate safety and seizure precautions.
5. Monitor the potassium level closely; as metabolic acidosis resolves, potassium moves back into the cells, and the potassium level decreases.

⚠ Monitor the client experiencing severe diarrhea for manifestations of metabolic acidosis.

E. Interventions for diabetes mellitus and diabetic ketoacidosis

1. Give insulin as prescribed to hasten the movement of serum glucose into the cell, thereby decreasing the concurrent ketosis.
2. When glucose is being properly metabolized, the body stops converting fats to glucose.
3. Monitor for circulatory collapse caused by polyuria, which may result from the hyperglycemic state; osmotic diuresis may lead to extracellular volume deficit and may require fluid and electrolyte replacement.

Nursing Sciences

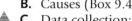

BOX 9.4   Causes of Metabolic Alkalosis

- Diuretics
- Excessive vomiting or gastrointestinal suctioning
- Hyperaldosteronism
- Ingestion and/or infusion of excess sodium bicarbonate
- Massive transfusion of whole blood

F. Interventions in kidney disease

1. Dialysis may be used to remove protein and waste products, thereby decreasing the acidotic state.
2. A diet low in protein and high in calories decreases the amount of protein waste products, which in turn lessens the acidosis.

VI. Metabolic Alkalosis

A. Description: A deficit of carbonic acid and a decrease in hydrogen ion concentration that results from the accumulation of base or from a loss of acid without a comparable loss of base in the body fluids

B. Causes (Box 9.4)

 C. Data collection: To compensate, respiratory rate and depth decrease to conserve CO_2 (see Table 9.2).

> ⚠ Monitor the client experiencing excessive vomiting or the client with gastrointestinal suctioning for manifestations of metabolic alkalosis.

D. Interventions

1. Monitor for signs of respiratory distress.
2. Monitor potassium and calcium levels.
3. Institute safety precautions.
4. Medications and intravenous fluids to promote the kidney excretion of bicarbonate may be prescribed.
5. Prepare to assist with potassium replacement as prescribed.
6. The underlying cause of the alkalosis needs to be treated.

VII. Arterial Blood Gases (Table 9.3)

A. Assisting with the collection of an arterial blood gas specimen

1. Obtain vital signs.
2. Allen's test is performed to determine the presence of collateral circulation (see **Priority Nursing Actions**).
3. Identify factors that may affect the accuracy of the results, such as changes in the O_2 settings on respiratory assistive devices, suctioning within the past 20 minutes, and client activities.
4. Provide emotional support to the client.
5. Assist with the specimen draw; a heparinized syringe is used (this syringe may be prepackaged in the specimen kit).

⚡ PRIORITY NURSING ACTIONS

Allen's Test Done Before Radial Artery Puncture

1. The procedure is explained to the client.
2. Pressure is applied over the ulnar and radial arteries simultaneously.
3. The client is asked to open and close the hand repeatedly.
4. Pressure is released from the ulnar artery while compressing the radial artery.
5. The color of the extremity distal to the pressure point is checked.
6. The findings are documented.

TABLE 9.3   Normal Arterial Blood Gas Values

Laboratory Test	Normal Range Conventional Units
pH	7.35–7.45
Paco₂	35–45 mm Hg
Bicarbonate (HCO₃)	21–28 mEq/L
Pao₂	80–100 mm Hg

Paco₂, Partial pressure of carbon dioxide in arterial blood; *Pao₂*, Partial pressure of oxygen in arterial blood. Note: Because ABG values are influenced by altitude, the value for Pao₂ decreases as the altitude increases.

6. Apply pressure immediately to the puncture site following the blood draw; maintain pressure for 5 minutes or for 10 minutes if the client is taking anticoagulants.
7. Record the client's temperature and the type of supplemental O_2 that the client is receiving on the laboratory form.
8. Appropriately label the specimen and transport it on ice to the laboratory.

B. Respiratory acid–base imbalances (Table 9.4)

1. Remember that the respiratory function indicator is the $Paco_2$.
2. During a respiratory imbalance, you will find an opposite relationship between the pH and the $Paco_2$. In other words, the pH will be elevated when the $Paco_2$ is decreased (alkalosis), or the pH will be decreased in the presence of an elevated $Paco_2$ (acidosis).
3. Look at the pH and the $Paco_2$ to determine whether the condition is a respiratory problem.
4. Respiratory acidosis: The pH is decreased; the $Paco_2$ is elevated.
5. Respiratory alkalosis: The pH is elevated; the $Paco_2$ is decreased.

C. Metabolic acid–base imbalances (see Table 9.4)

1. Remember that the metabolic function indicator is the bicarbonate ion (HCO_3^-).

TABLE 9.4   Acid–Base Imbalances: Usual Laboratory Value Changes

Imbalance	pH	HCO_3^-	Pao_2	$Paco_2$	K^+
Respiratory acidosis	Decreased	Normal or increased	Decreased	Increased	Increased
Respiratory alkalosis	Increased	Normal or decreased	Normal	Decreased	Decreased
Metabolic acidosis	Decreased	Decreased	Normal	Normal or decreased	Increased
Metabolic alkalosis	Increased	Increased	Normal	Normal or increased	Decreased

HCO_3^-s, Bicarbonate; K^+, potassium; $Paco_2$, partial pressure of carbon dioxide in arterial blood; Pao_2, partial pressure of oxygen in arterial blood.

2. During a metabolic imbalance, you will find a corresponding relationship between the pH and the HCO_3^-. In other words, the pH will be elevated and the HCO_3^- will be elevated (alkalosis), or the pH will be decreased and the HCO_3^- will be decreased (acidosis).
3. Look at the pH and the HCO_3^- concentration to determine whether the condition is a metabolic problem.
4. Metabolic acidosis: The pH is decreased; the HCO_3^- is decreased.
5. Metabolic alkalosis: The pH is elevated; the HCO_3^- is elevated.

⚠ During a respiratory imbalance, the ABG result indicates an opposite relationship between the pH and the $Paco_2$. During a metabolic imbalance, the ABG result indicates a corresponding relationship between the pH and the HCO_3^-.

D. Steps for interpreting ABG results (Box 9.5)

BOX 9.5   Interpreting Arterial Blood Gas Results

If you can remember the following pyramid points and steps, you will be able to interpret any blood gas report.

Pyramid Points
In acidosis, the pH is down.
In alkalosis, the pH is up.
The respiratory function indicator is the partial pressure of carbon dioxide (Pco_2) value.
The metabolic function indicator is the bicarbonate (HCO_3^-) level.

Pyramid Steps
Pyramid Step 1
Look at the arterial blood gas (ABG) report. Look at the pH. Is the pH elevated or decreased? If the pH is elevated, it reflects alkalosis. If the pH is decreased, it reflects acidosis.

Pyramid Step 2
Look at the Pco_2. Is the Pco_2 elevated or decreased? If the Pco_2 reflects an opposite relationship to the pH, then the condition is a respiratory imbalance. If the Pco_2 does not reflect an opposite relationship to the pH, go to Pyramid Step 3.

Pyramid Step 3
Look at the HCO_3^-. Does the HCO_3^- reflect a corresponding relationship with the pH? If it does, then the condition is a metabolic imbalance.

WHAT WOULD YOU DO?

Answer: Failure to determine the presence of adequate collateral circulation could result in severe ischemic injury to the hand if damage to the radial artery occurs with arterial puncture. Upon release of pressure on the ulnar artery, if pinkness fails to return within 6–7 seconds, the ulnar artery blood flow to the hand is insufficient, indicating that the radial artery should not be used for obtaining a blood specimen. Another site would need to be selected for the arterial puncture. The nurse would report this finding to the registered nurse, and the primary health care provider should also be notified of the finding.

PRACTICE QUESTIONS

1. A client has the following laboratory values: a pH of 7.55, an HCO_3^- level of 22 mEq/L, and a Pco_2 of 30 mm Hg. Which action would the nurse plan to take?
   1. Perform Allen's test
   2. Prepare the client for dialysis
   3. Administer insulin as prescribed
   4. Encourage the client to slow down breathing

2. The nurse is told that the arterial blood gas (ABG) results indicate a pH of 7.50 and a Pco_2 of 32 mm Hg. The nurse determines that these results are indicative of which acid–base disturbance?
   1. Metabolic acidosis
   2. Metabolic alkalosis
   3. Respiratory acidosis
   4. Respiratory alkalosis

3. A client is scheduled for blood to be drawn from the radial artery for an arterial blood gas (ABG) determination. The nurse assists with performing an Allen's test before drawing the blood to determine the adequacy of which?
   1. Ulnar circulation
   2. Carotid circulation
   3. Femoral circulation
   4. Brachial circulation

4. The nurse is caring for a client with a nasogastric tube that is attached to low suction. The nurse monitors the client closely for which acid–base disorder that is **most likely** to occur in this situation?
   1. Metabolic acidosis
   2. Metabolic alkalosis
   3. Respiratory acidosis
   4. Respiratory alkalosis

5. The nurse is caring for a client with severe diarrhea. The nurse monitors the client closely, understanding that this client is at risk for developing which acid–base disorder?
   1. Metabolic acidosis
   2. Metabolic alkalosis
   3. Respiratory acidosis
   4. Respiratory alkalosis

6. The nurse observes that a client with diabetic ketoacidosis is experiencing abnormally deep, regular, rapid respirations. How would the nurse correctly document this observation in the medical record?
   1. Apnea
   2. Bradypnea
   3. Cheyne-Stokes
   4. Kussmaul's respirations

7. The nurse is caring for a client with a diagnosis of chronic obstructive pulmonary disease (COPD). The nurse would monitor the client for which acid–base imbalance?
   1. Metabolic acidosis
   2. Metabolic alkalosis
   3. Respiratory acidosis
   4. Respiratory alkalosis

❖ 8. Which clients would the nurse determine to be at risk for development of metabolic alkalosis? **Select all that apply.**
   ❑ 1. Client with emphysema
   ❑ 2. Client who is hyperventilating
   ❑ 3. Client with chronic kidney disease
   ❑ 4. Client admitted with aspirin overdose
   ❑ 5. Client who has been vomiting for 2 days
   ❑ 6. Client receiving oral furosemide 40 mg daily

9. The nurse is caring for a client with respiratory insufficiency. The arterial blood gas (ABG) results indicate a pH of 7.50 and a P_{CO_2} of 30 mm Hg, and the nurse is told that the client is experiencing respiratory alkalosis. Which additional laboratory value would the nurse expect to note?
   1. A sodium level of 145 mEq/L
   2. A potassium level of 3.0 mEq/L
   3. A magnesium level of 1.3 mEq/L
   4. A phosphorus level of 3.0 mg/dL

10. The registered nurse (RN) reviews the results of the arterial blood gas (ABG) values with the licensed practical nurse (LPN) and tells the LPN that the client is experiencing respiratory acidosis. The LPN would expect to note which on the laboratory result report?
   1. pH 7.50, P_{CO_2} 52 mm Hg
   2. pH 7.35, P_{CO_2} 40 mm Hg
   3. pH 7.25, P_{CO_2} 50 mm Hg
   4. pH 7.50, P_{CO_2} 30 mm Hg

ANSWERS

1. 4

Rationale: The client is experiencing respiratory alkalosis based on the laboratory results of a high pH and a low Pco_2 level. Interventions for respiratory alkalosis are the voluntary holding of breath or slowed breathing and the rebreathing of exhaled CO_2 by methods such as using a paper bag or a rebreathing mask as prescribed. Performing an Allen's test would be incorrect, because the blood specimen has already been drawn, and the laboratory results have been completed. Dialysis and insulin administration are interventions for metabolic acidosis.

Test-Taking Strategy: Focus on the data in the question. Because the pH is high and the Pco_2 level is low, a respiratory problem is occurring. Then, applying the ABCs—airway, breathing, and circulation—you can determine that only one intervention deals with respirations.

2. 4

Rationale: The normal pH is 7.35 to 7.45. If a respiratory condition exists, an opposite relationship will be seen between the pH and the Pco_2, as is seen in the correct option. If an alkalotic condition exists, the pH is increased. During an acidotic condition, the pH is decreased so both metabolic acidosis and respiratory acidosis can be eliminated. Metabolic alkalosis can also be eliminated because both pH and HCO_3^- are increased above normal values with this condition.

Test-Taking Strategy: Focus on the data in the question. Remember that with a respiratory condition, you will find an opposite relationship between the pH and the Pco_2 level. Recalling that pH is increased in an alkalotic condition helps direct you to select respiratory alkalosis and eliminate respiratory acidosis. With metabolic conditions, pH and HCO_3^- are altered and either increase or decrease in the same direction.

3. 1

Rationale: Before performing a radial puncture to obtain an arterial specimen for ABG values, an Allen's test should be performed to determine adequate ulnar circulation. Failure to assess collateral circulation could result in severe ischemic injury to the hand if damage to the radial artery occurs with arterial puncture. The remaining options are not associated with this test.

Test-Taking Strategy: Focus on the subject, radial artery puncture and the purpose of the Allen's test. Visualize the location of each of the vessels in the options. First, eliminate carotid and femoral circulations, realizing their distance from the radial artery. From the remaining options, select the ulnar artery, realizing it runs parallel to the radial artery and supplies blood flow to the hand.

4. 2

Rationale: The loss of gastric fluid via nasogastric suction or vomiting causes a metabolic condition. This also results in an alkalotic condition as a result of the loss of hydrochloric acid through gastrointestinal fluid losses. Also, the options denoting a respiratory problem—respiratory acidosis and alkalosis—can be easily eliminated.

Test-Taking Strategy: Focus on the subject, nasogastric tube to low suction. Remember that hydrochloric acid is lost when the client is receiving nasogastric suctioning. This will direct you to the options that identify an alkalotic condition. Because the question addresses a situation other than a respiratory one, the acid–base disorder would be a metabolic condition.

5. 1

Rationale: Intestinal secretions high in bicarbonate may be lost through enteric drainage tubes, an ileostomy, or diarrhea. The decreased bicarbonate level creates the actual base deficit of metabolic acidosis. The remaining options are unlikely to occur in a client with severe diarrhea.

Test-Taking Strategy: Focus on the subject, diarrhea. Knowing that this condition is a gastrointestinal disorder will direct you to think about a metabolic imbalance. Remembering that intestinal fluids are primarily alkaline will assist you with selecting the correct option. When excess bicarbonate is lost, acidosis will result.

6. 4

Rationale: Abnormally deep, regular, and rapid respirations observed in the client with diabetic ketoacidosis are documented as Kussmaul's respirations. During apnea (no breathing), respirations cease for several seconds. During bradypnea, respirations are regular but abnormally slow. Cheyne-Stokes respirations gradually become shallower and are followed by periods of apnea, with repetition of the pattern.

Test-Taking Strategy: Knowledge regarding the description of alterations in breathing patterns is required to answer this question. Focus on options that are comparable or alike, such as apnea and Cheyne-Stokes respirations, where there are periods of apnea to help you eliminate these two options. Next, note the client's diagnosis and remember that Kussmaul's respirations occur in clients with diabetic ketoacidosis.

7. 3

Rationale: Respiratory acidosis most often occurs as a result of primary defects in the function of the lungs or changes in normal respiratory patterns from secondary problems. Chronic respiratory acidosis is most commonly caused by chronic obstructive pulmonary disease (COPD). Acute respiratory acidosis also occurs in clients with COPD when superimposed respiratory infection or concurrent respiratory disease increases the work of breathing. The remaining options are not likely to occur unless other conditions complicate the COPD.

Test-Taking Strategy: Focus on the subject, COPD, to assist with guiding you to select a respiratory acid–base balance. Then remembering that primary defects in the function of the lungs result in respiratory acidosis will direct you to the correct option.

8. 4, 6

Rationale: Metabolic alkalosis is caused by any condition that creates the acid–base imbalance through either an increase in bases or a deficit of acids, such as the client who has been vomiting for 2 days and the client receiving furosemide daily. Recall that clients with emphysema and hyperventilation are at risk for a respiratory acid–base disturbance. Chronic kidney disease and aspirin overdose will result in metabolic acidosis.

Test-Taking Strategy: Focus on the subject, those at risk for metabolic alkalosis. Eliminate options that are comparable or alike and refer to respiratory conditions. From the remaining metabolic conditions, determine whether there is an increase in bases or a deficit in acids to answer correctly.

9. 2

Rationale: Signs/symptoms of respiratory alkalosis include tachypnea, change in mental status, dizziness, pallor around the mouth, spasms of the muscles of the hands, and hypokalemia. The remaining options identify normal laboratory results.

Test-Taking Strategy: Recalling the clinical manifestations of respiratory alkalosis and the normal laboratory values will assist you with answering this question. Eliminate options that are comparable or alike in that they reflect normal laboratory values. You can then determine that the only abnormal laboratory value is the potassium level.

10. 3

Rationale: The normal pH is 7.35 to 7.45, and the normal P_{CO_2} value is 35 mm Hg to 45 mm Hg. In respiratory acidosis, the pH is down, and the P_{CO_2} is up. Therefore, the pH of 7.25 and the P_{CO_2} of 50 mm Hg option is the only one that reflects an acidotic condition. Options with an elevated pH (options 1 and 4) indicate an alkalotic condition. Option 2 identifies normal values for pH and P_{CO_2}.

Test-Taking Strategy: Focus on the subject, respiratory acidosis. Remember that with a respiratory imbalance, you will find an opposite relationship between the pH and the P_{CO_2} value. In addition, remember that the pH is down in an acidotic condition.

CHAPTER **10**

Vital Signs and Laboratory Reference Intervals

PRIORITY CONCEPTS Cellular Regulation; Perfusion

WHAT WOULD YOU DO?

A client arrives from the postanesthesia care unit (PACU) and the nurse is assisting in monitoring the client's vital signs. On arrival to the unit, the client's temperature was 37.2°C (98.9°F) orally, the blood pressure (BP) was 142/78 mm Hg, the heart rate was 98 beats per minute, the respiratory rate was 14 breaths per minute, and the oxygen saturation was 95% on 3 L of oxygen via nasal cannula. The nurse returns to the room 30 minutes later to find the client's temperature to be 36.8°C (98.2°F) orally, the BP 95/54 mm Hg, the heart rate 118 beats per minute, the respiratory rate 18 breaths per minute, and the oxygen saturation 92% on 3 L of oxygen via nasal cannula. On the basis of this data, what actions would the nurse take?
Answer is located on p. 110.

I. Vital Signs
A. Description: Vital signs include temperature, pulse, respirations, blood pressure (BP), oxygen saturation (pulse oximetry), and pain assessment.
B. Guidelines for measuring vital signs
   1. Initial measurement of vital signs provides baseline data on a client's health status and is used to help identify changes in the client's health status.
   2. Some vital sign measurements (temperature, pulse, respirations, BP, pulse oximetry) may be delegated to assistive personnel (AP), but the AP is not responsible for interpreting the findings.
   3. The primary health care provider (PHCP) determines the frequency of vital sign assessment; the nurse can make independent decisions regarding their frequency on the basis of the client's status.

⚠ The nurse always documents vital sign measurements and reports abnormal findings to the registered nurse (RN) and PHCP.

C. When vital signs are measured
   1. On initial contact with a client (e.g., when a client is admitted to a health care facility)
   2. During physical data collection procedures of a client
   3. Before and after an invasive diagnostic procedure or surgical procedure
   4. During the administration of medication that affects the cardiac, respiratory, or temperature-controlling functions (e.g., in a client who has a fever); may be required before, during, and after administration of the medication
   5. Before, during, and after a blood transfusion
   6. Whenever a client's condition changes or the client verbalizes unusual feelings such as nonspecific symptoms of physical distress (e.g., feeling funny or different)
   7. Whenever an intervention (e.g., ambulation) may affect a client's condition
   8. When a fever or known infection is present (every 2–4 hours)

II. Temperature
A. Description
   1. Normal body temperature ranges from 36.4°C to 37.5°CC (97.5°F–99.5°F); the average in a healthy young adult is 37.0°C (98.6°F).
   2. Common measurement sites are the mouth, rectum, axilla, ear, and across the forehead (temporal artery site); various types of electronic measuring devices are commonly used to measure temperature.
   3. Rectal temperatures are usually 1°F (0.5°C) higher and tympanic and axillary temperatures about 1°F (0.5°C) lower than the normal oral temperature.
   4. Know how to convert a temperature to a Fahrenheit or Celsius value (Box 10.1).

101

BOX 10.1   Body Temperature Conversion

To convert Fahrenheit to Celsius: Degrees Fahrenheit − 32 ×
5/9 = Degrees Celsius
Example: 98.2° F − 32 × 5/9 = 36.7°C
To convert Celsius to Fahrenheit: Degrees Celsius × 9/5 +
32 = Degrees Fahrenheit
Example: 38.6° C × 9/5 + 32 = 101.5° F

B. Nursing considerations
   1. Time of day
      a. Temperature is generally in the low-normal range at the time of awakening as a result of muscle inactivity.
      b. Afternoon body temperature may be high normal as a result of the metabolic process, activity, and environmental temperature.
   2. Environmental temperature: Body temperature is lower in cold weather and higher in warm weather.
   3. Age: Temperature may fluctuate during the first year of life because the infant's heat-regulating mechanism is not fully developed.
   4. Physical exercise: Use of the large muscles creates heat, causing an increase in body temperature.
   5. Menstrual cycle: Temperature decreases slightly just before ovulation, but may increase to 1°F above normal during ovulation.
   6. Pregnancy: Body temperature may consistently stay at high normal because of an increase in the woman's metabolic rate.
   7. Stress: Emotions increase hormonal secretion, leading to increased heat production and a higher temperature.
   8. Illness: Infective agents and the inflammatory response may cause an increase in temperature.
   9. The inability to obtain a temperature reading must not be ignored because it could represent a condition of hypothermia, a life-threatening condition in very young and older clients.
C. Methods of measurement
   1. Oral
      a. If the client has recently consumed hot or cold foods or liquids or has smoked or chewed gum, the nurse must wait 15 to 30 minutes before taking the temperature orally.
      b. The thermometer is placed under the tongue in one of the posterior sublingual pockets; ask the client to keep the tongue down and the lips closed and to not bite down on the thermometer.
   2. Rectal
      a. Provide privacy.
      b. Place the client in the Sims position.
      c. The temperature is taken rectally when an accurate temperature cannot be obtained orally or via other methods including by an electronic method, or when the client has nasal

congestion, has undergone nasal or oral surgery or had the jaws wired, has a nasogastric tube in place, is unable to keep the mouth closed, or is at risk for seizures.
      d. The thermometer is lubricated and inserted into the rectum, toward the umbilicus, about 1.5 inches (3.8 cm) (no more than 0.5 inch [1.25 cm] in an infant).

⚠️ The temperature is not taken rectally in cardiac clients; the client who has undergone rectal surgery; or the client with diarrhea, fecal impaction, or rectal bleeding, or who is at risk for bleeding.

   3. Axillary
      a. This method of taking the temperature is used when the oral or rectal temperature measurement is contraindicated.
      b. Axillary measurement is not as accurate as the oral, rectal, tympanic, or temporal artery method but is used when other methods of measurement are not possible.
      c. The thermometer is placed in the client's dry axilla, and the client is asked to hold the arm tightly against the chest, resting the arm on the chest; follow the instructions accompanying the measurement device for the amount of time the thermometer remains in the axillary area.
   4. Tympanic
      a. The auditory canal is checked for the presence of redness, swelling, discharge, or the presence of a foreign body before the probe is inserted; the probe must not be inserted if the client has an inflammatory condition of the auditory canal or if there is discharge from the ear.
      b. The reading may be affected by an ear infection or excessive wax blocking the ear canal.
   5. Temporal artery
      a. Ensure that the client's forehead is dry.
      b. The thermometer probe is placed flush against the skin and slid across the forehead or placed in the area of the temporal artery and held in place.
      c. If the client is diaphoretic, the temporal artery thermometer probe may be placed on the neck, just behind the earlobe.

III. Pulse

A. Description
   1. Pulse is a palpable bounding of blood flow in a peripheral artery; it is an indirect indicator of circulatory status.
   2. The average adult pulse (heart) rate is 60 to 100 beats per minute.
   3. Changes in pulse rate are used to evaluate the client's tolerance of interventions such as ambulation, bathing, dressing, and exercise.

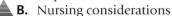

> **BOX 10.2   Grading Scale for Pulses**
>
> 4 + = strong and bounding
> 3 + = full pulse, increased
> 2 + = normal, easily palpable
> 1 + = weak, barely palpable
> 0 = absent, not palpable

4. Pedal pulses are checked to determine whether the circulation is blocked in the artery up to that pulse point.
5. When the pedal pulse is difficult to locate, a Doppler ultrasound stethoscope (ultrasonic stethoscope) may be needed to amplify the sounds of pulse waves.

B. Nursing considerations
1. The heart rate slows with age.
2. Exercise increases the heart rate.
3. Emotions stimulate the sympathetic nervous system, increasing the heart rate.
4. Pain increases the heart rate.
5. Increased body temperature causes the heart rate to increase.
6. Stimulant medications increase the heart rate; depressants and medications affecting the cardiac system slow it.
7. When the BP is low, the heart rate is usually increased.
8. Hemorrhage increases the heart rate.

C. Checking pulse qualities
1. When the pulse is being counted, note the rate, rhythm, strength (force or amplitude), and equality.
2. Once you have checked these parameters, use the grading scale for pulses to assess the information you have elicited (Box 10.2).

D. Pulse points and locations
1. The temporal artery can be palpated anterior to or in the front of the ear.
2. The carotid artery is located in the groove between the trachea and sternocleidomastoid muscle, medial to and alongside the muscle.
3. The apical pulse may be detected at the left midclavicular, fifth intercostal space.
4. The brachial pulse is located above the elbow at the antecubital fossa, between the biceps and triceps muscles.
5. The radial pulse is located in the groove along the radial or thumb side of the client's inner wrist.
6. The femoral pulse is located below the inguinal ligament, midway between the symphysis pubis and the anterosuperior iliac spine.
7. The popliteal pulse is located behind the knee.
8. The posterior tibial pulse is located on the inner side of the ankle, behind and below the medial malleolus (ankle bone).

9. The dorsalis pedis pulse is located on the top of the foot, in line with the groove between the extensor tendons of the great and first toes.

⚠ The apical pulse is counted for 1 full minute and is assessed in clients with an irregular radial pulse or a heart condition, before the administration of cardiac medications such as digoxin and beta-blockers, and in children younger than 2 years.

E. Pulse deficit
1. In this condition, the peripheral pulse rate (radial pulse) is less than the ventricular contraction rate (apical pulse).
2. A pulse deficit indicates a lack of peripheral perfusion; it can be an indication of cardiac dysrhythmias.
3. One-examiner technique: Auscultate and count the apical pulse first, and then immediately count the radial pulse.
4. Two-examiner technique: One person counts the apical pulse, and the other counts the radial pulse simultaneously.
5. A pulse deficit indicates that cardiac contractions are ineffective, failing to send pulse waves to the periphery.
6. If a difference in pulse rate is noted, the PHCP is notified.

IV. Respirations

A. Description
1. Respiration is a mechanism the body uses to exchange gases between atmosphere and the blood and between the blood and the cells.
2. Respiratory rates vary with age.
3. The normal adult respiratory rate is 12 to 20 breaths per minute.

B. Nursing considerations
1. Many of the factors that affect the pulse rate also affect the respiratory rate.
2. An increased level of carbon dioxide or a lower level of oxygen in the blood results in an increase in respiratory rate.
3. Head injury or increased intracranial pressure will depress the respiratory center in the brain, resulting in shallow respiration or slowed breathing.
4. Medications such as opioid analgesics depress respiration.

C. Measuring respiratory rate
1. Count the client's respirations after measuring the radial pulse. (Continue holding the client's wrist while counting the respirations, or position the hand on the client's chest.)
2. One respiration includes both inspiration and expiration.
3. The rate, depth, pattern, and sounds are assessed.

Nursing Sciences

 The respiratory rate may be counted for 30 seconds and multiplied by 2, except in a client who is very ill or is exhibiting irregular respirations, in which case respirations are counted for 1 full minute.

V. Blood Pressure

A. Description
   1. BP is the force on the walls of an artery exerted by the pulsating blood under pressure from the heart.
   2. The heart's contraction forces blood under high pressure into the aorta; the peak of maximum pressure when ejection occurs is the systolic pressure; the blood remaining in the arteries when the ventricles relax exerts a force known as the diastolic pressure.
   3. The difference between the systolic and diastolic pressures is called the pulse pressure.
   4. For an adult (age 18 years and older), a normal BP is a systolic pressure below 120 mm Hg and a diastolic pressure below 80 mm Hg.
   5. Classifications of hypertension (Box 10.3).
   6. In postural (orthostatic) hypotension, a normotensive client exhibits symptoms such as dizziness and lightheadedness and a low BP when rising to an upright position.
   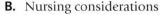
   7. To obtain orthostatic vital sign measurements, check the BP and pulse with the client supine, sitting, and standing; readings are obtained 1 to 3 minutes after the client changes position.

B. Nursing considerations

   1. Factors affecting BP
      a. BP tends to increase as the aging process progresses.
      b. Stress results in sympathetic stimulation that increases the BP.
      c. The incidence of high BP is higher among African Americans than among Americans of European descent.
      d. Antihypertensive medications and opioid analgesics can decrease BP.
      e. BP is typically lowest in the early morning, gradually increases during the day, and peaks in the late afternoon and evening.
      f. After puberty, males tend to have higher BP than females; after menopause, women tend to have higher BP than men of the same age.

   2. Guidelines for measuring BP
      a. Determine the best site for assessment.
      b. Avoid applying a cuff to an extremity into which intravenous (IV) fluids are infusing, where an arteriovenous shunt or fistula is present, on the side on which breast or axillary surgery has been performed, or on an extremity that has been traumatized or is diseased.
      c. The leg may be used if the brachial artery is inaccessible; the cuff is wrapped around the thigh and the stethoscope is placed over the popliteal artery.
      d. Ensure that the client has not smoked or exercised in the 30 minutes before measurement because both can yield falsely high readings.
      e. Have the client assume a sitting (with the feet flat on floor) or lying position and then rest for 5 minutes before the measurement; ask the client not to speak during the measurement.
      f. Ensure that the cuff is fully deflated, then wrap it evenly and snugly around the extremity.
      g. Ensure that the stethoscope being used fits the examiner and does not impair hearing.
      h. Document the first Korotkoff sound at phase 1 (heard as the blood pulsates through the vessel when air is released from the BP cuff and pressure on the artery is reduced) as the systolic pressure and the beginning of the fifth Korotkoff sound at phase 5 as the diastolic pressure.

⚠ When taking a BP, select the appropriate cuff size; a cuff that is too small will yield a falsely high reading, and a cuff that is too large will yield a falsely low reading.

VI. Pulse Oximetry

A. Description
   1. Pulse oximetry is a noninvasive test that registers the oxygen saturation of the client's hemoglobin.
   2. The capillary oxygen saturation (Sao_2) is recorded as a percentage.
   3. The normal value is 95% to 100%.
   4. After a hypoxic client uses up the readily available oxygen (measured as the arterial oxygen pressure, Pao_2, on arterial blood gas [ABG] testing), the reserve oxygen, that oxygen attached to the hemoglobin (Sao_2), is drawn on to provide oxygen to the tissues.
   5. A pulse oximeter reading can alert the nurse to hypoxemia before clinical signs occur.
   6. If pulse oximetry readings are below normal, instruct the client in deep breathing technique and recheck the pulse oximetry.

B. Procedure
   1. A sensor is placed on the client's finger, toe, nose, ear lobe, or forehead to measure oxygen saturation, which then is displayed on a monitor.

2. Maintain the transducer at heart level.

3. Do not select an extremity with an impediment to blood flow.

⚠ A usual pulse oximetry reading is between 95% and 100%. A pulse oximetry reading lower than 90% necessitates PHCP notification; values below 90% are acceptable only in certain chronic conditions. Agency procedures and PHCP prescriptions are followed regarding actions to take for specific readings.

VII. Pain

A. Types of pain

1. Acute/transient: Usually associated with an injury, medical condition, or surgical procedure; lasts hours to a few days

2. Chronic/persistent noncancer pain: Usually associated with long-term or chronic illnesses or disorders; may continue for months or even years

3. Chronic/episodic pain: Occurs sporadically over an extended period of time. Pain episodes last for hours, days, or weeks. Examples are migraine, headaches, and pain related to sickle cell crisis.

4. Cancer pain: Not all people with cancer have pain. Cancer pain is usually caused by tumor progression and related pathological processes, invasive procedures, treatment toxicities, infection, and physical limitations.

5. Idiopathic pain: This is chronic pain in the absence of identifiable physical or psychological cause or pain perceived as excessive for the extent of an organic pathological condition.

6. Phantom: Occurs after the loss of a body part (amputation); may be felt in the amputated part for years after the amputation

B. Data collection

1. Pain is a highly individual experience.

2. Ask the client to describe pain in terms of timing, location, severity, quality, aggravating and precipitating factors, and relief measures.

3. Ask the client about the use of complementary and alternative therapies to alleviate pain.

4. Pain experienced by the older client may be manifested differently than pain experienced by members of other age groups (e.g., sleep disturbances, changes in gait and mobility, decreased socialization, depression).

5. Clients with cognitive disorders (e.g., a client with dementia, a comatose client) may not be able to describe their pain experiences.

6. The nurse must be alert to nonverbal indicators of pain (Box 10.4).

7. Ask the client to use a number-based pain scale, such as a number scale of 1 to 10 with the number 10 indicating severe pain (a picture-based scale may be used in children or clients who cannot verbally describe their pain), to rate the degree of pain.

8. Evaluate client response to nonpharmacological interventions.

⚠ Consider the client's culture and spiritual and religious beliefs in assessing pain; some cultures frown on the outward expression of pain.

C. Conventional nonpharmacological interventions

1. Cutaneous stimulation

a. Techniques include heat, cold, pressure, and vibration. Therapeutic touch and massage are also cutaneous stimulation and may be considered complementary/alternative techniques.

b. Such treatments may require a PHCP's prescription.

2. Transcutaneous electrical nerve stimulation (TENS)

a. TENS is also referred to as percutaneous electrical nerve stimulation (PENS).

b. This technique, which requires a PHCP's prescription, involves the application of a battery-operated device that delivers a low electrical current to the skin and underlying tissues to block pain.

3. Binders, slings, and other supportive devices

a. Cloths or other materials or devices wrapped around a limb or body part can ease the pain of strains, sprains, and surgical incisions.

b. Such devices may require a PHCP's prescription.

c. Elevation of the affected body part is another intervention that can reduce swelling; supporting an extremity on a pillow may lessen discomfort.

4. Heat and cold

a. The application of heat and cold or alternating application of the two can soothe pain resulting from muscle strain; cold reduces swelling.

b. In some conditions, such treatment may require a PHCP's prescription.

c. Heat applications may include warm-water compresses, warm blankets, thermal pads, and tub and whirlpool baths.

BOX 10.4 **Nonverbal Indicators of Pain**

- Moaning
- Crying
- Irritability
- Restlessness
- Grimacing or frowning
- Inability to sleep
- Rigid posture
- Increased blood pressure, heart rate, or respiratory rate
- Nausea
- Diaphoresis

Nursing Sciences

d. The temperature of the application must be monitored carefully to help prevent burns; the skin of very young and older clients is extra sensitive to heat.

e. The application of cold can reduce swelling and muscle spasms and ease pain in joints and muscles.

f. The client is advised to remove the source of heat or cold if changes in sensation or discomfort occur. If the change in sensation or discomfort is not relieved after removal of the application, the PHCP would be notified.

> ⚠ Ice or heat needs to be applied with a towel or other barrier between the pack and the skin but must not be left in place for more than 15 to 30 minutes.

D. Complementary and alternative therapies
   1. Description: Therapies are used in addition to conventional treatment to provide healing resources and focus on the mind-body connection.
   2. Nursing considerations
      a. Some complementary and alternative therapies require a PHCP's prescription.
      b. Herbal remedies are considered pharmacological therapy by some PHCPs; because of the risk for interaction with prescription medications, it is important that the nurse ask the client about the use of such therapies.
      c. If cultural or spiritual measures are to be employed, the nurse must elicit from the client the preferred forms of spiritual expression and learn when they are practiced so that they may be integrated into the plan of care.

VIII. Pharmacological Interventions

A. Nonopioid analgesics
   1. Nonsteroidal anti-inflammatory drugs (NSAIDs) and acetylsalicylic acid (Box 10.5)
      a. These medication types are contraindicated if the client has gastric irritation or ulcer disease or an allergy to the medication.
      b. Bleeding is a concern with the use of these medication types.
      c. Instruct the client to take oral doses with milk or a snack to reduce gastric irritation.
      d. NSAIDs can amplify the effects of anticoagulants.
      e. Hypoglycemia may result for the client taking ibuprofen if the client is concurrently taking an oral antidiabetic agent.
      f. A high risk of toxicity exists if the client is taking ibuprofen concurrently with a calcium-channel blocker.
   2. Acetaminophen
      a. Acetaminophen is contraindicated in clients with hepatic or renal disease, alcoholism, or hypersensitivity.

BOX 10.5 **Side and Adverse Effects of Nonsteroidal Anti-inflammatory Drugs and Acetylsalicylic Acid**

Nonsteroidal Anti-inflammatory Drugs
- Gastric irritation
- Hypotension
- Sodium and water retention
- Blood dyscrasia
- Dizziness
- Tinnitus
- Pruritus

Acetylsalicylic Acid
- Gastric irritation
- Flushing
- Tinnitus
- Drowsiness
- Headache
- Change in vision

---

b. Determine whether the client has a history of liver dysfunction.
c. Monitor the client for signs of hepatic damage (e.g., nausea and vomiting, diarrhea, abdominal pain).
d. Monitor liver function parameters.
e. Tell the client that self-medication must not continue longer than 10 days in an adult or 5 days in a child because of the risk of hepatotoxicity.
f. The antidote to acetaminophen is acetylcysteine.

> ⚠ The major concern with acetaminophen is hepatotoxicity.

B. Opioid analgesics
   1. Description
      a. These medications suppress pain impulses but can also suppress respiration and coughing by acting on the respiratory and cough center, located in the medulla of the brainstem.
      b. Intravenous route administration produces a faster effect than other routes, but the effect lasts shorter to relieve pain.
      c. Opioids, which produce euphoria and sedation, can cause physical dependence.
      d. Administer the medication 30 to 60 minutes before painful activities.
      e. Monitor the respiratory rate; if it is slower than 12 breaths per minute in an adult, withhold the medication and notify the RN who will notify the PHCP.
      f. Monitor the pulse; if bradycardia develops, withhold the medication and notify the RN who will notify the PHCP.
      g. Monitor the BP for hypotension.

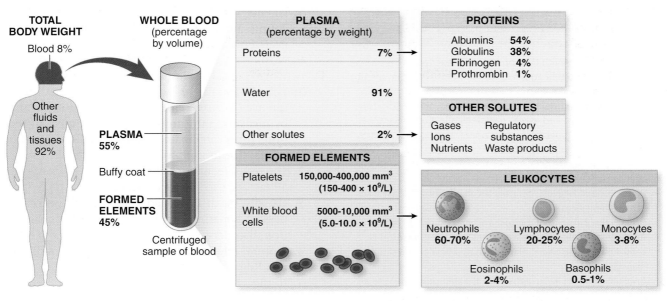

FIGURE 10.1 Approximate values for the components of blood in a normal adult.

h. Auscultate the lungs for normal breath sounds.
i. Encourage activities such as turning, deep breathing, and incentive spirometry to help prevent atelectasis and pneumonia.
j. Monitor the client's level of consciousness.
k. Initiate safety precautions.
l. Monitor intake and output and check for urine retention; also, constipation is common with opioid use.
m. Reinforce instructions to the client to take oral doses with milk or a snack to reduce gastric irritation.
n. Reinforce instructions to the client to avoid activities that require alertness.
o. Check the effectiveness of the medication.
p. Have an opioid antagonist (e.g., naloxone), oxygen, and resuscitation equipment available.

⚠ An electronic infusion device is always used for continuous or dose-demand intravenous infusion of opioid analgesics.

2. Codeine sulfate
a. This medication is also used in low doses as a cough suppressant.
b. It may cause constipation.
c. Common medications in this class are hydrocodone and oxycodone (synthetic forms).
3. Hydromorphone
a. The primary concern is respiration depression.
b. Other effects include drowsiness, dizziness, and orthostatic hypotension.
c. Monitor vital signs, especially the respiratory rate and BP.

4. Morphine sulfate
a. Morphine sulfate is used to ease acute pain resulting from myocardial infarction or cancer, for dyspnea resulting from pulmonary edema, and as a preoperative medication.
b. The major concern is respiratory depression, but postural hypotension, urine retention, constipation, and pupillary constriction may also occur; monitor the client for adverse effects.
c. Morphine may cause nausea and vomiting by increasing vestibular sensitivity.
d. It is contraindicated in severe respiratory disorders, head injuries, severe renal disease, or seizure activity and in the presence of increased intracranial pressure.
e. Monitor the client for urine retention.
f. Monitor bowel sounds for decreased peristalsis; constipation may occur.
g. Monitor the pupil for changes; pinpoint pupils may indicate overdose.

IX. Laboratory Reference Intervals

⚠ For reference throughout the chapter, please see Fig. 10.1.

A. Procedure for drawing blood (Box 10.6)
B. Serum sodium
1. A major cation of extracellular fluid
2. Maintains osmotic pressure and acid-base balance, and assists in the transmission of nerve impulses
3. Is absorbed from the small intestine and excreted in the urine in amounts dependent on dietary intake
4. Normal reference interval: 135 to 145 mEq/L

Nursing Sciences

BOX 10.6 Performing Venipuncture for a Blood Sample

- Check primary health care provider's prescription.
- Identify foods, medications, or other factors that may affect the procedure or results.
- Gather needed supplies, including gloves, the needle (appropriate gauge and size), transfer/collection device per agency policy, specimen containers per agency policy, tourniquet, antiseptic swabs, 2 × 2 inch gauze, tape, tube label(s), biohazard bag, requisition form or bar code per agency policy.
- Perform hand hygiene. Identify the client with at least 2 accepted identifiers.
- Explain the purpose of the test and procedure to the client.
- Apply clean gloves. Place the client in a lying position or a semi-Fowler's position. Place a small pillow or towel under the extremity.
- Apply tourniquet 5–10 cm above the venipuncture site so that it can be removed in one motion.
- Ask the client to open and close the fist several times, then clench the fist.
- Inspect to determine the vein to be used for venipuncture. Select the vein based on size and quality (use the most distal site in the nondominant arm if possible). Palpate the vein with the index finger for resilience.
- Clean site with antiseptic swabs or per agency policy, using a circular scrubbing motion, inward to outward for 30 seconds. Insert the needle bevel up at a 15- to 30-degree angle. Collect blood in collection device per agency policy.
- Release tourniquet. Apply 2 × 2 inch gauze over insertion site. Remove needle and engage safety on needle. Apply pressure for 2 minutes. If the client is taking anticoagulants, apply pressure for several minutes. Perform hand hygiene.
- Be certain that all blood tubes are labeled with the client's name and any other required information per agency policy. Send specimen to the laboratory in biohazard bag with associated requisition forms or bar codes per agency policy.

⚠️ Drawing blood specimens from an extremity in which an intravenous solution is infusing can produce an inaccurate result, depending on the test being performed and the type of solution infusing. Prolonged use of a tourniquet before venous sampling can increase the blood level of potassium, producing an inaccurate result.

C. Serum potassium

1. A major intracellular cation, potassium regulates cellular water balance, electrical conduction in muscle cells, and acid-base balance.
2. The body obtains potassium through dietary ingestion, and the kidneys preserve or excrete potassium, depending on cellular need.
3. Potassium levels are used to evaluate cardiac function, renal function, gastrointestinal function, and the need for IV replacement therapy.
4. If the client is receiving potassium supplementation, this needs to be noted on the laboratory form.

5. Clients with elevated white blood cell (WBC) counts and platelet counts may have falsely elevated potassium levels.
6. Normal reference interval: 3.5 to 5.0 mEq/L

D. Activated partial thromboplastin time (aPTT)

1. The aPTT evaluates how well the coagulation sequence (intrinsic clotting system) is functioning by measuring the amount of time it takes in seconds for recalcified citrated plasma to clot after partial thromboplastin is added to it.
2. The test screens for deficiencies and inhibitors of all factors, except factors VII and XIII.
3. Usually, the aPTT is used to monitor the effectiveness of heparin therapy and screen for coagulation disorders.
4. Normal reference interval: 30 to 40 seconds, depending on the type of activator used
5. If the client is receiving intermittent heparin therapy, the blood sample is drawn 1 hour before the next scheduled dose.
6. Blood samples are not drawn from an arm into which heparin is infusing.
7. Transport specimen to the laboratory immediately.
8. Provide direct pressure to the venipuncture site for 3 to 5 minutes.
9. The aPTT needs to be between 1.5 and 2.5 times normal when the client is receiving heparin therapy.

⚠️ If the aPTT value is prolonged (longer than 87.5 seconds or per agency policy) in a client receiving IV heparin therapy or in any client at risk for thrombocytopenia, initiate bleeding precautions.

E. Prothrombin time (PT) and international normalized ratio (INR)

1. Prothrombin is a vitamin K–dependent glycoprotein produced by the liver that is necessary for fibrin clot formation.
2. Each laboratory establishes a normal or control value based on the method used to perform the PT test.
3. The PT measures the amount of time it takes in seconds for clot formation and is used to monitor response to warfarin sodium therapy or to screen for dysfunction of the extrinsic clotting system resulting from liver disease, vitamin K deficiency, or disseminated intravascular coagulation.
4. A PT value within 2 seconds (plus or minus) of the control is considered normal.
5. The INR is a frequently used test to measure the effects of some anticoagulants.
6. The INR standardizes the PT ratio and is calculated in the laboratory setting by raising the observed PT ratio to the power of the international sensitivity index specific to the thromboplastin reagent used.
7. If a PT is prescribed, a baseline specimen would be drawn before anticoagulation therapy is started; note the time of collection on the laboratory form.

8. Provide direct pressure to the venipuncture site for 3 to 5 minutes.
9. Concurrent warfarin therapy with heparin therapy can lengthen the PT for up to 5 hours after dosing.
10. Diets high in green leafy vegetables can increase the absorption of vitamin K, which shortens the PT.
11. Orally administered anticoagulation therapy usually maintains the PT at 1.5 to 2 times the laboratory control value.
12. Normal reference intervals
    a. PT: 11 to 12.5 seconds
    b. INR: 0.81 to 1.2
    c. INR: 2 to 3 for standard warfarin therapy; 3 to 4.5 for high-dose warfarin therapy

⚠ If the PT value is longer than 32 seconds and the INR is greater than 3.0 in a client receiving standard warfarin therapy (or per agency policy), initiate bleeding precautions.

F. Platelet count
1. Platelets function in hemostatic plug formation, clot retraction, and coagulation factor activation.
2 Platelets are produced by the bone marrow to function in hemostasis.
3. Normal reference interval: 150,000 to 400,000 mm³
4. Monitor the venipuncture site for bleeding in clients with known thrombocytopenia.
5. High altitudes, chronic cold weather, acute infections, chronic granulocytic leukemia, chronic pancreatitis, cirrhosis, collagen disorders, polycythemia, and postsplenectomy can increase platelet counts.
6. Acute leukemia, chemotherapy, hemorrhage, infection, systemic lupus erythematosus, and thrombocytopenic purpura can decrease platelet counts.
7. Bleeding precautions must be instituted in clients with a low platelet count; the specific value for implementing bleeding precautions usually is determined by agency policy.

⚠ Monitor the platelet count closely in clients receiving chemotherapy because of the risk for thrombocytopenia. In addition, any client who will be having an invasive procedure (such as a liver biopsy or thoracentesis) must have coagulation studies and platelet counts done before the procedure.

G. Hemoglobin and hematocrit
1. Hemoglobin is the main component of erythrocytes and serves as the vehicle for transporting oxygen and carbon dioxide.
2. Hematocrit represents red blood cell (RBC) mass and is an important measurement in the presence of anemia or polycythemia (Table 10.1).
3. Fasting is not required for this test.

TABLE 10.1   Hemoglobin and Hematocrit: Reference Intervals

Blood Component	Reference Interval
Hemoglobin (Altitude Dependent)	
Male adult	*Male:* 14–18 g/dL
Female adult	*Female:* 12–16 g/dL
Hematocrit (Altitude Dependent)	
Male adult	*Male:* 42%–52%
Female adult	*Female:* 37%–47%

TABLE 10.2   Lipids: Reference Intervals

Blood Component	Reference Interval
Cholesterol	<200 mg/dL
High-density lipoproteins (HDLs)	*Male:* >40 mg/dL *Female:* >50 mg/dL
Low-density lipoproteins (LDLs)	*Recommended:* <100 mg/dL *Near optimal:* 100–129 mg/dL *Moderate risk for coronary artery disease (CAD):* 130–159 mg/dL *High risk for CAD:* >160 mg/dL
Triglycerides	<150 mg/dL

H. Lipids
1. Blood lipids consist primarily of cholesterol, triglycerides, and phospholipids.
2. Lipid assessment includes total cholesterol, high-density lipoprotein (HDL), low-density lipoprotein (LDL), and triglycerides.
3. Cholesterol is present in all body tissues and is a major component of LDLs, brain and nerve cells, cell membranes, and some gallbladder stones.
4. Triglycerides constitute a major part of very low-density lipoproteins and a small part of LDLs.
5. Triglycerides are synthesized in the liver from fatty acids, protein, and glucose, and are obtained from the diet.
6. Increased cholesterol levels, LDL levels, and triglyceride levels place the client at risk for coronary artery disease.
7. HDL helps protect against the risk of coronary artery disease.
8. Oral contraceptives may increase the lipid level.
9. Instruct the client to abstain from foods and fluid, except for water, for 12 to 14 hours and from alcohol for 24 hours before the test.
10. Instruct the client to avoid consuming high-cholesterol foods with the evening meal before the test.
11. Normal reference intervals (Table 10.2)
I. Fasting blood glucose
1. Glucose is a monosaccharide found in fruits and is formed from the digestion of carbohydrates and the conversion of glycogen by the liver.

2. Glucose is the main source of cellular energy for the body and is essential for brain and erythrocyte function.
3. Fasting blood glucose levels are used to help diagnose diabetes mellitus and hypoglycemia.
4. Instruct the client to fast for 8 to 12 hours before the test.
5. Instruct a client with diabetes mellitus to withhold morning insulin or oral hypoglycemic medication until after the blood is drawn.
6. Normal reference interval: Glucose (fasting) 70 to 99 mg/dL

J. Glycosylated hemoglobin (HgbA1C)
1. HgbA1C is blood glucose bound to hemoglobin.
2. Hemoglobin A1C (glycosylated hemoglobin A; HbA1C) is a reflection of how well blood glucose levels have been controlled for the past 3 to 4 months.
3. Hyperglycemia in clients with diabetes is usually a cause of an increase in the HbA1C.
4. Fasting is not required before the test.
5. Normal reference intervals (dependent on HCP preference): 4.0% to 6.0%
6. HgbA1C and estimated average glucose (eAG) (Table 10.3).

K. Renal function studies
1. Serum creatinine
   a. Creatinine is a specific indicator of renal function.
   b. Increased level of creatinine indicates a slowing of the glomerular filtration rate.
   c. Instruct the client to avoid excessive exercise for 8 hours and excessive red meat intake for 24 hours before the test.
   d. Normal reference interval: Male: 0.6 to 1.2 mg/dL; female: 0.5 to 1.1 mg/dL
2. Blood urea nitrogen (BUN)
   a. Urea nitrogen is the nitrogen portion of urea, a substance formed in the liver through an enzymatic protein breakdown process.
   b. Urea is normally freely filtered through the renal glomeruli, with a small amount reabsorbed in the tubules and the remainder excreted in the urine.

   c. Elevated levels indicate a slowing of the glomerular filtration rate.
   d. BUN and creatinine ratios would be analyzed when renal function is evaluated.
   e. Normal reference interval: 10 to 20 mg/dL

L. WBC count
1. WBCs function in the immune defense system of the body.
2. The WBC differential provides specific information on WBC types.
3. A "shift to the left" means that an increased number of immature neutrophils is present in the blood.
4. A low total WBC count with a left shift indicates a recovery from bone marrow depression or an infection of such intensity that the demand for neutrophils in the tissue is higher than the capacity of the bone marrow to release them into the circulation.
5. A high total WBC count with a left shift indicates an increased release of neutrophils by the bone marrow in response to an overwhelming infection or inflammation.
6. An increased neutrophil count with a left shift is usually associated with bacterial infection.
7. A "shift to the right" means that cells have more than the usual number of nuclear segments; found in liver disease, Down syndrome, and megaloblastic and pernicious anemia.
8. Normal reference interval: 5000 to 10,000 mm^3

⚠ Monitor the WBC count and differential closely in clients receiving chemotherapy because of the risk for neutropenia; neutropenia places the client at risk for infection.

WHAT WOULD YOU DO?

Answer: The client's vital signs are showing a significant change, particularly the blood pressure, heart rate, and oxygen saturation levels. The nurse would first compare the vital signs to the set of baseline vital signs obtained when the client arrived at the unit. This provides information about how much of a change has occurred in these parameters. The nurse must quickly consider the following when determining the next action: is the equipment working properly?; is the correct equipment being used?; is there a condition or procedure in the client's history that can be attributed to this change?; are there environmental factors that could influence the change in the client's vital signs?; does this change necessitate contacting the primary health care provider? Given the significant change from the baseline vital signs, and after checking equipment to ensure it is working properly, the nurse must then determine that it is necessary to notify the registered nurse of this change, especially considering the client recently had surgery and there is a potential for bleeding. The surgeon may also need to be notified.

TABLE 10.3 Glycosylated Hemoglobin (HgbA1C) and Estimated Average Glucose (eAG)

HgbA1C %	eAG mg/dL
4	65
5	100
6	135
7	170
8	205

Reference: Pagana, Pagana, Pagana (13th ed), p. 450.

PRACTICE QUESTIONS

1. A client with atrial fibrillation who is receiving maintenance therapy of warfarin sodium has a prothrombin time (PT) of 35 seconds and an international normalized ratio (INR) of 3.5. On the basis of these laboratory values, the nurse anticipates which prescription?
   1. Adding a dose of heparin sodium
   2. Holding the next dose of warfarin
   3. Increasing the next dose of warfarin
   4. Administering the next dose of warfarin

2. A licensed practical nurse (LPN) is precepting a student assigned to care for a client with chronic pain. Which statement, if made by the student, indicates the **need for further teaching** regarding pain management?
   1. "I will be sure to ask my client what their pain level is on a scale of 0 to 10."
   2. "I know that I need to follow up after giving medication to make sure it is effective."
   3. "I know that pain in the older client might manifest as sleep disturbance or depression."
   4. "I will be sure to cue in to any indicators that the client may be exaggerating their pain."

3. A client has been admitted to the hospital for urinary tract infection and dehydration. The nurse determines that the client has received adequate volume replacement if the blood urea nitrogen (BUN) level drops to which value?
   1. 3 mg/dL
   2. 15 mg/dL
   3. 29 mg/dL
   4. 35 mg/dL

4. A licensed practical nurse is explaining the appropriate methods for measuring an accurate temperature to an assistive personnel (AP). Which method, if noted by the AP as being an appropriate method, indicates the **need for further teaching?**
   1. Taking a rectal temperature for a client who has undergone nasal surgery
   2. Taking an oral temperature for a client with a cough and nasal congestion
   3. Taking an axillary temperature on a client who has just consumed hot coffee
   4. Taking a temporal temperature on the neck behind the ear on a client who is diaphoretic

5. A client is receiving a continuous intravenous infusion of heparin sodium to treat deep vein thrombosis. The client's activated partial thromboplastin (aPTT) time is 65 seconds. The licensed practical nurse reviews the laboratory results with the registered nurse, anticipating that which action is needed?
   1. Discontinuing the heparin infusion
   2. Increasing the rate of the heparin infusion
   3. Decreasing the rate of the heparin infusion
   4. Leaving the rate of the heparin infusion as is

6. A client with a history of cardiac disease is due for a morning dose of furosemide. Which serum potassium level, if noted in the client's laboratory report, would be reported before administering the dose of furosemide?
   1. 3.2 mEq/L
   2. 3.8 mEq/L
   3. 4.2 mEq/L
   4. 4.8 mEq/L

7. Several laboratory tests are prescribed for a client, ❖ and the nurse reviews the results of the tests. Which laboratory test results would the nurse report? **Select all that apply.**
   - ❑ 1. Platelets 35,000 mm^3
   - ❑ 2. Sodium 150 mEq/L
   - ❑ 3. Potassium 5.0 mEq/L
   - ❑ 4. Segmented neutrophils 40%
   - ❑ 5. Serum creatinine, 1 mg/dL
   - ❑ 6. White blood cells, 3000 mm^3

8. The nurse is caring for a client who takes ibuprofen ❖ for pain. The nurse is gathering information on the client's medication history and determines it is necessary to consult with the registered nurse if the client is also taking which medications? **Select all that apply.**
   - ❑ 1. Warfarin
   - ❑ 2. Glimepiride
   - ❑ 3. Amlodipine
   - ❑ 4. Simvastatin
   - ❑ 5. Hydrochlorothiazide

9. A client with diabetes mellitus has a glycosylated hemoglobin A1C level of 9%. On the basis of this test result, the nurse plans to reinforce teaching the client about the need for which measure?
   1. Avoiding infection
   2. Taking in adequate fluids
   3. Preventing and recognizing hypoglycemia
   4. Preventing and recognizing hyperglycemia

10. The nurse is caring for a client with a diagnosis of cancer who is immunosuppressed. The nurse would suggest to the registered nurse the need for implementing neutropenic precautions if the client's white blood cell count was which value?
    1. 2000 mm^3
    2. 5800 mm^3
    3. 8400 mm^3
    4. 11,500 mm^3

11. A client brought to the emergency department states that he has accidentally been taking two times his prescribed dose of warfarin for the past week. After noting that the client has no evidence of obvious bleeding, the nurse plans to assist the registered nurse with which action?
1. Administering an antidote
2. Drawing a sample for type and crossmatching and transfusing the client
3. Drawing a sample for an activated partial thromboplastin time (aPTT) level
4. Drawing a sample for prothrombin time (PT) and international normalized ratio (INR)

12. A licensed practical nurse is caring for a postoperative client who is receiving demand-dose hydromorphone via a patient-controlled analgesia (PCA) pump for pain control. The nurse enters the client's room and finds the client drowsy and records the following vital signs: temperature 36.2°C (97.2°F) orally, pulse 52 beats per minute, blood pressure 101/58 mm Hg, respiratory rate 11 breaths per minute, and SpO$_2$ of 93% on 3 liters of oxygen via nasal cannula. Which action must the nurse take **first**?
1. Document the findings
2. Attempt to arouse the client
3. Contact the registered nurse immediately
4. Check the medication administration history on the PCA pump

13. An adult female client has a hemoglobin level of 10.8 g/dL. The nurse interprets that this result is **most likely** caused by which condition noted in the client's history?
1. Dehydration
2. Heart failure
3. Iron deficiency anemia
4. Chronic obstructive pulmonary disease

14. A client with a history of gastrointestinal bleeding has a platelet count of 300,000 mm^3. The nurse needs to take which action after seeing the laboratory results?
1. Report the abnormally low count
2. Report the abnormally high count
3. Place the client on bleeding precautions
4. Place the normal report in the client's medical record

15. A client with diabetes mellitus has a blood sample drawn for the determination of a fasting blood glucose level. When reviewing the client's results, the nurse determines that which requires a call to the primary health care provider for intervention?
1. 75 mg/dL
2. 92 mg/dL
3. 120 mg/dL
4. 240 mg/dL

ANSWERS

1. 2

Rationale: The normal prothrombin time (PT) is 11 seconds to 12.5 seconds. The normal INR is 0.81 to 1.2; 2 to 3 for standard warfarin therapy, which is used for the treatment of atrial fibrillation, and 3 to 4.5 for high-dose warfarin therapy, which is used for clients with mechanical heart valves. A therapeutic PT level is 1.5 to 2 times higher than the normal level. Because the values of 35 seconds and 3.5 are high, the nurse would anticipate that the client would not receive further doses at this time. Therefore, the prescriptions noted in the remaining options are incorrect.

Test-Taking Strategy: Focus on the subject, a PT of 35 seconds and an INR of 3.5. Recall the normal ranges for these values and remember that a PT greater than 32 seconds and an INR greater than 3 for standard warfarin therapy places the client at risk for bleeding; this will direct you to the correct option.

2. 4

Rationale: Pain is a highly individual experience, and the nurse would not assume that the client is exaggerating the pain. Rather, the nurse must frequently assess the pain and intervene accordingly through the use of both nonpharmacological and pharmacological interventions. The nurse would assess pain using a number-based scale or a picture-based scale for clients who cannot verbally describe their pain to rate the degree of pain. The nurse must follow up with the client after giving medication to ensure the medication is effective in managing the pain. Pain experienced by the older client may be manifested differently than pain experienced by members of other age groups, and they may have sleep disturbances, changes in gait and mobility, decreased socialization, and depression; the nurse needs to be aware of this attribute of this population.

Test-Taking Strategy: Note the strategic words *need for further teaching*. These words indicate a negative event query and the need to select the incorrect statement as the answer. Recall that pain is a highly individual experience, and the nurse must not assume the client is exaggerating pain.

3. 2

Rationale: The normal blood urea nitrogen (BUN) level is 10 mg/dL to 20 mg/dL. Values of 29 mg/dL and 35 mg/dL reflect continued dehydration. A value of 3 mg/dL reflects a lower than normal value, which may occur with fluid volume overload, among other conditions.

Test-Taking Strategy: Focus on the subject, adequate fluid replacement and the normal blood urea nitrogen level. The correct option is the only option that identifies a normal value.

4. 2

Rationale: An oral temperature needs to be avoided if the client has nasal congestion. One of the other methods of measuring the temperature would be used according to the equipment available. Taking a rectal temperature for a client who has undergone nasal surgery is appropriate. Other, less invasive measures would be used if available; if not available, a rectal temperature is acceptable. Taking an axillary temperature on a client who just consumed coffee is also acceptable; however, the axillary method of measurement is the least reliable, and other methods would be used if available. If temporal equipment is available and the client is diaphoretic, it is acceptable to measure the temperature on the neck behind the ear, avoiding the forehead.

Test-Taking Strategy: Note the strategic words *need for further teaching*. These words indicate a negative event query and the need to select the incorrect action as the answer. Recall that nasal congestion is a reason to avoid taking an oral temperature as the nasal congestion will cause problems with breathing while the temperature is being taken.

5. 4

Rationale: The normal activated partial thromboplastin time (aPTT) varies between 30 seconds and 40 seconds, depending on the type of activator used in testing. The therapeutic dose of heparin for treatment of deep vein thrombosis is to keep the aPTT between 1.5 and 2.5 times normal. This means that the client's value would not be less than 45 seconds or greater than 100 seconds. Thus, the client's aPTT is within the therapeutic range, and the dose would remain unchanged.

Test-Taking Strategy: Focus on the subject, the expected aPTT for a client receiving a heparin sodium infusion. Remember that the normal range is 30 seconds to 35 seconds and that the aPTT needs to be between 1.5 and 2.5 times normal when the client is receiving heparin therapy. Simple multiplication of 1.5 and 2.5 by 30 and 40 will yield a range of 45 to 100 seconds. This client's value is 65 seconds.

6. 1

Rationale: The normal serum potassium level in the adult is 3.5 mEq/L to 5.0 mEq/L. The correct option is the only value that falls below the therapeutic range. Administering furosemide to a client with a low potassium level and a history of cardiac problems could precipitate ventricular dysrhythmias. The remaining options are within the normal range.

Test-Taking Strategy: Note the subject of the question, the level that must be reported. This indicates that you are looking for an abnormal level. Remember, the normal serum potassium level in the adult is 3.5 mEq/L to 5.0 mEq/L. This will direct you to the correct option.

7. 1, 2, 4, 6

Rationale: The normal values include the following: platelets 150,000 mm³ to 400,000 mm³; sodium 135 mEq/L to 145 mEq/L; potassium, 3.5 mEq/L to 5.0 mEq/L; segmented neutrophils 62% to 68%; serum creatinine, 0.6 mg/dL to 1.2 mg/dL; and white blood cells 5000 mm³ to 10,000 mm³. The platelet level noted is low; the sodium level noted is high; the potassium level noted is normal; the segmented neutrophil level noted is low; the serum creatinine level noted is normal; and the white blood cell level is low.

Test-Taking Strategy: Focus on the subject, the abnormal laboratory values that need to be reported. Recalling the normal laboratory values for the blood studies identified in the options will assist in answering this question.

8. 1, 2, 3

Rationale: Nonsteroidal anti-inflammatory drugs (NSAIDs) can amplify the effects of anticoagulants; therefore, these medications would not be taken together. Hypoglycemia may result for the client taking ibuprofen if the client is concurrently taking an oral hypoglycemic agent such as glimepiride; these medications would not be combined. A high risk of toxicity exists if the client is taking ibuprofen concurrently with a calcium-channel blocker such as amlodipine; therefore, this combination must be avoided. There is no known interaction between ibuprofen and simvastatin or hydrochlorothiazide.

Test-Taking Strategy: Note the subject of the question, data provided by the client necessitating consulting with the registered nurse. Determining that ibuprofen is classified as an NSAID will help you to determine that it would not be combined with anticoagulants. Also recalling that hypoglycemia can occur as an adverse effect will help you to recall that these medications would not be combined. From the remaining options, it is necessary to remember that toxicity can result if NSAIDs are combined with calcium-channel blockers.

9. 4

Rationale: The normal reference range for the glycosylated hemoglobin A1C (HgbA1C) is 4.0% to 6.0%. This test measures the amount of glucose that has become permanently bound to the red blood cells from circulating glucose. Elevations in the blood glucose level will cause elevations in the amount of glycosylation. Thus, the test is useful in identifying clients who have periods of hyperglycemia that are undetected in other ways. Therefore, an HgbA1C of 9% is elevated. Elevations indicate continued need for teaching related to the prevention of hyperglycemic episodes.

Test-Taking Strategy: Focus on the subject, a HgbA1C level of 9%. Recalling the normal value and that an elevated value indicates hyperglycemia will assist in directing you to the correct option.

10. 1

Rationale: The normal white blood cell count ranges from 5000 mm³ to 10,000 mm³. The client who has a decrease in the number of circulating white blood cells is immunosuppressed. The nurse implements neutropenic precautions when the client's values fall sufficiently below the normal level. The specific value for implementing neutropenic precautions usually is determined by agency policy. The remaining options are normal values.

Test-Taking Strategy: Focus on the subject, the need to implement neutropenic precautions. Recalling that the normal white blood cell count ranges from 5000 mm³ to 10,000 mm³ will direct you to the correct option.

11. 4

Rationale: The action that the nurse must take is to draw a sample for PT and INR level to determine the client's anticoagulation status and risk for bleeding. These results will provide information as to how to best treat this client (e.g., if an antidote such as vitamin K or a blood transfusion is needed). The aPTT monitors the effects of heparin therapy.

Test-Taking Strategy: Focus on the subject, client who has taken an excessive dose of warfarin. Eliminate the option with aPTT first because it is unrelated to warfarin therapy and relates to heparin therapy. Next, eliminate the options indicating to administer an antidote and to transfuse the client because these therapies would not be implemented unless the PT and INR levels were known.

12. 2

Rationale: The primary concern with opioid analgesics is respiratory depression and hypotension. Based on the findings, the nurse would suspect opioid overdose. The nurse needs to first attempt to arouse the client and then reassess the vital signs. The vital signs may begin to normalize once the client is aroused because sleep can also cause decreased heart rate, blood pressure, respiratory rate, and oxygen saturation. The nurse would also check to see how much medication has been taken via the PCA pump and would continue to monitor the client closely to determine whether further action is needed. The nurse must notify the registered nurse as the next step after attempting to arouse the client. The nurse would also then document the findings after all data is collected, the client is stabilized, and if an abnormality still exists after arousing the client.

Test-Taking Strategy: First, focus on the data in the question and determine whether an abnormality exists. It is clear that an abnormality exists because the client is drowsy and the vital sounds are outside of the normal range. Next, note the strategic word, *first*. Recall that attempting to arouse the client would come before further checking the pump. The client must always be checked before the equipment and before documentation.

13. 3

Rationale: The normal hemoglobin level for an adult female client is 12 g/dL to 16 g/dL. Iron deficiency anemia can result in lower hemoglobin levels. Dehydration may increase the hemoglobin level by hemoconcentration. Heart failure and chronic obstructive pulmonary disease may increase the hemoglobin level as a result of the body's need for more oxygen-carrying capacity.

Test-Taking Strategy: Note the strategic words *most likely*. Evaluate each of the conditions in the options in terms of their pathophysiology and whether each is likely to raise or lower the hemoglobin level. Also, note the relationship between hemoglobin level in the question and the correct option.

14. 4

Rationale: A normal platelet count ranges from 150,000 mm^3 to 400,000 mm^3. The nurse would place the report containing the normal laboratory value in the client's medical record. A platelet count of 300,000 mm^3 is not an elevated count. The count also is not low; therefore, bleeding precautions are not needed.

Test-Taking Strategy: Focus on the subject, a platelet count of 300,000 mm^3. Remember, options that are comparable or alike are not likely to be correct. With this in mind, eliminate options indicating to report the abnormally low count and placing the client on bleeding precautions first. From the remaining options, recalling the normal range for this laboratory test will direct you to the correct option.

15. 4

Rationale: The normal fasting blood glucose level is 70 mg/dL to 99 mg/dL in the adult client. Values above the normal range must be evaluated to determine whether further intervention is needed. The most critical value is 240 mg/dL.

Test-Taking Strategy: First, eliminate options that are comparable or alike—75 mg/dL and 92 mg/dL—because they are both within the normal fasting blood glucose range. Next, consider the blood glucose level of 120 mg/dL and realize it is just above normal range and can be eliminated. A fasting blood glucose of 240 mg/dL would require contacting the primary health care provider for further prescriptions.

CHAPTER **11**

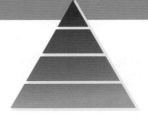

Nutritional Components of Care

PRIORITY CONCEPTS Health Promotion; Nutrition

WHAT WOULD YOU DO?

A client has been placed on fluid restriction because of an acute kidney injury. The client complains of thirst and asks what can be done to relieve this discomfort. What measures can the nurse tell the client to take to relieve thirst while adhering to the fluid restriction?
Answer is located on p. 124.

I. Nutrients

A. Carbohydrates
1. Carbohydrates are the preferred source of energy and provide 4 cal/g.
2. Carbohydrates promote normal fat metabolism, spare protein, and enhance lower gastrointestinal (GI) function.
3. Major food sources of carbohydrates include milk, grains, fruits, and vegetables.
4. Inadequate carbohydrate intake affects metabolism.

B. Fats
1. Fats provide a concentrated source and a stored form of energy and 9 cal/g.
2. Fats protect internal organs and maintain body temperature.
3. Fats enhance the absorption of fat-soluble vitamins.
4. Inadequate intake of essential fatty acids leads to clinical manifestations of sensitivity to cold, skin lesions, increased risk of infection, and amenorrhea in women.
5. Diets high in fat can lead to obesity and increase the risk of cardiovascular disease and some cancers.

C. Proteins
1. Amino acids, which make up proteins, are critical to all aspects of the growth and development of body tissues and provide 4 cal/g.

2. Proteins build and repair body tissues, regulate fluid balance, maintain acid-base balance, produce antibodies, provide energy, and produce enzymes and hormones.
3. Essential amino acids (EAAs) are required in the diet because the body cannot manufacture them.
4. Complete proteins contain all EAAs; incomplete proteins lack some of the essential fatty acids.
5. Inadequate protein intake can cause protein energy malnutrition and severe wasting of fat and muscle tissue.

D. Vitamins (Box 11.1)
1. Vitamins facilitate metabolism of proteins, fats, and carbohydrates, and act as catalysts for metabolic functions.
2. Vitamins promote life and growth processes, and maintain and regulate body functions.
3. Fat-soluble vitamins A, D, E, and K can be stored in the body, so an excess can cause toxicity.
4. The B vitamins and vitamin C are water soluble, are not stored in the body, and can be excreted in the urine.

 Major stages of the lifespan with specific nutritional needs are pregnancy, lactation, infancy, childhood, and adolescence. Adults and older adults may experience physiological aging changes, which influence individual nutritional needs.

E. Minerals and electrolytes (Box 11.2)
1. Minerals are components of hormones, cells, tissues, and bones.
2. Minerals act as catalysts for chemical reactions and enhancers of cell function.
3. Almost all foods contain some form of minerals.
4. A deficiency of minerals can develop in chronically ill or hospitalized clients.
5. Electrolytes play a major role in osmolality and body water regulation, acid-base balance, en-

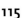

BOX 11.1   Examples of Food Sources of Vitamins

Water Soluble
- Folic acid: green, leafy vegetables; liver, beef, and fish; legumes
- Niacin: meats, poultry, fish, beans, peanuts, grains
- Vitamin B_1 (thiamine): pork, nuts, whole-grain cereals, legumes
- Vitamin B_2 (riboflavin): milk, lean meats, fish, grains
- Vitamin B_6 (pyridoxine): yeast, corn, meat, poultry, fish
- Vitamin B_{12} (cobalamin): meat, liver
- Vitamin C (ascorbic acid): citrus fruits, tomatoes, broccoli, cabbage

Fat Soluble
- Vitamin A: liver, egg yolk, whole milk, green or orange vegetables, fruits
- Vitamin D: fortified milk, fish oils, cereals
- Vitamin E: vegetable oils; green, leafy vegetables; cereals; apricots; apples; peaches
- Vitamin K: green, leafy vegetables; cauliflower; cabbage

BOX 11.2   Examples of Food Sources of Minerals

Calcium
Cheese
Collard greens
Milk and soy milk
Rhubarb
Sardines
Tofu
Yogurt

Chloride
Salt

Iron
Breads and cereals
Dark green vegetables
Dried fruits
Egg yolk
Legumes
Liver
Meats

Magnesium
Avocados
Canned white tuna
Cauliflower
Cooked rolled oats
Green, leafy vegetables
Milk
Peanut butter
Peas
Pork, beef, chicken
Potatoes
Raisins
Yogurt

Phosphorus
Fish
Nuts
Organ meats
Pork, beef, chicken
Whole-grain breads and cereals

Potassium
Avocado
Bananas
Cantaloupe
Carrots
Fish
Mushrooms
Oranges
Pork, beef, veal
Potatoes
Raisins
Spinach
Strawberries
Tomatoes

Sodium
Bacon
Butter
Canned food
Cheese
Cottage cheese
Cured pork
Hot dogs
Ketchup
Lunch meat
Milk
Mustard
Processed food
Snack food
Soy sauce
Table salt
White and whole-wheat bread

Zinc
Eggs
Green, leafy vegetables
Meats
Protein-rich foods

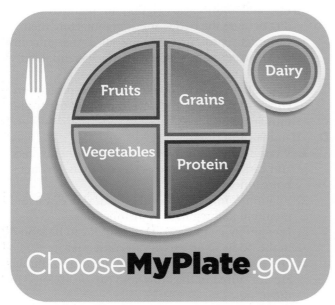

FIGURE 11.1 MyPlate. From US Department of Agriculture. http://www.choosemyplate.gov.

zyme reactions, and neuromuscular activity (see Chapter 8 for additional information on electrolytes).

⚠️ Always check the client's ability to eat and swallow and promote independence in eating as much as is possible.

II. MyPlate (Fig. 11.1)
A. Provides a description of a balanced diet that includes grains, vegetables, fruits, dairy products, and protein foods (refer to http://www.choosemyplate.gov/)

B. A nutritionist would be consulted for individualized dietary recommendations.
C. Guidelines
1. Avoid eating oversized portions of foods.
2. Fill half of the plate with fruits and vegetables.
3. Vary the type of vegetables and fruits eaten.
4. Select at least half of the grains as whole grains.
5. Ensure that foods from the dairy group are high in calcium.
6. Drink milk that is fat-free or low fat (1%).
7. Eat protein foods that are lean.
8. Select fresh foods over frozen or canned foods.
9. Drink water rather than liquids that contain sugar.

⚠ Always consider the client's cultural, spiritual, and personal choices when planning nutritional intake.

III. Therapeutic Diets

A. Clear liquid diet
  1. Indications
     a. Provides fluids and electrolytes to prevent dehydration
     b. Used as initial feeding after complete bowel rest
     c. Used initially to feed a malnourished person or a person who has not had any oral intake for some time
     d. Used for bowel preparation for surgery or diagnostic tests, as well as postoperatively and in clients with fever, vomiting, or diarrhea
     e. Used in gastroenteritis
  2. Nursing considerations
     a. Clear liquid diet is deficient in energy (calories) and many nutrients
     b. The body digests and absorbs clear liquids easily
     c. Contributes to little or no residue in the GI tract
     d. Can be unappetizing and boring
     e. As a transition diet, clear liquids are intended for short-term use only.
     f. Clear liquids and foods that are relatively transparent to light and are liquid at body temperature are considered "clear liquids," such as water, bouillon, clear broth, carbonated beverages, gelatin, hard candy, lemonade, ice pops, and regular or decaffeinated coffee or tea.
     g. By limiting caffeine intake, an upset stomach and sleeplessness may be prevented.
     h. Client may have salt or sugar.
     i. Dairy products and fruit juices with pulp are not clear liquids.

⚠ Monitor the client's hydration status by checking intake and output, checking weight, monitoring for edema, and monitoring for signs of dehydration. Each kilogram (2.2 lb) of weight gained or lost is equal to 1 L of fluid retained or lost.

B. Full liquid diet
  1. Indication: May be used as a transition diet after clear liquids after surgery or for clients who have difficulty chewing, swallowing, or tolerating solid foods
  2. Nursing considerations
     a. A full liquid diet is nutritionally deficient in energy (calories) and many nutrients.
     b. The diet includes both clear and opaque liquid foods and those that are liquid at body temperature.
     c. Foods include all clear liquids and items such as plain ice cream, sherbet, breakfast drinks, milk, pudding and custard, soups that are strained, refined cooked cereals, fruit juices, and strained vegetable juices.
     d. Use of a complete nutritional liquid supplement is often necessary to meet nutrient needs for clients on a full liquid diet for more than 3 days.

⚠ Provide nutritional supplements such as those high in protein, as prescribed for the client on a liquid diet.

C. Mechanical soft diet
  1. Indications
     a. Provides foods that have been mechanically altered in texture to require minimal chewing
     b. Used for clients who have difficulty chewing but who can tolerate more variety in texture than a liquid diet offers
     c. Used for clients who have dental problems, surgery of the head or neck, or dysphagia (requires swallowing evaluation and may require thickened liquids if the client has swallowing difficulties)
  2. Nursing considerations
     a. Degree of texture modification depends on individual need, including puréed, mashed, ground, or chopped.
     b. Foods to be avoided in mechanically altered diets include nuts; dried fruit; raw fruits and vegetables; fried foods; chocolate candy; tough, smoked, or salted meats; and foods with coarse textures.

D. Soft diet
  1. Indications
     a. Used for clients with difficulty chewing or swallowing
     b. Used for clients with ulcerations of the mouth or gums, broken jaws, or dysphagia, and for those who have experienced oral surgery, plastic surgery of the head or neck, or stroke
  2. Nursing considerations
     a. Clients with mouth sores would be served foods at cooler temperatures.
     b. Clients who have difficulty chewing and swallowing because the reduced flow of saliva can increase salivary flow by sucking on sour candy.
     c. Encourage the client to eat a variety of foods.
     d. Provide plenty of fluids with meals to ease chewing and swallowing of foods.
     e. Drinking fluids through a straw may be easier than drinking from a cup or glass; a straw may not be allowed for a client with dysphagia (because of the risk of aspiration).
     f. All foods and seasonings are permitted; however, liquid, chopped, or puréed foods or regular foods with a soft consistency are tolerated best.

g. Foods that contain nuts or seeds, which can easily become trapped in the mouth and cause discomfort, would be avoided.

h. Raw fruits and vegetables, fried foods, and whole grains would be avoided.

 Consider the client's disease or illness, and how it may affect his or her nutritional status.

E. Low-fiber (low-residue) diet
   1. Indications
      a. Supplies foods that are least likely to form an obstruction when the intestinal tract is narrowed by inflammation or scarring or when GI motility is slowed
      b. Used for inflammatory bowel disease, partial obstructions of the intestinal tract, gastroenteritis, diarrhea, or other GI disorders
   2. Nursing considerations
      a. Foods that are low in residue include white bread, refined cooked cereals, cooked potatoes without skins, white rice, and refined pasta.
      b. Foods to limit or avoid are raw fruits (except bananas), vegetables, nuts and seeds, plant fiber, and whole grains.
      c. Dairy products would be limited to 2 servings a day.

F. High-fiber (high-residue) diet
   1. Indications: Used for clients with constipation; irritable bowel syndrome, when the primary symptom is alternating constipation and diarrhea; and asymptomatic diverticular disease
   2. Nursing considerations
      a. Provides 25 g to 35 g of dietary fiber daily
      b. Adds volume and weight to the stool and speeds the movement of undigested materials through the intestine
      c. Consists of fruits, vegetables, and whole-grain products
      d. Increase fiber gradually and provide adequate fluids to reduce possible undesirable side effects such as abdominal cramps, bloating, diarrhea, and dehydration.
      e. Gas-forming foods would be limited (Box 11.3).

G. Cardiac diet
   1. Indications
      a. Indicated for atherosclerosis, diabetes mellitus, hyperlipidemia, hypertension, myocardial infarction, nephrotic syndrome, and renal failure
      b. Reduces the risk of heart disease
      c. Dietary Approaches to Stop Hypertension (DASH) diet: recommended to prevent and control hypertension, hypercholesterolemia, and obesity
      d. The DASH diet includes fruits, vegetables, whole grains, and low-fat dairy foods; meat, fish, poultry, nuts, and beans; and is limited

---

BOX 11.3   Gas-Forming Foods

- Apples
- Artichokes
- Barley
- Beans
- Bran
- Broccoli
- Brussels sprouts
- Cabbage
- Celery
- Figs

- Melons
- Milk
- Molasses
- Nuts
- Onions
- Radishes
- Soybeans
- Wheat
- Yeast

---

in sugar-sweetened foods and beverages, red meat, and added fats.
   2. Nursing consideration: Restricts total amounts of fat, including saturated, trans, polyunsaturated, and monounsaturated; cholesterol; and sodium (Box 11.4)

H. Fat-restricted diet
   1. Indications
      a. Used to reduce symptoms of abdominal pain, steatorrhea, flatulence, and diarrhea associated with a high intake of dietary fat, and to decrease nutrient losses caused by the ingestion of dietary fat in individuals with malabsorption disorders
      b. Used for clients with malabsorption disorders, pancreatitis, gallbladder disease, and gastroesophageal reflux
   2. Nursing considerations
      a. Restricts the total amount of fat, including saturated fats, trans fats, polyunsaturated fats, and monounsaturated fats
      b. Clients with malabsorption may also have difficulty tolerating fiber and lactose.
      c. Vitamin and mineral deficiencies may occur in clients with diarrhea or steatorrhea.
      d. A fecal-fat test may be prescribed and indicates fat malabsorption with the excretion of more than 6 g to 8 g of fat (or more than 10% of the fat consumed) per day during the 3 days of specimen collection.

I. High-calorie, high-protein diet
   1. Indications: Severe stress, burns, cancer, human immunodeficiency virus (HIV) infection, acquired immunodeficiency syndrome (AIDS), chronic obstructive pulmonary disease, respiratory failure, or any other type of debilitating disease
   2. Nursing considerations
      a. Encourage nutrient-dense, high-calorie, high-protein foods such as whole milk and milk products, peanut butter, nuts, seeds, beef, chicken, fish, pork, and eggs.
      b. Encourage snacks between meals, such as milkshakes, instant breakfasts, and nutritional supplements.

BOX 11.4 Sodium-Free Spices and Flavorings

- Allspice
- Almond extract
- Bay leaves
- Caraway seeds
- Cinnamon
- Curry powder
- Garlic powder or garlic
- Ginger
- Lemon extract
- Maple extract
- Marjoram
- Mustard powder
- Nutmeg

! Calorie counts assist in determining the client's total nutritional intake and can identify a deficit or excess intake.

J. Carbohydrate-consistent diet
  1. Indications: Diabetes mellitus, hypoglycemia, hyperglycemia, and obesity
  2. Nursing considerations
     a. The Exchange System for Meal Planning, developed by the Academy of Nutrition and Dietetics and the American Diabetes Association, is a food guide that may be recommended.
     b. The Exchange System groups foods according to the amounts of carbohydrates, fats, and proteins that they contain; major food groups include the carbohydrate, the meat and meat substitute, and the fat groups.
     c. A carbohydrate consistent diet focuses on maintaining a consistent amount of carbohydrate intake each day and with each meal; also known as "carb counting." For additional information, refer to http://www.livestrong.com/article/436101-the-consistent-carbohydrate-diet-for-diabetics/.
     d. The MyPlate diet may also be recommended.
K. Sodium-restricted diet (see Box 11.4)
  1. Indications: Used for hypertension, heart failure, kidney disease, cardiac disease, and liver disease
  2. Nursing considerations
     a. Individualized; can include 4 g of sodium daily (no-added-salt diet), 2 to 3 g of sodium daily (moderate restriction), 1 g of sodium daily (strict restriction), or 500 mg of sodium daily (severe restriction and seldom prescribed)
     b. Encourage the intake of fresh rather than processed foods, which contain higher amounts of sodium.
     c. Canned, frozen, instant, smoked, pickled, and boxed items usually contain higher amounts of sodium. Lunch meats, soy sauce, salad dressings, fast foods, soups, and snacks such as potato chips and pretzels also contain large amounts of sodium.
     d. Certain medications contain significant amounts of sodium.
     e. Salt substitutes may be used to improve palatability. Most salt substitutes contain large amounts of potassium and would not be used by clients with renal disease.

L. Protein-restricted diet
  1. Indications: Used for renal disease and end-stage liver disease
  2. The nutritional status of critically ill clients with protein-losing renal diseases, malabsorption syndromes, and continuous renal replacement therapy or dialysis would have their protein needs assessed by estimating the protein equivalent of total nitrogen appearance (PNA); a nutritionist would be consulted.
  3. Nursing considerations
     a. Provide enough protein to maintain nutritional status but not an amount that will allow for the buildup of waste products from protein metabolism (40–60 g of protein daily).
     b. The less protein allowed, the more important it becomes that all protein in the diet be of high biological value (contain all EAAs in recommended proportions).
     c. An adequate total energy intake from foods is critical for clients on protein-restricted diets. (Protein will be used for energy rather than for protein synthesis.)
     d. Special low-protein products, such as pastas, bread, cookies, wafers, and gelatin made with wheat starch, can improve energy intake and add variety to the diet.
     e. Carbohydrates in powdered or liquid form can also provide additional energy.
     f. Vegetables and fruits contain some protein. For very low-protein diets, these foods must be calculated into the diet.
     g. Foods from the milk, meat, bread, and starch groups are limited.
M. Gluten-free diet: A treatment for celiac disease and gluten sensitivity for clients needing the protein fraction "gluten" eliminated from their diet. See Chapter 31 for information on this diet.

! Fluid restriction may be prescribed for clients with hyponatremia, severe extracellular fluid volume excess, and renal disorders. Ask client specifically about preferences regarding types of oral fluids and temperature preference of fluids.

N. Renal diet (see Box 11.2)
  1. Indications: Used for the client with acute kidney injury and chronic kidney disease, and those requiring hemodialysis or peritoneal dialysis
  2. Nursing considerations
     a. Controlled amounts of protein, sodium, phosphorus, calcium, potassium, and fluids may be prescribed; may also require modifications of the amounts of fiber, cholesterol, and fat based on individual requirements; clients receiving peritoneal dialysis usually have diets prescribed that are less restrictive with fluid and protein intake than those receiving hemodialysis.
     b. Most clients who are receiving dialysis need to restrict fluids (Box 11.5).

> **BOX 11.5** **Measures to Relieve Thirst**
>
> Chew gum or suck hard candy.
> Freeze fluids so that they take longer to consume.
> Add lemon juice to water to make it more refreshing.
> Gargle with refrigerated mouthwash.

> ⚠ Initial data collection includes identifying allergies and food and medication interactions.

O. Potassium-modified diet (see Box 11.2)
  1. Indications
    a. A low-potassium diet is indicated for hyperkalemia, which may be the result of impaired renal function, hypoaldosteronism, Addison's disease, angiotensin-converting enzyme inhibitor medications, immunosuppressive medications, potassium-retaining diuretics, and chronic hyperkalemia.
    b. A high-potassium diet is indicated for hypokalemia, which may be the result of renal tubular acidosis, GI losses (diarrhea, vomiting), intracellular shifts, potassium-wasting diuretics, antibiotics, mineralocorticoid or glucocorticoid excess resulting from primary or secondary aldosteronism, Cushing's syndrome, or exogenous corticosteroid use.

  2. Nursing considerations
    a. Foods that are low in potassium include applesauce, green beans, cabbage, lettuce, peppers, grapes, blueberries, cooked summer squash, cooked turnip greens, fresh pineapple, and raspberries.
    b. Box 11.2 lists foods that are high in potassium.
P. High-calcium diet
  1. Indications: Calcium is needed during bone growth and in adulthood to prevent osteoporosis and facilitate vascular contraction and vasodilation, muscle contraction, and nerve transmission.
  2. Nursing considerations
    a. Primary dietary sources of calcium are dairy products (see Box 11.2 for food items high in calcium).
    b. Clients with lactose intolerance need to incorporate nondairy sources of calcium into their diet regularly.
Q. Low-purine diet
  1. Indications: Used for gout, kidney stones, and elevated uric acid levels
  2. Nursing considerations
    a. Purine is a precursor of uric acid, which forms stones and crystals.
    b. Foods to restrict include anchovies, herring, mackerel, sardines, scallops, organ meats, gravies, meat extracts, wild game, goose, and sweetbreads.

R. High-iron diet
  1. Indication: Used for anemia
  2. Nursing considerations
    a. The high-iron diet replaces an iron deficit caused by inadequate intake or loss.
    b. The diet includes organ meats; meat; egg yolks; whole-wheat products; dark green, leafy vegetables; dried fruit; and legumes.
    c. Inform the client that concurrent intake of vitamin C with iron foods enhances the absorption of iron.

IV. Vegan and Vegetarian Diets

A. Vegan
  1. Vegans follow a strict vegetarian diet and consume no animal foods.
  2. Eat only foods of plant origin (e.g., whole or enriched grains, legumes, nuts, seeds, fruits, vegetables).
  3. The use of soybeans, soy milk, soybean curd (tofu), and processed soy protein products enhance the nutritional value of the diet.
B. Lacto-vegetarian
  1. Lacto-vegetarians eat milk, cheese, and dairy foods but avoid meat, fish, poultry, and eggs.
  2. A diet of whole or enriched grains, legumes, nuts, seeds, fruits, and vegetables in sufficient quantities to meet energy needs provides a balanced diet.
C. Lacto-ovo-vegetarian
  1. Lacto-ovo-vegetarians follow a food pattern that allows for the consumption of dairy products and eggs.
  2. Consumption of adequate plant and animal food sources that excludes meat, poultry, pork, and fish poses no nutritional risks.
D. Ovo-vegetarians: The only animal foods that the ovo-vegetarian consumes are eggs, which are an excellent source of complete proteins.
E. Nursing considerations
  1. Vegan and vegetarian diets are not usually prescribed but are a diet choice made by a client.
  2. Ensure that the client eats a sufficient amount of varied foods to meet nutrient and energy needs.
  3. Clients need to be educated about consuming complementary proteins over the course of each day to ensure that all EAAs are provided.
  4. Potential deficiencies in vegetarian diets include energy, protein, vitamin B_{12}, zinc, iron, calcium, omega-3 fatty acids, and vitamin D (if limited exposure to sunlight).
  5. To enhance the absorption of iron, vegetarians would consume a good source of iron and vitamin C with each meal.
  6. Foods eaten may include tofu, tempeh, soy milk and soy products, meat analogs, legumes, nuts and seeds, sprouts, and a variety of fruits and vegetables.

7. Soy protein is considered equivalent in quality to animal protein.

⚠️ Body mass index (BMI) can be calculated by dividing the client's weight in kilograms by height in meters squared. For example, a client who weighs 75 kg (165 lbs) and is 1.8 m (5 feet, 9 inches) tall has a BMI of 23.15 ($75 \div$ by $1.8^2 = 23.15$). From Potter et al. (2013), p. 1008.

V. Enteral Nutrition

A. Description: Provides liquefied foods to the GI tract via a tube
B. Indications
   1. When the GI tract is functional but oral intake is not meeting estimated nutrient needs
   2. Used for clients with swallowing problems, burns, major trauma, liver or other organ failure, or severe malnutrition
C. Nursing considerations
   1. Clients with lactose intolerance (diarrhea, bloating, cramping) need to be placed on lactose-free formulas.
   2. See Chapter 18 for information regarding the administration of GI tube feedings and associated complications.

VI. Parenteral Nutrition

A. Description
   1. Parenteral nutrition (PN) (also termed *hyperalimentation or total parenteral nutrition [TPN]*) supplies nutrients via the veins.
   2. PN consists of both partial parenteral nutrition (PPN) and TPN. The indication of the type used depends on the client's nutritional needs.
   3. Supplies carbohydrates in the form of dextrose; fats in a special emulsified form; proteins in the form of amino acids; vitamins; minerals; electrolytes; and water.
   4. Prevents subcutaneous fat and muscle protein from being catabolized by the body for energy.
   5. PN solutions are hypertonic because of their higher concentration of glucose and the addition of amino acids.
B. Indications
   1. Clients with a severely dysfunctional or nonfunctional GI tracts who are unable to process nutrients may benefit from PN.
   2. Clients who can take some oral nutrition (but not enough to meet their nutrient requirements) may benefit from PN.
   3. Clients with multiple GI surgeries, GI trauma, severe intolerance to enteral feedings, intestinal obstructions, or those who need to rest the bowel for healing may benefit from PN.
   4. Clients with severe nutritionally deficient conditions, such as AIDS, cancer, burn injuries, or mal-

nutrition, or clients receiving chemotherapy, may benefit from PN.

⚠️ PN is a form of nutrition and is used when there is no other nutritional alternative. Other routes of administering nutrition, such as oral or via a GI tube, are initiated first.

C. Administration of PN
   1. PPN
      a. PPN: usually administered through a large distal vein in the arm with a standard peripheral (intravenous [IV]) catheter or midline or through a peripherally inserted central catheter (PICC).
      b. If a PICC cannot be established, the subclavian vein or internal or external jugular veins can be used for PPN.
   2. TPN: Administered through a central vein; the use of a PICC is acceptable.
   3. If the bag of PN is empty and the nurse needs to wait for the delivery of a new bag of solution from the pharmacy, a 10% dextrose solution in water would be infused at the prescribed rate to prevent hypoglycemia.

⚠️ The delivery of hypertonic solutions into peripheral veins can cause sclerosis, phlebitis, or swelling. Monitor closely for these complications.

D. Fat emulsion (lipids)
   1. Lipids provide up to 30% of calorie (energy) needs, nonprotein calories, and prevent or correct fatty-acid deficiency.
   2. Lipid solutions are isotonic and therefore can be administered through a peripheral or central vein.
   3. Most fat emulsions are prepared from soybean or  safflower oil with egg yolk to provide emulsification. The primary components are linoleic, oleic, palmitic, linolenic, and stearic acids (assess the client for allergies).
   4. Glucose-intolerant clients or those with diabetes mellitus may benefit from receiving a larger percentage of their PN from lipids, which helps control blood glucose levels and lower insulin requirements caused by infused dextrose.
   5. The bottle is examined for the separation of the emulsion into layers, fat globules, and the accumulation of froth. If observed, it is not used and is returned to the pharmacy.
   6. Additives would not be put into the fat emulsion solution.
   7. Monitor vital signs every 10 minutes, and observe for adverse reactions for the first 30 minutes of administration. If signs of an adverse reaction occur, stop the infusion and notify the registered nurse (Box 11.6).
   8. Serum lipids are checked 4 hours after discontinuing the infusion.

BOX 11.6   Signs of an Adverse Reaction to Lipids

- Chest and back pain
- Chills
- Cyanosis
- Diaphoresis
- Dyspnea
- Fever
- Flushing; rash
- Headache
- Nausea and vomiting
- Pressure over the eyes
- Thrombophlebitis
- Vertigo

⚠ Fat emulsions (lipids) contain egg yolk phospholipids and must not be given to clients with egg allergies.

E. Additional additives to PN solutions
1. Vitamins are usually added to meet needs and prevent deficiencies.
2. Minerals and trace elements may be added to promote normal metabolism.
3. Electrolytes may be added to correct losses related to organ dysfunction and disease processes.
4. Water amounts in PN are determined by electrolyte balance and fluid requirements.
5. Insulin may be added to control blood glucose levels because of the high concentration of glucose in the PN solution.
6. Heparin may be added to reduce the buildup of a fibrinous clot at the tip of centrally inserted catheters.

VII. Complications of Parenteral Nutrition and Nursing Considerations

A. See Table 11.1
B. The PN solution is checked with the primary health care provider's (PHCP's) prescription to ensure that the prescribed components are contained in the solution.
C. To prevent infection and solution incompatibility, IV medications and blood are not given through the PN line.
D. The partial thromboplastin time and prothrombin time are monitored for clients receiving anticoagulants.
E. Laboratory studies such as electrolyte and albumin levels and liver and renal function studies will be prescribed and monitored on a regular basis.
F. In severely dehydrated clients, the albumin level may drop initially after beginning PN, because the treatment restores hydration.
G. With severely malnourished clients, monitor for "refeeding syndrome" (a rapid drop in potassium, magnesium, and phosphate serum levels); monitor for shallow respirations, confusion, weakness, bleeding tendencies, and seizures (the RN is notified immediately if these signs occur and the primary HCP will be contacted).
H. Abnormal liver function values may indicate intolerance to, or an excess of, fat emulsion or problems with the metabolism of glucose and protein.

I. Abnormal renal function tests may indicate an excess of amino acids.
J. PN solutions need to be refrigerated and administered within 24 hours from the time that they were prepared. (They are removed from the refrigerator 0.5–1 hour before use.)
K. PN solutions that are cloudy or darkened must not be used and need to be returned to the pharmacy.
L. Additions to PN solutions need to be made in the pharmacy and not in the nursing unit.
M. Consultation with the nutritionist must be done on a regular basis (as prescribed or per agency protocol).
N. Discontinuing PN therapy
1. Evaluation of nutritional status by a nutritionist is done before PN is discontinued.
2. If discontinuation is prescribed, the flow rate is gradually decreased for 1 to 2 hours while increasing oral intake (this assists in preventing hypoglycemia).
3. After the IV catheter is removed, the dressing is changed daily until the insertion site heals.
4. Encourage oral nutrition.
5. Record oral intake, body weight, and laboratory results of serum electrolyte and glucose levels.

⚠ Abrupt discontinuation of a PN solution can result in hypoglycemia. The flow rate needs to be decreased gradually when the PN is discontinued.

VIII. Reinforcement of Home-Care Instructions (Box 11.7)

BOX 11.7   Home-Care Instructions

- Reinforce to the client and caregiver how to administer and maintain parenteral nutrition fluids.
- Reinforce to the client and the caregiver how to change a sterile dressing.
- Obtain a daily weight at the same time of day in the same clothes.
- Stress that weight gain of more than 3 lb/week may indicate excessive fluid intake and needs to be reported.
- Monitor the blood glucose level, and report abnormalities immediately.
- Check for signs and symptoms of infection, thrombosis, air embolism, and catheter displacement.
- Teach the client and caregiver about the signs and symptoms of side or adverse effects such as infection, thrombosis, air embolism, and catheter displacement.
- Teach the client and caregiver the actions to take if a complication arises and about the importance of reporting complications to the primary health care provider.
- For symptoms of thrombosis, the client must report edema of the arm or at the catheter insertion site, neck pain, and jugular vein distention.
- The leakage of fluid from the insertion site or pain or discomfort as the fluids are infused may indicate the displacement of the catheter. This must be reported immediately.
- Reinforce to the client and caregiver the importance of follow-up care.
- Teach the client to keep electronic infusion devices fully charged in case of electrical power failure.

TABLE 11.1   Complications of Parenteral Nutrition

Complication	Possible Cause	Signs/Symptoms	Intervention	Prevention
Air embolism	▪ Catheter system is opened or IV tubing is disconnected ▪ Air entry occurs on IV tubing changes	▪ Apprehension ▪ Chest pain ▪ Dyspnea ▪ Hypotension ▪ Loud churning sound heard over the pericardium on auscultation ▪ Rapid and weak pulse ▪ Respiratory distress	▪ Catheter is clamped ▪ The client placed in a left-side-lying position with the head lower than the feet ▪ Notify the RN and PHCP ▪ Administer oxygen	▪ Make sure all catheter connections are secure ▪ The catheter is clamped when not in use ▪ The client is instructed in Valsalva's maneuver for tubing and cap changes ▪ For tubing and cap changes, the client is placed in Trendelenburg's position (if not contraindicated), with the head turned in the opposite direction of the insertion site
Hyperglycemia	▪ Client is receiving solution too quickly ▪ Not enough insulin	▪ Restlessness ▪ Weakness ▪ Confusion ▪ Diaphoresis ▪ Elevated blood glucose level >200 mg/dL ▪ Excessive thirst ▪ Fatigue ▪ Kussmaul's respirations	▪ Notify the RN and PHCP ▪ May need to slow the infusion rate ▪ Administer regular insulin as prescribed ▪ Monitor blood glucose level	▪ Check the client for a history of glucose intolerance ▪ Check the client's medication history
Hypervolemia	▪ Excessive fluid administration or administration of fluid too rapidly ▪ Renal dysfunction ▪ Heart failure ▪ Hepatic failure	▪ Bounding pulse ▪ Crackles on lung auscultation ▪ Headache ▪ Increased blood pressure ▪ Jugular vein distention ▪ Weight gain greater than desired	▪ The IV infusion is slowed or stopped ▪ Restrict fluids as prescribed ▪ Diuretics ▪ Dialysis (in extreme cases)	▪ Check the client's history for risk for hypervolemia ▪ Ensure proper function of the electronic infusion device ▪ Monitor weight daily and intake and output
Hypoglycemia	▪ PN abruptly discontinued ▪ Too much insulin is being administered	▪ Anxiety ▪ Diaphoresis ▪ Hunger ▪ Low blood glucose level <70 mg/dL ▪ Shakiness ▪ Weakness	▪ The RN and PHCP is notified ▪ Assist to administer IV dextrose ▪ Monitor blood glucose level	▪ PN solution is gradually decreased when discontinuing it ▪ 10% dextrose is infused at the same rate as the PN to prevent hypoglycemia when the PN solution is discontinued ▪ Monitor glucose level when insulin is being given
Infection	▪ Poor aseptic technique ▪ Catheter contamination ▪ Contamination of solution	▪ Chills ▪ Fever ▪ Elevated white blood cell count ▪ Redness or drainage at the insertion site	▪ Notify the RN and PHCP ▪ Assist with removal of catheter ▪ Send the catheter tip to the laboratory for culture ▪ Prepare to assist to obtain blood cultures ▪ Prepare to assist with antibiotic administration	▪ Use strict aseptic technique ▪ Monitor temperature ▪ Check the IV site for signs of infection ▪ Assist to change site dressing, solution, and tubing as specified by agency policy ▪ Avoid disconnecting tubing unnecessarily
Pneumothorax	▪ Inexact catheter placement	▪ Chest or shoulder pain ▪ Sudden shortness of breath ▪ Tachycardia ▪ Cyanosis ▪ Absence of breath sounds on affected side	▪ The RN and PHCP are notified ▪ Prepare to obtain a chest x-ray ▪ Small pneumothorax may resolve ▪ Larger pneumothorax may require chest tube	▪ Monitor for signs of pneumothorax ▪ A chest x-ray is obtained after the insertion of the catheter to ensure proper placement ▪ PN is not initiated until correct catheter placement is verified and the absence of pneumothorax is confirmed

IV, Intravenous; *PHCP*, primary health care provider; *PN*, parenteral nutrition; *RN*, registered nurse.
Adapted from Ignatavicius D, Workman M: Medical-surgical nursing: patient-centered collaborative care, ed 7, St. Louis, 2013, Saunders.

Nursing Sciences

WHAT WOULD YOU DO?

Answer: The client with acute kidney injury may be placed on fluid restriction because of decreased renal function and glomerular filtration rate, resulting in fluid volume excess. To allow the kidneys to rest, decreased fluid consumption may be indicated. When a client is placed on this restriction, increased thirst may be a problem. The nurse would instruct the client in measures to relieve thirst in order to promote adherence to the fluid restriction. These measures include chewing gum or sucking hard candy, freezing fluids so they take longer to consume, adding lemon juice to water to make it more refreshing, and gargling with refrigerated mouthwash.

PRACTICE QUESTIONS

1. A client is having problems with blood clotting. Which food item would the nurse encourage the client to eat?
1. Legumes
2. Citrus fruits
3. Vegetable oils
4. Green, leafy vegetables

❖ **2.** When reinforcing dietary instructions to a client with irritable bowel syndrome whose primary symptom is alternating constipation and diarrhea, the nurse would tell the client that which foods are **best** to include in the diet for this disorder? **Select all that apply.**
☐ 1. Beans
☐ 2. Apples
☐ 3. Cabbage
☐ 4. Brussels sprouts
☐ 5. Whole-grain bread

3. A hospitalized client is a lacto-vegetarian. Which food item would the nurse remove from the meal tray?
1. Eggs
2. Milk
3. Cheese
4. Broccoli

4. A low-sodium diet has been prescribed for a client with hypertension. Which food selected from the menu by the client indicates an understanding of this diet?
1. Baked turkey
2. Tomato soup
3. Boiled shrimp
4. Chicken gumbo

5. The nurse is providing dietary instructions to a client with gout. The nurse needs to tell the client that which food item will exacerbate the condition?
1. Scallops
2. Chocolate
3. Cornbread
4. Macaroni products

6. A clear liquid diet has been prescribed for a client with gastroenteritis. Which item is appropriate to offer to the client?
1. Soft custard
2. Orange juice
3. Clam chowder
4. Fat-free beef broth

7. A client with heart disease is instructed regarding a low-fat diet. The nurse determines that the client understands the diet if the client states it is acceptable to eat which food item?
1. Steak
2. Apples
3. Cheese
4. Pizza without pepperoni

8. The nurse reinforces instructions to a client to increase the amount of riboflavin in the diet. The nurse would tell the client to select which food item that is high in riboflavin?
1. Milk
2. Tomatoes
3. Citrus fruits
4. Green, leafy vegetables

9. A client with a burn injury is transferred to the nursing unit, and a regular diet has been prescribed. The nurse encourages the client to eat which dietary items to promote wound healing?
1. Veal, potatoes, gelatin, and orange juice
2. Chicken breast, broccoli, strawberries, and milk
3. Peanut butter and jelly sandwich, cantaloupe, and tea
4. Spaghetti with tomato sauce, garlic bread, and ginger ale

10. The nurse has completed diet teaching for a client who has been prescribed a low-sodium diet to treat hypertension. The nurse determines that there is a

need for further teaching when the client makes which statement?
1. "This diet will help lower my blood pressure."
2. "Fresh foods such as fruits and vegetables are high in sodium."

3. "This diet is not a replacement for my antihypertensive medications."
4. "The reason I need to lower my salt intake is to reduce fluid retention."

ANSWERS

1. 4
Rationale: Green, leafy vegetables are high in vitamin K, which acts as a catalyst for facilitating blood-clotting factors. Legumes are high in folic acid and thiamine. Citrus fruits are high in vitamin C, which helps with wound healing. Vegetable oil is high in vitamin E, which acts as an antioxidant.
Test-Taking Strategy: First, focus on the subject, problems with blood clotting, and recall that vitamin K is involved in the clotting process. Next, determine the food sources that are high in vitamin K.

❖ **2. 2, 5**
Rationale: A high-fiber, high-residue diet is used for constipation; irritable bowel syndrome, when the primary symptom is alternating constipation and diarrhea; and asymptomatic diverticular disease. High-fiber foods include fruits and vegetables and whole-grain products. Gas-forming foods such as beans, cabbage, and Brussels sprouts need to be limited.
Test-Taking Strategy: Note the strategic word, *best*, and focus on the data in the question. Note that the client has irritable bowel syndrome whose primary symptom is alternating constipation and diarrhea. Think about the food items that would increase irritability in the bowel to direct you to the correct option.

3. 1
Rationale: Lacto-vegetarians eat milk, cheese, and dairy foods, but avoid meat, fish, poultry, and eggs.
Test-Taking Strategy: Focus on the subject, lacto-vegetarian. With that in mind, immediately eliminate broccoli. From the remaining options, note that milk and cheese are dairy products, making them comparable or alike, so they can be eliminated. Eggs are the food items that are not consumed by lacto-vegetarians; however, they are eaten by lacto-ovo vegetarians.

4. 1
Rationale: Regular soup (1 cup) contains 900 mg of sodium. Fresh shellfish (1 oz) contains 50 mg of sodium. Poultry (1 oz) contains 25 mg of sodium.
Test-Taking Strategy: Eliminate tomato soup and chicken gumbo first, because they are comparable or alike. Also, recall that canned foods are high in sodium. From the remaining

options, select baked turkey, remembering that shellfish is also high in sodium, even if it is boiled.

5. 1
Rationale: Scallops would be omitted from the diet of a client who has gout because of the high purine content; this food item would exacerbate the condition. The food items identified in the remaining options have negligible purine content and may be consumed by the client with gout.
Test-Taking Strategy: Focus on the subject, the food item that will exacerbate the condition. Note the client's diagnosis of gout, and think about the pathophysiology associated with this condition. Recalling the food items that are high in purine will direct you to the correct option.

6. 4
Rationale: A clear liquid diet consists of foods that are relatively transparent. Soft custard and orange juice would be included in a full liquid diet because they are opaque, not clear. Clam chowder is opaque and also includes pieces of clams, thus eliminating it from a full liquid diet.
Test-Taking Strategy: Focus on the subject, clear liquid diet. Remember that a clear liquid diet consists of foods that are relatively transparent. This will direct you to fat-free beef broth, because this is the only food item that is transparent.

7. 2
Rationale: Fruits contain minimal amounts of fat so apples are acceptable to eat. Steak, cheese, and pizza are high in fat. Even though pepperoni is removed from the pizza, the cheese and ingredients in the crust make pizza high in fat.
Test-Taking Strategy: Focus on the subject, the food item low in fat that is acceptable to eat. First note that cheese and pizza are comparable or alike in that pizza has cheese on it, so they can be eliminated. From the remaining options, recall that apples contain minimal fat as compared with steak, which is high in fat.

8. 1
Rationale: Food sources of riboflavin include milk, lean meats, fish, and grains. Tomatoes and citrus fruits are high in vitamin C. Green leafy vegetables are high in folic acid.
Test-Taking Strategy: Focus on the subject, food sources high in riboflavin. Knowledge regarding food items that are high in riboflavin is required to answer this question. Remember that milk is a food source of riboflavin, so this will help you eliminate the remaining options.

9. 2

Rationale: Protein and vitamin C are necessary for wound healing. Poultry and milk are good sources of protein. Broccoli and strawberries are good sources of vitamin C. Peanut butter is a source of niacin. Gelatin and jelly have no nutrient value. Spaghetti is a complex carbohydrate.

Test-Taking Strategy: Focus on the subject, promoting wound healing, and recall that protein and vitamin C are necessary for wound healing. Eliminate options containing gelatin and jelly first, because they have no nutrient value related to healing. From the remaining options, select chicken breast, broccoli, strawberries, and milk over the remaining option because of the greater nutrient value of the foods.

10. 2

Rationale: A low-sodium diet is used as an adjunct to antihypertensive medications for the treatment of hypertension. Sodium retains fluid, which leads to hypertension, secondary to increased fluid volume. Fresh foods such as fruits and vegetables are low in sodium.

Test-Taking Strategy: Note the strategic words, *need for further teaching*. These words indicate a negative event query and ask you to select an option that is an incorrect statement. Remember that fresh foods are low in sodium, so they would be incorporated in the diet. Eliminate the remaining options because these are accurate statements related to the management of hypertension.

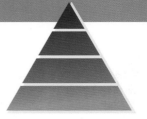

CHAPTER **12**

Intravenous Therapy and Blood Administration

Nursing Sciences

PRIORITY CONCEPTS Fluids and Electrolytes; Perfusion

WHAT WOULD YOU DO?

The nurse is monitoring a client receiving packed red blood cells (PRBCs) who has never received a blood transfusion. The client suddenly becomes apprehensive and complains of back pain after the first 10 minutes of administration. What would the nurse do?
Answer is located on p. 136.

I. Intravenous Therapy (see Chapter 8 and Table 8.1)

A. Used to sustain clients who are unable to take substances orally

B. Replaces water, electrolytes, and nutrients more rapidly than oral administration

C. Provides immediate access to the vascular system for the rapid delivery of specific solutions without the time required for gastrointestinal tract absorption

D. Provides a vascular route for the administration of medication or blood components

II. Intravenous (IV) Devices

A. IV cannulas
  1. Butterfly sets
    a. Wing-tipped needle with a metal cannula and plastic wings; the needle is 0.5 inches to 1.5 inches in length, with needle gauge sizes from 16 to 26
    b. Infiltration is more common with these devices as a result of their stiffness.
    c. May be used with children and older clients, whose veins are likely to be small or fragile, and in outpatient settings; may be used for drawing blood
  2. Plastic cannulas
    a. Used primarily for short-term therapy, especially if rapid infusion is necessary; more comfortable for the client

  b. Can cause a catheter embolism if the tip of the cannula breaks

B. IV gauges
  1. The gauge refers to the diameter of the lumen of the needle or cannula.
  2. The smaller the gauge number, the larger the diameter of the cannula.
  3. The size of the gauge used depends on the solution to be administered and the diameter of the available vein.
  4. Large-diameter lumens (smaller gauge numbers) allow for a higher fluid rate than smaller-diameter lumens and allow for the administration of higher concentrations of solutions.
  5. For rapid emergency fluid administration, blood products, or anesthetics, a large needle (e.g., 14-, 16-, 18-, or 19-gauge) is used.
  6. For standard IV fluid infusion and clear liquid IV medications, a 20- or 22-gauge needle is used.
  7. If the client has very small veins, a 24- to 25-gauge needle is used.

C. IV containers
  1. May be glass or plastic
  2. Squeeze the plastic bag to ensure intactness and check glass bottles for any cracks. Check the solution for any cloudiness or discoloration.
  3. The expiration date of IV fluid and all supplies would be checked. Medications would be reconstituted per agency protocol and pharmacy instruction.

  ⚠ Do not write on a plastic IV bag with a marker because the ink may be absorbed through the plastic into the solution. Use a label and a ballpoint pen for writing on the label, placing the label onto the bag.

D. IV tubing (Fig. 12.1)
  1. Contains a spike end for the bag or bottle, a drop (drip) chamber, a roller clamp, a Y site, and an adapter end for attachment to the cannula or needle

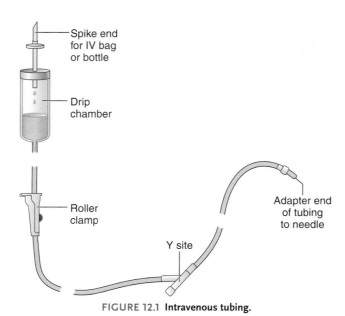

FIGURE 12.1 **Intravenous tubing.**

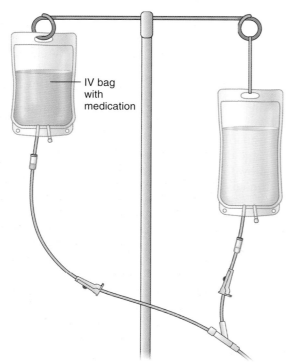

FIGURE 12.2 **Secondary bag with medication.**

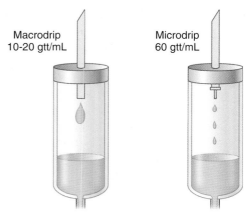

FIGURE 12.3 **Macrodrip and microdrip sizes.**

that is inserted into the client's vein. May also contain an area for insertion into an IV pump.

2. Shorter secondary tubing is used for piggyback solutions, connecting them to the injection sites nearest to the drop chamber (Fig. 12.2).

3. Special tubing is used for medication that absorbs into plastic. (Check specific medication administration guidelines when administering IV medications.)

4. Vented and nonvented tubing are available.
    a. A vent allows air to enter the IV container as the fluid leaves.

b. A vented adapter can be used to add a vent to a nonvented IV tubing system.
c. Use nonvented tubing for flexible containers.
d. Use vented tubing for glass or rigid plastic containers to allow air to enter and displace the fluid as it leaves. Fluid will not flow from a rigid IV container unless it is vented.

⚠ Extension tubing can be added to an IV tubing set to provide extra length to the tubing. Add extension tubing to the IV tubing set for children, clients who are restless, or clients who have special mobility needs.

E. Drip chambers (Fig. 12.3)
    1. Macrodrip chamber
        a. Used if the solution is thick or needs to infuse rapidly
        b. Drop factor varies from 10 to 20 drops (gtt)/mL, depending on the manufacturer
        c. Read the tubing package to determine how many drops per milliliter are delivered (drop factor).
    2. Microdrip chamber
        a. Normally, the chamber has a short, vertical, metal piece (stylet) where the drop forms.
        b. The chamber delivers about 60 gtt/mL.
        c. Read the tubing package to determine the drop factor (gtt/mL).
        d. Microdrip chambers are used if fluid will be infused at a slow rate (less than 50 mL/hour) or if the solution contains a potent medication that needs to be titrated, such as in a critical care setting or in the pediatric client.

F. Filters: May be used in IV lines to trap small particles and provide protection by preventing particles from entering the client's veins. Filters are also used for blood administration and with neutropenic clients.

G. Needleless infusion devices: Include recessed needles, plastic cannulas, or one-way valves; these devices decrease exposure to contaminated needles.

H. Intermittent infusion devices: Used when intravascular accessibility is desired for the intermittent administration of medications by IV push or piggyback.

1. Require periodic flushing with normal saline as well as before and after medication administration to maintain patency.

2. Normal saline is typically used to flush intermittent infusion sets. Hospital policy needs to be reviewed regarding amount of flush solution to instill.

I. Electronic infusion devices: Control the amount of fluid or medication infusing (for example, an infusion pump or controller, syringe pump, or patient-controlled analgesia [PCA])

⚠ Check electronic IV infusion devices frequently. Although these devices are electronic, this does not ensure that they are infusing solutions and medications accurately.

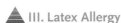

III. Latex Allergy

A. Ask the client about an allergy to latex.

1. IV supplies that may contain latex include IV catheters, IV tubing, IV ports (particularly IV rubber injection ports), rubber stoppers on multidose vials, and adhesive tape. Manufacturers typically label packaging when the item is latex-free.

2. Latex-free IV supplies need to be used for clients with latex allergy; most agencies carry these types of supplies, but this still needs to be checked.

3. Refer to Chapter 59 for additional information about latex allergy.

IV. Peripheral IV Sites

A. The most frequently used sites are the veins of the forearm, because the bones of the forearm act as a natural support and splint.

B. Veins in the lower extremities are not suitable because of the risk of thrombus formation and possible pooling in areas of decreased venous return (Box 12.1).

C. Veins in the scalp and feet may be suitable sites for infants.

D. Bending the elbow on the arm with an IV may easily obstruct the flow of the solution, thereby causing infiltration.

E. Avoid checking the blood pressure on the arm receiving the IV infusion.

F. Do not place restraints over the venipuncture site.

BOX 12.1   Peripheral Intravenous Sites to Avoid

- Edematous extremity
- The lower extremities
- An arm that is weak, traumatized, or paralyzed
- The arm on the same side as a mastectomy
- An arm that has an arteriovenous fistula or a shunt for dialysis
- A skin area that is infected

G. An arm board may be prescribed when the venipuncture site is located in an area of flexion.

⚠ In an adult, the most frequently used sites for inserting an IV cannula/needle are the veins of the forearm because the bones of the forearm act as a natural support and splint.

V. Administering IV Solutions

A. The IV solution must be checked against the primary health care provider's (PHCP's) prescription for the type, amount, percentage of solution, and rate of flow. The Rights for Medication Administration must be followed.

B. Check the health status and medical disorders of the client and identify client conditions that contraindicate the use of a particular IV solution or IV equipment, such as an allergy to a cleansing solution, any adhesive materials, or latex. Check the compatibility of IV solutions as appropriate.

C. Check the client's identification by two identifiers and explain the procedure to the client; assess the client's previous experience with IV therapy and preference for insertion site.

D. Wash hands thoroughly and put on a pair of nonsterile gloves.

E. Use sterile technique when inserting an IV line and when changing the dressing over the IV site.

F. The venipuncture site is changed every 72 to 96 hours or with a change in the venipuncture site in accordance with the Centers for Disease Control and Prevention (CDC) recommendations and agency policy.

G. The IV dressing is changed when the dressing is wet or contaminated, or as specified by the agency policy.

H. Do not let an IV bag or bottle of solution hang for more than 24 hours, to diminish the potential for bacterial contamination and possibly sepsis.

I. Do not allow the IV tubing to touch the floor to prevent potential bacterial contamination.

J. The LPN/LVN scope of practice regarding IV medications and/or IV initiation varies by state and facility. See Priority Nursing Actions for instructions on removing an IV.

VI. Precautions for IV Lines

A. On insertion, an IV line can cause initial pain and discomfort for the client.

B. An IV puncture provides a route of entry for microorganisms into the body.

C. Medications administered by the IV route enter the blood immediately, and any adverse reactions or allergic responses can occur immediately.

D. Fluid (circulatory) overload or electrolyte imbalances can occur from an excessive or too-rapid infusion of fluids.

E. Incompatibilities between certain solutions and medications can occur.

⚡ PRIORITY NURSING ACTIONS

Removing a Peripheral Intravenous Line

1. Check the primary health care provider's (PHCP's) prescription and explain the procedure to the client. Ask the client to hold the extremity still during cannula/needle removal.
2. Turn the intravenous (IV) tubing clamp off and apply a pair of nonsterile gloves. Remove the dressing and tape covering the site while stabilizing the catheter.
3. Apply light pressure with sterile gauze or other material as specified by agency procedure over the site, and withdraw the catheter using a slow, steady movement, keeping the hub parallel to the skin.
4. Apply pressure for 2 to 3 minutes using dry, sterile gauze (apply pressure for a longer period of time if the client has a bleeding disorder or is taking anticoagulant medication).
5. Inspect the site for redness, drainage, or swelling, and check the catheter for intactness.
6. Document the procedure and the client's response.

⚠ If IV fluids are administered for a client with heart failure, monitor the rate of administration very carefully because any excess of fluid could exacerbate heart failure by increasing the fluid overload.

F. Complications (Table 12.1)
G. Air embolism
  1. Description: A bolus of air enters the vein through an inadequately primed IV line, from a loose connection, during a tubing change, or during the removal of the IV.

  2. Prevention and interventions
    a. Prime the tubing with fluid before use and monitor for any air bubbles.
    b. Secure all connections.
    c. Replace IV fluid before the bag or bottle is empty.
    d. If an air embolism is suspected, the registered nurse (RN) is notified immediately, the tubing is clamped, the client is turned on his or her left side with the head of the bed lowered (Trendelenburg position) to trap the air in the right atrium, and the PHCP is notified.
H. Catheter embolism
  1. Description: An obstruction that results from the breakage of the catheter tip during IV insertion or removal
  2. Prevention and interventions
    a. Inspect the catheter before insertion.
    b. Remove the IV catheter carefully and inspect the catheter when removed.
    c. If the catheter tip has broken off, the RN notifies the PHCP immediately. A tourniquet is

placed high on the limb of the IV site as prescribed, an x-ray study is obtained, and the client may require surgery to remove the catheter pieces.
I. Circulatory overload
  1. Description: Also known as *fluid overload*; results from the administration of fluids too rapidly or in a client who is at risk for fluid overload
  2. Prevention and interventions
    a. Identify clients at risk for circulatory overload.
    b. Calculate and monitor the drip (flow) rate frequently.

TABLE 12.1   Signs of Complications of Intravenous Therapy

Complication	Signs
Air embolism	Tachycardia
	Chest pain and dyspnea
	Hypotension
	Cyanosis
	Decreased level of consciousness
Catheter embolism	Decrease in blood pressure
	Pain along the vein
	Weak, rapid pulse
	Cyanosis of the nail beds
	Loss of consciousness
Circulatory overload	Increased blood pressure
	Distended jugular veins
	Rapid breathing
	Dyspnea
	Moist cough and crackles
Electrolyte overload	Signs depend on the specific electrolyte overload imbalance
Infection	Local—redness, swelling, and drainage at the site
	Systemic—chills, fever, malaise, headache, nausea, vomiting, backache, tachycardia
Infiltration	Edema, pain, and coolness at the site; may or may not have a blood return
Phlebitis	Heat, redness, tenderness at the site
	Not swollen or hard
	Intravenous infusion sluggish
Thrombophlebitis	Hard and cord-like vein
	Heat, redness, tenderness at site
	Intravenous infusion sluggish
Tissue damage	Change in skin color; sloughing of the skin, discomfort at the site

c. Use an electronic IV infusion device and frequently check the drip rate or setting (at least every hour for an adult).

d. Monitor for signs of circulatory overload. If circulatory overload occurs, decrease the flow rate to a minimum, at a keep-vein-open rate; elevate the head of the bed; keep the client warm; check lung sounds; assess for edema; and the RN and PHCP are notified immediately.

⚠️ Clients with respiratory, cardiac, renal, or liver disease, older clients, and very young persons are at risk for circulatory overload and cannot tolerate an excessive fluid volume.

J. Electrolyte overload
   1. Description: An electrolyte imbalance caused by too-rapid or excessive infusion or use of an inappropriate IV solution
   2. Prevention and interventions
      a. Review laboratory value reports.
      b. Verify the correct solution and additives with the PHCP prescriptions.
      c. Calculate and monitor the flow rate closely.
      d. Use an electronic infusion device and frequently check the settings.
      e. A medication sticker is placed on the bag or bottle if a medication has been added to the IV solution.
      f. Monitor for signs of an electrolyte imbalance, and notify the PHCP if they occur.

⚠️ Lactated Ringer's solution contains potassium and must not be administered to clients with acute kidney injury or chronic kidney disease.

K. Hematoma
   1. Description: The collection of blood in the tissues after an unsuccessful venipuncture or after the venipuncture site is discontinued and blood continues to ooze from the tissue
   2. Prevention and interventions
      a. When starting an IV, avoid piercing the posterior wall of the vein.
      b. Do not apply a tourniquet to the extremity immediately after an unsuccessful venipuncture.
      c. When discontinuing an IV, apply pressure to the site for 2 to 3 minutes and elevate the extremity; apply pressure longer for clients with a bleeding disorder or who are taking anticoagulants.
      d. If a hematoma develops, elevate the extremity and apply pressure and ice as prescribed.
      e. Document accordingly, including taking pictures of the IV site if indicated by agency policy.

L. Infection
   1. Description
      a. The entry of microorganisms into the body through the venipuncture site
      b. Venipuncture interrupts the integrity of the skin, which is the first line of defense against infection.
      c. The longer the therapy continues, the greater the risk of infection.
      d. Infection can occur locally at the IV insertion site or systemically from the entry of microorganisms into the body.
   2. At-risk clients
      a. Clients who are immunocompromised as a result of diseases such as cancer or acquired immunodeficiency syndrome
      b. Clients receiving treatments such as chemotherapy who have an altered or lowered white blood cell (WBC) count
      c. Older clients, because aging alters the effectiveness of the immune system
      d. Clients with diabetes mellitus are at risk for infection
   3. Prevention and interventions
      a. Determine the client's risk for infection.
      b. Maintain strict asepsis when caring for the IV site.
      c. Monitor for signs of local or systemic infection.
      d. Monitor WBC counts.
      e. Check fluid containers for cracks, leaks, cloudiness, or other evidence of contamination.
      f. IV tubing is changed per CDC recommendations and agency policy; the IV site dressing is changed when soiled or contaminated and according to agency policy.
      g. Ensure that the IV site, bag or bottle, and tubing are labeled with the date and time to ensure that these are changed on time according to agency policy.
      h. Ensure that the IV solution is not hanging for more than 24 hours.
      i. If signs of infection occur, the RN and PHCP are notified; the IV is discontinued and the venipuncture device is placed in a sterile container for possible culture.
      j. Assist to obtain blood cultures as prescribed if infection is suspected.
      k. The IV is restarted in the opposite arm to differentiate sepsis (systemic infection) from local infection at the IV site.
      l. Document accordingly, taking pictures of the IV site if indicated by agency policy.

⚠️ A client with diabetes mellitus usually does not receive dextrose (glucose) solutions because the solution can increase the blood glucose level.

M. Infiltration
1. Description
   a. Seepage of the IV fluid out of the vein and into the surrounding tissues
   b. Occurs when an IV device has become dislodged or perforates the wall of the vein
2. Prevention and interventions
   a. Avoid venipuncture over an area of flexion.
   b. Anchor the cannula and loop of tubing securely with tape.
   c. Use an arm board or splint as prescribed if the client is restless or active.
   d. Monitor the IV rate for a decrease or cessation of flow.
   e. If infiltration has occurred, the IV device is removed immediately; the extremity is elevated, and compresses (warm or cool, depending on the IV solution that was infusing and the PHCP's prescription) are applied over the affected area.
   f. Do not rub an infiltrated area because this can cause the development of a hematoma.
   g. Document accordingly, including taking pictures of the IV site if indicated by agency policy.

N. Phlebitis and thrombophlebitis
1. Description
   a. Phlebitis is an inflammation of the vein that can occur from mechanical or chemical (medication) trauma or local infection.
   b. Phlebitis can cause the development of a clot (thrombophlebitis).
2. Prevention and interventions
   a. An IV cannula smaller than the vein is used. Very small veins are avoided when administering irritating solutions. Veins over an area of flexion are avoided.
   b. Using the lower extremities as an access area for the IV should be avoided.
   c. Anchor the cannula and loop of tubing securely with tape.
   d. Use an arm board or splint as prescribed if the client is restless or active.
   e. Change the venipuncture site every 72 to 96 hours in accordance with CDC recommendations and agency policy.
   f. If phlebitis occurs, the IV device is removed immediately.
   g. The RN and PHCP are notified if phlebitis is suspected and warm, moist compresses are applied as prescribed.
   h. Document accordingly, including taking pictures if indicated by agency policy.

O. Tissue damage
1. Description:
   a. Tissues most commonly damaged include the skin, veins, and subcutaneous tissue.
   b. Tissue damage can be uncomfortable and can cause permanent negative effects.
   c. Extravasation is a form of tissue damage caused by seepage of a vesicant or irritant solution into the tissues; this occurrence requires immediate PHCP notification so that treatment can be prescribed to prevent tissue necrosis.
2. Prevention and interventions:
   a. A careful and gentle approach is used when applying a tourniquet.
   b. Tapping the skin over the vein when an IV is started is avoided.
   c. Monitor for ecchymosis when penetrating the skin with the cannula.
   d. Check for allergies to tape or dressing adhesives.
   e. Monitor for any change in skin color, sloughing of the skin, or discomfort at the IV site.
   f. Notify the PHCP if tissue damage is suspected.
   g. Document accordingly, including taking pictures if indicated by agency policy.

⚠️ Always document the occurrence of a complication, data collection findings, actions taken, and the client's response.

VII. Central Venous Catheters (Fig. 12.4)
A. Description
1. Used to deliver hyperosmolar solutions, measure central venous pressure, infuse parenteral nutrition, or multiple IV solutions or medications
2. Catheter position is determined by radiography after insertion.
3. May have a single, double, or triple lumen
4. May be inserted peripherally and threaded through the basilic or cephalic vein into the superior vena cava, inserted centrally through the internal jugular or subclavian veins, or surgically tunneled through subcutaneous tissue
5. With multilumen catheters, more than one medication can be administered at the same time without incompatibility problems, and only one insertion site is present.

⚠️ For central line insertion, tubing change, and line removal, the client is placed in the Trendelenburg's position, if not contraindicated or in the supine position; instruct the client to perform Valsalva's maneuver to increase pressure in the central veins when the IV system is open.

B. Tunneled central venous catheters
1. A more permanent type of catheter (e.g., Hickman, Broviac, Groshong) used for long-term IV therapy
2. May be single or multilumen
3. Inserted in the operating room. The catheter is threaded into the lower part of the vena cava at

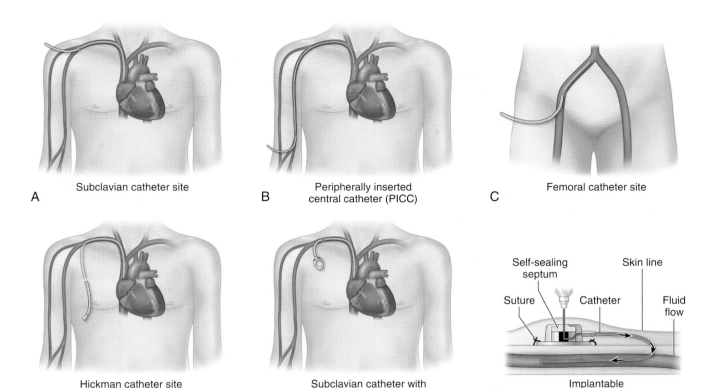

FIGURE 12.4 Central venous access sites. (A) Subclavian catheter. (B) Peripherally inserted central catheter (PICC). (C) Femoral catheter. (D) Hickman catheter. (E) Subclavian catheter with implantable vascular access port. (F) Implantable vascular access port.

the entrance of the right atrium and tunneled under the skin to the exit site where the catheter comes out of the chest. The catheter at the exit site is secured by means of a "cuff" just under the skin at the exit site.

4. The catheter is fitted with an intermittent infusion device to allow access as needed and to keep the system closed and intact.

5. Patency is maintained by flushing with a diluted heparin solution or a normal saline solution, depending on the type of catheter and according to agency policy.

C. Vascular access ports (implantable ports)
1. Surgically implanted under the skin (e.g., Port-a-Cath, Mediport, Infusaport); used for the long-term administration of repeated IV therapy
2. For access, the port requires palpation and injection through the skin into the self-sealing port with a noncoring needle, such as a Huber-point needle.
3. Patency is maintained by periodic flushing with a diluted heparin solution as prescribed and per agency policy.

D. Peripherally inserted central catheter line (PICC)
1. Used for long-term IV therapy, frequently in the home
2. The basilic vein is usually used, but the median cubital and cephalic veins in the antecubital area can also be used.

3. Threaded so that the catheter tip may terminate in the subclavian vein or the superior vena cava
4. A small amount of bleeding may occur at the time of insertion and may continue for 24 hours, but bleeding thereafter is not expected.
5. Phlebitis is a common complication.
6. Insertion is below the heart level; therefore, air embolism is not common.

VIII. Blood Administration

A. Types of blood components
1. Packed red blood cells (PRBCs)
   a. Used to replace erythrocytes; infusion time for 1 unit is usually between 2 and 4 hours
   b. Evaluation of an effective response is based on the resolution of the symptoms of anemia and an increase of the erythrocyte, hemoglobin, and hematocrit count.

Washed RBC (depleted of plasma, platelets, and leukocytes) may be prescribed for a client with a history of allergic transfusion reactions or those who underwent hematopoietic stem cell transplant. Leukocyte depletion (leukoreduction) by filtration, washing, or freezing is the process used to decrease the amount of WBCs in a unit of packed cells. This method is used to restore oxygen-carrying capacity of blood and intravascular volume.

TABLE 12.2 Compatibility Chart for Red Blood Cell Transfusions

Donor	Recipient			
	A	B	AB	O
A	X		X	
B		X	X	
AB			X	
O	X	X	X	X

The ABO type of the donor must be compatible with the recipient's. Type A can receive from type A or O; type B from type B or O; type AB can receive from type A, B, AB, or O; type O only from type O.
From Ignatavicius D, Workman ML: *Medical-surgical nursing: patient centered collaborative care*, ed 7, Philadelphia, 2013, Saunders.

2. Platelet transfusion
   a. Platelets are used to treat thrombocytopenia and platelet dysfunctions.
   b. Crossmatching is not required but is usually done (platelet concentrates contain few RBCs).
   c. Platelets are administered rapidly, usually over 15 to 30 minutes.
   d. Evaluation of an effective response is based on the improvement of the platelet count.
3. Fresh-frozen plasma
   a. May be used to provide clotting factors or volume expansion; contains no platelets
   b. Rh factor and ABO compatibility are required for the transfusion of plasma products
   c. Fresh frozen plasma is infused after thawing and administered rapidly, usually over 15 to 30 minutes.
   d. Evaluation of an effective response is assessed by monitoring coagulation studies, particularly the prothrombin time and the partial thromboplastin time, and the resolution of hypovolemia.
B. Compatibility (Table 12.2)
   1. Client (the recipient) blood samples are drawn and labeled at the bedside at the time the blood sample is drawn. The client is asked to state his or her name, which is compared with the identification band or bracelet. A witness may be required according to agency policy.
   2. The recipient's ABO and Rh factor are identified.
   3. An antibody screen is done to determine the presence of antibodies other than anti-A and anti-B.
   4. To determine compatibility, crossmatching is done, in which donor RBCs are combined with the recipient's serum and Coombs's serum; the crossmatch is compatible if no RBC agglutination occurs.
   5. The universal RBC donor is O negative. The universal recipient is AB positive.
   6. Clients with Rh-positive blood can receive an RBC transfusion from a Rh-negative donor if necessary; however, a Rh-negative client must not receive Rh-positive blood.

⚠️ The donor's blood and the recipient's blood must be tested for compatibility. If the blood is not compatible, a life-threatening transfusion reaction can occur.

C. Precautions and nursing responsibilities (Box 12.2)
D. Transfusion reactions
   1. Description: A transfusion reaction is an adverse reaction that happens as a result of receiving a blood transfusion. Types of transfusion reactions include hemolytic, allergic, febrile or bacterial reactions (septicemia), or transfusion-associated graft-versus-host disease (GVHD).
   2. Signs of an immediate transfusion reaction
      a. Chills and diaphoresis
      b. Muscle aches, back pain, or chest pain
      c. Rashes, hives, itching, and swelling
      d. Rapid, thready pulse
      e. Dyspnea, cough, or wheezing
      f. Pallor and cyanosis
      g. Apprehension
      h. Tingling and numbness
      i. Headache
      j. Nausea, vomiting, abdominal cramping, and diarrhea
   3. Signs of transfusion reaction in an unconscious client
      a. Weak pulse
      b. Fever
      c. Tachycardia or bradycardia
      d. Hypotension
      e. Visible hemoglobinuria
      f. Oliguria or anuria
   4. Delayed transfusion reaction
      a. Reactions can occur days to years after a transfusion.
      b. Signs include fever, mild jaundice, and a decreased hematocrit level.

⚠️ Stay with the client for the first 15 minutes of the infusion of the blood and monitor the client for signs and symptoms of a transfusion reaction. The first 15 minutes of the transfusion are the most critical, and this is the most likely time a transfusion reaction will occur. Vital signs are monitored every 30 minutes to 1 hour according to agency protocol.

BOX 12.2 Blood Administration Precautions and Nursing Responsibilities

General Precautions

- A large volume of refrigerated blood infused rapidly through a central venous catheter into the ventricle of the heart can cause cardiac dysrhythmias.
- Medications are never added to blood components or piggybacked into a blood transfusion; no solution other than normal saline would be added to blood components.
- To avoid the risk of septicemia, infusions (1 unit) must not exceed the prescribed time for administration (2–4 hours for packed red blood cells [PRBCs]); the blood administration set would also be changed with each unit. Follow evidence-based practice guidelines and agency procedure.
- Always check the blood bag for the date of expiration; components expire at midnight on the day marked on the bag unless otherwise specified.
- Inspect the blood bag for leaks, abnormal color, clots, and bubbles.
- Blood must be administered as soon as possible, within 20 to 30 minutes—the maximum allowable time out of monitored storage—from its being received from the blood bank. If the blood is not administered within that time, return it to the blood bank.
- Never refrigerate blood in refrigerators other than those used in blood banks.
- The recommended rate of infusion varies with the blood component being transfused and depends on the client's condition; generally, blood is infused as quickly as the client's condition allows; caution must be taken to avoid circulatory overload.
- The nurse would measure vital signs and check the lung sounds before the transfusion and again after the first 15 minutes and every hour until 1 hour after the transfusion is completed.

Blood Bank Precautions

- Blood will be released from the blood bank only to personnel specified by agency policy.
- The name and identification number of the intended recipient must be provided to the blood bank, and a documented permanent record of this information must be maintained.
- Blood must be transported from the blood bank to only one client at a time to prevent blood delivery to the wrong client.

Client Identity and Compatibility

- The most critical phase of the transfusion is confirming product compatibility and verifying client identity.
- Two licensed nurses (follow agency policy) need to check the PHCP's prescription. At the bedside, check the client's identity—ask the client to state his/her name—and compare the name to the client's identification band or bracelet and number, verifying that the name and number are identical to those on the blood component tag.
- The nurse checks the blood bag tag, label, and blood requisition form to ensure that ABO and Rh types are compatible.
- If the nurse notes any inconsistencies when verifying client identity and compatibility, the nurse notifies the blood bank immediately.

Client Data Collection

- Determine any cultural or religious beliefs regarding blood transfusions (e.g., a Jehovah's Witness cannot receive blood or blood products; this group believes that blood transfusions have eternal consequences).
- Ensure that informed consent has been obtained.
- Explain the procedure to the client and determine whether the client has ever received a blood transfusion or experienced any previous reactions to blood transfusions.
- Check the client's vital signs, and check renal, circulatory, and respiratory status and the client's ability to tolerate intravenously administered fluids.
- If the client's temperature is elevated, the PHCP is notified before beginning the transfusion; a fever may be a cause for delaying the transfusion in addition to masking a possible symptom of an acute transfusion reaction.

Administration of the Transfusion

- Maintain standard and transmission-based precautions and surgical asepsis as necessary.
- Assist the registered nurse in administering the blood.
- Always check the bag for the volume of the blood component.
- Blood products must be infused through administration sets designed specifically for blood; use a Y-tubing or straight tubing blood administration set that contains a filter designed to trap fibrin clots and other debris that accumulate during blood storage.
- Premedicate the client with acetaminophen or diphenhydramine, as prescribed, if the client has a history of adverse reactions; if prescribed, oral medications must be administered 30 minutes before the transfusion is started, and intravenously administered medications may be given immediately before the transfusion is started.
- Reinforce instructions to the client to report anything unusual immediately.
- Determine the rate of infusion by the PHCP's prescription or, if not specified, by agency policy.
- Begin the transfusion slowly under close supervision; stay with the client and monitor for signs and symptoms of a transfusion reaction. If no reaction is noted within the first, most critical, 15 minutes, the flow can be increased to the prescribed rate.
- If a major ABO incompatibility exists or a severe allergic reaction occurs, the reaction is usually evident within the first 50 mL of the transfusion.
- Document the client's tolerance to the administration of the blood product.
- Monitor appropriate laboratory values and document effectiveness of treatment related to the specific type of blood product.

Reactions to the Transfusion

- If a transfusion reaction occurs, stop the transfusion, change the intravenous (IV) tubing down to the IV site, keep the IV line open with normal saline, and ensure that the PHCP is notified immediately, the blood bank is notified, and the blood bag and tubing are returned the blood bank. (Refer to Priority Nursing Actions.)
- Do not leave the client alone and monitor the client for any life-threatening symptoms.
- Obtain appropriate laboratory samples according to agency policies, such as blood and urine samples. (Free hemoglobin indicates that red blood cells were hemolyzed.)

Refer to Priority Nursing Actions for caring for a client experiencing a transfusion reaction.

⚡ PRIORITY NURSING ACTIONS

Care of a Client Experiencing a Transfusion Reaction

1. Stop the transfusion.
2. Assist to change the intravenous (IV) tubing down to the IV site and keep the IV line open with normal saline.
3. Notify the registered nurse (RN) and primary health care provider (PHCP) and blood bank.
4. Stay with the client, observing signs and symptoms and monitoring vital signs as often as every 5 minutes.
5. Assist to administer emergency medications as prescribed.
6. Obtain a urine specimen for laboratory studies (and perform any other laboratory studies as prescribed).
7. Return blood bag, tubing, attached labels, and transfusion record to the blood bank.
8. Document the occurrence, actions taken, and the client's response.

WHAT WOULD YOU DO?

Answer: Signs of an immediate transfusion reaction include the following: chills and diaphoresis; muscle aches, back pain, or chest pain; rash, hives, itching, and swelling; rapid, thready pulse; dyspnea, cough, or wheezing; pallor and cyanosis; apprehension; tingling and numbness; headache; and nausea, vomiting, abdominal cramping, and diarrhea. In the event that a transfusion reaction is suspected, the nurse immediately calls for the registered nurse and stops the infusion. The nurse would then assist to change the intravenous (IV) tubing down to the IV site and keep the IV line open with normal saline. The primary health care provider is notified, as is the blood bank, and the blood bag and the tubing are returned to the blood bank. The nurse must also collect a urine specimen. The nurse would assist to implement prescriptions and always stays with the client and monitors the client closely until the client is stabilized.

PRACTICE QUESTIONS

1. The nurse is assisting with caring for a client who will receive a unit of blood. Just before the infusion, it is **most important** for the nurse to check which item?
   1. Vital signs
   2. Skin color
   3. Oxygen saturation
   4. Latest hematocrit level

2. A client who is receiving a blood transfusion pushes the call light for the nurse. When entering the room, the nurse notes that the client is flushed, dyspneic, and complaining of generalized itching. How would the nurse correctly interpret these findings?
   1. Bacteremia
   2. Fluid overload
   3. Hypovolemic shock
   4. Transfusion reaction

3. A client who was receiving a blood transfusion has experienced a transfusion reaction. The nurse sends the blood bag that was used for the client to which area?
   1. The pharmacy
   2. The laboratory
   3. The blood bank
   4. The risk-management department

4. The nurse takes a client's temperature before giving a blood transfusion. The temperature is 100°F (37.7°C) orally. The nurse reports the finding to the registered nurse (RN) and anticipates that which action will take place?
   1. The transfusion will begin as prescribed.
   2. The transfusion will begin after the administration of an antihistamine.
   3. The transfusion will begin after the administration of 650 mg of acetaminophen.
   4. The blood will be held, and the primary health care provider (PHCP) will be notified.

5. Which of these clients is/are **most likely** to develop fluid (circulatory) overload? **Select all that apply**.
   - ❑ 1. A premature infant
   - ❑ 2. A 101-year-old man
   - ❑ 3. A client with heart failure
   - ❑ 4. A client with diabetes mellitus
   - ❑ 5. A client receiving renal dialysis
   - ❑ 6. A 29-year-old client with pneumonia

6. A client has a prescription to receive 1000 mL of 5% dextrose in 0.45% sodium chloride. After gathering the appropriate equipment, the nurse takes which action first before spiking the intravenous (IV) bag with the tubing?
   1. Uncaps the distal end of the tubing
   2. Uncaps the spike portion of the tubing
   3. Opens the roller clamp on the IV tubing
   4. Closes the roller clamp on the IV tubing

7. The nurse is doing a routine assessment of a client's peripheral intravenous (IV) site. The nurse notes that the site is cool, pale, and swollen and that the IV has stopped running. The nurse determines that which complication has probably occurred?
   1. Phlebitis
   2. Infection
   3. Infiltration
   4. Thrombosis

8. The nurse is assigned to care for a client with a peripheral intravenous (IV) infusion. The nurse is providing hygiene care to the client and would take which actions while changing the client's hospital gown? **Select all that apply.**
   - ❑ 1. Using a hospital gown with snaps at the sleeves
   - ❑ 2. Disconnecting the IV tubing from the catheter in the vein
   - ❑ 3. Checking the IV flow rate immediately after changing the hospital gown
   - ❑ 4. Putting the bag and tubing through the sleeve, followed by the client's arm
   - ❑ 5. Cutting the sleeves of the hospital gown and using safety pins to hold the sleeves together

9. The nurse is making a worksheet and listing the tasks that need to be performed for assigned adult clients during the shift. The nurse writes on the plan to check the intravenous (IV) site of an assigned client who is receiving fluid replacement therapy how frequently?
   1. Every hour
   2. Every 2 hours
   3. Every 3 hours
   4. Every 4 hours

10. The nurse is checking the insertion site of a peripheral intravenous (IV) catheter. The nurse notes the site to be reddened, warm, painful, and slightly edematous in the area of the vein proximal to the IV catheter. The nurse interprets that this is most likely the result of which complication?
    1. Phlebitis of the vein
    2. Infiltration of the IV line
    3. Hypersensitivity to the IV solution
    4. An allergic reaction to the IV catheter material

11. The nurse has been instructed to remove an intravenous (IV) line. The nurse removes the catheter by withdrawing the catheter while applying pressure to the site with which item?
    1. Band-Aid
    2. Alcohol swab
    3. Betadine swab
    4. Sterile 2 × 2 gauze

12. The nurse is preparing an intravenous (IV) solution and tubing for a client who requires IV fluids. While preparing to prime the tubing, the tubing drops and hits the top of the medication cart. The nurse would plan to take which action?
    1. Change the IV tubing.
    2. Wipe the tubing with Betadine.
    3. Scrub the tubing with an alcohol swab.
    4. Scrub the tubing before attaching it to the IV bag.

13. A client is going to be transfused with a unit of packed red blood cells (PRBCs). The nurse understands that it is necessary to remain with the client for what time period after the transfusion is started?
    1. 5 minutes
    2. 15 minutes
    3. 30 minutes
    4. 45 minutes

14. The nurse is assisting with caring for a client who is receiving a unit of packed red blood cells (PRBCs). The nurse would tell the client that it is **most important** to report which sign(s) **immediately?**
    1. Sore throat or earache
    2. Chills, itching, or rash
    3. Unusual sleepiness or fatigue
    4. Mild discomfort at the catheter site

15. The nurse is assisting with caring for a client who has received a transfusion of platelets. The nurse determines that the client is benefiting most from this therapy if the client exhibits which finding?
    1. An increased hematocrit level
    2. An increased hemoglobin level
    3. A decline of the temperature to normal
    4. A decrease in oozing from puncture sites and gums

ANSWERS

1. 1

Rationale: A change in the vital signs may indicate that a transfusion reaction is occurring. The nurse assesses the client's vital signs before the procedure to obtain a baseline every 15 minutes for the first half hour after beginning the transfusion and every half hour thereafter. Skin color, oxygen saturation, and most recent hematocrit may be checked but are not the most important.

Test-Taking Strategy: Note the strategic words, *most important*. This tells you that more than one option may be partially or totally correct. Recalling the signs of a blood transfusion reaction will direct you to vital signs. In addition, vital signs are the umbrella option.

2. 4

Rationale: The signs and symptoms exhibited by the client are consistent with a transfusion reaction. With bacteremia, the client would have a fever, which is not part of the clinical picture presented. With fluid (circulatory) overload, the client would have crackles in addition to dyspnea. There is no correlation between the signs mentioned in the question and hypovolemic shock. The signs identified in the question are indicative of an allergic reaction, which is one type of blood transfusion reaction.

Test-Taking Strategy: Focus on the subject, interpretation of the client findings. Focus on this data. Recalling signs and symptoms of transfusion reaction will direct you to the correct option.

3. 3

Rationale: The nurse prepares to return the blood transfusion bag containing any remaining blood to the blood bank. This allows the blood bank to complete any follow-up testing procedures that are needed after a transfusion reaction has been documented. The remaining options are incorrect.

Test-Taking Strategy: Focus on the subject, actions to take if a blood transfusion reaction occurs. Recalling that blood is obtained from the blood bank will help you eliminate each of the incorrect options.

4. 4

Rationale: If the client has a temperature of 100°F (37.7°C) or more, the unit of blood would be held until the primary health care provider (PHCP) is notified and has the opportunity to give further prescriptions. The other options are incorrect actions.

Test-Taking Strategy: Eliminate the options that are comparable or alike in that they all involve the initiation of the transfusion. Remember that if the temperature is elevated, the PHCP needs to be notified before a blood transfusion is initiated.

5. 1, 2, 3, 5

Rationale: Clients with cardiac, respiratory, renal, or liver diseases and older and very young clients cannot tolerate an excessive fluid volume. The risk of fluid (circulatory) overload exists with these clients.

Test-Taking Strategy: Note the strategic words, *most likely*. Focus on the subject, those at risk for fluid (circulatory) overload. Thinking about the physiology associated with each client described in the options will assist you with answering correctly.

6. 4

Rationale: The nurse would first clamp the tubing to prevent the solution from running freely through the tubing after it is attached to the intravenous (IV) bag. The nurse would next uncap the proximal (spike) portion of the tubing and attach it to the IV bag. The IV bag is elevated, the roller clamp is then opened slowly, and the fluid is allowed to flow through the tubing in a controlled fashion to prevent air from remaining in parts of the tubing.

Test-Taking Strategy: Note the strategic words, *first*. This question tests a specific procedure related to IV therapy. Visualize this procedure to answer the question correctly.

7. 3

Rationale: An infiltrated IV is one that has dislodged from the vein and is lying in subcutaneous tissue. The pallor, coolness, and swelling are the result of IV fluid being deposited into the subcutaneous tissue. When the pressure in the tissues exceeds the pressure in the tubing, the flow of the IV solution will stop. The other options identify complications that are likely to be accompanied by warmth at the site rather than coolness.

Test-Taking Strategy: Focus on the data in the question, and note the word *cool*. Recalling that coolness occurs at the site of IV infiltration will direct you to the correct option. Also note that options 1, 2, and 4 are comparable or alike and are accompanied by warmth at the IV site.

8. 1, 3, 4

Rationale: The tubing would not be removed from the intravenous (IV) catheter. With each break in the system, there is an increased chance of introducing bacteria into the system, which can lead to infection. Using gowns with snaps and inserting the IV bag and tubing through the sleeve of the gown first are appropriate. The flow rate must be checked immediately after changing the hospital gown, because the position of the roller clamp may have been affected during the change. Cutting the sleeves of the hospital gown and using safety pins to hold the sleeves together is not an appropriate action; this is not cost-effective since the gown would need to be discarded after use and additionally safety pins can be unsafe if they accidentally open.

Test-Taking Strategy: Focus on the subject, the actions to take when changing a hospital gown of a client with an IV. Visualize this procedure and use your knowledge of the basic principles related to IV therapy, asepsis, and safety to direct you to the correct options.

9. 1

Rationale: Safe nursing practice includes monitoring an intravenous (IV) infusion at least once every 1 hour for an adult client. The remaining options do not provide time frames that are safe or acceptable.

Test-Taking Strategy: Focus on the subject, frequency of observation of the IV infusion. To answer this question accurately, it is necessary to be familiar with the specific time frames indicated for this nursing procedure. For questions similar to this one, it is best to select the most frequently occurring time frame.

10. 1

Rationale: Phlebitis at an intravenous (IV) site results in discomfort at the site and redness, warmth, and swelling proximal to the IV catheter. The IV catheter would be removed, and a new IV line would be inserted at a different site. The remaining options are incorrect; the signs and symptoms in the question are not associated with these conditions.

Test-Taking Strategy: Remember that comparable or alike options are not likely to be correct. In this case, hypersensitivity to the IV solution and an allergic reaction to the IV catheter material are comparable or alike and are therefore eliminated. Recalling that warmth occurs at the site of phlebitis directs you to the correct option.

11. 4

Rationale: A dry, sterile dressing such as sterile 2 × 2 gauze is used to apply pressure to the site while the catheter is discontinued and removed. This material is absorbent, sterile, and nonirritating to the site. A Band-Aid may be used to cover the site after hemostasis has occurred. An alcohol swab or Betadine would irritate the opened puncture site and would not stop the blood flow.

Test-Taking Strategy: Focus on the subject, the procedure for removing an intravenous (IV). Visualize this procedure and think about each of the items identified in the options to answer the question. Noting the word *sterile* will assist with directing you to the correct option.

12. 1

Rationale: The nurse must change the intravenous (IV) tubing. The tubing has become contaminated, and if used, it could result in a systemic infection in the client. Wiping or scrubbing the tubing is insufficient to prevent systemic infection.

Test-Taking Strategy: Use your knowledge of basic infection control measures and IV therapy concepts to answer this question. Note that three of the options are comparable or alike in that they involve wiping the end of the tubing.

13. 2

Rationale: The nurse must remain with the client for the first 15 minutes of a transfusion, which is the most likely time that a transfusion reaction will occur. This enables the nurse to detect a reaction and intervene quickly. The nurse engages in safe nursing practice by obtaining coverage for the other clients during this time. Five minutes is too short of a time period, while 30 and 45 minutes are lengthy time periods.

Test-Taking Strategy: Focus on the subject, length of time to remain with the client after initiation of a transfusion. Use knowledge regarding blood transfusion procedures to answer this question. Remember, the client must be directly monitored for the first 15 minutes of the transfusion.

14. 2

Rationale: The client is told to report chills, itching, or rash immediately, because these could be signs of a possible transfusion reaction. Mild discomfort at the catheter site may be indicative of a problem, or it could result from the size of the intravenous (IV) catheter required to infuse the blood product. Sore throat, earache, sleepiness, and fatigue are unrelated to a transfusion reaction.

Test-Taking Strategy: Note the strategic words, *most important* and *immediately*. These tell you that more than one or all of the options may be partially or totally correct. With the knowledge that a transfusion reaction is of greatest concern to the nurse, prioritize and select the option that characterizes this problem.

15. 4

Rationale: Platelets are necessary for proper blood clotting. The client with insufficient platelets may exhibit frank bleeding or the oozing of blood from puncture sites, wounds, and mucous membranes. The client's temperature would decline to normal after the infusion of granulocytes if those transfused cells were then instrumental in fighting infection in the body. Increased hemoglobin and hematocrit levels would be seen when the client has received a transfusion of red blood cells.

Test-Taking Strategy: Focus on the subject, expected outcome, and note the strategic word, *most*. Recalling that bleeding is a concern when the platelets are low will direct you to the correct option.

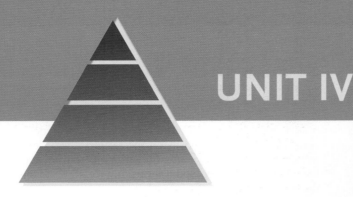

Foundations of Care

▲ Pyramid to Success

On the NCLEX-PN®, safety and infection control concepts, including standard precautions and transmission-based precautions related to client care, are a priority focus. Medication or intravenous (IV) calculation questions are also a focus on the NCLEX-PN examination. Fill-in-the-blank questions may require that you calculate a medication dose or an IV flow rate. Use the on-screen calculator for these medications and IV problems, and then recheck the calculation before selecting an option or typing the answer.

The Pyramid to Success also focuses on the data collection procedures for a health and physical assessment of the adult client and collecting both subjective and objective data. Perioperative nursing care and monitoring for postoperative complications is a priority. Client safety related to positioning and ambulation, and care to the client with a tube such as a gastrointestinal tube or chest tube, are important concepts addressed on the NCLEX. Because many surgical procedures are performed through ambulatory care units (one-day-stay units), Pyramid Points also focus on preparing the client for discharge, assisting with teaching related to the prescribed treatments and medications, follow-up care, and the mobilization of home care support services.

▲ Client Needs: Learning Objectives

- **Safe and Effective Care Environment**
  Acting as an advocate regarding the client's wishes
  Collaborating with health care members in other disciplines
  Ensuring environmental, personal, and home safety
  Ensuring that the client's rights, including informed consent, are upheld
  Establishing priorities of assessment and interventions

Following advance directives regarding the client's documented requests
Following guidelines regarding the use of safety devices
Handling hazardous and infectious materials safely
Informing the client of the surgical process and ensuring that informed consent for a surgical procedure and other procedures has been obtained
Knowing the emergency response plan and actions to take for exposure to biological and chemical warfare agents
Maintaining confidentiality
Maintaining continuity of care and initiating referrals to home care and other support services
Maintaining precautions to prevent errors, accidents, and injury
Positioning the client appropriately and safely
Preparing and administering medications, using the rights of medication administration
Preventing a surgical infection
Protecting the medicated client from injury
Upholding the client's rights
Using equipment safely
Using ergonomic principles and body mechanics when moving a client
Using standard and transmission-based precautions and surgical asepsis procedures

- **Health Promotion and Maintenance**
  Assisting clients and families to identify environmental hazards in the home
  Discussing high-risk behaviors and lifestyle choices
  Performing home safety assessments
  Performing the techniques associated with the health and physical assessment of the client
  Providing health and wellness teaching to prevent complications
  Respecting lifestyle choices and health care beliefs and preferences

Teaching clients and families about accident prevention

Teaching clients and families about measures to be implemented in an emergency situation

Teaching clients and families about preventing the spread of infection and preventing diseases

Teaching the client about prescribed medication(s) or IV therapy

- **Psychosocial Integrity**

Collecting data and managing the client with sensory and perception alterations

Discussing expected body image changes and situational role changes

Facilitating client and family coping

Identifying support systems

Identifying the cultural, religious, and spiritual factors influencing health

Keeping the family informed of client progress

Providing emotional support to significant others

- **Physiological Integrity**

Administering medications and IV therapy safely

Assisting the client with activities of daily living

Calculating medication doses and IV flow rates

Determining the mobility and immobility level of the client

Handling medical emergencies as appropriate

Identifying client allergies and sensitivities

Identifying the adverse effects of, and contraindications to, pharmacological therapy

Implementing priority nursing actions in an emergency situation

Initiating nursing interventions when surgical complications arise

Managing and providing care to clients with infectious diseases

Monitoring for alterations in body systems

Monitoring for surgical complications

Monitoring for wound infection

Observing for expected and unexpected effects of pharmacological therapy

Preparing for diagnostic tests to confirm accurate placement of a tube

Preventing the complications of immobility

Promoting an environment that will allow the client to express concerns

Providing comfort and assistance to the client

Providing interventions compatible with the client's age; cultural, religious, and health care beliefs; education level; and language

Providing nutrition and oral intake

Providing personal hygiene as needed

Recognizing changes in the client's condition that indicate a potential complication and intervening appropriately

Using assistive devices to prevent injury safely

Using special equipment safely

Client Needs lists modified from: National Council of State Boards of Nursing, Inc. (NCSBN). *NCLEX-PN Examination: Test Plan for the National Council Licensure Examination for Practical Nurses,* effective April 2020. Chicago: NCSBN.

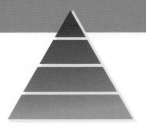

CHAPTER **13**

Health and Physical Assessment of the Adult Client

PRIORITY CONCEPTS Clinical Judgment; Health Promotion

WHAT WOULD YOU DO?

The nurse is collecting cardiovascular data from a client. The nurse notes an irregular beat when auscultating the heart rate. What would the nurse do?
Answer is located on p. 158.

⚠ Health and physical assessment techniques that can be performed by the licensed practical nurse/licensed vocational nurse may vary depending on the scope of practice defined by the employment agency and State Board of Nursing Practice Act. The content in this chapter is comprehensive and some of the physical examination techniques would be performed by the registered nurse (RN) or other primary health care provider (PHCP) rather than the licensed practical nurse/licensed vocational nurse.

I. Environment/Setting

A. Establish a relationship and explain the procedure to the client.
B. Ensure privacy and make the client feel comfortable (comfortable room temperature and sufficient lighting; remove distractions such as noise or objects; and avoid interruptions).
C. Sit down for the interview (avoid barriers such as a desk or staring at computer continuously), maintain an appropriate social distance, and maintain eye level.
D. Use therapeutic communication techniques and open-ended questions to obtain information about the client's symptoms and concerns. Allow time for the client to ask questions.
E. Consider religious, spiritual, and cultural characteristics such as language (the need for an interpreter), values and beliefs, health practices, eye contact, and touch.

F. Keep note-taking to a minimum so the client is the focus of attention.
G. Types of health and physical data collections (Box 13.1)

II. Health History

A. General state of health: Body features and physical characteristics, body movements, body posture, level of consciousness, nutritional status, speech
B. Chief complaint and history of present illness (direct client quotes) that directs the client to seek care
C. Family history: The health status of direct blood relatives, as well as the client's spouse
D. Social history
  1. Data about the client's lifestyle, with a focus on factors that may affect health
  2. Information about alcohol, drug, and tobacco use; sexual practices; tattoos; body piercing; travel history; and work setting to identify occupational hazards
E. Domestic violence screening
  1. Done to determine whether the client is experiencing any form of domestic violence
  2. Conducted during a one-to-one interview with client while obtaining the health history

III. Mental Status Examination

A. The mental status can be checked while obtaining subjective data from the client during the health history interview.
B. Appearance
  1. Note appearance, including posture, body movements, dress, hygiene, and grooming.
  2. An inappropriate appearance and poor hygiene may be indicative of depression, manic disorder, dementia, organic brain disease, or another disorder.

C. Behavior
1. Level of consciousness: Check alertness and awareness and the client's ability to interact appropriately with the environment.
2. Facial expression and body language: Check for appropriate eye contact and determine whether facial expression and body language are appropriate to the situation. This data collection technique also provides information regarding the client's mood and affect.
3. Speech: Check speech pattern for articulation and appropriateness of conversation.

D. Cognitive level of functioning (Box 13.2)

IV. Physical Assessment

A. Overview
1. Gather equipment needed for the examination.
2. Use the senses of sight, smell, touch, and hearing to collect data.
3. Data collection includes inspection, palpation, percussion, and auscultation. These skills are

---

BOX 13.1   Types of Health and Physical Assessment

Complete assessment: Includes a complete health history and physical examination and forms a baseline database
Focused assessment: Focuses on a limited or short-term problem, such as the client's complaint
Episodic/follow-up assessment: Focuses on evaluating a client's progress
Emergency assessment: Involves the rapid collection of data, often during the provision of lifesaving measures

---

BOX 13.2   The Mental-Status Examination: Cognitive Level of Functioning

Orientation: Check the client's orientation to person, place, and time.
Attention span: Check the client's ability to concentrate.
Recent memory: This is checked by asking the client to recall a recent occurrence (e.g., the means of transportation used to get to the health care agency for the physical assessment).
Remote memory: This is checked by asking the client about a verifiable past event (e.g., a vacation).
New learning: This is used to checked the client's ability to recall unrelated words identified by the examiner. The examiner selects four words and asks the client to recall the words 5, 10, and 30 minutes later.
Judgment: This determines whether the client's actions or decisions regarding discussions during the interview are realistic.
Thought processes and perceptions: The way the client thinks and what the client says needs to be logical, coherent, and relevant. The client must be consistently aware of reality.

---

performed one at a time, in this order (except for the abdominal assessment).

B. Assessment techniques

⚠ Data collection techniques primarily used by the licensed practical nurse/licensed vocational nurse include inspection, some palpation procedures, and auscultation.

1. Inspection
   a. The first data collection technique uses vision and smell senses while observing the client.
   b. Requires good lighting, adequate body exposure, and possibly the use of certain instruments by the registered nurse (RN) or primary health care provider (PHCP) (examiners), such as an otoscope or ophthalmoscope.
2. Palpation
   a. Uses the sense of touch
   b. Warm the hands before touching the client.
   c. Identify tender areas and palpate them last.
   d. The examiner will start with light palpation (done with one hand pressing the skin gently with the tips of two to three fingers held close together) to detect surface characteristics and then perform deeper palpation (done by placing one hand on top of the other and pressing down with fingertips of both hands).
   e. Check texture, temperature, and moisture of the skin, as well as organ location and size and symmetry if appropriate.
   f. Check for swelling, vibration or pulsation, rigidity or spasticity, and crepitation.
   g. Check for the presence of lumps or masses, as well as the presence of tenderness or pain.
3. Percussion
   a. The examiner will tap the client's skin to check underlying structures and to determine the presence of vibrations and sounds, and if present, their intensity, duration, pitch, quality, and location.
   b. Provides information related to the presence of air, fluid, or solid masses, as well as organ size, shape, and position.
   c. Description of findings include resonance, hyperresonance, tympany, dullness, or flatness.
4. Auscultation: Involves listening with a stethoscope to sounds produced by the body, such as heart, lung, or bowel sounds

C. Vital signs
1. Includes temperature, radial pulse (apical pulse may be measured during the cardiovascular data collection process), respirations, blood pressure, pulse oximetry, and presence of pain
2. Height and weight and nutritional status may also be checked with vital sign measurement.

V. Body Systems: Assessment Process

A. Integumentary system: Involves inspection and palpation of skin, hair, and nails
   1. Subjective data: Self-care behaviors, history of skin disease, medications being taken, environmental or occupational hazards and exposure to toxic substances, change in skin color or pigmentation, change in a mole or a sore that does not heal, presence of tattoos
   2. Objective data: Color, temperature (hypothermia or hyperthermia); excessive dryness or moisture; skin turgor; texture (smoothness, firmness); excessive bruising, itching, rash; hair loss (alopecia) or nail abnormalities such as pitting; lesions (may be inspected by the examiner with a magnifier and light or with the use of a wood's lamp [ultraviolet light used in a darkened room]); scars or birthmarks; edema; capillary filling time (Boxes 13.3 and 13.4, and Table 13.1)

⚠ To test skin turgor, gently pinch a large fold of skin and check the ability of the skin to return to its place when released. (Poor turgor occurs with severe dehydration or extreme weight loss.)

   3. Dark-skinned client
      a. Cyanosis: Check lips and tongue for a gray color; nailbeds, palms, and soles for a blue color; and conjunctivae for pallor.
      b. Jaundice: Check oral mucous membranes for a yellow color; check the sclera nearest to the iris for a yellow color.
      c. Bleeding: Look for skin swelling and darkening, and compare the affected side with the unaffected side.
      d. Inflammation: Check for warmth, a shiny or taut and pitting skin area, and compare with the unaffected side.
   4. Refer to Chapter 39 for diagnostic tests related to the integumentary system. ▲
   5. Reinforce client teaching ▲
      a. Provide information about factors that can be harmful to the skin, such as the sun.
      b. Encourage performing self-examination of the skin monthly using the ABCDE (asymmetry, border irregularity, color variance, diameter greater than 6 mm, evolving size, shape, and color) mnemonic.

B. Head, neck, and lymph nodes: Involves inspection and palpation of the head, neck, and lymph nodes
   1. Ask the client about headaches; episodes of dizziness (lightheadedness) or vertigo (spinning sensation); history of head injury; loss of consciousness; seizures; episodes of neck pain; limitations of range of motion; numbness or tingling in the shoulders, arms, or hands; lumps or swelling in the neck; difficulty swallowing; medications

---

BOX 13.3	Characteristics of Skin Color

Cyanosis: Mottled bluish coloration
Erythema: Redness
Pallor: Pale, whitish coloration
Jaundice: Yellow coloration

BOX 13.4	Checking Capillary Filling Time

Depress the nail bed to produce blanching.
Release and observe for the return of color.
Color will return within 3 seconds if arterial capillary perfusion is normal.

TABLE 13.1   Pitting Edema Scale

Scale	Description	"Measurement"[a]	
1 +	A barely perceptible pit	2 mm (3/32 in)	
2 +	A deeper pit, rebounds in a few seconds	4 mm (6/32 in)	
3 +	A deep pit, rebounds in 10–20 seconds	6 mm (1/4 in)	
4 +	A deeper pit, rebounds in >30 seconds	8 mm (5/16 in)	

[a]"Measurement" is in quotation marks because depth of edema is rarely actually measured but is included as a frame of reference.
Description column data from Kirton C: Assessing edema. Nursing 96 26(7):54, 1996.
Data from Wilson AF, Giddens JF: Health assessment for nursing practice, ed 5, St. Louis, 2013, Mosby.

being taken; and history of surgery in the head and neck region.

2. Head
   a. Inspect and palpate: Size, shape, masses or tenderness, and symmetry of the skull
   b. Palpate temporal arteries, located above the cheekbone between the eye and the top of the ear.
   c. Palpate frontal and maxillary sinuses for tenderness.
   d. Temporomandibular joint: The client is asked to open his or her mouth. The examiner will look for any crepitation, tenderness, or limited range of motion.
   e. Face: Inspect facial structures for shape, symmetry, involuntary movements, or swelling such as periorbital edema (swelling around the eyes).

3. Neck
   a. Inspect for symmetry of accessory neck muscles.
   b. Check the range of motion.
   c. Test cranial nerve XI (spinal accessory nerve) to check muscle strength: Ask the client to push against resistance applied to the side of the chin (tests sternocleidomastoid muscle); also ask the client to shrug the shoulders against resistance (tests trapezius muscle).
   d. The trachea is palpated: It would be midline, without any deviations.
   e. Thyroid gland: the neck is inspected as the client takes a sip of water and swallows (thyroid tissue moves up with a swallow). Palpation is done using an anterior-and-posterior approach. (Usually the normal adult thyroid cannot be palpated. If it is enlarged, auscultate for a bruit.)

4. Lymph nodes
   a. The examiner will palpate using a gentle pressure and a circular motion of the finger pads.
   b. Begins with the pre-auricular lymph nodes (in front of the ear); move to the posterior auricular lymph nodes and then downward toward the supraclavicular lymph nodes.
   c. Palpation is done with both hands, comparing the two sides for symmetry.
   d. If nodes are palpated, their size, shape, location, mobility, consistency, and tenderness are noted.

5. Reinforce client teaching: The client is instructed to notify the PHCP if persistent headache, dizziness, or neck pain occurs; swelling or lumps are noted in the head/neck region; or a neck or head injury occurs.

 Neck movements are never performed if the client has sustained a neck injury or a neck injury is suspected.

Checking and Documenting Pupillary Responses

Pupillary Light Reflex
Darken the room (to dilate the client's pupils) and ask the client to look forward.
Test each eye.
Advance a light in from the side to note constriction of the same-side pupil (direct light reflex) and simultaneous constriction of the other pupil (consensual light reflex).

Accommodation
Ask the client to focus on a distant object (dilates the pupil).
Ask the client to shift gaze to a near object held about 3 inches from the nose.
Normal response includes pupillary constriction and convergence of the axes of the eye.

Documenting Normal Findings: PERRLA
P = pupils
E = equal
R = round
RL = reactive to light
A = reactive to accommodation

C. Eyes: Includes inspection, palpation, vision-testing procedures, and the use of an ophthalmoscope
   1. Subjective data: Difficulty with vision (e.g., decreased acuity, double vision, blurring, blind spots); pain, redness, swelling, watery or other discharge from the eyes; use of glasses or contact lenses; medications being taken; history of eye problems
   2. Objective data
      a. The external eye structures are inspected, including the eyebrows for symmetry; eyelashes for even distribution; eyelids for ptosis (drooping); eyeballs for exophthalmos (protrusion) or enophthalmos (recession into the orbit, sunken eye).
      b. Structures inspected include the conjunctiva (would be clear), sclera (would be white), and lacrimal apparatus (check for excessive tearing, redness, tenderness, or swelling), cornea and lens (would be smooth and clear), iris (would be flat, with a round, regular shape and even coloration), eyelids, and pupils (Box 13.5).
   3 Snellen eye chart
      a. A simple tool to measure distance vision
      b. Position the client in a well-lit spot 20 feet from the chart, with the chart at eye level, and ask the client to read the smallest line he or she can discern. (The client is instructed to leave glasses on or contact lenses in. If the glasses are for reading only, they are removed because they blur distant vision.)
      c. One eye at a time is tested; cover the eye not being tested.

d. Results are recorded using the fraction at the end of the last line successfully read on the chart. Normal visual acuity is 20/20 (distance in feet at which the client is standing from the chart/distance in feet at which a normal eye could have read that particular line).

4. Near vision

a. Tested using a handheld vision screener (held about 14 inches from the eye) that contains various sizes of print, or the client is asked to read from a magazine

b. Each eye is tested separately with the client's glasses on or contact lenses in; normal result is 14/14 (distance in inches at which the subject holds the card from the eye/distance in inches at which a normal eye could have read that particular line)

5. Confrontation test

a. Used to measure peripheral vision and compare the client's peripheral vision with the examiner's (under the assumption that the examiner's peripheral vision is normal)

b. The client covers one eye and looks straight ahead. The examiner, positioned 2 feet away, covers his or her eye opposite the client's covered eye.

c. The examiner advances a finger or other small object in from the periphery from several directions. The client needs to see the object at the same time the examiner does.

6. Corneal light reflex

a. Used to check for parallel alignment of the axes of the eye

b. The client is asked to gaze straight ahead as the examiner holds a light about 12 inches from the client.

c. The examiner looks for reflection of the light on the corneas in exactly the same spot in each eye.

7. Cover/uncover test

a. Used to check for slight degrees of deviated alignment

b. Each eye is tested separately.

c. The examiner asks the client to gaze straight ahead and cover one eye.

d. The examiner observes the uncovered eye, expecting to note a steady, fixed gaze.

8. Diagnostic positions test (six cardinal positions of gaze) (Fig. 13.1)

a. The six muscles that attach the eyeball to its orbit and serve to direct the eye to points of interest are tested.

b. Client holds head still and is asked to move the eyes and follow a small object.

c. The examiner notes any parallel movements of the eye or nystagmus: an involuntary, rhythmic, rapid twitching of the eyeballs.

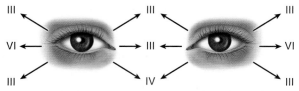

FIGURE 13.1 Checking extraocular muscles in the six cardinal positions. This indicates the functioning of cranial nerves III, IV, and VI.

9. Color vision

a. Tests for color vision involve picking numbers or letters out of a complex and colorful picture.

b. The Ishihara chart is used for testing and consists of numbers composed of colored dots located within a circle of colored dots.

c. The client is asked to read the numbers on the chart.

d. Each eye is tested separately.

e. Reading the numbers correctly indicates normal color vision.

f. The test is sensitive for the diagnosis of red-green blindness but cannot detect discrimination of blue.

⚠ The first slide on the Ishihara chart is one that everyone can discriminate; failure to identify numbers on this slide suggests a problem with performing the test, not a problem with color vision.

10. Pupils (see Box 13.5)

a. The pupils are round and of equal size.

b. Increasing light causes pupillary constriction.

c. Decreasing light causes pupillary dilation.

d. Constriction of both pupils is a normal response to direct light.

11. Sclera and cornea

a. Normal sclera color is white.

b. A yellow color to the sclera may indicate jaundice or systemic problems.

c. In a dark-skinned person, the sclera may normally appear yellow; pigmented dots may be present.

d. The cornea is transparent, smooth, shiny, and bright.

e. Cloudy areas or specks on the cornea may be the result of an accident or eye injury.

12. Ophthalmoscopy or funduscopy

a. The ophthalmoscope, or funduscope, is an instrument used to examine the external structures and the interior of the eye.

b. The room is darkened so that the pupil will dilate.

c. The examiner inspects the size, color, and clarity of the disc; the integrity of the vessels; and the appearance of the macula and fovea; and looks for retinal lesions.

13. Refer to Chapter 53 for diagnostic tests related to the eye.
14. Reinforce client teaching.
    a. Instruct the client to notify the PHCP if alterations in vision occur or any redness, swelling, or drainage from the eye is noted.
    b. Inform the client of the importance of regular eye examinations.
D. Ears: Includes inspection, palpation, hearing tests, vestibular assessment, and the use of an otoscope
    1. Subjective data: Difficulty hearing, earaches, drainage from the ears, dizziness, ringing in the ears, exposure to environmental noise, use of a hearing aid, medications being taken, history of ear problems or infections
    2. Objective data
        a. Inspect and palpate the external ear, noting size, shape, symmetry, skin color, and the presence of pain.
        b. Inspect the external auditory meatus for size, swelling, redness, discharge, and foreign bodies. Some cerumen (ear wax) may be present.
    3. Auditory assessment
        a. Sound is transmitted by air conduction and bone conduction.
        b. Air conduction takes two or three times longer than bone conduction.
        c. Hearing loss is categorized as conductive, sensorineural, or mixed conductive and sensorineural.
        d. Conductive hearing loss is caused by any physical obstruction to the transmission of sound waves.
        e. Sensorineural hearing loss is caused by a defect in the cochlea, 8th cranial nerve, or the brain itself.
        f. A mixed hearing loss is a combination of a conductive and sensorineural hearing loss; it results from problems in the inner ear, the outer ear, or the middle ear.
    4. Voice (Whisper) test
        a. Used to determine whether hearing loss has occurred
        b. One ear is tested at a time (the ear not being tested is occluded by the client).
        c. The examiner stands 1 to 2 feet from the client, covers his or her mouth so that the client cannot read the lips, exhales fully, and softly whispers two-syllable words in the direction of the unoccluded ear. The client points a finger up during the test when the examiner's voice is heard (a ticking watch may also be used to test hearing acuity).
    5. Watch test
        a. A ticking watch is used to test for high-frequency sounds.
        b. The examiner holds a ticking watch about 5 inches from each ear and asks the client if the ticking is heard.
    6. Tuning fork tests
        a. Used to measure hearing on the basis of air conduction or bone conduction; includes the Weber and Rinne tests.
        b. To activate the tuning fork, the nurse holds the base and lightly taps the tines against the other hand, setting the fork in vibration.
    7. Weber test
        a. Stem of the vibrating tuning fork is placed in the midline of the client's skull, and the client is asked if the tone sounds the same in both ears or better in one ear.
        b. The client hears the tone by bone conduction, and the sound would be heard equally in both ears.
    8. Rinne test
        a. Stem of the vibrating tuning fork is placed on the client's mastoid process.
        b. When the client no longer hears the sound, the tuning fork is quickly inverted and placed near the ear canal; the client would still hear a sound.
        c. Normally the sound is heard twice as long by way of air conduction (near the ear canal) than by way of bone conduction (at the mastoid process).
    9. Vestibular assessment (Box 13.6)
    10. Otoscopic examination
        a. An otoscope is used. For best visualization, the largest speculum that fits comfortably into the client's ear canal would be used.
        b. The client's head is tilted slightly away, to the opposite shoulder. Next the examiner pulls the pinna up and back (on an adult or older child), holds the otoscope upside down, and inserts the speculum slightly down and forward, approximately ½ inch into the ear canal.
        c. The normal tympanic membrane is translucent, shiny, and pearly gray.

⚠ Before performing an otoscopic examination and inserting the speculum, the examiner checks the auditory canal for foreign bodies. The client is instructed not to move the head during the examination to avoid the risk of perforating the tympanic membrane.

    11. Refer to Chapter 53 for diagnostic tests related to the ear.
    12. Reinforce client teaching.
        a. Instruct the client to notify the PHCP if an alteration in hearing, ear pain, or ringing in the ears occurs, or redness, swelling, or drainage from the ear is noted.

BOX 13.6 **Vestibular Assessment**

Test for Falling

1. The examiner asks the client to stand with the feet together, arms hanging loosely at the sides, and eyes closed.
2. The client normally remains erect, with only slight swaying.
3. A significant sway is a positive Romberg sign.

Test for Past Pointing

1. The client sits in front of the examiner.
2. The client closes the eyes and extends the arms in front, pointing both index fingers at the examiner.
3. The examiner holds and touches his or her own extended index fingers under the client's extended index fingers to give the client a point of reference.
4. The client is instructed to raise both arms and then lower them, attempting to return to the examiner's extended index fingers.
5. The normal test response is that the client can easily return to the point of reference.
6. The client with a vestibular function problem lacks a normal sense of position and cannot return the extended fingers to the point of reference; instead, the fingers deviate to the right or left of the reference point.

Gaze Nystagmus Evaluation

1. The client's eyes are examined as the client looks straight ahead, 30 degrees to each side, upward and downward.
2. Any spontaneous nystagmus—an involuntary, rhythmic, rapid twitching of the eyeballs—represents a problem with the vestibular system.

Dix-Hallpike Maneuver

1. The client starts in a sitting position; the examiner lowers the client to the examination table and rather quickly turns the client's head to the 45 degrees position.
2. If after about 30 seconds there is no nystagmus, the client is returned to a sitting position, and the test is repeated on the other side.

---

  b. Instruct the client in the proper method of cleaning the ear canal.
  c. The client needs to cleanse the ear canal with the corner of a moistened washcloth and must never insert sharp objects or cotton-tipped applicators into the ear canal.
E. Nose, mouth, and throat: Includes inspection and palpation
  1. Subjective data
   a. Nose: The examiner checks for discharge or nosebleed (epistaxis), facial or sinus pain, history of frequent colds, altered sense of smell, allergies, medications being taken, history of nose trauma or surgery.
   b. Mouth and throat: The examiner checks for the presence of sores or lesions, bleeding from the gums or elsewhere, altered sense of taste, toothaches, use of dentures or other appliances, tooth- and mouth-care hygiene habits, at-risk behaviors (e.g., smoking, alcohol consumption), history of infection, trauma, or surgery.
  2. Objective data
   a. External nose would be midline and in proportion to other facial features.
   b. Patency of the nostrils can be tested by pushing each nasal cavity closed and asking the client to sniff inward through the other nostril.
   c. A nasal speculum and penlight or a short, wide-tipped speculum attached to an otoscope head is used to inspect for redness, swelling, discharge, bleeding, or foreign bodies. The nasal septum is checked for deviation.
   d. The examiner presses the frontal sinuses (below the eyebrows) and over the maxillary sinuses (below the cheekbones). The client would feel firm pressure but no pain.
   e. The external and inner surfaces of the lips are checked for color, moisture, cracking, or lesions.
   f. The teeth are inspected for condition and number (would be white, spaced evenly, straight, clean, and free of debris and decay).
   g. The alignment of the upper and lower jaw is checked by having the client bite down.
   h. The gums are inspected for swelling, bleeding, discoloration, and retraction of gingival margins (gums normally appear pink).
   i. The tongue is inspected for color, surface characteristics, moisture, white patches, nodules, and ulcerations (dorsal surface is normally rough; ventral surface is smooth and glistening, with visible veins).
   j. The examiner retracts the cheek with a tongue depressor to check the buccal mucosa for color and for the presence of nodules or lesions. Normal mucosa is glistening, pink, soft, moist, and smooth.
   k. Using a penlight and tongue depressor, the examiner inspects the hard and soft palates for color, shape, texture, and defects. The hard palate (roof of the mouth), which is located anteriorly, would be white and dome-shaped; the soft palate, which extends posteriorly, would be light pink and smooth. The pharyngeal (gag) reflex can also be tested.
   l. The uvula is inspected for midline location. The examiner asks the client to say "Ahhh" and watches for the soft palate and uvula to rise in the midline. (This tests 1 function of cranial nerve X, the vagus nerve.)
   m. Using a penlight and tongue depressor, the examiner inspects the throat for color, presence of tonsils, and the presence of exudate or lesions. One of the techniques to test cranial nerve XII (the hypoglossal nerve) is asking the

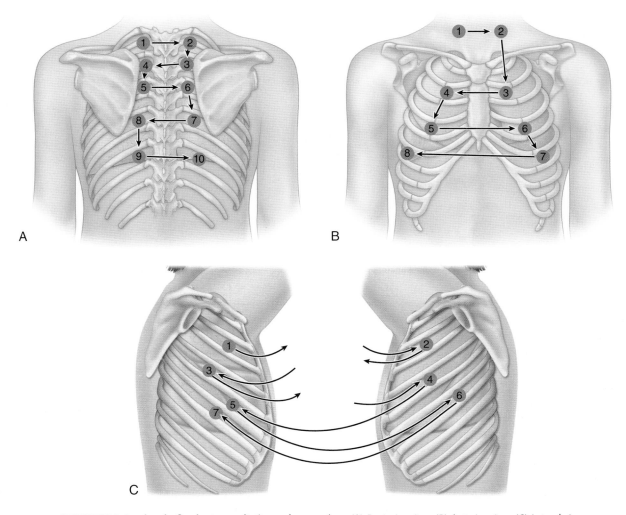

FIGURE 13.2 **Landmarks for chest auscultation and percussion.** (A) Posterior view. (B) Anterior view. (C) Lateral view.

client to stick out the tongue (would protrude in the midline).

   3. Reinforce client teaching

      a. Emphasize the importance of hygiene and tooth care, as well as regular dental examinations and the use of fluoridated water or fluoride supplements.

      b. Encourage the client to avoid at-risk behaviors (e.g., smoking, alcohol consumption).

      c. Stress the importance of reporting pain or abnormal occurrence (e.g., nodules, lesions, signs of infection).

F. Lungs

   1. Subjective data: Cough; expectoration of sputum; shortness of breath or dyspnea; chest pain on breathing; environmental exposure to pollution or chemicals; medications being taken; history of respiratory disease or infection; last tuberculosis test; chest x-ray; pneumonia and any influenza immunizations. Record the smoking history in pack/years (the number of packs per day times the number of years smoked). For example, a client who has smoked one half-pack a day for 20 years has a 10 pack/year smoking history.

   2. Objective data: Includes inspection, palpation, percussion, and auscultation

   3. Inspection of the anterior and posterior chest: Note skin color and condition and the rate and quality of respirations, look for lumps or lesions, note the shape and configuration of the chest wall, and note the position the client takes to breathe.

   4. Palpation: The examiner will palpate the entire chest wall, noting skin temperature and moisture and looking for areas of tenderness and lumps, lesions, masses, or tenderness; chest excursion and tactile or vocal fremitus are assessed.

   5. Percussion

      a. Starting at the apices, the examiner percusses across the top of the shoulders, moving to the interspaces, making a side-to-side comparison all the way down the lung area (Fig. 13.2).

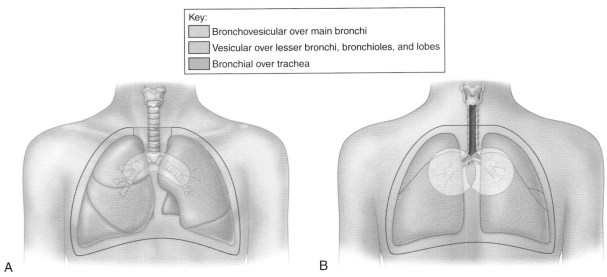

FIGURE 13.3 **Auscultatory sounds.** (A) Anterior thorax. (B) Posterior thorax.

TABLE 13.2   **Characteristics of Adventitious Sounds**

Adventitious Sounds	Characteristics	Clinical Examples
Crackles (previously called *rales*)	*Fine crackles:* high-pitched crackling and popping noises (discontinuous sounds) heard during the end of inspiration. Not cleared by cough. *Medium crackles:* medium-pitched moist sound heard about halfway through inspiration; not cleared by cough. *Coarse crackles:* low-pitched, bubbling or gurgling sounds that start early during inspiration and extend into the first part of expiration.	*Fine crackles:* may be heard in pneumonia, heart failure, asthma, and restrictive pulmonary diseases. *Medium crackles:* same as fine, but condition is worse. *Coarse crackles:* same as fine and medium as noted above; may be heard in terminally ill clients with diminished gag reflex and in individuals with pulmonary edema or pulmonary fibrosis.
Wheeze (also called *sibilant* wheeze)	High-pitched, musical sound similar to a squeak. Heard more commonly during expiration, but may also be heard during inspiration. Occurs in small airways.	Heard in narrowed airway diseases such as asthma.
Rhonchi (also called *sonorous* wheeze)	Low-pitched, coarse, loud, low snoring or moaning tone. Actually sounds like snoring. Heard primarily during expiration, but may also be heard during inspiration. Coughing may clear.	Heard in disorders causing obstruction of the trachea or bronchus, such as chronic bronchitis.
Pleural friction rub	A superficial, low-pitched, coarse rubbing or grating sound. Sounds like two surfaces rubbing together. Heard throughout inspiration and expiration. Loudest over the lower anterolateral surface. Not cleared by cough.	Heard in individuals with pleurisy (inflammation of the pleural surfaces).

Data from Wilson AF, Giddens JF: Health assessment for nursing practice, ed 4, St. Louis, 2009, Mosby.

b. The examiner will determine the predominant note. Resonance is noted in healthy lung tissue.

c. Hyperresonance is noted when excessive air is present, and a dull note indicates lung density.

 6. Auscultation

    a. Use the flat diaphragm end piece of the stethoscope and hold it firmly against the chest wall and listen for at least one full respiration in each location (anterior, posterior, and lateral).

    b. Posterior: Start at the apices and move side to side for comparison (see Fig. 13.2).

    c. Anterior: Auscultate the lung fields from the apices in the supraclavicular area down to the sixth rib. Avoid auscultation over female breast tissue (displace this tissue) because a dull sound will be produced (see Fig. 13.2).

    d. Compare findings on each side.

7. Normal breath sounds: Three types of breath sounds are considered normal in certain parts of the thorax. These include vesicular, bronchovesicular, and bronchial. Breath sounds would be clear to auscultation (Fig. 13.3).

8. Abnormal breath sounds: Also known as adventitious sounds (Table 13.2)

9. Voice sounds (Box 13.7)

    a. Performed when a pathological lung condition is suspected

    b. Auscultate the spoken word over the chest wall.

BOX 13.7 Voice Sounds During Lung Auscultation

Bronchophony
Ask the client to repeat the words "ninety-nine."
Normal voice transmission is soft, muffled, and indistinct.

Egophony
Ask the client to repeat a long "ee-ee-ee" sound.
Normally the nurse would hear the "ee-ee-ee" sound.

Whispered Pectoriloquy
Ask the client to whisper the word "ninety-nine."
Normal voice transmission is faint, muffled, and almost inaudible.

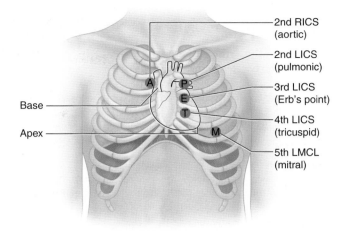

FIGURE 13.4 **Auscultation areas of the heart.** *LICS,* Left intercostal space; *LMCL,* left midclavicular line; *RICS,* right intercostal space.

c. The client is asked to vocalize words or a phrase while the examiner listens to the chest.

d. Normal voice transmission is soft and muffled. The examiner can hear the sound but is unable to distinguish exactly what is being said.

 When auscultating breath sounds, instruct the client to breathe through the mouth, and monitor the client for dizziness.

10. Refer to Chapter 47 for diagnostic tests related to the respiratory system.
11. Reinforce client teaching
    a. Encourage the client to avoid exposure to environmental hazards, including smoking. (Discuss smoking-cessation programs as appropriate.)
    b. The client needs to undergo periodic examinations as prescribed (e.g., chest x-ray, tuberculosis skin testing).
    c. Encourage the client to obtain pneumonia and influenza immunizations.
    d. The PHCP needs to be notified if the client experiences persistent cough, shortness of breath, or other respiratory symptoms.

G. The heart and peripheral vascular system
1. Subjective data: Chest pain, dyspnea, cough, fatigue, edema, nocturia, leg pain or cramps (claudication), changes in skin color, obesity, medications being taken, cardiovascular risk factors, family history of cardiac or vascular problems, personal history of cardiac or vascular problems
2. Objective data: May include inspection, palpation, percussion, and auscultation
3. Inspection: Inspect the anterior chest for pulsations (apical impulse) created as the left ventricle rotates against the chest wall during systole; not always visible.

4. Palpation
   a. The examiner may palpate the apical impulse at the fourth or fifth interspace, or medial to the midclavicular line (not palpable in obese clients or clients with thick chest walls).
   b. The examiner may palpate the apex, left sternal border, and base for pulsations; normally none are present.
5. Percussion: May be performed to outline the heart's borders and check for cardiac enlargement (denoted by resonance over the lung and dull notes over the heart).
6. Auscultation
   a. Auscultation areas of the heart (Fig. 13.4)
   b. Auscultate heart rate and rhythm. Check for a pulse deficit (auscultate the apical heartbeat while palpating an artery) if an irregularity is noted.
   c. Check for S1 ("lub") and S2 ("dub") sounds. If abnormalities such as irregularities in the beat, extra heart sounds, or the presence of gentle blowing or swooshing sounds (murmurs) are noted, the RN or PHCP is notified.
7. Peripheral vascular system
   a. Check for adequacy of blood flow to the extremities by palpating arterial pulses for equality and symmetry and checking the condition of the skin and nails.
   b. Check for pretibial edema and measure calf circumference (see Table 13.1).
   c. Measure blood pressure.
   d. The examiner may palpate superficial inguinal nodes (using firm but gentle pressure), beginning in the inguinal area and moving down toward the inner thigh.
   e. An ultrasonic stethoscope may be needed to amplify the sounds of a pulse wave if the pulse cannot be palpated.

BOX 13.8 **Arterial Pulse Points and Grading the Force of Pulses**

Arteries in the Arms and Hands
Radial pulse: Located at the radial side of the forearm at the wrist
Ulnar pulse: Located on the opposite side of the location of the radial pulse at the wrist
Brachial pulse: Located above the elbow at the antecubital fossa, between the biceps and triceps muscles

Arteries in the Legs
Femoral pulse: Located below the inguinal ligament, midway between the symphysis pubis and the anterosuperior iliac spine
Popliteal pulse: Located behind the knee
Dorsalis pedis pulse: Located at the top of the foot, in line with the groove between the extensor tendons of the great and first toes
Posterior tibial pulse: Located inside of the ankle, behind and below the medial malleolus (ankle bone)

Grading the Force
4 + = strong and bounding
3 + = full pulse, increased
2 + = normal, easily palpable
1 + = weak, barely palpable

---

    f. Carotid artery: Located in the groove between the trachea and sternocleidomastoid muscle, medial to and alongside the muscle
    g. Palpate one carotid artery at a time to avoid compromising blood flow to the brain. The examiner will also auscultate each carotid artery for the presence of a bruit (a blowing, swishing sound, which indicates blood-flow turbulence). Normally a bruit is not present.
    h. Palpate the arteries in the extremities (Box 13.8).
  8. Refer to Chapter 49 for diagnostic tests related to the cardiovascular system.

  9. Reinforce client teaching.
    a. Advise the client to modify lifestyle for risk factors associated with heart and vascular disease.
    b. Encourage the client to seek regular physical examinations.
    c. Client must seek medical assistance for signs of heart or vascular disease.

H. The breasts
  1. Subjective data: Pain or tenderness, lumps or thickening, swollen axillary lymph nodes, nipple discharge, rash or swelling, medications being taken, personal or family history of breast disease, trauma or injury to the breasts, previous surgery on the breasts, breast self-examination (BSE) compliance, mammograms as prescribed

  2. Objective data: Includes inspection and palpation

⚠️ An important role of the nurse is to teach the client how to perform the BSE, which involves inspection and palpation.

  3. Inspection
    a. Performed with the client's arms raised above the head, the hands pressed against the hips, and the arms extended straight ahead while the client sits and leans forward
    b. Check size and symmetry (one breast is often larger than the other); masses, flattening, retraction, or dimpling; color and venous pattern; size, color, shape, and discharge in the nipple and areola; and the direction in which nipples point.
  4. Palpation
    a. Client lies supine with the arm on the side being examined behind the head and a small pillow under the shoulder.
    b. The examiner uses the pads of the first three fingers to compress the breast tissue gently against the chest wall, noting tissue consistency.
    c. Palpation is performed systematically, ensuring that the entire breast and tail are palpated.
    d. The examiner notes the consistency of the breast tissue, which normally feels dense, firm, and elastic.
    e. The examiner gently palpates the nipple and areola, and compresses the nipple, noting any discharge.
  5. Axillary lymph nodes
    a. The examiner faces the client and stands on the side being examined, supporting the client's arm in a slightly flexed position, and abducts the arm away from the chest wall.
    b. The examiner places the free hand against the client's chest wall and high in the axillary hollow; then, with the fingertips, gently presses down, rolling soft tissue over the surface of the ribs and muscles.
    c. Lymph nodes are normally not palpable.
  6. Reinforce client teaching.
    a. Encourage and teach the client to perform BSE. (Refer to Chapter 41 for information on performing BSE.)
    b. BSE must be performed 7 to 10 days after the menses. Postmenopausal clients or those who have had a hysterectomy would select a specific day of the month and perform BSE monthly on that day.
    c. Regular physical examinations and mammograms would be obtained as prescribed.
    d. The client needs to report lumps or masses to the PHCP immediately.

I. The abdomen
1. Subjective data: Changes in appetite or weight, difficulty swallowing, dietary intake, intolerance to certain foods, nausea or vomiting, pain, bowel habits, medications being taken, history of abdominal problems or abdominal surgery
2. Objective data
   a. The client is asked to empty the bladder.
   b. Be sure to warm the hands and the end piece of the stethoscope.
   c. Painful areas are examined last.

⚠ When performing an abdominal assessment, the specific order for assessment techniques is inspection, auscultation, percussion, and palpation.

3. Inspection
   a. Contour: The examiner will look down at the abdomen and then across the abdomen from the rib margin to the pubic bone; described as flat, rounded, concave, or protuberant.
   b. Symmetry: Note any bulging or masses.
   c. Umbilicus: Would be midline and inverted
   d. Skin surface: Would be smooth and even
   e. Pulsations from the aorta may be noted in the epigastric area, and peristaltic waves may be noted across the abdomen.
4. Auscultation
   a. Perform auscultation before percussion and palpation, which can increase peristalsis.
   b. Hold the stethoscope lightly against the skin and listen for bowel sounds in all four quadrants. Begin in the right lower quadrant (as bowel sounds are normally heard here).
   c. Note the character and frequency of normal bowel sounds: high-pitched gurgling sounds occurring irregularly from 5 to 30 times a minute.
   d. Identify as normal, hypoactive, or hyperactive (borborygmus).
   e. Absent sounds: Auscultate for 5 minutes before determining that sounds are absent.
5. Percussion
   a. All four quadrants are percussed lightly by the examiner.
   b. Borders of the liver and spleen are percussed and measured.
   c. Tympany would predominate over the abdomen with dullness over the liver and spleen.
   d. Percussion over the kidney at the 12th rib (costovertebral angle) would produce no pain. This is also known as costovertebral tenderness.
6. Palpation
   a. The examiner will begin with light palpation of all four quadrants, using the fingers to depress the skin about 1 cm. Next, the examiner

will perform deep palpation, depressing 5 to 8 cm.
   b. The examiner will palpate the liver and spleen (which may not be palpable).
   c. The examiner will palpate the aortic pulsation in the upper abdomen slightly to the left of midline. Normally it pulsates in a forward direction. (Pulsation expands laterally if an aneurysm is present.)
7. Refer to Chapter 45 for diagnostic tests related to the gastrointestinal system.
8. Reinforce client teaching.
   a. Encourage the client to consume a balanced diet.
   b. Substances that can cause gastric irritation must be avoided.
   c. The regular use of laxatives is discouraged.
   d. Lifestyle behaviors that can cause gastric irritation (e.g., smoking, spicy foods) would be avoided.
   e. Regular physical examinations are important.
   f. The client must report gastrointestinal problems to the PHCP.

J. Musculoskeletal system
1. Subjective data: Joint pain or stiffness; redness, swelling, or warm joints; limited motion of joints; muscle pain, cramps, or weakness; bone pain; limitations in activities of daily living; exercise patterns; exposure to occupational hazards (e.g., heavy lifting, prolonged standing or sitting); medications being taken; history of joint, muscle, or bone injuries; history of surgery of the joints, muscles, or bones
2. Objective data: Inspection and palpation
3. Inspection: Inspect gait and posture and for cervical, thoracic, and lumbar curves (Box 13.9).
4. Palpation: The examiner will palpate all bones, joints, and surrounding muscles.
5. Range of motion
   a. Perform active and passive range-of-motion exercises of each major joint.
   b. Check for pain, limited mobility, spastic movement, joint instability, stiffness, and contractures.
   c. If range of motion is unable to be performed, clarify with client whether it is because of muscle weakness or pain.
   d. Normally joints are nontender, without swelling, and move freely.

BOX 13.9 **Common Postural Abnormalities**

Lordosis (swayback): Increased lumbar curvature
Kyphosis (hunchback): Exaggeration of the posterior curvature of the thoracic spine
Scoliosis: Lateral spinal curvature

6. Muscle tone and strength
   a. This will be checked during measurement of range of motion
   b. The client is asked to flex the muscle to be examined and then to resist while applying opposing force against the flexion.
   c. Check for increased tone (hypertonicity) or little tone (hypotonicity).
7. Grading muscle strength (Table 13.3)
8. Refer to Chapter 57 for diagnostic tests related to the musculoskeletal system.
9. Reinforce client teaching.
   a. The client needs to consume a balanced diet, including foods high in calcium and vitamin D.
   b. Activities that cause muscle strain or stress to the joints must be avoided.

   c. Encourage the client to maintain a normal weight.
   d. Participation in a regular exercise program is beneficial.
   e. The client must contact the PHCP if joint or muscle pain or problems occur, or if limitations in range of motion or muscle strength develop.
K. Neurological system (refer to Chapter 55 for additional information)
   1. Subjective data: Headache, dizziness or vertigo, tremors, weakness, incoordination, numbness or tingling in any area of the body, difficulty speaking or swallowing, medication(s) being taken, history of seizure, history of head injury or surgery, exposure to environmental or occupational hazard(s) (e.g., chemicals, alcohol, drugs)
   2. Objective data: Include assessment of cranial nerves, level of consciousness, pupils, motor function, cerebellar function, coordination, sensory function, and reflexes.
   3. Note mental and emotional status, behavior and appearance, language ability, and intellectual functioning, including memory, knowledge, abstract thinking, association, and judgment.
   4. Vital signs: Check temperature, pulse, respirations, and blood pressure; monitor for blood pressure or pulse changes, which may indicate increased intracranial pressure (ICP) in a client with a neurological disorder. (See Chapter 47 for abnormal respiratory patterns.)
   5. Cranial nerves: Assessed by the examiner (Table 13.4)
   6. Level of consciousness
      a. Check the client's behavior to determine level of consciousness (e.g., alertness, confusion, delirium, unconsciousness, stupor,

TABLE 13.3   Criteria for Grading and Recording Muscle Strength

Functional Level	Lovett Scale	Grade	Percentage of Normal
No evidence of contractility	Zero (0)	0	0
Evidence of slight contractility	Trace (T)	1	10
Complete range of motion with gravity eliminated	Poor (P)	2	25
Complete range of motion with gravity	Fair (F)	3	50
Complete range of motion against gravity with some resistance	Good (G)	4	75
Complete range of motion against gravity with full resistance	Normal (N)	5	100

Data from Wilson AF, Giddens JF: Health assessment for nursing practice, ed 4, St. Louis, 2009, Mosby.

TABLE 13.4   Cranial Nerves: Function and Testing

Cranial Nerve	Function of Nerve	Testing the Nerve
Cranial nerve I: Olfactory	Sensory: Controls the sense of smell	The client is asked to close his or her eyes and occlude one nostril with a finger. Then, the client is asked to identify nonirritating and familiar odors (e.g., coffee, tea, cloves, soap, chewing gum, peppermint). The test is repeated on the other nostril.
Cranial nerve II: Optic	Sensory: Controls vision	Visual acuity is assessed with a Snellen chart and an ophthalmoscopic examination. Peripheral vision is checked by confrontation. Color vision is checked.
Cranial Nerves III, IV, and VI		
Cranial nerve III: Oculomotor	Motor: Controls pupillary constriction, upper-eyelid elevation, and most eye movement	The motor functions of these nerves overlap; therefore, they would be tested together. The eyelids are inspected for ptosis (drooping); then ocular movements are assessed, noting any eye deviation.

TABLE 13.4 Cranial Nerves: Function and Testing—cont'd

Cranial Nerve	Function of Nerve	Testing the Nerve
Cranial nerve IV: Trochlear	Motor: Controls downward and inward eye movement	Accommodation and direct and consensual light reflexes are tested.
Cranial nerve VI: Abducens	Motor: Controls lateral eye movement	
Cranial nerve V: Trigeminal	Sensory and motor: Controls sensation in the cornea, nasal and oral mucosa, and facial skin, as well as mastication	To test motor function, the client is asked to clench the teeth, and the muscles of mastication are assessed; then the examiner tries to open the client's jaw after asking client to keep it tightly closed. The corneal reflex is tested by lightly touching the client's cornea with a cotton wisp. (This test may be omitted if the client is alert and blinking normally.) Sensory function is checked by asking the client to close the eyes; the examiner lightly touches forehead, cheeks, and chin, noting whether the touch is felt equally on the two sides.
Cranial nerve VII: Facial	Sensory and motor: Controls movement of the face and taste sensation	Taste perception is tested on the anterior two thirds of the tongue; the client would be able to taste salty and sweet. The client is asked to smile, frown, and show the teeth, and asked to puff out the cheeks. The examiner attempts to close the client's eyes against resistance.
Cranial nerve VIII: Acoustic or vestibulocochlear	Sensory: Controls hearing and vestibular function	Assessing the client's ability to hear tests the cochlear portion. Assessing the client's sense of equilibrium tests the vestibular portion. The client's hearing is checked using acuity tests. Observe the client's balance and watch for swaying when he or she is walking or standing. Assessment of sensorineural hearing loss may be done by the examiner with the Weber or Rinne test.
Cranial Nerve IX and X Cranial nerve IX: Glosso-pharyngeal	Sensory and motor: Controls swallowing ability, sensation in the pharyngeal soft palate and tonsillar mucosa, taste perception on the posterior third of the tongue, and salivation	Usually cranial nerves IX and X are tested together. The client's taste perception is tested on the posterior one third of the tongue or pharynx; the client would be able to taste bitter and sour tastes. The soft palate is inspected, and the examiner watches for symmetrical elevation when the client says "Aaah."
Cranial nerve X: Vagus	Sensory and motor: Controls swallowing and phonation, sensation in the exterior ear's posterior wall, and sensation behind the ear Controls sensation in the thoracic and abdominal viscera	The posterior pharyngeal wall is touched with a tongue depressor to elicit the gag reflex.
Cranial nerve XI: Spinal accessory	Motor: Controls strength of neck and shoulder muscles	The examiner palpates and inspects the sternocleidomastoid muscle as the client pushes the chin against the examiner's hand. The examiner palpates and inspects the trapezius muscle as the client shrugs the shoulders against the examiner's resistance.
Cranial nerve XII: Hypo-glossal	Motor: Controls tongue movements involved in swallowing and speech	The examiner observes the tongue for asymmetry, atrophy, deviation to one side, and fasciculations (uncontrollable twitching). The client is asked to push the tongue against a tongue depressor, and then the client is asked to move the tongue rapidly in and out and from side to side.

coma). The data collection process becomes increasingly invasive as the client is less responsive.
b. Speak to client.
c. Determine appropriateness of behavior and conversation.
d. Lightly touch the client (as culturally appropriate).

7. Pupils
a. Check size, equality, and reaction to light (brisk, slow, or fixed), and note any unusual eye movements (check direct light and consensual light reflex).
b. This component of the neurological examination may be performed during the data collection process of the eye.

8. Motor function
   a. Check muscle tone, including strength and equality.
   b. Monitor for voluntary and involuntary movements and purposeful and nonpurposeful movements.
   c. This component of the neurological examination may be performed during the data collection process of the musculoskeletal system.
9. Cerebellar function
   a. Monitor gait as the client walks in a straight line, heel to toe (tandem walking).
   b. Romberg test: The client is asked to stand with the feet together and the arms at the sides and to close the eyes and hold the position. Normally the client can maintain posture and balance.
   c. If appropriate, the client is asked to perform a shallow knee bend or hop in place on one leg and then the other.
10. Coordination
    a. This is checked by asking the client to perform rapid alternating movements of the hands (e.g., turning the hands over and patting the knees continuously).
    b. The examiner asks the client to touch the examiner's finger, then his or her own nose. The client keeps the eyes open, and the examiner moves the finger to different spots to ensure that the client's movements are smooth and accurate.
    c. Heel-to-shin test: The client is assisted into a supine position, then asked to place the heel on the opposite knee and run it down the shin. Normally the client moves the heel down the shin in a straight line.
11. Sensory function
    a. Pain: Checked by applying an object with a sharp point and one with a dull point to the client's body in random order; the client is asked to identify the sharp and dull feelings.
    b. Light touch: A piece of cotton is brushed over the client's skin at various locations in a random order, and the client is asked to say when the touch is felt.
    c. Position sense (kinesthesia): The client's finger or toe is moved up or down, and the client is asked which way it has been moved. This tests the client's ability to perceive passive movement.
    d. Stereognosis: Tests the client's ability to recognize objects placed in his or her hand
    e. Graphesthesia: Tests the client's ability to identify a number traced on the client's hand
    f. Two-point discrimination: Tests the client's ability to discriminate two simultaneous pinpricks on the skin

---

BOX 13.10   Scoring Deep Tendon Reflex Activity

0 = No response
1 + = Sluggish or diminished
2 + = Active or expected response
3 + = Slightly hyperactive, more brisk than normal; not necessarily pathological
4 + = Brisk, hyperactive with intermittent clonus associated with disease

Adapted from Wilson AF, Giddens JF: Health assessment for nursing practice, ed 4, St. Louis, 2009, Mosby.

12. Deep tendon reflexes
    a. Includes testing the following reflexes: biceps, triceps, brachioradialis, patella, Achilles
    b. Limb would be relaxed.
    c. The tendon is tapped quickly with a reflex hammer, which would cause contraction of muscle.
    d. Scoring deep tendon reflex activity (Box 13.10)
13. Plantar reflex
    a. A cutaneous (superficial) reflex; is tested with a pointed, but not sharp, object
    b. The sole of the client's foot is stroked from the heel, up the lateral side, and then across the ball of the foot to the medial side.
    c. The normal response is plantar flexion of all toes.

⚠️ Dorsiflexion of the great toe and fanning of the other toes (Babinski's sign) are abnormal in anyone older than 2 years and indicate the presence of central nervous system disease, suggestive of an upper motor neuron lesion.

14. Testing for meningeal irritation
    a. A positive Brudzinski's sign or Kernig's sign indicates meningeal irritation.
    b. Brudzinski's sign is tested with the client in the supine position. The nurse flexes the client's head (gently moves the head to the chest), and there would be no reports of pain or resistance to the neck flexion; a positive Brudzinski's sign is observed if the client passively flexes the hip and knee in response to neck flexion and reports pain in the vertebral column.
    c. Kernig's sign is positive when the client flexes the legs at the hip and knee and complains of pain along the vertebral column when the leg is extended.
15. Refer to Chapter 55 for diagnostic tests related to the neurological system.
16. Reinforce client teaching.
    a. The client must avoid exposure to environmental hazards (e.g., insecticides, lead).
    b. High-risk behaviors that can result in head and spinal cord injuries must be avoided.

c. Protective devices (e.g., a helmet, body pads) must be worn when participating in high-risk behaviors; seat belts would always be worn.

L. Female genitalia and reproductive tract

1. Subjective data: Urinary difficulties or symptoms such as frequency, urgency, or burning; vaginal discharge; pain; menstrual and obstetrical histories; onset of menopause; medications being taken; sexual activity and the use of contraceptives; history of sexually transmitted infections

2. Objective data
   a. Use a calm and relaxing approach. The examination is embarrassing for many women and may be a difficult experience for an adolescent.
   b. Consider the client's cultural background and her beliefs with regard to examination of the genitalia.
   c. Consider sexual orientation in these types of exams, such as transgendered individual and the sensitivity required in caring for this special population.
   d. A complete examination will include the external genitalia and a vaginal examination.
   e. The nurse's role is to prepare the client for the examination and assist the PHCP.
   f. The client is asked to empty her bladder before the examination.
   g. The client is placed in the lithotomy position, and a drape is placed across the client.

3. External genitalia
   a. Quantity and distribution of hair
   b. Characteristics of labia majora and minora (no inflammation, edema, lesions, or lacerations would be noted)
   c. Urethral orifice is observed for color and position.
   d. Vaginal orifice (introitus) is inspected for inflammation, edema, discoloration, discharge, and lesions.
   e. The examiner may check Skene's and Bartholin's glands for tenderness or discharge (if discharge is present, color, odor, and consistency are noted and a culture of the discharge is obtained).
   f. The client is checked for the presence of a cystocele (a portion of the vaginal wall and bladder prolapse or fall into the orifice anteriorly) or a rectocele (bulging of the posterior wall of the vagina caused by prolapse of the rectum).

4. Speculum examination of the internal genitalia
   a. Performed by the PHCP
   b. Permits visualization of the cervix and vagina
   c. Papanicolaou (Pap) smear test: A painless screening test for cervical cancer is done; the specimen is obtained during the speculum examination, and the nurse helps prepare the specimen for laboratory analysis.

5. Reinforce client teaching.
   a. Stress the importance of personal hygiene.
   b. Explain the purpose and recommended frequency of Pap tests.
   c. Explain the signs of sexually transmitted infections.
   d. Educate the client on measures to take for the prevention of sexually transmitted infections.
   e. Inform the client with a sexually transmitted infection that she must inform her sexual partner of the need for an examination.

M. Male genitalia

1. Subjective data: Urinary difficulty (e.g., frequency, urgency, hesitancy or straining, dysuria, nocturia); pain, lesions, or discharge on or from the penis; pain or lesions in the scrotum; medications being taken; sexual activity and the use of contraceptives; history of sexually transmitted infections

2. Objective data
   a. Includes assessment (inspection and palpation) by the examiner of the external genitalia and inguinal ring and canal
   b. The client may stand or lie down for this examination.
   c. Genitalia are manipulated gently to avoid causing erection or discomfort.
   d. Sexual maturity is checked by noting the size and shape of the penis and testes, the color and texture of the scrotal skin, and the character and distribution of pubic hair.
   e. The penis is checked for the presence of lesions or discharge. A culture is obtained if a discharge is present.
   f. The scrotum is inspected for size, shape, and symmetry (normally the left testicle hangs lower than the right) and palpated for the presence of any lumps.
   g. Inguinal ring and canal: Inspection (asking the client to bear down) and palpation are performed by the PHCP to check for the presence of a hernia.

3. Reinforce client teaching.
   a. Stress the importance of personal hygiene.
   b. Teach the client how to perform testicular self-examination (TSE). A day of the month is selected, and the examination is performed on the same day each month after a shower or bath when the hands are warm and soapy and the scrotum is warm. (Refer to Chapter 41 for information on performing TSE.)
   c. Explain the signs of sexually transmitted infections.
   d. Educate the client on measures to prevent sexually transmitted infections.
   e. Inform the client with a sexually transmitted infection that he must inform his sexual partner of the need for an examination.

N. Rectum and anus
1. Subjective data: Usual bowel pattern; any change in bowel habits; rectal pain, bleeding from the rectum, or black or tarry stools; dietary habits; problems with urination; previous screening for colorectal cancer; medications being taken; history of rectal or colon problems; family history of rectal or colon problems
2. Objective data
   a. Examination can detect colorectal cancer in its early stages. In men, the rectal examination can also detect prostate tumors.
   b. Women may be examined in the lithotomy position after examination of the genitalia.
   c. A man is best examined by having the client bend forward with his hips flexed and upper body resting over the examination table.
   d. A nonambulatory client may be examined in the left lateral (Sims') position.
   e. The external anus is inspected for lumps or lesions, rashes, inflammation or excoriation, scars, or hemorrhoids.
   f. Digital examination is performed by the PHCP
   g. Digital examination is performed to assess sphincter tone; check for tenderness, irregularities, polyps, masses, or nodules in the rectal wall; and assess the prostate gland.
   h. The prostate gland is normally firm, without bogginess, tenderness, or nodules. (Hardness or nodules may indicate the presence of a cancerous lesion.)
3. Reinforce client teaching.
   a. The diet would include high-fiber and low-fat foods and plenty of liquids.
   b. The client would obtain regular digital examinations.
   c. The client needs to be able to identify the symptoms of colorectal cancer or prostatic cancer (men).
   d. The client would follow the American Cancer Society's guidelines for screening for colorectal cancer and prostate cancer.

VI. Documenting Health and Physical Assessment Findings

A. Documentation findings may be recorded either written or electronically (depending on agency protocol).

B. Whether written or electronic, the documentation is a legal document and permanent record of the client's health status.

C. Principles of documentation need to be followed, and data need to be recorded accurately, concisely, completely, legibly, and objectively without bias or opinions. Also, always follow agency protocol for documentation.

D. Documentation findings serve as a source of client information for other PHCPs. Procedures for maintaining confidentiality are always followed.

E. Record findings about the client's health history and physical examination as soon as possible after completion of the health assessment.

F. Refer to Chapter 6 for additional information about documentation guidelines.

WHAT WOULD YOU DO?

Answer: If the nurse notes an irregular beat when auscultating the heart rate, the nurse needs to be sure to listen for 1 full minute to obtain adequate information. The nurse would also note the client's appearance and notify the registered nurse (RN). The RN will then perform a complete cardiac assessment and notify the primary health care provider. The nurse would also document the findings.

PRACTICE QUESTIONS

❖ **1.** The nurse is assisting to perform a focused data collection process on a client who is complaining of symptoms of a cold, a cough, and lung congestion. Which would the nurse include for this type of data collection? **Select all that apply.**
   ❏ **1.** Listening to lung sounds
   ❏ **2.** Obtaining the client's temperature
   ❏ **3.** Checking the strength of peripheral pulses
   ❏ **4.** Obtaining information about the client's respirations
   ❏ **5.** Performing a musculoskeletal and neurological examination
   ❏ **6.** Asking the client about a family history of any illness or disease

2. A client with a diagnosis of asthma is admitted to the hospital with respiratory distress. Which signs would the nurse expect to note in the health record when collecting data related to the respiratory system for this client?
   1. Stridor and cyanotic lips
   2. Diminished breath sounds and fever
   3. Wheezes and use of accessory muscles
   4. Pleural friction rub and inspirational chest pain

❖ **3.** The nurse is reviewing the client's health record and notes that the client elicited a positive Romberg sign. Based on this finding, the nurse would institute which intervention? **Select all that apply.**
   ❏ **1.** Collect data to determine factors for fall risk.
   ❏ **2.** Close the blinds and turn off the overhead light.
   ❏ **3.** Instruct the client to ask for assistance when getting up to walk.
   ❏ **4.** Teach the client to lift legs high while walking, as if walking over planks.

❑ 5. Ensure the client is upright when eating and swallows twice after each bite.

4. The nurse learns in report that a client is exhibiting Cheyne-Stokes respirations. Based on these data, which action is **most appropriate** for the nurse to take **initially**?
   1. Listen to the client's heart sounds.
   2. Determine whether the client has a pulse deficit.
   3. Instruct the client to use an incentive spirometer.
   4. Determine the client's ability to follow verbal commands.

❖ 5. The nurse notes documentation that a client has conductive hearing loss. The nurse plans care knowing that this kind of hearing loss can be caused by which circumstances? **Select all that apply.**
   ❑ 1. A defect in the cochlea
   ❑ 2. Acute otitis media with effusion
   ❑ 3. A defect in the 8th cranial nerve
   ❑ 4. A physical obstruction to the transmission of sound waves
   ❑ 5. A defect in the sensory fibers that lead to the cerebral cortex

6. While collecting data related to the cardiac system on a client, the nurse hears a murmur. Which **best** describes the sound of a heart murmur?
   1. Lub-dub sounds
   2. Scratchy, leathery heart noise
   3. Gentle, blowing or swooshing noise
   4. Abrupt, high-pitched snapping noise

7. The nurse is preparing to assist the health care provider to test the extraocular movements in a client and muscle weakness in the eyes. The nurse anticipates that which physical assessment technique will be done?
   1. Testing using the Ishihara chart
   2. Testing using a Snellen eye chart
   3. Testing the corneal light reflexes
   4. Testing the six cardinal positions of gaze

❖ 8. The nurse is reinforcing instructions for a client in how to perform a testicular self-examination (TSE). Which instructions would the nurse include? **Select all that apply.**
   ❑ 1. Perform TSE after a shower or bath.
   ❑ 2. Perform TSE after emptying the bladder.
   ❑ 3. Perform TSE on the same day each month.
   ❑ 4. Observe for urethral discharge after performing TSE.
   ❑ 5. Perform TSE by rolling each testicle between the thumb and fingers.

❖ 9. The nurse notes the physical assessment findings for a client with a diagnosis of possible meningitis. Which findings would the nurse expect to observe because of meningeal irritation? **Select all that apply.**
   ❑ 1. Pupils are unequal and react slowly to light.
   ❑ 2. The client reports stiffness and soreness in the neck area.
   ❑ 3. The client reports pain in the vertebral column and passively flexes the hip and knee in response to neck flexion.
   ❑ 4. The client flexes a leg at the hip and knee and reports pain in the vertebral column when the leg is extended.
   ❑ 5. The client's upper arms are flexed and held tightly to the sides of the body, and the legs are extended and internally rotated.

10. A Spanish-speaking client arrives at the triage desk in the emergency department and states to the nurse, "No speak English, need interpreter." Which action must the nurse take?
   1. Have one of the client's family members interpret.
   2. Have the Spanish-speaking triage receptionist interpret.
   3. Seek an interpreter from the hospital's interpreter services.
   4. Obtain a Spanish–English dictionary and attempt to triage the client.

ANSWERS

❖ **1. 1, 2, 4**

Rationale: A focused data collection process is centered around a limited or short-term problem, such as the client's complaint. Because the client is complaining of symptoms of a cold, a cough, and lung congestion, the nurse would focus on the respiratory system and the presence of an infection. A complete data collection includes a complete health history and physical examination and forms a baseline database. Checking the strength of peripheral pulses relates to a vascular assessment, which is not related to this client's complaints. A musculoskeletal and neurological examination also is not related to this client's complaints. However, strength of peripheral pulses and a musculoskeletal and neurological examination would be included in a complete data collection. Likewise, asking the client about a family history of any illness or disease would be included in a complete assessment.

Test-Taking Strategy: Focus on the data in the question. Noting the subject, how the client's symptoms relate to the respiratory system, and the presence of an infection will direct you to options 1, 2, and 4.

2. 3

Rationale: Asthma is a respiratory disorder characterized by recurring episodes of dyspnea, constriction of the bronchi, and wheezing. Wheezes are described as high-pitched musical sounds heard when air passes through an obstructed or narrowed lumen of a respiratory passageway. Clients with respiratory distress use other chest muscles to breathe. Muscle retraction is observed at the sternum and between the ribs. Stridor is a harsh crowing sound noted with an upper airway obstruction and often signals a life-threatening emergency. Cyanosis is bluish coloration of the lips occurring as a result of poor oxygenation of the circulating blood. Diminished lung sounds are heard over lung tissue where poor oxygen exchange is occurring. Fever (elevated temperature) occurs with a respiratory infection such as pneumonia. A pleural friction rub is heard in individuals with pleurisy (inflammation of the pleural surfaces) and often causes chest discomfort with inspiration.

Test-Taking Strategy: Focus on the subject, signs observed with acute asthma. Think about the pathophysiology that occurs in this disorder. Recalling that bronchial constriction occurs with asthma will assist in directing you to option 3. Also, thinking about the definition of the lung sounds and the signs identified in the choices will direct you to the correct option.

❖ **3. 1, 3**

Rationale: In the Romberg test, the client is asked to stand with the feet together, the arms at the sides, and to close the eyes and hold the position for 20 to 30 seconds. Normally the client can maintain posture and balance. A positive Romberg is a vestibular neurological sign that is found when a client elicits a loss of balance when closing the eyes. This may occur with cerebellar ataxia, loss of proprioception, and loss of vestibular function. The nurse would determine the client's risk for falling by collecting data. Because the client has difficulty maintaining balance, the nurse would instruct the client to ask for assistance when getting up or walking. Decreasing the light in the environment is done if a client has photophobia (sensitive to light). Clients with a shuffling gait as with Parkinson's disease need to lift their legs high when walking. Clients experiencing dysphagia, which often occurs with stroke, must eat sitting upright and perform double swallowing.

Test-Taking Strategy: Focus on the subject, the Romberg test. Specific knowledge regarding the significance of a positive Romberg test is needed to answer this question. Recall that a positive result means the client is experiencing problems with balance. This will lead you to select the options that relate to client safety and fall prevention.

4. 4

Rationale: Cheyne-Stokes respirations, rhythmic respirations with periods of apnea, occur with disorders affecting the respiratory center of the pons in the central nervous system such as a metabolic dysfunction in the cerebral hemisphere or basal ganglia. The nurse would initially obtain data about neurological functioning, starting with determining the client's ability to respond to verbal stimuli. Listening to heart sounds is important but is secondary to determining the neurological status. There is no information related to the need to check for a pulse deficit (difference between the apical and radial pulse). The use of incentive spirometry is indicated for shallow breathing and postoperatively.

Test-Taking Strategy: Focus on the strategic words, *most appropriate* and *initially*. Use the steps of the nursing process to eliminate use of the incentive spirometer because this is an intervention. Next, recall that Cheyne-Stokes respirations occur in clients with problems involving the central nervous system. Eliminate the options dealing with data collection of the circulation system. Select the option that details basic data collection of the nervous system.

5. 2, 4

Rationale: A conductive hearing loss is as a result of a physical obstruction to the transmission of sound waves. Acute otitis media with effusion, a fluid buildup in the middle ear, can block the transmission of sound waves. A sensorineural hearing loss occurs as a result of a pathological process in the inner ear, a defect in the 8th cranial nerve, or a defect of the sensory fibers that lead to the cerebral cortex.

Test-Taking Strategy: Focus on the subject, a conductive hearing loss. First, recall that this type of hearing loss is a result of a physical obstruction to the transmission of sound waves. Next, select the options that identify the conditions that obstruct transmission of sound, effusion, and physical blockage.

6. 3

Rationale: A heart murmur is an abnormal heart sound and is described as a gentle, blowing, swooshing sound. It occurs from increased or abnormal blood flow through the valves of the heart. Lub-dub sounds are normal and represent the S1 (first heart sound) and S2 (second heart sound), respectively. A pericardial friction rub is described as a scratchy, leathery heart sound that occurs with pericarditis. A click is described as an abrupt, high-pitched snapping sound.

Test-Taking Strategy: Focus on the subject, characteristics of a murmur, and note the strategic word, *best*. Eliminate option 1 because it describes normal heart sounds. Next, recall that a murmur occurs as a result of the manner in which the blood is flowing through the cardiac chambers and valves. This will direct you to the correct option.

7. 4

Rationale: Testing the six cardinal positions of gaze is done to check for muscle weakness in the eyes. The client is asked to hold the head steady, then to follow movement of an object through the positions of gaze. The client would follow the object in a parallel manner with the two eyes. The Ishihara chart is used to detect color blindness. A Snellen eye chart is used to determine visual acuity and cranial nerve II (optic nerve) functioning. Testing the corneal light reflex, shining a penlight in the eyes of a client gazing straight ahead, would demonstrate the corneal reflection in the exact position in each eye and parallel alignment.

Test-Taking Strategy: Focus on the subject, checking for eye movement and muscle strength in the eyes. Note the relationship between the words *extraocular movements* in the question and *positions of gaze*.

❖ **8. 1, 3, 5**

Rationale: The nurse needs to teach the client how to perform a testicular self-examination (TSE). The nurse needs to instruct the client that the best time to perform TSE is after a shower or bath when the hands are warm and soapy and the scrotum is warm. This will provide ease in palpating, and the client will be better able to identify any abnormalities. The nurse would instruct the client to select a day of the month and perform the examination on the same day each month to avoid forgetting to do the examination. TSE is done by the client rolling each testicle between the thumb and fingers. The client must seek medical attention if a lump, mass, or swelling of the testicle is detected. The bladder does not have to be empty to complete the examination. There is no connection between urethral discharge and TSE.

Test-Taking Strategy: Think about the subject, reinforcing how to perform TSE, and visualize this data collection technique. Eliminate options 2 and 4 because voiding before and checking for urethral discharge afterward are unrelated to performing TSE. Select the options that relate to regularity in performing the examination.

❖ **9. 2, 3, 4**

Rationale: Meningitis is the inflammation of the meninges, the membranes covering the brain and spinal cord. It is caused by organisms such as bacteria, viruses, or fungi. The client with meningitis experiences discomfort when pressure is placed on certain areas that irritate the inflamed meninges. Neck stiffness (nuchal rigidity) is an early sign of meningitis. A positive Brudzinski's sign is observed if the supine client passively flexes the hip and knee in response to neck flexion by the examiner and the client reports pain in the vertebral column. Kernig's sign also tests for meningeal irritation and is positive when the client flexes the legs at the hip and knee and complains of pain along the vertebral column when the leg is extended. Unequal pupils and slowed pupillary response to light is a sign of increased intracranial pressure. This may occur in clients who are critically ill, but it is not a sign of meningeal irritation. Decorticate posturing is abnormal flexion and is noted when the client's upper arms are flexed and held tightly to the sides of the body and the legs are extended and internally rotated. This posturing occurs with severe brain damage and the client requires emergency medical attention.

Test-Taking Strategy: Focus on the subject, signs/symptoms of meningeal irritation. Recall that the meninges are the membranes covering the brain and spinal cord. Select the options that put pressure on the meningeal area. Eliminate the options that are not specifically related to the meninges.

10. 3

Rationale: The nurse would have a professional hospital-based interpreter translate for the client. English-speaking family members may not appropriately understand what is asked of them and may paraphrase what the client is actually saying. Also, client confidentiality and accurate information may be compromised when a family member or a non-health care provider acts as interpreter. Using a Spanish-English dictionary is time-consuming and not the best action; accurate interpretation is best done by a professional hospital-based interpreter.

Test-Taking Strategy: Focus on the subject of the question: translator for the non-English-speaking client. Initially focus on what the client needs. In this case the client needs and asks for an interpreter. Next, keep in mind the issue of confidentiality and making sure that information is obtained in the most efficient and accurate way. This will assist in eliminating the incorrect options.

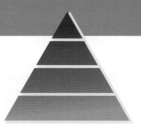

CHAPTER **14**

Hygiene and Safety

PRIORITY CONCEPTS Infection; Safety

WHAT WOULD YOU DO?

The nurse is working in a long-term care facility that has a "no restraint policy." An assigned client is disoriented and unsteady and continually attempts to climb out of bed. What would the nurse do with regard to instituting safety precautions for this client?
Answer is located on p. 170.

I. **Hygiene**
A. Description
   1. The activity of providing care or promoting self-care, which includes bathing and grooming
   2. Includes care of the skin, hair, nails, mouth, teeth, eyes, ears, nasal cavities, and perineal and genital areas
   3. Personal hygiene is the activity of self-care, including bathing and grooming.
B. General principles
   1. Ensure privacy.
   2. Wash hands and wear gloves.
   3. Explain procedures to the client.
   4. Determine and treat pain.
   5. Determine the client's health status and readiness for hygiene procedures.
   6. Determine the client's routine hygiene practices.
   7. Use proper body mechanics during bathing and hygiene activities.
   8. Use time spent with client as an opportunity to determine the client's mental health status and implement communication and teaching.
   9. Maintain and encourage independence as much as possible.

II. **Environmental Safety**
A. Fire safety (see Priority Nursing Actions)
   1. Keep open spaces free of clutter.
   2. Clearly mark fire exits.
   3. Know the locations of all fire alarms, exits, and extinguishers (Table 14.1).
   4. Know the telephone number for reporting fires.
   5. Know the agency's fire drill and evacuation plan.
   6. Never use the elevator in the event of a fire.
   7. Turn off oxygen and appliances in the vicinity of the fire.
   8. In the event of a fire, if a client is on life support, maintain the client's respiratory status manually with an Ambu bag (resuscitation bag) until the client is moved away from the threat of the fire and placed back on life support.
   9. In the event of a fire, ambulatory clients can be directed to walk by themselves to a safe area. In some cases, they may be able to assist with moving clients who are in wheelchairs.
   10. Bedridden clients are generally moved from the scene of a fire by stretcher, bed, or wheelchair.
   11. If a client must be carried from the area of a fire, appropriate transfer techniques would be used; **ergonomic principles** and good body mechanics should be instituted to prevent injury. Institutions may have specific equipment designed to evacuate clients who are unable to walk.
   12. If fire department personnel are at the scene of the fire, they will supervise and can help evacuate clients.

   ⚠ Remember the mnemonic RACE (Rescue clients, Activate the fire alarm, Confine the fire, Extinguish the fire) to set priorities in the event of a fire and the mnemonic PASS (Pull the pin, Aim at the base of the fire, Squeeze the handle, Sweep from side to side) to use a fire extinguisher.

B. Electrical safety
   1. Electrical equipment must be maintained in good working order and would be grounded; otherwise, it is a **physical hazard**; remove equipment that is not in proper working order and notify appropriate staff.
   2. Use a three-pronged electrical cord.

TABLE 14.1 Types of Fire Extinguishers

Type	Class of Fires
A	Wood, cloth, upholstery, paper, rubbish, and plastic
B	Flammable liquids or gases; grease, tar, and oil-based paint
C	Electrical equipment

Note: Certain extinguishers may be appropriate for more than one type of fire. These type are placed in health care facilities.

3. In a three-pronged electrical cord, the third, longer prong of the cord is the ground. The other two prongs carry the power to the piece of electrical equipment.
4. Check electrical cords and outlets for exposed, frayed, or damaged wires.
5. Avoid overloading any circuit.
6. Read warning labels on all equipment. Never operate unfamiliar equipment.
7. Use safety extension cords only when absolutely necessary, and tape them to the floor with electrical tape.
8. Never run electrical wiring under carpets.
9. Never pull a plug by using the cord. Always grasp the plug itself.
10. Never use electrical appliances near sinks, bathtubs, or other water sources.
11. Always disconnect a plug from the outlet before cleaning equipment or appliances.
12. If a client receives an electrical shock, turn off the electricity before touching the client.

⚡ PRIORITY NURSING ACTIONS

Event of a Fire

1. Rescue clients and remove those in immediate danger.
2. Activate the fire alarm.
3. Confine the fire.
4. Extinguish the fire: obtain the fire extinguisher.
5. Pull the pin on the fire extinguisher.
6. Aim at the base of the fire.
7. Squeeze the extinguisher handle.
8. Sweep extinguisher from side to side to coat the area of the fire evenly.

⚠ Any electrical equipment that the client brings into the health care facility must be inspected for safety by maintenance personnel before use.

C. Radiation safety (refer to Chapter 41 for additional information on radiation safety)
   1. Know the health care agency's protocols and guidelines.
   2. Label potentially radioactive material.
   3. To reduce exposure to radiation (agency policies would also be followed):

BOX 14.1 Physiological Changes in the Older Client That Increase the Risk of Accidents

Musculoskeletal Changes
- Strength and function of muscles decrease.
- Joints become less mobile, and bones become brittle.
- Postural changes and limited range of motion occur.

Nervous System Changes
- Voluntary and autonomic reflexes become slower.
- Decreased ability to respond to multiple stimuli occurs.
- Decreased sensitivity to touch occurs.

Sensory Changes
- Decreased vision and lens accommodation and cataracts develop.
- Delayed transmission of hot and cold impulses occurs.
- Impaired hearing develops, with high-frequency tones less perceptible.

Genitourinary Changes
- Increased nocturia and occurrences of incontinence may occur.

Adapted from Potter A, Perry P, Stockert P, Hall A: *Fundamentals of nursing*, ed 8, St. Louis, 2013, Mosby; and Touhy T, Jett K: *Ebersole and Hess' toward healthy aging*, ed 8, St. Louis, 2012, Mosby.

   a. The time spent near the source would be limited.
   b. The distance from the source would be as great as possible.
   c. A shielding device such as a lead apron would be used.
4. Monitor radiation exposure with a film (dosimeter) badge.
5. Place the client who has a radiation implant in a private room.
6. Keep all linens and dressings in the client's room until the implant is removed.
7. Never touch dislodged implants.
D. Disposal of infectious wastes
   1. Handle all infectious materials as a hazard.
   2. Dispose of waste in designated areas only, and use proper containers for disposal.
   3. Ensure that infectious material is properly labeled.
   4. Dispose of all sharps immediately after use in closed, puncture-resistant disposal containers that are leak-proof and labeled or color coded.

⚠ Needles (sharps) would not be recapped, bent, or broken because of the risk of accidental injury (needle-stick).

E. Physiological changes in the older client that increase the risk of accidents (Box 14.1)
F. Risk for falls assessment (Box 14.2 lists measures to prevent falls)

Foundations of Care

BOX 14.2   Measures to Prevent Falls

- Determine the client's risk for falling.
- Ensure that the client at risk for falling is in a room near the nurses' station.
- Be alert to clients who are at risk for falling.
- Check to see if there is a notation on the door to the room indicating a fall risk.
- Orient the client to his or her physical surroundings.
- Instruct the client to seek assistance when getting up.
- Explain the use of the call-bell system.
- Keep the bed in the low position; the use of side rails is based on state and agency policies and procedures and must be followed.
- Lock wheels on all beds, wheelchairs, and stretchers.
- Keep personal items within reach.
- Eliminate clutter and obstacles in the client's room.
- Provide adequate lighting, including subdued lighting at night.
- Reduce bathroom hazards.
- Maintain the client's toileting schedule throughout the day.

1. Assessment would be client-centered and include the use of a fall risk scale per agency procedures.
2. Include the client's own perceptions of their risk factors for falls and their method to adapt to these factors. Areas of concern may include gait, stability, muscle strength and coordination, balance, and vision.
3. Assess for any previous accidents.
4. Assess with the client any concerns about their immediate environment, including stairs, use of throw rugs, grab bars, or a raised toilet seat.
5. Review the medications that the client is taking that could have side/adverse effects or that could place the client at risk for a fall.
6. Determine any scheduled procedures that pose risks to the client.

G. Measures to promote safety in ambulation for the client
1. Gait belt may be used to keep the center of gravity midline.
   a. Place the belt on the client before ambulation.
   b. Encircle the client's waist with the belt.
   c. Hold on to the side or back of the belt so that the client does not lean to one side.
   d. Return the client to bed or a nearby chair if the client develops dizziness or becomes unsteady.
   e. When finished safely ambulating the client, remove belt and place it in its appropriate storage area.

▲ **H.** Steps to prevent injury to the health care worker (Box 14.3)

I. National Patient Safety Goals 2019: Access the following link for The Joint Commission's National Patient Safety Goals: https://www.jointcommission.org/standards_information/npsgs.aspx.

BOX 14.3   Steps to Prevent Injury to the Health Care Worker

- Keep the weight to be lifted as close to the body as possible.
- Bend at the knees.
- Tighten abdominal muscles and tuck the pelvis.
- Maintain the trunk erect and knees bent so that multiple muscle groups work together in a coordinated manner.

Adapted from Potter A, Perry P, Stockert P, Hall A: *Fundamentals of nursing*, ed 8, St. Louis, 2013, Mosby.

J. Restraints (safety devices)   ▲
1. Restraints are protective devices used to limit the physical activity of a client or immobilize a client or an extremity.
   a. The agency policy would be checked when applying side rails.
   b. The use of side rails is not considered a restraint when they are used to prevent a sedated client from falling out of bed.
   c. The client must be able to exit the bed easily in case of an emergency when using side rails. Only the top two side rails would be used.
   d. The bed must be kept in the lowest position when using side rails.
2. Physical restraints: Restrict client movement through the application of a device
3. Chemical restraints: Medications given to inhibit a specific behavior or movement
4. Interventions
   a. Use alternative devices whenever possible, such as pressure-sensitive beds or chair pads with alarms or other types of bed or chair alarms.
   b. If safety devices are necessary, the primary health care provider's (PHCP's) prescriptions would state the type of restraint, identify specific client behaviors for which restraints are to be used, and identify a limited time frame for use.
   c. The PHCP's prescriptions for safety devices would be renewed within a specific time frame according to the policy of the agency.
   d. Safety devices are not to be prescribed PRN (as needed).
   e. The reason for the safety device would be given to the client and the family, and their permission would be sought and documented.
   f. Safety devices would not interfere with any treatments or affect the client's health problem.
   g. Use a half-bow or safety knot (quick-release tie) to secure the device to the bed frame or chair, not to the side rails or movable parts of the bed.
   h. Ensure that enough slack is on the straps to allow some movement of the body part.

    i. Assess skin integrity and neurovascular and circulatory status every 30 minutes, and remove the safety device at least every 2 hours to permit muscle exercise and to promote circulation (follow agency policies).

    j. Continually assess and document the need for safety devices (Box 14.4).

⚠ A PHCP's prescription for use of a safety device is needed. Alternative measures for safety devices would always be used first.

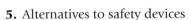

5. Alternatives to safety devices
    a. Orient the client and family to surroundings.
    b. Explain all procedures and treatments to the client and family.
    c. Encourage family and friends to stay with the client, and use sitters for clients who need supervision.
    d. Assign confused and disoriented clients to rooms near the nurses' station.
    e. Provide appropriate visual and auditory stimuli to the client (e.g., clock, calendar, television, radio); leave the client's room door open.
    f. Place familiar items (e.g., family pictures) near the client's bedside.
    g. Maintain toileting routines.
    h. Eliminate bothersome treatments (e.g., tube feedings) as soon as possible.
    i. Check all medications that the client is receiving.
    j. Use relaxation techniques with the client.
    k. Institute exercise and ambulation schedules as the client's condition allows.
    l. Assess for pain and adequate pain control.
    m. Collaborate with the registered nurse to evaluate oxygenation status, vital signs, electrolyte/laboratory values, and other pertinent assessment findings that may provide information about the cause of the client's confusion.

K. Poisons
    1. Any substance that impairs health or destroys life when ingested, inhaled, or otherwise absorbed by the body

    2. Specific antidotes or treatments are available for only some types of poisons.
    3. The capability of body tissue to recover from a poison determines the reversibility of the effect.
    4. Poison can impair the respiratory, circulatory, central nervous, hepatic, gastrointestinal, and renal systems.
    5. Toddlers, preschoolers, and young school-age children must be protected from accidental poisoning.
    6. In older adults, diminished eyesight and impaired memory may result in the accidental ingestion of poisonous substances or an overdose of prescribed medications.
    7. A poison control center phone number would be visible on the telephone in homes with small children. In all cases of suspected poisoning, the number would be called immediately. Health care institutions have material data sheets that list substances (poisons) used commonly in the area, and associated risks and interventions in case of exposure.
    8. Interventions
      a. Remove any obvious materials from the mouth, eye, or body area immediately.
      b. Identify the type and amount of substance ingested.
      c. Call the poison control center before attempting an intervention.
      d. If the victim vomits or vomiting is induced, save the vomitus if requested to do so, and deliver it to the poison control center.
      e. If instructed by the poison control center to take the poisoned victim to the emergency department, call an ambulance.
      f. Vomiting is never induced after the ingestion of lye, household cleaners, grease, or petroleum products.
      g. Vomiting is never induced in an unconscious victim.

⚠ The Poison Control Center would be called first before attempting an intervention.

III. Health Care–Associated (Nosocomial) Infections

A. Health care–associated (nosocomial) infections are also referred to as hospital-acquired infections.
B. These infections are acquired in a hospital or other health care facility and were not present or incubating at the time of a client's admission.
C. *Clostridium difficile* (*C. difficile*) is spread mainly by hand-to-hand contact in a health care setting. Clients taking multiple antibiotics for a prolonged period are most at risk.
D. Common drug-resistant infections: Vancomycin-resistant enterococci, methicillin-resistant *Staphylococcus aureus*, multidrug-resistant tuberculosis, carbapenem-resistant enterobacteriaceae.

E. Illness impairs the normal defense mechanisms of the body.

F. The hospital environment provides exposure to a variety of virulent organisms that the client has not been exposed to in the past; therefore, the client has not developed resistance to these organisms.

G. Infections can be transmitted by health care personnel who fail to practice proper standard precautions (i.e., hand-washing procedures and/or fail to change gloves between client contacts).

H. At many health care agencies, dispensers containing an alcohol-based solution for hand sanitization are mounted at the entrance to each client's room; it is important to note that alcohol-based sanitizers are not effective against some infectious agents such as *C. difficile* spores.

IV. Standard Precautions

 A. Description
1. Must be practiced with all clients in any setting, regardless of the diagnosis or presumed infectiousness.
2. Standard precautions include hand washing and the use of gloves, masks, eye protection, and gowns, when appropriate, during client contact.
3. These precautions apply to blood, all body fluids, secretions, and excretions (whether or not they contain blood), nonintact skin, or mucous membranes.

 B. Interventions
1. Wash hands between client contacts; after contact with blood, body fluids, secretions or excretions, nonintact skin, or mucous membranes; after contact with equipment or contaminated articles; and immediately after removing gloves.
2. Wear gloves when touching blood, body fluids, secretions, excretions, nonintact skin, mucous membranes, or contaminated items; remove gloves and wash hands between client care contacts.
3. For routine decontamination of hands, alcohol-based hand rubs may be used when hands are not visibly soiled, but the use of alcohol-based hand rubs is not always effective; for example, alcohol-based hand sanitizer is ineffective against the spores of *C. difficile*. For more information on hand hygiene from the Centers for Disease Control and Prevention (CDC), please see www.cdc.gov/handhygiene/.
4. Wear masks and eye protection, or face shields if client care activities may generate splashes or sprays of blood or body fluid.
5. Wear gowns if soiling of clothing is likely from blood or body fluid; wash hands after removing a gown.
6. Steps for donning and removing personal protective equipment (PPE) (Table 14.2)
7. Clean and reprocess client care equipment properly and discard single-use items.
8. Place contaminated linen in leak-proof bags and limit handling to prevent skin and mucous membrane exposure. Dispose according to agency policy.

TABLE 14.2 Steps for Donning and Removing (Doffing) Personal Protective Equipment

Donning of PPE	Removal (Doffing) of PPE
Gown	**Gloves**
Fully cover front of body from neck to knees and upper arms to end of wrist	Grasp outside of glove with opposite hand with glove still on and peel off
Wrap around the back; fasten in the back at neck and waist	Hold on to removed glove in gloved hand
Mask or respirator	Slide fingers of ungloved hand under clean side of remaining glove at wrist and peel off
Secure ties or elastic band at neck and middle of head	**Goggles/face shield**
Fit snug to face and below chin	Remove by touching clean band or inner part
Fit to nose bridge	**Gown**
Respirator fit would be checked per agency policy	Unfasten at neck, then at waist
Goggles/face shield	Remove using a peeling motion, pulling gown from each shoulder toward the hands
Adjust to fit according to agency policy	Allow gown to fall down, and roll into a bundle to discard
Gloves	**Mask or respirator**
Select appropriate size and extend to cover wrists of gown	Grasp bottom ties then top ties to remove

aNote: Hand hygiene is performed before donning, after removing the gown, and after removal of the mask or respirator. All equipment is considered contaminated on the outside. *PPE*, Personal protective equipment. Adapted from the Centers for Disease Control and Prevention at https://www.cdc.gov/coronavirus/2019-ncov/downloads/A_FS_HCP_COVID19_PPE_11x17.pdf

9. Use needleless devices or special needle safety devices whenever possible to reduce the risk of needle sticks and sharps injuries to health care workers.
10. Discard all sharp instruments and needles in a puncture-resistant container; dispose of needles uncapped or engage the safety mechanism on the needle if available.
11. Clean spills of blood or body fluids with a solution of bleach and water (diluted 1:10) or agency-approved disinfectant.

 Handle all blood and body fluids from all clients as if they were contaminated.

V. Transmission-Based Precautions

A. Transmission-based precautions include airborne, droplet, and contact precautions.
B. Airborne precautions
1. Diseases
   a. Measles
   b. Chickenpox (varicella)
   c. Disseminated varicella zoster
   d. Pulmonary or laryngeal tuberculosis
   e. SARS-CoV-2; Coronavirus (COVID-19)

2. Barrier protection for airborne precautions
   a. Single room maintained under negative pressure; door remains closed except upon entering or exiting
   b. Negative airflow pressure is used in the room, with a minimum of 6 to 12 air exchanges per hour via high-efficiency particulate air (HEPA) filtration mask or according to agency protocol.
   c. Ultraviolet germicide irradiation or HEPA filter is used in the room.
   d. Health care workers wear a respiratory mask (N95 or higher level). In cases of COVID clients, both airborne and droplet precautions may be instituted. Follow agency protocols; healthcare workers must wear eye protection (i.e. face shield or goggles). Place a surgical mask on the client when the client needs to leave the room; the client leaves the room only if necessary.

C. Droplet precautions
   1. Diseases
      a. Adenovirus
      b. Diphtheria (pharyngeal)
      c. Epiglottitis
      d. Influenza (flu)
      e. Meningitis
      f. Mumps
      g. Mycoplasmal pneumonia or meningococcal pneumonia
      h. Parvovirus B19
      i. Pertussis
      j. Pneumonia
      k. Pneumonic plague
      l. Rubella
      m. Scarlet fever
      n. Streptococcal pharyngitis
      o. SARS-CoV-2; Coronavirus (COVID-19)
   2. Barrier protection for droplet precautions
      a. Private room or cohort client (a client whose body cultures contain the same organism)
      b. Wear a surgical mask when within 3 feet of a client. Health care workers wear a respiratory mask (N95 or higher level). In cases of COVID clients, both airborne and droplet precautions may be instituted. Follow agency protocols; healthcare workers must wear eye protection (i.e. face shield or goggles). Place a mask on the client if the client must leave the room.

D. Contact precautions
   1. Diseases
      a. Colonization or infection with a multidrug-resistant organism
      b. Enteric infections such as *C. difficile*
      c. Respiratory infections such as respiratory syncytial virus
      d. Influenza: Infection can occur by touching something with flu viruses on it and then touching the mouth or nose.
      e. Wound infections

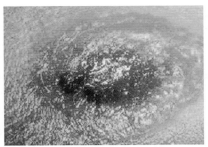

FIGURE 14.1 **Anthrax.** From Swartz M: *Textbook of physical diagnosis*, ed 6, Philadelphia, 2010, Saunders.

   f. Skin infections, such as cutaneous diphtheria, herpes simplex, impetigo, pediculosis, scabies, staphylococci, and varicella zoster
   g. Eye infections, such as conjunctivitis
   h. Indirect contact transmission may occur when contaminated object, instrument, or hand(s) are encountered.
   i. SARS-CoV-2; Coronavirus (COVID-19)
   2. Barrier protection
      a. Private room or cohort client
      b. Use gloves and a gown whenever entering the client's room.
      c. With *C. difficile*: gloves and gown when in room, use of soap and water for handwashing when exiting, no sharing of equipment between clients, and room cleaned with chlorine (bleach) to kill spores and spread of infection

VI. Emergency Response Plan and Disasters
A. Know the emergency response plan of the agency.
B. Internal disasters are those that occur within the health care facility.
C. External disasters occur in the community, and victims will be brought to the health care facility for care.
D. When the health care agency is notified of a disaster, the nurse would follow the guidelines specified in the agency's emergency response plan.
E. See Chapter 7 for additional information about disasters and emergency responseplanning.

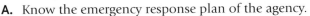 In the event of a disaster, the emergency response plan is immediately activated.

VII. Biological Warfare Agents
A. A warfare agent is a biological or chemical substance that can cause mass casualty destruction or fatality.
B. Anthrax (Fig. 14.1)
   1. The disease is caused by *Bacillus anthracis* (*B. anthracis*) and can be contracted through the digestive system, abrasions in the skin, or inhalation.
   2. Anthrax is transmitted by direct contact with the bacteria and its spores; spores are dormant encapsulated bacteria that become active when they enter a living host (no person-to-person spread) (Box 14.5).

BOX 14.5 **Anthrax: Transmission and Symptoms**

Skin

Spores enter the skin through cuts and abrasions and are contracted by handling contaminated animal skin products.

The infection starts with an itchy bump like a mosquito bite that progresses to a small, liquid-filled sac.

The sac becomes a painless ulcer with an area of black, dead tissue in the middle.

Toxins destroy the surrounding tissue.

Gastrointestinal System

Infection occurs after the ingestion of contaminated, undercooked meat.

Symptoms begin with nausea, loss of appetite, and vomiting.

The infection progresses to severe abdominal pain, the vomiting of blood, and severe diarrhea.

Inhalation

Infection is caused by the inhalation of bacterial spores, which multiply in the alveoli.

Symptoms begin with the same symptoms as influenza, including fever, muscle aches, and fatigue.

Symptoms suddenly become more severe with the development of breathing problems and shock.

Toxins cause hemorrhage and the destruction of lung tissue.

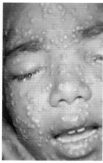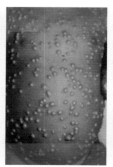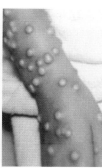

FIGURE 14.2 Smallpox. Courtesy of Centers for Disease Control and Prevention [CDC]: Evaluating patients for smallpox. Atlanta, 2002, CDC. Available online at https://www.cdc.gov/smallpox/clinicians/algorithm-protocol.html.

3. The infection is carried to the lymph nodes and then spread to the rest of the body via the blood and lymph; high levels of toxins lead to shock and death.

4. In the lungs, anthrax can cause a buildup of fluid, tissue decay, and death (fatal if untreated).

5. A blood test is available to detect anthrax (detects and amplifies *B. anthracis* DNA if present in the blood sample).

6. Anthrax is usually treated with antibiotics such as ciprofloxacin, doxycycline, or penicillin.

7. The vaccine for anthrax has limited availability.

⚠ Anthrax is transmitted by direct contact with bacteria and spores and can be contracted through the digestive system, abrasions in the skin, or inhalation through the lungs.

C. Smallpox (Fig. 14.2)

1. Smallpox is transmitted in air droplets and by handling contaminated materials and is highly contagious.

2. Symptoms begin 7 to 17 days after exposure and include fever, back pain, vomiting, malaise, and headache.

3. Papules develop 2 days after symptoms develop and progress to pustular vesicles that are abundant on the face and extremities initially.

4. A vaccine is available to those at risk for exposure to smallpox.

D. Botulism

1. Botulism is a serious paralytic illness caused by a nerve toxin produced by the bacterium *Clostridium botulinum* (death can occur within 24 hours).

2. Its spores are found in the soil and can spread through the air or food (particularly improperly canned food) or via a contaminated wound.

3. Cannot be spread from person to person.

4. Symptoms include abdominal cramps, diarrhea, nausea, vomiting, double vision, blurred vision, drooping eyelids, difficulty swallowing or speaking, dry mouth, and muscle weakness.

5. Neurological symptoms begin 12 to 36 hours after ingestion of food-borne botulism and 24 to 72 hours after inhalation and can progress to paralysis of the arms, legs, trunk, or respiratory muscles (mechanical ventilation is necessary).

6. If diagnosed early, food-borne and wound botulism can be treated with an antitoxin that blocks the action of toxin circulating in the blood.

7. No vaccine is available.

E. Plague

1. Plague is caused by *Yersinia pestis*, a bacteria found in rodents and fleas.

2. Contracted by being bitten by a rodent or flea carrying the plague bacterium, the ingestion of contaminated meat, or the handling of an animal infected with the bacteria

3. Transmitted by direct person-to-person spread

4. Forms include bubonic (most common), pneumonic, and septicemic (most deadly).

5. Symptoms usually begin within 1 to 3 days and include fever, chest pain, lymph node swelling, and a productive cough (hemoptysis).

6. The disease rapidly progresses to dyspnea, stridor, and cyanosis; death occurs from respiratory failure, shock, and bleeding.

7. Antibiotics are effective only if administered immediately; the usual medications of choice include streptomycin or gentamicin.

8. A vaccine is available.

F. Tularemia

1. Tularemia is an infectious disease of animals caused by the bacillus *Francisellatularensis*; also called deerfly fever or rabbit fever.
2. Transmitted by ticks, deerflies, or contact with an infected animal
3. Symptoms include fever, headache, ulcerated skin lesion with localized lymph node enlargement, eye infection, gastrointestinal ulceration, and pneumonia.
4. Treated with antibiotics
5. Recovery produces lifelong immunity (a vaccine is available).

G. Hemorrhagic fever

1. Hemorrhagic fever is caused by several viruses, including Marburg, Lassa, Junin, and Ebola.
2. Virus is carried by rodents and mosquitoes.
3. Can be transmitted by direct person-to-person spread via body fluids.
4. Symptoms include fever, headache, malaise, conjunctivitis, nausea, vomiting, hypotension, hemorrhage of tissues and organs, and organ failure.
5. No known specific treatment is available; treatment is symptomatic.

H. Ebola virus disease (EVD)

1. Previously known as Ebola hemorrhagic fever
2. Caused by infection with a virus of the family *Filoviridae, genus Ebolavirus*
3. First discovered in 1976 in the Democratic Republic of the Congo. Outbreaks have appeared in Africa.
4. The natural reservoir host of *Ebolavirus* remains unknown. It is believed that the virus is animal borne, and bats are the most likely reservoir.
5. Spread of the virus is through contact with objects (such as clothes, bedding, needles, syringes/sharps, or medical equipment) that have been contaminated with the virus.
6. Symptoms similar to hemorrhagic fever may appear from 2 to 21 days after exposure.
7. Assessment: Ask the client if he or she traveled to an area with EVD such as Guinea, Liberia, or Sierra Leone within the last 21 days or if he or she has had contact with someone with EVD and had any of the following symptoms:
   a. Fever at home or a current temperature of 38°C (100.4°F) or greater
   b. Severe headache
   c. Muscle pain
   d. Weakness
   e. Fatigue
   f. Diarrhea
   g. Vomiting
   h. Abdominal pain
   i. Unexplained bleeding or bruising
8. Interventions
   a. If the assessment indicates possible infection with EVD, the client needs to be isolated in a private room with a private bathroom or a covered bedside commode with the door closed.
   b. Health care workers need to wear the proper PPE and follow updated procedures designated by the CDC for donning (putting on) and doffing (removing) PPE. Refer to the following website for updated information: http://www.cdc.gov/vhf/ebola/healthcare-us/ppe/guidance.html.
   c. The number of health care workers entering the room would be limited, and a log of everyone who enters and leaves the room would be kept.
   d. Only necessary tests and procedures would be performed, and aerosol-generating procedures must be avoided.
   e. Refer to the CDC guidelines for cleaning, disinfecting, and managing waste (www.cdc.gov/vhf/ebola/healthcare-us/cleaning/hospitals.html).
   f. The agency's infection control program must be notified, and state and local public health authorities must be notified. A list of the state and local health department numbers is available at https://www.cdc.gov/coronavirus/2019-ncov/php/open-america/hd-search/index.html

VIII. Chemical Warfare Agents

A. Sarin

1. Sarin is a highly toxic nerve gas that can cause death within minutes of exposure.
2. Enters the body through the eyes and skin; acts by paralyzing the respiratory muscles

B. Phosgene: Colorless gas normally used in chemical manufacturing; if inhaled at high concentrations for a long enough period, it leads to severe respiratory distress, pulmonary edema, and death.

C. Mustard gas: Yellow to brown in color and has a garlic-like odor that irritates the eyes and causes skin burns and blisters

D. Ionizing radiation

1. Acute radiation poisoning develops after substantial exposure to radiation.
2. Can occur from external radiation or internal absorption
3. Symptoms depend on the amount of exposure to the radiation; range from nausea and vomiting, diarrhea, fever, electrolyte imbalances, and neurological and cardiovascular impairment to leukopenia, purpura, hemorrhage, and death.

IX. Nursing Role in Exposure to Warfare Agents

A. Be aware that, initially, a bioterrorism attack may resemble a naturally occurring outbreak of an infectious disease.

B. Nurses and other health care workers must be prepared to assess and determine what type of event occurred, the number of clients who may be affected, and how and when clients will be expected to arrive at the health care agency.

C. It is essential to know about any change in the microorganism that may increase its virulence or make it resistant to conventional antibiotics or vaccines.

D. See Chapter 7 for additional information on disasters and emergency response planning.

WHAT WOULD YOU DO?

Answer: Many facilities implement a "no restraint policy," which requires health care workers to implement other safety strategies for clients who pose a risk for falls. There are several strategies that can be implemented to ensure safety, as safety is the nurse's primary concern. These strategies include orienting the client and family to the surroundings; explaining all procedures and treatments to the client and family; encouraging family and friends to stay with the client as appropriate and using sitters for clients who need supervision; assigning confused and disoriented clients to rooms near the nurses' station; providing appropriate visual and auditory stimuli to the client, such as clocks, calendars, a television, and a radio; maintaining toileting routines; eliminating bothersome treatments, such as tube feedings, as soon as possible; evaluating all medications that the client is receiving; using relaxation techniques with the client; and instituting exercise and ambulation schedules as the client's condition allows.

PRACTICE QUESTIONS

1. A mother calls a neighborhood nurse and tells the nurse that her 3-year-old child has just ingested liquid furniture polish. Which action would the nurse instruct the mother to take **first**?
1. Induce vomiting.
2. Call an ambulance.
3. Call the poison control center.
4. Bring the child to the emergency department.

2. The emergency department nurse receives a telephone call and is informed that a tornado has hit a local residential area and numerous casualties have occurred. The victims will be brought to the emergency department. Which would be the **initial** nursing action?
1. Prepare the triage rooms.
2. Activate the agency emergency response plan.
3. Obtain additional supplies from the central supply department.
4. Obtain additional nursing staff to assist with treating the casualties.

❖ **3.** The nurse is caring for a client with a health care associated infection caused by methicillin-resistant

Staphylococcus aureus. Contact precautions are prescribed for the client. The nurse prepares to irrigate the wound and apply a new dressing. Which protective interventions would the nurse use to perform this procedure? **Select all that apply.**
☐ 1. Put on a mask.
☐ 2. Don gown and gloves.
☐ 3. Apply shoe protectors.
☐ 4. Wear a pair of protective goggles.
☐ 5. Have the client wear a mask and goggles.

4. The nurse would institute which interventions for ❖ a client diagnosed with *Clostridium difficile* (*C. difficile*)? **Select all that apply.**
☐ 1. Wear a mask if within 3 feet of the client.
☐ 2. Place a mask on the client when client is outside the room.
☐ 3. Wear gloves and gown while in the room caring for the client.
☐ 4. Use soap and water, not alcohol-based hand rub, for hand hygiene.
☐ 5. Keep the door of the room shut except when entering or exiting the client's room.

5. The nurse enters a client's room and finds that the wastebasket is on fire. The nurse quickly assists the client out of the room. Which is the **next** nursing action?
1. Call for help.
2. Extinguish the fire.
3. Activate the fire alarm.
4. Confine the fire by closing the room door.

6. A licensed practical nurse (LPN) attends a session about bioterrorism agents including anthrax. Which statement by an attendee demonstrates the **need for further teaching** about anthrax?
1. Anthrax is treated with antibiotic medications.
2. The most lethal form of anthrax is contacted by inhalation of the spores.
3. Anthrax can be transmitted by consumption of meat from an infected animal.
4. Anthrax bacteria produces a neurotoxin leading to a serious, possibly fatal paralysis.

7. The nurse obtains a prescription to restrain a client using a belt (safety) restraint and instructs the assistive personnel (AP) to apply the restraint. Which observation, if made by the nurse, indicates unsafe application of the restraint?
1. A safety knot is made in the restraint strap.
2. The restraint straps are safely secured to the side rails.
3. The restraint strap does not tighten when force is applied against it.
4. The restraint is secure, and the client is able to turn from back to side.

8. The nurse applies wrist restraints, prescribed to prevent a client from pulling out a nasogastric tube. How would the nurse determine that the restraints are not too constrictive?
   1. Observe the skin in the wrist area for redness.
   2. Check the temperature of the skin in the hands.
   3. Remove the restraint and exercise the extremity in 2 hours.
   4. Place two fingers under the restraint to determine snugness.

❖ 9. The nurse is assisting with creating a plan of care for a client with an internal radiation implant. Which would be included in the plan of care? **Select all that apply.**
   ❑ 1. Wearing gloves when emptying the client's bedpan.
   ❑ 2. Keeping all linens in the room until the implant is removed.
   ❑ 3. Wearing a film (dosimeter) badge when in the client's room.
   ❑ 4. Wearing a lead apron when providing direct care to the client.
   ❑ 5. Placing the client in a semiprivate room at the end of the hallway.

10. The nurse enters the nursing lounge and discovers that a chair is on fire. The nurse activates the alarm, closes the lounge door, and obtains the fire extinguisher to extinguish the fire. The nurse pulls the pin on the fire extinguisher. Which is the **next** action the nurse must perform?
   1. Aim at the base of the fire.
   2. Squeeze the handle on the extinguisher.
   3. Sweep the fire from side to side with the extinguisher.
   4. Sweep the fire from top to bottom with the extinguisher.

ANSWERS

1. 3

Rationale: If a suspected poisoning occurs, the poison control center must be contacted immediately. The nurse can assist the mother with contacting the poison control center. Vomiting would not be induced without instructions from the poison control center. Inducing vomiting is not done if the client is unconscious or the substance ingested is a strong corrosive or petroleum product. Bringing the child to the emergency department or calling an ambulance would delay treatment. The poison control center may advise the mother to bring the child to the emergency department; if this is the case, the mother would call an ambulance.

Test-Taking Strategy: Note the strategic word, *first*, in the question. Recall that persons at the poison control center have expertise and resources. Eliminate options 2 and 4, because these options would delay treatment. Recalling that vomiting must not be induced if a corrosive substance was ingested will assist you with eliminating option 1.

2. 2

Rationale: During a widespread disaster, many people will be brought to the emergency department for treatment. Health care institutions are required to have an emergency response plan in place and perform practice drills. The initial nursing action would be to activate the emergency response plan. The plan entails the other options, which include preparing triage rooms to take casualties, and obtaining sufficient supplies and medical personnel.

Test-Taking Strategy: Note the strategic word, *initial*, and note that option 2 is the umbrella option.

3. 1, 2, 4

Rationale: Contact precautions are in place, which include wearing gloves and a gown while providing care to the client. The mask and goggles are indicated because of the potential of splash contact during the wound irrigation procedure. Goggles are worn to protect the mucous membranes of the eye during interventions that may produce splashes of blood, body fluids, secretions, and excretions. Shoe protectors are not necessary and are used in operating rooms in the surgical departments. If the client is under airborne or droplet precautions, a mask is worn by the client when going outside of the room. Goggles are not worn by clients.

Test-Taking Strategy: Focus on the subject, protective items needed for performing irrigation and contact precautions. Visualize the procedure for performing a wound irrigation to determine the items required to protect the nurse while providing care for this client.

4. 3, 4

Rationale: Contact precautions are necessary for colonization or infection with a multidrug-resistant organism. This includes enteric infection with *Clostridium difficile*. Measures used to prevent the spread of *C. difficile* are wearing gowns and gloves while in the room (not just during care) because the spores are on surfaces in the room. Washing with soap and water for hand hygiene is indicated because alcohol-based sanitizers are ineffective against the spores. The use of a mask by the nurse, or the client when outside the client's room, is unnecessary because *C. difficile* is not transmitted by the respiratory route. The door does not need to be kept shut.

Test-Taking Strategy: Focus on the subject, route of transmission of *C. difficile*. Recall that the organism forms spores that are difficult to destroy. Think about the route of transmission of this organism and select the options that are aimed at eliminating the bacteria on surfaces. Also, eliminate options that are used with infections spread by the respiratory route.

5. 3

Rationale: The order of priority in the event of a fire is to rescue the clients who are in immediate danger. The next step is to activate the fire alarm. The fire is then confined by closing all doors. Finally, the fire is extinguished.

Test-Taking Strategy: Note the strategic word, *next*. Remember the mnemonic *RACE* to help you prioritize in the event of a fire: R = Rescue clients who are in immediate danger; A = Alarm, activate the alarm; C = Confine the fire by closing all doors; E = Extinguish or evacuate.

6. 4

Rationale: Anthrax is caused by *Bacillus anthracis*, and it can be contracted through the digestive system, abrasions in the skin, or inhalation. Antibiotics are administered. Botulism is caused by a neurotoxin that causes severe paralysis and can be fatal.

Test-Taking Strategy: Focus on the subject, the types, transmission, and treatment of anthrax and the strategic words, *need for further teaching*. These words indicate a negative event query and the need to select the incorrect statement about anthrax.

7. 2

Rationale: The restraint strap is secured to the bed frame (never to the side rail) to avoid accidental injury in case the side rail is released. The nurse recognizes that tying the strap to the side rail is not correct and is unsafe. A half-bow or safety knot must be used when applying a restraint, because it does not tighten when force is applied against it and allows for the quick and easy removal of the restraint in case of an emergency. The belt restraint would be secure, and one to two fingers must easily slide between the restraint and the client's skin. The client needs to be able to turn from back to side while in the restraint. A purpose of a restraint is to remind the client not to get out of bed alone.

Test-Taking Strategy: Focus on the subject, application of restraints, and note that the question is asking to identify the unsafe intervention. Visualize each action in the options to determine the unsafe action. Recall how to safely apply a restraint and select the incorrect intervention: tying the restraint to the side rail.

8. 4

Rationale: Limb restraints are often prescribed to prevent clients from pulling out tubes and injuring themselves. The restraint is prescribed for 24 hours, and the nurse must verify that the restraint is protecting the client from self-injury but not too constrictive to impair circulation or harm the skin. Limb restraints are made with padding to protect the client's skin. The nurse determines the tightness of the wrist restraint by placing two fingers under the restraint. Observing the skin

and checking the temperature of the skin is not as thorough or accurate as checking the tightness of the restraint manually. Restraints need to be removed at least every 2 hours, but this does not evaluate how tight the restraint is around the wrist.
Test-Taking Strategy: Note the subject, verification that a restraint is not too constrictive. Visualize the action in each of the options to determine which would verify that the restraint is not too constrictive.

9. 1, 2, 3, 4
Rationale: The nurse must follow standard precautions when caring for any client and wear gloves when emptying a bedpan. Linens are kept in the room as a safety precaution in case there is contamination or part of the implant is lost. The film badge dosimeter allows the nurse to visualize the estimated amount of radiation exposure during the shift. The nurse wears a lead apron to protect oneself and block the radiation waves emitted when close to the client. A private room with a private bath is essential if a client has an internal radiation implant. This is necessary to prevent the accidental exposure of other clients to radiation.

Test-Taking Strategy: Focus on the subject, interventions to be included in the plan of care for a client with an internal radiation implant. Read each option carefully and think about the concerns related to exposure. Noting the word *semiprivate* will assist in eliminating this option.

10. 1
Rationale: A fire can be extinguished by using a fire extinguisher. To use the extinguisher, the pin is pulled first. The extinguisher would then be aimed at the base of the fire. The handle of the extinguisher is squeezed, and the fire is extinguished by sweeping from side to side to coat the area evenly. Remember that the safety of anyone present is more important than extinguishing the fire. Remember the mnemonic *RACE: R* = Rescue; *A* = Alarm; *C* = Confine; *E* = Extinguish.
Test-Taking Strategy: Note the strategic word, *next*. Remember the mnemonic *PASS* to prioritize in the use of a fire extinguisher: *P* = Pull the pin; *A* = Aim at the base of the fire; *S* = Squeeze the handle; *S* = Sweep from side to side to coat the area evenly.

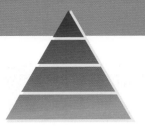
CHAPTER 15

Calculation of Medication and Intravenous Dosages

PRIORITY CONCEPTS Clinical Judgment; Safety

WHAT WOULD YOU DO?

The nurse is preparing to administer 30 mL of a liquid medication to an assigned client. What would the nurse do when preparing this medication?
Answer is located on p. 179.

I. **Medication Administration (Box 15.1)**

II. **Drug-Measurement Systems**

A. Metric system (Box 15.2)
   1. The basic units of metric measurement are meter, liter, and gram.
   2. Meter measures length; liter measures volume; gram measures mass.
B. Apothecary and household systems
   1. Apothecary measures such as dram, grain, and minim are not commonly used in the clinical setting.
   2. Commonly used household measures include drop, teaspoon, tablespoon, ounce, pint, and cup.

⚠ The NCLEX will not likely present questions that require you to convert from the apothecary system of measurement to the metric system; however, this system is still important to know because, although it is not common, you may encounter it in the clinical setting.

C. Additional common drug measures
   1. Milliequivalent (mEq)
      a. The milliequivalent is an expression of the number of grams of a medication contained in 1 mL of a solution.
      b. For example: the measure of potassium is given in milliequivalents, such as 5 mEq of potassium loose.

2. Unit
   a. Measures a medication in terms of its action rather than its physical weight
   b. For example: penicillin, heparin, and insulin are measured in units.

III. **Conversions**

A. Conversion between metric units (Box 15.3)
   1. The metric system is a decimal system; therefore, conversions between the units in this system can be done by either dividing or multiplying by 1000 or by moving the decimal point three places to the right or three places to the left.
   2. In the metric system, to convert larger to smaller, multiply by 1000 or move the decimal point three places to the right; for example, 1 g = 1000 mg.
   3. In the metric system, to convert smaller to larger, divide by 1000 or move the decimal point three places to the left; for example, 1000 mg = 1 g.
B. Conversion between household and metric systems
   1. Conversions between the metric and household systems are equivalent—not equal—measures.
   2. Conversion to equivalent measures between systems is necessary when a medication prescription is written in one system but the medication label is given in another.
   3. Medications are not always prescribed and prepared in the same system of measurement. Therefore, it is necessary to convert units from one system to another. However, the metric system is the most commonly used system in the clinical setting.
   4. Calculating equivalents between two systems may be done by using the method of ratio and proportion (Boxes 15.4 and 15.5).

⚠ Conversion is the first step in the calculation of dosages.

BOX 15.1 Medication Administration

Check the medication prescription.
Compare the client's medication prescription with all the medications that the client was previously taking (medication reconciliation).
Ask the client about a history of allergies.
Determine the client's current condition and the purpose of the prescribed medication or intravenous solution.
Determine the client's understanding regarding the purpose of the prescribed medication or intravenous solution.
Plan to reinforce teaching to the client about the medication and about self-administration at home.
Identify and address social, cultural, and religious concerns that the client may have about taking the medication.
Determine the need for conversion when preparing a dose of medication for administration to the client.
Check the medication administration rights: some rights include right medication, right dose, right client, right route, right time and frequency, right indication, and right documentation.
Check the client's vital signs, check significant laboratory results, and identify any potential interactions (food or medication interactions) before administering medication, when appropriate.
Identify any food or medication interactions before administering the medication.
Document the administration of the prescribed therapy and client's response to the therapy.

BOX 15.2 Metric System

Abbreviations
meter: m
liter: L
milliliter: mL
kilogram: kg
gram: g
milligram: mg
microgram: mcg

Equivalents
1 mcg = 0.000001 g
1 mg = 1000 mcg or 0.001 g
1 g = 1000 mg
1 kg = 1000 g
1 kg = 2.2 lb
1 mL = 0.001 L

IV. Medication Labels

A. A medication label will usually contain both the generic name and the trade name of the medication.

B. Always check expiration dates on medication labels.

> ⚠ The NCLEX® now tests you only on generic names of medications. Trade names will not be available for most medications, so be sure to learn the medications by their generic names for the examination. However, you will likely still encounter the trade names in the clinical setting.

BOX 15.3 Conversion Between Metric Units

Problem 1
Convert 2 g to milligrams.

Solution
Change a larger unit to a smaller unit.
2 g = 2000 mg (moving decimal point three places to right)

Problem 2
Convert 250 mL to liters.

Solution
Change a smaller unit to a larger unit.
250 mL = 0.25 L (moving decimal point three places to left)

BOX 15.4 Ratio and Proportion

Ratio: The relationship between two numbers, separated by a colon; for example, 1:2
Proportion: The relationship between two ratios, separated by a double colon (::) or an equal sign (=)
Formula: H (on hand): V (vehicle):: (=) desired dose: X (unknown)
To solve a ratio and proportion problem: The middle numbers (means) are multiplied, and the end numbers (extremes) are multiplied.

Sample Problem
H = 1
V = 2
Desired dose = 3
X = unknown
Set up the formula: 1: 2:: 3: X
Solve: Multiply means and extremes.
1X = 6
X = 6

BOX 15.5 Calculating Equivalents Between Two Systems

Calculating equivalents between two systems may be done by using the method of ratio and proportion.

Problem
The primary health care provider prescribes nitroglycerin, grain (gr) 1/150. The medication label reads 0.4 milligram (mg) per tablet. The nurse prepares to administer how many tablets to the client?
    If you know that 1/150 gr is equal to 0.4 mg, you know that you need to administer 1 tablet. Otherwise, use the ratio and proportion formula.

Ratio and Proportion Formula
H (on hand): V (vehicle):: (=) desired dose: X
1 gr: 60 mg:: 1/150 gr: X mg
60 × 1/150 = 60/150 = X
X = 0.4 mg (1 tablet)

BOX 15.6   Medication Prescriptions

Name of client
Date and time when prescription is written
Name of medication to be given
Dosage of medication
Medication route
Time and frequency of administration
Signature of person who wrote the prescription

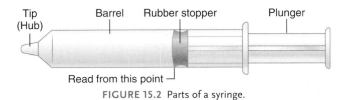

FIGURE 15.2 Parts of a syringe.

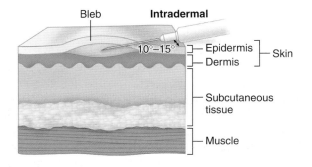

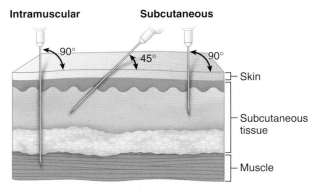

FIGURE 15.1 Angles of injection.

V. Medication Prescriptions (Box 15.6)

A. In a medication prescription, the name of the medication is written first, followed by the dosage, route, and frequency (depending on the frequency of the prescription, times of administration are usually established by the health care agency and written in an agency policy).

B. Medication prescriptions need to be written using accepted abbreviations, acronyms, and symbols approved by The Joint Commission; also follow agency guidelines.

⚠ If the nurse has any questions about, or sees inconsistencies in, the written prescription, the nurse must contact the person who wrote the prescription immediately and must verify it.

VI. Oral Medications

A. Scored tablets contain an indented mark to be used for breaking the tablet into partial dosages. When necessary, scored tablets (those marked for division)

can be divided into halves or quarters. Use of a pill cutter is recommended.

B. Enteric coated tablets and sustained-released capsules delay absorption until the medication reaches the small intestine. These medications should not be crushed.

C. Capsules contain a powdered or oily medication in a gelatin cover.

D. Oral liquids are supplied in solution form and contain a specific amount of medication in a given amount of solution, as stated on the label. ▲

E. The medicine cup
   1. The medicine cup has a capacity of 30 mL or 1 oz and is used for orally administered liquids.
   2. The medicine cup is calibrated to measure teaspoons, tablespoons, and ounces.
   3. To pour accurately, place the medication cup on a level surface at eye level and then pour the liquid while reading the measuring markings.
   4. Volumes of less than 5 mL are measured by using a syringe (with the needle removed) specifically designed for oral administration

⚠ A calibrated dropper is used for giving medicine to children.

VII. Parenteral Medications

A. *Parenteral* means injection route, and parenteral medications are administered by intravenous (IV), intramuscular, intradermal, or subcutaneous routes (Fig. 15.1, angles of injection).

B. Parenteral medications are packaged in single-use ampules, single- and multiple-use rubber-stoppered vials, and premeasured syringes and cartridges.

C. The nurse should not administer more than 3 mL per intramuscular injection site (2 mL for the deltoid) or 0.5 mL to 1.5 mL per subcutaneous injection site; larger volumes are difficult for an injection site to absorb and, if prescribed, need to be verified. Variations for pediatric clients are discussed in the pediatric sections of this book.

D. The standard 3-mL syringe is used to measure most injectable medications. It is calibrated in tenths (0.1) of a milliliter.

E. The syringe is filled by drawing in solution until the top ring of the rubber stopper on the plunger (i.e., the ring closest to the needle), not the middle section and not the bottom ring of the rubber stopper, is aligned with the desired calibration (Fig. 15.2).

⚠ Always question and verify excessively large or small volumes of medication.

F. Prefilled medication cartridge
   1. The medication cartridge slips into the cartridge holder, which provides a plunger for its injection.
   2. Designed to provide sufficient capacity to allow for the addition of a second medication when combined dosages are prescribed
   3. The prefilled medication cartridge is to be used once and discarded. If the nurse is to give less than the full single dose provided, he or she needs to discard the extra amount before giving the client the injection, in accordance with agency policies and procedures. Always read instructions with commercial medications of prefilled syringes to determine removing air from the syringe.
G. In general, standard medication doses for adults are to be rounded to the nearest tenth (0.1) of a milliliter and measured on the milliliter scale; for example, 1.28 mL is rounded to 1.3 mL (follow agency policy for rounding medication doses).
H. When volumes of more than 3 mL are required, a 5-mL syringe may be used. These syringes are calibrated in fifths (0.2 mL) (Fig. 15.3).
I. Other syringes that may be available are 10, 20, and 50 mL and may be used for medication administration requiring dilution.
J. Tuberculin syringe (Fig. 15.4)
   1. Holds a total capacity of 1 mL; used to measure small or critical amounts of medication, such as allergen extract, vaccine, or a child's medication.
   2. It is calibrated in hundredths (0.01) of a milliliter, with each one-tenth (0.1) marked on the metric scale.
K. Insulin syringe (Fig. 15.5)
   1. The standard unit-100 insulin syringe is used to measure unit-100 insulin only. It is calibrated for

a total of 100 units or 1 mL. Low-dose insulin syringes, such as a 30-unit insulin syringe or a 50-unit insulin syringe, may be used when administering smaller doses.
   2. Insulin should not be measured in any other type of syringe.

⚠ If the insulin prescription states to administer regular and NPH insulin, combine both types of insulin in the same syringe. Use the mnemonic RN: draw Regular insulin into the insulin syringe first, and then draw the NPH insulin.

   3. Insulin is also administered using insulin pens with disposable needles, which are usually primed before administering a dose. Each pen is used for an individual client. The dosage is dialed into the pen. Many clients use these pens for administering insulin at home.
L. Safety needles contain shielding devices that are attached to the syringe and slipped over the needle; their use reduces the incidence of needle-stick injuries.

VIII. Injectable Medications in Powder Form

A. Some medications become unstable when stored in solution form and are therefore packaged in powder form.
B. Powders must be dissolved with a sterile diluent before use. Usually sterile water or normal saline is used according to instructions from the supplier of the medication. The dissolving procedure is called "reconstitution" (Box 15.7).

IX. Calculating the Correct Dosage (Box 15.8)

A. When calculating dosages of oral medications, check the calculation and question the prescription if the calculation calls for more than three tablets.
B. When calculating dosages of parenteral medications, check the calculation and question the prescription if the amount to be given is too large a dose.
C. Be sure that all measures are in the same system and that all units are in the same size, converting them when necessary. Carefully consider the reasonable amount of the medication that would be administered.
D. Round standard adult injection doses to tenths, and measure in a 3-mL syringe (follow agency policy).
E. Round small, critical, or children's doses to hundredths, and measure in a 1-mL tuberculin syringe (follow agency policy).

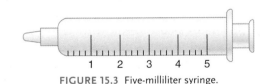

FIGURE 15.3 Five-milliliter syringe.

FIGURE 15.4 Tuberculin syringe.

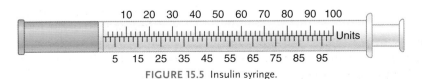

FIGURE 15.5 Insulin syringe.

BOX 15.7 Reconstitution

- When reconstituting a medication, locate the instructions on the label or in the vial package insert and read and follow the directions carefully.
- The instructions will state the volume of diluent to be used and the resulting volume of the reconstituted medication.
- Often a powdered medication adds volume to the solution in addition to the amount of diluent added.
- The total volume of the prepared solution will always exceed the volume of the diluent added.
- When reconstituting a multiple-dose vial, label the medication vial with the date and time of preparation, your initials, and the date of expiration.
- Indicating the strength per volume on the medication label also is important.

BOX 15.8 Standard Formula for Calculating a Medication Dosage

$$\frac{D}{A} \times Q = X$$

D (desired) is the dosage that the health care provider prescribed.

A (available) is the dosage strength as stated on the medication label.

Q (quantity) is the volume or form in which the dosage strength is available, such as tablets, capsules, or milliliters.

F. In addition to using the standard formula (see Box 15.8), calculations can be done through the use of dimensional analysis; the required elements of a dimensional analysis equation include the desired answer units, conversion formula that includes the desired answer units and the units that need to be converted, and the original factors to convert, including quantity and units.

⚠ Regardless of the source of the error, if the nurse gives an incorrect dose, he or she is legally responsible for the action.

X. Percentage and Ratio Solutions

A. Percentage solutions
  1. Express the number of grams of the medication per 100 mL of solution.
  2. For example, calcium gluconate 10% is 10 g of pure medication per 100 mL of solution.

B. Ratio solutions
  1. Express the number of grams of the medication per total milliliters of solution.
  2. For example, epinephrine 1:1000 is 1 g of pure medication per 1000 mL of solution.

BOX 15.9 Formulas for Intravenous Calculations

Flow Rates

$$\frac{Total\ volume \times drop\ factor}{Time\ in\ minutes} = drops\ per\ minute$$

Infusion Time

$$\frac{Total\ volume\ to\ infuse}{Milliliters\ per\ hour\ being\ infused} = infusion\ time$$

Number of Milliliters per Hour

$$\frac{Total\ volume\ in\ milliliters}{Number\ of\ hours} = number\ of\ milliliters\ per\ hour$$

XI. Intravenous Flow Rates (Box 15.9)

A. Monitor IV flow rate frequently even if the IV solution is being administered through an electronic infusion device (follow agency policy regarding frequency).

B. If an IV infusion is running behind schedule, collaborate with the primary health care provider (PHCP) to determine the client's ability to tolerate an increased flow rate, particularly if the client has cardiac, pulmonary, renal, or neurological conditions.

⚠ The nurse would never increase (speed up) the rate of an IV infusion to catch up if the infusion is running behind schedule. Any IV fluid administered has to be included in the intake portion of the client's assessment.

C. Whenever a prescribed IV rate is increased, the nurse needs to monitor the client for increased heartrate, increased respiration, or increased lung congestion, which could indicate fluid overload.

D. IV fluids are most frequently prescribed on the basis of milliliters per hour (mL/hr) to be administered. The volume per hour prescribed is administered by adjusting the rate at which the IV infuses, which is counted in drops per minute (gtt/min).

E. Most flow-rate calculations involve changing mL/hr into gtt/min.

F. IV tubing
  1. Calibrated in gtts/mL. This calibration is needed for calculating flow rates.
  2. A standard or macrodrip set is used for routine adult IV administrations. Depending on the manufacturer and type of tubing, it requires 10, 15, or 20 drops (gtt) to equal 1 mL.
  3. A minidrip or microdrip set is used when more exact measurements are needed, such as in intensive care and pediatric units.
  4. In a minidrip or microdrip set, 60 gtts is equal to 1 mL.
  5. The calibration, in gtts/mL, is written on the IV tubing package.

WHAT WOULD YOU DO?

Answer: When preparing to administer a liquid medication, the nurse must use a medicine cup, pouring liquids into it after placing it on a flat surface at eye level, with the thumbnail at the medicine cup line indicating the desired amount. Liquids would not be mixed with tablets or with other liquids in the same container. The nurse would be sure not to return poured medication to its container and must properly discard poured medication if not used. The nurse needs to pour liquids from the side opposite the bottle's label to avoid spilling medicine on the label. Medications that irritate the gastric mucosa, such as potassium products, must be diluted or be taken with meals. Ice chips would be offered before administering unpleasant-tasting medications, to numb the client's taste buds.

PRACTICE QUESTIONS

❖ **1.** The medication prescribed is hydromorphone hydrochloride 3 mg intramuscularly, every 4 hours as needed. The medication label reads hydromorphone hydrochloride 4 mg/1 mL. The nurse would prepare to administer how many mL to the client? **Fill in the blank.**

Answer: _____ mL

❖ **2.** The medication prescribed is digoxin 0.25 mg orally, daily. The medication label reads digoxin 0.125 mg/tablet. The nurse would prepare how many tablet(s) to administer the dose? **Fill in the blank.**

Answer: _____ tablet(s)

❖ **3.** The medication prescribed is heparin 5000 units subcutaneously, every 12 hours. The medication vial reads heparin 10,000 units/mL. The nurse prepares how many mL to administer one dose? **Fill in the blank.**

Answer: _____ mL

❖ **4.** The medication prescribed is metoclopramide hydrochloride 10 mg intramuscularly times one dose. The medication label reads metoclopramide hydrochloride 5 mg/mL. The nurse prepares how much medication to administer the dose? **Fill in the blank.**

Answer: _____ mL

❖ **5.** The medication prescribed is morphine sulfate 6 mg subcutaneously. The medication label states morphine sulfate 10 mg/1 mL. The nurse plans to prepare how much medication to administer the dose? **Fill in the blank.**

Answer: _____ mL

❖ **6.** The medication prescribed is prochlorperazine 5 mg intramuscularly, every 4 hours as needed. The medication label states prochlorperazine 10 mg/mL. The nurse prepares how much medication to administer the dose? **Fill in the blank.**

Answer: _____ mL

❖ **7.** The medication prescribed is haloperidol, 4 mg intramuscularly, immediately. The medication label states 5 mg/1 mL. The nurse prepares how much medication to administer the dose? **Fill in the blank.**

Answer: _____ mL

❖ **8.** The medication prescribed is levodopa 1 g orally, daily. The medication label states levodopa, 500-mg tablets. The nurse prepares to administer how many tablets for one dose? **Fill in the blank.**

Answer: _____ tablet(s)

❖ **9.** The medication prescribed is zidovudine, 0.2 g orally, three times daily. The medication label states zidovudine, 100-mg tablets. The nurse prepares to administer how many tablets for one dose? **Fill in the blank.**

Answer: _____ tablet(s)

❖ **10.** The medication prescribed is methylprednisolone acetate 60 mg intramuscularly. The medication label states methylprednisolone acetate 40 mg/1 mL. How many milliliters will the nurse prepare to administer to the client? **Fill in the blank.**

Answer: _____ mL

11. The medication prescription states to administer acetaminophen 650 mg orally for a temperature of more than 38°C. The medication bottle states acetaminophen 325-mg tablets. The nurse takes the client's temperature and notes that it is 101°F. The nurse plans to take which action?
   1. Administer two tablets of acetaminophen.
   2. Administer three tablets of acetaminophen.
   3. Do not administer acetaminophen at this time.
   4. Check the client's temperature in 30 minutes.

❖ **12.** The medication prescription reads phenytoin 0.2 g orally, twice daily. The medication label states 100-mg capsules. The nurse prepares how many capsule(s) to administer one dose? **Fill in the blank.**

Answer: _____ capsule(s)

❖ **13.** The intravenous prescription is 1000 mL of 0.9% NaCl (normal saline) to run over 12 hours. The drop factor is 15 gtts/1 mL. The nurse plans to adjust the flow rate to how many gtts/minute? **Fill in the blank and record the answer to the nearest whole number.**

Answer: _____ gtts/minute

❖ **14.** The medication is an intramuscular dose of 400,000 units of penicillin G benzathine. The medication label reads penicillin G benzathine 300,000 units/mL. The nurse prepares how much medication to administer the correct dose? **Fill in the blank and record the answer using one decimal place.**

Answer: _____ mL

❖ **15.** The intravenous prescription is 3000 mL of 5% dextrose in water (D5W) to run over a 24-hour period. The drop factor is 10 gtts/1 mL. The nurse plans to adjust the flow rate to how many gtts/minute? **Fill in the blank and record the answer to the nearest whole number.**

Answer: _____ gtts/minute

ANSWERS

❖ **1. 0.75**
Rationale: Follow the formula for dosage calculation.

Formula:

$$\frac{Desired \times mL}{Available} = mL \ per \ dose$$

$$\frac{3 \ mg \times 1 \ mL}{4 \ mg} = 0.75 \ mL$$

Test-Taking Strategy: Focus on the subject, a dosage calculation. Follow the formula for the calculation of the correct medication dose. Once you have performed the calculation, verify your answer using a calculator and make sure that the answer makes sense.

❖ **2. 2**
Rationale: Follow the formula for dosage calculation.

Formula:

$$\frac{Desired \times tablet(s)}{Available} = tablet(s) \ per \ dose$$

$$\frac{0.25 \ mg \times 1 \ tablet}{0.125 \ mg} = 2 \ tablets$$

Test-Taking Strategy: Focus on the subject, a dosage calculation. Follow the formula for the calculation of the correct medication dose. Once you have performed the calculation, verify your answer using a calculator and make sure that the answer makes sense.

❖ **3. 0.5**
Rationale: Follow the formula for dosage calculation.

Formula:

$$\frac{Desired \times mL}{Available} = mL \ per \ dose$$

$$\frac{5000 \ units \times 1 \ mL}{10,000 \ units} = 0.5 \ mL$$

Test-Taking Strategy: Focus on the subject, a dosage calculation. Follow the formula for the calculation of the correct medication dose. Once you have performed the calculation, verify your answer using a calculator and make sure that the answer makes sense.

❖ **4. 2**
Rationale: Follow the formula for dosage calculation.

Formula:

$$\frac{Desired \times mL}{Available} = mL \ per \ dose$$

$$\frac{10 \ mg \times 1 \ mL}{5 \ mg} = 2 \ mL$$

Test-Taking Strategy: Focus on the subject, a dosage calculation. Follow the formula for the calculation of the correct medication dose. Once you have performed the calculation, verify your answer using a calculator and make sure that the answer makes sense.

❖ **5. 0.6**
Rationale: Follow the formula for dosage calculation.

Formula:

$$\frac{Desired \times mL}{Available} = mL \ per \ dose$$

$$\frac{6 \ mg \times 1 \ mL}{10 \ mg} = 0.6 \ mL$$

Test-Taking Strategy: Focus on the subject, a dosage calculation. Follow the formula for the calculation of the correct medication dose. Once you have performed the calculation, verify your answer using a calculator and make sure that the answer makes sense.

❖ **6. 0.5**
Rationale: Follow the formula for dosage calculation.

Formula:

$$\frac{Desired \times mL}{Available} = mL \ per \ dose$$

$$\frac{5 \ mg \times 1 \ mL}{10 \ mg} = 0.5 \ mL$$

Test-Taking Strategy: Focus on the subject, a dosage calculation. Follow the formula for the calculation of the correct medication dose. Once you have performed the calculation, verify your answer using a calculator and make sure that the answer makes sense.

❖ **7. 0.8**

Rationale: Follow the formula for dosage calculation.

Formula:

$$\frac{Desired \times mL}{Available} = mL \ per \ dose$$

$$\frac{4 \ mg \times 1 \ mL}{5 \ mg} = 0.8 \ mL$$

Test-Taking Strategy: Focus on the subject, a dosage calculation. Follow the formula for the calculation of the correct medication dose. Once you have performed the calculation, verify your answer using a calculator and make sure that the answer makes sense. Remember to round the answer and record to one decimal place.

❖ **8. 2**

Rationale: Convert 1 g to milligrams. In the metric system, to convert larger to smaller, multiply by 1000, or move the decimal three places to the right; therefore, 1 g = 1000 mg.

Formula:

$$\frac{Desired \times tablet(s)}{Available} = Tablet(s) \ per \ dose$$

$$\frac{1000 \ mg \times tablet}{500 \ mg} = 2 \ tablets$$

Test-Taking Strategy: Focus on the subject, a medication calculation. For this medication calculation problem, it is necessary to first convert grams to milligrams. Follow the formula for conversion, and read the question carefully. After you have performed the calculation, verify your answer using a calculator.

❖ **9. 2**

Rationale: Convert 0.2 g to milligrams. In the metric system, to convert larger to smaller, multiply by 1000, or move the decimal three places to the right; therefore, 0.2 g = 200 mg.

Formula:

$$\frac{Desired \times tablet(s)}{Available} = tablet(s) \ per \ dose$$

$$\frac{200 \ mg \times tablet}{100 \ mg} = 2 \ tablets$$

Test-Taking Strategy: Focus on the subject, a medication calculation. For this medication calculation problem, it is necessary to first convert grams to milligrams. Follow the formula for conversion, and read the question carefully. After you have performed the calculation, verify your answer using a calculator.

❖ **10. 1.5**

Rationale: Follow the formula for dosage calculation.

Formula:

$$\frac{Desired \times mL}{Available} = mL \ per \ dose$$

$$\frac{60 \ mg \times 1 \ mL}{40 \ mg} = 1.5 \ mL$$

Test-Taking Strategy: Focus on the subject, a dosage calculation. Follow the formula for the calculation of the correct medication dose. Once you have performed the calculation, verify your answer using a calculator and make sure that the answer makes sense.

❖ **11. 1**

Rationale: Convert Fahrenheit to Celsius, and then calculate the dose to be administered.

Step 1: Conversion of Fahrenheit to Celsius

Formula: To convert Fahrenheit to Celsius, subtract 32, and divide the result by 1.8:

$$C = (101 - 32) = 69, \ divided \ by \ 1.8 = 38.3°\ C$$

Step 2: Dosage calculation

Formula:

$$\frac{Desired \times tablet(s)}{Available} = tablet(s) \ per \ dose$$

$$\frac{650 \ mg \times 1 \ tablet}{325 \ mg} = 2 \ tablets$$

The temperature meets the criteria to administer acetaminophen. The medication would be administered. Therefore, option 1 is the correct option.

Test-Taking Strategy: Focus on the subject, a medication calculation. For this medication calculation problem, it is necessary to convert Fahrenheit to Celsius. Follow the formula for conversion, and then perform the medication calculation. The temperature meets the criteria to administer acetaminophen. The medication would be administered. The nurse may want to recheck the temperature, but that option is secondary to administration of the acetaminophen. After you have performed the calculation, verify the calculation using a calculator. This will direct you to the correct option of administering two Tylenol tablets.

❖ **12. 2**

Rationale: You must convert 0.2 g to milligrams. In the metric system, to convert larger to smaller, multiply by 1000 or move the decimal three places to the right. Therefore, 0.2 g equals 200 mg. After conversion from grams to milligrams, use the formula to calculate the correct dose.

Formula:

$$\frac{Desired \times capsule(s)}{Available} = capsule(s) \ per \ dose$$

$$\frac{200 \ mg \times capsule}{100 \ mg} = 2 \ capsules$$

Test-Taking Strategy: Focus on the subject, a medication calculation. In this medication calculation problem, first you must convert grams to milligrams. Once you have done the conversion and reread the medication calculation problem, you will know that two capsules is the correct answer. Recheck your work using a calculator and make sure that the answer makes sense.

❖ **13. 21**

Rationale: Use the intravenous (IV) flow rate formula.

Formula:

$$\frac{Total\ volume \times drop\ factor}{Time\ in\ minutes} = drops\ per\ minute$$

$$\frac{1000\ mL \times 15\ gtt}{720\ minutes} = \frac{15,000}{720} = 20.8,\ or\ 21\ gtts\ /\ minute$$

Test-Taking Strategy: Focus on the subject, an IV calculation. Follow the formula for calculating an infusion rate for an IV. Be sure to change 12 hours to minutes (1 hour = 60 minutes; $60 \times 12 = 720$ minutes). After you have performed the calculation, verify your answer using a calculator and remember to record the answer to the nearest whole number.

❖ **14. 1.3**

Rationale: Follow the formula for dosage calculation.

Formula:

$$\frac{Desired \times mL}{Available} = mL\ per\ dose$$

$$\frac{400,000\ units \times 1\ mL}{300,000\ units} = 1.3\ mL$$

Test-Taking Strategy: Focus on the subject, a dosage calculation. Follow the formula for the calculation of the correct medication dose. Once you have performed the calculation, verify your answer using a calculator and make sure that the answer makes sense. Remember to record the answer using one decimal place.

❖ **15. 21**

Rationale: Use the intravenous (IV) flow rate formula.

Formula:

$$\frac{Total\ volume \times drop\ factor}{Time\ in\ minutes} = gtts/minute$$

$$\frac{3000\ mL \times 10\ gtt}{1440\ minutes} = \frac{30,000}{1440} = 20.8,\ or\ 21\ gtts/minute$$

Test-Taking Strategy: Focus on the subject, an IV calculation. Follow the formula for calculating the infusion rate for an IV. Be sure to change 24 hours to minutes. After you have performed the calculation, verify your answer using a calculator, and remember to record the answer to the nearest whole number.

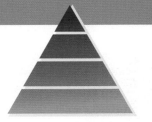

CHAPTER **16**

Perioperative Nursing Care

PRIORITY CONCEPTS Infection; Safety

WHAT WOULD YOU DO?

The nurse is assisting a surgeon in obtaining informed consent from a client for a scheduled surgical procedure. The client signs the consent, and after the surgeon leaves the nursing unit, the client informs the nurse that he or she is unclear about certain aspects of the surgical procedure. What would the nurse do?
Answer is located on p. 192.

I. Preoperative Care

⚠️ A client may return home shortly after having a surgical procedure because many are done through ambulatory care or 1-day-stay surgical units. Perioperative care procedures apply even if the client returns home the same day.

A. Obtaining informed consent
1. The surgeon is responsible for obtaining the informed consent for surgery. Often, the nurse is responsible for obtaining the client's signature on the consent form for surgery, which indicates the client's agreement to the procedure based on the surgeon's explanation.
2. The nurse may witness the client's signing of the consent form, but the nurse must be sure that the client has understood the surgeon's explanation of the surgery.
3. The nurse typically signs as a witness of the client's signature on the consent form after the client acknowledges understanding of the procedure.
4. The nurse's signature indicates that it was the client, and not another person, who signed the informed consent form.
5. Minors (clients younger than 18 years old) may need a parent or legal guardian to sign the informed consent form, unless they are an emancipated minor.

6. Older clients may need a legal guardian to sign the consent form.
7. Psychiatric clients have a right to refuse treatment until a court has legally determined that they are unable to make decisions for themselves.
8. No sedation would be administered to the client before he or she signs the consent form.
9. Obtaining a telephone consent from a legal guardian or power of attorney for health care is an acceptable practice if clients are unable to give consent themselves. The nurse must engage another nurse as a witness to the consent given over the telephone.

B. Nutrition
1. Check the surgeon's prescriptions regarding nothing by mouth (NPO) status before surgery.
2. Solid foods and liquids are generally withheld for 6 to 8 hours before general anesthesia and for 3 hours before surgery with local anesthesia to avoid aspiration.
3. An intravenous (IV) line is inserted, and IV fluids are administered, if prescribed; per agency policy, the IV catheter size must be large enough to administer blood products if they are required.

C. Elimination
1. If the client is to have intestinal or abdominal surgery, the surgeon may prescribe an enema, laxative, or both the day or evening before surgery.
2. The client needs to be asked to void immediately before surgery.
3. Prepare to insert an indwelling urinary catheter, if prescribed; if there is a Foley catheter in place, it would be emptied immediately before surgery, and the amount and quality of urine output must be documented.

D. Surgical site
1. Prepare to clean the surgical site with a mild antiseptic soap the night before surgery, as prescribed.
2. Inform the client about the procedure for hair removal on the operative site; shaving with a special shaver or hair clipping may be done in the operative

BOX 16.1 **Client Teaching**

Deep Breathing and Coughing Exercises

Instruct the client that a sitting position provides the best lung expansion for coughing and deep breathing exercises.

Instruct the client to breathe deeply three times by inhaling through the nostrils and exhaling slowly through pursed lips.

Instruct the client that the third breath needs to be held for 3 seconds; then the client can cough deeply three times, splinting the operative site if necessary.

The client needs to perform this exercise every 1 to 2 h.

Incentive Spirometry

Instruct the client to assume a sitting or upright position.

Instruct the client to place the mouth tightly around the mouthpiece.

Instruct the client to inhale slowly to raise and maintain the flow rate indicator between the 600 and 900 marks or at a point prescribed.

Instruct the client to hold their breath for 5 seconds and then to exhale through pursed lips.

Instruct the client to repeat this process 10 times every hour.

Leg and Foot Exercises

Gastrocnemius (calf) pumping: Instruct the client to move both ankles by pointing the toes up and then down.

Quadriceps (thigh) setting: Instruct the client to press the back of the knees against the bed and then to relax the knees. This contracts and relaxes the thigh and calf muscles to prevent thrombus formation.

Foot circles: Instruct the client to rotate each foot in a circle.

Hip and knee movements: Instruct the client to flex the knee and thigh, straighten the leg, and hold the position for 5 seconds before lowering. (This would not be performed if the client is having abdominal surgery or has a back problem.)

Splinting the Incision

If the surgical incision is abdominal or thoracic, instruct the client to brace the incisional area with a pillow, folded blanket, or extended hand.

During deep breathing and coughing, the client presses gently against the area of the incision to splint or support it.

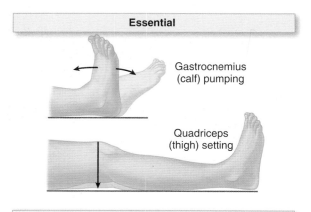

Essential

Gastrocnemius (calf) pumping

Quadriceps (thigh) setting

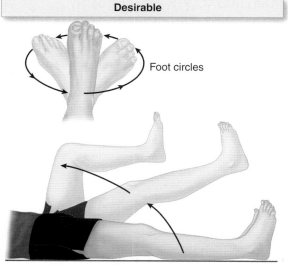

Desirable

Foot circles

Hip and knee movements

FIGURE 16.1 Postoperative leg exercises.

area. Shaving the operative site with a razor is associated with an increase in surgical site infections.

⚠ The hair on the head or face (including eyebrows) is removed only if it will interfere with the surgical procedure and only if prescribed.

▲ **E.** Reinforcing preoperative instructions

1. The client is informed about what to expect postoperatively.
2. Tell the client to notify the nurse if he or she experiences any postoperative pain and that pain medication will be prescribed to be given as the client requests according to the surgeon's prescription. Instruct client to report pain on a pain scale, 0 being no pain and 10 the worst pain ever experienced. Pain will be treated to a tolerable level.

3. The client is informed that requesting an opioid after surgery will not make them a drug addict.
4. Reinforce instructions about the use of a patient-controlled analgesia (PCA) pump if its use is prescribed.
5. The client is instructed to use noninvasive pain relief techniques such as relaxation or guided imagery before the pain occurs and as soon as the pain is noticed.
6. The client needs to be instructed not to smoke for at least 24 hours before surgery; discuss smoking cessation and treatments and programs.
7. Inform the client that the surgeon will need to be consulted about taking daily prescribed medications, aspirin, selected vitamins, and herbal products before surgery and when these products need to be stopped.
8. The client is instructed in deep breathing and coughing techniques, the use of incentive spirometry, and the importance of performing the techniques after surgery to prevent the development of pneumonia and atelectasis (Box 16.1).
9. The client is instructed in leg and foot exercises to prevent venous stasis of blood and facilitate venous blood return (Fig. 16.1; also see Box 16.1).

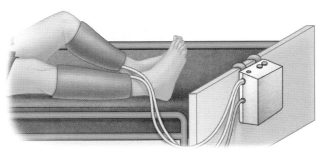

FIGURE 16.2 **Intermittent pulsatile compression device.**

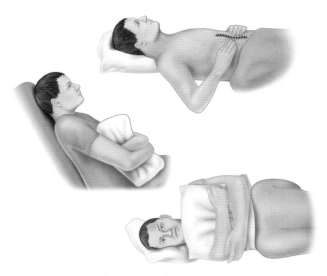

FIGURE 16.3 **Techniques for splinting a wound when coughing.**

Also instruct the client about the use of sequential compression devices (SCDs) to prevent venous stasis (Fig. 16.2).

10. The client is instructed about how to splint an incision and how to turn and reposition (Fig. 16.3; also see Box 16.1).

11. The client is informed of any invasive devices that may be needed after surgery, such as tubes, drains, indwelling urinary catheters, or IV lines.

12. The client is instructed not to pull on any of the invasive devices and that they will be removed as soon as possible.

▲ **F.** Psychosocial preparation
1. Be alert to the client's anxiety level.
2. Encourage the client to talk about feelings.
3. Answer questions or address concerns that the client may have regarding surgery.
4. Allow time for privacy for the client to prepare psychologically for surgery.
5. Provide support and assistance as needed.
6. Consider any cultural aspects when providing care (Box 16.2).

G. Preoperative checklist
▲ 1. Ensure that the client is wearing an identification bracelet.
2. Check for client allergies (see Chapter 59 for information about latex allergy).

BOX 16.2 **Cultural Aspects of Perioperative Nursing Care**

Cultural assessment includes questions related to:
- Primary language spoken and cultural practices
- Feelings related to surgery and pain
- Pain management
- Expectations
- Support systems
- Feelings toward self

Allow a family member to be present, if appropriate.

Secure the help of a professional interpreter to communicate with non–English-speaking clients.

Encourage the client to express any personal needs; be supportive.

Use pictures or phrase cards to communicate and assess the non–English-speaking client's perception of pain or other feelings.

Provide preoperative and postoperative educational materials in the appropriate language.

Adapted from Potter P, Perry A, Stockel P, Hall A: *Fundamentals of nursing*, ed 8, St. Louis, 2013, Mosby.

BOX 16.3 **Medical Conditions That Increase the Risk of Surgery**

- Bleeding disorders, such as thrombocytopenia and hemophilia
- Diabetes mellitus
- Chronic pain
- Heart disease, such as a recent myocardial infarction, dysrhythmia, heart failure, and peripheral vascular disease
- Obstructive sleep apnea
- Upper respiratory infection
- Liver disease
- Fever
- Chronic respiratory disease, such as emphysema, bronchitis, or asthma
- Immunological disorders, such as leukemia, acquired immunodeficiency syndrome, bone marrow depression, and the use of chemotherapy or immunosuppressive agents
- The abuse of street drugs

Adapted from Potter P, Perry A, Stockel P, Hall A: *Fundamentals of nursing*, ed 8, St. Louis, 2013, Mosby.

3. Review the preoperative checklist to be sure that ▲ each item is addressed before the client is transported to surgery.

4. Follow agency policies regarding preoperative procedures, including informed consents, preoperative checklists, prescribed laboratory or radiological tests, pregnancy screening, or any other preoperative procedure.

5. Ensure that consent forms have been signed for ▲ the operative procedure, anesthesia, any blood transfusions, the disposal of a limb, or surgical sterilization procedures.

6. Ensure that a history and physical examination ▲ were completed and documented in the client's record (Box 16.3).

BOX 16.4	Substances That Can Affect the Surgical Client

Analgesics

These potentiate the action of anesthetic agents.

Antibiotics

Prescribed before and after surgery as a prophylactic measure to prevent infection.

Anticholinergics

Medications with anticholinergic effects increase the potential for confusion.

Anticoagulants, Antiplatelets, and Thrombolytics

These alter normal clotting factors and increase the risk of hemorrhage.

Aspirin (acetylsalicylic acid) and nonsteroidal anti-inflammatory drugs are commonly used medications that can alter platelet aggregation.

These medications need to be discontinued at least 48 hours before surgery or as specified by the surgeon; clopidogrel usually has to be discontinued 5 days before surgery.

Complementary remedies such as garlic and ginseng may also alter normal clotting factors.

These medications need to also be discontinued at least 48 hours before surgery or as prescribed.

Anticonvulsants

The long-term use of certain anticonvulsants can alter the metabolism of anesthetic agents.

Antidepressants

These may lower the blood pressure during anesthesia.

Antidysrhythmics

These reduce cardiac contractility and impair cardiac conduction during anesthesia.

Antihypertensives

These can interact with anesthetic agents and cause bradycardia, hypotension, and impaired circulation.

Corticosteroids

These cause adrenal atrophy and reduce the body's ability to withstand stress.

Before and during surgery, dosages may be temporarily increased.

Diuretics

These potentiate electrolyte imbalances after surgery.

Herbal Substances

These can interact with anesthesia and cause a variety of adverse effects. These substances may need to be stopped at a specific time before surgery. During the preoperative period, clients need to be asked if they are taking any herbal substances.

Insulin

The need for insulin after surgery in a diabetic client may either be reduced, because the client's nutritional intake is decreased, or be increased, because of the stress response and the intravenous administration of glucose solutions.

Adapted from Potter P, Perry A, Stockel P, Hall A: *Fundamentals of nursing*, ed 8, St. Louis, 2013, Mosby.

7. Ensure that any screenings and clearances are noted in the client's record, such as a pregnancy test or cardiology clearance.

8. Ensure that any consultation reports that were prescribed are completed and documented in the client's record.

9. Ensure that the prescribed laboratory test results are documented in the client's record.

10. Ensure that any prescribed electrocardiography and chest radiography reports are noted in the client's record.

11. Ensure that blood type and screen or crossmatch are noted in the client's record and are within the established time frame per agency policy.

12. Remove, according to the agency's policy, the client's jewelry, makeup, dentures, hairpins, nail polish, contact lenses, and any prostheses.
    a. Hearing aids or glasses may be removed at the last possible moment before surgery.
    b. Clients with language or hearing concerns need to have access to agency-approved medical interpreters until anesthesia induction.

13. Document that valuables were given to the client's family members or locked in the hospital safe.

14. Monitor and document the client's vital signs.

15. Document the last time that the client ate or drank.

16. Document that the client has voided before surgery.

17. Document that the prescribed preoperative medication was given (Box 16.4).

H. Preoperative medications

1. Prepare to assist to administer preoperative medications as prescribed or to have them be administered in the operating room immediately before the surgery.

2. The client is instructed about the desired effects of the preoperative medication.

⚠ After administering the preoperative medications, keep the client in bed with the side rails up (per agency policy). Place the call bell next to the client; instruct the client not to get out of bed and to call for assistance if needed.

I. Arrival in the operating room

1. Guidelines to eliminate wrong site and wrong procedure surgery
   a. The surgeon meets with the client in the preoperative area and uses indelible ink to mark the operative site.
   b. In the operating room, the nurse and surgeon ensure and reconfirm that the operative site has been appropriately marked.

c. Just before starting the surgical procedure, a time-out is conducted with all members of the operative team present to identify the appropriate surgical site again.

2. When the client arrives in the operating room, the operating room nurse will verify the identification bracelet with the client's verbal response and will review the client's chart.

3. The client's chart will be checked for completeness and reviewed for informed consent forms, history and physical examination, and allergic reaction information.

4. The surgeon's prescriptions will be verified and implemented.

5. The IV line may be initiated at this time (or in the preoperative area), if prescribed.

6. The anesthesia team will administer the prescribed anesthesia.

 Verification of the client and the surgical operative site is critical.

II. Postoperative Care

A. Description:
   1. Postoperative care is the management of a client after surgery and includes care given during the immediate postoperative period as well as during the days following surgery.
   2. The goal of postoperative care is to prevent complications, to promote healing of the surgical incision, and to return the client to a healthy state.

B. Respiratory system

 Monitor breath sounds. Stridor, wheezing, or a crowing sound can indicate partial obstruction, bronchospasm, or laryngospasm; crackles or rhonchi may indicate pulmonary edema.

   1. Monitor vital signs, noting presurgical baseline vital signs.
   2. Monitor airway patency and ensure adequate ventilation (prolonged mechanical ventilation during anesthesia may affect postoperative lung function).
   3. Remember that extubated clients who are lethargic may not be able to maintain an airway.
   4. Monitor for secretions; if the client is unable to clear the airway by coughing, suction the secretions from the client's airway.
   5. Observe chest movement for symmetry and the use of accessory muscles.
   6. Monitor oxygen administration if prescribed.
   7. Monitor pulse oximetry and end-title carbon dioxide (CO_2) as prescribed.
   8. Encourage deep breathing and coughing exercises and the use of the incentive spirometer as soon as possible after surgery.
   9. Note the rate, depth, and quality of respirations; the respiratory rate needs to be higher than 10 and lower than 20 breaths/minute.
   10. Monitor for signs of respiratory distress, atelectasis, or other respiratory complications.

C. Cardiovascular system
   1. Monitor circulatory status, such as skin color, peripheral pulses, capillary refill, and the absence of edema, numbness, and tingling.
   2. Monitor for bleeding.
   3. Check the pulse for rate and rhythm (a bounding pulse may indicate hypertension, fluid overload, or client anxiety).
   4. Monitor for cardiac dysrhythmias.
   5. Monitor for signs of thrombophlebitis, particularly in clients who were in the lithotomy position during surgery.
   6. Encourage the use of antiembolism stockings, if prescribed, to promote venous return, strengthen muscle tone, and prevent pooling of blood in the extremities.

D. Musculoskeletal system
   1. Monitor the client for movement of the extremities.
   2. Review surgeon's prescriptions regarding client positioning or restrictions.
   3. Encourage ambulation if prescribed; before ambulation, instruct the client to sit at the edge of the bed with his or her feet supported to assume balance. Have enough personnel and/or equipment for safety of client.
   4. Unless contraindicated, place the client in a low Fowler position after surgery to increase the size of the thorax for lung expansion.
   5. Avoid positioning the postoperative client in a supine position until pharyngeal reflexes have returned; if the client is comatose or semicomatose, position on the side (in addition, an oral airway may be needed).
   6. If the client is unable to get out of bed, turn the client every 1 to 2 hours.

E. Neurological system
   1. Monitor level of consciousness.
   2. Frequent periodic attempts to awaken the client must continue until the client awakens.
   3. Orient the client to the environment.
   4. Speak in a soft tone; filter out extraneous noises in the environment.
   5. Maintain body temperature and prevent heat loss by providing the client with warm blankets and raising the room temperature as necessary.

F. Temperature control
   1. Monitor temperature.
   2. Monitor for signs of hypothermia that may result from anesthesia, a cool operating room, or exposure of the skin and internal organs during surgery.
   3. Apply warm blankets, continue oxygen, and administer medications as prescribed if the client experiences shivering.

G. Integumentary system

1. Check the surgical site, drains, and wound dressings (serous drainage may occur from an incision, but if excessive bleeding occurs from the site, the surgeon is notified).
2. Check the skin for redness, abrasions, or breakdown that may have resulted from surgical positioning.
3. Monitor body temperature and wound for signs of infection.
4. Maintain a dry, intact dressing.
5. Change dressings as prescribed, noting the amount of bleeding or drainage, odor, and intactness of sutures or staples. Commonly used dressings include 4 × 4 inch gauze, nonadherent pads, abdominal pads, gauze roles, and split gauze commonly referred to as drain sponges.
6. Wound drains must be patent; prepare to assist with the removal of drains (as prescribed by the surgeon) when the drainage amount becomes insignificant. Notify surgeon for excessive drain output, and if there is a sudden decrease in output.
7. An abdominal binder may be prescribed for obese and debilitated individuals to prevent dehiscence of the incision.

H. Fluid and electrolyte balance
1. Monitor IV fluid administration as prescribed.
2. Record intake and output.

3. Monitor for signs of fluid or electrolyte imbalances and electrolyte blood levels.
4. Replace electrolytes per protocol as prescribed.

I. Gastrointestinal system
1. Monitor intake and output and for nausea and vomiting.
2. Maintain patency of the nasogastric tube if present, and monitor placement-prescribed suction, and drainage per agency procedure.
3. Monitor for abdominal distention.

4. Monitor for passage of flatus and return of bowel sounds.
5. Administer frequent oral care, at least every 2 hours.
6. Maintain the NPO status until the gag reflex and peristalsis return.
7. When oral fluids are permitted, start with ice chips and water.
8. Ensure that the client advances to clear liquids and then to a regular diet, as prescribed and as the client can tolerate.

 To prevent aspiration, turn the client to a side-lying position if vomiting occurs and have suctioning equipment available and ready to use.

J. Renal system
1. Assess the bladder for distention by palpation or bladder scan if retention is expected.
2. Monitor urine output (urinary output must be at least 30 mL/hr).

3. If the client does not have an indwelling Foley catheter, the client is expected to void within 6 to 8 hours postoperatively, depending on the type of anesthesia administered; ensure that the amount is at least 200 mL.

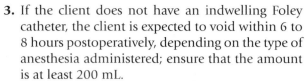

K. Pain management
1. Assess the type of anesthetic used and preoperative medication that the client received, and note whether the client received any pain medications in the postanesthesia period.
2. Assess for pain and inquire about the type and location of pain; ask the client to rate the degree of pain on a scale of 0 to 10, with 0 being no pain and 10 being the most severe.
3. If the client is unable to rate the pain with a numerical pain scale, then use a descriptor scale that lists words that describe different levels of pain intensity, such as *no pain, mild pain, moderate pain,* and *severe pain.*
4. Monitor for objective data related to pain, such as facial expressions, or use a picture pain scale such as the Wong-Baker FACES Pain Rating Scale, body gestures, increased pulse rate, increased blood pressure, and increased respirations.

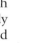

5. Assess respiratory rate, blood pressure, heart rate, oxygen saturation, and level of consciousness, and note if and when the last pain medication was given priori to administering another dose. Inquire about the effectiveness of the last pain medication.
6. Administer pain medication as prescribed.
7. Ensure that the client with a PCA pump understands how to use it; reinforce instructions as needed.
8. If an opioid has been prescribed, during the initial administration monitor vital signs first, especially blood pressure and respiratory rate; assess the client every 30 minutes for respiratory rate and pain relief.
9. Use noninvasive measures to relieve postoperative pain, including distractions, comfort measures, positioning, back rubs, and providing a quiet and restful environment.
10. Document effectiveness of the pain medication and noninvasive pain relief measures.

 Consider cultural practices and beliefs when planning pain management.

III. Pneumonia and Atelectasis (Fig. 16.4 and Box 16.5)

A. Description
1. Pneumonia, an inflammation of the alveoli caused by an infectious process, may develop 3 to 5 days after the surgical procedure because of infection, aspiration, unresolved atelectasis, or immobility.
2. Atelectasis, which is a collapse of the alveoli with retained mucous secretions, is the most common postoperative complication. It usually occurs 1 to 2 days after the surgical procedure.

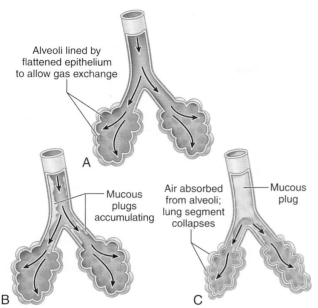

FIGURE 16.4 Postoperative atelectasis. (A) Normal bronchiole and alveoli. (B) Mucous plug in bronchiole. (C) Collapse of alveoli as a result of atelectasis after the absorption of air.

B. Data collection
1. Dyspnea and increased respiratory rate
2. Elevated temperature
3. Productive cough and chest pain
4. Crackles over involved lung area

C. Interventions
1. Monitor lung sounds and temperature.
2. Encourage fluid intake and early ambulation.
3. Reposition the client every 1 to 2 hours.
4. Encourage the client to deep breathe, cough, and use an incentive spirometer.
5. Suction to clear secretions if the client is unable to cough.
6. Provide chest physiotherapy and postural drainage, as prescribed.

IV. Hypoxemia (see Box 16.5)

A. Description: An inadequate concentration of oxygen in arterial blood; in the postoperative client, hypoxemia can be as a result of shallow breathing from the effects of anesthesia or medications.

B. Data collection
1. Restlessness
2. Dyspnea
3. Diaphoresis
4. Tachycardia
5. Hypertension
6. Cyanosis
7. Low pulse oximetry readings

C. Interventions
1. Monitor for signs of hypoxemia, eliminate the cause of hypoxemia, and notify the registered nurse (RN) and/or surgeon immediately.
2. Monitor lung sounds and pulse oximetry.

BOX 16.5 **Postoperative Complications**

Note: The licensed practical/vocational nurse always notifies the registered nurse and/or the surgeon if signs of complications are noted.
- Pneumonia and atelectasis
- Hypoxemia
- Pulmonary embolism
- Hemorrhage
- Shock
- Thrombophlebitis
- Urinary retention
- Constipation
- Paralytic ileus
- Wound infection
- Wound dehiscence
- Wound evisceration

3. Administer oxygen, as prescribed.
4. Encourage coughing, deep breathing, and the use of incentive spirometry.
5. Turn and reposition the client frequently; encourage ambulation. Reassess pulse oximetry after measures are implemented.

V. Pulmonary Embolism (see Box 16.5)

A. Description: An embolus blocking the pulmonary artery and disrupting the blood flow to one or more lobes of the lung that usually results from a thrombus in a leg and/or pelvic vein

B. Data collection
1. Sudden dyspnea
2. Sudden sharp chest or upper abdominal pain
3. Cyanosis
4. Tachycardia
5. A drop in blood pressure

C. Interventions
1. Notify the RN and/or surgeon immediately because pulmonary embolism may be life threatening and requires emergency action.
2. Monitor vital signs.
3. Administer oxygen and medications as prescribed.

VI. Hemorrhage (see Box 16.5)

A. Description: The loss of a large amount of blood externally or internally during a short period of time

B. Data collection
1. Restlessness
2. Weak, rapid pulse
3. Hypotension
4. Tachypnea
5. Cool, clammy skin
6. Reduced urine output

C. Interventions
1. Apply pressure to the site of bleeding.
2. Notify the RN and/or surgeon immediately.
3. Administer oxygen, as prescribed.

4. Administer IV fluids and blood, as prescribed.

5. Prepare the client for a surgical procedure, if necessary.

VII. Shock (see Box 16.5)

A. Description: A loss of circulatory fluid volume that is usually caused by hemorrhage

B. Data collection: Similar to data collection findings of hemorrhage

C. Interventions

1. Notify the RN and/or surgeon immediately.
2. Administer oxygen, as prescribed.
3. Determine and treat the cause of shock.
4. Administer oxygen, as prescribed.
5. Monitor the level of consciousness.
6. Monitor vital signs for an increased pulse and decreased blood pressure.
7. Monitor intake and output.
8. Monitor color, temperature, turgor, and moisture of the skin and mucous membranes.
9. Assist with the administration of IV fluids, blood, and colloid solutions as prescribed.

VIII. Thrombophlebitis (see Box 16.5)

A. Description

1. An inflammation of a vein, often accompanied by clot formation
2. Veins in the legs are most commonly affected.

B. Data collection

1. Aching or cramping leg pain
2. Vein inflammation; vein feels hard and cord-like and is tender to touch.
3. Elevated temperature
4. Swelling in one extremity

C. Interventions

1. Monitor legs for swelling, inflammation, cyanosis, pain, tenderness, and venous distention; the RN is notified immediately.
2. Elevate the extremity 30 degrees without allowing any pressure on the popliteal area as prescribed.

3. Encourage the use of antiembolism stockings as prescribed; remove stockings twice a day to wash and inspect the legs.
4. Use an intermittent pulsatile compression device as prescribed to prevent thrombophlebitis (see Fig. 16.2).
5. Prepare to perform passive range-of-motion exercises every 2 hours if the client is confined to bed rest.
6. Encourage early ambulation, as prescribed.
7. Do not allow the client to dangle the legs.
8. Instruct the client not to sit in one position for an extended period of time.
9. Anticoagulants such as heparin sodium may be prescribed for prevention of thrombophlebitis or as treatment.

IX. Urinary Retention (see Box 16.5)

A. Description

1. The involuntary accumulation of urine in the bladder from a loss of muscle tone
2. Occurs as a result of the effects of anesthetics and opioid analgesics and appears approximately 6 to 8 hours after surgery

B. Data collection

1. Inability to void
2. Restlessness and diaphoresis
3. Lower abdominal pain
4. Distended bladder and urinary retention on bladder scan
5. Elevated blood pressure
6. During percussion, the bladder sounds like a drum.

C. Interventions

1. Monitor for voiding and check for a distended bladder by palpation and bladder scanning if indicated.
2. Encourage ambulation when prescribed.
3. Encourage fluid intake unless contraindicated.
4. Assist the client to void by helping the client stand.
5. Provide privacy.
6. Pour warm water over the perineum or allow the client to hear running water to promote voiding.
7. Prepare to catheterize the client, as prescribed, after all noninvasive techniques have been attempted.

X. Constipation (see Box 16.5)

A. Description

1. The abnormal and infrequent passage of stool
2. When the client resumes a solid diet after surgery, failure to pass stool within 48 hours may indicate constipation.

B. Data collection

1. Absence of bowel movements
2. Abdominal distention
3. Anorexia, headache, and nausea

C. Interventions

1. Check bowel sounds.
2. Encourage fluid intake up to 3000 mL/day unless contraindicated.
3. Encourage early ambulation.
4. Encourage the consumption of fiber-rich foods unless contraindicated.
5. Provide privacy and adequate time for bowel elimination.
6. Administer stool softeners and laxatives as prescribed, particularly if opioid pain medications are used.

XI. Paralytic Ileus (see Box 16.5)

A. Description

1. A failure of the appropriate forward movement of bowel contents
2. May occur as a result of anesthetic medications or the manipulation of the bowel during the surgical procedure, hypokalemia, and opioid analgesics.

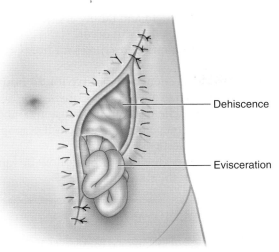

FIGURE 16.5 **Complications of wound healing.**

B. Data collection
1. Postoperative nausea and vomiting
2. Abdominal distention
3. Absence of bowel sounds, bowel movement, or flatus

C. Interventions
1. Maintain NPO status until bowel sounds return.
2. Insert and maintain the patency of the nasogastric tube, if present.
3. Encourage ambulation.
4. Monitor IV fluids and parenteral nutrition, as prescribed.
5. Assist to administer medications, as prescribed, to increase gastrointestinal motility and secretions.
6. If ileus occurs, it is usually first treated nonsurgically with bowel decompression by the insertion of a nasogastric tube attached to intermittent or constant suction.

⚠ Postoperative vomiting, abdominal distention, and/or absence of bowel sounds may be signs of paralytic ileus.

XII. Wound Infection (see Box 16.5)

A. Description
1. Wound infection may be caused by poor aseptic technique or a contaminated wound before surgical exploration; existing client conditions such as diabetes mellitus or immunocompromise may place the client at risk.
2. Infection usually occurs 3 to 6 days after surgery.
3. Purulent material may exit from the drains or separated wound edges.

B. Data collection
1. Fever and chills
2. Warm, tender, painful, and inflamed incision site
3. Edematous skin at the incision and tight skin sutures
4. Elevated white blood cell count

C. Interventions
1. Monitor the temperature.

2. Monitor the incision site for approximation of the suture line, edema, bleeding, and signs of infection (*REEDA*: *R*edness, *E*dema, *E*cchymosis, *D*rainage, and *A*pproximation of the wound edges); the RN and surgeon are notified if signs of infection are present.
3. Maintain patency of drains, and assess drainage amount, color, and consistency.
4. Maintain asepsis and change the dressing, as prescribed.
5. Assist to administer antibiotics, as prescribed.

XIII. Wound Dehiscence and Evisceration (Fig. 16.5; ▲ also see Box 16.5)

A. Description
1. Wound dehiscence is separation of the wound edges at the suture line; it usually occurs 6 to 8 days after surgery.
2. Wound evisceration is protrusion of the internal organs through an incision; it usually occurs 6 to 8 days after surgery.
3. Evisceration is most common among obese clients, clients who have had abdominal surgery, or those who have poor wound-healing ability, such as clients with a chronic illness treated with corticosteroids.
4. Wound evisceration is an emergency.

B. Data collection: Dehiscence
1. Increased drainage
2. Opened wound edges
3. The appearance of underlying tissues through the wound

C. Data collection: Evisceration
1. Discharge of serosanguineous fluid from a previously dry wound
2. The appearance of loops of bowel or other abdominal contents through the wound
3. Client reports feeling a popping sensation after coughing or turning.

D. Interventions (see Priority Nursing Actions)

⚡ PRIORITY NURSING ACTIONS

Evisceration Occurs

1. Call for help; the registered nurse (RN) will contact the surgeon and ask that needed supplies be brought to the client's room.
2. Stay with the client.
3. While waiting for supplies to arrive, place the client in a low Fowler position with the knees bent.
4. Cover the wound with a sterile normal saline dressing and keep the dressing moist.
5. Take vital signs and monitor the client closely for signs of shock.
6. Prepare the client for surgery as necessary.
7. Document the occurrence, the actions taken, and the client's response.

BOX 16.6 Reinforcing Discharge Instructions

- Determine the client's readiness to learn, educational level, and desire to change or modify their lifestyle.
- Determine the need for resources for home care.
- Demonstrate how to care for the incision and how to change the dressing.
- Instruct the client to cover the incision with plastic, as prescribed, if showering is allowed.
- Be sure that the client is provided with a 48-hour supply of dressings for home use.
- Instruct the client about the importance of returning to the surgeon's office for follow-up visits.
- Instruct the client that sutures and staples are usually removed in the surgeon's office 7–10 days after surgery and that the skin may become slightly reddened when they are ready to be removed.
- Sterile adhesive strips (e.g., Steri-Strips) may be applied to provide extra support after the sutures are removed. Instruct the client to not remove the strips until they are close to falling off.
- Instruct the client regarding the use of medications and their purpose, dose, administration, and side effects.
- Instruct the client regarding proper diet and to drink 6–8 glasses of liquid per day.
- Instruct the client regarding activity levels and to resume normal activities gradually.
- Instruct the client to avoid lifting for 6 weeks if a major surgical procedure was performed.
- Instruct the client with an abdominal incision to not lift anything weighing 10 lb or more and to not engage in any activities that involve pushing or pulling.
- Clients usually can return to work after 6–8 weeks, as prescribed by the surgeon.
- Instruct the client regarding the signs/symptoms of complications and when to call the surgeon.

3. Instruct the client and family about postoperative complications that can occur.
4. Suggest appropriate resources for home-care support.
5. Instruct the client not to drive for 24 hours if he or she has had a general anesthetic.
6. Inform the client to call the surgeon, ambulatory center, or emergency department if postoperative problems occur.
7. Instruct the client to keep follow-up appointments with the surgeon.

WHAT WOULD YOU DO?

Answer: With regard to informed consent for a surgical procedure, the nurse can act as a witness to the client's signing of the consent form, but the nurse must be sure that the client has understood the surgeon's explanation of the surgery. The nurse needs to witness the signing of the consent form after the client acknowledges understanding of the procedure. If the client informs the nurse that the explanation was not fully understood, the nurse must notify the surgeon, and the surgeon will need to clarify anything that was not understood by the client.

PRACTICE QUESTIONS

❖ **1.** The nurse is assisting in creating a plan of care for a client who is scheduled for surgery. The nurse would include which activities in the nursing care plan for the client on the day of surgery? **Select all that apply.**
- ☐ **1.** Have the client void before surgery.
- ☐ **2.** Avoid oral hygiene and rinsing with mouthwash.
- ☐ **3.** Verify that the client has not eaten for the last 24 hours.
- ☐ **4.** Determine that the client has signed the informed consent for the surgical procedure.
- ☐ **5.** Report immediately any slight increase in blood pressure or pulse from the client's baseline vital signs.

2. The nurse is caring for a client who is scheduled for surgery. The client states concern about the surgical procedure. How would the nurse **initially** address the client's concerns?
1. Tell the client that preoperative fear is normal.
2. Explain all nursing care and possible discomfort that may result.
3. Ask the client to discuss information known about the planned surgery.
4. Provide explanations about the procedures involved in the planned surgery.

XIV. Ambulatory Surgery

A. General criteria for client discharge
1. Is alert and oriented
2. Has voided
3. Has no respiratory distress
4. Vital signs and oxygen saturation are within normal limits.
5. Is able to ambulate, swallow, and cough
6. Has minimal pain
7. Is not vomiting
8. Has minimal (if any) bleeding from the incision site
9. A responsible adult is available to drive the client home.
10. The surgeon has signed a release form.

 B. Reinforce discharge instructions (Box 16.6).
1. Would be performed before the date of the scheduled procedure
2. Provide written instructions to the client and family regarding the specifics of care.

❖ 3. The nurse is collecting data from a client who is scheduled for surgery in 1 week in the ambulatory care surgical center. Which pertinent client data would the nurse report to the surgeon before the surgery? **Select all that apply.**
   ❑ 1. Is allergic to penicillin
   ❑ 2. Quit smoking 3 months earlier
   ❑ 3. History of tonsillectomy at the age of 7 years
   ❑ 4. Wonders if the surgery could cause incontinence
   ❑ 5. Takes daily multivitamin and calcium supplement
   ❑ 6. History of deep venous thrombosis (DVT) in right leg 10 years earlier

❖ 4. The nurse obtains the vital signs on a postoperative client who just returned to the nursing unit. The client's blood pressure (BP) is 100/60 mm Hg, the pulse is 90 beats per minute, and the respiration rate is 20 breaths per minute. On the basis of these findings, which actions would the nurse take? **Select all that apply.**
   ❑ 1. Ask if the client is thirsty, and assist with drinking a glass of water.
   ❑ 2. Ask how the client feels, and inquire about any feelings of dizziness.
   ❑ 3. Review the client record to determine time and type of analgesia last received.
   ❑ 4. Assist the client to perform leg exercises, and then recheck the blood pressure and pulse rate.
   ❑ 5. Review the client record to note the vital signs taken in the post anesthesia care unit (PACU).
   ❑ 6. Review the client record to determine whether the client has voided postoperatively.

5. A client arrives to the surgical nursing unit after surgery. What would be the **initial** nursing action after surgery?
   1. Assess patency of the airway.
   2. Check tubes or drains for patency.
   3. Check dressing for bleeding or drainage.
   4. Obtain vital signs to compare with those recorded preoperatively.

6. The nurse is monitoring an adult client for postoperative complications. Which is most indicative of a potential postoperative complication that requires further observation?
   1. A urinary output of 20 mL/hour
   2. A temperature of 37.6°C (99.6°F)
   3. A blood pressure of 100/70 mm Hg
   4. Serous drainage on the surgical dressing

7. The nurse monitors the 4-day postoperative client who underwent abdominal surgery. Vital signs are: temperature: 37.9°C (100.2°F), pulse 104 beats per minute, respirations 22 breaths per minute, blood pressure 128/74 mm Hg. Oxygen saturation is 93% on room air. The client feels tired and has a productive cough. Fine crackles are audible in the bases of the lungs posteriorly. The nurse considers the client has developed which postoperative problem?
   1. Hypoxia
   2. Atelectasis
   3. Pneumonia
   4. Fluid overload

❖ 8. The nurse is caring for a postoperative client who has a Jackson-Pratt drain inserted into the surgical wound. Which actions would the nurse take in the care of the drain? **Select all that apply.**
   ❑ 1. Check the drain for patency.
   ❑ 2. Check that the drain is decompressed.
   ❑ 3. Observe for bright red, bloody drainage.
   ❑ 4. Maintain aseptic technique when emptying.
   ❑ 5. Empty the drain when it is half full and every 8 to 12 hours.
   ❑ 6. Secure the drain by curling or folding it and taping it firmly to the body.

9. The nurse checks the postoperative client for signs of infection. Which observations are indicative of a potential infection? **Select all that apply.**
   ❑ 1. Slight redness along the incision
   ❑ 2. The presence of purulent drainage
   ❑ 3. A temperature of 98.8°F (37.1°C)
   ❑ 4. The client states that he feels cold.
   ❑ 5. The client states that the incision itches.
   ❑ 6. Tender firmness palpable around the incision

10. The nurse is checking a client's surgical incision and notes an increase in the amount of drainage, a separation of the incision line, and the appearance of underlying tissue. Which actions would the nurse take to deal with this event? **Select all that apply.**
   ❑ 1. Turn the client to the side with the knees bent.
   ❑ 2. Notify the registered nurse (RN) and the surgeon.
   ❑ 3. Apply a sterile dressing soaked with normal saline to the wound.
   ❑ 4. Explain to the client that obesity is a risk factor and weight loss would be a future goal.
   ❑ 5. Gently explore the wound with a cotton-tipped applicator to determine whether evisceration has occurred.

ANSWERS

❖ **1. 1, 4**

Rationale: The nurse caring for clients who will be having surgery must ensure that the client is properly identified and prepared according to the prescription(s) by the surgeon and anesthesiologist. The nurse would assist the client with voiding before surgery so that the bladder is empty at the beginning of the procedure. The nurse must verify that the client has signed the consent for the procedure. If the client has not signed a consent, no preoperative medications can be given, and the surgeon can obtain the consent before proceeding. Oral hygiene is allowed, but the client cannot swallow any water. The client usually has a restriction of food and fluids for 8 hours before surgery rather than 24 hours (often nothing by mouth [NPO] after midnight). A slight increase in blood pressure and pulse is common during the preoperative period; this is generally the result of anxiety. The nurse would verify what the normal blood pressure and pulse rate are for this client.

Test-Taking Strategy: Focus on the subject, preoperative care. Recall that the purpose of preoperative preparation is to promote a successful surgical outcome and lower the risk of complications from surgery and anesthesia. Evaluate each option according to that standard, and you will select the answers that assure a positive surgical outcome.

2. 3

Rationale: The client is concerned about having surgery and needs to discuss it. This will offer the client the opportunity to verbalize his or her current and specific understanding. Explanations need to begin with the information that the client knows. Option 1 is a block to communication and minimizes the client's feelings. Giving unsolicited explanations may produce additional anxiety and not address the real concerns of the client.

Test-Taking Strategy: Note the strategic word, *initially*, and realize the question asks for the first response of the nurse. Use therapeutic communication techniques of open-ended questions, active listening questions and active listening, and focus on the client's feelings first. Option 3 is the only option that addresses data collection, which follows the steps of the nursing process.

3. 1, 2, 4, 6

Rationale: The nurse conducts an interview and reviews current health practices and health history preoperatively with clients. Specific client data that are likely to affect a surgery is communicated promptly. The nurse reports any client allergies, especially an antibiotic allergy to avoid an allergic reaction perioperatively. The fact that the client was a smoker until recently is pertinent because it may affect how the client tolerates and recovers from anesthesia. The nurse would communicate any client concerns about the effects of the surgery so that the matter can be discussed and understood clearly before the surgery (informed consent). A history of a deep venous thrombosis (DVT) is pertinent because of an increased risk for DVT after the planned surgery, and precautions would be prescribed. A history of a childhood tonsillectomy and routine vitamin and mineral supplementation are part of the client history but are not pertinent data that needs to be reported specifically.

Test-Taking Strategy: Focus on the subject, reporting pertinent client data that affects surgery. Considering each option

and its effect on the client having the surgery will assist in answering the question.

4. 2, 3, 5

Rationale: In a clinical situation, the nurse must evaluate the vital signs of each postoperative client individually. If complications such as hemorrhage or shock are developing, early intervention is extremely important. Determining how the client feels and asking about dizziness lets the nurse evaluate how the client is tolerating these vital signs. Accessing the medical record to determine the most recent analgesic administration is pertinent because hypotension is a frequent side/adverse effect of analgesics, especially opioids. Reviewing the client's record gives the nurse data on the client's vital signs during and after surgery in the PACU, and the nurse can evaluate whether there has been a change. Giving the client oral fluids is an intervention if the client has a fluid volume deficit, and this has not been established. Oral fluids would not correct the problem as quickly as administering intravenous (IV) fluids would. Collecting data about the client voiding is not directly related to the vital signs. Encouraging leg exercises is a correct postoperative intervention but is not appropriate for evaluating the vital signs.

Test-Taking Strategy: Focus on the data in the question, and select the options in which the nurse gathers additional data to determine whether the vital signs are within the normal range for this individual client. Determining whether the client has voided is not pertinent to evaluating the vital signs. Eliminate the options that are interventions: giving oral fluids or having the client exercise.

5. 1

Rationale: If the airway is not patent, immediate measures must be taken for the survival of the client. After checking the client's airway, the nurse would then check the client's vital signs, followed by the dressings, tubes, and drains.

Test-Taking Strategy: Note the strategic word, *initial*. Use the ABCs—airway, breathing, and circulation. Maintaining the airway patency is the first action to be taken. The other options are all nursing actions that can be performed after a patent airway has been established.

6. 1

Rationale: Urine output is maintained at a minimum of at least 30 mL/hr for an adult. An output of less than 30 mL/hr for each of 2 consecutive hours must be reported to the surgeon. A temperature more than 37°C (100°F) or less than 36.1°C (97°F) and a falling systolic blood pressure less than 90 mm Hg are to be reported. The client's preoperative or baseline blood pressure is used to make informed postoperative comparisons. Moderate or light serous drainage from the surgical site is considered normal.

Test-Taking Strategy: Note the strategic word, *most*, and focus on the subject, normal assessment data in a postoperative client. Use knowledge of normal expected postoperative ranges to determine that the urinary output is the only finding that is not within normal range.

7. 3

Rationale: Pneumonia is a postoperative condition caused by inflammation and infection in the lungs. Frequently it results from shallow breathing that leads to atelectasis (the alveoli partially collapse and eventually become fluid filled). This fluid is good medium for bacteria. Pneumonia usually occurs 3 to 7 days postoperatively. Signs and symptoms include fever, productive cough, painful breathing, and an increased respiratory effort and rate. Fine crackles may be audible over the lung area involved. Treatment includes coughing up the purulent sputum, deep breathing, antibiotics, and adequate hydration. Hypoxia is inadequate concentration of oxygen in the blood and usually occurs as an acute process, such as respiratory depression as a result of anesthesia or analgesia, or the pulmonary oxygen saturation is relatively below normal, less than 92%. Atelectasis occurs 1 to 2 days postoperatively, and auscultation reveals diminished breath sound and/or crackles that clear with coughing. Fluid overload is excessive blood volume with too much fluid in the circulation. It causes coarse crackles and severe dyspnea.

Test-Taking Strategy: Focus on the data in the question, and determine if an abnormality exists in the client's signs and symptoms. Eliminate option 1 because the pulse oximetry reading is 93%. Next note that the client is 4 days postoperative to assist in eliminating option 2. Compare the client situation with the usual signs and symptoms that occur with the problems in the remaining options. This will direct you to the correct option.

❖ **8. 1, 2, 3, 4, 5**
Rationale: A drain is a tube that is placed to drain out fluid and blood near the surgical site and could lead to infection. The tube is connected to a bulb, which is compressed to create a vacuum and pull out the fluid. The nurse would check for patency and that fluid is being pulled out. The bulb would be decompressed in order to create the vacuum. The drainage usually is dark red as a result of blood content but may be pale yellow with serous fluid. Aseptic technique must be used when emptying the drainage container to avoid contamination of the wound. The bulb of the drain would be emptied when it is half full and at least every 8 to 12 hours. The amount of drainage is documented in the client medical record under intake and output. Curling or folding the drain prevents the flow of the drainage.

Test-Taking Strategy: Focus on the subject, caring for a surgical drain. Remember that the nurse needs to ensure that drainage flows freely from a drain. Consider each option and whether it promotes flow and does not lead to infection.

❖ **9. 2, 6**
Rationale: A wound infection occurs when healing is delayed and pathogens such as bacteria grow in the wound. Signs and symptoms of a wound infection include warmth, redness, swelling, and tenderness of skin around the incision. The client may have fever and chills. Purulent material may exit from drains or from separated wound edges. Infection may be caused by poor aseptic technique or a wound that was contaminated before surgical exploration; it appears 3 to 6 days after surgery. Slight redness along an incision is a sign of inflammation and would be monitored to determine whether it progresses. A temperature of 98.8°F (37.1°C) is not an abnormal finding in a postoperative client. Itching around a wound may be from irritation or dryness and is not associated with infection. The fact that a client feels cold is not indicative of an infection, although chills and fever are signs of infection. The room temperature may be too cold for client comfort.

Test-Taking Strategy: Focus on the subject, wound infection. Noting the words *purulent*, *tender*, and *hardness* will direct you to the correct options.

❖ **10. 2, 3**
Rationale: Wound dehiscence is the separation of the wound edges at the suture line. Signs and symptoms include increased drainage and the appearance of underlying tissues. It usually occurs as a complication 6 to 8 days after surgery. The client would be instructed to remain quiet and avoid coughing or straining, and he or she needs to be positioned to prevent further stress on the wound. Sterile dressings soaked with sterile normal saline need to be used to cover the wound. The registered nurse (RN) and surgeon need to be notified. The client needs to assume a low Fowler position with knees bent to avoid further stress on the incision. Obesity is a risk factor for dehiscence, but now is not the appropriate time for this teaching. The nurse would not explore the wound because this may actually cause evisceration, a more serious complication.

Test-Taking Strategy: Note the subject, the postoperative complication of wound dehiscence. Consider that the client may need to return to surgery, and keeping the underlying tissues moist and sterile is the priority. The RN and surgeon are responsible to provide the urgent care the client needs.

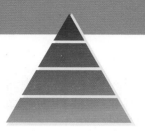

Foundations of Care

CHAPTER **17**

Positioning Clients

PRIORITY CONCEPTS **Mobility; Safety**

WHAT WOULD YOU DO?

The nurse is caring for a client who is receiving intermittent tube feedings via a nasogastric tube. In maintaining proper positioning for this client, what actions would the nurse take? *Answer is located on p. 200.*

⚠ Always review the primary health care provider's (PHCP's) prescription(s), especially after treatments or procedures, and take note of instructions regarding positioning and mobility. PHCP's prescriptions are always followed.

I. Guidelines for Client Positioning.
A. Principles of body movement for clients
  1. Body movement and alignment are important for clients. Many clients are unable to change position or move in bed independently.
  2. Basic principles include maintaining correct anatomical position and changing the position frequently.
B. Position in a safe and appropriate manner to provide safety, alignment, and comfort.

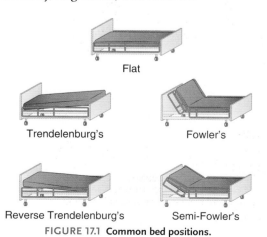

FIGURE 17.1 Common bed positions.

Flat

Trendelenburg's

Fowler's

Reverse Trendelenburg's

Semi-Fowler's

C. Select a position that will prevent the development of complications related to an existing condition, a prescribed treatment, or a medical or surgical procedure.
D. Ergonomic principles related to body mechanics ▲ (Box 17.1)
II. Positions to Ensure Safety and Comfort (see Figures 17.1 to 17.4)
A. Integumentary system
  1. Autograft: After surgery, the site is immobilized for approximately 3 to 7 days or as prescribed to provide the time needed for the graft to adhere and attach to the wound bed.
  2. Burns of the face and head: Elevate the head of ▲ the bed to prevent or reduce facial, head, and tracheal edema.
  3. Circumferential burns of the extremities: Check ▲ PHCP prescription. If compartment syndrome is a concern or suspected the extremity is not elevated and kept at heart level.
  4. Skin graft: Elevate and immobilize the graft site to prevent the movement and shearing of the graft and the disruption of tissue; avoid weight bearing.
B. Reproductive system
  1. Mastectomy
    a. Position the client with the head of the bed elevated at least 30 degrees (semi-Fowler's position), with the affected arm elevated on a pillow to promote lymphatic fluid return after the removal of axillary lymph nodes.

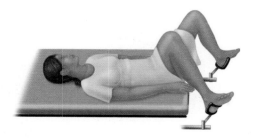

FIGURE 17.2 Lithotomy position for examination.

⚡ PRIORITY NURSING ACTIONS

Client Undergoing a Liver Biopsy

1. Explain the procedure to the client.
2. Ensure that informed consent has been obtained.
3. Position the client supine, with the right side of the upper abdomen exposed; the client's right arm is raised and extended behind the head and over the left shoulder.
4. Remain with the client during the procedure.
5. After the procedure, assist the client into a right lateral (side-lying) position and place a small pillow or folded towel under the puncture site.
6. Monitor vital signs closely after the procedure and monitor for signs of bleeding.
7. Document appropriate information about the procedure, client's tolerance, and postprocedure assessment findings.

   b. Turn the client only to the back and the unaffected side.
   2. Perineal and vaginal procedures: Place the client in the lithotomy position. (Fig 17.2).

C. Endocrine system
   1. Hypophysectomy: Elevate the head of the bed to prevent increased intracranial pressure.
   2. Thyroidectomy
      a. Place the client in the semi-Fowler's or Fowler's position to reduce swelling and edema in the neck area.
      b. Sandbags or pillows may be used to support the client's head or neck.
      c. Avoid neck extension to decrease tension on the suture line.

D. Gastrointestinal system
   1. Hemorrhoidectomy: Assist the client to a lateral (side-lying) position to prevent pain and bleeding.
   2. Gastroesophageal reflux disease: Reverse Trendelenburg position may be prescribed to promote gastric emptying and prevent esophageal reflux. This is done by elevating the head of the bed 6 to 12 inches, either by blocks under the head of the bed or use of a wedge pillow.
   3. Liver biopsy (see Priority Nursing Actions)
   4. Paracentesis: The client is positioned in a semi-Fowler's position in bed, or sitting upright on the side of the bed, or in a chair with the feet supported. The client is assisted to a position of comfort following the procedure. (The procedure may be done under fluoroscopy in the radiology department.)
   5. Nasogastric tube: insertion
      a. Position the client in a high Fowler's position with the head tilted forward.
      b. This position will help close the trachea and open the esophagus.

   ⚠️ If the client receiving a continuous tube feeding needs to be placed in a supine position when providing care, such as when giving a bed bath or changing linens, shut the feeding off to prevent aspiration. Remember to turn the feeding back on and check the rate of flow when the client is placed back into the semi-Fowler's or Fowler's position.

   6. Nasogastric tube: irrigations and feedings
      a. Keep the head of the bed elevated 30 degrees (semi-Fowler's position) to prevent aspiration.

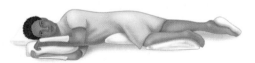

Lateral (side-lying) position

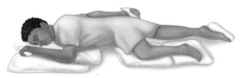

Semiprone (forward side-lying) position

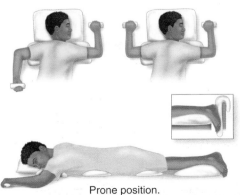

Prone position.
The client's arms and shoulders may be positioned in internal or external rotation.

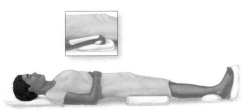

Supine position

FIGURE 17.3 Common client positions.

b. Maintain head elevation for 30 minutes to 1 hour (per agency procedure) after an intermittent feeding.

c. The head of the bed needs to remain elevated for continuous feedings.

7. Rectal enemas or irrigations: Place the client in Sims' (left-lateral) position to allow the solution to flow by gravity in the natural direction of the colon.

8. Sengstaken-Blakemore and Minnesota tubes

a. Not commonly used because they are uncomfortable for the client and can cause compli-

---

BOX 17.1   **Body Mechanics for Health Care Workers**

- When planning to move a client, arrange for adequate help.
- Use mechanical aids as much as possible, including ceiling-mounted lifts and air-assisted devices.
- Encourage the client to assist as much as possible.
- Keep your back, neck, pelvis, and feet aligned. Avoid twisting.
- Flex your knees, and keep your feet wide apart.
- Raise the client's bed so that the client's weight is at the level of the nurse's center of gravity.
- Position yourself close to the client or to the object being lifted.
- Use your arms and legs rather than your back.
- Slide the client toward you using a pull sheet. When transferring a client onto a stretcher, a slide board is more appropriate.
- Set (tighten) your abdominal and gluteal muscles in preparation for the move.
- The person with the heaviest load needs to coordinate the efforts of the team involved by counting to 3.

Adapted from Potter P, Perry A, Stockert P, et al: *Fundamentals of nursing*, ed 8, St. Louis, 2013, Mosby.

---

cations, but their use may be necessary when other interventions are not feasible.

b. If prescribed, maintain elevation of the head of the bed to enhance lung expansion and reduce portal blood flow, permitting effective esophagogastric balloon tamponade.

E. Respiratory system

1. Chronic obstructive pulmonary disease: For the client with advanced disease, place the client in a sitting position, leaning forward with the arms over several pillows or on an overbed table. This position will help the client to breathe easier.

2. Laryngectomy (radical neck dissection): Place the client in a semi-Fowler's or Fowler's position to maintain a patent airway and minimize edema.

3. Bronchoscopy postprocedure: Place the client in a semi-Fowler's position to prevent choking or aspiration resulting from an impaired ability to swallow.

4. Postural drainage: The lung segment to be drained must be in the uppermost position. Trendelenburg position may be used.

5. Thoracentesis (may be done under fluoroscopy in radiology department)

a. During the procedure: To facilitate the removal of fluid from the pleural space, position the client sitting on the edge of the bed and leaning over the bedside table with the feet supported on a stool or lying in bed on the unaffected side with the head of the bed elevated approximately 45 degrees (Fowler's position). The procedure includes administration of a local anesthetic, insertion of a needle into the pleural space where fluid has collected, and connecting the needle to a vacuum bottle to remove the fluid.

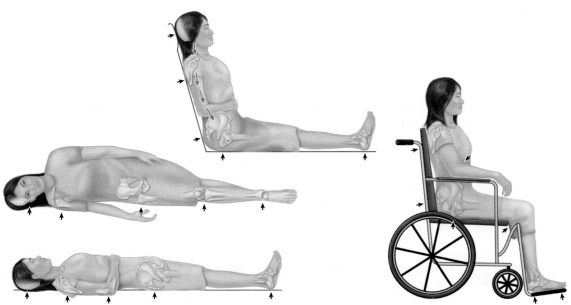

FIGURE 17.4 **Pressure points of lying and sitting positions.**

b. After the procedure: Assist the client to a position of comfort.

6. Thoracotomy: Check the surgeon's prescription(s) regarding positioning.

⚠ Always check the surgeon's prescription(s) regarding positioning for the client who had a thoracotomy, lung wedge resection, lobectomy of the lung, or pneumonectomy.

F. Cardiovascular system

1. Abdominal aneurysm resection

a. After open aneurysm repair surgery, check the surgeon's prescriptions for positioning; usually head elevation is limited to some degree to avoid flexion of the graft.

b. The client may be turned from side to side.

c. Clients with endovascular repair have fewer restrictions and shorter hospitalization times.

2. Amputation of the lower extremity

a. During the first 24 hours after amputation, elevate the foot of the bed to reduce edema. The residual limb is supported with pillows but not elevated because of the risk of flexion contractures.

b. Consult with the surgeon and, if prescribed, position the client in a prone position twice a day for a 20- to 30-minute period to stretch muscles and prevent flexion contractures of the hip.

3. Arterial vascular grafting of an extremity

a. To promote graft patency after the procedure, bed rest is usually maintained for approximately 24 hours, and the client's affected extremity is kept straight.

b. Limit movement and avoid flexion of the client's hip and knee.

4. Cardiac catheterization

a. If the femoral artery was used, the client is maintained on bed rest for approximately 4 to 6 hours (time for bed rest may vary depending on PHCP preference and if a vascular closure device was used); the client may turn from side to side.

b. The client's affected extremity is kept straight and the head elevated no more than 30 degrees (some PHCPs prefer a lower head position or the flat position) until hemostasis is adequately achieved.

5. Heart failure and pulmonary edema: Position the client upright, preferably with the legs dangling over the side of the bed, to decrease venous return and lung congestion.

⚠ Most often, clients with respiratory and cardiac disorders need to be positioned with the head of the bed elevated.

6. Peripheral arterial disease

a. Obtain the PHCP's prescription for positioning.

b. Because swelling can prevent arterial blood flow, clients may be advised to place their legs at heart level when at rest. They must not raise their legs above the level of the heart, because elevation slows arterial blood flow. Some clients may be advised to maintain a slightly dependent position to promote perfusion.

7. Deep vein thrombosis

a. If the extremity is red, edematous, and painful, traditional heparin therapy may be initiated. Bed rest with leg elevation may also be prescribed for the client.

b. Clients receiving low-molecular-weight heparin can usually be out of bed after 24 hours, if prescribed and if the pain level permits.

8. Varicose veins: Leg elevation is usually prescribed. The client is also advised to minimize prolonged sitting or standing during daily activities.

9. Venous insufficiency and leg ulcers: Leg elevation is usually prescribed.

G. Sensory system

1. Cataract surgery: Postoperatively, elevate the head of the bed (semi-Fowler's to Fowler's position), and position the client on the back or the nonoperative side to prevent the development of edema at the operative site. Client needs to avoid activities that increase intraocular pressure, such as lifting heavy objects or bending from the waist.

2. Retinal detachment

a. If the detachment is large, bed rest and bilateral eye patching may be prescribed to minimize eye movement and prevent the extension of the detachment.

b. Restrictions in activity and positioning after the repair of the detachment depend on the PHCP's preference and the surgical procedure performed.

H. Neurological system

1. Autonomic dysreflexia: Elevate the head of the bed to a high Fowler position to help with adequate ventilation and prevent hypertensive stroke.

⚠ If autonomic dysreflexia occurs, immediately place the client in a high Fowler position.

2. Cerebral aneurysm: Bed rest is maintained with the head of the bed elevated 30 to 45 degrees to prevent pressure on the aneurysm site.

3. Cerebral angiography

a. Maintain bed rest for the length of time, as prescribed.

b. The extremity into which the contrast medium is injected is kept straight and immobilized for approximately 6 to 8 hours.

4. Stroke (brain attack)

a. In clients with hemorrhagic strokes, the head of the bed is usually elevated 30 degrees to reduce intracranial pressure and facilitate venous drainage.

b. For clients with ischemic strokes, the head of the bed is minimally elevated to promote cerebral perfusion.

c. Maintain the client's head in a midline, neutral position to facilitate venous drainage from the head.

d. Avoid extreme hip and neck flexion; extreme hip flexion may increase intrathoracic pressure, whereas extreme neck flexion prohibits venous drainage from the brain.

5. Craniotomy

a. The client would not be positioned on the site that was operated on, especially if the bone flap has been removed, because the brain has no bony covering over the affected site.

b. Elevate the head of the bed 30 to 45 degrees (semi-Fowler's to Fowler's position) and maintain the head in a midline, neutral position to facilitate venous drainage from the head.

c. Avoid extreme hip and neck flexion.

6. Laminectomy and other vertebral surgery

a. Clients are often out of bed postoperatively with a back brace if prescribed.

b. When the client is out of bed, the client's back is kept straight (the client is placed in a straight-backed chair) with the feet resting comfortably on the floor.

7. Increased intracranial pressure

a. Elevate the head of the bed 30 to 45 degrees (semi-Fowler's to Fowler's position) and maintain the head in a midline, neutral position to facilitate venous drainage from the head.

b. Avoid extreme hip and neck flexion.

⚠ Do not place a client with a head injury in a flat or Trendelenburg position because of the risk of increased intracranial pressure.

8. Lumbar puncture (may be done under fluoroscopy in radiology department)

a. During the procedure: Assist the client to the lateral (side-lying) position, with the back bowed at the edge of the examining table, the knees flexed up to the abdomen, and the head bent so that the chin is resting on the chest.

b. After the procedure: Place the client in the supine position for 4 to 12 hours, as prescribed.

9. Spinal cord injury

a. Immobilize the client on a spinal backboard with the head in a neutral position to prevent an incomplete injury from becoming complete.

b. Prevent head flexion, rotation, or extension. The head is immobilized with a firm, padded cervical collar.

c. Logroll the client. No part of the body would be twisted or turned, and the client would not be allowed to assume a sitting position.

d. Once a potential spinal cord injury has been ruled out, the client will be prescribed activity according to any other injuries.

e. A spinal cord injury client who had surgery or Halo traction applied to stabilize the fracture will have prescribed activity beyond logrolling.

I. Musculoskeletal system

1. Total hip replacement

a. Positioning depends on the surgical techniques used (anterior or posterior approach), the method of implantation, and the prosthesis; however, always follow the surgeon's prescription(s).

b. Avoid extreme internal and external rotation.

c. Avoid adduction; in most cases side-lying is permissible as long as an abduction pillow is in place; some surgeons allow turning to only one side.

d. Maintain abduction when the client is in a supine position or positioned on the nonoperative side.

e. Place a wedge (abduction) pillow between the client's legs to maintain abduction; instruct the client not to cross the legs (Box 17.2).

f. Check the surgeon's prescriptions regarding elevation of the head of the bed and hip flexion.

2. Devices used to promote proper positioning (see Box 17.2)

WHAT WOULD YOU DO?

Answer: For the client receiving intermittent tube feedings via a nasogastric tube, the nurse needs to position the client in an upright (semi-Fowler's or high Fowler's) position during the feeding and for 30 minutes to 1 hour following the feeding, per agency policy. Positioning the client in an upright position prevents aspiration of the formula. For the client receiving a continuous tube feeding, an upright position needs to be maintained at all times.

BOX 17.2 Devices Used for Proper Positioning

Bed Boards
These plywood boards are placed under the entire surface area of the mattress. They are useful for increasing back support and body alignment Some special beds can provide this firmness.

Foot Boots
Foot boots are made of rigid plastic or heavy foam, and they keep the foot flexed at the proper angle. They would be removed two or three times a day to assess skin integrity and joint mobility.

Hand Rolls
Hand rolls maintain the fingers in a slightly flexed and functional position, and they keep the thumb slightly adducted in opposition to the fingers.

Hand–Wrist Splints
These splints are individually molded for the client to maintain the proper alignment of the thumb in slight adduction and the wrist in slight dorsiflexion.

Pillows
Pillows provide support, elevate body parts, splint incisional areas, and reduce postoperative pain during activity, coughing, or deep breathing. They need to be the appropriate size for the body part to be positioned.

Sandbags
Sandbags are soft devices filled with a substance that can be shaped to body contours to provide support. They immobilize extremities and maintain specific body alignment.

Side Rails
These bars, positioned along the sides of the length of the bed, ensure client safety and are useful for increasing mobility. They also provide assistance in rolling from side to side or sitting up in bed. Agency policies regarding the use of side rails must always be followed.

Trapeze Bar
This bar descends from a securely fastened overhead bar attached to the bed frame. It allows the client to use the upper extremities to raise the trunk off of the bed, to assist with transfer from the bed to a wheelchair, and to perform upper-arm strengthening exercises.

Trochanter Rolls
These rolls prevent the external rotation of the legs when the client is in the supine position. To form a roll, use a cotton bath blanket or a sheet folded lengthwise to a width that extends from the greater trochanter of the femur to the lower border of the popliteal space.

Wedge Pillow
This triangular-shaped pillow is made of heavy foam, and it is used to maintain the legs in abduction after total hip replacement surgery.

Adapted from Potter P, Perry A, Stockert P, et al: *Fundamentals of nursing*, ed 8, St. Louis, 2013, Mosby.

PRACTICE QUESTIONS

❖ 1. The nurse is preparing to reposition a dependent client who weighs more than 250 lb. Which interventions would the nurse use to move this client? **Select all that apply.**
   - ❑ 1. Use a friction-reducing slide sheet.
   - ❑ 2. Use a mechanical lift to move the client.
   - ❑ 3. Place the client in Trendelenburg position.
   - ❑ 4. Keep elbows close and work close to the body.
   - ❑ 5. Administer oral pain medication 5 minutes before moving the client.
   - ❑ 6. Obtain assistance of a second caregiver to assist with mechanical aids.

2. The nurse is assigned to assist with caring for a client after cardiac catheterization performed through the left femoral artery. The nurse needs to plan to maintain bed rest for this client in which position?
   1. High Fowler's position
   2. Supine with no head elevation
   3. Left lateral (side-lying) position
   4. Supine with head elevation no greater than 30 degrees

❖ 3. The nurse is reinforcing home-care instructions to a client and family regarding care after left cataract surgery with lens implant. Which statements made by the client indicate an understanding of the instructions? **Select all that apply.**
   - ❑ 1. "I will bend over to tie my shoes."
   - ❑ 2. "I will not sleep lying on my left side."
   - ❑ 3. "I will sit at the table to eat breakfast."
   - ❑ 4. "I will sit in my recliner with my feet elevated."
   - ❑ 5. "I will not lift anything heavy according to my surgeons' order."
   - ❑ 6. "I will resume my exercise routine including pushups."

4. After a client undergoes a liver biopsy, the nurse places the client in the prescribed right-side-lying position. The nurse understands that the purpose of this intervention is to accomplish which outcome?
   1. Promote bile flow
   2. Limit client discomfort
   3. Promote hepatic glucose storage
   4. Limit bleeding from the biopsy site

5. The nurse is administering a cleansing enema to a client with a fecal impaction. Before administering the enema, the nurse asks the client to assume a left Sims' position. The nurse explains that this positioning is preferred because of which reason?

1. The nurse is right-handed.
2. The rectal sphincter will relax.
3. The enema will flow into the bowel easily.
4. The client is more likely to retain the enema solution.

❖ 6. A client is being prepared for a thoracentesis. The nurse reinforces instructions with the client given by the registered nurse. Which points would be included in the instructions? **Select all that apply.**
   ❑ 1. The client leans over a bedside table.
   ❑ 2. The client would sit on the edge of the bed.
   ❑ 3. The procedure involves obtaining a biopsy.
   ❑ 4. A time-out is performed before the procedure.
   ❑ 5. The procedure is performed during a bronchoscopy.
   ❑ 6. A local anesthetic is administered before the procedure.

7. The nurse is assisting with the insertion of a nasogastric tube into a client. The nurse needs to place the client in which position for insertion?
   1. Right side
   2. Low Fowler's position
   3. High Fowler's position
   4. Supine, with the head flat

❖ 8. The nurse is assisting with caring for a client after a craniotomy. Which are the positions that would be used for the client? **Select all that apply.**
   ❑ 1. Prone position
   ❑ 2. Supine position
   ❑ 3. Semi-Fowler's position
   ❑ 4. Dorsal recumbent position
   ❑ 5. With the foot of the bed flat
   ❑ 6. With the foot of the bed elevated 30 degrees

9. The nurse is caring for a client following a craniotomy in which a large tumor was removed from the left side. In which position would the nurse safely place the bed for the client? Refer to Figures 17.1 to 17.4.

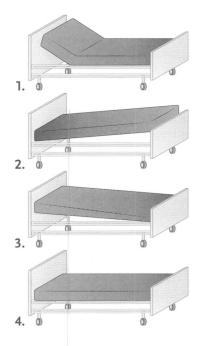

1.
2.
3.
4.

10. A client has just returned to a nursing unit after an above-knee amputation of the right leg. The nurse needs to plan to place the client in which position?
   1. Prone
   2. Reverse Trendelenburg's
   3. Supine, with the residual limb flat on the bed
   4. Supine, with the residual limb supported with pillows

ANSWERS

❖ **1. 1, 2, 4, 6**

Rationale: Manually lifting or transferring clients can result in work-related injuries and back problems for health care workers. In addition, the shearing of the client's skin over bony prominences may occur when health care workers move clients independently. The nurse would seek the assistance of another caregiver, and use correct body mechanics while utilizing mechanical aids, such as a ceiling lift or friction-reducing slide sheet. Placing the client in Trendelenburg is not a useful technique for repositioning and could be harmful to the client because of the pressure this position places on the diaphragm. Administering oral pain medication may be necessary, but oral medications need to be given at least 30 minutes before the activity to provide time for the medication to work and provide relief of pain.

Test-Taking Strategy: Focus on the subject, safely moving a client. Next, focus on the data in the question. This client's dependent condition and weight require extra help and use of mechanical aids.

2. 4

Rationale: After cardiac catheterization, the extremity into which the catheter was inserted is kept straight for the prescribed time period to prevent arterial occlusion or bleeding and hematoma. With a femoral approach, the client's affected extremity is kept straight and the head elevated no more than 30 degrees (some primary health care providers prefer a lower head position or the flat position) until hemostasis is adequately achieved. The client may turn from side to side. Bathroom privileges are not allowed during the immediate postcatheterization period. High Fowler's (90-degree elevation), flat, and side lying on the puncture site are not effective in preventing complications or allowing for client comfort.

Test-Taking Strategy: Focus on the subject, positioning after cardiac catheterization. Recalling that concerns after this procedure are bleeding and arterial occlusion will direct you to the correct option.

❖ **3.** 2, 3, 4, 5

Rationale: After cataract surgery, the client would not assume positions that will increase the intraocular pressure. This could lead to injury to the surgical site and damage the lens implant. The client would not sleep on the side of the body that was operated on. The client may resume activities such as sitting upright at a table or sitting in a recliner with the feet elevated. The client would be instructed to avoid lifting heavy objects, per surgeon's order. The client also is instructed to avoid activities that would increase the pressure within the eye, such as bending over to tie shoes or performing pushups.

Test-Taking Strategy: Focus on the subject, activity and positioning after cataract surgery. Consider each option and determine whether the action would increase pressure within the eye. This will lead you to answer correctly.

4. 4

Rationale: After a liver biopsy, the client is assisted with assuming a right side-lying position with a small pillow or folded towel under the puncture site for at least 3 hours to apply pressure and limit bleeding from the biopsy site. The liver produces bile that flows through the common bile duct; client discomfort may be decreased; and the liver does store glucose as glycogen, but this is not the purpose of the right side-lying position.

Test-Taking Strategy: Focus on the subject, the purpose of client positioning after a liver biopsy. Think about the vascularity of the liver. Remember that the liver is on the right side of the body and that the application of pressure on the right side will minimize the escape of blood or bile through the puncture site.

5. 3

Rationale: When administering an enema, the client is placed in a left Sims' position so that the enema solution can flow by gravity in the natural direction of the colon. The anatomy of the colon consists of ascending on the right, transverse across, with descending on the left leading to the sigmoid and rectum. If the client lies on the left side, the enema solution will flow easily into the bowel. The hand dominance of the nurse is not a factor. The nurse assists the client to relax the rectal sphincter by asking the client to take a deep breath. The nurse assists the client to retain the enema solution by administering the enema slowly. The nurse would also use teach-back to determine the client's understanding about the reason for the enema.

Test-Taking Strategy: Focus on the subject, enema administration. Recalling the anatomy of the bowel will assist you with selecting the correct option.

❖ **6.** 1, 2, 4, 6

Rationale: A thoracentesis is a procedure in which fluid is removed from the pleural space. The procedure involves insertion of a needle percutaneously and then removal of the fluid by connecting the needle to a vacuum bottle. Before the thoracentesis, the nurse needs to check for allergies because a local anesthetic is administered. A time-out is performed in which the client identification, coagulation studies, and area of the pleural effusion are verified. A chest x-ray is performed after the procedure. A potential complication is a pneumothorax. The client sits on the bedside and leans over a bedside table, which exposes the area between the ribs. A lung biopsy is often done during a bronchoscopy.

Test-Taking Strategy: Focus on the subject, thoracentesis. Recall that the procedure is performed percutaneously and removes pleural fluid. Consider that the area for the needle insertion is best exposed by the client sitting at the bedside while leaning over the bedside table and a local anesthetic is indicated.

7. 3

Rationale: Before insertion of a nasogastric tube the nurse places the client in a sitting or high Fowler's position to reduce the risk of pulmonary aspiration if the client begins to vomit. A pillow may be placed behind the head and shoulders to promote the client's ability to swallow during the procedure. Options 1, 2, and 4 do not facilitate the insertion of the tube or prevent aspiration.

Test-Taking Strategy: Focus on the subject, insertion of a nasogastric tube. Visualize this procedure. Use the ABCs—airway, breathing, and circulation—because pulmonary aspiration is a concern with insertion of a nasogastric tube. Select the option that promotes safe insertion.

❖ **8.** 3, 5

Rationale: After a craniotomy, the client is at risk for developing complications of increased intracranial pressure and cerebral edema. The head of the bed is elevated 30 degrees (semi-Fowler's position), and the client's head is maintained in a midline, neutral position to facilitate venous drainage. The foot of the bed must be flat because flexion at the hips will impair venous drainage. Blocking venous drainage increases the risk for increased intracranial pressure and cerebral edema. Remember there are no valves in the veins that drain the head.

Test-Taking Strategy: Focus on the subject, positioning after craniotomy. Use knowledge about the anatomy and physiology and effects of gravity and the development of edema to answer correctly.

❖ **9.** 1

Rationale: Clients who have undergone craniotomy must have the head of the bed elevated 30 degrees to promote venous drainage from the head. The client is positioned to avoid extreme hip or neck flexion and the head is maintained in a midline, neutral position. If a large tumor has been removed, the client needs to be placed on the nonoperative side to prevent displacement of the cranial contents. A flat position or

Trendelenburg's position would increase intracranial pressure. A reverse Trendelenburg's position would not be helpful and may be uncomfortable for the client.

Test-Taking Strategy: Focus on the subject, positioning following a supratentorial craniotomy. Remember that a primary concern is the risk for increased intracranial pressure. Therefore, use concepts related to preventing increased intracranial pressure to answer this question.

10. 4

Rationale: The residual limb is usually supported on pillows for the first 24 hours following surgery to promote venous return and decrease edema. After the first 24 hours, the residual limb usually is placed flat on the bed to reduce hip contracture. Edema is controlled by limb-wrapping techniques. In addition, it is important to check the surgeon's prescription(s) regarding positioning following amputation.

Test-Taking Strategy: Focus on the subject, positioning following amputation, and note that the client has just returned from surgery. Using basic principles related to immediate postoperative care and preventing edema will assist in directing you to the correct option.

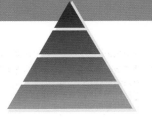

CHAPTER **18**

Care of a Client With a Tube

PRIORITY CONCEPTS **Clinical Judgment; Safety**

WHAT WOULD YOU DO?

The nurse is assisting in monitoring a client with a closed chest tube drainage system. During inspection, the nurse notes that the system is cracked. What would the nurse do? *Answer is located on p. 215.*

I. Nasogastric (NG) Tubes

A. Description
   1. Tubes used to intubate the stomach
   2. Inserted from the nose to the stomach
B. Purpose
   1. To decompress the stomach by removing fluids or gas to promote abdominal comfort
   2. To allow surgical anastomoses to heal without distention
   3. To decrease the risk of aspiration
   4. To administer medications in clients who are unable to swallow
   5. To provide nutrition by acting as a temporary feeding tube
   6. To irrigate the stomach and remove toxic substances, such as in poisonings
C. Types of tubes and routes (Fig. 18.1)

   ⚠ The air vent on a Salem sump tube is not to be clamped and is to be kept above the level of the stomach. If leakage occurs through the air vent, instill 30 mL of air into the air vent and irrigate the main lumen with normal saline (NS). Salem sump tubes are available with an antireflux valve that is placed in the air vent. The valve allows air in one way and prevents leakage.

D. Intubation procedures (Box 18.1)
E. Irrigation
   1. Check placement before irrigating (see Box 18.1).
   2. Perform irrigation every 4 hours to monitor and maintain the patency of the tube.

   3. Gently instill 30 to 50 mL of water or NS (depending on agency policy) with an irrigation syringe. Irrigation must be specifically prescribed if the client underwent gastric surgery.
   4. Pull back on the syringe plunger to withdraw the fluid to check patency; repeat if the tube flow is sluggish.
F. Removal of an NG tube: Irrigate the tube with NS before removal to prevent aspiration. Ask the client to take a deep breath and hold; remove the tube slowly and evenly over the course of 3 to 6 seconds (coil the tube around the hand while removing it).

II. Gastrointestinal Tube Feedings

A. Types of tubes and anatomical placement
   1. NG: Nose to stomach
   2. Nasoduodenal-nasojejunal: Nose to duodenum or jejunum
   3. Gastrostomy: Stomach
   4. Jejunostomy: Jejunum
B. Types of administration
   1. Bolus
      a. Resembles normal meal feeding patterns
      b. Formula is administered over a 30- to 60-minute period every 3 to 6 hours; the amount of formula is prescribed by the primary health care provider (PHCP).
   2. Continuous
      a. Administered continuously for 24 hours
      b. A feeding pump regulates the flow.
   3. Cyclical
      a. Feeding is administered either during the daytime or nighttime for approximately 8 to 16 hours.
      b. A feeding pump regulates the flow.
      c. Feedings at night allow for more freedom during the day.
C. Administering feedings
   1. Check the PHCP's prescription and agency policy regarding residual amounts; usually, if the residual

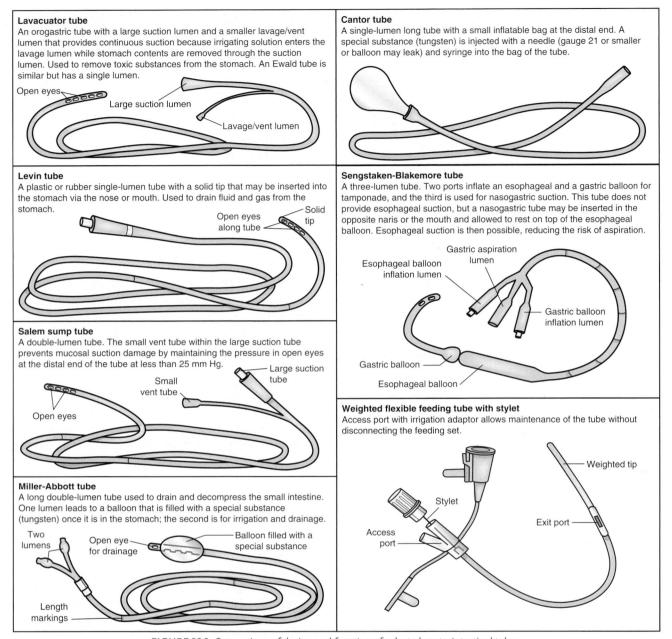

Lavacuator tube
An orogastric tube with a large suction lumen and a smaller lavage/vent lumen that provides continuous suction because irrigating solution enters the lavage lumen while stomach contents are removed through the suction lumen. Used to remove toxic substances from the stomach. An Ewald tube is similar but has a single lumen.

Open eyes

Large suction lumen

Lavage/vent lumen

Cantor tube
A single-lumen long tube with a small inflatable bag at the distal end. A special substance (tungsten) is injected with a needle (gauge 21 or smaller or balloon may leak) and syringe into the bag of the tube.

Levin tube
A plastic or rubber single-lumen tube with a solid tip that may be inserted into the stomach via the nose or mouth. Used to drain fluid and gas from the stomach.

Solid tip

Open eyes along tube

Sengstaken-Blakemore tube
A three-lumen tube. Two ports inflate an esophageal and a gastric balloon for tamponade, and the third is used for nasogastric suction. This tube does not provide esophageal suction, but a nasogastric tube may be inserted in the opposite naris or the mouth and allowed to rest on top of the esophageal balloon. Esophageal suction is then possible, reducing the risk of aspiration.

Gastric aspiration lumen

Esophageal balloon inflation lumen

Gastric balloon inflation lumen

Gastric balloon

Esophageal balloon

Salem sump tube
A double-lumen tube. The small vent tube within the large suction tube prevents mucosal suction damage by maintaining the pressure in open eyes at the distal end of the tube at less than 25 mm Hg.

Large suction tube

Small vent tube

Open eyes

Weighted flexible feeding tube with stylet
Access port with irrigation adaptor allows maintenance of the tube without disconnecting the feeding set.

Weighted tip

Stylet

Access port

Exit port

Miller-Abbott tube
A long double-lumen tube used to drain and decompress the small intestine. One lumen leads to a balloon that is filled with a special substance (tungsten) once it is in the stomach; the second is for irrigation and drainage.

Two lumens

Open eye for drainage

Balloon filled with a special substance

Length markings

FIGURE 18.1 Comparison of design and function of selected gastrointestinal tubes.

is less than 100 mL, feeding is administered; large-volume aspirates indicate delayed gastric emptying and place the client at risk for aspiration.

2. Assess bowel sounds; hold the feeding and notify the registered nurse (RN) or PHCP if bowel sounds are absent.

3. Position the client in a high Fowler's position; if comatose, place in high Fowler's and on the right side.

4. Assess tube placement by aspirating gastric contents and measuring the pH (needs to be 3.5 or lower), or per agency policy.

5. Aspirate all stomach contents (residual), measure the amount, and return the contents to the stomach to prevent electrolyte imbalance, unless the color or characteristics of the residual are abnormal or the amount is greater than 250 mL.

6. Warm the feeding to room temperature to prevent diarrhea and cramps.

7. Use a feeding pump for continuous or cyclic feedings.

8. For bolus feeding, maintain the client in a high Fowler's position for 30 minutes after the feeding. Use a feeding pump or allow the feeding to infuse via gravity. Do not plunge the feeding into the stomach.

9. For a continuous feeding, keep the client in a semi-Fowler's position at all times.

BOX 18.1 Nasogastric Tubes: Insertion Procedures

1. Follow agency procedures.
2. Explain the procedure and its potential discomfort to the client.
3. Position the client with pillows behind the shoulders.
4. Determine which nostril is more patent.
5. Measure the length of the tube from the bridge of the nose to the earlobe to the xiphoid process and indicate this length with a piece of tape on the tube.
6. If the client is conscious and alert, have him or her swallow or drink water (follow agency procedure).
7. Lubricate the tip of the tube with water-soluble lubricant.
8. Gently insert the tube into the nasopharynx and advance the tube.
9. When the tube nears the back of the throat (first black measurement on the tube), instruct the client to swallow or drink sips of water (unless contraindicated). If resistance is met, then slowly rotate and aim the tube downward and toward the closer ear; in the intubated or semiconscious client, flex the head toward the chest while passing the tube.
10. Immediately withdraw the tube if any change is noted in the client's respiratory status.
11. Secure the tube to the client's nose with adhesive tape and to the client's gown (follow agency procedure and check for client allergy to tape).
12. Obtain an abdominal x-ray study to confirm placement of the tube.
13. Connect the tube to suction, to either the intermittent or continuous suction setting, as prescribed.
14. Observe the client for nausea, vomiting, abdominal fullness, or distention, and monitor output.
15. Check residual volumes every 4 hours, before each feeding, and before giving medications. Aspirate all stomach contents (residual) and measure the amount. Reinstill residual contents to prevent excessive fluid and electrolyte losses, unless the residual contents appear abnormal and the volume is large (follow agency procedure). Withhold the feeding if the amount is more than 100 mL or according to agency or nutritional consult recommendations.
16. Before the instillation of any substance through the tube (i.e., irrigation solution, feeding, medications), aspirate stomach contents and test the pH (a pH of 3.5 or lower indicates that the tip of the tube is in a gastric location).
17. If irrigation is indicated, use normal saline solution (check agency procedure).
18. Observe the client for fluid and electrolyte balance.
19. Instruct the client about movement to prevent nasal irritation and dislodgment of the tube.
20. On a daily basis, remove the adhesive tape that is securing the tube to the nose and clean and dry the skin, assessing for excoriation or pressure areas that can cause pressure ulcers; then reapply the tape.

Note: Gastrostomy or jejunostomy tubes are surgically inserted. A dressing is placed at the site of insertion. The dressing needs to be removed, the skin needs to be cleansed (with a solution determined by the primary health care provider [PHCP] or agency procedure), and a new sterile dressing needs to be applied every 8 hours (or as specified by agency policy). The skin at the insertion site is checked for signs of excoriation, infection, or other abnormalities, such as leakage of the feeding solution.

From Potter P, Perry AG, Stockert PA, Hall AM: *Fundamentals of nursing,* ed 8, St. Louis, 2013, Mosby, p. 594.

 D. Precautions

 Always check the placement of a gastrointestinal tube before instilling feeding solutions, medications, or any other solution. If the tube is incorrectly placed, the client is at risk for aspiration.

1. Change the feeding container and tubing every 24 hours or per agency policy.
2. Do not hang more solution than required for a 4-hour period; this prevents bacterial growth unless it is a closed system with a container of formula that is to be infused over the 24-hour period.
3. Check the expiration date on the formula before administering it.
4. Shake the formula well before pouring it into the container or feeding bag. Some feedings require the use of a bag in which formula is added, or require the use of bottles that feeding tubing can be attached to directly. The tubing sometimes has a Y-site connection so a regular flush can be programmed using the pump rather than using a piston syringe.
5. Always check the bowel sounds. Feedings cannot be administered if bowel sounds are absent.

6. Administer the feeding at the prescribed rate or via gravity flow (intermittent bolus feedings) with a 50- to 60-mL syringe with the plunger removed.
7. Gently flush with 30 to 50 mL of water or normal saline (depending on agency policy) with the irrigation syringe after the feeding. Clients receiving continuous feedings are given set amounts of sterile water every 4 hours to prevent clogging of the tube.

E. Prevention of complications
1. Diarrhea
   a. Monitor the client for lactose intolerance.
   b. Fiber-containing feedings may be prescribed.
   c. Administer feeding slowly and at room temperature. When feedings are initiated, the feeding are begun at a slow rate and gradually increased according to client toleration.
2. Aspiration
   a. Verify tube placement.
   b. Do not administer the feeding if residual is more than 100 mL (check with the RN and PHCP's prescription and agency policy).
   c. Keep the head of the bed elevated.
   d. If aspiration occurs, suction as needed, monitor respiratory rate, auscultate lung sounds,

monitor temperature for aspiration pneumonia, and prepare to obtain chest radiograph.

3. Clogged tube
   a. Use liquid forms of medication, if possible; if liquid forms cannot be used, medications need to be crushed.
   b. Flush the tube with 30 to 50 mL of water or NS (depending on agency policy) before and after medication administration and before and after bolus feeding.
   c. Flush with water every 4 hours for continuous feeding.
   d. If tube becomes clogged, attempt to irrigate to remove the obstruction. Notify the PHCP if unable to unclog the tube.
4. Vomiting
   a. Administer feedings slowly and, for bolus feedings, make feeding last for at least 30 minutes.
   b. Measure abdominal girth.
   c. Do not allow the feeding bag to empty.
   d. Do not allow air to enter the tubing.
   e. Administer the feeding at room temperature.
   f. Elevate the head of the bed.
   g. Administer antiemetics as prescribed.
5. Additional complications can include sinusitis, gastric erosion, or pulmonary infections and the nurse must monitor for signs of these complications.

⚠ If the client vomits, stop the tube feeding and place the client in a side-lying position; suction the client as needed.

F. Administration of medications (see Priority Nursing Actions)

⚡ PRIORITY NURSING ACTIONS

Administering Medications via a Nasogastric or Gastrostomy Tube

1. Check the primary health care provider's (PHCP's) prescription(s).
2. Prepare the medication for administration.
3. Ensure that the medication prescribed can be crushed or (if it is a capsule) that it can be opened; use elixir forms of medications if available.
4. Dissolve crushed medication or capsule contents in 15 to 30 mL of water.
5. Verify the client's identity and explain the procedure to the client.
6. Check tube placement and residual contents before instilling the medication; check for bowel sounds.
7. Draw up the medication into a catheter tip syringe, clear excess air from the syringe, and insert the medication into the tube.
8. Flush with 30 to 50 mL of water or NS (depending on agency policy).
9. Clamp the tube for 30 to 60 minutes (depending on medication and agency policy).
10. Document the administration of the medication and any other appropriate information.

III. Intestinal Tubes
A. Description
   1. Passed nasally into the small intestine
   2. Used to decompress the bowel or to remove intestinal secretions when other interventions to decompress the bowel are not effective
   3. Designed to enter the small intestine through the pyloric sphincter with the use of the weight of a small bag containing a special substance (tungsten) at the end
B. Types of tubes include the Cantor tube (single lumen) and the Miller-Abbott tube (double lumen) (see Fig. 18.1).
C. Interventions
   1. Check the PHCP's prescription(s) and agency policy for advancement and removal of the tube and tungsten; assist the RN.
   2. Position the client on the right side to facilitate passage of the weighted bag in the tube through the pylorus of the stomach and into the small intestine.
   3. Do not secure the tube to the face with tape until it has reached final placement (may take several hours) in the intestines.
   4. Check the abdomen during the procedure by monitoring drainage from the tube and the abdominal girth.
   5. If the tube becomes blocked, notify the RN and the PHCP.
   6. When the tube is removed, the tungsten is removed from the balloon portion of the tube with a syringe; the tube is removed gradually (6 inches every hour) as prescribed by the PHCP.

IV. Esophageal and Gastric Tubes
A. Description
   1. May be used to apply pressure against bleeding esophageal veins to control the bleeding when other interventions are not effective or they are contraindicated.
   2. Not used if the client has ulceration or necrosis of the esophagus or has had previous esophageal surgery because of the risk of rupture. Clients may have treatment of esophageal varices with sclerosing therapy during gastroscopy procedure done by gastroenterologist.
   3. Examples are the Sengstaken-Blakemore tube or Minnesota tube (a modified Sengstaken-Blakemore tube with an additional lumen for aspirating esophagopharyngeal secretions). These tubes are uncomfortable for the client and can cause complications, but their use may be necessary when other interventions are not feasible (see Fig. 18.1).
B. Interventions
   1. The patency and integrity of all balloons are checked before insertion and each lumen is labeled.

2. The client is placed in an upright or Fowler's position for insertion.
3. Prepare the client for an x-ray study of chest or abdomen as prescribed, immediately after insertion to verify placement.
4. Maintain head elevation after the tube is in place.
5. The balloon ports are double-clamped to prevent air leaks.
6. Scissors are kept at the bedside at all times. The scissors are available in case the gastric balloon of the tube ruptures and the tube moves upward, occluding the client's airway. Cutting the tube below the bifurcation will deflate all balloons and allow the tube to be removed manually.
7. The client is monitored for respiratory distress. If it occurs, notify the RN immediately. The tubes will be cut to deflate the balloons.
8. Monitor for increased bloody drainage that may indicate persistent bleeding.
9. Monitor for signs of esophageal rupture, including a drop in blood pressure, increased heart rate, and back and upper abdominal pain. (Esophageal rupture is an emergency and signs of its occurrence must be reported immediately to the RN and PHCP.)

V. Lavage Tubes
A. Description: Used to remove toxic substances from the stomach
B. Types of tubes
   1. Lavacuator (see Fig. 18.1)
   2. Ewald tube: A single-lumen large tube used for rapid one-time irrigation and evacuation

VI. Urinary and Renal Tubes
A. Types of urinary catheters
   1. Single lumen: Usually used for straight catheterization to empty the client's bladder, obtain sterile urine specimens, or to check the residual amount of urine after the client voids (amount of urine may be obtained by portable bladder ultrasound [bladder scan]).
   2. Double lumen: Used when an indwelling catheter is needed for continuous bladder drainage; one lumen is for drainage, and the other is for balloon inflation.
   3. Triple lumen: Used when bladder irrigation and drainage is necessary; one lumen is for instilling the bladder irrigant solution, one lumen is for continuous bladder drainage, and one lumen is for balloon inflation.
   4. Strict aseptic technique is necessary for insertion and care of the catheter.
B. Routine urinary catheter care
   1. Use gloves and wash the perineal area with warm soapy water.
   2. With the nondominant hand, pull back the labia or foreskin to expose the meatus (in the adult male, return the foreskin to its normal position).

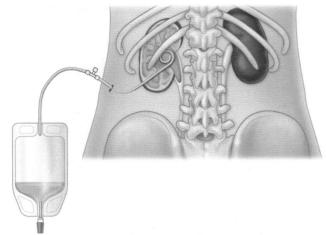

FIGURE 18.2 Ureteral and nephrostomy tubes.

3. Cleanse along the catheter with soap and water.
4. Anchor the catheter to the thigh according to agency policy.
5. Maintain the catheter bag below the level of the bladder.
6. Empty the drainage bag when it is ½ to ⅔ full.
7. Preventing catheter-associated urinary tract infection: Discontinue catheter when no longer indicated, avoid dependent loops in tubing, utilize commercial catheter holder.
C. Ureteral and nephrostomy tubes (Fig. 18.2)
   1. Never clamp the tubes.
   2. Maintain patency.
   3. Monitor output closely.
   4. Tube irrigation may be prescribed by the PHCP and will be done by the RN as per prescription.
D. Catheter insertion and removal (Box 18.2)

⚠ If the client has a ureteral or nephrostomy tube, monitor output closely. Urine output of less than 30 mL/hour or lack of output for more than 15 minutes must be reported to the RN and PHCP immediately.

VII. Respiratory Airway Tubes
A. Endotracheal tube (Fig. 18.3)
   1. Description
      a. Used to maintain a patent airway
      b. Indicated when the client needs mechanical ventilation
      c. If the client requires an artificial airway for longer than 10 to 14 days, a tracheostomy may be created to avoid the mucosal and vocal cord damage that can be caused by the endotracheal tube.
      d. The cuff (located at the distal end of the tube), when inflated, produces a seal between the trachea and the cuff to prevent aspiration and ensure delivery of set tidal volume when mechanical ventilation is used; an inflated cuff also prevents air from passing to the vocal cords, nose, or mouth.

BOX 18.2 **Urinary Catheters: Insertion and Removal Procedures**

Urinary Catheters: Insertion Procedure

1. Follow agency procedures.
2. Explain the procedure and its potential discomfort to the client.
3. Place in position for catheterization:
   a. *Female:* Assist to dorsal recumbent position (supine with knees flexed). Support legs with pillows to reduce muscle tension and promote comfort.
   b. *Male:* Assist to supine position with thighs slightly abducted.
4. Wearing clean gloves, wash perineal area with soap and water as needed; dry thoroughly. Remove and discard gloves; perform hand hygiene.
5. Open outer wrapping of the catheter kit, remembering that all components of the catheterization tray are sterile (all supplies are arranged in the box in order of sequence of use).
6. Apply waterproof sterile drape (when packed as first item in tray).
7. Foley catheter procedure with specifics for male and female:
   a. *Female:* With nondominant hand, fully expose urethral meatus by spreading labia. Using forceps in sterile dominant hand, pick up cotton ball or swab sticks saturated with antiseptic solution, wiping from front to back (from clitoris toward anus). Using a new cotton ball or swab for each area you clean, wipe far labial fold, near labial fold, and directly over center of urethral meatus. Open packet containing lubricant and lubricate catheter tip. Advance catheter a total of 7.5 cm (3 inches) in adult or until urine flows out of catheter end. When urine appears, advance catheter another 2.5 to 5 cm (1–2 inches). Do not use force to insert catheter.
   b. *Male:* Use of square sterile drape is optional; you may apply fenestrated drape with fenestrated slit resting over penis. Open package of sterile antiseptic solution. Pour solution over sterile cotton balls. Grasp penis at shaft just below glans. (If client is not circumcised,

retract foreskin with nondominant hand.) With dominant hand, pick up antiseptic-soaked cotton ball with forceps or swab stick, and clean penis. Move cotton ball or swab in circular motion from urethral meatus down to base of glans. Repeat cleaning 3 more times, using clean cotton ball/stick each time. Pick up catheter with gloved dominant hand and insert catheter by lifting penis to position perpendicular to the client's body and apply light traction. Advance catheter to the bifurcation of the catheter 17 to 22.5 cm (7–9 inches) in adult or until urine flows out of catheter end. Lower penis, and hold catheter securely in nondominant hand.
8. Inflate balloon fully per manufacturer's directions.
9. Secure catheter tubing to inner thigh with strip of nonallergenic tape (use paper tape if allergic to silk tape or a multipurpose tube holder with a Velcro strap).
10. Record type and size of catheter inserted, amount of fluid used to inflate the balloon, characteristics and amount of urine, specimen collection if appropriate, client's response to procedure, and that teaching is completed.

Urinary Catheters: Removal Procedure

1. Follow agency procedures.
2. Explain the procedure and its potential discomfort to the client.
3. Position the client in the same position as during catheterization.
4. Remove the tape and place the towel between a female client's thighs or over a male client's thighs.
5. Insert a 10-mL syringe into the balloon injection port. Slowly withdraw all of the solution to deflate the balloon totally.
6. After deflation, explain to the client that they may feel a burning sensation as the catheter is withdrawn. Pull the catheter out smoothly and slowly.
7. Monitor the client's urinary function by noting the first voiding after catheter removal and documenting the time and amount of voiding for the next 24 hours.

From Potter P, Perry A, Stockert P, Hall A: *Fundamentals of nursing*, ed 8, St. Louis, 2013, Mosby.

---

   e. The pilot balloon permits air to be inserted into the cuff, prevents air from escaping, and it is used as a guideline for determining the presence or absence of air in the cuff.
   f. Types of tubes: Orotracheal and nasotracheal
2. Orotracheal
   a. Inserted through the mouth; allows for the use of a larger-diameter tube and reduces the work of breathing
   b. Indicated when the client has a nasal obstruction or a predisposition to epistaxis
   c. Uncomfortable for the client and can be manipulated by the tongue, causing airway obstruction; an oral airway may be needed to prevent the client from biting on the tube.
3. Nasotracheal
   a. Inserted through the nose; this smaller tube increases both resistance and the client's work of breathing.

   b. Use of this type of tube is avoided in clients with bleeding disorders.
   c. More comfortable for the client, and the client is unable to manipulate the tube with the tongue
4. Interventions
   a. Placement is confirmed by a chest x-ray study (correct placement is 1 to 2 cm above the carina) and by auscultating both sides of the chest while manually ventilating with resuscitation (Ambu) bag. If breath sounds and chest wall movement are absent on the left side, the tube may be in the right main stem bronchus.
   b. Perform auscultation over the stomach to rule out esophageal intubation.
   c. If the tube is in the stomach, louder breath sounds will be heard over the stomach than over the chest and abdominal distention will be present.

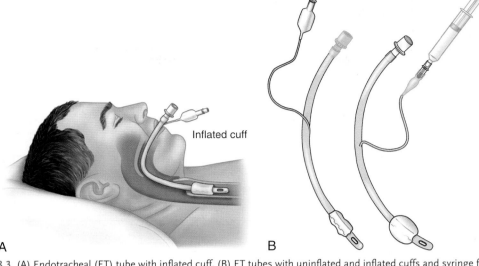

Inflated cuff

A

B

FIGURE 18.3 (A) Endotracheal (ET) tube with inflated cuff. (B) ET tubes with uninflated and inflated cuffs and syringe for inflation.

   d. The tube is secured immediately after intubation with adhesive tape or commercial device to hold endotracheal tube in place.

   e. Monitor the position of the tube at the lip or nose.

   f. Monitor the skin and mucous membranes.

   g. Suction the tube only when needed.

   h. The oral tube needs to be moved to the opposite side of the mouth daily to prevent pressure and necrosis of the lip and mouth area, prevent nerve damage, and facilitate the inspection and cleaning of the mouth. Moving the tube to the opposite side of the mouth would be done by two PHCPs.

   i. Prevent dislodgment and pulling or tugging on the tube. Suction, coughing, and speaking attempts by the client place extra stress on the tube and can cause dislodgment.

   j. Check the pilot balloon to ensure that the cuff is inflated; maintain cuff inflation, which creates a seal and allows complete mechanical control of respiration.

   k. Interventions to prevent ventilator-associated pneumonia: position head of bed higher than 30 degrees, suction the oropharynx, use endotracheal tubes that have continuous subglottic suction ports.

⚠ A resuscitation (Ambu) bag needs to be kept at the bedside of a client with an endotracheal tube or tracheostomy tube at all times.

5. Extubation

   a. Hyperoxygenate the client, and suction the endotracheal tube and the oral cavity.

   b. Place the client in semi-Fowler's position.

   c. The cuff is deflated. The client is asked to inhale. At peak inspiration, the tube is removed, and the airway is suctioned through the tube as it is pulled out.

   d. After removal, instruct the client to cough and deep breathe to assist with the removal of accumulated secretions from the throat.

   e. Apply oxygen therapy, as prescribed.

   f. Monitor for respiratory difficulty. Contact the RN and PHCP if respiratory difficulty occurs.

   g. Inform the client that hoarseness or a sore throat is normal and that he or she needs to limit talking if it occurs.

B. Tracheostomy

  1. Description

   a. A tracheostomy is an opening made surgically, directly into the trachea to establish an airway; a tracheostomy tube is inserted into the opening, and the tube attaches to the mechanical ventilator or another type of oxygen delivery device (Fig. 18.4).

   b. The tracheostomy can be temporary or permanent.

  2. Interventions

   a. Monitor respiration and check for bilateral breath sounds.

   b. Monitor the pulse oximetry; arterial blood gas results are also monitored.

   c. Encourage coughing and deep breathing.

   d. Maintain a semi-Fowler's to high Fowler's position.

   e. Monitor for bleeding, difficulty breathing (pneumothorax), and crepitus (subcutaneous emphysema), which are indications of hemorrhage or pneumothorax.

   f. Provide respiratory treatments, as prescribed.

   g. Maintain cuff inflation with prescribed air amount.

   h. Suction as needed; hyperoxygenate the client before suction (see Chapter 47 for the suctioning procedure).

   i. If the client is allowed to eat, sit him or her up for meals, and ensure that the cuff is inflated

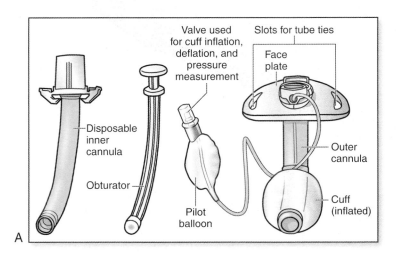

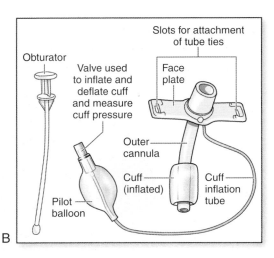

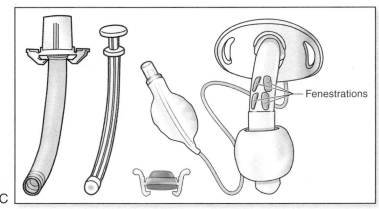

FIGURE 18.4 Tracheostomy tubes. (A) Double-lumen cuffed tracheostomy tube with disposable inner cannula. (B) Single-lumen cannula cuffed tracheostomy tube. (C) Double-lumen cuffed fenestrated tracheostomy tube with plug (red cap).

(if the tube is not capped) for meals and for 1 hour after meals.

j. Check the stoma and secretions for blood or purulent drainage.

k. Follow the PHCP's prescriptions and agency policy for cleaning the tracheostomy site and inner cannula (many inner cannulas are disposable); usually, half-strength hydrogen peroxide is used.

l. Administer humidified oxygen, as prescribed. The normal humidification process is bypassed in a client with a tracheostomy.

m. Obtain assistance with changing the tracheostomy ties. After placing the new ties, cut and remove the old ties that are holding the tracheostomy tube in place (some securing devices are soft and made with Velcro to hold the tube in place).

n. Keep a resuscitation (Ambu) bag, an obturator, clamps, and a spare tracheotomy set at the bedside.

o. Provide frequent mouth care to reduce the risk of pneumonia.

3. Complications of a tracheostomy (Table 18.1)

 Never insert a decannulation plug into a tracheostomy tube until the cuff is deflated and the inner cannula is removed. Prior insertion prevents airflow to the client.

VIII. Chest-Tube Drainage System

A. Description
1. Returns negative pressure to the intrapleural space
2. Used to remove abnormal accumulations of air and fluid from the pleural space
3. Chest-tube placement (Fig. 18.5)

B. Drainage collection chamber (Fig. 18.6)
1. Located where the chest tube from the client connects to the system
2. Drainage from the tube drains into and collects in a series of calibrated columns in this chamber.

C. Water-seal chamber (see Fig. 18.6)
1. The tip of the tube is underwater, allowing fluid and air to drain from the pleural space and preventing air from entering the pleural space.
2. Water oscillates (moves up as the client inhales and moves down as the client exhales).
3. Excessive, continuous bubbling indicates an air leak in the chest-tube system.

TABLE 18.1 **Complications of a Tracheostomy**

Complications and Description	Manifestations	Management	Prevention
Tracheomalacia: Constant pressure exerted by the cuff causes tracheal dilation and erosion of cartilage.	An increased amount of air is required in the cuff to maintain the seal. A larger tracheostomy tube is required to prevent an air leak at the stoma. Food particles are seen in tracheal secretions. The client does not receive the set tidal volume on the ventilator.	No special management is needed unless bleeding or airway problems occur.	Use an uncuffed tube as soon as possible. Monitor cuff pressure and air volume closely to detect changes.
Tracheal stenosis: Narrowed tracheal lumen is the result of scar formation from irritation of tracheal mucosa by the cuff.	Stenosis is usually seen after the cuff is deflated or the tracheostomy tube is removed. The client has increased coughing, inability to expectorate secretions, or difficulty in breathing and talking.	Tracheal dilation or surgical intervention is used.	Prevent pulling of, and traction on, the tracheostomy tube. Properly secure the tube in the midline position. Maintain cuff pressure. Minimize oronasal intubation time.
Tracheoesophageal fistula (TEF): Excessive cuff pressure causes erosion of the posterior wall of the trachea. A hole is created between the trachea and the anterior esophagus. The client at highest risk also has a nasogastric tube present.	Similar to tracheomalacia: • Food particles are seen in tracheal secretions. • Increased air in cuff is needed to achieve a seal. • The client has increased coughing and choking while eating. • The client does not receive the set tidal volume on the ventilator.	Manually administer oxygen by mask to prevent hypoxemia. Use a small, soft feeding tube instead of a nasogastric tube for tube feedings. A gastrostomy or jejunostomy may be performed. Monitor the client with a nasogastric tube closely; assess for TEF and aspiration.	Maintain cuff pressure. Monitor the amount of air needed for inflation to detect changes. Progress to a deflated or cuffless tube as soon as possible.
Trachea–innominate artery fistula: A malpositioned tube causes its distal tip to push against the lateral wall of the trachea. Continued pressure causes necrosis and erosion of the innominate artery. *This is a medical emergency.*	The tracheostomy tube pulsates in synchrony with the heartbeat. There is heavy bleeding from the stoma. *This is a life-threatening complication.*	Remove the tracheostomy tube immediately. Apply direct pressure to the innominate artery at the stoma site. Prepare the client for immediate repair surgery.	Use the correct tube size and length, and maintain the tube in midline position. Prevent pulling or tugging of the tracheostomy tube. Immediately notify the primary health care provider of a pulsating tube.
Tube obstruction	Difficulty in breathing Noisy respirations Difficulty in inserting the suction catheter Thick, dry secretions Unexplained peak pressures if client is on a mechanical ventilator	The primary health care provider repositions or replaces the tube if obstruction occurs as a result of cuff prolapse over the end of the tube.	Assist the client to cough and deep breathe. Provide humidification and suctioning. Clean the inner cannula regularly.
Tube dislodgment	Difficulty in breathing Noisy respirations Restlessness Excessive coughing Audible wheeze or stridor	Be familiar with institutional policy regarding replacement of a tracheostomy tube as a nursing procedure. During the first 72 hours following surgical placement of the tracheostomy, the nurse manually ventilates the client by using a manual resuscitation (Ambu) bag, while another nurse calls the Rapid Response team for help. 72 hours following surgical placement of the tracheostomy: • Extend the client's neck and open the tissues of the stoma to secure the airway. • Grasp the retention sutures (if they are present) to spread the opening.	Secure the tube in place. Minimize manipulation and traction on the tube. Ensure that the client does not pull on the tube. Ensure that a tracheostomy tube of the same type and size is at the client's bedside.

Continued

TABLE 18.1   Complications of a Tracheostomy—cont'd

Complications and Description	Manifestations	Management	Prevention
		▪ Use a tracheal dilator (curved clamp) to hold the stoma open. ▪ Prepare to insert a tracheostomy tube; place the obturator into the tracheostomy tube, replace the tube, and remove the obturator. ▪ Maintain ventilation by resuscitation (Ambu) bag. ▪ Assess airflow and bilateral breath sounds. ▪ If unable to secure an airway, call the Rapid Response team and the anesthesiologist.	

Adapted from Ignatavicius D, Workman ML: *Medical-surgical nursing: patient centered collaborative care*, ed 7, Philadelphia, 2013, Saunders.

D. Suction-control chamber (see Fig. 18.6)
1. Provides suction, which can be controlled to provide negative pressure to the chest
2. Filled with various levels of water to achieve the desired level of suction; without this control, lung tissue could be sucked into the chest tube.
3. Gentle bubbling indicates that there is suction. It does not indicate that air is escaping from the pleural space.

E. Dry-suction system (see Fig. 18.6)
1. This is another type of chest drainage system, and because this is a dry suction system, absence of bubbling is noted in the suction control chamber.
2. A knob on the collection device is used to set the prescribed amount of suction; then the wall suction source dial is turned until a small orange floater valve appears in the window on the device (when the orange floater valve is in the window, the correct amount of suction is applied).

F. Portable chest drainage system
1. Small and portable chest drainage systems are also available and are dry systems that use a control flutter valve to prevent the backflow of air into the client's lung.
2. Principles of gravity and pressure, and the nursing care involved, are the same for all types of systems, and these systems allow greater ambulation and allow the client to go home with the chest tubes in place.

G. Interventions
1. Collection chamber
   a. Monitor the drainage. The RN and PHCP is notified if the drainage is more than 70 to 100 mL/hour or the drainage becomes bright red or increases suddenly. A client who returns from lung resection may have increased amounts of drainage initially.
   b. Mark the chest-tube drainage in the collection chamber at 1- to 4-hour intervals with the use of a piece of tape.

2. Water-seal chamber
   a. Monitor for the fluctuation of the fluid level in the water-seal chamber.
   b. Fluctuation in the water-seal chamber stops if the tube is obstructed, if a dependent loop exists, if the suction is not working properly, or if the lung has reexpanded.
   c. If the client has a known pneumothorax, intermittent bubbling in the water-seal chamber is expected as air is drained from the chest. Continuous bubbling indicates an air leak in the system.
   d. Notify the RN and PHCP if there is continuous bubbling in the water-seal chamber.
3. Suction-control chamber: Gentle (not vigorous) bubbling would be noted in the suction-control chamber. Vigorous bubbling indicates an air leak, and the RN and PHCP must be notified.
4. An occlusive sterile dressing is maintained at the insertion site.
5. A chest radiograph assesses the position of the tube and determines whether the lung has reexpanded.
6. Monitor the respiratory status and listen to the lung sounds.
7. Monitor for signs of an extended pneumothorax or hemothorax (respiratory distress, crepitus [subcutaneous emphysema], increase in bloody drainage, or a change to bright red drainage).
8. Keep the drainage system below the level of the chest, and the tubes free of kinks, dependent loops, or other obstructions.
9. Ensure that all connections are secure.
10. Encourage coughing and deep breathing.
11. Change the client's position frequently to promote drainage and ventilation.
12. Stripping or milking a chest tube is not done unless specifically prescribed by a PHCP and agency policy allows.

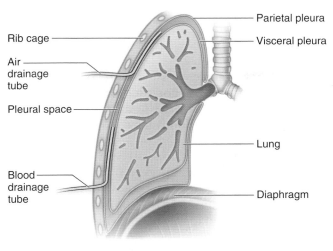

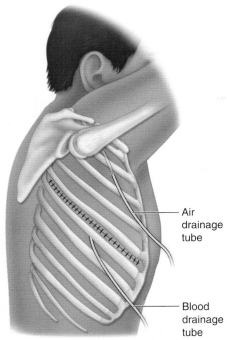

FIGURE 18.5 Chest tube placement.

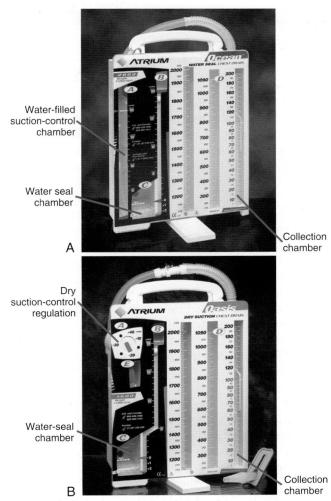

FIGURE 18.6 The Pleur-evac drainage system, a commercial three-bottle chest drainage device. A, Wet suction water seal chest drainage system. B, Dry suction control chest drainage system.

⚠ If the chest tube is pulled out of the chest accidentally, pinch the skin opening together, apply an occlusive sterile dressing, cover the dressing with overlapping pieces of 2-inch tape, and call the RN and PHCP immediately.

13. Keep a clamp (may be needed if the system needs to be changed) and a sterile occlusive dressing at the bedside at all times.
14. A chest tube is never clamped without a written prescription from the PHCP. Also, determine agency policy for clamping chest tubes.
15. If the drainage system cracks or breaks, the RN is notified immediately, and the chest tube is inserted into a bottle of sterile water. The cracked or broken system is removed and replaced with a new system.
16. Depending on the PHCP's preference, when the chest tube is to be removed, the client may be asked to take a deep breath and hold it, or exhale and bear down (i.e., Valsalva maneuver).
17. A dry sterile dressing, petroleum gauze dressing, or Telfa dressing (depending on the PHCP's preference) is taped in place after the removal of the chest tube.

WHAT WOULD YOU DO?

Answer: If the nurse notes that the chest tube drainage system is cracked, the nurse must immediately notify the RN. The chest tube would be disconnected from the system and submerged in a bottle of sterile water in order to maintain the water seal. The system will then need to be replaced, and this can be done by the RN, depending on agency policy. A clamp needs to be kept at the bedside in case the system needs to be changed. However, the nurse would never clamp a chest tube without a written prescription from the PHCP and per agency policy. The drainage system (chest tube and bottle of sterile water) must also be maintained below the level of the chest if this complication occurs.

PRACTICE QUESTIONS

1. The nurse is preparing to administer an intermittent tube feeding to a client. The nurse aspirates 90 mL of residual from the tube. What would the nurse do? **Select all that apply.**
   - ❏ 1. Hold the feeding.
   - ❏ 2. Document the amount of residual.
   - ❏ 3. Place it into a container for laboratory analysis.
   - ❏ 4. Reinstill the residual and administer the feeding.
   - ❏ 5. Deduct the amount of the residual from the new feeding before administering.

2. The nurse is providing endotracheal suctioning to a client who is mechanically ventilated when the client becomes restless and tachycardic. Which actions would the nurse take? **Select all that apply.**
   1. Notify the registered nurse (RN).
   2. Notify the Rapid Response team.
   3. Finish the suctioning as quickly as possible.
   4. Discontinue suctioning until the client is stabilized.
   5. Contact the respiratory department to suction the client.

3. The nurse has assisted in inserting a nasogastric (NG) tube in a client and is checking for the correct placement of a NG tube. Which is the **most** reliable data to ensure that the end of the tube is in the stomach?
   1. Placement is verified on x-ray.
   2. The pH of the aspirated fluid is 5.
   3. The aspirated fluid is bile green in color.
   4. Air injection is auscultated in the left upper quadrant.

4. A licensed practical nurse (LPN) is preparing to assist a registered nurse (RN) with removing a nasogastric (NG) tube from the client. Which interventions would be included in the procedure? **Select all that apply.**
   - ❏ 1. Remove the air from the balloon.
   - ❏ 2. Explain the procedure to the client.
   - ❏ 3. Ask the client to take a deep breath and hold.
   - ❏ 4. Pull the tube out in one continuous steady motion.
   - ❏ 5. Remove the device or tape securing the tube from the nose.

5. The nurse is assisting with monitoring the functioning of a chest-tube drainage system in a client who just returned from the recovery room after a thoracotomy with wedge resection. Which findings would the nurse expect to note? **Select all that apply.**
   - ❏ 1. Excessive bubbling in the water-seal chamber
   - ❏ 2. Vigorous bubbling in the suction-control chamber

   - ❏ 3. 50 mL of drainage in the drainage-collection chamber
   - ❏ 4. The drainage system is maintained below the client's chest.
   - ❏ 5. An occlusive dressing is in place over the chest-tube insertion site.
   - ❏ 6. Fluctuation of water in the tube of the water-seal chamber during inhalation and exhalation

6. The nurse is assigned to assist with caring for a client with esophageal varices who had a Sengstaken-Blakemore tube inserted because other treatment measures were unsuccessful. The nurse would check the client's room to ensure that which **priority** item is at the bedside?
   1. An obturator
   2. A Kelly clamp
   3. An irrigation set
   4. A pair of scissors

7. The nurse is inserting an indwelling urinary catheter into a male client. As the catheter is inserted into the urethra, urine begins to flow into the tubing. When would the nurse inflate the balloon?
   1. Immediately
   2. When resistance is met
   3. After inserting the catheter an additional 2.5 to 5 cm
   4. When the catheter is advanced to the point of bifurcation

8. The nurse is assigned to assist with caring for a client who has a chest tube. The nurse notes fluctuations of the fluid level in the water-seal chamber. Based on this observation, which action would be appropriate?
   1. Empty the drainage.
   2. Continue to monitor.
   3. Encourage the client to deep breathe.
   4. Encourage the client to hold his or her breath periodically.

9. The nurse is assigned to assist the primary health care provider (PHCP) with the removal of a chest tube. Which interventions would the nurse anticipate performing during this process? **Select all that apply.**
   - ❏ 1. Reinforce instructions to breathe deeply while the tube is removed.
   - ❏ 2. Cover the site with an occlusive dressing after the tube is removed.
   - ❏ 3. Clamp the chest tube near the insertion site just before the removal.
   - ❏ 4. Raise the drainage system to the level of the chest tube insertion site.
   - ❏ 5. Have the client perform the Valsalva maneuver as the chest tube is pulled out.

10. The nurse is planning to begin a continuous tube feeding on a client with a nasogastric (NG) tube. Which interventions would the nurse perform before initiating the feeding? **Select all that apply.**
- ❏ **1.** Irrigate the NG tube with saline.
- ❏ **2.** Explain the procedure to the client.
- ❏ **3.** Elevate the head of the bed to 45 degrees.
- ❏ **4.** Aspirate all stomach contents and discard.
- ❏ **5.** Ensure that the end of the NG tube is in the esophagus.
- ❏ **6.** Have a pair of scissors for emergency use at the bedside.

11. The nurse is preparing to administer an intermittent tube feeding to a client with a nasogastric (NG) tube. The nurse checks the residual and obtains an amount of 200 mL. Which actions would the nurse take? **Select all that apply.**
- ❏ **1.** Listen to the client's bowel sounds.
- ❏ **2.** Document and discard the residual.
- ❏ **3.** Offer the client sips of water to drink.
- ❏ **4.** Question the client regarding nausea.
- ❏ **5.** Determine whether the client has abdominal distension.
- ❏ **6.** Hold the feeding after flushing the tubing with 30 mL saline.

12. The nurse is assisting in planning care for a client with a chest tube. The nurse would suggest to include which interventions in the plan? **Select all that apply.**
- ❏ **1.** Pin the tubing to the bed linens.
- ❏ **2.** Be sure all connections remain airtight.
- ❏ **3.** Be sure all connections are taped and secure.
- ❏ **4.** Monitor closely for tubing that is kinked or obstructed.
- ❏ **5.** Empty the drainage from the drainage collection chamber daily.

13. The nurse is assigned to care for a client who has a chest tube. The nurse is told to monitor the client for crepitus (subcutaneous emphysema). Which method would be used to monitor the client for crepitus?
- **1.** Auscultating the posterior breath sounds
- **2.** Asking the client about pain upon inspiration
- **3.** Placing the hands over the rib area and observing expansion
- **4.** Palpating the skin around the chest and neck for a crackling sensation

14. The nurse is told that an assigned client will have a fenestrated tracheostomy tube inserted. The nurse plans care knowing that which facts are true with the use of a fenestrated tracheostomy tube? **Select all that apply.**
- ❏ **1.** Enables the client to speak
- ❏ **2.** Is necessary for mechanical ventilation
- ❏ **3.** Must have the cuff deflated when capped
- ❏ **4.** Eliminates the need for tracheostomy care
- ❏ **5.** Prevents air from being inhaled through the tracheostomy opening

15. The nurse is preparing to administer a medication through a nasogastric (NG) tube that is connected to suction. Which interventions would be included to accurately administer the medication? **Select all that apply.**
- ❏ **1.** Position the client supine to assist with medication absorption.
- ❏ **2.** Clamp the NG tube for 30 minutes after medication administration.
- ❏ **3.** Before medication administration, verify correct placement of tube.
- ❏ **4.** Flush the NG tube with saline before and after medication administration.
- ❏ **5.** Discontinue the suction from the tube during administration of medication.

ANSWERS

1. 2, 4
Rationale: Unless otherwise instructed or if the residual contents appear abnormal, an amount of less than 100 mL is reinstilled; then a normal amount of prescribed tube feeding is administered. The amount of residual would be documented. It is important to return the contents to the stomach to prevent electrolyte imbalances. The feeding is not held, and the residual is not sent to the laboratory. The tube feeding would continue at the prescribed rate.
Test-Taking Strategy: Note the subject, residual from a nasogastric tube. Generally the residual is always reinstilled to prevent electrolyte and nutritional imbalance. There is **no data in the question** that indicates that laboratory analysis is necessary. To prevent dehydration, clients need to get the correct amount of feeding prescribed.

2. 1, 4
Rationale: When suctioning a client with an endotracheal tube, the nurse removes the secretions and clears the airway. If a client becomes cyanotic or restless or develops tachycardia, bradycardia, or another abnormal heart rhythm, the nurse must discontinue suctioning until the client is stabilized. The nurse would also notify the RN. It is also important to monitor the vital signs and the pulse oximetry. If the client's condition continues to deteriorate, then the respiratory department and primary health care provider (PHCP) may need to be notified. There is no data in the question that indicates that the Rapid Response team needs to be notified.
Test-Taking Strategy: Focus on the subject, the client becomes restless and tachycardic during suctioning. Use the ABCs—airway, breathing, circulation—to direct you to the correct option.

3. 1

Rationale: The end of the NG tube needs to be in the stomach. An x-ray is the most reliable method of determining correct placement. The radiologist may recommend moving the tube backward or forward for a preferable placement. A low pH, such as 4.5, of the fluid aspirated is likely to be from the stomach, but pH is affected by tube feeding formulas and prescribed proton-pump inhibitors. The characteristic bile green is highly suggestive that the tube is in the stomach. Auscultation of the air injection is not recommended as a reliable method to establish correct placement.

Test-Taking Strategy: Focus on the strategic word, *most*. Focus on the fact that an x-ray gives objective proof as to placement of the end of the NG tube. The other methods are done but are not the most reliable. The air injection auscultation is not recommended but is sometimes in addition to one of the other methods.

4. 2, 3, 4, 5

Rationale: Before removing the tube, the client would be told about the procedure and review the instructions. The tape or securing device needs to be removed from the client's nose. When the NG tube is removed, the client is instructed to take and hold a deep breath. This will close the epiglottis, and the airway will be temporarily obstructed during the tube removal. This allows for the easy withdrawal of the tube through the esophagus into the nose. The tube is removed with one very smooth, continuous pull. There is no balloon that needs to be deflated on a NG tube.

Test-Taking Strategy: Focus on the subject, the procedure for removing an NG tube. Think about the procedure and consider what each client action identified in the options would produce. This will help direct you to the correct options.

5. 3, 4, 5, 6

Rationale: In a thoracotomy the lung is opened and exposed, and a wedge resection is the removal of part of the lung. The chest tube is placed during the surgery to remove fluid and air so the remaining lung can reinflate. The bubbling of water in the water-seal chamber would be gentle and indicates air drainage from the client. This is usually seen when intrathoracic pressure is greater than atmospheric pressure, and it may occur during exhalation, coughing, or sneezing. The fluctuation of water in the tube in the water-seal chamber during inhalation and exhalation is expected. An absence of fluctuation may indicate that the chest tube is obstructed, the lung has reexpanded, or no more air is leaking into the pleural space. Gentle (not vigorous) bubbling would be noted in the suction-control chamber. A total of 50 mL of drainage is not excessive in a client returning to the nursing unit from the recovery room; however, drainage of more than 70 to 100 mL/hour is considered excessive and requires RN and PHCP notification. The chest-tube insertion site is covered with an occlusive (airtight) dressing to prevent air from entering the pleural space. Positioning the drainage system below the client's chest allows gravity to drain the pleural space. Excessive and/or vigorous bubbling in the water-seal chamber may indicate an air leak, which is an unexpected finding.

Test-Taking Strategy: Focus on the subject, expected findings in a chest-tube drainage system. The words *excessive bubbling* and *vigorous bubbling* in options 1 and 2 are comparable or alike and would be eliminated. Also, think about the physi-

ology associated with chest tube drainage systems to answer correctly.

6. 4

Rationale: When the client has a Sengstaken-Blakemore tube, a pair of scissors must be kept at the client's bedside at all times. If the gastric balloon of the tube ruptures, the tube will move upward and potentially occlude the client's airway. The client needs to be observed for sudden respiratory distress. If this occurs, the RN is notified immediately, and the balloon lumens will be cut. An obturator and a Kelly clamp are kept at the bedside of a client with a tracheostomy. An irrigation set may also be kept at the bedside, but it is not the priority item.

Test-Taking Strategy: Note the strategic word, *priority*. Use ABCs—airway, breathing, circulation—to lead you to the emergency equipment to protect the client's airway if there is a malfunction with the Sengstaken-Blakemore tube. Use your knowledge of the structure, function, and placement of a Sengstaken-Blakemore tube to assist you in answering this question.

7. 4

Rationale: Urinary catheterization is a sterile procedure. When inserting an indwelling catheter, the nurse would ensure the balloon is in the bladder before inflating it. If the balloon is inflated in the urethra of the male client, trauma may occur. When catheterizing a male client, the nurse observes the tubing for the flow of urine and then continues to advance the catheter to the point of bifurcation and then inflates the balloon. The nurse then pulls the catheter back until slight resistance is felt and applies a catheter tube holder onto the thigh to hold the catheter in place. The balloon would not be inflated when urine is first observed, after advancing several more centimeters, or when resistance is felt.

Test-Taking Strategy: Focus on the subject, when to inflate the balloon when inserting an indwelling urinary catheter in a male client. Visualize the proper procedure for inserting an indwelling urinary catheter. Recalling that the catheter's balloon is behind the opening of the tip and that the male urethra is approximately 20 cm or 8 inches long will assist in answering correctly.

8. 2

Rationale: The presence of fluctuations in the fluid level in the water-seal chamber indicates a patent drainage system. With normal breathing, the water level rises with inspiration and falls with expiration. The apparatus and all connections must remain airtight at all times, and the drainage is never emptied because of the risk of disruption in the closed system, which can result in lung collapse. Encouraging the client to deep breathe is unrelated to this observation. The client is not told to hold his or her breath.

Test-Taking Strategy: Focus on the subject, the fluctuation of the fluid level in the water-seal chamber. Eliminate option 2 first because drainage is not emptied. Options 3 and 4 are comparable or alike and can be eliminated.

9. 2, 5

Rationale: A chest tube is removed when the lung has fully reexpanded or there is limited drainage. When the chest tube is removed, the client is asked to perform a Valsalva maneuver

(i.e., take a deep breath, exhale, and bear down), the tube is quickly withdrawn, and an airtight (occlusive) dressing is taped in place. An alternative instruction is to ask the client to take a deep breath and hold the breath while the tube is removed. After the tube is removed, the client needs to take deep breaths to ensure adequate lung expansion. The tube is not usually clamped before it is removed, and the drainage apparatus must always be lower than the chest tube site.
Test-Taking Strategy: Focus on the subject, removal of a chest tube. Visualize the procedure, client instructions, and the effect of each of the actions in the options to answer correctly.

10. 1, 2, 3
Rationale: When a tube feeding is initiated, the most important intervention is to make sure the NG tube is properly placed in the stomach to prevent aspiration of the formula. After explaining the procedure to the client and assessing placement of the tube, the nurse would irrigate the tube with saline to ensure the formula flows well through the tube. When a tube feeding is administered, the client is placed in a high Fowler's position for a bolus feeding and in a semi-Fowler's position (30–45 degrees) for a continuous feeding to allow gravity to help the flow of formula and to prevent reflux and aspiration. There is no need to aspirate contents because the formula has not been given and the contents are gastric secretions. Scissors are not kept at the bedside with a NG tube. Scissors are kept at the bedside with the Sengstaken-Blakemore tube that is used to treat bleeding esophageal varices; if respiratory distress occurs, the scissors are used to immediately cut the tube to deflate the balloons. The correct placement for the end of the NG tube is in the stomach, not the esophagus.
Test-Taking Strategy: Focus on the subject, intervention before initiation of tube feeding administration through a NG tube. Visualize the procedure. Note that the nurse would always explain a nonemergent procedure to the client before initiating the intervention. Read the options carefully and note that the feeding was not imitated to eliminate the need to aspirate residual. Note that the NG tube is nasal gastric and gastric refers to the stomach, not esophagus in medical terminology.

11. 1, 4, 5, 6
Rationale: Large-volume aspirates in clients receiving intermittent tube feedings indicate delayed gastric emptying and place the client at risk for aspiration. The nurse would obtain data concerning the presence of nausea, bowel sounds, and abdominal distention indicating possible bowel obstruction. When 200 mL of residual formula is obtained, the feeding is held and the RN is notified because this is an indication that the feeding is not being absorbed. If the residual is less than 100 mL, the feeding is usually administered. If the feeding will be held, the tube needs to be flushed with 30 mL saline to decrease the risk of the tube clogging from residual formula. In addition, the nurse would always check the PHCP's prescriptions and agency policy regarding residual amounts. The residual amount would be documented, but the residual aspirated is returned to the client to avoid electrolyte imbalance. There is no indication to give the client sips of water.
Test-Taking Strategy: Focus on the subject, the action to take with a high residual intermittent tube feeding. Also use the

steps of the nursing process to determine that additional data, the first step, would be gathered to determine why the client has such a large residual. Recalling that the feeding is sometimes held when more than 100 mL of residual are obtained will direct you to the correct options.

12. 2, 3, 4
Rationale: The chest-tube system must be maintained as a closed system in order for the air to be removed by suction and for the lungs to reexpand to a normal state. The connections must be air tight (no leaks), and all connections must be taped and secure. It is important that the tubes to the suction and the chest tube be patent (without kinks or obstructions). Chest-tube tubing is never pinned to the bed linens because this presents the risk of accidental dislodgment of the tube when the client moves. The chest tube system is not opened and emptied because a closed system must be maintained; if the system is opened, air pressure causes air to rush in, and lung collapse can occur.
Test-Taking Strategy: Focus on the subject, interventions for the client with a chest tube. Think about the principles associated with maintaining a closed chest-tube drainage system and its purpose.

13. 4
Rationale: Air caught under the skin in the subcutaneous tissues is known as crepitus or subcutaneous emphysema. It presents as a "puffed-up" appearance that is caused by the leakage of air into the subcutaneous tissues. It is monitored by palpating, and it feels like bubble wrap when palpated. Auscultation of posterior breath sounds gives data about adequate depth of respirations. Pain upon inspiration can occur with pleurisy (inflammation of the pleurae) or pericarditis. Placing the hands over the rib area is a method of determining equal chest expansion on each side.
Test-Taking Strategy: Note the subject, monitoring for crepitus (subcutaneous emphysema). Think about what this condition entails to answer correctly. Also note the word *subcutaneous* in the question and that it relates to the area just under the skin. This will assist you in selecting the correct option.

14. 1, 3
Rationale: A fenestrated tracheostomy tube is used when a client is being weaned from breathing through the tracheostomy to breathing normally through the nose and mouth. A fenestrated tube has a small opening in the outer cannula that allows some air to escape through the larynx; this type of tube enables the client to speak. The cuff of the tracheostomy tube must always be deflated before the fenestrated tube is capped. When the cuff is inflated, the tracheostomy tube can be used for mechanical ventilation. When the cuff is deflated and the cap is applied, the client can breathe around the tracheostomy tube. The client continues to need cleaning of the tracheostomy site. The client is unable to breathe through the tracheal opening or at all if the cuff is inflated and the opening capped.
Test-Taking Strategy: Focus on the subject, a fenestrated tracheostomy tube. Recall that the term *fenestrated* means there is an opening in the object like a fenestrated drape in a catheterization kit. Knowledge regarding the design and purpose of a fenestrated tracheostomy tube will direct you to the correct option.

15. 2, 3, 4, 5

Rationale: Oral medications are sometimes administered to a client who is prescribed suction through a nasogastric (NG) tube. The nurse must verify that the tube has correct placement by checking drainage characteristics and pH to avoid aspiration of the medication into the trachea. The NG tube must be flushed with saline before and after medication administration to facilitate delivery and promote absorption. The suction must be stopped during administration and then the tube is clamped for 30 minutes afterward. The client needs to be in an upright position at least 30 degrees, but higher is better to avoid aspiration. Medications would not be given in the supine position.

Test-Taking Strategy: Focus on the **subject**, medication administration to a client with an NG tube. Visualize the interventions in a stepwise manner. Evaluate each option regarding promoting medication absorption and safe practice. Recall that the risk of aspiration is great with the supine position.

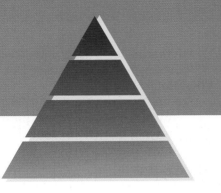

UNIT V

Growth and Development Across the Life Span

 Pyramid to Success

Normal growth and development proceed in an orderly, systematic, and predictable pattern, which provides a basis for identifying and assessing an individual's abilities. Understanding the normal path of growth and development across the life span assists the nurse with identifying appropriate and expected human behavior. The Pyramid to Success focuses on Sigmund Freud's theory of psychosexual development, Jean Piaget's theory of cognitive development, Erik Erikson's psychosocial theory, and Lawrence Kohlberg's theory of moral development. Growth and development concepts also focus on the aging process; and on physical characteristics, nutritional behaviors, skills, play, and specific safety measures relevant to a particular age group that will ensure a safe and hazard-free environment. When a question is presented on the NCLEX-PN® examination, if an age is identified in the question, note the age and think about the associated growth and developmental concepts to answer the question correctly.

Client Needs: Learning Objectives

Safe and Effective Care Environment
Acting as a client advocate
Communicating with the interprofessional health care team
Ensuring home safety and security plans
Ensuring that informed consent has been obtained for invasive treatments or procedures
Establishing priorities of care
Maintaining confidentiality
Preventing accidents and errors

Providing care in accordance with ethical and legal standards
Providing care using a nonjudgmental approach
Respecting client and family needs, based on their preferences
Implementing standard precautions and other transmission-based precautions as appropriate
Upholding the client's rights

Health Promotion and Maintenance
Assisting with client and family education
Discussing high-risk behaviors and lifestyle choices
Identifying changes that occur as a result of the aging process
Identifying developmental stages and transitions
Maintaining health and wellness and self-care measures
Monitoring growth and development
Performing the necessary health and physical data collection techniques
Respecting health care beliefs and preferences

Psychosocial Integrity
Assessing for abuse and neglect
Considering grief and loss issues and end-of-life care
Identifying coping mechanisms
Identifying cultural practices and beliefs of the client and appropriate support systems
Identifying loss of quantity and quality of relationships with the older client
Monitoring for adjustment to potential deterioration in physical and mental health and well-being in the older client
Monitoring for changes and adjustment in role function in the older client (threat to independent functioning)

Monitoring for sensory and perceptual alterations

Providing resources for the client and family

Physiological Integrity

Administering medication safely and assisting with teaching the client about prescribed medications

Identifying practices or restrictions related to procedures and treatments

Monitoring for alterations in body systems and the related risks associated with the client's age

Providing basic care and comfort needs

Providing interventions compatible with the client's age; cultural, religious, and health care beliefs; education level; and language

Client Needs lists modified from: National Council of State Boards of Nursing, Inc. (NCSBN). *NCLEX-PN Examination: Test Plan for the National Council Licensure Examination for Practical Nurses*, effective April 2020. Chicago: NCSBN.

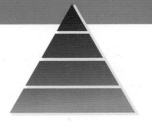

CHAPTER 19

Theories of Growth and Development

PRIORITY CONCEPTS Development; Health Promotion

I. Psychosocial Development: Erik Erikson

A. The theory

1. Erikson's theory of psychosocial development describes the human life cycle as a series of eight ego developmental stages from birth to death.
2. Each stage presents a psychosocial crisis, the goal of which is to integrate physical, maturational, and societal demands.
3. The result of one stage may not be permanent, but it can be changed by experience(s) later in life.
4. The theory focuses on psychosocial tasks that are accomplished throughout the lifecycle.

B. Psychosocial development: Occurs through a life-long series of crises affected by social and cultural factors.

⚠ According to Erikson's theory of psychosocial development, each psychosocial crisis needs to be resolved for the child or adult to progress emotionally. Unsuccessful resolution may leave the person emotionally weakened.

C. Stages of psychosocial development (Table 19.1)
D. Interventions to assist the client in achieving Erikson's stages of development (Box 19.1)

II. Cognitive Development: Jean Piaget

A. The theory

1. Piaget's theory defines cognitive acts as the ways in which the mind organizes and adapts to its environment (i.e., "mental mapping").

2. Schema: Refers to an individual's cognitive structure or framework of thought
3. Schemata
   a. Schemata are categories that an individual forms in his or her mind to organize and understand the world.
   b. A young child has only a few schemata with which to understand the world; gradually these are increased.
   c. Adults use a wide variety of schemata to understand the world.
4. Assimilation
   a. Assimilation is the ability to incorporate new ideas, objects, and experiences into the framework of one's thoughts.
   b. The growing child will perceive and give meaning to new information according to what is already known and understood.
5. Accommodation
   a. Accommodation is the ability to change a schema to introduce new ideas, objects, or experiences.
   b. Accommodation changes the mental structure so that new experiences can be added.

B. Stages of cognitive development

1. Sensorimotor stage
   a. Birth to 2 years
   b. Development proceeds from reflex activity to imagining and solving problems through the senses and movement.
   c. The infant or toddler learns about reality and how it works.
   d. The infant or toddler does not recognize that objects continue to exist, even if out of the visual field.
2. Preoperational stage
   a. 2 to 7 years
   b. The child learns to think in terms of past, present, and future.

TABLE 19.1 Erik Erikson's Stages of Psychosocial Development

Age	Psychosocial Crisis	Task	Successful Resolution of Crisis	Unsuccessful Resolution of Crisis
Infancy (birth to 18 months)	Trust vs. mistrust	Attachment to the mother	Trust in other people; faith and hope about the environment and the future	General difficulties relating to others effectively; suspicion; trust/fear conflict; fear of the future
Early childhood (18 months to 3 years)	Autonomy vs. shame and doubt	Gaining some basic control over the self and the environment	Sense of self-control and adequacy; willpower	Independence/fear conflict; severe feelings of self-doubt; lack of self-control
Late childhood (3–6 years)	Initiative vs. guilt	Becoming purposeful and directive	Ability to initiate one's own activities; sense of purpose	Aggression/fear conflict; sense of inadequacy or guilt
School age (6–12 years)	Industry vs. inferiority	Developing social, physical, and learning skills	Competence; ability to learn and work	Sense of inferiority; difficulty learning and working
Adolescence (12–20 years)	Identity vs. role confusion	Developing a sense of identity	Sense of personal identity	Unsure about one's identity; have a weak sense of self, experience role confusion, and are confused about the future
Early adulthood (20–35 years)	Intimacy vs. isolation	Establishing intimate bonds of love and friendship	Ability to love deeply and commit oneself	Emotional isolation; egocentricity
Middle adulthood (35–65 years)	Generativity vs. stagnation	Fulfilling life goals that involve family, career, and society	Ability to give and care for others	Self-absorption; inability to grow as a person
Later (65 years to death)	Integrity vs. despair	Looking back over one's life and accepting its meaning	Sense of integrity and fulfillment	Dissatisfaction with life

Adapted from Halter MJ: *Varcarolis' foundations of psychiatric mental health nursing*, ed 7, St. Louis, 2014, Saunders.

BOX 19.1 Interventions to Assist the Client in Achieving Erikson's Stages of Development

Infancy
Hold the infant often.
Offer comfort after painful procedures.
Meet the infant's needs for food and hygiene.
Encourage parents to room in while infant is hospitalized.

Early Childhood
Allow self-feeding opportunities.
Encourage child to remove and put on own clothes.
Allow for choice.

Late Childhood
Offer medical equipment for play.
Respect the child's choices and expressions of feelings.

School Age
Encourage the child to continue schoolwork while hospitalized.
Encourage the child to bring favorite leisure activities, such as board games, electronic games, or books to the hospital.

Adolescence
Take the health history and perform examinations without parents present.
Allow adolescent a choice in the plan of care.

Early Adulthood
Include support from client's partner or significant other.
Assist with rehabilitation and contacting support services as needed before returning to work.

Middle Adulthood
Assist in choosing creative ways to foster social development.
Encourage volunteer activities.

Later Adulthood
Listen attentively to reminiscent stories about their life's accomplishments.
Assist with making changes to living arrangements.

---

   c. The child moves from knowing the world through sensation and movement to prelogical thinking and finding solutions to problems.

   d. The child is egocentric.

   e. The child is unable to conceptualize and requires concrete examples.

3. Concrete operational

   a. 7 to 11 years

   b. The child is able to classify, order, and sort facts.

   c. The child moves from prelogical thought to solving concrete problems through logic.

   d. The child begins to develop abstract thinking.

    e. The child is less egocentric and thinks about how others may view a situation.

  4. Formal operations

    a. 11 years to adulthood

    b. The person is able to think abstractly and logically.

    c. Logical thinking is expanded to include solving abstract and concrete problems.

III. Moral Development: Lawrence Kohlberg

A. Moral development

  1. Moral development is a complicated process involving the acceptance of the values and rules of society in a way that shapes behavior.

  2. Moral development is classified into a series of levels and behaviors.

  3. Moral development is sequential, but people do not automatically go from one stage or level to the next as they mature.

  4. Stages or levels of moral development cannot be skipped.

B. Levels of moral development (Box 19.2)

IV. Psychosexual Development: Sigmund Freud

A. Components of the theory (Box 19.3)

BOX 19.2   Moral Development and Lawrence Kohlberg

Level One: Preconventional Morality

Stage 0 (Birth to 2 Years): Egocentric Judgment

The infant has no awareness of right or wrong.

Stage 1 (2–4 Years): Punishment–Obedience Orientation

At this stage, children cannot reason as mature members of society.

Children view the world in a selfish way, with no real understanding of right or wrong.

The child obeys rules and demonstrates acceptable behavior to avoid punishment and to avoid displeasing those who are in power, and because he or she fears punishment from a superior force, such as a parent.

A toddler typically is at the first substage of the preconventional stage. This involves a punishment–obedience orientation in which the toddler makes judgments on the basis of avoiding punishment or obtaining a reward.

Physical punishment and withholding privileges tend to give the toddler a negative view of morals.

Withdrawing love and affection as punishment leads to feelings of guilt in the toddler.

Appropriate discipline includes providing simple explanations of why certain behaviors are not acceptable, praising appropriate behavior, and using distractions when the toddler is headed for danger.

Stage 2 (4–7 Years): Instrumental Relativist Orientation

The child conforms to rules to obtain rewards or have favors returned.

The child's moral standards are those of others, and the child observes them to avoid punishment or obtain rewards.

A preschooler is in the preconventional stage of moral development.

During this stage, the conscience emerges, and the emphasis is on external control.

Level Two: Conventional Morality

The child conforms to rules to please others.

The child has an increased awareness of others' feelings.

A concern for social order begins to emerge.

A child views good behavior as that of which those in authority will approve.

If the behavior is not acceptable, the child feels guilty.

Stage 3 (7–10 Years): Good Boy–Nice Girl Orientation

Conformity occurs to avoid disapproval or dislike by others.

This stage involves living up to what is expected by individuals close to the child or what individuals generally expect of others in their roles as son, brother, friend, and so on.

Being good is important and is interpreted as having good motives and showing concern about others.

It also means maintaining mutual relationships with the use of such characteristics as trust, loyalty, respect, and gratitude.

Stage 4 (10–12 Years): Law-and-Order Orientation

The child has more concern with society as a whole.

The emphasis is on obeying laws to maintain social order.

Moral reasoning develops as the child shifts the focus of living to society.

The school-age child is at the conventional level of the role-conformity stage and has an increased desire to please others.

The child observes, and to some extent internalizes, the standards of others.

The child wants to be considered "good" by those individuals whose opinions matter to him or her.

Level Three: Postconventional Morality

The individual focuses on individual rights and principles of conscience.

The focus is a concern regarding what is best for all.

Stage 5 (12 Years and Older): Social Contract and Legalistic Orientation

The adolescent is aware that people hold a variety of values and opinions, and most values and rules are relative to the group.

The adolescent in this stage gives, as well as takes, and does not expect to get something without paying for it.

At this stage, the adolescent may disobey rules if they feel they are inconsistent with their personal values.

Stage 6: Universal Ethical Principles Orientation

Conformity is based on universal principles of justice and occurs to avoid self-condemnation.

This stage involves following self-chosen ethical principles.

The development of the postconventional level of morality occurs in the adolescent at about the age of 13 years. It is marked by the development of an individual conscience and a defined set of moral values.

The adolescent can now acknowledge a conflict between two socially accepted standards and try to decide between them.

The control of conduct is now internal, both in standards observed and in reasoning about right and wrong.

> **BOX 19.3** **Components of Sigmund Freud's Psychosexual Development Theory**
>
> - Levels of awareness
> - Agencies of the mind: id, ego, and superego
> - Concept of anxiety and defense mechanisms
> - Psychosexual stages of development

B. Levels of awareness

1. Unconscious level of awareness
   a. The unconscious is not logical and is governed by the Pleasure Principle, which refers to seeking immediate tension reduction.
   b. Memories, feelings, thoughts, and wishes are repressed and are not available to the conscious mind.
   c. These repressed memories, thoughts, or feelings, if made prematurely conscious, can cause anxiety.
2. Preconscious level of awareness
   a. The preconscious is also called the *subconscious*.
   b. Preconscious includes experiences, thoughts, feelings, or desires that might not be in an individual's immediate awareness but that can be recalled to consciousness.
   c. The subconscious can help repress unpleasant thoughts or feelings and examine and censor certain wishes and thinking.
3. Conscious level of awareness
   a. The conscious mind is logical and regulated by the Reality Principle.
   b. Consciousness includes all experiences that are within an individual's awareness and that the individual is able to control and includes all information that is easily remembered and immediately available to an individual.

C. Agencies of the mind: id, ego, and superego

 The id, ego, and superego are the three systems of personality. These psychological processes follow different operating principles. In a mature and well-adjusted personality, they work together as a team under the leadership of the ego.

1. The id
   a. Source of all drives, present at birth, operates according to the Pleasure Principle
   b. Does not tolerate uncomfortable states and seeks to discharge the tension and return to a more comfortable, constant level of energy
   c. Acts immediately in an impulsive, irrational way and pays no attention to the consequences of its actions; therefore, often behaves in ways harmful to self and others
   d. The primary process is a psychological activity in which the id attempts to reduce tension.

   e. The primary process by itself is not capable of reducing tension; therefore, a secondary psychological process must develop if the individual is to survive. When this occurs, the structure of the second system of the personality, the ego, begins to take form.
2. The ego
   a. Functions include reality testing and problem solving; follows the Reality Principle
   b. Begins its development during the fourth or fifth month of life
   c. Emerges out of the id and acts as an intermediary between the id and the external world
   d. Emerges because the needs, wishes, and demands of the id require appropriate exchanges with the outside world of reality
   e. Distinguishes between things in the mind and things in the external world
3. The superego
   a. Necessary part of socialization that develops during the phallic stage of 3 to 6 years of age
   b. Develops from the interactions with one's parents during the extended period of childhood dependency
   c. Includes the internalization of the values, ideals, and moral standards of society
   d. The superego consists of the conscience and the ego ideal.
   e. The conscience refers to the capacity for self-evaluation and criticism. When moral codes are violated, the conscience punishes the individual by instilling guilt.

D. Anxiety and defense mechanisms
1. The ego develops defenses or defense mechanisms to fight off anxiety.
2. Defense mechanisms operate on an unconscious level (except for suppression), so the individual is not aware of their operation.
3. Defense mechanisms deny, falsify, or distort reality to make it less threatening.
4. An individual cannot survive without defense mechanisms; however, if they become too extreme in distorting reality, then interference in healthy adjustment and personal growth may occur.

E. Psychosexual stages of development (Box 19.4)
1. Human development proceeds through a series of stages from infancy to adulthood.
2. Each stage is characterized by the inborn tendency of all individuals to reduce tension and seek pleasure.
3. Each stage is associated with a particular conflict that must be resolved before the child can move successfully to the next stage.
4. Experiences during the early stages determine an individual's adjustment patterns and the personality traits that the individual has as an adult.

BOX 19.4 Freud's Psychosexual Stages of Development

Oral Stage (Birth to 1 Year)
During this stage, the infant is concerned with self-gratification.

The infant is all id, operating on the Pleasure Principle and striving for the immediate gratification of needs.

When the infant experiences the gratification of basic needs, a sense of trust and security begins.

The ego begins to emerge as the infant begins to see self as separate from the mother. This marks the beginning of the development of a sense of self.

Anal Stage (1–3 Years)
Toilet training occurs during this period, and the child gains pleasure from both the elimination and retention of feces.

The conflict of this stage is between demands from society and parents and the sensations of pleasure associated with the anus.

The child begins to gain a sense of control over instinctive drives and learns to delay immediate gratification to gain a future goal.

Phallic Stage (3–6 Years)
The child experiences both pleasurable and conflicting feelings associated with the genital organs.

The pleasures of masturbation and the fantasy life of children set the stage for the Oedipus complex.

The child's unconscious sexual attraction to, and wish to possess, the parent of the opposite sex; the hostility toward, and desire to remove the parent of the same sex; and the subsequent guilt regarding these wishes comprise the conflict that the child faces.

The conflict is resolved when the child identifies with the parent of the same sex.

The emergence of the superego is both the solution to and the result of these intense impulses.

Latency Stage (6–12 Years)
During this stage, there is a tapering off of conscious biological and sexual urges.

The sexual impulses are channeled and elevated into a more culturally accepted level of activity.

The growth of ego functions and the ability to care about and relate to others outside of the home are the tasks of this stage of development.

Genital Stage (12 Years and Beyond)
This emerges at adolescence with the onset of puberty, when the genital organs mature.

The individual gains gratification from his or her own body.

During this stage, the individual develops satisfying sexual and emotional relationships with members of the opposite sex.

The individual plans life goals and gains a strong sense of personal identity.

WHAT WOULD YOU DO?

Answer: According to Freud's psychosexual stages of development, between the ages of 3 and 6 years the child is in the phallic stage. At this time, the child devotes much energy to examining genitalia, masturbating, and expressing interest in sexual concerns. Therefore, the nurse would alleviate the mother's concern by telling the mother that this behavior is normal.

PRACTICE QUESTIONS

1. Which statement by a nursing student about Kohlberg's theory of moral development indicates the **need for further teaching** about the theory?
   1. "All individuals move through all six stages in a sequential fashion."
   2. "Moral development progresses in relation to cognitive development."
   3. "A person's ability to make moral judgments develops over a period of time."
   4. "It provides a framework for understanding how individuals determine a moral code to guide his or her behavior."

2. The parents of an 8-year-old child tell the nurse that they are concerned about the child because the child seems to be more attentive to friends than anyone else. Which is the appropriate nursing response?
   1. "You need to be concerned."
   2. "You need to monitor the child's behavior closely."
   3. "You need to praise the child more often to stop this behavior."
   4. "At this age, the child is developing his or her own personality."

3. The nurse notes that a 6-year-old child does not recognize that objects exist even when the objects are outside of the visual field. Based on this observation, which action would the nurse take?
   1. Move the objects in the child's direct field of vision.
   2. Teach the child how to visually scan the environment.
   3. Report the observation to the primary health care provider.
   4. Provide additional lighting for the child during play activities.

4. The nurse is providing instructions to a new parent regarding the psychosocial development of the infant. Using Erikson's psychosocial development theory, which instruction would the nurse reinforce to the parents?
   1. Allow the infant to signal a need.
   2. Anticipate all of the needs of the infant.
   3. Attend to the crying infant immediately.
   4. Avoid the infant during the first 10 minutes of crying.

5. The parent of a 3-year-old tells the nurse that the child is constantly rebelling and having temper tantrums. Which instruction would the nurse reinforce to the parent?
   1. Set limits on the child's behavior.
   2. Ignore the child when this behavior occurs.
   3. Allow the behavior, because this is normal at this age period.
   4. Punish the child every time the child says "no" to change the behavior.

6. The nurse is caring for an older client who is reminiscing about past life experiences in a positive manner. The nurse plans care with the understanding that this behavior indicates which of the following?
   1. A mental status alteration
   2. A normal psychosocial response
   3. A need for psychiatric consultation
   4. A sensory deficit requiring social activities

7. The nurse is observing a parent and 3-year-old child interacting in the clinic waiting room. The child begins to bounce on the couch. The parent removes the child from the couch stating firmly, "Couches are for sitting, not for jumping." The parent then gives the child a toy to play with on the carpet. The child plays with the toy until called by the nurse. The nurse determines the child is acting within which Kohlberg stage of moral development?
   1. Egocentric judgment
   2. Law-and-order orientation
   3. Punishment–obedience stage
   4. Good boy–nice girl orientation

8. The nurse determines a child is in the "preoperational" phase of Piaget's cognitive developmental theory when the child makes which statement?
   1. "I know all of my multiplication tables by memory."
   2. "The ball is gone," when a ball disappears out of sight.
   3. "I'll use a map to help me find my way in a new town."
   4. "The moon follows me, and goes to bed when I go to bed."

9. A child remarks, "I share my toys and snacks with my friends so they will like me more." The nurse determines the child is in which stage of moral development?
   1. Egocentric judgment
   2. Law-and-order orientation
   3. Good boy–nice girl orientation
   4. Social contract and legalistic orientation

10. The nursing student is preparing a conference on Freud's psychosexual stages of development, specifically the anal stage. Which appropriately relates to this stage?
   1. Gratification of self
   2. Beginning of toilet training
   3. Tapering off of conscious biological and sexual urges
   4. Association with pleasurable and conflicting feelings about the genital organs

ANSWERS

1. 1
Rationale: Kohlberg's theory states that individuals move through the six stages of development in a sequential fashion but that not everyone reaches stages 5 or 6 as part of their development of personal morality. The other options are correct statements regarding Kohlberg's theory.
Test-Taking Strategy: Note the strategic words, *need for further teaching*. These words indicate a negative event query and ask you to select an option that is an incorrect statement. Also, note the closed-ended word, "all" in the answer.

2. 4
Rationale: According to Erikson, at ages 7 to 12 years, the child begins to move toward receiving support from peers and friends and away from that of parents. The child also begins to develop special interests that reflect his or her own developing personality instead of those of the parents. Therefore, the other options identify incorrect responses.
Test-Taking Strategy: Note the subject, Erikson's psychosocial development for a school-age child, and remember the importance of peer groups. You can eliminate options 1 and 2 because there is no reason to be concerned or to monitor the child's behavior. Eliminate option 3 next; although praising the child for accomplishments is important at this age, the behavior that the child is exhibiting is normal.

3. 3
Rationale: According to Jean Piaget's theory of cognitive development, it is normal for the infant or toddler not to recognize that objects continue to be in existence, even if out of the visual field; however, this is abnormal for a 6-year-old. If a 6-year old child does not recognize that objects still exist even when outside the visual field, the child is not progressing normally through the developmental stages. The nurse

must report this finding to the primary health care provider. Options 1, 2, and 4 delay necessary follow-up and treatment. **Test-Taking Strategy:** Focus on the data in the question. Also, note the age of the child and think about developmental concepts related to this age. Noting that the child is not able to recognize that objects continue to be in existence, even if out of the visual field, will direct you to the correct option. Also, note that options 1, 2, and 4 are comparable or alike and are interventions that will delay follow-up for an abnormal observation.

4. 1
Rationale: According to Erikson, the caregiver would not try to anticipate the infant's needs at all times but rather allow the infant to signal his or her needs. If an infant is not allowed to signal a need, the infant will not learn how to control the environment. Erikson believed that a delayed or prolonged response to an infant's signal would inhibit the development of trust and lead to the mistrust of others. Therefore, the remaining options are incorrect.
Test-Taking Strategy: Note the subject, Erikson's stage of development for an infant. This stage is to develop trust. First, eliminate options 3 and 4 with the words *immediately* and *avoid*. Additionally, eliminate option 2 with the closed-ended word, "all."

5. 1
Rationale: According to Erikson, the child focuses on independence between the ages of 1 and 3 years. Gaining independence often means that the child has to rebel against the parents' wishes. Saying things like "no" and "mine" and having temper tantrums are common during this period of development. Being consistent and setting limits on the child's behavior are necessary elements. Punishing the child every time the child says "no" is likely to produce a negative response.
Test-Taking Strategy: Note the subject, actions to take for "temper tantrums." Options mentioning ignoring or allowing behavior can be eliminated first because they are comparable or alike. Eliminate the option of punishment next because this action is likely to produce a negative response during this normal developmental pattern.

6. 2
Rationale: According to Erikson, the later years of life are from 65 years of age until death. The adult reminisces about past life experiences, often viewing them in a positive way. The adult needs to feel good about his or her accomplishments, see successes in his or her life, and feel that he or she has made a contribution to society.
Test-Taking Strategy: Use your knowledge of the subject, Erikson's theory of psychosocial development, in regard to late adulthood, to answer the question. Note that options 1, 3, and 4 are comparable or alike; this will direct you to the correct option.

7. 3
Rationale: Kohlberg's theory states that individuals move through the six stages of development in a sequential fashion, but not everyone reaches stages 5 and 6 during his or her development of personal morality. The theory provides a framework for understanding how individuals determine a moral code to guide their behavior. It also states that moral development progresses in relation to cognitive development, and a person's ability to make moral judgments develops over a period of time. In stage 1 (ages 2–3 years; punishment–obedience orientation), children cannot reason as mature members of society because they are too young to do so. A child obeys rules to avoid punishment. It is appropriate for a parent to explain limitations, and to provide distractions. In the egocentric stage, an infant has no concept of right or wrong. A child who is in the law-and-order orientation stage obeys laws to maintain social order. In the good boy–nice girl orientation stage, a child behaves in a way to avoid displeasing others.
Test-Taking Strategy: Focus on the information in the question, parents remove the child from the couch and then redirect the child's attention. The punishment–obedience stage is when parents explain limitations and provide distractions. Recall the ages associated with each stage and that the theory provides a framework for understanding how individuals determine a moral code to guide their behavior.

8. 4
Rationale: In the preoperational stage, the child is demonstrating egocentric thinking by believing the moon's actions revolve around the child. In the sensorimotor stage, a child does not believe an object exists if it is not in sight. A child in the concrete operations stage is able to classify, order, and sort facts, such as the multiplication tables. A child in the formal operations stage is able to solve more complex problems, such as using a map to determine location and directions.
Test-Taking Strategy: Focus on the subject, Piaget's theory. Use knowledge regarding the characteristics of cognitive developmental theory for a child in the preoperational stage. Remember, in the preoperational stage, the child is egocentric and believes other objects exist for the purpose of the child.

9. 3
Rationale: According to Kohlberg's theory of moral development, during the good boy–nice girl orientation, the child acts in a way to please other people. Sharing is an example of this behavior. A child in the egocentric judgment stage has no awareness of right or wrong. A person in the law-and-order orientation stage obeys laws to maintain social order. During the social contract and legalistic orientation stage, a person is aware that others may have another set of values and opinions.
Test-taking Strategy: Focus on the information in the question, the child shares toys and snacks with friends. This will lead you to the option of the child being in the good boy–nice girl orientation. The options of law-and-order, egocentric judgment, and legalistic do not describe the child's behavior and statements.

10. 2
Rationale: Toilet training generally occurs during this period. According to Freud, the child gains pleasure from both the elimination and retention of feces. Self-gratification relates to the oral stage. Tapering off of conscious biological and sexual urges relates to the latency period. Association with pleasurable and conflicting feelings about genital organs relates to the phallic stage.
Test-Taking Strategy: Focus on the subject, Freud's stages of psychosexual development. Note the relationship between the words *anal* in the question and *toilet training* in the correct option.

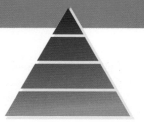

CHAPTER 20

Growth, Development, and Stages of Life

PRIORITY CONCEPTS Development, Family Dynamics

WHAT WOULD YOU DO ?

The nurse is caring for a hospitalized preschool child who is very apprehensive. What would the nurse do to assist with promoting comfort for the child?
Answer located on p. 242.

I. The Hospitalized Infant and Toddler

A. Separation anxiety
  1. Protest
     a. Cries, screams, searches for a parent; avoids and rejects contact with strangers
     b. Verbal attacks on others
     c. Physical fighting: kicks, fights, hits, and pinches
  2. Despair
     a. Withdrawn, depressed, and uninterested in the environment
     b. Loss of newly learned skills
  3. Detachment
     a. Detachment is uncommon and occurs only after lengthy separations from the parent.
     b. Superficially, the toddler appears to have adjusted to the loss.
     c. During the detachment phase, the toddler again becomes more interested in the environment, plays with others, and seems to form new relationships. This behavior is a form of resignation and is not a sign of contentment.
     d. The toddler detaches from the parents in an effort to escape the emotional pain of desiring the parent's presence.
     e. The toddler copes by forming shallow relationships with others, becoming increasingly self-centered, and attaching primary importance to material objects.
     f. Detachment is the most concerning phase, because the reversal of the potential adverse effects is less likely to occur after detachment is established.
     g. In most situations, the temporary separation imposed by hospitalization does not cause such prolonged parental absence that the toddler enters into detachment.
B. Fear of injury and pain: Affected by previous experiences, separation from parents, and preparation for the experience
C. Loss of control
  1. Hospitalization with its own set of rituals and routines can severely disrupt the life of a toddler.
  2. The lack of control is often exhibited in behaviors related to feeding, toileting, playing, and bedtime.
  3. The toddler may demonstrate regression.
D. Interventions
  1. Provide cuddling and touch and talk softly to the infant.
  2. Provide opportunities for sucking and oral stimulation for the infant using a pacifier if the infant is not to receive anything by mouth.
  3. Provide stimulation for the infant, if appropriate, with the use of objects of contrasting colors and textures.
  4. Provide choices to the toddler as possibilities to enable him or her to have some control.
  5. Approach the toddler with a positive attitude.
  6. Allow the toddler to express feelings of protest.
  7. Encourage the toddler to talk about parents or others in his or her life.
  8. Accept regressive behavior without ridiculing the toddler.
  9. Provide the toddler with favorite and comforting objects.
  10. Utilize **play** therapy for the toddler.
  11. Allow the toddler as much mobility as possible.
  12. Anticipate temper tantrums from the toddler and maintain a safe environment for physical acting out.
  13. Employ pain-reduction techniques, as appropriate.

⚠ For the hospitalized toddler, provide routines and rituals as close as possible to what he or she is used to at home.

II. The Hospitalized Preschooler

A. Separation anxiety
   1. Separation anxiety is generally less obvious and less concerning than in the toddler.
   2. As stress increases, the preschooler's ability to separate from the parents decreases.
   3. Protest
      a. Protest is less direct and more aggressive than seen in the toddler.
      b. The preschooler may displace feelings onto others.
   4. Despair
      a. The preschooler reacts in a manner similar to the toddler.
      b. The preschooler is quietly withdrawn, depressed, and uninterested in the environment.
      c. The child exhibits loss of newly learned skills.
      d. The preschooler becomes generally uncooperative, refusing to eat or take medication.
      e. The preschooler repeatedly asks when the parents will be visiting.
      f. Detachment: Similar to the toddler

B. Fear of injury and pain
   1. The preschooler has a general lack of understanding of body integrity.
   2. The child fears invasive procedures and mutilation.
   3. The child imagines things to be much worse than they are.
   4. Preschoolers believe they are ill because of something they did or thought.

C. Loss of control
   1. The preschooler likes familiar routines and rituals, and may show regression if not allowed to maintain some control.
   2. Preschoolers' egocentric and magical thinking limits their ability to understand events because they view all experiences from their own self-referenced (egocentric) perspective.
   3. The child has attained a good deal of independence and self-care at home. The child may expect that to continue in the hospital.

D. Interventions
   1. Provide a safe and secure environment.
   2. Take time for communication.
   3. Allow the preschooler to express anger.
   4. Acknowledge fears and anxieties.
   5. Accept regressive behavior. Assist the preschooler to move from regressive to appropriate behaviors according to age.
   6. Encourage rooming-in or leaving a favorite toy.
   7. Allow mobility, and provide play and diversional activities.
   8. Place the preschooler with other children of the same age if possible.
   9. Encourage the preschooler to be independent.
   10. Explain procedures simply, on the preschooler's level.
   11. Avoid intrusive procedures when possible.
   12. Allow for the wearing of underpants.

III. The Hospitalized School-Age Child

A. Separation anxiety
   1. The school-age child is accustomed to periods of separation from the parents, but as stressors are added, the separation becomes more difficult.
   2. The child is more concerned with missing school and the fear that friends will forget him or her.
   3. Usually, the stages of behavior related to protest, despair, and detachment do not occur with the school-age child.

B. Fear of injury and pain
   1. The school-age child fears bodily injury and pain.
   2. The child fears illness itself, disability, death, and intrusive procedures in genital areas.
   3. The child is uncomfortable with any type of sexual examination.
   4. The child groans or whines, holds rigidly still, and communicates about pain.

C. Loss of control
   1. The child is usually highly social, independent, and involved with activities.
   2. The child seeks information and asks relevant questions about tests, procedures, and the illness.
   3. The child associates his or her actions with the cause of the illness.
   4. The child may feel helpless and dependent if physical limitations occur.

D. Interventions
   1. Encourage rooming-in.
   2. Focus on the school-age child's abilities and needs.
   3. Encourage the school-age child to become involved with his or her own care.
   4. Accept regression, but encourage independence.
   5. Provide choices to the school-age child.
   6. Allow for the expression of feelings, both verbally and nonverbally.
   7. Acknowledge fears and concerns and allow for discussion.
   8. Explain all procedures with the use of body diagrams or outlines.
   9. Provide privacy.
   10. Avoid intrusive procedures, if possible.
   11. Allow the school-age child to wear underpants.
   12. Involve the school-age child in activities that are appropriate to his or her developmental level and illness.
   13. Encourage the school-age child to contact friends.
   14. Provide for educational needs.
   15. Employ appropriate interventions to relieve pain.

IV. The Hospitalized Adolescent

A. Separation anxiety
   1. Adolescents are not sure whether they want their parents with them when they are hospitalized.

> **BOX 20.1** **General Guidelines for Communication**
>
> - Allow the child time to feel comfortable with the nurse.
> - Communicate through the use of objects.
> - Allow the child to express fears and concerns.
> - Speak clearly and in a quiet, unhurried voice.
> - Offer choices when possible.
> - Be honest with the child.
> - Set limits with the child as appropriate.

    2. Adolescents become upset if friends go on with their lives, excluding them.

> ⚠ For the hospitalized adolescent, separation from friends is a source of anxiety.

 B. Fear of injury and pain
1. Adolescents fear being different from others and their peers.
2. Adolescents may give the impression that they are not afraid, although they are terrified.
3. Adolescents become guarded when any areas related to sexual development are examined.

C. Loss of control
1. Behaviors exhibited include anger, withdrawal, and uncooperativeness.
2. Adolescents seek help and then reject it.

 D. Interventions
1. Encourage questions about appearance and the effects of the illness on the future.
2. Explore feelings about the hospital and the significance that the illness might have with regard to relationships.
3. Encourage the adolescent to wear his or her own clothes and perform normal grooming activities.
4. Allow favorite foods to be brought in to the hospital, if possible.
5. Provide privacy.
6. Use body diagrams to prepare for procedures.
7. Introduce to other adolescents in the nursing unit.
8. Encourage the maintenance of contact with peer groups.
9. Provide for educational needs.
10. Identify the formation of future plans.
11. Help develop positive coping mechanisms.

 V. Communication Approaches

A. General guidelines (Box 20.1)

 B. Infant
1. Infants respond to the nonverbal communication behaviors of adults, such as holding, rocking, patting, cuddling, and touching.
2. Use a slow approach; allow the infant to get to know the nurse.
3. Use a calm, soft, soothing voice.
4. Be responsive to cries.
5. Talk and read to infants.
6. Allow security objects such as blankets and pacifiers, if the infant has them.

C. Toddler
1. Approach the toddler cautiously.
2. Remember that toddlers accept the verbal communications of others literally.
3. Learn the toddler's words for common items and use them in conversation.
4. Use short, concrete terms.
5. Prepare the toddler for procedures immediately before the event.
6. Repeat explanations and descriptions.
7. Use play for demonstrations.
8. Use visual aids such as picture books, puppets, and dolls.
9. Allow the toddler to handle the equipment or instruments. Explain what the equipment or instrument does and how it feels.
10. Encourage the use of comfort objects.

D. Preschooler
1. Seek opportunities to offer choices.
2. Speak in simple sentences.
3. Be concise. Limit the length of explanations.
4. Allow for the asking of questions.
5. Describe the procedures as they are about to be performed.
6. Use play to explain procedures and activities.
7. Allow the handling of equipment or instruments, which will ease fear and help answer questions.

E. School-age child
1. Establish limits.
2. Provide reassurance to help with alleviating fears and anxieties.
3. Engage in conversations that encourage thinking.
4. Use medical play techniques.
5. Use photographs, books, dolls, DVDs, and other appropriate videos to explain procedures.
6. Explain in clear terms.
7. Allow time for composure and privacy.

F. Adolescent
1. Remember that the adolescent may be preoccupied with body image.
2. Encourage and support independence.
3. Provide privacy.
4. Use photographs, books, CDs, DVDs, videos, and the internet to explain procedures.
5. Engage in conversation about the adolescent's interests.
6. Avoid becoming too abstract, too detailed, and too technical.
7. Avoid responding to less-than-desirable social behaviors by prying, confrontation, or judgmental attitudes.

VI. Car Safety Seats and Guidelines

A. The safest place for all children to ride, regardless of age, is in the backseat of the car.

BOX 20.2	Preventative Service and Screening: Infancy through Adolescents

- History
- Measurements
  - Length/height/weight
  - Head circumference
  - Body mass index (BMI)
  - Blood pressure
- Sensory screening
  - Vision
  - Hearing
- Developmental/behavioral health
  - Developmental screenings
  - Autism spectrum disorder screening
  - Developmental surveillance
  - Psychosocial/behavioral assessment
  - Depression screening
  - Maternal depression screening (as appropriate)
- Physical examination
  - Procedures
    - Newborn blood
    - Newborn bilirubin
    - Critical congenital heart defect
    - Immunizations
    - Anemia
    - Lead
    - Tuberculosis
    - Dyslipidemia
    - Sexually transmitted infections
    - Human immunodeficiency virus (HIV)
    - Cervical dysplasia
  - Oral health
    - Fluoride varnish
    - Fluoride supplementation
  - Anticipatory guidance

BOX 20.3	Preventative Services and Screenings: Well-check Schedule

- Prenatal visit
- Newborn visit
- First week visit (3–5 days)
- 1-month visit
- 2-month visit
- 3-month visit
- 4-month visit
- 6-month visit
- 9-month visit
- 12-month visit
- 15-month visit
- 18-month visit
- 2-year visit
- 2½-year visit
- 3-year visit
- Annual visits from 4 years of age to 18 years of age; thereafter, the child would begin to visit a general practitioner

B. Lock the car doors; four-door cars would be equipped with child safety locks on the back doors.

C. There are different types of car safety seats and the manufacturer's guidelines need to be followed.

D. Refer to the American Academy of Pediatrics (2020). Car seats: Information for families. https://www.healthychildren.org/English/safety-prevention/on-the-go/Pages/Car-Safety-Seats-Information-for-Families.aspx.

VII. Preventative Pediatric Health Care

A. The American Academy of Pediatrics (AAP) and Bright Futures have developed guidelines regarding the recommended ages children need to receive certain assessments and screenings. See Box 20.2 for more information regarding the recommended types of assessments and screenings and see Box 20.3 for suggested timeline for preventive services also known as well-child checks. For detailed information on these screenings and the timeline, access the following links: https://brightfutures.aap.org/Pages/default.aspx https://www.aap.org/en-us/Documents/periodicity_schedule.pdf

B. Well-checks are important in promoting health early in childhood and preventing diseases later in life. Childhood obesity, type 2 diabetes mellitus, and hyperlipidemia should also be a focus of screening and prevention.

VIII. Developmental Characteristics

A. Infant

   1. Physical

   a. Height increases by 1 inch per month in the first 6 months, and by 1 year, the length has increased by 50%.

   b. Weight is doubled at 5 to 6 months and tripled at 12 months.

   c. At birth, head circumference is 33 cm to 35 cm (13.2–14 inches), approximately 2 cm to 3 cm more than chest circumference.

   d. By 1 to 2 years of age, head circumference and chest circumference are equal.

   e. The anterior fontanel (soft and flat in a normal infant) closes by 12 to 18 months.

   f. The posterior fontanel (soft and flat in a normal infant) closes by the end of the second month.

   g. The first primary teeth to erupt are the lower central incisors at approximately 6 to 10 months of age.

   h. Sleep patterns vary among infants; in general, by 3 to 4 months of age, most infants have developed a nocturnal pattern of sleep that lasts 9 to 11 hours.

   2. Vital signs (Box 20.4)

   3. Nutrition

   a. The infant may breast-feed or bottle-feed (with iron-fortified formula), depending on the mother's choice; however, human milk is the preferred form of nutrition for all infants, especially during the first 6 months.

BOX 20.4 **Vital Signs: The Newborn and 1-Year-Old Infant**

Newborn

- *Temperature:* Axillary, 96.8°F–99°F (36°C–37.2°C)
- *Apical rate:* 120–160 beats per minute
- *Respirations:* 30–60 (average 40) breaths per minute
- *Blood pressure:* 80–90 mm Hg/40–50 mm Hg

1-Year-Old Infant

- *Temperature:* Axillary, 97°F–99°F (36.1°C–37.2°C)
- *Apical rate:* 90–130 beats per minute
- *Respirations:* 20–40 breaths per minute
- *Blood pressure:* Average, 90/56 mm Hg

TABLE 20.1 **Infant Skills**

Age	Skills
2–3 Months	Smiles Turns head from side to side Follows objects Holds head in midline
4–5 Months	Grasps objects Switches objects from hand to hand Rolls over for the first time Enjoys social interaction Begins to show memory Aware of unfamiliar surroundings
6–7 Months	Creeps Sits with support Imitates Exhibits fear of strangers Holds arms out Frequent mood swings Waves "bye-bye"
8–9 Months	Sits steadily unsupported Crawls May stand while holding on Begins to stand without help
10–11 Months	Can change from a prone to a sitting position Walks while holding onto furniture Stands securely Entertains self for periods of time
12–13 Months	Walks with one hand held Can take a few steps without falling Can drink from a cup
14–15 Months	Walks alone Can crawl up stairs Shows emotions such as anger and affection Will explore away from mother in familiar surroundings

b. Exclusively breast-fed infants and infants ingesting less than 1000 mL of vitamin D–fortified formula or milk per day would receive daily vitamin D supplementation (400 IU) starting in the first few days of life to prevent rickets and vitamin D deficiency.

c. Iron stores from birth are depleted by 4 months; if the infant is being only breast-fed, iron supplementation usually with iron-fortified cereal is needed.

d. Whole milk, low-fat milk, skim milk, other animal milk, or imitation milk would not be given to infants as a primary source of nutrition because these food sources lack the necessary components needed for growth and have limited digestibility.

e. Fluoride supplementation may be needed at about 6 months of age, depending on the infant's intake of fluoridated tap water.

f. Solid foods (strained, pureed, or finely mashed) are introduced at about 5 to 6 months of age. Introduce solid foods one at a time, usually at intervals of 4 to 5 days, to identify food allergens.

g. The sequence of introduction of solid foods varies depending on the health care provider's preference and usually begins with iron-fortified rice cereal, then fruits and vegetables, and then meats.

h. At 12 months of age, eggs can be given (introduce egg whites in small quantities to detect an allergy); cheese may be used as a substitute for meat.

i. Avoid solid foods that place the infant at risk for choking, such as nuts, foods with seeds, raisins, popcorn, grapes, and pieces of hot dog.

j. Avoid microwaving baby bottles and baby food because of the potential for uneven heating and risk of scalding the infant.

k. Never mix food and/or medications with formula.

l. Avoid adding honey to formula, water, or other fluids because of the risk of botulism.

m. Offer fruit juice from a cup (12–13 months or at a prescribed age) rather than a bottle to prevent nursing (bottle-mouth) caries; fruit juice is limited because of its high sugar content.

4. Skills (Table 20.1)

5. Play

a. Solitary

b. Birth to 3 months: Verbal, visual, and tactile stimuli

c. 4 to 6 months: Initiates actions and recognizes new experiences

d. 6 to 12 months: Aware of self, imitates, and repeats pleasurable actions

e. Enjoys soft stuffed animals, crib mobiles with contrasting colors, squeeze toys, rattles, musical toys, water toys during the bath, large picture books, and push toys after the child begins to walk

6. Safety

 The parents need to be instructed to keep the poison control number available and to contact the poison control center immediately in the event of a poisoning.

a. Parents must baby-proof the home.

b. Guard the infant when on a bed or changing table.

   c. Do not allow the infant to sleep in bed with the parents due to risk of suffocation.

   d. Use gates to protect the infant from stairs.

   e. Be sure that bathwater is not hot. Do not leave the infant unattended in the bath.

   f. Do not hold the infant while drinking or working near hot liquids or items such as a stove.

   g. Cool vaporizers would be used rather than steam vaporizers to prevent burn injuries.

   h. Avoid offering food that is round and similar in size to the airway to prevent choking.

   i. Be sure that toys have no small pieces.

   j. Toys or mobiles hanging over the crib would be well out of reach to prevent strangulation.

   k. Avoid placing large toys in the crib. An older infant may use them as steps to climb out.

   l. Cribs would be positioned away from curtains and blind cords.

   m. Cover electrical outlets.

   n. Remove hazardous objects from low, reachable places.

   o. Remove chemicals, medications, poisons, and plants from the infant's reach.

   p. Keep Poison Control Center telephone number available.

⚠ Never shake an infant because of the risk of causing a closed head injury; this is known as shaken baby syndrome, which is a life-threatening injury.

B. Toddler

  1. Physical

   a. Height and weight increase in phases, reflecting growth spurts and lags.

   b. The head circumference increases about 1 inch between the ages of 1 and 2 years. Thereafter, head circumference increases about ½ inch per year until the age of 5 years.

   c. Anterior fontanel closes between ages 12 and 18 months.

   d. Weight gain is slower than in infancy. By 2 years of age, the average weight is 22 to 27 pounds (10–12 kg).

   e. Normal height changes include a growth of about 3 inches per year. The average height of a toddler is 34 inches at 2 years old.

   f. Lordosis, also known as a potbelly, is evident.

   g. The toddler would see a dentist soon after the first teeth erupt (usually around 1 year of age), and oral hygiene measures would be instituted. Regular dental care is essential, and the toddler will require assistance with brushing and flossing the teeth. (Fluoride supplements may be necessary if the water is not fluoridated.)

> **BOX 20.5   The Toddler's Vital Signs**
>
> ▪ *Temperature:* Axillary, 97.5°F–98.6°F (36.4°C–37°C)
> ▪ *Apical rate:* 80–120 beats per minute
> ▪ *Respirations:* 20–30 breaths per minute
> ▪ *Blood pressure:* Average, 92/55 mm Hg

   h. A toddler would never be allowed to fall asleep with a bottle containing milk, juice, soda, or sweetened water because of the risk of nursing (bottle-mouth) caries.

   i. A toddler typically sleeps through the night, has one daytime nap; the daytime nap normally is discontinued at about the age of 3.

   j. A consistent bedtime ritual helps prepare the toddler for sleep.

   k. Security objects at bedtime may assist with sleep.

  2. Vital signs (Box 20.5)

  3. Nutrition

   a. The MyPlate food guide provides dietary guidelines and applies to children as young as 2 years of age (see www.choosemyplate.gov).

   b. The toddler would average an intake of two to three servings of milk daily (24–30 oz) to ensure an adequate amount of calcium and phosphorus (low-fat milk may be given after 2 years of age).

   c. Trans fatty acids and saturated fats need to be restricted; otherwise, fat restriction is not appropriate for a toddler (mothers would be taught about the types of food that contain fat that would be selected).

   d. Iron-fortified cereal and a high-iron diet, adequate amounts of calcium and vitamin D, and vitamin C (4–6 oz of juice daily) are essential components of the toddler's diet.

   e. Most toddlers prefer to feed themselves.

   f. The toddler generally does best by eating several small nutritious meals each day rather than three large meals.

   g. Offer a limited number of foods at any one time.

   h. Offer finger foods and avoid concentrated sweets and empty calories.

   i. The toddler is at risk for aspiration of small foods that are not chewed easily, such as nuts, foods with seeds, raisins, popcorn, grapes, and hot dog pieces.

   j. Physiological anorexia may occur and is normal because of the alternating stages of fast and slow growth.

   k. Sit the toddler in a high chair at the family table for meals.

   l. Allow sufficient time to eat, but remove food when the toddler begins to play with it.

BOX 20.6 Signs of Readiness for Toilet Training

- Able to stay dry for 2 hours
- Waking dry from a nap
- Able to sit, squat, and walk
- Able to remove clothing
- Recognizes urge to defecate or urinate
- Expresses willingness to please parent
- Able to sit on toilet for 5–10 minutes without fussing or getting off

Data from Hockenberry M, Wilson D: *Nursing care of infants and children*, ed 9, St. Louis, 2011, Mosby.

m. The toddler drinks well from a cup held with both hands.

n. Avoid using food as a reward or punishment.

4. Skills

  a. The toddler begins to walk with one hand held by the age of 12 to 13 months.

  b. The toddler runs by the age of 2 years and walks backward and hops on one foot by the age of 3 years.

  c. The toddler usually cannot alternate feet when climbing stairs.

  d. The toddler begins to master fine motor skills for building, undressing, and drawing lines.

  e. The young toddler often uses the word "no," even when he or she (toddler or child) means "yes," to assert independence.

  f. The toddler begins to use short sentences and has a vocabulary of about 300 words by the age of 2 years.

5. Bowel and bladder control

  a. Certain signs indicate a toddler is ready for toilet training (Box 20.6).

  b. Bowel control develops before bladder control.

  c. By the age of 3 years, the toddler achieves fairly good bowel and bladder control.

  d. The toddler may stay dry during the day but may need a diaper at night until about the age of 4 years.

6. Play

  a. The major socializing mechanism is parallel play. Therapeutic play can begin at this age.

  b. The toddler has a short attention span that causes him or her (toddler) to change toys often.

  c. The toddler explores the body parts of self and others.

  d. Typical toys include push-pull toys, blocks, sand, finger paints, bubbles, large balls, crayons, trucks, dolls, Play-Doh, toy telephones, cloth books, and wooden puzzles.

7. Safety

  Toddlers are eager to explore the world around them. They need to be supervised during play to ensure their safety.

  a. Use back burners on the stove to prepare a meal and turn pot handles inward and toward the middle of the stove.

  b. Keep dangling cords from small appliances away from the toddler.

  c. Place inaccessible locks on windows and doors and keep furniture away from windows.

  d. Secure screens on all windows.

  e. Place safety gates at stairways.

  f. Do not allow the toddler to sleep or play in an upper bunk bed.

  g. Never leave the toddler alone near a bathtub, pail of water, swimming pool, or any other body of water.

  h. Keep toilet lids closed.

  i. Keep all medicines, poisons, household plants, and toxic products high and locked out of reach.

  j. Keep Poison Control Center telephone number available.

C. Preschooler

1. Physical

  a. Grows 2½ to 3 inches per year

  b. Average height is 37 inches at the age of 3 years, 40½ inches at the age of 4 years, and 43 inches at the age of 5 years.

  c. Gains 5 pounds per year; average weight of 35 to 40 pounds at the age of 5 years

  d. Requires about 12 hours of sleep each day

  e. A security object and a nightlight help with sleeping.

  f. At the beginning of the preschool period, the eruption of the deciduous (primary) teeth is complete.

  g. Regular dental care is essential and the preschooler requires assistance with brushing and flossing his/her teeth. Fluoride supplements may be necessary if the water is not fluoridated.

2. Vital signs (Box 20.7)

3. Nutrition

  a. Nutritional needs are similar to those required for the toddler, although the daily amounts of minerals, vitamins, and protein may increase with age.

  b. The MyPlate food guide is appropriate for preschoolers (see www.choosemyplate.gov).

  c. The preschooler exhibits food fads and certain taste preferences and may exhibit finicky eating.

  d. By 5 years old, the child tends to focus on social aspects of eating, table conversations, manners, and willingness to try new foods.

BOX 20.7   The Preschooler's Vital Signs

- *Temperature:* Axillary, 97.5°F–98.6°F (36.4°C–37°C)
- *Apical rate:* 70–110 beats per minute
- *Respirations:* 16–22 breaths per minute
- *Blood pressure:* Average, 95/57 mm Hg

---

4. Skills
   a. Has good posture
   b. Develops fine motor coordination
   c. Can hop, skip, and run more smoothly
   d. Athletic abilities begin to develop
   e. Demonstrates increased balancing skills
   f. Alternates feet when climbing stairs
   g. Can tie shoelaces by the age of 6 years
   h. May talk continuously and ask many "why" questions
   i. Vocabulary increases to about 900 words by the age of 3 years and to about 2100 words by the age of 5 years.
   j. By the age of 3 years, the preschooler usually talks in three- or four-word sentences and speaks in short phrases.
   k. By the age of 4 years, the preschooler uses five- or six-word sentences. By the age of 5 years, the preschooler speaks in longer sentences that contain all parts of speech.
   l. The preschooler can be readily understood by others and can clearly understand what others are saying.

5. Bowel and bladder control
   a. By the age of 4 years, the preschooler has daytime control of bowel and bladder, but may experience bed-wetting accidents at night.
   b. By the age of 5 years, the preschooler achieves both bowel and bladder control, although accidents may occur in stressful situations.
6. Play
   a. Cooperative
   b. Imaginary playmates
   c. Likes to build and create things; play is simple and imaginative.
   d. Understands sharing and is able to interact with peers
   e. Requires regular socialization with children of the same age
   f. Play activities include a large space for running and jumping.
   g. Likes dress-up clothes, paints, paper, and crayons for creative expression
   h. Swimming and sports aid with growth and development.
   i. Puzzles and toys aid with fine motor development.

7. Safety
   a. Preschoolers are active and inquisitive.
   b. Because of their magical thinking, they may believe that daring feats seen in cartoons are possible and may attempt them.
   c. Preschoolers can learn simple safety practices, because they can follow simple and verbal directions, and their attention span is longer.
   d. Reinforce instructions to the preschooler and basic safety rules to ensure safety when playing in a playground near swings and ladders.
   e. Reinforce instructions to the preschooler to never play with matches or lighters.
   f. The preschooler would be taught what to do in the event of a fire or if clothes catch fire. Fire drills would be practiced with the preschooler.
   g. Guns must be stored unloaded and secured under lock and key, regardless of the age of the child (ammunition must be locked in a separate place).
   h. Teach the preschooler his or her full name, address, parents' names, and telephone number.
   i. Teach the preschooler how to dial 911 in an emergency situation.
   j. Keep Poison Control Center telephone number available.

⚠ Teach a preschooler and school-age child to leave an area immediately if a gun is visible and to tell an adult. The child must also be taught never to point a toy gun at another person.

D. School-age child
   1. Physical
      a. Girls usually grow faster than boys.
      b. Growth of about 2 inches per year between the ages of 6 and 12 years
      c. Height ranges from 45 inches at the age of 6 years to 59 inches at the age of 12 years.
      d. Weight gain of 4½ to 6½ pounds (2–3 kg) per year
      e. Average weight of 46 pounds (21 kg) at the age of 6 years and 88 pounds (40 kg) at the age of 12 years
      f. The first permanent (secondary) teeth erupt around the age of 6 years and the deciduous teeth are gradually lost.
      g. Regular dentist visits are necessary, and the school-age child needs to be supervised during the brushing and flossing of teeth. Fluoride supplements may be necessary if the water is not fluoridated.
      h. For school-age children with primary and permanent dentition, the best toothbrush is one with soft nylon bristles and an overall length of about 6 inches.
      i. Sleep requirements range from 10 to 12 hours per night.

BOX 20.8   The School-Age Child's Vital Signs

- *Temperature:* Oral, 97.5°F–98.6°F (36.4°C–37°C)
- *Apical rate:* 60–100 beats per minute
- *Respirations:* 18–20 breaths per minute
- *Blood pressure:* Average, 107/64 mm Hg

2. Vital signs (Box 20.8)
3. Nutrition
    a. School-age children have increased growth needs.
    b. Children require a balanced diet from foods in the MyPlate food guide; healthy snacks would continue to be emphasized to prevent childhood obesity (see www.choosemyplate.gov).
    c. School-age children may still be picky eaters but are willing to try new foods.
4. Skills
    a. School-age children exhibit refinement of fine motor skills.
    b. Development of gross motor skills continues.
    c. Strength and endurance increase.
5. Play
    a. Play is more competitive.
    b. Rules and rituals are important aspects of play and games.
    c. The school-age child enjoys drawing, collecting items, dolls, pets, guessing games, board games, listening to the radio, television, reading, videos or DVDs, and computer games.
    d. The child participates in team sports.
    e. The child participates in secret clubs, peer-group activities, and scout organizations.
6. Safety
    a. The school-age child experiences less fear during play activities and frequently imitates real life with the use of tools and household items.
    b. Major causes of injuries include bicycles, skateboards, and team sports as the child increases motor abilities and independence.
    c. Children would always wear a helmet when riding a bike or using in-line skates or skateboards.
    d. Teach the school-age child regarding water safety rules.
    e. Teach the school-age child to avoid teasing or playing roughly with animals.
    f. Teach the school-age child never to play with matches or lighters.
    g. The school-age child would be taught what to do in the event of a fire or if clothes catch fire. Fire drills would be practiced with the school-age child.
    h. Guns must be stored unloaded and secured under lock and key, regardless of the age of the child (ammunition must be locked in a separate place).
    i. Teach the school-age child regarding traffic safety rules.
    j. Teach the school-age child how to dial 911 in an emergency situation.
    k. Keep Poison Control Center telephone number available.

⚠ Teach the child that if another person touches his or her body in an inappropriate way, an adult must be told. Also teach the child to avoid speaking to strangers and never to accept a ride, toys, or gifts from a stranger.

E. Adolescent
1. Physical
    a. Puberty: The maturational, hormonal, and growth process that occurs when the reproductive organs begin to function and the secondary sex characteristics develop
    b. Body mass increases to adult size.
    c. Sebaceous and sweat glands become active and fully functional.
    d. Body hair distribution occurs.
    e. Increases in height, weight, breast development, and pelvic girth occur in girls.
    f. Menstrual periods usually occur about 2½ years after the onset of puberty.
    g. In boys, increases in height, weight, muscle mass, and penis and testicle size occur.
    h. The voice deepens in boys.
    i. Normal weight gain during puberty: Girls gain 15 to 55 pounds (7–25 kg), and boys gain 15 to 65 pounds (7–30 kg).
    j. Careful brushing and care of the teeth are important, and many adolescents need to wear braces.
    k. Sleep patterns include a tendency to stay up late; therefore, in an attempt to catch up on missed sleep, adolescents sleep late whenever possible. An overall average of 8 hours per night is recommended.
2. Vital signs (Box 20.9)
3. Nutrition
    a. Reinforcing instructions about the MyPlate food guide is important (see www.choosemyplate.gov).
    b. Adolescents typically eat whenever they have a break in activities.
    c. Calcium, zinc, iron, folic acid, and protein are especially important nutritional needs.
    d. Adolescents tend to snack on empty calories, and the importance of adequate and healthy nutrition needs to be stressed.
    e. Body image is important.
4. Skills
    a. Gross and fine motor skills are well developed.
    b. Strength and endurance increase.

BOX 20.9   The Adolescent's Vital Signs

- *Temperature:* Oral, 97.5°F–98.6°F (36.4°C–37°C)
- *Apical rate:* 55–90 beats per minute
- *Respirations:* 12–20 breaths per minute
- *Blood pressure:* Average, 120/70 mm Hg

---

5. Play
   a. Games and athletics are the most common forms of play.
   b. Competition and strict rules are important.
   c. Adolescents enjoy activities such as sports, videos, movies, reading, parties, dancing, hobbies, computer games, music, communicating via the internet and other social media platforms, and experimenting, such as with makeup, hairstyles, tattoos, and piercings.
   d. Friends are important. Adolescents like to gather in small groups.
6. Safety
   a. Adolescents are risk takers.
   b. Adolescents have a natural urge to experiment and be independent.
   c. Reinforce instructions to adolescents regarding the dangers related to drugs, alcohol, cigarettes, caffeine ingestion, and motor vehicles of any type.
   d. Help adolescents to recognize that they have choices when difficult or potentially dangerous situations arise.
   e. Ensure that the adolescent uses a seat belt.
   f. Reinforce instructions to adolescents regarding the consequences of injuries that motor vehicle crashes can cause.
   g. Reinforce instructions to adolescents regarding water safety. Emphasize that they would enter the water feet first, as opposed to diving, especially when the depth of the water is unknown.
   h. Reinforce instructions to adolescents about the dangers associated with guns, violence, and gangs.
   i. Reinforce instructions to adolescents about the complications associated with body piercing, tattooing, and sun tanning.

⚠ Discuss issues such as acquaintance rape, sexual relationships, and transmission of sexually transmitted infections with the adolescent. Also discuss the dangers of the internet and other social media platforms related to communicating and setting up meetings (dates) with unknown persons.

F. Early adulthood
   1. Description: Period between the late teens and the mid- to late 30s

2. Physical changes
   a. The person has completed physical growth by the age of 20 years.
   b. The person is quite active.
   c. Severe illnesses are less common than those seen among older age groups.
   d. The person tends to ignore physical symptoms and postpones seeking health care.
   e. Lifestyle habits such as smoking, stress, lack of exercise, poor personal hygiene, and family history of disease increase the risk of future illness.
3. Cognitive changes
   a. The person has rational thinking habits.
   b. Conceptual, problem-solving, and motor skills increase.
   c. The person identifies preferred occupational areas.
4. Psychosocial changes
   a. The person separates from the family of origin.
   b. The person gives much attention to occupational and social pursuits to improve socioeconomic status.
   c. The person makes decisions regarding career, marriage, and parenthood.
   d. The person needs to adapt to new situations.
5. Sexuality
   a. The person has the emotional maturity to develop mature sexual relationships.
   b. The person is at risk for sexually transmitted infections.
G. Middle adulthood
   1. Description: Period between the mid- to late 30s and the mid-60s
   2. Physical changes
   a. Occur between the ages of 40 and 65 years
   b. The individual becomes aware that changes in reproductive and physical abilities signify the beginning of another stage in life.
   c. Menopause occurs in women; climacteric occurs in men.
   d. Physiological changes often have an effect on self-concept and body image.
   e. Physiological concerns include stress, level of wellness, and the formation of positive health habits.
3. Cognitive changes
   a. The person may be interested in learning new skills.
   b. The person may become involved with educational or vocational programs for entering the job market or changing careers.
4. Psychosocial changes
   a. These may include expected events, such as children moving away from home (post parental family stage), or unexpected events, such as the death of a close friend.

    b. Time and financial demands decrease as children move away from home and the couple faces redefining their relationship.

    c. Adults may become grandparents.

    d. Adults are achieving generativity.

  5. Sexuality

    a. Many couples renew their relationships and find increased marital and sexual satisfaction.

    b. The onset of menopause and climacteric may affect sexual health.

    c. Stress, health, and medications can affect sexuality.

H. Later adulthood (period between 65 years to death): refer to Chapter 21.

IX. Gender Identity

A. Gender identity

  1. Gender identity is one's personal sense of one's own gender.

  2. It can be the same as the assigned sex at birth or it can be different.

B. Gender expression

  1. Gender expression is how one expresses their gender to others.

  2. Characteristics in personality, appearance, behavior, or the name one chooses to be called can relate to gender expression.

C. Sexual orientation

  1. Sexual orientation refers to the gender to whom one is typically sexually attracted.

  2. A person can be attracted to someone of the same gender and/or different gender(s).

D. Children

  1. Children become aware of their physical difference from those of the opposite gender around age 2 and think of themselves as either a boy or a girl by age 3.

  2. Children express their gender by their choices of toys, sports, preferred name, clothing, hairstyle, social behavior, and manner of behavior, such as through physical gestures.

E. Adolescents

  1. Adolescents continue to develop their gender identity through their own personal sense of gender and from involvement with their social environment, such as family and friends.

  2. Some adolescents are confident in their gender identity whereas others need time to develop their identity.

  3. At puberty, some adolescents may realize that their gender identity is different from their assigned birth sex and sometimes the they need to figure out who they are and their place in the world.

F. Family support interventions

  1. Encourage the child to express themselves as to their sense of gender; avoid pressuring the child to change who they are.

  2. Encourage love and unconditional support for the child and accept the child for who they are.

  3. Suggest that the parents ask the school about how they support gender expression and what is taught about gender identity.

  4. Support the child and prepare them for possible negative reactions or bullying from other children and the importance of sharing if these negative reactions or bullying surfaces against them.

  5. Watch for signs of depression, anxiety, or other behaviors that affect the emotional health of the child.

  6. Seek out medical professional assistance if concerned about the child's emotional health or if family members are having difficulty accepting the child's decision about one's own gender.

  7. For additional information refer to: Rafferty, J. (2020). *Gender identity in children.* American Academy of Pediatrics at https://www.healthychildren.org/English/ages-stages/gradeschool/Pages/Gender-Identity-and-Gender-Confusion-In-Children.aspx

X. End-of-Life Care

A. Description: End-of-life care relates to death and dying.

B. Cultural and religious issues (Box 20.10)

C. Legal and ethical issues

  1. Outcomes related to care during illness and the dying experience would be based on the client's wishes.

  2. Issues for consideration may include organ and tissue donations, advance directives or other legal documents, withholding or withdrawing treatment, and cardiopulmonary resuscitation.

D. Palliative and hospice care

  1. Focuses on caring interventions and symptom management rather than cure for diseases or conditions that no longer respond to treatment and can be required at any age depending on the condition and prognosis.

  2. Pain and symptoms are controlled; the dying client would be as pain-free and as comfortable as possible.

  3. Provides support and care for clients in the last phases of incurable diseases so that they might live as fully and as comfortably as possible; client and family needs are the focus of any intervention.

E. Near-death physiological manifestations

  1. As death approaches, metabolism is reduced and the body gradually slows down until all functions end.

  2. Sensory: The client experiences blurred vision, decreased sense of taste and smell, decreased pain and touch perception, loss of blink reflex, and appears to stare (hearing is believed to be the last sense lost).

  3. Respirations

    a. Respirations may be rapid or slow, shallow, and irregular.

    b. Respirations may be noisy and wet sounding (death rattle).

    c. Cheyne-Stokes respiration refers to alternating periods of apnea and deep, rapid breathing.

BOX 20.10	Religion and End-of-Life Care.

End-of-life care and practices may vary among members of each religious group. Therefore, culturally competent care requires that the nurse identify the specific preferences and needs of each individual. The nurse must ask the client and/or family what these preferences are and develop a plan of care that addresses these individualized preferences.

Buddhism

The decision to forego life-sustaining efforts is an individual matter that requires consultation with the person concerned and their family.

Disposition of the body varies with the culture and denomination and the family needs to be consulted.

Beliefs on autopsy vary; therefore, the individual or the individual's family must be consulted.

Guidelines for health care providers interacting with patients of the Buddhist religion and their families at: https://www.advocatehealth.com/assets/documents/faith/cgbuddhist.pdf.

Catholic

Members look to a priest for prayers and support and comfort.

Sacraments before death include reconciliation and Holy Communion.

The teachings of the Catholic church: caring for people at the end of life at: https://www.chausa.org/docs/default-source/ethics/3058_cha_end-of-life-guide_tcc_lores.pdf?sfvrsn=6.

Church of Jesus Christ of Latter-Day Saints (Mormons)

Members look to church leaders for support and comfort.

Some may want to be blessed by the Mormon priesthood.

Caring for a Mormon Patient at: https://sites.google.com/site/culturalsensitivitytomormons/home/values-beliefs-norms/health-practices/caring-for-a-mormon-patient.

Islam

A Muslim chaplain, a volunteer, or an Imam may be preferred to be present at the time of death and offer support to the family, read the Quran, and comfort the dying client.

Preference may be that the client face Mecca (west or southwest in the United States).

Ziyara, Muslim spiritual care: end-of-life care at: https://ziyara.org/programs/end-of-life-care/.

Jehovah's Witnesses

Likely to refuse a blood transfusion whatever the possible consequences.

Congregational support is important.

Caring for the Jehovah witness patient at: https://www.ashfordstpeters.info/images/other/PAS09.pdf.

Judaism

A dying person should not be left alone (a rabbi's presence is desired).

If a client is mentally competent, Jewish tradition encourages them to reflect on their life, pass on wisdom, make amends if needed and say goodbye.

The culture connection: Judaism at end-of-life at: https://www.crossroadshospice.com/hospice-palliative-care-blog/2015/august/10/the-culture-connection-judaism-at-end-of-life/.

Hinduism

Special prayers are said and often a relative must be present at the moment of death. A pandit (priest) may be called in to do a puja (prayer). Pujas may involve adorning the person's head with sandalwood paste, holy ash, and red kum kum powder.

A red or yellow string may be tied around the wrist. After death, close family members will wash the body, close the eyes, and straighten the legs. A death needs to be registered as soon as possible and the body cremated within 24 hours.

Health care providers handbook on Hindu patients: https://www.health.qld.gov.au/__data/assets/pdf_file/0024/156255/hbook-hindu.pdf).

Protestant

Some prefer specific rituals and practices at the time of one's dying and death.

Many prefer family members, friends, and their own clergy to be present for comfort and prayers at this time. Consult with the family regarding their preference.

Guidelines for health care providers interacting with patients and their families who are members of Protestant religious groups at: https://www.advocatehealth.com/assets/documents/faith/cgprotestant.pdf.

---

4. Circulation
   a. Heart rate slows and blood pressure falls progressively.
   b. Skin is cool to touch and the extremities become pale, mottled, and cyanotic.
   c. Skin is wax-like very near death.
5. Urinary output decreases; incontinence may occur.
6. Gastrointestinal motility and peristalsis diminish, leading to constipation, gas accumulation, and distention; incontinence may occur.
7. Musculoskeletal system: The client gradually loses ability to move, has difficulty speaking and swallowing, and loses the gag reflex.

F. Death
   1. Death occurs when all vital organs and body systems cease to function.
   2. In general, respirations cease first, and then the heartbeat stops a few minutes thereafter.
   3. Brain death occurs when the cerebral cortex stops functioning or is irreversibly damaged.
G. Nursing care
   1. Frequency of assessment depends on the client's stability (at least every 4 hours); as changes occur, assessment needs to be done more frequently.
   2. Physical care (Box 20.11)

BOX 20.11   Physical Care of the Dying Client

Pain
- Assist to administer pain medication.
- Do not delay or deny pain medication.

Dyspnea
- Elevate the head of the bed or position the client on his or her side.
- Supplemental oxygen may be administered for comfort.
- Suction fluids from the airway as needed.
- Assist to administer medications as prescribed.

Skin
- Check color and temperature.
- Check for breakdown.
- Implement measures to prevent breakdown.

Dehydration
- Maintain regular oral care.
- Encourage taking ice chips and sips of fluid.
- Do not force the client to eat or drink.
- Use moist cloths to provide moisture to the mouth.
- Apply lubricant to the lips and oral mucous membranes.

Anorexia, Nausea, and Vomiting
- Provide antiemetics before meals.
- Have family members provide the client's favorite foods.
- Provide frequent small portions of favorite foods.

Elimination
- Monitor urinary and bowel elimination.
- Place absorbent pads under the client and check frequently.

Weakness and Fatigue
- Provide rest periods.
- Assess tolerance for activities.
- Provide assistance and support as needed for maintaining bed or chair positions.

Restlessness
- Maintain a calm, soothing environment.
- Do not restrain.
- Limit the number of visitors at the client's bedside (consider cultural practices).
- Allow a family member to stay with the client.

BOX 20.12   Fear Associated with Dying

Fear of Pain
- Fear of pain may occur, based on anxieties related to dying.
- Do not delay or deny pain relief measures to a terminally ill client.

Fear of Loneliness and Abandonment
- Allow family members to stay with the client.
- Holding hands, touching (if culturally acceptable), and listening to the client are important.

Fear of Being Meaningless
- Client may feel hopeless and powerless.
- Encourage life reviews and focus on the positive aspects of the client's life.

Adapted from Lewis S, Dirksen S, Heitkemper M, Bucher L: *Medical-surgical nursing: assessment and management of clinical problems*, ed 9, St. Louis, 2014, Mosby.

BOX 20.13   General Postmortem Procedures

- Close the client's eyes.
- If the client wore dentures, place them in the mouth.
- Wash the body and change bed linens if needed.
- Place pads under the perineum.
- Remove tubes and dressings.
- Straighten the body and place a pillow under the head in preparation for family viewing.

---

d. Prepare the body for immediate viewing by the family.
e. Provide privacy and time for the family to be with the deceased person.
f. Medical examiner jurisdiction guidelines are determined by each state and usually include non-natural, traumatic, or question of criminal involvement deaths; any forensic evidence is preserved and the body is not cleaned or prepared before transfer to the morgue.

3. Psychosocial care
   a. Monitor for anxiety and depression.
   b. Monitor for fear (Box 20.12).
   c. Encourage the client and family to express feelings.
   d. Provide support and advocacy for the client and family.
   e. Provide privacy for the client and family.
   f. Provide a private room for the client.
4. See Chapter 64 for information on grief and loss.
5. Postmortem care (Box 20.13)
   a. Maintain respect and dignity for the client.
   b. Determine whether the client is an organ donor; if so, follow appropriate procedures related to the donation.
   c. Consider cultural rituals, state laws, and agency procedures when performing postmortem care.

WHAT WOULD YOU DO?

Answer: When caring for a child who is apprehensive, the nurse would provide a safe and secure environment. The nurse would also take time to communicate with the child; allow the child to express feelings such as anxiety, fear, or anger; accept any regressive behavior; and assist the preschooler with moving from regressive to appropriate behaviors. Additional interventions include encouraging rooming-in with the parents or leaving a favorite toy; allowing mobility and providing play and diversional activities; placing the preschooler with other children of the same age if possible; and encouraging the preschooler to be independent. The nurse would also explain procedures simply on the preschooler's level, avoid intrusive procedures when possible, and allow the child to wear underpants.

PRACTICE QUESTIONS

1. The parents of a 16-year-old child tell the nurse that they are concerned because the child sleeps until noon every weekend. Which is the **most appropriate** nursing response?
   1. "Adolescents love to sleep late in the morning."
   2. "The child shouldn't be staying up so late at night."
   3. "If the child eats properly, that shouldn't be happening."
   4. "The child needs to have a blood test to check for anemia."

2. A 16-year-old child is admitted to the hospital for acute appendicitis, and an appendectomy is performed. Which intervention is **most appropriate** to facilitate normal growth and development?
   1. Encourage the child to rest and read.
   2. Encourage the parents to room-in with the child.
   3. Allow the family to bring in favorite computer games.
   4. Allow the child to participate in activities with other individuals in the same age group when the condition permits.

3. The nurse is reinforcing discharge instructions to the parents of a 2-year-old child who sustained accidental burns from a hot cup of coffee. The nurse determines that the parents have correctly understood the teaching when they make which statement?
   1. "We will be sure not to leave hot liquids unattended."
   2. "I guess my child needs to understand what the word 'hot' means."
   3. "We will be sure that our child stays in his room when we work in the kitchen."
   4. "We will install a safety gate as soon as we get home so that our child can't get into the kitchen."

❖ 4. Which interventions are appropriate for the care of an infant? **Select all that apply.**
   ❑ 1. Provide swaddling.
   ❑ 2. Talk in a loud voice.
   ❑ 3. Provide the infant with a bottle of juice at naptime.
   ❑ 4. Hang mobiles with black-and-white contrast designs.
   ❑ 5. Caress the infant while bathing or during diaper changes.
   ❑ 6. Allow the infant to cry for at least 10 minutes before responding.

❖ 5. The nurse is preparing to care for a dying client and several family members are at the client's bedside. Which therapeutic techniques would the nurse use when communicating with the family? **Select all that apply.**

❑ 1. Discourage reminiscing.
❑ 2. Make the decisions for the family.
❑ 3. Encourage expression of feelings, concerns, and fears.
❑ 4. Explain everything that is happening to all family members.
❑ 5. Touch and hold the client's or family member's hand if appropriate.
❑ 6. Be honest and let the client and family know that they will not be abandoned by the nurse.

6. The parents of a 2-year-old arrive at the hospital to visit their child. The child is in the play room and ignores the parents during the visit. The nurse tells the parents that this behavior in a 2-year-old child indicates which characteristic about the child?
   1. The child is withdrawn.
   2. The child is upset with the parents.
   3. The child is exhibiting a normal pattern.
   4. The child has adjusted to the hospitalized setting.

7. When caring for a 3-year-old child, the nurse would provide which toy for the child?
   1. A puzzle
   2. A wagon
   3. A golf set
   4. A miniature farm set

8. Upon palpation of the fontanel of a 3-month-old newborn, the nurse notes that the anterior fontanel has not closed and is soft and flat. Which action would the nurse take?
   1. Increase oral fluids.
   2. Document the findings.
   3. Notify the registered nurse.
   4. Elevate the head of the bed to 90 degrees.

9. The nurse is caring for a 5-year-old child who has been placed in traction after a fracture of the femur. Which is the **most appropriate** activity for this child?
   1. Blocks
   2. A music video
   3. A 10-piece puzzle
   4. Large picture books

10. The parent of a 4-year-old child expresses concern because her hospitalized child has started sucking his thumb. The mother states that this behavior began 2 days after hospital admission. Which is the appropriate nursing response?
    1. "Your child is acting like a baby."
    2. "The doctor will need to be notified."
    3. "This is common during hospitalization."
    4. "A 4-year-old is too old for this type of behavior."

ANSWERS

1. 1
Rationale: The sleep patterns of the adolescent vary some according to individual needs. However, in general, adolescents love to sleep late in the morning, but they would be encouraged to be responsible for waking themselves, particularly in time to get ready for school. Options 2, 3, and 4 are incorrect.
Test-Taking Strategy: Note the strategic words, *most appropriate*. The options that suggest comments about the child's sleeping and eating habits can be eliminated first, because they are inappropriate responses and are not helpful or therapeutic. From the remaining options, there is no indication that a physiological alteration is present; therefore, the sleeping late option is most appropriate.

2. 4
Rationale: Adolescents are not often sure they want their parents with them when they are hospitalized. Because of the importance of the peer group, separation from friends is a source of anxiety. Ideally, the peer group will support the ill friend. The other options isolate the child from the peer group.
Test-Taking Strategy: Note the strategic words, *most appropriate*. Consider the psychosocial needs of the adolescent when answering the question. The other options are comparable or alike in that they isolate the child from their own peer group.

3. 1
Rationale: Toddlers, with their increased mobility and developing motor skills, can reach hot water, open fires, or hot objects placed on counters and stoves above their eye level. Parents would be encouraged to remain in the kitchen when preparing a meal and reminded to use the back burners of the stove. Pot handles must be turned inward and toward the middle of the stove. Hot liquids must never be left unattended, and the toddler must always be supervised. The other options do not reflect an adequate understanding of the principles of safety.
Test-Taking Strategy: The option about the child understanding the word "hot" can be easily eliminated considering the development level of a 2-year-old. Next eliminate options 3 and 4 because they are comparable or alike in that they isolate the child from the environment.

4. 1, 4, 5
Rationale: Holding, caressing, and swaddling provide warmth and tactile stimulation for the infant. To provide auditory stimulation, the nurse would talk to the infant in a soft voice and would instruct the mother to also do so. Additional interventions include playing a music box, radio, or television or having a ticking clock or metronome nearby. Hanging a bright, shiny object within 20 cm to 25 cm of the infant's face in the midline and hanging mobiles with contrasting colors (e.g., black and white) provide visual stimulation. Crying is an infant's way of communicating; therefore, the nurse would respond to the infant's crying. The mother is taught to do so also. An infant or child must never be allowed to fall asleep with a bottle containing milk, juice, soda, or sweetened water because of the risk of nursing (bottle-mouth) caries.
Test-Taking Strategy: Focus on the subject, the care of the infant. Noting the word *loud* in option 2 and the words *at least*

10 minutes before responding in option 6 will assist you with eliminating these interventions. Recalling the concerns related to dental caries will assist you with eliminating option 3.

5. 3, 5, 6
Rationale: The nurse must determine whether there is a spokesperson for the family and how much the client and family want to know. The nurse needs to allow the family and client the opportunity for informed choices and assist with the decision-making process if asked. The nurse would encourage expression of feelings, concerns, and fears and reminiscing. The nurse needs to be honest and let the client and family know that they will not be abandoned. The nurse would touch and hold the client's or family member's hand, if appropriate.
Test-Taking Strategy: Use therapeutic communication techniques, and recall client and family rights to assist in directing you to the correct options.

6. 3
Rationale: The toddler is particularly vulnerable to separation. A toddler often shows anger at being left by ignoring the parent or pretending to be more interested in play than in going home. The parents of hospitalized toddlers are frequently distressed by such behavior. The toddler normally engages in parallel play and plays alongside (but not with) other children. Options 1, 2, and 4 are incorrect.
Test-Taking Strategy: Focus on the subject, separation anxiety, and use the concepts of growth and development. The option mentioning adjustment can be easily eliminated first, because there is no indication that the child has adjusted. There is no information in the question to support the option that the child is withdrawn, so eliminate this option. From the remaining options, knowledge regarding separation anxiety in the toddler will direct you to the correct option.

7. 2
Rationale: Toys for the toddler must be strong, safe, and too large to swallow or place in the ear or nose. Toddlers need supervision at all times. Push-pull toys, large balls, large crayons, trucks, and dolls are some appropriate toys. A puzzle, with large pieces only, may be appropriate. A miniature farm set and a golf set may contain items that the child could swallow.
Test-Taking Strategy: Focus on the subject, appropriate toys for a 3-year-old. A golf set and a miniature farm set can be easily eliminated because they contain items that could be swallowed by the child. From the remaining options, the appropriate toy is a wagon. Remember that large and strong toys are safest for the toddler.

8. 2
Rationale: The anterior fontanel is diamond shaped and located on the top of the head. It needs to be soft and flat in a normal infant, and it normally closes by 12 to 18 months of age. The posterior fontanel closes by 2 to 3 months of age. Therefore, because the findings are normal, the nurse must document the findings.
Test-Taking Strategy: Note the subject, findings for an infant's fontanelles. Because they are "soft and flat," this would provide you with the clue that this is a normal finding. A bulging or tense fontanel may result from crying or increased intracranial pressure.

9. 3

Rationale: In the preschooler, play is simple and imaginative, and it includes activities such as dressing up, paints, crayons, and simple board and card games. Ten-piece puzzles are also appropriate and aid with fine motor development. Blocks are most appropriate for the toddler. A music video is most appropriate for the adolescent. Large picture books are most appropriate for the infant.

Test-Taking Strategy: Note the strategic words, *most appropriate*. Also note the subject, play activity and the age of the child, and then think about the age-related activity that would be appropriate. Eliminate the music video, knowing that it is most appropriate for the adolescent. From the remaining options, the words *blocks* and *large* in the remaining option would provide you with the clue that these activities would be more appropriate for a child who is less than 5 years old.

10. 3

Rationale: In the hospitalized preschooler, it is best to accept regression, such as thumb sucking if it occurs, because it is most often caused by the stress of the hospitalization. Parents may be overly concerned about regression and would be told that their child may continue the behavior at home. There is no need to call the health care provider. Telling the parents the child is acting like a baby or being too old to act this way is inappropriate.

Test-Taking Strategy: Focus on the subject, regression because of hospitalization. The incorrect options will cause additional stress and concern for the parent.

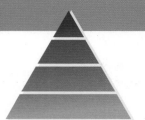

CHAPTER **21**

Care of the Older Client

PRIORITY CONCEPTS Development, Safety

WHAT WOULD YOU DO?

The home care nurse is caring for an older female client who lives with her son and is physically and financially dependent on her son. The nurse notes multiple bruises on the client's arms and asks the client how these bruises occurred. The client confides in the nurse that her son takes out his anger on her sometimes. What would the nurse do?

Answer is located on p. 250.

I. Aging and Gerontology

A. Aging is the biopsychosocial process of change that occurs in a person between birth and death.

B. Gerontology is the study of the aging process.

II. Physiological Changes

A. Integumentary system
1. Loss of pigment in hair and skin
2. Wrinkling of the skin
3. Thinning of the epidermis; easy bruising and tearing of the skin
4. Decreased skin turgor, elasticity, and subcutaneous fat
5. Increased nail thickness and decreased nail growth
6. Decreased perspiration
7. Dry, itchy, and scaly skin
8. Seborrheic dermatitis and keratosis formation (overgrowth and thickening of the skin)

B. Neurological system
1. Slowed reflexes
2. Slight tremors and difficulty with fine motor movement
3. Loss of balance
4. An increased incidence of awakening after sleep onset
5. Increased susceptibility to hypothermia and hyperthermia
6. Short-term memory may decline.
7. Long-term memory usually maintained.

C. Musculoskeletal system
1. Muscle mass and strength decrease; muscles atrophy.
2. Decreased mobility, range of motion, flexibility, coordination, and stability
3. Change of gait, with a shortened step and a wider base
4. Posture and stature changes that cause a decrease in height (Fig. 21.1)
5. Increased brittleness of the bones
6. Deterioration of joint capsule components
7. Kyphosis of the dorsal spine (increased convexity in the curvature of the spine)

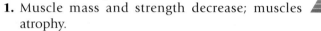 The older client is at risk for falls because of the changes that occur in the neurological and musculoskeletal systems.

D. Cardiovascular system
1. Diminished energy and endurance, with lowered tolerance to exercise
2. Decreased compliance of the heart muscle causing increase in heart size; heart valves become thicker and more rigid.
3. Decreased cardiac output; decreased efficiency of blood return to the heart due to less elasticity of blood vessels
4. Decreased compensatory response, so less able to respond to increased demands on the cardiovascular system
5. Decreased resting heart rate
6. Weak peripheral pulses
7. Increased blood pressure related to the aorta becoming thicker, stiffer, and less flexible; susceptible to postural hypotension

E. Respiratory system
1. Decreased stretch and compliance of the chest wall related to decreased vital capacity and tidal volume

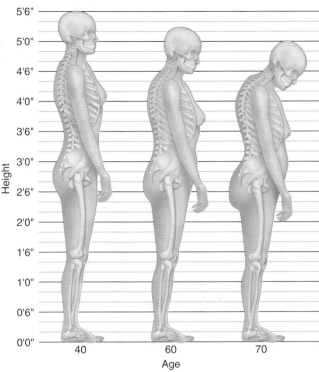

FIGURE 21.1 A normal spine at 40 years of age and osteoporotic changes at 60 and 70 years of age. These changes can cause a loss of as much as 6 inches in height and can result in the so-called dowager's hump (*far right*) in the upper thoracic vertebrae.

2. Decreased strength and function of the respiratory muscles
3. Decreased size and number of alveoli
4. Respiratory rate usually unchanged
5. Decreased depth of respirations and oxygen intake
6. Decreased ability to cough and expectorate sputum

F. Hematological system
   1. Hemoglobin and hematocrit levels average toward the low end of normal.
   2. Prone to increased blood clotting due to less water in vasculature
   3. Decreased protein available for protein-bound medications

G. Immune system
   1. Tendency for lymphocyte counts to be low with altered immunoglobulin production
   2. Decreased resistance to infection and disease

H. Gastrointestinal system
   1. Decreased need for calories because of lowered basal metabolic rate
   2. Decreased appetite, thirst, and oral intake
   3. Decreased lean body mass
   4. Decreased stomach-emptying time
   5. Increased tendency toward constipation
   6. Increased susceptibility to dehydration
   7. Prone to gum disease, dental decay, oral cancer, mouth infection, and tooth loss
   8. Difficulty with chewing and swallowing food

I. Endocrine system
   1. Decreased secretion of hormones, with specific changes related to each hormone function
   2. Decreased metabolic rate
   3. Decreased glucose tolerance, with resistance to insulin in the peripheral tissues

J. Renal system
   1. Decreased kidney size, function, and ability to concentrate urine
   2. Decreased glomerular filtration rate
   3. Decreased capacity of the bladder
   4. Increased residual urine; increased incidence of infection and possibly incontinence
   5. Impaired medication excretion

K. Reproductive system
   1. Decreased testosterone production and size of testes
   2. Changes in the prostate gland, leading to urinary problems
   3. Decreased secretion of hormones, with the cessation of menses
   4. Vaginal changes, including decreased muscle tone and lubrication
   5. Impotence or sexual dysfunction for both genders; sexual function varies and depends on general physical condition, mental health status, and medications.

L. Special senses
   1. Decreased visual acuity
   2. Decreased accommodation in eyes, which requires increased time for adjustment to changes in light
   3. Decreased peripheral vision and increased sensitivity to glare
   4. Presbyopia and cataract formation
   5. Possible loss of hearing ability; low-pitched tones are more easily heard
   6. Inability to discern taste of food
   7. Decreased sense of smell
   8. Change in touch sensation
   9. Decreased pain awareness

III. Psychosocial Concerns

   A. Adjustment to deterioration in physical and mental health and well-being
   B. Threat to independent functioning; fear of becoming a burden to loved ones
   C. Adjustment to retirement and loss of income
   D. Loss of skills and competencies developed early in life
   E. Coping with changes in role function and social life
   F. Diminished quantity and quality of relationships and coping with loss
   G. Dependence on governmental and social systems
   H. Access to social support systems
   I. Costs of health care and medications
   J. Loss of independence in living, driving, and their daily functions

TABLE 21.1   Differentiating Delirium, Depression, and Dementia

Characteristic	Delirium	Depression	Dementia
Onset	Sudden, abrupt	Recent; may relate to life change	Insidious, slow, over years and often unrecognized until deficits obvious
Course over 24 hours	Fluctuating, often worse at night	Fairly stable; may be worse in the morning	Fairly stable; may see changes with stress; sundowning may occur
Consciousness	Reduced	Clear	Clear
Alertness	Increased, decreased, or variable	Normal	Generally normal
Psychomotor activity	Increased, decreased, or mixed	Variable, agitation, or retardation	Normal; may have apraxia or agnosia; agitation can occur
Duration	Hours to weeks	Variable and may be chronic	Years
Attention	Disordered, fluctuates	Little impairment	Generally normal but may have trouble focusing; overwhelmed with multiple stimuli
Orientation	Usually impaired, fluctuates	Usually normal; may answer "I don't know" to questions or may not try to answer	Often impaired; may make up answers or answer close to the right thing, or may confabulate but tries to answer
Speech	Often incoherent, slow or rapid; may call out repeatedly or repeat the same phrase	May be slow	Difficulty finding word, perseveration
Affect	Variable but may look disturbed, frightened	Flat	Slowed response; may be labile

Modified from Rapp CG, Mentes J, Titler M: Acute confusion/delirium protocol, *J Gerontol Nurse* 27(4):21–33, 2001. Reprinted with permission from SLACK, Inc., Thorofare, NJ.

 IV. Mental Health Concerns

A. Depression: The increased dependency that older adults may experience can lead to hopelessness, helplessness, a lowered sense of self-control, and decreased self-esteem and self-worth. These changes can interfere with daily functioning and lead to depression.

B. Grief: Client reacts to the perception of loss, including physical, psychological, social, and spiritual aspects.

C. Isolation: Client is alone and desires contact with others but is unable to make that contact.

D. Suicide: Depression can lead to thoughts of self-harm.

E. Depression differs from delirium and dementia (Table 21.1).

⚠ Any suicide threat from an older client must be taken seriously.

 V. Pain

A. Description
1. Pain can come about from numerous causes and most often occurs from degenerative changes in the musculoskeletal system.
2. The nurse needs to monitor the older client closely for signs of pain; failure to alleviate pain in the older client can lead to functional limitations that affect the client's ability to be independent.

B. Data collection
1. Restlessness
2. Verbal reporting of pain
3. Agitation
4. Moaning
5. Crying

C. Interventions
1. Monitor the client for signs of pain.
2. Identify the pattern of pain.
3. Identify the precipitating factor(s) for the pain.
4. Monitor the effect of the pain on the client's activities of daily living.
5. Provide pain relief through measures such as distraction, relaxation, massage, and biofeedback.
6. Administer pain medications, as prescribed. Instruct the client in their use.
7. Evaluate the effects of pain-reducing measures.

VI. Infection

A. Altered mental status is a common sign of infection in the older adult, especially infection of the urinary tract.

B. Carefully monitor the older adult with an infection because of diminished and altered immune response.

C. Nonspecific symptoms may indicate illness or infection (Box 21.1).

VII. Medications

A. Major problems with prescription medications include adverse effects, medication interactions, medication errors, noncompliance, polypharmacy, and

BOX 21.1 Nonspecific Symptoms That May Indicate Illness or Infection

- Altered mental status, including delirium
- Anorexia
- Apathy
- Blood pressure below baseline
- Change in functional status
- Dyspnea
- Falling
- Fatigue
- Hyperglycemia
- Incontinence
- Self-neglect
- Shortness of breath
- Tachypnea

BOX 21.2 Medications to Avoid in the Older Client

Analgesics
- Indomethacin
- Ketorolac
- Nonsteroidal antiinflammatory drugs (NSAIDs)
- Meperidine

Antidepressants
- First-generation tricyclic antidepressants

Antihistamines
- First-generation antihistamines

Antihypertensives
- α_1-blockers
- Centrally acting α_2-agonists

Urge Incontinence Medications
- Oxybutynin
- Tolterodine

Muscle Relaxants
- Carisoprodol
- Cyclobenzaprine
- Metaxalone
- Methocarbamol

Sedative-Hypnotics
- Barbiturates
- Benzodiazepines

Based on Beers Criteria from the American Geriatrics Society. Information on this criteria and a full list of medications to avoid can be located at https://geriatricscareonline.org/ProductAbstract/american-geriatrics-society-updated-beers-criteria-for-potentially-inappropriate-medication-use-in-older-adults/CL001.

cost. See Box 21.2 for information on medications to avoid in the older adult client. This information is based on Beers Criteria from the American Geriatrics Society. Information on this criteria and a full list of medications to avoid can be located at https://www.guideline.gov/summaries/summary/49933.

 B. Determine the use of over-the-counter medications.

 C. Polypharmacy
1. Routinely monitor the number of prescription and nonprescription medications used and determine whether any can be eliminated or combined.
2. Keep the use of medications to a minimum.
3. Overprescribing medications leads to increased problems with more side effects, increased interaction between medications, duplication of medication treatment, diminished quality of life, and increased costs.

D. Medication dosages normally are prescribed at one third to one half of the normal adult doses.

 E. Closely monitor the client for side effects and adverse effects and response to therapy because of the increased risk for medication toxicity (see Box 21.2).

F. Check for medication interactions in the client who is taking multiple medications.

 G. Advise the client to use one pharmacy and notify the consulting primary health care providers of the medications taken.

⚠ A common sign of an adverse reaction to a medication in the older client is an acute change in mental status.

 H. Safety measures for administration of medications (see Priority Nursing Actions Box)
1. Place the client in a sitting position when administering medication.
2. Check for mouth dryness, because medication may stick and dissolve in the mouth.
3. Administer liquid preparations if the client has difficulty swallowing tablets.

4. Crush tablets if necessary and give with textured food (e.g., applesauce), if not contraindicated.
5. Enteric-coated tablets are not crushed and capsules are not opened.
6. If administering a suppository, avoid inserting it immediately after removal from the refrigerator. A suppository may take a while to dissolve because of a decreased body core temperature.
7. When administering parenteral medication, monitor the site, because it may ooze medication or bleed as a result of decreased tissue elasticity. An immobile limb is not used for administering parenteral medication.
8. Monitor client compliance with the taking of prescribed medications.
9. Monitor the client for safety with regard to correctly taking medications, including an assessment of the client's ability to read the instructions and discriminate among the pills and their color and shape.
10. Use a medication cassette to facilitate the proper administration of medication.
11. Encourage clients to keep an up-to-date list of medications with them at all times.
12. Educate the client on each medication, common side effects, and when to notify the primary health care provider.

⚡ PRIORITY NURSING ACTIONS

Administering Oral Medications to a Client at Risk for Aspiration

1. Check the medication prescription and compare against the medical record. Clarify any incomplete prescriptions before administration. Check the rights of medication administration.
2. Review pertinent information related to the medication and any related nursing considerations, such as laboratory parameters.
3. Assess for any contraindications to the administration, such as NPO (nothing by mouth) status or decreased level of consciousness.
4. Place the client in a high Fowler's position. Assess aspiration risk using a screening tool or per agency policy. Check for an ability to swallow and cough on command. Check for the presence of a gag reflex. Following this assessment, if aspiration is a serious concern, the nurse would collaborate with the registered nurse (RN) or primary health care provider (PHCP) and speech therapist before administering the medication.
5. Prepare the medication in the form that is easiest to swallow, checking the rights of medication administration again. Mix medications whole, or crush medications and mix with applesauce or pudding if indicated (use sugar-free products for clients with diabetes). Do not crush sustained-release tablets and use liquid preparations when possible. Thicken liquids when indicated and avoid the use of straws.
6. Check the rights of medication administration for the last time and administer the medications one at a time in the prepared form, ensuring that the client has effectively swallowed everything. Ensure that the client is comfortable and safe and document the medications given using an electronic system or per agency policy.

VIII. Mistreatment of the Older Adult

A. Domestic mistreatment takes place in the home of the older adult and is usually carried out by a family member or significant other; this can include physical maltreatment, neglect, or abandonment.

B. Institutional mistreatment takes place when an older adult experiences abuse when hospitalized or living somewhere other than at their home (e.g., long-term care facility).

C. Self-neglect is the choice by a mentally competent individual to avoid medical care or other services that could improve optimal function, not to care for oneself, and engage in actions that negatively affect his or her personal safety; unless declared legally incompetent, an individual has the right to refuse care.

> ⚠ Individuals at most risk for abuse include those who are dependent because of their immobility or altered mental status.

D. For additional information about abuse of the older client, see Chapter 64.

WHAT WOULD YOU DO?

Answer: If the nurse suspects or knows for certain that elder abuse is occurring, the nurse must report this abuse to the appropriate authorities and follow state and agency guidelines in doing so. The nurse would then perform a thorough assessment of physical injuries, while providing confidentiality during the assessment with an empathetic and nonjudgmental approach. The nurse would reassure the victim that she or he has done nothing wrong. The nurse would also assist the victim in developing self-protective and problem-solving skills. Even if the victim is not ready to leave the situation, encourage them to develop a specific safety plan (a fast escape if the violence returns) and where to obtain help (hotlines, safe houses, and shelters); an abused person is usually reluctant to call the police.

PRACTICE QUESTIONS

1. An older client has been prescribed digoxin. The nurse determines that which age-related change would place the client at risk for digoxin toxicity?
1. Decreased salivation and gastrointestinal motility
2. Decreased muscle strength and loss of bone density
3. Decreased lean body mass and glomerular filtration rate
4. Decreased cardiac output and decreased efficiency of blood return to the heart

2. The nurse would plan which to encourage autonomy in the client who is a resident in a long-term care facility?
1. Choosing meals
2. Decorating the room
3. Scheduling haircut appointments
4. Allowing the client to choose social activities

❖ 3. Which data indicate to the nurse that a client is experiencing **effective** coping following the loss of a spouse? **Select all that apply.**
- ❑ 1. Looks at old snapshots of family
- ❑ 2. Constantly neglects personal grooming
- ❑ 3. Visits the spouse's grave once a month
- ❑ 4. Visits the senior citizens' center once a month
- ❑ 5. Prefers to spend time alone and avoids contact with others

4. The nurse is preparing to communicate with an older client who is hearing impaired. Which intervention would be implemented **initially**?
1. Stand in front of the client.
2. Exaggerate lip movements.
3. Obtain a sign-language interpreter.
4. Pantomime and write the client notes.

5. Which intervention needs to be implemented for the older client with presbycusis who has a hearing loss?
   1. Speak louder
   2. Speak more slowly
   3. Use low-pitched tones
   4. Use high-pitched tones

❖ 6. When the nurse is collecting data from the older adult, which findings would be considered normal physiological changes? **Select all that apply.**
   ❑ 1. Increased heart rate
   ❑ 2. Decline in visual acuity
   ❑ 3. Decreased respiratory rate
   ❑ 4. Decline in long-term memory
   ❑ 5. Increased susceptibility to urinary tract infections
   ❑ 6. Increased incidence of awakening after sleep onset

7. The nurse is planning to feed an older client who is at risk for aspiration of food. During the meal how would the nurse position the client?
   1. Upright in a chair
   2. On the left side in bed
   3. On the right side in bed
   4. In a low Fowler's position, with the legs elevated

8. The nurse is providing an education class to healthy older adults. Which exercise will **best** promote health maintenance?
   1. Gardening every day for an hour
   2. Sculpting once a week for 40 minutes
   3. Cycling three times a week for 20 minutes
   4. Walking three to five times a week for 30 minutes

9. The nurse would implement which activity to promote reminiscence among older clients?
   1. Having storytelling hours
   2. Setting up pet therapy sessions
   3. Displaying calendars and clocks
   4. Encouraging client participation in a pottery class

10. Which client is **most likely** at risk to become a victim of elder abuse?
   1. A 75-year-old man with moderate hypertension
   2. A 68-year-old man with newly diagnosed cataracts
   3. A 90-year-old woman with advanced Alzheimer's disease
   4. A 70-year-old woman with early diagnosed Lyme disease

ANSWERS

1. 3

Rationale: The older client is at risk for medication toxicity because of decreased lean body mass and an age-associated decreased glomerular filtration rate. Although the other changes identify age-related changes that occur in the older client, they are not specifically associated with this risk.

Test-Taking Strategy: Focus on the subject, age-related body change that could place the client at risk for medication toxicity. Note that option 3 is the only choice that addresses renal excretion.

2. 4

Rationale: Autonomy is the personal freedom to direct one's own life as long as it does not impinge on the rights of others. An autonomous person is capable of rational thought. This individual can identify problems, search for alternatives, and choose solutions that allow for continued personal freedom as long as the rights and property of others are not harmed. The loss of autonomy—and, therefore, independence—is a very real fear among older clients. The correct option is the only choice that allows the client to be a decision maker.

Test-Taking Strategy: Focus on the subject, encouraging autonomy. Recalling the definition of autonomy will direct you to the correct option. Remember that to promote independence in clients, it is essential to give the client choices.

3. 1, 3, 4

Rationale: Coping mechanisms are behaviors that are used to decrease stress and anxiety. Visiting a spouse's grave, visiting the senior citizens' center, and looking at snapshots of the family are effective coping mechanisms. Neglecting grooming and preferring to spend time alone and avoiding contact with others are behaviors that identify ineffective coping with the grieving process.

Test-Taking Strategy: Note the strategic word, *effective*, and choose behaviors that indicate positive coping mechanisms. Visiting the grave, visiting the senior citizens' center, and looking at snapshots of family are positive activities that indicate an individual is getting on with life.

4. 1

Rationale: The nurse needs to ensure that the hearing-impaired client can see the nurse when the nurse is speaking by providing adequate lighting and standing in front of the client. The nurse would enunciate words clearly, but not exaggerate lip movements. If the client is profoundly hearing impaired and uses signing, a sign-language interpreter needs to be obtained. If a client cannot understand by reading lips, the nurse would try using gestures, pantomiming, or writing notes.

Test-Taking Strategy: Note the strategic word, *initially*. To communicate effectively with a client who is hearing impaired, the nurse first makes sure that the client can see the nurse.

5. 3

Rationale: Presbycusis refers to the age-related, irreversible, degenerative changes of the inner ear that lead to decreased hearing acuity. As a result of these changes, the older client has a decreased response to high-frequency sounds. Low-pitched tones of voice are more easily heard and interpreted by the older client. Speaking loudly, softly, or slowly is not helpful.

Test-Taking Strategy: Focus on the subject, interventions for a client with hearing loss. Recalling that the client with a hearing loss responds better to low-pitched tones will direct you to the correct option.

6. 2, 5, 6

Rationale: Anatomical changes to the eye affect the individual's visual ability, which leads to potential problems with activities of daily living. Light adaptation and visual fields are reduced. Respiratory rates are usually unchanged. The heart rate decreases, and the heart valves thicken. Age-related changes that affect the urinary tract increase an older client's susceptibility to urinary tract infections. Short-term memory may decline with age, but long-term memory is usually maintained. Changes in sleep patterns are consistent, age-related changes. Older persons experience an increased incidence of awakening after sleep onset.

Test-Taking Strategy: Focus on the subject, normal physiological changes. Read each characteristic carefully, and think about the physiological changes that occur with aging to select the correct items.

7. 1

Rationale: It is preferable to get clients out of bed and sitting in a chair for meals. This position facilitates chewing and swallowing and prevents the reflux of stomach contents and aspiration. The other options do not identify positions that will reduce the risk of aspiration.

Test-Taking Strategy: Focus on the subject, reducing the risk of aspiration. Read each option and think about how the position can affect swallowing. This would direct you to the correct option.

8. 4

Rationale: Exercise and activity are essential for health promotion and maintenance in the older adult and for achieving an optimal level of functioning. One of the best exercises for an older adult is walking, with the goal of progressing to 30-minute sessions three to five times each week. Gardening for an hour each day may not be practical. Not all clients have access to sculpting, and performing the activity once a week for 40 minutes would not provide enough activity. Cycling three times a week for 20 minutes would not provide enough activity, and not all clients have access to cycling.

Test-Taking Strategy: Note the strategic word, *best*. The options of gardening, sculpting and cycling, although possible, are not the best activities. Remember that walking is one of the best forms of exercise.

9. 1

Rationale: Clients who like to retell stories or to describe past events need to be provided with the opportunity to do so. This phenomenon is called life review or reminiscence. In a sense, it is a way for the older client to relive and restructure life experiences, and it is a part of achieving ego identity. Displaying calendars and clocks indicates reality orientation techniques. Pet therapy and pottery classes describe socialization and physical activities.

Test-Taking Strategy: Focus on the subject, reminiscence. Recalling its definition will direct you to option 1.

10. 3
Rationale: Elder abuse is widespread and occurs among all subgroups of the population. It includes physical and psychological abuse, the misuse of property, and the violation of rights. The person at highest risk of abuse is an elder with dementia that occurs with Alzheimer's disease.

Test-Taking Strategy: Focus on the strategic words, *most likely*, and read each option carefully to identify the client who is most defenseless as a result of the disease process.

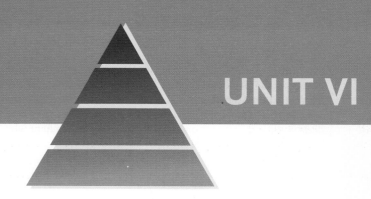

UNIT VI

Maternity Nursing

Pyramid to Success

The Pyramid to Success focuses on the physiological and psychosocial aspects related to the experience of pregnancy, birth, and the postpartum period. Pyramid Points begin with the assessment and knowledge of expected findings of the pregnant client and fetus during the antepartum period. Instructing the pregnant client in measures that promote a healthy environment for the mother and the fetus is included. The focus is on the importance of antepartum follow-up, nutrition, and interventions for common discomforts that occur during pregnancy. Knowledge of the purpose of the commonly prescribed diagnostic tests and procedures in the antepartum period is also part of the Pyramid to Success. The focus is on disorders that can occur during pregnancy, particularly gestational hypertension and diabetes mellitus. The labor and birth process and the immediate interventions for conditions in which the maternal or fetal status is compromised, such as prolapsed cord or altered fetal heart rate, are a part of the Pyramid to Success. Review of the fetus of a mother with human immunodeficiency virus or acquired immunodeficiency syndrome or a substance-abusing mother is recommended. The Pyramid to Success also includes a focus on the normal expectations of the postpartum period and the complications that can occur during this time. Additionally, focus on the normal physical assessment findings and early identification of disorders in the neonate and on maternity and newborn medications.

Client Needs: Learning Objectives

Safe and Effective Care Environment

Consulting with the interprofessional health care team

Ensuring that informed consent for diagnostic tests and procedures has been obtained

Establishing priorities of care

Handling hazardous and infectious materials safely

Maintaining confidentiality

Providing continuity of client care

Promoting a safe environment from potential teratogenic threats

Upholding client's rights

Using surgical asepsis when providing care

Using standard and transmission-based precautions when providing care

Health Promotion and Maintenance

Discussing expected body image changes with the client

Discussing family planning and birthing and parenting issues

Identifying at-risk clients during pregnancy

Identifying health and wellness concepts and providing health care screening

Identifying lifestyle choices and high-risk behaviors

Monitoring growth and development patterns

Performing techniques of physical assessment and data collection

Providing antepartum, intrapartum, postpartum, and newborn care

Teaching regarding antepartum, intrapartum, and postpartum care, and care to the newborn

Psychosocial Integrity

Considering cultural, religious, and spiritual influences regarding birth and motherhood

Discussing situational role changes in the family

Ensuring therapeutic interactions within the family

Identifying available support systems

Identifying coping mechanisms

Physiological Integrity

Instructing the client about prescribed diagnostic tests and procedures

Monitoring for expected outcomes and effects related to prescribed pharmacological and parenteral therapies

Monitoring for normal expectations during pregnancy

Monitoring for side effects and adverse effects related to prescribed pharmacological and parenteral therapies

Monitoring the client during the labor and birth process

Providing interventions for unexpected events during pregnancy

Providing nonpharmacological comfort interventions and prescribed pharmacological pain management during labor

Supporting families who are experiencing fertility issues

Teaching the client about nutrition during pregnancy and in the postpartum period

Teaching the client about the physiological changes that occur during pregnancy

Client Needs lists modified from: National Council of State Boards of Nursing, Inc. (NCSBN). *NCLEX-PN Examination: Test Plan for the National Council Licensure Examination for Practical Nurses,* effective April 2020. Chicago: NCSBN.

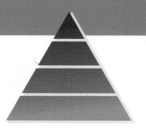

CHAPTER **22**

Reproductive System

PRIORITY CONCEPTS Reproduction; Sexuality

WHAT WOULD YOU DO?

The nurse is collecting data for the first time from a pregnant adolescent who reports consuming small amounts of alcohol on a daily basis. On the basis of the information provided, what would the nurse do?
Answer is located on p. 260.

I. Female Reproductive Structures

A. Ovaries
  1. Form and expel ova
  2. Secrete estrogen and progesterone
B. Fallopian tubes
  1. Muscular tubes (oviducts) lying near the ovaries and connected to the uterus
  2. Tubes that propel the ova from the ovaries to the uterus
C. Uterus
  1. Muscular, pear-shaped cavity in which the fetus develops
  2. Cavity from which menstruation occurs
D. Cervix
  1. Internal os of the cervix opens into the body of the uterine cavity.
  2. The cervical canal is located between the internal cervical os and the external cervical os.
  3. The external cervical os opens into the vagina.
E. Vagina
  1. Muscular tube that extends from the cervix to the vaginal opening in the perineum
  2. Known as the *birth canal*
  3. Passageway for menstrual blood flow, for penis during intercourse, and for the fetus

II. Male Reproductive Structures

A. Penis
  1. Structures include the body or shaft, glans penis, and urethra.
  2. Primary functions include pathway for urination and it is the organ for intercourse.
B. Scrotum
  1. Structures include the testes, epididymis, and vas deferens.
  2. Normal temperature within the scrotum is slightly cooler than body temperature for optimum sperm production.
C. Prostate gland
  1. Secretes a milky alkaline fluid
  2. Enhances sperm movement and neutralizes acidic vaginal secretions

III. Menstrual Cycle (Box 22.1)

A. Ovarian hormones
  1. Ovarian hormones, released by the anterior pituitary gland, include follicle-stimulating hormone (FSH) and luteinizing hormone (LH).
  2. The hormones produce changes in the ovaries and in the endometrium.
  3. The menstrual cycle, the regularly recurring physiological changes in the endometrium that culminate in its shedding, may vary in length, with the average length being about 28 days.
B. Ovarian and uterine phases (see Box 22.1)

IV. Female Pelvis and Measurement

A. True pelvis
  1. Lies below the pelvic brim
  2. Consists of the pelvic inlet, the mid pelvis, and the pelvic outlet
B. False pelvis
  1. The shallow portion above the pelvic brim
  2. Supports the abdominal viscera
C. Types of pelvis
  1. Gynecoid
    a. Normal female pelvis
    b. Transversely rounded or blunt

BOX 22.1   Menstrual Cycle

Ovarian Changes
Preovulatory Phase
The hypothalamus releases gonadotropin-releasing hormone through the portal system to the anterior pituitary system.

Secretion of follicle-stimulating hormone (FSH) by the anterior lobe of the pituitary gland stimulates growth of follicles.

Most follicles die, leaving one to mature into a large Graafian follicle.

Estrogen produced by the follicle stimulates increased secretions of luteinizing hormone (LH) by the anterior lobe of the pituitary gland.

The follicle ruptures and releases an ovum into the peritoneal cavity.

Luteal Phase
The luteal phase begins with ovulation.

Body temperature drops and then rises by 0.5°F–1°F around the time of ovulation.

Corpus luteum is formed from follicle cells that remain in the ovary following ovulation.

Corpus luteum secretes estrogen and progesterone during the remaining 14 days of the cycle.

Corpus luteum degenerates if the ovum is not fertilized, and secretion of estrogen and progesterone declines.

The decline of estrogen and progesterone stimulates the anterior pituitary to secrete more FSH and LH, initiating a new reproductive cycle.

Uterine Changes
Menstrual Phase
The menstrual phase consists of 4–6 days of bleeding as the endometrium breaks down because of the decreased levels of estrogen and progesterone.

The level of FSH increases, enabling the beginning of a new cycle.

Proliferative Phase
The proliferative phase lasts about 9 days.

Estrogen stimulates proliferation and growth of the endometrium.

As estrogen increases, it suppresses secretion of FSH and increases secretion of LH.

Secretion of LH stimulates ovulation and the development of the corpus luteum.

Ovulation occurs between days 12 and 16.

The estrogen level is high and the progesterone level is low.

Secretory Phase
The secretory phase lasts about 12 days and follows ovulation.

This phase is initiated in response to the increase in LH level.

The Graafian follicle is replaced by the corpus luteum.

The corpus luteum secretes progesterone and estrogen.

Progesterone prepares the endometrium for pregnancy if a fertilized ovum is implanted.

⚠ The gynecoid pelvis is most favorable for successful labor and birth. If cephalopelvic disproportion (CPD) exists, the normal labor process will be delayed and most likely result in a cesarean delivery.

2. Anthropoid
   a. Oval shape
   b. The outlet is adequate, with a normal or moderately narrow pubic arch.
3. Android
   a. Heart-shaped or angulated
   b. Resembles a male pelvis
   c. Not favorable for labor and birth
   d. Narrow pelvic planes can cause slow descent and midpelvic arrest
4. Platypelloid
   a. Flat shape with an oval inlet
   b. Wide transverse diameter, but short anteroposterior diameter, making labor and vaginal birth difficult
D. Pelvic inlet diameters
   1. Anteroposterior diameters
      a. Diagonal conjugate: Distance from the lower margin of the symphysis pubis to the sacral promontory
      b. True conjugate or conjugate vera: Distance from the upper margin of the symphysis pubis to the sacral promontory

     c. Obstetrical conjugate: Extends from the sacral promontory to the top of the symphysis pubis. It is the smallest front-to-back distance through which the fetal head must pass in moving through the pelvic inlet.
   2. Transverse diameter: The largest of the pelvic inlet diameters; located at right angles to the true conjugate
   3. Oblique (diagonal) diameter: Not clinically measurable
   4. Posterior sagittal diameter: Distance from the point where the anteroposterior and transverse diameters cross each other to the middle of the sacral promontory
E. Pelvic midplane diameters
   1. Transverse (interspinous diameter)
   2. Midplane normally is the largest plane and has the longest diameter.
F. Pelvic outlet diameters
   1. Transverse (intertuberous diameter)
   2. Outlet presents the smallest plane of the pelvic canal.

V. Fertilization and Implantation

A. Fertilization
   1. Fertilization occurs in the ampulla of the fallopian (uterine) tube when sperm and ova unite.
   2. When fertilized, the membrane of the ovum undergoes changes that prevent entry of other sperm.

BOX 22.2   Fetal Development

Preembryonic Period
First 2 weeks after conception

Embryonic Period
Beginning day 15 through approximately week 8 after conception

Fetal Period
Week 9 after conception to birth

Week 1
Blastocyst is free-floating.

Weeks 2–3
Embryo is 1.5–2 mm in length.
Lung buds appear.
Blood circulation begins.
Heart is tubular and begins to beat.
Neural plate becomes brain and spinal cord.

Week 5
Embryo is 0.4–0.5 cm in length.
Embryo is 0.4 g.
Double heart chambers are visible.
Heart is beating.
Limb buds form.

Week 8
Embryo is 3 cm in length.
Embryo is 2 g.
Eyelids begin to fuse.
Circulatory system through umbilical cord is well established.
Every organ system is present.

Week 12
Fetus is 6–9 cm in length.
Fetus is 19 g.
Face is well formed
Limbs are long and slender.
Kidneys begin to form urine.
Spontaneous movements occur.
Heartbeat is detected by Doppler transducer between 10 and 12 weeks.

Week 16
Fetus is 11.5–13.5 cm in length.
Fetus is 100 g.
Active movements are present.
Fetal skin is transparent.
Lanugo hair begins to develop.
Skeletal ossification occurs.

Week 20
Fetus is 16–18.5 cm in length.
Fetus is 300 g.
Lanugo covers the entire body.
Fetus has nails.
Muscles are developed.
Enamel and dentin are depositing.
Heartbeat is detected by regular (nonelectronic) fetoscope.
Gender can be determined about 18 to 20 weeks.

Week 24
Fetus is 23 cm in length.
Fetus is 600 g.
Hair on head is well formed.
Skin is reddish and wrinkled.
Reflex hand grasp functions.
Vernix caseosa covers entire body.
Fetus has ability to hear.

Week 28
Fetus is 27 cm in length.
Fetus is 1100 g.
Limbs are well flexed.
Brain is developing rapidly.
Eyelids open and close.
Lungs are developed sufficiently to provide gas exchange (lecithin forming).
If born, neonate can breathe at this time.

Week 32
Fetus is 31 cm in length.
Fetus is 1800–2100 g.
Bones are fully developed.
Subcutaneous fat has collected.
The L/S (lecithin-to-sphingomyelin) ratio is 1.2:1.

Week 36
The fetus is 35 cm in length.
The fetus is 2200–2900 g.
The skin is pink and the body is rounded.
The skin is less wrinkled.
Lanugo is disappearing.
The L/S ratio is higher than 2:1.

Week 40
The fetus is 40 cm in length.
The fetus is 3200+ g.
The skin is pinkish and smooth.
Lanugo present on upper arms and shoulders.
Vernix caseosa decreases.
Fingernails extend beyond fingertips.
Sole (plantar) creases run down to the heel.
The testes are in the scrotum.
The labia majora are well developed.

  3. Each reproductive cell carries 23 chromosomes.
  4. Sperm carry an X or a Y chromosome—XY, male; XX, female.
B. Implantation
  1. The zygote is propelled toward the uterus and implants 6 to 8 days after ovulation.

  2. The blastocyst secretes chorionic gonadotropin to ensure that the corpus luteum remains viable and secretes estrogen and progesterone for the first 2 to 3 months of gestation.

VI. Fetal Development (Box 22.2)

VII. Fetal Environment

A. Amnion
  1. Encloses the amniotic cavity
  2. Inner cell membrane that forms around the second week of embryonic development
  3. Forms a fluid-filled sac that surrounds the embryo and later the fetus

B. Chorion
  1. Outer membrane enclosing the amniotic cavity
  2. Becomes vascularized and forms the fetal part of the placenta

C. Amniotic fluid
  1. Consists of 800 to 1200 mL by the end of pregnancy
  2. Surrounds, cushions, and protects the fetus and allows for fetal movement
  3. Maintains the body temperature of the fetus
  4. Contains fetal urine and is a measure of fetal kidney function
  5. The fetus modifies the amniotic fluid through the processes of swallowing, urinating, and moving the fluid through the respiratory tract.

D. Placenta
  1. The placenta provides for exchange of nutrients and waste products between the fetus and the mother.
  2. Begins to form at implantation; structure is complete by week 12.
  3. It produces hormones to maintain pregnancy and assumes full responsibility for the production of these hormones by the twelfth week of gestation.
  4. In the third trimester, transfer of maternal immunoglobulin provides the fetus with passive immunity to certain diseases for the first few months after birth.
  5. By week 10 and 12, genetic testing can be done via chorionic villus sampling (CVS).

> Nutrients, medications, alcohol, antibodies, viruses, and some bacteria can pass through the placenta.

VIII. Fetal Circulation

A. Umbilical cord
  1. It contains two arteries and one vein.
  2. The arteries carry deoxygenated blood and waste products from the fetus.
  3. The vein carries oxygenated blood and provides oxygen and nutrients to the fetus.

B. Fetal heart rate (FHR)
  1. FHR depends on gestational age: FHR is 160 to 170 beats per minute during the first trimester, but slows with fetal growth to 110 to 160 beats per minute near or at term.
  2. FHR is about twice the maternal heart rate.

C. Fetal circulation bypass (Fig. 22.1)
  1. Fetal circulation bypass is present as a result of nonfunctioning lungs.
  2. Bypasses must close after birth to allow for blood to flow through the lungs and liver.
  3. The ductus arteriosus connects the pulmonary artery to the aorta, bypassing the lungs.
  4. The ductus venosus connects the umbilical vein and the inferior vena cava, bypassing the liver.
  5. The foramen ovale is the opening between the right and left atria of heart, bypassing the lungs.

IX. Family Planning

A. Description
  1. Involves choosing when to have children
  2. Includes contraception, prevention of pregnancy, and methods to achieve pregnancy

B. Birth control
  1. The focus of counseling on contraception must meet the needs and feelings of the woman and her partner.
  2. Several factors would be considered when choosing a method of birth control, including effectiveness, safety, and personal preference.
  3. The woman's preferences are most important, and cultural practices and beliefs and religious or other personal beliefs may affect the choice of contraceptives.
  4. Other factors that bear on selection of a contraceptive method include family-planning goals, age, frequency of intercourse, and the individual's capacity for compliance.
  5. If family planning goals have already been met, sterilization of either the male or female partner may be desirable (it is important for the couple to understand that tubal reconstruction may be unsuccessful).
  6. For women who frequently engage in coitus, oral contraceptives or a long-term method such as implants or an intrauterine device (IUD) may be considered.
  7. When sexual activity is limited, use of spermicide, condoms, or a diaphragm may be most appropriate.
  8. Because some methods have adverse effects, a signed informed consent form may be needed.
  9. For additional information on the use of contraceptives, see Chapter 44.

C. Infertility
  1. Infertility is the involuntary inability to conceive when desired.
  2. Some factors contributing to infertility in men include abnormalities of the sperm, abnormal erections or ejaculations, or abnormalities of seminal fluid.
  3. Some factors that contribute to infertility in women include disorders of ovulation or abnormalities of the uterus, fallopian tubes, or cervix.
  4. Several diagnostic tests are available to determine the probable cause of infertility, and the therapy recommended may depend on the cause of infertility.
  5. Infertility options
     a. Options include medication, surgical procedures, and therapeutic insemination.

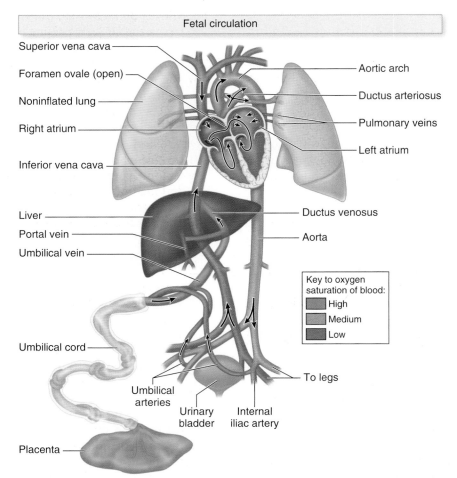

| Fetal circulation |

Superior vena cava
Foramen ovale (open)
Noninflated lung
Right atrium
Inferior vena cava
Liver
Portal vein
Umbilical vein
Umbilical cord
Umbilical arteries
Urinary bladder
Internal iliac artery
Placenta

Aortic arch
Ductus arteriosus
Pulmonary veins
Left atrium
Ductus venosus
Aorta
To legs

Key to oxygen saturation of blood:
- High
- Medium
- Low

FIGURE 22.1 Fetal circulation. Three shunts (ductus venosus, ductus arteriosus, and foramen ovale) allow most blood from the placenta to bypass the fetal lungs and liver.

b. Other therapies are available, such as *in vitro* fertilization, surrogate mothers, and embryo hosts.

c. Adoption may also be an option.

6. The nurse needs to provide support to the couple in their decision-making process and during therapy.

WHAT WOULD YOU DO?

Answer: Adolescent pregnancies are considered high risk because of the immaturity of the reproductive system and the high-risk behaviors that some adolescents engage in. The nurse would provide information to the adolescent regarding the risks associated with drug and alcohol consumption during pregnancy. The nurse would explain to the adolescent that large particles such as bacteria cannot pass through the placenta, but nutrients, drugs, antibodies, and viruses can pass through; therefore, measures must be taken to minimize exposure to substances that can cross the placental barrier and affect the health of the fetus. Follow-up regarding this high-risk behavior is also necessary.

PRACTICE QUESTIONS

1. The nurse is collecting data from a pregnant client when the client asks the nurse about the purpose of the fallopian tubes. Which is the accurate response the nurse would make?
1. The organ of copulation
2. Where the fetus develops
3. Where fertilization occurs
4. The organ that secretes estrogen and progesterone

❖ **2.** The nursing instructor asks a nursing student to list the functions of the amniotic fluid. The student **needs further teaching** if which responses are made? **Select all that apply.**
❑ **1.** Allows for fetal movement
❑ **2.** Is a measure of kidney function
❑ **3.** Surrounds, cushions, and protects the fetus
❑ **4.** Maintains the body temperature of the fetus
❑ **5.** Prevents large particles such as bacteria from passing to the fetus
❑ **6.** Provides an exchange of nutrients and waste products between the mother and the fetus

❖ **3.** The nurse working in a prenatal clinic reviews a client's chart and notes that the primary health care provider documents that the client has a gynecoid pelvis. The nurse plans care understanding that which findings are characteristic of this type of pelvis? **Select all that apply.**
- ❑ 1. Round shape
- ❑ 2. Shallow depth
- ❑ 3. Narrow pubic arch
- ❑ 4. Diagonal conjugate measures 12.5 to 13 cm
- ❑ 5. Blunt, somewhat widely separated ischial spines

4. The client asks the nurse about the purpose of the placenta. The nurse plans to respond to the client knowing which about the placenta?
1. Cushions and protects the fetus
2. Maintains the body temperature of the fetus
3. Surrounds the fetus and allows for fetal movement
4. Provides an exchange of nutrients and waste products between the mother and the fetus

5. The nurse is describing the process of fetal circulation to a client during a prenatal visit. The nurse needs to tell the client that fetal circulation consists of which components?
1. Two umbilical veins and one umbilical artery
2. Two umbilical arteries and one umbilical vein
3. Arteries that carry oxygenated blood to the fetus
4. Veins that carry deoxygenated blood to the fetus

6. A nursing student is assigned to a client in labor. The nursing instructor asks the student to describe fetal circulation, specifically the ductus venosus. The instructor determines that the student understands the structure of the ductus venosus if the student states which about the ductus venosus?
1. Connects the pulmonary artery to the aorta
2. Is an opening between the right and left atria
3. Connects the umbilical vein to the inferior vena cava
4. Connects the umbilical artery to the inferior vena cava

7. During a prenatal visit, the nurse checks the fetal heart rate (FHR) of a client in the third trimester of pregnancy. The nurse determines that the FHR is normal if which heart rate is noted?
1. 80 beats per minute
2. 100 beats per minute
3. 150 beats per minute
4. 180 beats per minute

8. The nurse is reinforcing teaching to a pregnant woman about the physiological effects and hormonal changes that occur during pregnancy. The woman asks the nurse about the purpose of estrogen. The nurse bases the response on which purpose of estrogen?
1. It maintains the uterine lining for implantation.
2. It stimulates the metabolism of glucose and converts glucose to fat.
3. It stimulates uterine development to provide an environment for the fetus and stimulates the breasts to prepare for lactation.
4. It prevents the involution of the corpus luteum and maintains the production of progesterone until the placenta is formed.

9. The nursing student is asked to describe the size of the uterus in a nonpregnant client. Which response indicates an understanding of the anatomy of this structure?
1. "The uterus weighs about 2 ounces."
2. "The uterus weighs about 2.2 pounds."
3. "The uterus has a capacity of about 50 milliliters."
4. "The uterus is round in shape and weighs approximately 1000 grams."

10. A couple comes to the family planning clinic and asks about sterilization procedures. Which question by the nurse helps determine whether this method of family planning is appropriate?
1. "Have either of you ever had surgery?"
2. "Do you plan to have any other children?"
3. "Do either of you have diabetes mellitus?"
4. "Do either of you have problems with high blood pressure?"

ANSWERS

1. 3
Rationale: Each fallopian tube is a hollow muscular tube that transports a mature oocyte for final maturation and fertilization. Fertilization typically occurs near the boundary between the ampulla and the isthmus of the tube. The vagina is the organ of copulation, and the fetus develops in the uterus. Estrogen is a hormone that is produced by the ovarian follicles, the corpus luteum, the adrenal cortex, and the placenta during pregnancy. Progesterone is a hormone that is secreted by the corpus luteum of the ovary, the adrenal glands, and the placenta during pregnancy.
Test-Taking Strategy: Focus on the subject, anatomy and physiology of the female reproductive system, which will direct you to the correct option. Remember that fertilization occurs in the fallopian tube.

❖ **2. 5, 6**
Rationale: The amniotic fluid surrounds, cushions, and protects the fetus. The placenta, not the amniotic fluid, prevents large particles such as bacteria from passing to the fetus, and the placenta provides an exchange of nutrients and waste products between the mother and the fetus. Amniotic fluid allows the fetus to move freely, it maintains the body temperature of the fetus, and it helps to measure kidney function, because the amount of fluid is based on the amount of urination from the fetus.
Test-Taking Strategy: Note the strategic words, *needs further teaching*. These words indicate a negative event query and ask you to select an option that is an incorrect statement regarding amniotic fluid. Think about the functions of the amniotic fluid to assist in answering correctly.

❖ **3. 1, 4, 5**
Rationale: A gynecoid pelvis is a normal female pelvis, and it is the most favorable for successful labor and birth. Characteristics of a gynecoid pelvis include a round shape, blunted ischial spines that are widely separated, a diagonal conjugate of at least 12.5 to 13 cm, a wide pelvic arch, and an adequate depth.
Test-Taking Strategy: Focus on the subject, knowledge regarding pelvic types, to answer this question. Remember that the gynecoid pelvis is the normal female pelvis.

4. 4
Rationale: The placenta provides an exchange of nutrients and waste products between the mother and the fetus. The amniotic fluid surrounds, cushions, and protects the fetus and allows for fetal movement. The amniotic fluid also maintains the body temperature of the fetus.
Test-Taking Strategy: Focus on the subject, the purpose of the placenta. This knowledge is required to answer this question. Remember that the placenta provides nutrients.

5. 2
Rationale: Blood pumped by the fetus's heart leaves the fetus through two umbilical arteries. After the blood is oxygenated, it is then returned by one umbilical vein. The umbilical arteries carry deoxygenated blood and waste products from the fetus, and the umbilical vein carries oxygenated blood and provides oxygen and nutrients to the fetus.
Test-Taking Strategy: Focus on the subject, anatomy of fetal circulation. Remember that there are three umbilical vessels within an umbilical cord (two arteries and one vein).

6. 3
Rationale: The ductus venosus connects the umbilical vein to the inferior vena cava. The foramen ovale is a temporary opening between the right and left atria. The ductus arteriosus joins the aorta and the pulmonary artery.

Test-Taking Strategy: Focus on the subject, fetal circulation. Recall the anatomy of the fetal circulation to answer this question. Remember that the ductus venosus connects the umbilical vein to the inferior vena cava.

7. 3
Rationale: Fetal heart rate depends on gestational age. It is normally 160 to 170 beats per minute during the first trimester, but it slows with fetal growth to 110 to 160 beats per minute near or at term.
Test-Taking Strategy: Focus on the subject, the fetal heart rate in the third trimester of pregnancy. Think about the physiology associated with cardiac structures in fetal development to answer correctly.

8. 3
Rationale: Estrogen stimulates uterine development to provide an environment for the fetus and it stimulates the breasts to prepare for lactation. Progesterone maintains the uterine lining for implantation and relaxes all smooth muscle. Human placental lactogen stimulates the metabolism of glucose and converts the glucose to fat. Human chorionic gonadotropin prevents the involution of the corpus luteum and maintains the production of progesterone until the placenta is formed.
Test-Taking Strategy: Focus on the subject, functions of various hormones related to pregnancy. Remember that estrogen stimulates uterine development to provide an environment for the fetus and that it stimulates the breasts to prepare for lactation.

9. 1
Rationale: Before conception, the uterus is a small, pear-shaped organ that is contained entirely in the pelvic cavity. Before pregnancy, the uterus weighs approximately 60 g (2 oz) and it has a capacity of about 10 mL (⅓ oz). At the end of pregnancy, the uterus weighs approximately 1000 g (2.2 lb) and it has a capacity that is sufficient for the fetus, the placenta, and the amniotic fluid.
Test-Taking Strategy: Focus on the subject, size of the uterus, and note the word, *nonpregnant*. Visualizing each of the items identified in the options will direct you to the correct answer.

10. 2
Rationale: Sterilization is a method of contraception for couples who have completed their families. It would be considered a permanent end to fertility because reversal surgery is not always successful. The nurse would ask the couple about their plans for having children in the future. Options 1, 3, and 4 are unrelated to this procedure.
Test-Taking Strategy: Focus on the subject, sterilization procedure. Noting the relationship between the word *sterilization* and the correct option will direct you to this answer.

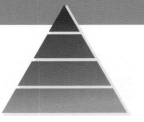

CHAPTER **23**

Prenatal Period and Risk Conditions

PRIORITY CONCEPTS Development, Reproduction

WHAT WOULD YOU DO?

The pregnant client tells the nurse that she is experiencing morning sickness. What information would the nurse provide to the client to assist with relief?

Answer is located on p. 289.

I. Gestation

A. Time from the fertilization of the ovum until the date of delivery

B. About 280 days

C. Nägele's rule for estimating date of delivery, also known as date of birth (Box 23.1)

  1. Use of Nägele's rule requires that the woman have a regular 28-day menstrual cycle

  2. Subtract 3 months and add 7 days to the first day of the last menstrual period; then add 1 year if appropriate. Alternatively, add 7 days to the first day of the last menstrual period and count forward 9 months.

II. Gravidity and Parity

A. Gravidity

  1. Gravida: A woman who is pregnant

  2. Gravidity: Number of pregnancies

  3. Nulligravida: A woman who has never been pregnant

  4. Primigravida: A woman who is pregnant for the first time

  5. Multigravida: A woman in at least her second pregnancy

B. Parity

  1. Parity: The number of births (not the number of fetuses [e.g., twins]) carried past 20 weeks' gestation, whether or not the fetus was born alive

  2. Nullipara: A woman who has not had a birth at more than 20 weeks of gestation

  3. Primipara: A woman who has had one birth that occurred after 20 weeks of gestation

  4. Multipara: A woman who has had two or more pregnancies to the stage of fetal viability

C. Use of GTPAL: Pregnancy outcomes can be described with the GTPAL acronym (Box 23.2).

  1. G = Gravidity; number of pregnancies, including the present one

  2. T = Term births; number of born at term (i.e., longer than 37 weeks' gestation)

  3. P = Preterm births; number born before 37 weeks' gestation

  4. A = Abortions or miscarriages; number of abortions/miscarriages (included in gravida if before 20 weeks' gestation)

  5. L = Live births; number of live births or living children. This number can be greater than the P if multiples were delivered, or less than the P if a loss occurred.

  6. *Note:* Multiples count as a 1 for gravidity, as well as 1 for term, preterm, or abortions, but are recorded as the actual number for living.

III. Pregnancy Signs

A. Presumptive signs

  1. Amenorrhea

  2. Nausea and vomiting

  3. Increased size and fullness of breasts

  4. Pronounced nipples

  5. Urinary frequency

  6. Fatigue

  7. Discoloration of vaginal mucosa

  8. Quickening: First perception of fetal movement by the mother may appear at the 16th to 20th week of gestation

B. Probable signs

  1. Uterine enlargement

  2. Goodell's sign: Softening of the cervix that occurs at the beginning of the second month of pregnancy

BOX 23.2 **GTPAL Acronym**

G = Gravidity
T = Term births
P = Preterm births
A = Abortions/miscarriages
L = Live births

Example: A woman is pregnant for the fourth time. She had one elective abortion during the first trimester, a daughter who was born at 40 weeks' gestation, and a son who was born at 36 weeks' gestation. Therefore, she is gravida (G) = 4; term (T) = 1 (the daughter born at 40 weeks' gestation). She is also preterm (P) = 1 (the son born at 36 weeks' gestation); abortion (A) = 1 (the abortion is counted in the gravida because it occurred before 20 weeks' gestation); and live births (L) = 2. Therefore, she would be considered GTPAL = 4, 1, 1, 1, 2.

3. **Chadwick's sign:** Violet coloration of the mucous membranes of the cervix, vagina, and vulva that occurs at about week 6
4. **Hegar's sign:** Compressibility and softening of the lower uterine segment that occurs at about week 6
5. **Ballottement:** The rebounding of the fetus against the examiner's fingers during palpation
6. Braxton Hicks contractions: Irregular painless contractions that may occur intermittently throughout pregnancy

C. Positive signs (diagnostic)
   1. Positive pregnancy test for determination of the presence of human chorionic gonadotropin
   2. Outline of the fetus via radiography or ultrasound
   3. Fetal heart rate detected by electronic device (Doppler transducer) at 10 to 12 weeks, and by nonelectronic device (fetoscope) at 20 weeks of gestation
   4. Active fetal movements palpated by the examiner

IV. Fundal Height (Box 23.3)

A. Measured to evaluate the gestational age of the fetus
B. During the second and third trimesters (weeks 18–30), the fundal height in centimeters approximately equals the fetus's age in weeks, plus or minus 2 cm (Fig. 23.1).
C. At 16 weeks, the fundus can be found approximately halfway between the symphysis pubis and the umbilicus.

BOX 23.3 **Measuring Fundal Height**

1. Place the client in a supine position.
2. Place the end of the tape measure at the level of the symphysis pubis.
3. Stretch the tape to the top of the uterine fundus.
4. Note and record the measurement.

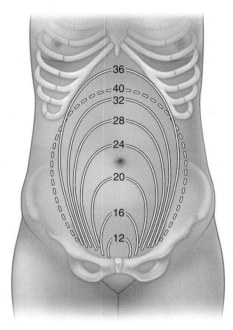

FIGURE 23.1 Height of fundus by weeks of normal gestation with a single fetus. *Dashed line*, Height after lightening.

D. At 20 to 22 weeks, the fundus is approximately at the location of the umbilicus.
E. At 36 weeks, the fundus is at the xiphoid process.

⚠ When assessing fundal height, monitor the client closely for supine hypotension when placed in the supine position.

V. Physiological Maternal Changes

⚠ Culture often determines health beliefs, values, and family expectations. Therefore, it is important to identify cultural beliefs during care of the maternity client.

A. Cardiovascular system
   1. Circulating blood volume increases, plasma increases, and total red blood cell volume increases (total volume increases by approximately 40%–50%).
   2. Physiological anemia may occur as the plasma increase exceeds the increase in the production of red blood cells.
   3. Heart size is increased, and the heart is elevated slightly upward and to the left because of displacement of the diaphragm as the uterus enlarges (Fig. 23.2).

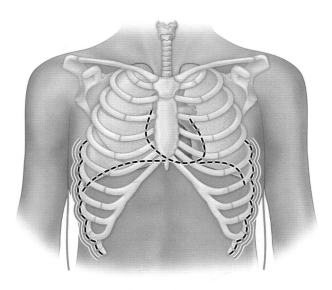

FIGURE 23.2 Changes in position of the heart, lungs, and thoracic cage in pregnancy. *Broken line,* nonpregnant state; *solid line,* change that occurs during pregnancy.

    4. There is an increase in the body's demand for iron.
    5. Sodium and water retention may occur.
B. Respiratory system
    1. Oxygen consumption increases by approximately 15% to 20%.
    2. Diaphragm is elevated as a result of the enlarged uterus (see Fig. 23.2).
    3. Shortness of breath may be experienced.

⚠ During pregnancy, a woman's pulse rate may increase about 10 to 15 beats per minute; the blood pressure slightly decreases in the second trimester, then increases in the third trimester but not above the prepregnancy level; and the respiratory rate remains unchanged or slightly increases.

C. Gastrointestinal (GI) system
    1. Nausea and vomiting, which usually subsides by the third month, may occur as a result of the secretion of human chorionic gonadotropin (hCG); hCG stabilizes or decreases around week 12.
    2. Poor appetite may occur because of decreased gastric motility.
    3. Alterations in taste and smell may occur.
    4. Constipation may occur because of an increase in progesterone production or pressure of the uterus, resulting in decreased gastrointestinal motility.
    5. Flatulence and heartburn may occur because of decreased gastrointestinal motility and slowed emptying of the stomach caused by an increase in progesterone production.
    6. Hemorrhoids may occur as a result of increased venous pressure.

    7. Gum tissue may become swollen and easily bleed because of increasing levels of estrogen.
    8. Ptyalism (excessive secretion of saliva) may occur because of increasing levels of estrogen.
D. Renal system
    1. Frequency of urination increases in the first and third trimesters because of increased bladder sensitivity and pressure of the enlarging uterus on the bladder.
    2. Decreased bladder tone may occur and is caused by an increase in progesterone and estrogen levels; bladder capacity increases in response to increasing levels of progesterone.
    3. The renal threshold for glucose may be reduced.
E. Endocrine system
    1. Basal metabolic rate and metabolic function increase.
    2. Anterior lobe of pituitary gland enlarges and produces serum prolactin needed for the lactation process.
    3. The posterior lobe of the pituitary gland produces oxytocin, which stimulates uterine contractions.
    4. Thyroid gland enlarges slightly and thyroid activity increases.
    5. Parathyroid gland increases in size.
    6. Aldosterone levels gradually increase.
    7. Body weight increases.
    8. Water retention is increased, which can contribute to weight gain.
F. Reproductive system
    1. Uterus
        a. Uterus enlarges, increasing in mass from approximately 60 to 1000 g as a result of hyperplasia (influence of estrogen) and hypertrophy.
        b. Size and number of blood vessels and lymphatics increase.
        c. Irregular contractions occur, typically beginning after 16 weeks' gestation.
    2. Cervix
        a. Cervix becomes shorter, more elastic, and larger in diameter.
        b. Endocervical glands secrete a thick mucus plug, which is expelled from the canal when dilation begins.
        c. Increased vascularization and an increase in estrogen causes a softening and a violet discoloration (Chadwick's sign), which occurs at about week 6.
    3. Ovaries
        a. Secrete progesterone for first 6 to 7 weeks of pregnancy
        b. Block maturation of new follicles
        c. Cease ovum production
    4. Vagina
        a. Hypertrophy and thickening of the muscle occurs.

b. Increase in vaginal secretions is experienced; secretions are usually thick, white, and acidic.

5. Breasts

a. Breast changes occur because of the increasing effects of estrogen and progesterone.

b. Breast size increases and breasts may be tender.

c. Nipples become more pronounced and the areolae become darker.

d. Superficial veins become prominent.

e. Montgomery's follicles become hypertrophied.

f. Colostrum may leak from the breasts.

G. Skin

1. Changes in skin occur because of increased levels of melanocyte-stimulating hormone, which increase secondary to increases in estrogen and progesterone; these changes include the following:

a. Increased pigmentation

b. A dark streak down the midline of the abdomen may appear (linea nigra).

c. Chloasma (mask of pregnancy), a blotchy, brownish hyperpigmentation, may occur over the forehead, cheeks, and nose.

d. Reddish-purple stretch marks (striae gravidarum) may occur on the abdomen, breasts, thighs, and upper arms.

2. Vascular spider nevi may occur on the neck, chest, face, arms, and legs.

3. The rate of hair growth may increase.

H. Musculoskeletal system

1. Changes in center of gravity begin in the second trimester and are caused by the hormones relaxin and progesterone.

2. The lumbosacral curve increases.

3. Aching, numbness, and weakness may result; walking becomes more difficult, and the woman develops a waddling gait and is at risk for falls.

4. Relaxation and increased mobility of pelvic joints occurs, which permits enlargement of pelvic dimensions.

5. Abdominal wall stretches with loss of tone throughout pregnancy, regained postpartum.

6. Umbilicus flattens or protrudes.

⚠ During pregnancy, postural changes occur as the increased weight of the uterus causes a forward pull of the bony pelvis. It is important for the nurse to encourage the client to implement measures that maintain safety and correct posture to prevent a backache.

VI. Psychological Maternal Changes

A. Ambivalence

1. May occur early in pregnancy, even when the pregnancy is planned.

2. Mother may experience a dependence-independence conflict and ambivalence related to role changes.

3. Partner may experience ambivalence related to assuming a new role, increased financial responsibilities, and having to share attention with the child.

B. Acceptance: Factors that may be related to the acceptance of the pregnancy are the woman's readiness for the experience and her identification with the motherhood role.

1. Specific developmental tasks must be accomplished successfully for positive maternal role adaptation.

2. These tasks include accepting the pregnancy, identifying with the mothering role, solidifying her relationship with her partner, establishing a relationship with her unborn infant, and preparing for her birth experience.

C. Emotional lability

1. Manifested by frequency in the change of emotional states or extremes in emotional states

2. These emotional changes are common, but the mother may believe that these changes are abnormal.

D. Body image changes

1. The changes in a woman's perception of her image during pregnancy occur gradually and may be positive or negative.

2. Physical changes and symptoms that the woman experiences during pregnancy contribute to her body image.

E. Relationship with the fetus

1. The woman may daydream to prepare for motherhood and think about the maternal qualities she would like to possess.

2. The woman first accepts the biological fact that she is pregnant.

3. The woman next accepts the growing fetus as distinct from herself and a person to nurture.

4. Finally, the woman prepares realistically for the birth and parenting of the child.

VII. Discomforts of Pregnancy

A. Nausea and vomiting

1. Occurs during the first trimester and usually subsides by the third month

2. Caused by elevated hCG levels and changes in carbohydrate metabolism

3. Interventions

a. Eating dry crackers before rising

b. Avoiding brushing the teeth immediately after rising

c. Eating small, frequent, low-fat meals during the day

d. Drinking liquids between meals rather than at meals

e. Avoiding fried and spicy foods

f. Asking the primary health care provider (PHCP) about acupressure (some types may require a prescription)

g. Asking the PHCP about the use of herbal remedies

h. Taking antiemetic medications as prescribed

B. Syncope

1. Usually occurs during the first trimester; supine hypotension occurs, particularly during the second and third trimesters.

2. May be hormonally triggered or caused by increased blood volume, anemia, fatigue, sudden position changes, or lying supine

3. Interventions

a. Sitting with the feet elevated

b. Changing positions slowly because of the risk for falls

⚠ The nurse needs to inform the pregnant client to avoid lying in the supine position, particularly in the second and third trimesters. The supine position places the woman at risk for supine hypotension, which occurs as a result of pressure of the uterus on the inferior vena cava.

C. Urinary urgency and frequency

1. Usually occurs during the first and third trimesters

2. Caused by the pressure of the uterus on the bladder

3. Interventions

a. Drinking no less than 2000 mL of fluid during the day

b. Limiting fluid intake during the evening

c. Voiding at regular intervals

d. Sleeping on the side at night

e. Wearing perineal pads, if necessary

f. Performing Kegel exercises

D. Breast tenderness

1. Can occur from the first through the third trimesters

2. Caused by increased levels of estrogen and progesterone

3. Interventions

a. Encouraging wearing a supportive bra

b. Avoiding the use of soap on the nipples and areolar area to prevent drying of skin

E. Increased vaginal discharge

1. Can occur from the first through the third trimesters

2. Caused by hypertrophy and thickening of the vaginal mucosa and increased mucus production

3. Interventions

a. Using proper cleansing and hygiene techniques

b. Wearing cotton underwear

c. Avoiding douching

d. Informing the client of the signs of infection and to consult the PHCP if an infection is suspected

F. Nasal stuffiness

1. Occurs during the first through the third trimesters

2. Occurs as a result of increased estrogen that causes swelling of the nasal tissues and dryness

3. Interventions

a. Encouraging the use of a humidifier

b. Avoiding the use of nasal sprays or antihistamines (the PHCP must always be consulted regarding their use)

G. Fatigue

1. Occurs usually during the first and third trimesters

2. Is usually the result of hormonal changes

3. Interventions

a. Arranging frequent rest periods throughout the day

b. Using correct posture and body mechanics

c. Obtaining regular exercise

d. Performing muscle relaxation and strengthening exercises for the legs and hip joints

e. Avoiding eating and drinking foods that contain stimulants throughout the pregnancy

H. Heartburn

1. Occurs during the second and third trimesters

2. Results from increased progesterone levels, decreased GI motility, esophageal reflux, and the displacement of the stomach by the enlarging uterus

3. Interventions

a. Eating small, frequent meals

b. Avoiding fatty and spicy food

c. Sitting upright for 30 minutes after a meal

d. Drinking milk between meals

e. Consulting with the PHCP about the use of antacids

f. Performing tailor-sitting exercises

I. Ankle edema

1. Usually occurs during the second and third trimesters

2. Occurs as a result of vasodilation, venous stasis, and increased venous pressure below the uterus

3. Interventions

a. Elevating the legs at least twice a day and when resting

b. Sleeping in a side-lying position

c. Wearing supportive stockings or supportive hose as prescribed

d. Avoiding sitting or standing in one position for long periods

J. Varicose veins

1. Usually occur during the second and third trimesters

2. Occur because of weakening walls of the veins or valves and venous congestion

3. Thrombophlebitis is rare, but it may occur.
4. Interventions
   a. Wearing supportive stockings or support hose
   b. Elevating the feet when sitting
   c. Lying with the feet and hips elevated
   d. Avoiding long periods of standing or sitting
   e. Moving about while standing to improve circulation
   f. Avoiding leg crossing
   g. Avoiding constricting articles of clothing such as knee-high stockings
   h. Teaching leg exercises
   i. Avoiding airline travel if possible, because of sitting position

K. Headaches
   1. Usually considered benign in the first trimester; may need investigation if occurring in the second and third trimesters
   2. Occur as a result of changes in blood volume and vascular tone
   3. Interventions
     a. Changing position slowly
     b. Applying a cool cloth to the forehead
     c. Eating a small snack
     d. Using acetaminophen only if prescribed by the PHCP

L. Hemorrhoids
   1. Usually occur during the second and third trimesters
   2. Occur as a result of increased venous pressure and constipation
   3. Interventions
     a. Soaking in a warm sitz bath
     b. Sitting on a soft pillow
     c. Eating high-fiber foods and drinking sufficient fluids to avoid constipation
     d. Increasing exercise, such as walking
     e. Applying ointments, suppositories, or compresses as prescribed by the PHCP

M. Constipation
   1. Usually occurs during the second and third trimesters
   2. Results from increased progesterone production, decreased intestinal motility, displacement of the intestines, pressure of the uterus, and taking iron supplements
   3. Interventions
     a. Eating high-fiber foods such as whole grains, fruits, and vegetables
     b. Drinking no less than 2000 mL/day
     c. Exercising regularly, such as a daily 20-minute walk
     d. Consulting with the PHCP about interventions such as the use of stool softeners, laxatives, or enemas

N. Backache
   1. Usually occurs during the second and third trimesters

2. Occurs as a result of the exaggerated lumbosacral curve, resulting from an enlarged uterus
3. Risk for falls; teach to move about slowly
4. Interventions
   a. Obtaining rest
   b. Using correct posture and body mechanics
   c. Wearing low-heeled, comfortable, and supportive shoes
   d. Performing pelvic tilt (rock) and conscious relaxation exercises
   e. Sleeping on a firm mattress

O. Leg cramps
   1. Usually occur during the second and third trimesters
   2. Occur as a result of an altered calcium-phosphorus balance, the pressure of the uterus on nerves, or from fatigue
   3. Interventions
     a. Getting regular exercise, such as walking
     b. Dorsiflexing the foot of the affected leg
     c. Increasing calcium intake

P. Shortness of breath
   1. Can occur during the second and third trimesters
   2. Occurs as a result of pressure on the diaphragm from the enlarged uterus
   3. Interventions
     a. Taking frequent rest periods
     b. Sitting and sleeping with the head elevated or on the side
     c. Avoiding overexertion

VIII. Maternal Risk Factors

A. Maternal age: Women younger than 20 years and older than 35 years are at risk for adverse perinatal outcomes.

B. Adolescent pregnancy
   1. Factors that result in adolescent pregnancy include the early onset of menarche, sexual behaviors in this age group, problems with family relationships, poverty, and a lack of knowledge of reproduction and birth control.
   2. Major concerns related to adolescent pregnancy include poor nutritional status, emotional and behavioral difficulties, lack of support systems, increased risk of stillbirth, low birth weight infants, fetal mortality, cephalopelvic disproportion, and increased risks of maternal complications such as hypertension, anemia, prolonged labor, and infections.
   3. The role of the nurse in reducing the risks and consequences of adolescent pregnancy is twofold: first, to encourage early and continued prenatal care, and second, to refer the adolescent, if necessary, for appropriate assistance, which can help to counter the effects of a negative socioeconomic environment.

C. Nutrition: Adequate nutrition is necessary for normal fetal growth and development. Nutrition needs are determined by the stage of the pregnancy and nutrition should support recommended weight gain during the various stages.

⚠ Women of childbearing age need to take folic acid supplements to prevent neural tube defects and orofacial clefts in the fetus.

D. Genetic considerations: Genetic abnormalities such as defective genes or transmissible inherited disorders can result in congenital anomalies; the nurse needs to collect data about genetic risks.

E. Health care: Failure to seek and obtain prenatal care, including dental care, increases the risk of preterm birth and low birth weight.

F. Abuse and violence: Physical abuse and violence can increase the risk for abruptio placentae, preterm birth, and infections from unwanted and forced sex.

G. Medical conditions: Concurrent medical conditions, such as, but not limited to, diabetes mellitus, hypertensive disorder, or cardiac disease, increase the risk of complications during pregnancy.

H. German measles (rubella): Maternal infection during the first 8 weeks of gestation carries the highest rate of fetal infection.

I. Sexually transmitted infections
  1. Syphilis
    a. Organism may cross the placenta.
    b. Infection usually leads to spontaneous abortions and increases the incidence of mental subnormality and physical deformities.
  2. Condylomata acuminata (human papillomavirus)
    a. Transmission may occur during vaginal birth.
    b. Infection is associated with the development of epithelial tumors of the mucous membranes of the larynx in children.
  3. Gonorrhea
    a. Fetus is contaminated at the time of birth.
    b. Maternal infection may result in postpartum infection of the neonate.
    c. Risks to the neonate include ophthalmia neonatorum, pneumonia, and sepsis.
  4. Chlamydial infection
    a. Transmission may occur during vaginal birth and can result in neonatal conjunctivitis or pneumonitis.
    b. Infection can cause premature rupture of the membranes, premature labor, and postpartum endometritis.
  5. Trichomoniasis: Associated with premature rupture of the membranes and postpartum endometritis
  6. Genital herpes simplex virus
    a. Characterized by painful lesions, fever, chills, malaise, and severe dysuria and may last 2 to 3 weeks

    b. Assessment includes questioning all women about signs/symptoms and inspecting the vulvar, perineal, and vaginal areas for vesicles or areas of ulceration or crusting; this is done during pregnancy and at the onset of labor.
    c. Vaginal birth may be acceptable; cesarean birth is required if visible lesions are present.
    d. Infants who are born through an infected vagina must be carefully observed, and skin cultures or blood testing needs to be done if suspected.

J. Human immunodeficiency virus (HIV)
  1. HIV is transmitted via blood, blood products, and other body fluids such as urine, semen, and vaginal secretions; the virus is also transmitted through exposure to infected secretions during birth and via breast milk.
  2. Repeated exposure to the virus during pregnancy through unsafe sex practices and/or intravenous drug use can increase the risk of transmission to the fetus.
  3. Perinatal administration of zidovudine may be recommended to decrease risk of transmission of HIV from mother to fetus.

K. Substance abuse
  1. Substance abuse threatens normal fetal growth and the successful term completion of the pregnancy.
  2. Substance abuse places the pregnancy at risk for fetal growth restriction, abruptio placentae, and fetal bradycardia.
  3. Many substances cross the placenta and can be teratogenic (drugs, tobacco, alcohol, medications, certain foods such as raw fish); no over-the-counter medications should be taken unless prescribed by the PHCP.
  4. Smoking (tobacco) can lead to low birth weight, a higher incidence of birth defects, and stillbirths.
  5. Physical signs of drug abuse may include dilated or contracted pupils, fatigue, track (needle) marks, skin abscesses, inflamed nasal mucosa, and inappropriate behavior by the mother.
  6. The consumption of alcohol during pregnancy may lead to fetal alcohol syndrome and can cause jitteriness, physical abnormalities, congenital anomalies, and growth deficits in the newborn.

L. Viral hepatitis: see Chapters 31 and 45 for information regarding hepatitis B infection.

IX. Antepartum Diagnostic Testing

⚠ The usual schedule for antepartum health care visits is every 4 weeks for the first 28 to 32 weeks, every 2 weeks from 32 to 36 weeks, and every week from 36 to 40 weeks.

A. Blood type and Rh factor
  1. ABO typing is performed to determine the woman's blood type in the ABO antigen system.

2. Rh typing is done to determine the woman's blood type in the rhesus antigen system (Rh positive indicates the presence of the antigen; Rh negative indicates the absence of the antigen).

3. If the client is Rh negative and has a negative antibody screen, the client will need repeat antibody screens and must receive $Rh_o(D)$ immune globulin (RhoGAM) at 28 weeks' gestation.

B. Rubella titer

1. If the client has a negative titer (less than 1:8), this indicates susceptibility to the rubella virus. The client would receive the appropriate immunization postpartum.

2. The client must be using effective birth control at the time of the immunization. She must be counseled not to become pregnant for 1 to 3 months after immunization (as specified by the PHCP) and to avoid contact with anyone who is immunocompromised.

3. If the rubella vaccine is administered at the same time as the $Rh_o(D)$ immune globulin, it may not be effective.

4. Rubella vaccine is administered postpartum (before discharge) via the subcutaneous route if the titer is less than 1:8; inquire about sensitivity to eggs.

⚠ Rubella vaccine is not given during pregnancy because the live attenuated virus may cross the placenta and present a risk to the developing fetus.

C. Hemoglobin and hematocrit levels

1. Hemoglobin and hematocrit levels decline during gestation as a result of increased plasma volume.

2. A decrease in the hemoglobin level below 10 g/dL or a decrease in the hematocrit level below 30% indicates anemia.

D. Papanicolaou (Pap) smear: Done during the initial prenatal examination to screen for cervical neoplasia if the woman has not had a screening before, or is beyond the recommended time frame since her last screening

E. Sexually transmitted infections (Table 23.1)

F. Sickle cell screening

1. Indicated for clients who are at risk for sickle cell disease

2. A positive test result may indicate a need for further screening.

G. Tuberculin skin test

1. The PHCP may prefer to perform this skin test after birth.

2. A positive skin test indicates the need for a chest radiograph (using an abdominal lead shield) to rule out active disease. In a pregnant client, a chest radiograph will not be performed until after 20 weeks' gestation (after the fetal organs are formed).

TABLE 23.1   Monitoring for Sexually Transmitted Infections

Disease	Laboratory Test
Gonorrhea	A vaginal culture or urine specimen is obtained during the initial prenatal examination to screen for gonorrhea. Culture may be repeated during the third trimester for high-risk clients.
Syphilis	A culture of lesions (if present) is done during the initial prenatal examination to screen for syphilis. Diagnosis is dependent on microscopic examination of primary and secondary lesion tissue and serology (Venereal Disease Research Laboratory [VDRL] or rapid plasma reagin [RPR]) test during latency and late infection. Culture may be repeated during the third trimester for high-risk clients.
Condyloma acuminatum (human papillomavirus)	Culture is indicated for clients with a positive history or with active lesions. Test is performed to determine route of delivery. Weekly cultures may be done at weeks 35 or 36 of pregnancy until delivery.
Chlamydia	Vaginal culture is indicated for all pregnant clients if client is in a high-risk group or if infants from previous pregnancies have developed neonatal conjunctivitis or pneumonia.
Trichomoniasis	Normal saline wet smear of vaginal secretions is checked for presence of protozoa. Associated with premature rupture of membranes and postpartum endometritis.
Genital herpes simplex virus (HSV-2)	Culture is done of lesions (if present) during initial prenatal examination to screen for HSV. Microscopic examination is done to determine presence of virus. Additional screening may be necessary as pregnancy progresses.
HIV	Testing may be done for high-risk client. Common tests to determine the presence of antibodies include ELISA, Western blot, and immunofluorescence assay (IFA).

ELISA, Enzyme-linked immunosorbent assay; *HIV,* human immunodeficiency virus.

3. Those who convert to positive may be referred for treatment with medication after birth.

H. Hepatitis B surface antigen

1. Testing for the hepatitis antigens is recommended for all women because of the prevalence of the disease in the general population.

2. Vaccination for hepatitis B antigen may be specifically indicated for the following:
   a. Health care workers
   b. Intravenous (IV) drug abusers
   c. Clients born in high-risk countries such as Asia, Africa, Haiti, or the Pacific islands
   d. Clients with previously undiagnosed jaundice or chronic liver disease
   e. Clients with tattoos
   f. Clients with histories of blood transfusions
   g. Clients with histories of multiple episodes of sexually transmitted infections

h. Clients who have been rejected previously as blood donors

i. Clients with histories of dialysis or renal transplantation

j. Clients from households having hepatitis B–infected members or hemodialysis clients

3. Hepatitis B vaccine is not contraindicated during pregnancy and may be recommended by the PHCP.

4. See Chapter 45 for additional information about hepatitis.

I. Glucose challenge test (GCT)

1. Screening for gestational diabetes mellitus (GDM) begins at the initial prenatal visit and is diagnosed by a fasting blood glucose greater than 126 mg/dL, A1C greater than 6.5%, or a random plasma glucose level greater than 200 mg/dL, then subsequently confirmed by an elevated fasting glucose level or A1C.

2. According to the American Congress of Obstetricians and Gynecologists (ACOG), a GCT using a two-step approach would be used in screening for GDM.

3. A 50-G oral glucose load without regard to time of day is given. After 1 hour a plasma or serum glucose level is drawn and is considered elevated if it is greater than 140 mg/dL and a 3-hour GCT would be done.

4. If the 3-hour GCT is above 130 to 140 mg/dL, it is considered a positive result and may be indicative of GDM.

5. It is important to note that the GCT has 86% sensitivity, and some false positives may be noted.

J. Urinalysis and urine culture

1. A urine specimen for glucose and protein determinations would be obtained at every prenatal visit.

2. Glycosuria is a common result of decreased renal threshold that occurs during pregnancy.

3. If glycosuria persists, this may indicate diabetes mellitus.

4. White blood cells in the urine may indicate infection.

5. Ketonuria may result from insufficient food intake or vomiting.

6. Protein levels of 2+ to 4+ in the urine may indicate infection or preeclampsia.

K. Ultrasonography

1. Outlines and identifies fetal and maternal structures

2. Assists with confirming gestational age and estimated date of delivery and evaluating amniotic fluid volume (amniotic fluid index), which is done via special measurements

3. May be done abdominally or transvaginally during pregnancy

4. Can be used to determine the presence of premature dilation of the cervix (incompetent cervix).

A transvaginal ultrasound is used during the first trimester to check the length of the cervix.

5. Interventions

a. If an abdominal ultrasound is being performed, the woman may be asked to drink water to fill the bladder before the procedure to obtain a better image of the fetus.

b. If a transvaginal ultrasound is being performed, a lubricated probe is inserted into the vagina.

c. Inform the client that the test presents no known risks to the client or the fetus.

L. Biophysical profile

1. Noninvasive assessment of the fetus that includes fetal breathing movements, fetal movements, fetal tone, amniotic fluid index, and fetal heart rate patterns via a nonstress test

2. Normal fetal biophysical activities indicate that the central nervous system is functional and the fetus is not hypoxemic.

M. Doppler blood flow analysis: noninvasive (ultrasonography) method of studying blood flow in the fetus and placenta

N. Percutaneous umbilical blood sampling

1. Performed if fetal blood sampling is necessary

2. Involves insertion of needle directly into fetal umbilical vessel under ultrasound guidance

3. Fetal heart rate monitoring is necessary for 1 hour after procedure, and a follow-up ultrasound to check for bleeding or hematoma formation is done 1 hour after the procedure.

O. Alpha-fetoprotein (AFP) screening

1. Assesses the quantity of fetal serum proteins; abnormal protein levels are associated with open neural tube and abdominal wall defects.

2. Can screen for spina bifida and Down syndrome

3. If abnormal, the test is repeated; a false-positive test result is common.

4. Interventions

a. The AFP level is determined by a maternal blood sample drawn between 16 and 18 weeks' gestation.

b. If the level is abnormal and the gestation is less than 18 weeks, a second sample is drawn and screened.

c. An ultrasound is performed for elevated levels to rule out fetal abnormalities or multiple gestation.

P. Deoxyribonucleic acid (DNA) genetic testing

1. Can be used to detect abnormalities related to an inherited condition

2. Assists with determining whether the woman is at risk for having a fetus with Down syndrome (trisomy 21), Edwards syndrome (trisomy 18), or Patau syndrome (trisomy 13)

3. Interventions: this type of testing can be done as early as 7 weeks' gestation and a blood sample is used.

Q. Chorionic villus sampling (CVS)
   1. Performed for the purpose of detecting genetic abnormalities; the PHCP aspirates a small sample of chorionic villus tissue at 10 to 13 weeks' gestation.
   2. Interventions
      a. Monitor that informed consent was obtained
      b. The client may need to drink water to fill the bladder before the procedure to aid in visualizing the uterus for catheter insertion.
      c. Obtain baseline vital signs and fetal heart rate; monitor frequently after the procedure.
      d. Rh-negative women may be given $Rh_o(D)$ immune globulin, because chorionic villus sampling increases the risk of Rh sensitization.

⚠ The nurse needs to ensure that an informed consent has been obtained for any procedure that is invasive, such as a chorionic villus sampling or amniocentesis.

R. Amniocentesis
   1. Aspiration of amniotic fluid; best performed between 15 and 20 weeks of pregnancy because amniotic fluid volume is adequate and many viable fetal cells are present in the fluid by this time
   2. Performed to determine genetic disorders, metabolic defects, and fetal lung maturity
   3. Risks
      a. Maternal hemorrhage
      b. Infection
      c. Rh isoimmunization
      d. Abruptio placentae
      e. Amniotic fluid emboli
      f. Premature rupture of the membranes
   4. Interventions
      a. If less than 20 weeks' gestation, the woman would have a full bladder to support the uterus. If more than 20 weeks' gestation, the woman would have an empty bladder to minimize the chance of puncture.
      b. Prepare the client for ultrasonography, which is performed to locate the placenta and avoid puncture of it.
      c. Obtain baseline vital signs and fetal heart rate. Monitor every 15 minutes.
      d. Position the client supine during the procedure and on the left side after the procedure.
      e. Be sure that informed consent was obtained.

⚠ After chorionic villus sampling and amniocentesis, instruct the client that if chills, fever, bleeding, leakage of fluid at the needle insertion site, decreased fetal movement, uterine contractions, or cramping occurs, she must notify the PHCP.

S. Kick counts (fetal movement counting)
   1. Beginning at 28 weeks' gestation, the client sits quietly or lies down on her side and counts fetal kicks for a specific period of time.
   2. Instruct the client to notify the PHCP if there are fewer than 10 kicks in two consecutive 2-hour periods or as instructed by her PHCP.

T. Fern test
   1. A microscopic slide test to determine the presence of amniotic fluid leakage
   2. Using sterile technique, a specimen is obtained from the external os of the cervix and vaginal pool and examined on a slide under a microscope.
   3. A fern-like pattern that results from the salts of the amniotic fluid indicates the presence of amniotic fluid; may be done in conjunction with the Nitrazine test
   4. Interventions
      a. Position the client in the dorsal lithotomy position.
      b. Instruct the client to cough. This causes the fluid to leak from the uterus if the membranes are ruptured.

U. Nitrazine test
   1. A Nitrazine test strip is used to detect the presence of amniotic fluid in vaginal secretions.
   2. Vaginal secretions have a pH of 4.5 to 5.5 and do not affect the color of the Nitrazine strip or swab.
   3. Amniotic fluid has a pH of 7.0 to 7.5 and turns the Nitrazine strip or swab blue in color.
   4. Interventions
      a. Position the client in the dorsal lithotomy position.
      b. Touch the test tape to the fluid.
      c. Check the test tape for a blue-green, blue-gray, or deep blue color, which indicates that the membranes are probably ruptured, causing leakage of amniotic fluid.

V. Fibronectin test
   1. Sampling of cervical and vaginal secretions for fetal fibronectin is done between week 22 and week 34 of pregnancy if the PHCP is concerned about preterm labor.
   2. Positive results indicate the onset of labor in 1 to 3 weeks; negative test results are more predictive that preterm labor will not begin.
   3. Test is used if the client is at risk for preterm labor, before 37 weeks' gestation.
   4. Interventions
      a. Client is placed in lithotomy position for a sterile speculum examination.
      b. Cervical secretions are obtained with a cotton swab.
      c. Laboratory tests are done for the presence of fibronectin.

W. Nonstress test (Box 23.4)
X. Contraction stress test (Box 23.5)
Y. Group B Streptococcus (GBS) testing; vaginal and rectal cultures are obtained and tested for the presence of bacteria.

BOX 23.4 Nonstress Test

Description
- Performed to assess placental function and oxygenation
- Determines fetal well-being
- Evaluates fetal heart rate (FHR) in response to fetal movement

Interventions
- An external ultrasound transducer and tocodynamometer are applied to the mother, and a tracing of at least 20 minutes' duration is obtained so that the FHR and the uterine activity can be observed.
- Obtain a baseline blood pressure reading and monitor frequently.
- Position the mother in the lateral (side-lying) position to avoid vena cava compression.
- The mother may be asked to press a button every time she feels fetal movement. The monitor records a mark at each point of fetal movement and this is used as a reference point to assess FHR response.

Results
Reactive Nonstress Test (Normal, Negative)
"Reactive" indicates a healthy fetus.
The result requires two or more FHR accelerations of at least 15 beats per minute and lasting at least 15 seconds from the beginning of the acceleration to the end, in association with fetal movement, during a 20-minute period.

Nonreactive Nonstress Test (Abnormal)
No accelerations or accelerations of less than 15 beats per minute or lasting less than 15 s in duration during a 40-minute observation

Unsatisfactory
The result cannot be interpreted because of the poor quality of the FHR tracing.

BOX 23.5 Contraction Stress Test

Description
- Assesses placental oxygenation and function
- Determines fetal ability to tolerate labor and determines fetal well-being
- Fetus is exposed to the stress of contractions to assess the adequacy of placental perfusion under simulated labor conditions.
- Performed if the nonstress test is abnormal

Interventions
- The external fetal monitor is applied to the mother, and a 20- to 30-minute baseline strip is recorded.
- The uterus is stimulated to contract, either by the administration of a dilute dose of oxytocin or by having the mother use nipple stimulation, until 3 palpable contractions with a duration of 40 seconds or more during a 10-minute period have been achieved.
- Frequent maternal blood pressure readings are obtained and the mother is monitored closely while increasing doses of oxytocin are given.

Results
Negative Contraction Stress Test (Normal)
Represented by no late decelerations of the fetal heart rate (FHR)

Positive Contraction Stress Test (Abnormal)
Represented by late decelerations of the FHR with 50% or more of the contractions in the absence of hyperstimulation of the uterus

Equivocal
Contains decelerations but with less than 50% of the contractions, or uterine activity shows a hyperstimulated uterus

Unsatisfactory
Adequate uterine contractions cannot be achieved, or the FHR tracing is not of sufficient quality for adequate interpretation.

X. Nutrition
A. General guidelines
1. Guidelines for health and nutrition information for breast-feeding and pregnant women are located at the US Department of Agriculture ChooseMyPlate website at https://www.choosemyplate.gov/browse-by-audience/view-all-audiences/adults/moms-pregnancy-breastfeeding. The client would be assisted with accessing this site and preparing a nutritional plan.
2. The average expected weight gain during pregnancy is 25 to 35 lb for women with a normal prepregnancy weight.
3. An increase of about 300 calories per day is needed during pregnancy. Calorie needs are greater in the last two trimesters than in the first.
4. An increase of about 500 calories per day is needed during lactation.
5. A diet high in folic acid and folic acid supplements is necessary for all women of childbearing age to prevent neural tube defects and orofacial clefts in the fetus.
6. Encourage the consumption of at least 8 to 10 (8-oz) glasses of fluid each day, of which 4 to 6 glasses would be water.
7. Sodium is not restricted unless specifically prescribed by the PHCP.
B. Vegan and vegetarian diets and other diets (see Chapter 11)
1. Ensure that the client eats a sufficient amount of varied foods to meet normal nutrient and energy needs.
2. Clients should be educated about consuming complementary proteins over the course of each day to ensure that all essential amino acids are provided.
3. Potential deficiencies in vegetarian diets include energy, protein, vitamin B_{12}, zinc, iron, calcium, omega-3 fatty acids, and vitamin D (if exposure to sunlight is limited).
4. Protein intake can be increased by consumption of a variety of vegetable protein sources based on

whole grains, legumes, seeds, nuts, and vegetables combined to provide essential amino acids.

5. To enhance absorption of iron, vegetarians should include a good source of iron and vitamin C with each meal.

6. Foods commonly eaten include tofu, tempeh, soy milk and soy products, meat analogs, legumes, nuts, seeds, sprouts, and a variety of fruits and vegetables.

C. Lactose intolerance diets

1. Lactose consumed by an individual with lactose intolerance can cause abdominal distention, discomfort, nausea, vomiting, cramps, and loose stools.

2. Clients who experience lactose intolerance need to regularly incorporate sources of calcium (other than dairy products) into their dietary patterns.

3. Milk may be tolerated in cooked form (e.g., custards, fermented dairy products).

4. Cheese and yogurt are sometimes tolerated.

5. Lactase, which is an enzyme, may be prescribed and taken before ingesting milk or milk products.

6. Lactase-treated milk and lactose-free products are also available commercially.

D. Pica

1. Definition: Eating nonfood substances such as dirt, clay, starch, and freezer frost

2. The cause is unknown. Cultural values, such as beliefs regarding a material's effect on the mother or fetus, may make pica a common practice.

3. Iron-deficiency anemia may occur as a result of pica.

XI. Bleeding During Pregnancy

A. Implantation bleeding: Bleeding that occurs 10 to 14 days after conception. Usually lasts 1 to 2 days and is lighter than the typical menstrual period. Often confused with a normal menstrual period. No treatment is necessary.

B. Other causes include abortion, malignancy, polyps, trauma, ectopic pregnancy, idiopathic, infection, molar pregnancy, subchorionic hemorrhage, vaginitis, urinary tract infection, cervicitis, cervical polyps, postcoital bleeding, placenta previa, and abruptio placentae.

XII. Abortion

A. Description: A pregnancy that ends before 20 weeks' gestation, either spontaneously or electively

B. Types (Box 23.6)

C. Risk factors

1. Advanced maternal age

2. Those who have experienced a previous miscarriage are at a higher risk

---

BOX 23.6 Types of Abortions

Spontaneous Pregnancy ends because of natural causes.

Induced Therapeutic or elective reasons exist for terminating pregnancy.

Threatened Spotting and cramping without cervical change occur.

Inevitable Spotting and cramping occur and the cervix begins to dilate and efface.

Incomplete Loss of some of the products of conception occurs, with part of the products retained (most often placenta is retained).

Complete Loss of all products of conception occurs.

Missed Products of conception are retained in utero after fetal death.

Habitual Spontaneous abortions occur in three or more successive pregnancies.

---

3. Previous elective abortion

4. Uterine abnormalities such as adhesions or fibroids

5. Prolonged time to achieve pregnancy

6. Low serum progesterone

7. Celiac disease

8. Polycystic ovarian syndrome

9. Thyroid dysfunction or Cushing's syndrome

10. Systemic lupus erythematosus

11. Infection, fever, trauma

12. Low body mass index (BMI), less than 18.5

13. Smoking, alcohol, cocaine use, certain medications, high caffeine intake

D. Data collection

1. Spontaneous vaginal bleeding with the passage of clots and tissue through the vagina

2. Low uterine cramping and contractions

3. Hemorrhage and shock can result if bleeding is excessive.

E. Interventions

1. Maintain bed rest as prescribed.

2. Monitor vital signs.

3. Monitor for cramping and bleeding.

4. Count perineal pads to evaluate blood loss. Save any expelled tissue and clots.

5. Maintain IV fluids as prescribed. Monitor for signs of hemorrhage or shock.

6. Prepare the client for dilation and curettage, as prescribed, for incomplete abortion.

7. Prepare to administer $Rh_o(D)$ immune globulin to an Rh-negative woman.

8. Provide psychological support.

XIII. Anemia

A. Description

1. Develops as a result of an inadequate amount of serum iron

2. Predisposes the client to postpartum infection

B. Data collection
1. Fatigue
2. Headache
3. Pallor
4. Tachycardia
5. Hemoglobin value usually less than 10 g/dL and hematocrit value usually less than 30%
C. Interventions
1. Hemoglobin and hematocrit levels are monitored every 2 weeks.
2. Administer and reinforce instructions about iron and folic acid supplements.
3. Instruct the client to take iron with a source of vitamin C to increase its absorption and to avoid taking iron with tea or milk products; absorbed best if taken between meals.
4. Instruct the client to eat foods high in iron, folic acid, and protein.
5. Teach the client to monitor for signs and symptoms of infection.
6. Prepare to assist with the administration of parenteral iron or blood transfusions, which may be prescribed for severe anemia.
7. Prepare to assist with the administration of oxytocic medications during the postpartum period if excessive bleeding is a concern.

XIV. Cardiac Disease

A. Description: A pregnant client with cardiac disease may be unable to physiologically cope with the added plasma volume and increased cardiac output that occur during pregnancy; blood volume peaks at weeks 32 to 34 and then declines slightly to week 40.
B. Data collection
1. Signs/symptoms of cardiac decompensation
   a. Cough and respiratory congestion
   b. Dyspnea and fatigue
   c. Palpitations and tachycardia
   d. Peripheral edema
   e. Chest pain
2. Signs of respiratory infection
3. Signs of heart failure and pulmonary edema
C. Interventions
1. Monitor vital signs, fetal heart rate, and condition of the fetus.
2. Limit physical activities and stress the need for sufficient rest.
3. Monitor for signs of cardiac stress and decompensation such as cough, fatigue, dyspnea, chest pain, and tachycardia; also monitor for signs of heart failure and pulmonary edema.
4. Encourage adequate nutrition to prevent anemia, which would worsen the cardiac status; in addition, a low-sodium diet may be prescribed to prevent fluid retention and heart failure.
5. Avoid excessive weight gain.
6. During labor, prepare to assist with the following:

a. Monitor the vital signs frequently.
b. Place the client on a cardiac monitor and an external fetal monitor.
c. Maintain bed rest, with the mother lying on her side and her head and shoulders elevated.
d. Administer oxygen and pain medication, as prescribed.
e. Manage pain early in labor. Cardiology clearance may be required for epidural, spinal, or general anesthetic agents.
f. Use controlled pushing efforts to decrease cardiac stress.

⚠ Excessive weight gain places stress on the heart. In addition, obesity places the client at increased risk for complications of pregnancy.

XV. Chorioamnionitis

A. Description
1. A bacterial infection of the amniotic cavity that can result from the premature rupture of the membranes, vaginitis, amniocentesis, or intrauterine procedures
2. It may result in the development of postpartum endometritis and neonatal sepsis.
B. Data collection
1. Uterine tenderness and contractions
2. Elevated temperature
3. Maternal or fetal tachycardia
4. Foul odor to amniotic fluid
5. Leukocytosis
C. Interventions
1. Monitor maternal vital signs and fetal heart rate.
2. Monitor for uterine tenderness, contractions, and fetal activity.
3. Monitor the results of blood cultures.
4. Prepare for amniocentesis to obtain amniotic fluid for Gram stain and leukocyte count and other testing as prescribed.
5. Administer antibiotics, as prescribed, after cultures are obtained.
6. Oxytocic medications may be prescribed to increase uterine tone.
7. Prepare to obtain neonatal cultures after birth, as prescribed.

XVI. Diabetes Mellitus

A. Description
1. Pregnancy places demands on carbohydrate metabolism and causes insulin requirements to change.
2. Insulin resistance and hyperinsulinemia may predispose some women to diabetes.
3. Maternal glucose crosses the placenta, but insulin does not.
4. The fetus produces its own insulin and pulls glucose from the mother, which predisposes the mother to hypoglycemic reactions.

5. The newborn of a diabetic mother may be large in size but will have functions related to gestational age rather than size.

6. The newborn of a diabetic mother is at risk for hypoglycemia, hyperbilirubinemia, respiratory distress syndrome, hypocalcemia, and congenital anomalies.

⚠ During the first trimester, maternal insulin needs decrease. During the second and third trimesters, increases in placental hormones cause an insulin-resistant state, requiring an increase in the client's insulin dose. After placental delivery, placental hormone levels abruptly decrease and insulin requirements decrease.

B. Gestational diabetes mellitus
1. Occurs during pregnancy (during the second or third trimester) among clients not previously diagnosed as diabetic. Occurs when the pancreas cannot respond to the demand for more insulin.
2. Women may be diagnosed with overt diabetes while pregnant as well, and as a result of personal risk factors such as being overweight or obese, there is an increased likelihood of overt, unrecognized diabetes. An HbA1C level may be helpful in making this determination.
3. There is an increased incidence of gestational diabetes when a woman also has polycystic ovarian syndrome.
4. Pregnant women would be screened for gestational diabetes between 24 and 28 weeks' gestation via the 1 hour glucose challenge test.
5. If the 1 hour glucose challenge test is abnormal, a 3 hour oral glucose tolerance test is performed to confirm gestational diabetes mellitus.
6. Gestational diabetes frequently can be treated by diet alone; however, some clients may need insulin (selected oral medications that are safe during pregnancy may be prescribed).
7. Most gestational diabetics convert to a euglycemic state after birth; however, these individuals have an increased risk for developing diabetes mellitus during their lifetimes.
8. Early screening at an initial prenatal visit is done if the client has predisposing conditions as risk factors.
9. The need for cesarean section is more likely in neonatal hypoglycemia, and macrosomia may be evident.

⚠ Some oral hypoglycemic agents are unsafe for use during pregnancy; usually insulin is prescribed.

C. Predisposing conditions for gestational diabetes
1. Older than 35 years old
2. Obese—BMI greater than 30
3. Non-white race
4. Previous unexplained perinatal loss
5. Previous child born with congenital anomalies
6. Polycystic ovarian syndrome
7. Multiple gestations
8. Family history of diabetes mellitus
9. Previous delivery of a fetus weighing greater than 9 lb
10. Maternal birth weight less than 6 lb or greater than 9 lb
11. Previous pregnancy with gestational diabetes
12. Glycosuria
13. Essential or pregnancy-related hypertension
14. Use of glucocorticoids

D. Data collection
1. Excessive thirst
2. Hunger
3. Weight loss
4. Frequent urination
5. Blurred vision
6. Recurrent urinary tract infections and vaginal yeast infections
7. Glycosuria and ketonuria
8. Signs/symptoms of gestational hypertension and preeclampsia
9. Polyhydramnios
10. Fetus is large for gestational age.

E. Interventions
1. Employ diet, medications (if diet cannot control blood glucose levels), exercise, and blood glucose determinations 4 times daily (fasting and 1 to 2 hours after meals) to maintain blood glucose levels as follows: fasting less than 95 mg/dL, 1 hour postprandial less than 130 to 140 mg/dL, 2 hour postprandial less than 120 mg/dL.
2. Encourage moderate physical activity.
3. Facilitate referral to a diabetic educator and nutritionist.
4. Observe for signs of hyperglycemia, glycosuria, ketonuria, and hypoglycemia.
5. Monitor weight.
6. Maintain calorie intake, as prescribed, with adequate oral medication or insulin therapy so that glucose will move into the cells.
7. Monitor for signs of maternal complications, such as preeclampsia, a serious blood pressure disorder that can affect all organs in the body (hypertension is characteristic of the condition).
8. Monitor for signs of infection.
9. Instruct the client to report burning and pain on urination, vaginal discharge or itching, or any other signs of infection to the PHCP.
10. Monitor the fetal status and for signs of fetal compromise.
11. Schedule visits every 2 weeks until 36 weeks, and then every week from 36 weeks and up.

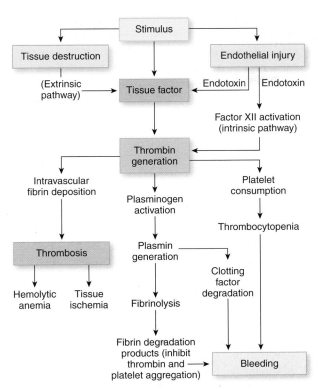

FIGURE 23.3 Pathophysiology of disseminated intravascular coagulation.

BOX 23.7 Predisposing Conditions for Disseminated Intravascular Coagulation

- Abruptio placentae
- Amniotic fluid embolism
- Gestational hypertension
- Intrauterine fetal death
- Liver disease
- Sepsis

F. Interventions during labor
1. Monitor the fetal status continuously for signs of distress; if noted, assist to prepare the client for immediate cesarean section.
2. Assist to carefully regulate insulin and provide IV glucose, as prescribed, because labor depletes glycogen.

G. Interventions during the postpartum period
1. Observe the client closely for a hypoglycemic reaction, because a precipitous drop in insulin requirements normally occurs. The mother may not require insulin for the first 24 hours.
2. Reregulate insulin needs, as prescribed, after the first day, according to blood glucose testing and PHCP's prescriptions.
3. Determine dietary needs on the basis of blood glucose and insulin requirements.
4. Monitor for signs of infection or postpartum hemorrhage.

XVII. Disseminated Intravascular Coagulation

A. Description: Disseminated intravascular coagulation (DIC) is a maternal condition in which the clotting cascade is activated, resulting in the formation of clots in the microcirculation (Fig. 23.3).

⚠ The rapid and extensive formation of clots that occurs in DIC causes the platelets and clotting factors to be depleted. This results in bleeding and potential vascular occlusion of organs from thromboembolus formation.

B. Predisposing conditions (Box 23.7)
C. Data collection
1. Uncontrolled bleeding
2. Bruising, purpura, petechiae, and ecchymosis
3. Presence of occult blood in excretions, such as stool (melena)
4. Hematuria, hematemesis, or vaginal bleeding
5. Signs of shock
6. Decreased fibrinogen level, platelet count, and hematocrit level
7. Increased prothrombin time, partial thromboplastin time, clotting time, and fibrin degradation products
D. Interventions
1. Eliminate by treating the underlying cause.
2. Monitor vital signs and look for bleeding and signs of shock.
3. Assist in preparing to administer oxygen therapy, volume replacement, blood-component therapy, and possibly heparin therapy.
4. Monitor for complications associated with fluid and blood replacement and heparin therapy.
5. Monitor the urine output, and maintain it at 30 mL/hour (renal failure is a complication of DIC).

XVIII. Ectopic Pregnancy

A. Description: Implantation of the fertilized ovum outside of the uterine cavity, commonly in the ampulla of the fallopian tube
B. Data collection
1. Missed menstrual period
2. Abdominal pain
3. Vaginal spotting to bleeding that is dark red or brown
4. Rupture: Increased pain, referred shoulder pain, and signs of shock
C. Interventions
1. Obtain vital signs.
2. Monitor bleeding and prepare to assist to initiate measures to prevent rupture and shock.
3. Methotrexate (a folic acid antagonist) may be prescribed to inhibit cell division in the developing embryo.
4. Prepare the client for laparotomy and the removal of the pregnancy and tube, if necessary, or repair of the tube.
5. Assist to administer antibiotics. $Rh_o(D)$ immune globulin is prescribed for Rh-negative women.

XIX. Fetal Death In Utero

A. Description

1. Death of a fetus after 20 weeks' gestation and before birth
2. DIC can develop if the dead fetus is retained in the uterus for 3 to 4 weeks or longer.

B. Data collection

1. Absence of fetal movement
2. Absence of fetal heart tones
3. Maternal weight loss
4. Lack of fetal growth or decrease in fundal height
5. No evidence of cardiac activity
6. Other characteristics suggestive of fetal death noted on the ultrasound

C. Interventions

1. Prepare for the birth of the fetus.
2. Support the client's decision about labor, birth, and the postpartum period.
3. Provide support and ask what can be helpful; provide assistance as appropriate and requested.
4. Accept behaviors such as sadness, anger, and hostility from the parents.
5. Refer parents to an appropriate support group.

⚠ Cultural, spiritual and religious practices and beliefs are important to consider when caring for the parents of a fetus who has died. Be aware of cultural, spiritual, and religious practices and beliefs and ensure that such beliefs are respected and implemented as appropriate.

XX. Hepatitis B

A. Description

1. The risks of prematurity, low birth weight, and neonatal death increase if the mother has hepatitis B infection.
2. It is transmitted through blood, saliva, vaginal secretions, semen, breast milk, and across the placental barrier.

B. Interventions

1. Minimize the risk for intrapartum ascending infections by limiting the number of vaginal examinations.
2. Remove the maternal blood from the neonate immediately after birth.
3. Suction the neonate immediately after birth.
4. Bathe the neonate before any invasive procedures, including injections.
5. Clean and dry the face and eyes of the neonate before instilling eye prophylaxis.
6. Infection of the neonate can be prevented by the administration of hepatitis B immune globulin and hepatitis B vaccine soon after birth but after newborn is bathed.

BOX 23.8   Hematoma: Assessment Findings

- Abnormal, severe pain
- Pressure in the peritoneal area (client states that she feels like she has to have a bowel movement)
- Palpable sensitive swelling in the peritoneal area, with discolored skin
- Inability to void
- Decreased hemoglobin and hematocrit levels
- Signs of shock, such as pallor, tachycardia, and hypotension, if significant blood loss has occurred

---

7. Discourage the mother from kissing the neonate until the neonate has received the vaccine.
8. Inform the mother that the hepatitis B vaccine will be administered to the neonate and that the second dose will be administered at 1 month after birth. The third dose is administered at 6 months.
9. Support breast-feeding after neonatal treatment for hepatitis B; breast-feeding is not contraindicated if the neonate has been vaccinated.

XXI. Hematoma

A. Description

1. Hematoma occurs following the escape of blood into the maternal tissue after birth.
2. Predisposing conditions include operative delivery with forceps or injury to a blood vessel.

B. Data Collection (Box 23.8)

C. Interventions

1. Monitor vital signs.
2. Monitor client for abnormal pain, especially when forceps delivery has been performed.
3. Apply ice to the hematoma site.
4. Administer analgesics as prescribed.
5. Monitor intake and output.
6. Encourage fluids and voiding; prepare for urinary catheterization if the client is unable to void.
7. Assist to administer blood replacements as prescribed.
8. Monitor for signs of infections, such as increased temperature, pulse rate, and white blood cell count.
9. Administer antibiotics as prescribed; infection is common after hematoma formation.
10. Prepare for incision and evacuation of the hematoma if necessary.

XXII. Human Immunodeficiency Virus and Acquired Immunodeficiency Syndrome

A. Description

1. The human immunodeficiency virus (HIV) is the causative factor of the development of acquired immunodeficiency syndrome (AIDS).
2. Women infected with the HIV virus may first demonstrate signs/symptoms at the time of pregnancy

or possibly develop life-threatening infections, because normal pregnancy involves some suppression of the maternal immune system.

3. Repeated exposure to the virus during pregnancy through unsafe sex practices or intravenous (IV) drug use can increase the risk of transmission to the fetus.

4. Three-drug combination HAART (highly active antiretroviral therapy) treatment, which is monitored by an infectious disease specialist, is recommended to reduce mother-to-child transmission (MTCT). Zidovudine is recommended for the prevention of MTCT. It is administered based on the following recommendations:

 a. Antepartum: Orally beginning after 12 weeks of gestation, maternal HAART is given to reduce the viral load to undetectable.

 b. Intrapartum: Intravenously during labor, zidovudine is given 1 hour before a vaginal birth and 3 hours before a cesarean section if the HIV RNA is greater than or equal to 400 copies per mL or unknown. Of note, this may not be required if the HIV RNA is less than 400 copies per mL but is given at the discretion of the provider. A vaginal birth is acceptable if the viral load is less than 1000 copies per mL; otherwise a cesarean section is recommended.

 c. Postpartum: In the form of syrup to the newborn 2 hours after birth and every 12 hours for 6 weeks; depending on agency procedures, the newborn may need to be placed in the newborn intensive care unit (NICU) to begin initial therapy.

B. Transmission

 1. Sexual exposure to genital secretions of an infected person

 2. Parenteral exposure to infected blood and tissue

 3. Perinatal exposure of an *infant* to infected maternal secretions through the birth process or breastfeeding

C. Risks to the mother: The mother with HIV is managed as high risk because she is vulnerable to infections.

D. Diagnosis

 1. Tests used to determine the presence of antibodies to HIV include enzyme-linked immunosorbent assay (ELISA), Western blot (WB), and immunofluorescence assay (IFA).

 2. A single reactive ELISA test result by itself cannot be used to diagnose HIV and would be repeated in duplicate with the same blood sample. If the result is repeatedly reactive, follow-up tests using WB or IFA would be performed.

 3. A positive WB or IFA is considered confirmatory for HIV.

 4. A positive ELISA that fails to be confirmed by WB or IFA would not be considered negative for HIV. Repeat testing must take place in 3 to 6 months.

> **BOX 23.9** **Stages of Acquired Immunodeficiency Syndrome**
>
> **Stage 1**
> - Fever
> - Headache
> - Myalgia
> - Lymphadenopathy
>
> **Stage 2**
> - Active infection but asymptomatic; may remain so for years
> - May experience an outbreak of herpes zoster (shingles)
> - May experience a transient thrombocytopenia
>
> **Stage 3**
> - Symptomatic
> - Evidence of immune dysfunction
> - All body systems can present with signs of immune dysfunction
> - Integumentary and gynecological problems are common
>
> **Stage 4**
> - Advanced human immunodeficiency virus infection
> - Vulnerable to common bacterial infections
> - Development of opportunistic infections
> - Serious immune compromise

5. See Chapter 59 for additional laboratory tests.

E. Data collection (Box 23.9)

F. Interventions

 1. Prenatal period

 a. Prevent opportunistic infections.

 b. Procedures that increase the risk of perinatal transmission are avoided, such as amniocentesis and fetal scalp sampling.

 2. Intrapartum period

 a. If the fetus has not been exposed to HIV in utero, the highest risk exists during delivery through the birth canal.

 b. The use of internal scalp electrodes for monitoring of the fetus is avoided.

 c. Episiotomy is avoided to decrease the amount of maternal blood in and around the birth canal.

 d. The administration of oxytocin is avoided, because oxytocin contractions can be strong, thus inducing vaginal tears or necessitating the need for an episiotomy.

 e. Place heavy absorbent pads under the mother's hips to absorb amniotic fluid and maternal blood.

 f. Minimize the neonate's exposure to maternal blood and body fluids. Promptly remove the neonate from the mother's blood after delivery.

 g. Suction fluids from the newborn promptly.

 h. Prepare to assist to administer zidovudine as prescribed to the mother during labor and delivery.

3. Postpartum period
   a. Monitor for signs of infection.
   b. Place the mother in protective isolation if she is immunosuppressed.
   c. Breast-feeding is usually restricted; follow PHCP's recommendations regarding breast-feeding.
   d. Instruct the mother to monitor for signs of infection and report any signs if they occur.
   e. The newborn can room with the mother; however, depending on agency procedures, the newborn may be placed in the NICU for first 24 hours of life to complete baseline laboratory studies and to receive initial treatment.
G. The neonate and HIV (see Chapter 26)

XXIII. Hydatidiform Mole

A. Description
   1. A form of gestational trophoblastic disease that occurs when the trophoblasts, the peripheral cells that attach the fertilized ovum to the uterine wall, develop abnormally.
   2. Presents as an edematous, grapelike cluster that may be nonmalignant or may develop into choriocarcinoma
B. Data collection
   1. Fetal heart rate not detectable
   2. Vaginal bleeding, which may occur as early as the fourth week or as late as the second trimester; it is usually bright red or dark brown in color, and it may be slight, profuse, or intermittent.
   3. Signs of preeclampsia, progressive blood pressure elevations may be present before gestational week 20. Preeclampsia usually occurs after 20 weeks of pregnancy, typically in the third trimester.
   4. Fundal height is greater than expected for gestational date.
   5. Elevated hCG levels
   6. Ultrasound shows a characteristic snowstorm pattern.
C. Interventions
   1. Assist to prepare the mother for uterine evacuation (before evacuation, diagnostic tests are done to detect metastatic disease).
   2. Evacuation of the mole is done by vacuum aspiration. Oxytocin may be administered after evacuation to contract the uterus.
   3. Tissue is sent to the laboratory for evaluation. Follow-up is important to detect changes that are suggestive of malignancy.
   4. Monitor for post-procedure hemorrhage and infection.
   5. Human chorionic gonadotropin levels are monitored every 1 to 2 weeks until normal prepregnancy levels are attained. The levels are then checked every 1 to 2 months for 1 year.

6. Instruct the client and her partner regarding birth control measures so that pregnancy can be prevented during the 1-year follow-up.

XXIV. Hyperemesis Gravidarum

A. Description: Intractable nausea and vomiting that persists beyond the first trimester and causes disturbance in nutrition and fluid and electrolyte balance
B. Data collection
   1. Nausea is most pronounced on arising; however, it can occur at other times during the day.
   2. Persistent vomiting
   3. Weight loss
   4. Signs of dehydration
   5. Fluid and electrolyte imbalances
C. Interventions
   1. Measures to alleviate nausea, including medication therapy, are initiated. If this is unsuccessful and weight loss and fluid and electrolyte imbalances occur, the administration of IV fluid and electrolyte replacement or parenteral nutrition may be necessary.
   2. Monitor the vital signs, intake, output, weight, and calorie count.
   3. Monitor the laboratory data and for signs of dehydration and electrolyte imbalance.
   4. Monitor urine for ketones.
   5. Monitor fetal heart rate, fetal activity, and fetal growth.
   6. Encourage the intake of small portions of food (low-fat, easily digestible carbohydrates, such as cereals, rice, and pasta).
   7. Liquids need to be taken between meals to avoid distending the stomach and triggering vomiting.
   8. Encourage the client to sit upright after meals.

XXV. Hypertensive Disorders of Pregnancy

A. Description and types: Four major categories include preeclampsia, chronic/preexisting hypertension, chronic hypertension with superimposed preeclampsia, and gestational hypertension.
B. Blood pressure elevations can lead to preeclampsia and then eclampsia (seizures) (Tables 23.2 and 23.3)
C. Women who have had preeclampsia, especially those who delivered preterm, have an increased risk later in life of cardiovascular disease and kidney disease, including heart attack, stroke, and high blood pressure.
D. Having preeclampsia once increases the risk of having it again in a future pregnancy.
E. Preeclampsia also can lead to eclampsia (seizures).
F. HELLP syndrome can result. HELLP stands for *h*emolysis, *e*levated *l*iver enzymes, and *l*ow *p*latelet count. In this condition, red blood cells are damaged or destroyed, blood clotting is impaired, and the liver can bleed internally, causing chest or abdominal pain.

TABLE 23.2 Classification of Hypertensive Stages of Pregnancy

Type of Hypertension	Description
Normal	Less than 120/80 mm Hg
Elevated	Systolic between 120 and 129 and diastolic less than 80 mm Hg
Stage 1 hypertension	Systolic between 130 and 139 or diastolic between 80 and 89 mm Hg
Stage 2 hypertension	Systolic at least 140 or diastolic at least 90 mm Hg
Chronic hypertension	Hypertension that is present and observable before pregnancy or that occurs in the first half (before 20 weeks) of the pregnancy
Gestational Hypertensive Disorders	
Gestational hypertension	Blood pressure elevation that first occurs in the second half (after 20 weeks) of pregnancy. Although gestational hypertension usually resolves after childbirth, it may increase the risk of developing hypertension in the future.
Preeclampsia	Usually occurs after 20 weeks of pregnancy, typically in the third trimester. When it occurs before 32 weeks of pregnancy, it is called early-onset preeclampsia. It also can occur in the postpartum period.
Eclampsia	Seizure occurring in pregnancy and linked to high blood pressure

From The American College of Obstetricians and Gynecologists, May 2018 at: https://www.acog.org/Patients/FAQs/Preeclampsia-and-High-Blood-Pressure-During-Pregnancy.

TABLE 23.3 Mild versus Severe Preeclampsia

Parameter Evaluated	Mild	Severe
Systolic blood pressure	≥140 mm Hg, but <160 mm Hg	≥160 mm Hg (two readings, 6 hours apart, while on bed rest)
Diastolic blood pressure	≥90 mm Hg, but <110 mm Hg	≥110 mm Hg
Proteinuria (a 24-hour specimen is preferred to eliminate hour-to-hour variations)	≥0.3 g, but <5 g in a 24-hour specimen (1 + on a random dipstick test)	≥5 g in a 24-hour specimen (≥3 g + on a random dipstick test)
Creatinine, serum (renal function)	Normal	Elevated (>1.0 mg/dL)
Platelets	Normal	Decreased (<100,000 mm³)
Liver enzymes (alanine aminotransferase or aspartate aminotransferase)	Normal or minimal increase in levels	Elevated levels
Urine output	Normal	Oliguria common, often <500 mL/day
Severe, unrelenting headache not attributable to other cause; mental confusion (cerebral edema)	Absent	Often present
Persistent right upper quadrant or epigastric pain or pain penetrating to the back (distention of the liver capsule); nausea and vomiting	Absent	May be present and often precedes seizure
Visual disturbances (spots or "sparkles," temporary blindness; photophobia)	Absent to minimal	Common
Pulmonary edema, heart failure, and cyanosis	Absent	May be present
Fetal growth restriction	Normal growth	Growth restriction; reduced amniotic fluid volume

Adapted from Lowdermilk D, Cashion MC, Perry S: *Maternity & women's health care*, ed 10, St. Louis, 2012, Mosby.

HELLP syndrome is a medical emergency; the woman can die from HELLP syndrome or have lifelong health problems as a result.

G. Data Collection (see Table 23.2)

⚠ Proteinuria is not a reliable indicator of preeclampsia. Evidence demonstrates that kidney or liver dysfunction can occur without signs of protein, and that the amount of protein in the urine does not predict how severely the disease will progress.

1. Persistent hypertension
2. Swelling of the face or hands
3. Headache
4. Changes in eyesight
5. Pain in the upper abdomen or shoulder

6. Nausea and vomiting (in the second half of pregnancy)

7. Sudden weight gain

8. Difficulty breathing

H. Risk factors

1. Previous preeclampsia or gestational hypertension, previous placental abruption, or fetal demise

2. Primigravida

3. Family history or first-degree relative with preeclampsia

4. Women who are 40 years or older

5. African American ethnicity

6. Women who are carrying more than one fetus

7. History of chronic hypertension, kidney disease, or both

8. Women who have medical conditions such as chronic hypertension, renal disease, connective tissue disease, diabetes mellitus, thrombophilia, or lupus erythematosus

9. BMI greater than 26

10. Metabolic syndrome

11. Multifetal pregnancy

12. Hydatidiform mole, hydrops fetalis, unexplained intrauterine growth retardation (IUGR)

13. Mother had IUGR as a newborn

14. Women who had in vitro fertilization

I. Complications of hypertension and gestational hypertension disorders

1. Abruptio placentae

2. Disseminated intravascular coagulopathy

3. Fetal growth restriction

4. Preeclampsia and eclampsia

5. Intracranial hemorrhage; maternal cerebral hemorrhage or infarction

6. Subcapsular hepatic hematoma

7. HELLP (*h*emolysis, *e*levated *l*iver enzyme levels, *l*ow *p*latelet count) syndrome

8. Oligohydramnios

9. Placental insufficiency

10. The need for preterm delivery or cesarean delivery

11. Maternal and/or fetal death

J. Interventions for hypertension and preeclampsia

1. Frequent blood pressure and weight monitoring throughout the pregnancy; the client may need to be taught how to take her blood pressure at home.

2. Weekly or twice-weekly health care visits may be necessary; delivery may be recommended at 37 weeks of gestation (earlier if there is evidence of fetal distress).

3. Monitor fetal activity (teach the client how to perform kick counts) and monitor fetal growth (ultrasounds will be prescribed).

4. Encourage frequent rest periods, instructing the client to lie in the lateral position; for

---

BOX 23.10 **Checking Reflexes**

Biceps Reflex

The thumb is placed over the client's biceps tendon, and the client's elbow is supported with the palm of the hand.

The examiner strikes a downward blow over the thumb with the percussion hammer.

Normal Response: Flexion of the arm at the elbow

Patellar Reflex

The client is positioned with the legs dangling over the edge of the examining table, or lying on her back, with the legs slightly flexed.

The examiner strikes the patellar tendon just below the kneecap with the percussion hammer.

Normal Response: Extension or kicking out of the leg

Clonus Reflex

The client is positioned with the legs dangling over the edge of the examining table.

The leg is supported with one hand, and the client's foot is sharply dorsiflexed with the other hand.

The dorsiflexed position is maintained for a few seconds; then the foot is released.

Normal Response (Negative Clonus Response)

The foot will remain steady in the dorsiflexed position.

No rhythmic oscillations or jerking of the foot will be felt.

When released, the foot will drop to a plantar-flexed position, with no oscillations.

Abnormal Response (Positive Clonus Response)

Rhythmic oscillations will occur when the foot is dorsiflexed.

Similar oscillations will be noted when the foot drops to the plantar-flexed position.

Grading the Response

0 = Reflex absent

1+ = Reflex present but hypoactive

2+ = Normal reflex

3+ = Hyperactive reflex

4+ = Hyperactive reflex with clonus present

---

preeclampsia with severe features, the client may be hospitalized and bedrest may be prescribed (client would be placed in the lateral position).

5. Administer medications as prescribed to reduce blood pressure; blood pressure must not be reduced rapidly because placental perfusion can be compromised.

6. Provide adequate fluids.

7. Monitor intake and output; a urinary output of 30 mL/hour indicates adequate renal perfusion.

8. Monitor neurological status because changes can indicate cerebral hypoxia or impending seizure.

9. Monitor deep tendon reflexes, and for the presence of hyperreflexia or clonus, because hyperreflexia indicates increased central nervous system irritability (Box 23.10).

10. Monitor for HELLP syndrome.

Seizure typically begins with twitching around the mouth.

Body then becomes rigid in a state of tonic muscular contractions that last 15–20 seconds.

Facial muscles and then all body muscles alternately contract and relax in rapid succession (clonic phase may last about 1 minute).

Respiration ceases during seizure because diaphragm tends to remain fixed (breathing resumes shortly after the seizure).

Postictal sleep occurs.

11. Evaluate renal function through prescribed studies such as blood urea nitrogen, serum creatinine, and 24-hour urine levels for creatinine clearance and protein.
12. Magnesium sulfate (use a controlled infusion device) may be prescribed to prevent seizures; magnesium sulfate may be continued for 24 to 48 hours postpartum.
13. Monitor for signs of magnesium toxicity with the administration of magnesium sulfate, including flushing, sweating, hypotension, depressed deep tendon reflexes, urine output, and central nervous system depression including respiratory depression; keep antidote (calcium gluconate) available for immediate use, if necessary.
14. Corticosteroids may be prescribed to promote fetal lung maturity.
15. Prepare the client for delivery as prescribed.

K. Eclampsia
1. Data collection: Characterized by generalized seizures (Box 23.11)
2. Interventions (see Priority Nursing Actions)

⚡ PRIORITY NURSING ACTIONS

Eclampsia Event

1. Remain with the client and call for help.
2. Ensure an open airway, turn the client on her side, and oxygen is administered by face mask at 8 L/minute to 10 L/minute.
3. Monitor fetal heart rate patterns.
4. Assist to administer medications to control the seizures as prescribed.
5. After the seizure has ended, insert an oral airway and suction the client's mouth as needed.
6. Prepare for delivery of the fetus after stabilization of the client, if warranted.
7. Document occurrence, client's response, and outcome.

XXVI. Incompetent Cervix

A. Description
1. Premature dilation of the cervix, which occurs most often during the fourth or fifth month of pregnancy and is associated with structural or functional defects of the cervix
2. Treatment involves surgical placement of a cervical cerclage.

B. Data collection
1. Vaginal bleeding
2. Fetal membranes are visible through the cervix.

C. Interventions
1. Provide bed rest, hydration, and assist with tocolysis, as prescribed, to inhibit uterine contractions.
2. Prepare for cervical cerclage (at 10–14 weeks' gestation as prescribed), in which a band of fascia or nonabsorbable ribbon is placed around the cervix beneath the mucosa to constrict the internal os of the cervix.
3. After cervical cerclage, the woman is told to refrain from intercourse and avoid prolonged standing and heavy lifting.
4. The cervical cerclage is removed at 37 weeks' gestation or left in place, and a cesarean birth is performed. If removed, the cerclage must be repeated with each successive pregnancy.
5. After the procedure, monitor for contractions, rupture of the membranes, and signs of infection.
6. Instruct the woman to report any post-procedure vaginal bleeding or increased uterine contractions immediately to the PHCP.

XXVII. Infections (TORCH Complex Acronym)

A. Toxoplasmosis ("T")
1. Caused by infection with the protozoan intracellular parasite *Toxoplasma gondii*
2. Produces a rash and symptoms of acute, flu-like infection in the mother
3. Transmitted to the mother through the consumption of raw meat or the handling of the cat litter of infected cats
4. Organism is transmitted to the fetus across the placenta.
5. Can cause miscarriage in the first trimester
6. Client education regarding preventing infection is critical.

B. Other infections ("O," includes HIV—discussed earlier; syphilis—discussed under Sexually Transmitted Infections; parvovirus; hepatitis B virus (HBV); West Nile, etc.)

C. Rubella (German measles) ("R")
1. Teratogenic during the first trimester
2. Transmitted to the fetus across the placenta
3. Causes congenital defects of the eyes, heart, ears, and brain
4. If not immune (titer of 1:8 or less), the mother must be vaccinated during the postpartum period. She must then wait 1 to 3 months (as specified by PHCP) before becoming pregnant again.

D. Cytomegalovirus ("C")
1. The organism is transmitted through close personal contact or across the placenta to the fetus,

or the fetus may be infected through the birth canal.

2. The mother may be asymptomatic, and most infants are asymptomatic at birth.

3. Cytomegalovirus causes low birth weight, intrauterine growth restriction, enlarged liver and spleen, jaundice, cognitive impairment, blindness, hearing loss, and seizures.

4. Antiviral medications may be prescribed for severe infections in the mother, but these medications are toxic and may only temporarily suppress the shedding of the virus.

5. Maintain contact precautions.

E. Herpes simplex virus ("H")

1. Herpes simplex virus affects the external genitalia, vagina, and cervix and causes draining, painful vesicles.

2. Acyclovir can be used to treat recurrent outbreaks during pregnancy or used as suppressive therapy late in pregnancy to prevent an outbreak during labor and birth.

3. Virus usually is transmitted to the fetus during birth through the infected vagina or via an ascending infection after rupture of the membranes.

4. No vaginal examinations are done in the presence of active vaginal herpetic lesions.

5. Herpes can cause death or severe neurological impairment in the newborn.

6. Delivery of the fetus is usually by cesarean section if active lesions are present in the vagina; delivery may be performed vaginally if the lesions are in the anal, perineal, or inner thigh area (strict precautions are necessary to protect the fetus during delivery).

7. Maintain contact precautions.

F. Group B *Streptococcus* (GBS) (may be indicated as an "O" under TORCH complex)

1. A leading cause of life-threatening perinatal infections

2. The gram-positive bacterium colonizes the rectum, vagina, cervix, and urethra of pregnant and nonpregnant women.

3. Meningitis, fasciitis, and intraabdominal abscess can occur in the pregnant client if she is infected at the time of birth.

4. Transmission occurs during vaginal delivery.

5. Early onset newborn GBS occurs within the first week after birth, usually within 48 hours. It can include infections such as sepsis, pneumonia, or meningitis, and permanent neurological disability can result.

6. Diagnosis of the mother is done via vaginal and rectal cultures between 35 and 37 weeks' gestation.

7. Antibiotics such as penicillin may be prescribed for the mother during labor and birth. IV antibiotics may be prescribed for infected infants.

8. Maintain contact precautions.

XXVIII. Multiple Gestation

A. Description

1. Results from the fertilization of more than one ova (fraternal or dizygotic) or a splitting of one fertilized ovum (identical or monozygotic)

2. Complications include miscarriage, anemia, congenital anomalies, hyperemesis gravidarum, intrauterine growth restriction, gestational hypertension, polyhydramnios, postpartum hemorrhage, premature rupture of membranes, and preterm labor and delivery.

B. Data collection

1. Excessive fetal activity

2. Uterus large for gestational age

3. Fetal movements felt in different parts of the abdomen at the same time

4. Auscultation of more than one fetal heart rate

5. Excessive weight gain

C. Interventions

1. Monitor vital signs.

2. Monitor fetal heart rates, fetal activity, and fetal growth.

3. Monitor for cervical changes.

4. Prepare the client for ultrasound, as prescribed.

5. Monitor for anemia. Administer supplemental vitamins, as prescribed.

6. Monitor for preterm labor and assist to treat it promptly.

7. Prepare for cesarean section for abnormal presentations.

8. Prepare to assist with administration of oxytocic medications after delivery to prevent postpartum hemorrhage from uterine overdistention.

XXIX. Placenta Accreta, Placenta Increta, Placenta Percreta

A. Description: Placenta accreta is an abnormally adherent placenta; placenta increta occurs when the placenta penetrates the uterine muscle itself; placenta percreta occurs when the placenta goes all the way through the uterus.

B. Data collection: May cause hemorrhage immediately after birth because placenta does not separate easily.

C. Intervention

1. Monitor for hemorrhage and shock.

2. Prepare the client for a hysterectomy if a large portion of the placenta is abnormally adherent.

XXX. Placenta Previa (Fig. 23.4)

A. Description

1. Placenta previa is an improperly implanted placenta in the lower uterine segment near or over the internal cervical os.

2. Total (complete): The internal cervical os is covered entirely by the placenta when the cervix is dilated fully.

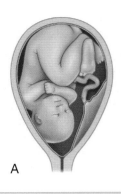 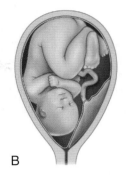 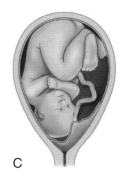

A	B	C
Marginal	Partial	Total
Placenta is implanted in its lower uterus but its lower border is >3 cm from internal cervical os.	Lower border of placenta is within 3 cm of internal cervical os but does not fully cover it.	Placenta completely covers internal cervical os.

FIGURE 23.4 The three classifications of placenta previa.

3. Partial: The lower border of the placenta is within 3 cm of the internal cervical os but does not fully cover it.

4. Marginal (low-lying): The placenta is implanted in the lower uterus, but its lower border is more than 3 cm from the internal cervical os.

5. Management depends on the classification of the placenta previa and the gestational age of the fetus.

B. Data collection

1. Sudden onset of painless bright red vaginal bleeding occurs in the last half of pregnancy.

2. Uterus is soft, relaxed, and nontender.

3. Fundal height may be more than expected for gestational age.

C. Interventions

1. Monitor maternal vital signs, fetal heart rate, and fetal activity.

2. Assist in preparation for ultrasound to confirm diagnosis.

3. Vaginal exams or any other actions that would stimulate uterine activity are avoided.

4. Maintain bedrest in a side-lying position as prescribed.

5. Monitor amount of bleeding (signs of shock are treated).

6. Assist RN to administer intravenous (IV) fluids, blood products, or tocolytic medications as prescribed.

7. If bleeding is heavy, a cesarean delivery may be performed.

⚠ Vaginal exams are contraindicated if the client is suspected of having or has a known placenta previa.

XXXI. Abruptio Placentae (Fig. 23.5)

A. Description: Premature separation of the placenta from the uterine wall after the 20th week of gestation and before the fetus is delivered

B. Data collection

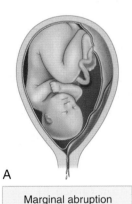

A

Marginal abruption with external bleeding

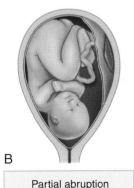 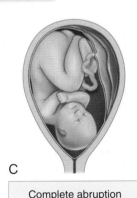

B

Partial abruption with concealed bleeding

C

Complete abruption with concealed bleeding

FIGURE 23.5 Types of abruptio placentae.

1. Dark red vaginal bleeding. If the bleeding is high in the uterus or is minimal, there can be an absence of visible blood.

2. Uterine pain or tenderness or both

3. Uterine rigidity

4. Severe abdominal pain

5. Signs of fetal distress

6. Signs of maternal shock if bleeding is excessive

C. Interventions

1. Monitor maternal vital signs and fetal heart rate.

Maternity Nursing

2. Assess for excessive vaginal bleeding, abdominal pain, and an increase in fundal height.
3. Maintain bedrest; administer oxygen, assist with IV fluids and blood products as prescribed.
4. Place the client in Trendelenburg position if indicated to decrease the pressure of the fetus on the placenta, or place in lateral position with the head of the bed flat and report any uterine activity.
5. Assist in monitoring any uterine activity.
6. Prepare for delivery of the fetus as quickly as possible, with vaginal delivery preferable if the fetus is healthy and stable and the presenting part is in the pelvis; emergency cesarean delivery is performed if the fetus is alive but shows signs of distress.
7. Monitor for signs of disseminated intravascular coagulation in the postpartum period.

⚠️ Know the difference between placenta previa and abruptio placentae. In placenta previa, there is painless, bright red vaginal bleeding, and the uterus is soft, relaxed and nontender. In abruptio placentae, there is dark red vaginal bleeding, uterine pain or tenderness or both, and uterine rigidity.

XXXII. Sexually Transmitted Infections (See Table 23.1)

A. Gonorrhea
1. Description
   a. An infection caused by *Neisseria gonorrhoeae*, which causes inflammation of the mucous membranes of the genital and urinary tracts
   b. Transmission of the organism is by sexual intercourse.
   c. Infection may be transmitted to the newborn's eyes during delivery, causing blindness (ophthalmia neonatorum).
2. Data collection: Usually asymptomatic. Vaginal discharge, urinary frequency, and lower abdominal pain are possible.
3. Interventions
   a. Obtain a vaginal culture for gonorrhea during the first prenatal visit. Prepare to repeat the culture during the third trimester in high-risk clients.
   b. Instruct the client that the treatment of her partner is necessary if infection is present.
   c. Complications are similar to those of chlamydia.

B. Syphilis
1. Description
   a. Chronic infectious disease caused by the organism *Treponema pallidum*
   b. Transmission is by physical contact with syphilitic lesions, which are usually found on the skin, mucous membranes of the mouth, and genitals.

BOX 23.12   Stages of Syphilis

Primary Stage
- Most infectious stage
- Appearance of ulcerative, painless lesions produced by spirochetes at the point of entry into the body

Secondary Stage
- Highly infectious stage
- Lesions appear about 6 weeks to 6 months after the primary stage and may occur anywhere on the skin and mucous membranes.
- Generalized lymphadenopathy

Tertiary Stage
- Spirochetes enter the internal organs and cause permanent damage; symptoms may occur 10–30 years after the occurrence of an untreated primary lesion.
- Disease invades the central nervous system, causing meningitis, ataxia, general paresis, and progressive mental deterioration.
- Affects the aortic valve and the aorta

---

   c. Infection may cause abortion or preterm labor. Passed to the fetus after the fourth month of pregnancy as congenital syphilis.
2. Data collection (Box 23.12)
3. Interventions
   a. A serum test (Venereal Disease Research Laboratory [VDRL] for syphilis is done on the first prenatal visit;). The serology test may be repeated at 36 weeks of gestation because the disease may be acquired after the initial visit.
   b. If the test result is positive, treatment with an antibiotic such as penicillin may be necessary.
   c. Sonographic evaluation is necessary to assess for signs of placental syphilis.
   d. Instruct the client that the treatment of her partner is necessary if an infection is present, and intercourse must be avoided until treatment is instituted.
   e. Complications include transmission to fetus (100% in primary and secondary stages), congenital anomalies, deafness, neurological impairment (mortality rate is 50%).
   f. Those with syphilis must also be treated for HIV.

C. Condylomata acuminata (*human papillomavirus*)
1. Description
   a. Caused by *human papillomavirus* (HPV)
   b. Infection affects the cervix, urethra, anus, penis, and scrotum.
   c. *Human papillomavirus* is transmitted through sexual contact.
2. Data collection
   a. Small to large wart-like growths on the genitals

b. Cervical cell changes may be noted, because HPV is associated with cervical malignancies.

3. Interventions

a. Lesions are removed with the use of cytotoxic agents, cryotherapy, electrocautery, and laser, but this is done for symptomatic relief only and is usually delayed until after birth. The genital warts often regress after delivery, and treatment outcomes may be poor until after delivery

b. Encourage a yearly Pap smear.

c. Sexual contact is avoided until the lesions are healed. (Condoms reduce transmission.)

d. Cesarean delivery is indicated only if genital warts are obstructing the pelvic outlet or if vaginal delivery would result in excessive bleeding.

D. Chlamydia

1. Description

a. Sexually transmitted pathogen associated with an increased risk of preterm birth, stillbirth, neonatal conjunctivitis, and newborn chlamydial pneumonia

b. Can cause salpingitis, pelvic abscesses, ectopic pregnancy, chronic pelvic pain, and infertility

c. Diagnostic test is a vaginal culture for *Chlamydia trachomatis*.

2. Data collection

a. Usually asymptomatic

b. Bleeding between periods or after coitus

c. Mucoid or purulent cervical discharge

d. Dysuria and pelvic pain

3. Interventions

a. The client is screened to determine whether the client is at high risk; this is indicated for all pregnant clients if the client is in a high risk group or if infants from previous pregnancies have developed neonatal conjunctivitis or pneumonia.

b. Instruct the client about the importance of rescreening, because reinfection can occur as the client nears term.

c. Ensure that the sexual partner is treated for the infection.

d. Treatment for both gonorrhea and chlamydia must be done in pregnancy, which includes antibiotics.

e. Complications may include septic spontaneous abortion or miscarriage, preterm delivery, premature rupture of membranes (PROM), chorioamnionitis, disseminated gonococcal infection, ophthalmia neonatorum, postpartum metritis.

E. Trichomoniasis

1. Description

a. Caused by *Trichomonas vaginalis* and is transmitted via sexual contact

b. Normal saline wet smear of vaginal secretions is checked for the presence of protozoa.

c. Infection is associated with premature rupture of membranes and postpartum endometritis.

2. Data collection

a. Yellowish to greenish, frothy, mucopurulent, copious, and malodorous vaginal discharge

b. Inflammation of the vulva, vagina, or both may be present.

3. Interventions

a. Metronidazole may be prescribed.

b. Sexual partner may need to be treated.

F. Bacterial vaginosis

1. Description

a. Caused by *Haemophilus vaginalis* (*Gardnerella vaginalis*) and transmitted via sexual contact

b. Associated with preterm labor and birth

2. Data collection

a. Client complains of "fishy odor" to vaginal secretions and increased odor after intercourse.

b. Microscopic examination of vaginal secretions identifies the infection.

3. Interventions

a. Treatment with oral metronidazole may be prescribed.

b. Sexual partner may need to be treated.

G. Vaginal candidiasis

1. Description

a. *Candida albicans* is the most common causative organism.

b. Predisposing factors include the use of antibiotics, diabetes mellitus, and obesity.

c. Diagnosis is by identifying the spores of *Candida albicans*.

2. Data collection

a. Vulvar and vaginal pruritus

b. White, lumpy, and cottage cheese–like discharge from the vagina

3. Interventions

a. An antifungal vaginal preparation such as miconazole may be prescribed.

b. For extensive irritation and swelling, sitz baths may be prescribed.

c. Sexual partner may need to be treated.

XXXIII. Tuberculosis

A. Description

1. A highly communicable disease caused by *Mycobacterium tuberculosis*

2. Transmitted by the airborne route

3. A multidrug-resistant strain can exist as a result of improper compliance, noncompliance with treatment programs, and the development of mutations in the tubercle bacilli.

B. Transmission

1. Transplacental transmission is rare.

2. Can occur during birth through the aspiration of infected amniotic fluid

3. Newborn can become infected from contact with infected individuals.

C. Risk to mother: Active disease during pregnancy has been associated with an increase in hypertensive disorders of pregnancy.

D. Diagnosis: If a chest radiograph is required for the mother, it is obtained only after 20 weeks' gestation, and a lead shield for the abdomen is required.

> ⚠ Tuberculin skin testing is safe during pregnancy; however, the PHCP may want to delay testing until after delivery.

E. Data collection
  1. Mother
    a. May be asymptomatic
    b. Fever and chills
    c. Night sweats
    d. Weight loss
    e. Fatigue
    f. Cough, hemoptysis, or green or yellow sputum
    g. Dyspnea
    h. Pleural pain
  2. Newborn
    a. Fever
    b. Lethargy
    c. Poor feeding
    d. Failure to thrive
    e. Respiratory distress
    f. Hepatosplenomegaly
    g. Meningitis
    h. Disease may spread to all major organs.

F. Interventions
  1. Pregnant client
    a. Administer isoniazid, pyrazinamide, and rifampin daily for 9 months, as prescribed. Ethambutol is added if medication resistance is probable.
    b. Pyridoxine must be administered along with isoniazid to pregnant women to prevent fetal neurotoxicity caused by the isoniazid.
    c. Promote breast-feeding only if the mother is noninfectious and per PHCP prescription.

G. Newborn
    a. Management focuses on preventing disease and treating early infection.
    b. The newborn is skin-tested at birth and may be placed on isoniazid therapy. The skin test is repeated in 3 to 4 months, and the isoniazid may be stopped if the skin test results remain negative.
    c. If the skin test result is positive, the newborn needs to receive isoniazid for at least 6 months (as prescribed).

d. If the mother's sputum is free of organisms, the newborn does not need to be isolated from the mother while in the hospital.

XXXIV. Urinary Tract Infection

A. Description: A urinary tract infection can occur during pregnancy (pregnancy is a predisposing factor). A urinary tract infection can be either lower urinary tract (cystitis) or upper urinary tract (pyelonephritis).

B. Women may also experience asymptomatic bacteriuria.

C. Predisposing conditions
  1. History of urinary tract infections
  2. Urinary tract anomalies
  3. Lower socioeconomic status
  4. Sexual activity
  5. Young age
  6. Sickle cell trait
  7. Poor hygiene
  8. Anemia
  9. Diabetes mellitus
  10. Obesity
  11. Urinary catheterization

D. Screening is done at the first prenatal visit or at 12 to 16 weeks' gestation. Rescreening is done based on risk factors.

E. Data collection and interventions (refer to Chapter 51): It is important to differentiate between cystitis and the progression to pyelonephritis. If progressed to pyelonephritis, hospitalization may be required for antibiotic therapy and possible tocolysis.

XXXV. Pyelonephritis

A. Description
  1. Results from bacterial infections that extend upward from the bladder through the blood vessels and lymphatics
  2. Frequently follows untreated urinary tract infections and is associated with increased incidence of anemia, low birth weight, gestational hypertension, preterm labor and delivery, and premature rupture of the membranes

B. Data collection and interventions (refer to Chapters 34 and 51)

XXXVI. Obesity in Pregnancy

A. Description: Obesity in every population, including adults and children, is a problem in the United States. Obesity in pregnancy places the client at risk for complications during pregnancy, including gestational hypertension, preeclampsia, and venous thromboembolism, and increases the need for cesarean birth.

B. Delivery complications can result from difficulty obtaining IV access, epidural access, intubation, and decreased oxygen consumption with associated increased cardiac output, stressing the heart.

C. Obesity in pregnancy can have negative effects on the newborn, including stillbirth, congenital anomalies, future obesity, heart disease, and difficulty with breast-feeding.

D. Obese women have lower prolactin response to suckling in the first week postpartum, contributing to high rates of breast-feeding failure in this population.

E. Potential postpartum complications and associated interventions
  1. Thromboembolism formation is a concern; as prescribed, thromboembolism stockings (TEDs), sequential compression devices (SCDs), and pharmacological venous thromboembolism prophylaxis may be necessary postdelivery.
  2. Postpartum hemorrhage is more common, as well as difficulty locating the fundus, predisposing further to this problem.
  3. Endometriosis is common in this population.

4. Early ambulation is encouraged to prevent venous thromboembolism formation.

5. Frequent monitoring and cleaning of surgical incisions (episiotomy or cesarean incision) is needed to prevent infection or dehiscence resulting from excess abdominal fat.

WHAT WOULD YOU DO?

Answer: Interventions for nausea and vomiting in the pregnant client include eating dry crackers before arising; avoiding brushing teeth immediately after arising; eating small, frequent, low-fat meals during the day; drinking liquids between meals rather than at meals; avoiding fried foods and spicy foods; asking the primary health care provider (PHCP) about acupressure (some types may require a prescription); and asking the PHCP about the use of herbal remedies.

PRACTICE QUESTIONS

1. The client arrives at the prenatal clinic for her first prenatal assessment. The client tells the nurse that the first day of her last menstrual period (LMP) was October 20, 2023. Using Nägele's rule, the nurse determines the estimated date of birth is which date?
  1. July 12, 2024
  2. July 27, 2024
  3. August 12, 2024
  4. August 27, 2024

2. The nurse is collecting data from a client who is pregnant with twins. The client has a healthy 5-year-old child who was delivered at 38 weeks, and she tells the nurse that she does not have a history of any type of abortion or fetal demise. The nurse would document which as the GTPAL for this client?
  1. G = 3, T = 2, P = 0, A = 0, L = 1
  2. G = 2, T = 1, P = 0, A = 0, L = 1
  3. G = 1, T = 1, P = 1, A = 0, L = 1
  4. G = 2, T = 0, P = 0, A = 0, L = 1

3. The nurse is collecting data from a client who is pregnant with triplets. The client also has a 3-year-old child who was born at 39 weeks' gestation. The nurse would document which gravida and para status on this client?
  1. Gravida I, para I
  2. Gravida II, para I
  3. Gravida II, para II
  4. Gravida III, para II

4. The nurse is reviewing the record of a client who has just been told that her pregnancy test is positive. The nurse notes that the primary health care provider has documented the presence of Goodell's sign. The nurse determines that this sign is indicative of which change that occurs with pregnancy?
  1. A softening of the cervix
  2. The presence of fetal movement
  3. The presence of human chorionic gonadotropin in the urine
  4. A soft blowing sound that corresponds with the maternal pulse that is heard while auscultating the uterus

5. A primipara is being evaluated in the clinic during her second trimester of pregnancy. Which occurrence indicates an abnormal physical finding that necessitates further testing?
  1. Quickening
  2. Braxton Hicks contractions
  3. Consistent increase in fundal height
  4. Fetal heart rate of 180 beats per minute

6. The nursing instructor asks a nursing student to describe the process of quickening. Which statement indicates an understanding of this term?
  1. "It is the fetal movement that is felt by the mother."
  2. "It is the compressibility of the lower uterine segment."

3. "It is the irregular, painless contractions that occur throughout pregnancy."
4. "It is the soft blowing sound that can be heard when the uterus is auscultated."

7. The client is undergoing an amniocentesis at 16 weeks' gestation to detect the presence of biochemical or chromosomal abnormalities. Which instructions would the nurse reinforce to the client?
1. The bladder must be full during the examination.
2. The bladder must be empty during the examination.
3. She should not eat or drink anything 4 to 6 hours before the examination.
4. She will be given $Rh_o(D)$ immune globulin because she is Rh positive.

8. The nurse is checking a client's record for probable signs of pregnancy. Which are the probable signs of pregnancy that the nurse would note? **Select all that apply.**
- ❑ 1. Ballottement
- ❑ 2. Chadwick's sign
- ❑ 3. Uterine enlargement
- ❑ 4. Braxton Hicks contractions
- ❑ 5. Outline of the fetus via radiography or ultrasound
- ❑ 6. Fetal heart rate detected by a nonelectronic device

9. The perinatal client is admitted to the obstetrical unit during an exacerbation of a heart condition. When planning for the nutritional requirements of the client, the nurse would consult with the dietitian to ensure which dietary measure?
1. A low-calorie diet to ensure the absence of weight gain
2. A diet that is high in fluids and fiber to decrease constipation
3. A diet that is low in fluids and fiber to decrease blood volume
4. Unlimited sodium intake to increase the circulating blood volume

10. The nurse caring for a client with abruptio placentae is monitoring the client for signs of disseminated intravascular coagulopathy (DIC). The nurse would suspect DIC if which is observed?
1. Rapid clotting times
2. Pain and swelling of the calf of one leg
3. Laboratory values that indicate increased platelets
4. Petechiae, oozing from injection sites, and hematuria

11. The nurse is assigned to assist with caring for a client who is at risk for eclampsia. If the client progresses from preeclampsia to eclampsia, the nurse would take which action **first**?
1. Administer oxygen by face mask.
2. Clear and maintain an open airway.
3. Check the blood pressure and the fetal heart tones.
4. Prepare for the administration of intravenous magnesium sulfate.

12. The nurse is reinforcing instructions to a pregnant client regarding measures to prevent heartburn. The nurse would instruct the client to take which **best** measure?
1. Eliminate between-meal snacks.
2. Drink decaffeinated coffee and tea.
3. Lie down for 30 minutes after eating.
4. Substitute salt in cooking for other spices.

13. The nurse is monitoring a client with mild gestational hypertension (GH). Which data indicate that GH is a concern?
1. Urinary output has increased.
2. There is no evidence of proteinuria.
3. The client complains of a headache and blurred vision.
4. The blood pressure reading has returned to the prenatal baseline.

ANSWERS

1. 2
Rationale: The accurate use of Nägele's rule requires that the woman have a regular 28-day menstrual cycle. Subtract 3 months from the first day of the last menstrual period, add 7 days, and then adjust the year as appropriate. In this case, the first day of the LMP was October 20, 2023. When you subtract 3 months, you get July 20, 2023. If you add 7 days, you get July 27, 2023. Add 1 year to this, and you get the estimated date of birth: July 27, 2024.
Test-Taking Strategy: Follow the subject, Nägele's rule, to answer this question. Read all of the options carefully, and use this rule. Then, note the dates and years in the options before selecting an answer.

2. 2
Rationale: Pregnancy outcomes can be described with the GTPAL acronym: G = gravidity (number of pregnancies); T = term births (number born after 37 weeks); P = preterm births (number born before 37 weeks' gestation); A = abortions/miscarriages (number of abortions/miscarriages); L = live births (number of live births or living children). Therefore, a woman who is pregnant with twins and who already has a child has a gravida of 2. Because the child was delivered at 38 weeks, the number of preterm births is 0, and the number of term births is 1. The number of abortions is 0, and the number of live births is 1.
Test-Taking Strategy: Specific knowledge about the subject, GTPAL, is needed to answer this question. Your knowledge and understanding will direct you to the correct option.

3. 2

Rationale: Gravida is a term that refers to a woman who is or who has been pregnant, regardless of the duration of the pregnancy. *Parity* is a term that means the number of births after 20 weeks' gestation; it does not reflect the number of fetuses or infants. Options 1, 3, and 4 are incorrect on the basis of these definitions.

Test-Taking Strategy: Focus on the subject, the terms *gravida* and *parity*, which are necessary to answer this question correctly. Remember that *gravida* refers to a woman who is or has been pregnant, regardless of the duration of the pregnancy. *Parity* means the number of births past 20 weeks' gestation.

4. 1

Rationale: During the early weeks of pregnancy, the cervix becomes softer as a result of pelvic vasoconstriction, which causes Goodell's sign. Cervical softening is noted by the examiner during a pelvic examination. Goodell's sign does not indicate the presence of fetal movement. Human chorionic gonadotropin is noted in maternal urine with a positive urine pregnancy test. A soft blowing sound that corresponds with the maternal pulse may be auscultated over the uterus; it is the result of blood circulating through the placenta.

Test-Taking Strategy: Focus on the subject, the physiological findings of Goodell's sign. Remember that Goodell's sign refers to a softening of the cervix.

5. 4

Rationale: The fetal heart rate depends on the gestational age. It is 160 to 170 beats per minute during the first trimester, and it slows with fetal growth to approximately 110 to 160 beats per minute. Options 1, 2, and 3 are normal expected findings.

Test-Taking Strategy: Focus on the subject, an abnormal physical finding. Recalling the normal fetal heart rate will direct you to the correct option.

6. 1

Rationale: Quickening is fetal movement that appears usually at weeks 16 to 20, when the expectant mother first notices subtle fetal movements that gradually increase in intensity. A compressibility of the lower uterine segment occurs at about 6 weeks' gestation and is called *Hegar's sign*. Braxton Hicks contractions are irregular, painless contractions that may occur throughout pregnancy. A soft blowing sound that corresponds with the maternal pulse may be auscultated over the uterus; this is known as *uterine souffle*. This sound is the result of blood circulation to the placenta, and it corresponds with the maternal pulse.

Test-Taking Strategy: Focus on the subject, a description of quickening. Remember that *quickening* is fetal movement.

7. 1

Rationale: Before 20 weeks' gestation, the bladder must be kept full during amniocentesis to support the weight of the uterus. After 20 weeks' gestation, the bladder would be emptied to minimize the chance of puncturing the placenta or fetus. Rh₀(D) immune globulin is administered to Rh-negative women because of the risk of contact with the fetal blood during the examination. There are no fluid or food restrictions.

Monitoring the fetal heart tones and the vital signs throughout and after the examination is an important intervention.

Test-Taking Strategy: Focus on the subject, an amniocentesis at 16 weeks' gestation. Remember that before 20 weeks' gestation, the bladder must be kept full to support the weight of the uterus.

8. 1, 2, 3, 4

Rationale: The probable signs of pregnancy include uterine enlargement; Hegar's sign (the compressibility and softening of the lower uterine segment that occurs at about week 6); Goodell's sign (the softening of the cervix that occurs at the beginning of the second month of pregnancy); Chadwick's sign (the violet coloration of the mucous membranes of the cervix, vagina, and vulva that occurs at about week 4); ballottement (the rebounding of the fetus against the examiner's fingers on palpation); Braxton Hicks contractions; and a positive pregnancy test that measures for human chorionic gonadotropin. Positive signs of pregnancy include a fetal heart rate that is detected by an electronic device (Doppler transducer) at 10 to 12 weeks' gestation and by a nonelectronic device (fetoscope) at 20 weeks' gestation; active fetal movements that are palpable by the examiner; and an outline of the fetus via radiography or ultrasound.

Test-Taking Strategy: Focusing on the subject, the probable signs of pregnancy, will assist you with answering this question. Remember that the detection of the fetal heart rate and an outline of the fetus via radiography or ultrasound are positive signs of pregnancy.

9. 2

Rationale: Constipation causes the client to use the Valsalva maneuver. This causes blood to rush to the heart and overload the cardiac system. The absence of weight gain is not recommended during pregnancy. Diets that are low in fluid and fiber cause a decrease in blood volume, which in turn deprives the fetus of nutrients. Too much sodium could cause an overload to the circulating blood volume and contribute to the cardiac condition.

Test-Taking Strategy: Focus on the subject, nutritional requirements for the pregnant client with a heart condition. Try to relate the situation to something with which you are familiar. Look for options that would apply to any heart condition, and think about the needs of a pregnant client.

10. 4

Rationale: DIC is a state of diffuse clotting in which clotting factors are consumed, which leads to widespread bleeding. Platelet counts are decreased, because they are consumed by the process. Coagulation studies show no clot formation (clotting times are thus prolonged), and fibrin plugs may clog the microvasculature diffusely rather than in an isolated area.

Test-Taking Strategy: Focus on the subject, the signs/symptoms of DIC. Eliminate option 2 on the basis of the knowledge that DIC is a widespread problem rather than a localized one. Eliminate options 1 and 3 next, because they are comparable or alike.

11. 2

Rationale: The first actions are to maintain an open airway and to prevent injuries to the client. The client needs to be turned to the side and monitored for airway compromise. Options 1, 3, and 4 may be components of care, but they are not the first actions.

Test-Taking Strategy: Note the strategic word, *first.* Use the ABCs—airway, breathing, and circulation—to answer this question. Airway is the first priority.

12. 2

Rationale: Caffeine, like spices, may cause heartburn and needs to be avoided. Spices tend to trigger heartburn. Eating smaller, more frequent portions is preferable to eating three large meals to control heartburn. Lying down after meals is likely to lead to the reflux of stomach contents and cause heartburn. Salt leads to the retention of fluid.

Test-Taking Strategy: Note the strategic word, *best,* and focus on the subject, measures to prevent heartburn. This will direct you to the correct option.

13. 3

Rationale: Options 1, 2, and 4 are all signs that gestational hypertension is not present. Option 3 is a symptom of the worsening of the gestational hypertension and is a concern that needs to be reported.

Test-Taking Strategy: Focus on the subject, a concern associated with gestational hypertension. Recalling the signs and symptoms associated with gestational hypertension will direct you to the correct option.

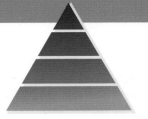

CHAPTER **24**

Labor and Birth and Associated Complications

PRIORITY CONCEPTS **Perfusion; Reproduction**

WHAT WOULD YOU DO?

A client is in active labor. The nurse is monitoring the fetal heart rate and notes that the heart rate is 180 beats per minute, lasting for longer than 10 minutes. What would the nurse do?
Answer is located on p. 304.

I. The Process of Labor: "The Four Ps"

A. Description
  1. Labor: A coordinated sequence of rhythmic involuntary intermittent uterine contractions
  2. Delivery: The actual event of birth
B. Four major factors (four *P*s) interact during normal childbirth; the four *P*s are interrelated and depend on one another for a safe birth and are *P*owers, *P*assageway, *P*assenger, and *P*syche.
C. Powers: Uterine contractions
  1. The forces acting to expel the fetus and placenta
  2. Effacement: The shortening and thinning of the cervix during the first stage of labor
  3. Dilation: The enlargement of the cervical os and cervical canal during the first stage of labor
  4. Pushing efforts of the mother during the second stage
D. Passageway: Composed of the mother's rigid bony pelvis and the soft tissues of the cervix, pelvic floor, vagina, and introitus (external opening to the vagina)
E. Passenger: The fetus, membranes, and placenta
F. Psyche: A woman's emotional structure that can determine her entire response to labor and influence physiological and psychological functioning; the mother may experience anxiety or fear.

G. Attitude
  1. The relationship of the fetal body parts to one another
  2. The normal intrauterine attitude is flexion, in which the fetal back is rounded, the head is forward on the chest, and the arms and legs are folded in against the body. The other attitude, extension, tends to present larger fetal diameters.
H. Lie
  1. Relationship of the spine of the fetus to the spine of the mother
  2. Longitudinal or vertical: (Fig. 24.1)
    a. Fetal spine is parallel to the mother's spine.
    b. The fetus is in either a cephalic or breech presentation.
  3. Transverse or horizontal:
    a. Fetal spine is at a right angle, or perpendicular, to the mother's spine.
    b. The presenting part is usually the shoulder.
    c. Delivery is by cesarean section (see Fig. 24.1).
I. Presentation
  1. Portion of the fetus that enters the pelvis first
  2. Cephalic: Fetal head presents first.
    a. The most common presentation
    b. Cephalic presentation has four variations: vertex, military, brow, and face.
  3. Breech: Buttocks present first.
    a. Delivery by cesarean section may be required, although vaginal birth is often possible.
    b. Breech presentation has three variations: frank, full (complete), and footling.
  4. Shoulder
    a. Fetus is in a transverse lie, or the arm, back, abdomen, or side could present.
    b. If the fetus does not spontaneously rotate or it is not possible to turn the fetus manually, a cesarean section may be performed.

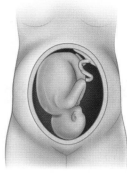
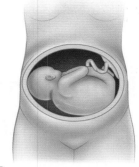

A   Longitudinal lie   B   Transverse lie

FIGURE 24.1 Fetal lie. (A) In a longitudinal lie, the long axis of the fetus is parallel to the long axis of the mother. (B) In a transverse lie, the long axis of the fetus is at a right angle to the long axis of the mother. The mother's abdomen has a wide, short appearance.

BOX 24.1 Fetal Positions

Vertex Presentations
- See Fig. 24.2.
- ROA: Right occipitoanterior
- LOA: Left occipitoanterior
- ROP: Right occipitoposterior
- LOP: Left occipitoposterior
- ROT: Right occipitotransverse
- LOT: Left occipitotransverse

Face Presentations
- RMA: Right mentoanterior
- LMA: Left mentoanterior
- RMP: Right mentoposterior

Breech Presentations
- LSA: Left sacroanterior
- LSP: Left sacroposterior

Other Presentations
- Brow presentation
- Shoulder presentation

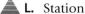

J. Presenting part: The specific fetal structure lying nearest to the cervix

K. Position: The relationship of the assigned area of the presenting part or landmark to the maternal pelvis (Box 24.1 and Fig. 24.2)

L. Station
1. The measurement of the progress of descent in centimeters above or below the midplane from the presenting part to the ischial spine
2. Station 0: At the ischial spine
3. Minus station: Above the ischial spine
4. Plus station: Below the ischial spine
5. Engagement: When the widest diameter of the presenting part has passed the inlet; corresponds to a 0 station.

II. Mechanisms of Labor (Box 24.2)

A. Data collection
1. Lightening or dropping: Is also known as engagement and occurs when the fetus descends into the pelvis about 2 weeks before birth. Lightening or dropping is most noticeable in first pregnancies.
2. Braxton Hicks contractions increase.
3. Vaginal mucosa congested, and vaginal discharge increases.
4. Brownish or blood-tinged cervical mucus is passed.
5. Cervix ripens and becomes soft and partly effaced; it may begin to dilate.
6. Sudden burst of energy experienced by the mother. This is also known as "nesting" and occurs 24 to 48 hours before the onset of labor.
7. Loss of 1 to 3 lb from water loss resulting from fluid shifts produced by changes in progesterone and estrogen levels 24 to 48 hours before the onset of labor.
8. Spontaneous rupture of the membranes occurs.
   a. True labor: Contractions may manifest as back pain in some women; contractions often resemble menstrual cramps during early labor (Box 24.3).
   b. False labor: Also known as *prodromal labor*, contractions are felt in the abdomen and groin and may be more annoying than painful (see Box 24.3).

⚠ In true labor, contractions increase in duration and intensity, and cervical dilation and effacement are progressive, with engagement and descent of the fetus. In false labor, contractions are irregular and do not produce dilation, effacement, or descent.

III. Leopold's Maneuvers

A. Description: A method of palpation for determining the presentation and position of the fetus; an aid for locating fetal heart sounds

B. If the head is in the fundus, a hard, round, movable object is felt. The buttocks feel soft and have an irregular shape, and they are more difficult to move.

C. The fetus's back, which is a smooth, hard surface, would be felt on one side of the abdomen.

D. Irregular knobs and lumps, which may be the hands, feet, elbows, and knees, are felt on the opposite side of the abdomen.

IV. Breathing Techniques (Box 24.4)

A. Provide a focus during contractions, thus interfering with pain sensory transmission

B. Promote relaxation and oxygenation

C. Begin with simple breathing patterns and progress to more complex ones as needed.

V. Fetal Monitoring

A. Description
1. The fetal monitor displays fetal heart rate (FHR).
2. Monitors uterine activity, frequency, and duration of contractions
3. Monitors FHR in relation to maternal contractions

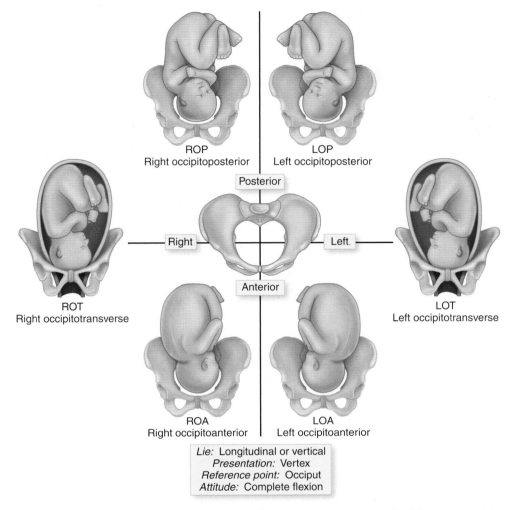

ROP
Right occipitoposterior

LOP
Left occipitoposterior

Posterior

Right

Left

Anterior

ROT
Right occipitotransverse

LOT
Left occipitotransverse

ROA
Right occipitoanterior

LOA
Left occipitoanterior

Lie: Longitudinal or vertical
Presentation: Vertex
Reference point: Occiput
Attitude: Complete flexion

FIGURE 24.2 Fetal vertex (occiput) presentations in relation to the front, back, or side of the maternal pelvis.

BOX 24.2   Mechanisms of Labor

Engagement
- Engagement is the mechanism by which the fetus nestles into the pelvis.
- Engagement occurs when the presenting part reaches the level of the ischial spines.

Descent
- Descent is the process that the fetal head undergoes as it begins its journey through the pelvis.
- It is a continuous process from prior to engagement until birth, and is assessed by the measurement called *station*.

Flexion
- Flexion is the process of nodding of the fetal head forward toward the fetal chest.

Internal Rotation
- The internal rotation of the fetus occurs most commonly from the occipitotransverse position, which is assumed at engagement into the pelvis, to the occipitoanterior position while continuously descending.

Extension
- Extension enables the head to emerge when the fetus is in a cephalic position.
- Extension begins after the head crowns.
- Extension is complete when the head passes under the symphysis pubis and occiput, and the anterior fontanel, brow, face, and chin pass over the sacrum and coccyx and are over the perineum.

Restitution
- Restitution is the realignment of the fetal head with the body after the head emerges.

External Rotation
- The shoulders externally rotate after the head emerges and restitution occurs, so that the shoulders are in the anteroposterior diameter of the pelvis.

Expulsion
- Expulsion is the birth of the entire body.

BOX 24.3 True Labor and False Labor

True Labor
- Contractions occur regularly. They become stronger, last longer, and occur closer together.
- Cervical dilation and effacement are progressive.
- The fetus usually becomes engaged in the pelvis and begins to descend.

False Labor
- False labor does not produce dilation, effacement, or descent.
- Contractions are irregular and without progression.
- Activity, such as walking, often relieves false labor.

Example
If a woman has been sleeping and wakes up with contractions, gets up, and moves around, and her contractions become stronger and closer together, this is true labor. If the contractions go away, this is false labor.

BOX 24.4 Breathing Techniques

First-Stage Breathing
Cleansing Breath
Each contraction begins and ends with a deep inspiration and expiration.

Slow-Paced Breathing
A slow-paced breathing that promotes relaxation
Used as long as possible during labor

Modified-Paced Breathing
Used when slow-paced breathing is no longer effective
Shallow, fast breathing

Pattern-Paced Breathing
Pattern-paced breathing sometimes is referred to as *pant–blow*. After a certain number of breaths (modified-paced breathing), the woman exhales with a slight blow and then begins the modified-paced breathing again.

Breathing to Prevent Pushing
The woman blows repeatedly using short puffs when the urge to push is strong.

Second-Stage Breathing
Several variations of breathing can be used in the pushing stage of labor, and the woman may grunt, groan, sigh, or moan as she pushes. Prolonged breath holding while pushing with a closed glottis may result in a decrease in cardiac output. If breath holding while pushing is used, the open glottis method or limiting breath holding to less than 6–8 seconds would be done.

4. Baseline FHR is measured between contractions. The normal FHR at term is 110 to 160 beats per minute.
B. External fetal monitoring
1. Noninvasive; performed with the use of a tocotransducer (uterine activity) or a Doppler ultrasonic transducer (FHR)
2. Leopold's maneuvers are performed to determine on which side the fetal back is located, and the ultrasound transducer is then placed over this area and fastened with a belt or stocking tubing.

3. The tocotransducer is placed over the fundus of the uterus, where contractions feel the strongest, and fastened with a belt or stocking tubing.
4. Allow the client to assume a comfortable position, avoiding vena cava compression (maternal supine hypotensive syndrome).
5. The preferred maternal position is to have her lie on her side to increase perfusion.
C. Internal fetal monitoring
1. Invasive; requires rupturing the membranes and attaching an electrode to the presenting part of the fetus
2. The client must be dilated 2 to 3 cm before internal monitoring can be performed.
D. Periodic patterns in the FHR
1. Fetal bradycardia and tachycardia
a. Bradycardia: FHR is less than 110 beats per minute for 10 minutes or longer.
b. Tachycardia: FHR is greater than 160 beats per minute for 10 minutes or longer.

⚠ If fetal bradycardia or tachycardia occurs, change the position of the mother, administer oxygen, and check the mother's vital signs. Notify the registered nurse immediately. The primary health care provider (PHCP) is also notified.

2. Variability
a. Fluctuations in the baseline FHR
b. Absence of variability or undetected variability is considered nonreassuring.
c. Decreased variability can result from fetal hypoxemia, acidosis, or certain medications.
d. A temporary decrease in variability can occur when the fetus is in a sleep state. (Sleep states do not usually last more than 30 minutes.)
3. Accelerations
a. Brief, temporary increases in the FHR of at least 15 beats per minute more than the baseline and lasting at least 15 seconds
b. Usually a reassuring sign that reflects a responsive, nonacidotic fetus
c. Usually occur with fetal movement
d. May be nonperiodic (having no relation to contractions) or periodic (with contractions)
e. May occur with uterine contractions, vaginal examinations, mild cord compression, or when the fetus is in a breech presentation
4. Early decelerations
a. Decrease in FHR below baseline. The rate at the lowest point of the deceleration usually remains greater than 100 beats/min.
b. Occur during contractions as the fetal head is pressed against the mother's pelvis or soft tissues, such as the cervix, and return to baseline FHR by the end of the contraction
c. Early decelerations are not associated with fetal compromise and require no intervention.

BOX 24.5 **Nonreassuring Fetal Heart Rate Patterns**

- Bradycardia
- Tachycardia
- Late decelerations
- Prolonged decelerations
- Hypertonic uterine activity
- Decreased or absent variability
- Variable decelerations falling to less than 70 beats per minute for longer than 60 seconds

---

⚡ PRIORITY NURSING ACTIONS

Nonreassuring Fetal Heart Rate Pattern

1. Call the registered nurse and stay with the client.
2. Identify the cause.
3. Stop the oxytocin infusion.
4. Change the mother's position.
5. Administer oxygen by face mask at 8 L/min to 10 L/min and assist to infuse intravenous fluids as prescribed.
6. Prepare to assist to initiate continuous electronic fetal monitoring with internal devices if not contraindicated.
7. Prepare for cesarean delivery if necessary.
8. Document the event, actions taken, and the mother's response.

---

5. Late decelerations
- **a.** Nonreassuring patterns that reflect impaired placental exchange or uteroplacental insufficiency
- **b.** Degree of the decline in the heart rate from baseline is not related to the amount of uteroplacental insufficiency.

⚠ Interventions for late decelerations include immediately improving placental blood flow and fetal oxygenation.

6. Variable decelerations
- **a.** Caused by conditions that restrict flow through the umbilical cord
- **b.** May be nonperiodic, occurring at times that are unrelated to contractions
- **c.** Are significant when the FHR repeatedly decreases to less than 70 beats per minute and persists at that level for at least 60 seconds before returning to baseline

⚠ If variable decelerations occur, the nurse would change the position of the mother, administer oxygen, discontinue oxytocin if infusing, and check the mother's vital signs. The registered nurse (RN) will notify the PHCP immediately. Amnioinfusion (intrauterine instillation of warmed saline to decrease compression on the umbilical cord) may be prescribed.

7. Hypertonic uterine activity
- **a.** Checking uterine activity includes frequency, duration, intensity of contractions, and uterine resting tone; assessment is performed either by palpating by hand or with an internal uterine pressure catheter (IUPC).
- **b.** Uterus would relax between contractions for 60 seconds or more.
- **c.** Uterine contraction intensity is about 50 to 75 mm Hg (with an IUPC) during labor and may reach 110 mm Hg with pushing during the second stage.
- **d.** Average resting tone is 5 to 15 mm Hg.
- **e.** In hypertonic uterine activity, the uterine resting tone between contractions is high, reducing uterine blood flow and decreasing fetal oxygen supply.

8. Nonreassuring FHR patterns (see Box 24.5)
9. Interventions for nonreassuring patterns (see Priority Nursing Actions)

VI. Four Stages of Labor (Table 24.1)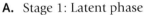

A. Stage 1: Latent phase
1. Description: Stage 1 is the longest.
2. Data collection
   - **a.** Cervical dilation of up to 1 to 4 cm
   - **b.** Uterine contractions occur every 15 to 30 minutes, 15 to 30 seconds in duration, and of mild intensity
3. Interventions
   - **a.** Encourage the mother and partner to participate in care.
   - **b.** Assist with comfort measures, changes in position, and ambulation.
   - **c.** Keep the mother and partner informed of progress.
   - **d.** Offer fluids and ice chips.
   - **e.** Encourage voiding every 1 to 2 hours.

B. Stage 1: Active phase
1. Data collection
   - **a.** Cervical dilation of 4 to 7 cm
   - **b.** Uterine contractions occur every 3 to 5 minutes, 30 to 60 seconds in duration, and of moderate intensity
2. Interventions
   - **a.** Encourage the maintenance of effective breathing patterns.
   - **b.** Provide a quiet environment.
   - **c.** Keep the mother and partner informed of progress.
   - **d.** Promote comfort with back rubs, sacral pressure, pillow support, and position changes.
   - **e.** Offer fluids, oral care, and ice chips, as prescribed; and ointment for dry lips.
   - **f.** Instruct the partner in effleurage (light stroking of abdomen).
   - **g.** Encourage voiding every 1 to 2 hours.

TABLE 24.1   Four Stages of Labor

First Stage	Second Stage	Third Stage	Fourth Stage
Effacement and dilation of the cervix	Expulsion of the fetus	Separation of the placenta	Physical recovery
Divided into three stages: latent, active, and transition	Pushing stage Latent phase—known as "laboring down" Active phase—pushing	Expulsion of the placenta	1–4 hours after the expulsion of the placenta
Mother is talkative and eager in the latent phase; becoming tired, restless, and anxious as labor intensifies and contractions become stronger	Mother has intense concentration during pushing with contractions; may fall asleep between contractions	Mother is relieved after birth of newborn; usually very tired	Mother is tired but is eager to become acquainted with her newborn

C. Stage 1: Transition phase
   1. Data collection
      a. Cervical dilation of 8 to 10 cm
      b. Uterine contractions occur every 2 to 3 minutes, 45 to 90 seconds in duration, and of strong intensity.
   2. Interventions
      a. Encourage rest between contractions.
      b. Wake mother at beginning of contraction so she can begin breathing pattern.
      c. Keep the mother and partner informed of progress.
      d. Provide privacy.
      e. Offer fluids, ice chips, and ointment for dry lips.
      f. Encourage voiding every 1 to 2 hours.
D. Interventions throughout stage 1
   1. Monitor maternal vital signs.
   2. Monitor FHR via ultrasound Doppler, fetoscope, or electronic fetal monitor.
   3. Check the FHR before, during, and after a contraction, noting that the normal FHR is 110 to 160 beats per minute.
   4. Assist with monitoring uterine contractions by palpation or tocodynamometer, and determine frequency, duration, and intensity.
   5. Assist with monitoring the status of cervical dilation and effacement.
   6. Assist with monitoring fetal station, presentation, and position by Leopold's maneuvers.
   7. Assist with pelvic examinations and prepare for a fern test.

   ⚠ If the membranes rupture, the priority is to check the FHR because of the risk of prolapsed umbilical cord. Then, check the color of the amniotic fluid because meconium-stained fluid can indicate fetal distress.

E. Stage 2
   1. Data collection
      a. Cervical dilation is complete.
      b. Progress of labor is measured by the descent of the fetal head through the birth canal (change in fetal station).
      c. Uterine contractions occur every 2 to 3 minutes and last 60 to 75 seconds, and are of strong intensity.

      d. Increase in bloody show occurs.
      e. The mother feels the urge to push (Ferguson reflex). Assist the mother with pushing efforts.
   2. Interventions
      a. Perform assessments every 5 minutes.
      b. Monitor maternal vital signs.
      c. Monitor FHR via ultrasound Doppler, fetoscope, or electronic fetal monitor.
      d. Monitor the FHR before, during, and after a contraction, noting that normal FHR is 110 to 160 beats per minute.
      e. Monitor the uterine contractions with palpation or tocodynamometer, determining the frequency, duration, and intensity.
      f. Provide the mother with encouragement and praise, and provide for rest between contractions.
      g. Keep the mother and partner informed of progress.
      h. Maintain privacy.
      i. Provide ice chips and ointment for dry lips.
      j. Assist mother into a position that promotes comfort and facilitates pushing efforts, such as lithotomy, semi-sitting, kneeling, side-lying, or squatting.
      k. Monitor for signs of approaching birth, such as perineal bulging or visualization of the fetal head.
      l. Prepare for birth (expulsion of fetus).
F. Stage 3
   1. Data collection
      a. Contractions occur until the placenta is expelled.
      b. Placental separation and expulsion occur.
      c. Expulsion of the placenta occurs 5 to 30 minutes after the birth of the infant.
      d. Schultze mechanism: Center portion of the placenta separates first, and its shiny fetal surface emerges from the vagina.
      e. Duncan mechanism: Margin of the placental separates, and the dull, red, rough maternal surface emerges from the vagina first.
      f. Method of placental presentation is of no clinical significance.
   2. Interventions
      a. Monitor maternal vital signs and uterine status.
      b. Provide the parents with explanation regarding expulsion of the placenta.

TABLE 24.2 Factors of the Bishop Score

Score	0	1	2	3
Dilation of cervix (cm)	0	1–2	3–4	>5
Effacement of cervix (%)	0–30	40–50	60–70	>80
Consistency of cervix	Firm	Medium	Soft	—
Position of cervix	Posterior	Midposition	Anterior	—
Station of presenting part	−3	−2	−1	+1, +2

   c. After the expulsion of the placenta, the uterine fundus remains firm and is located approximately two fingerbreadths below the umbilicus.

   d. Examine the placenta for cotyledons and membranes to verify that it is intact.

   e. Monitor the mother for shivering. Provide warmth.

   f. Promote parental–neonatal attachment.

G. Stage 4

  1. Description: The period of time from 1 to 4 hours after delivery

  2. Data collection

   a. Blood pressure returns to prelabor level.

   b. Pulse is slightly lower than during labor.

   c. Fundus remains contracted, in the midline, 1 or 2 fingerbreadths below the umbilicus.

⚠ Monitor lochia discharge. Lochia may be moderate in amount and red in color in stage 4.

  3. Interventions

   a. Maternal assessments are performed every 15 minutes for 1 hour, every 30 minutes for 1 hour, and hourly for 2 hours (or as per agency policy).

   b. Provide warm blankets.

   c. Apply ice packs to the perineum.

   d. Massage the uterus, if needed, and teach the mother to massage the uterus.

   e. Provide breast-feeding support, as needed.

   f. See Chapter 26 for information about caring for the newborn.

VII. Anesthesia

A. Local anesthesia

  1. Used for blocking the pain during episiotomy

  2. Administered just before the birth of the baby

  3. No effect on the fetus

B. Lumbar epidural block

  1. Injection site in the epidural space at L3–L4

  2. Administered as partial anesthesia after labor is established or just before a scheduled cesarean birth

  3. Relieves pain from contractions and numbs the vagina and perineum

  4. May cause hypotension, bladder distention, and a prolonged second stage

  5. Does not cause headache, because the dura mater is not penetrated

  6. Monitor maternal blood pressure and assist to assess bladder frequently.

  7. Maintain the mother in a side-lying position or place a rolled blanket beneath the right hip to displace the uterus from the vena cava.

  8. Intravenous (IV) fluids are administered, as prescribed.

  9. Increase fluids as prescribed if hypotension occurs.

  10. Observe for any adverse effects from opioid epidurals, such as nausea and vomiting, pruritus, or respiratory depression.

C. Intrathecal opioid analgesics

  1. Medication is injected into the subarachnoid space and has a rapid onset of action.

  2. May be used in combination with a lumbar epidural block

D. Subarachnoid (spinal) block

  1. Injection site is in the spinal subarachnoid space at L3–L5.

  2. The block is administered just before birth.

  3. Relieves uterine and perineal pain and numbs the vagina, perineum, and lower extremities

  4. May cause maternal hypotension

  5. Observe for postpartum headache—a headache that is worse when woman is upright and that may disappear when she is lying flat; the mother needs to lie flat 8 to 12 hours after spinal injection.

  6. IV fluids are administered, if prescribed.

E. General anesthesia

  1. May be used for some surgical interventions

  2. The mother is not awake.

⚠ General anesthesia presents a maternal danger of respiratory depression, vomiting, and aspiration.

VIII. Obstetrical Procedures

A. Bishop score (Table 24.2)

  1. Used to determine maternal readiness for labor induction and evaluates cervical status and fetal position

  2. Indicated before the induction of labor

  3. The five factors are assigned a score of 0 to 3, and the total score is calculated.

  4. A score of 8 or greater indicates that the chance of a successful vaginal delivery is good and the cervix is favorable for induction.

B. Induction

  1. Induction is a deliberate initiation of uterine contractions that stimulates labor.

  2. Elective induction may be accomplished by oxytocin infusion.

3. Baseline tracing of uterine contractions and FHR is obtained.

4. The IV dosage of oxytocin may be increased, as prescribed; contractions, FHR, and maternal blood pressure and pulse are assessed by the registered nurse before increasing the dose.

5. The rate of oxytocin is not increased when the desired contraction pattern is obtained (contraction frequency of 2–3 minutes and lasting 60 seconds).

⚠ An oxytocin infusion is discontinued if uterine contraction frequency is less than 2 minutes or duration is longer than 90 seconds, or if fetal distress is noted.

C. Amniotomy

1. Artificial rupture of membranes (AROM); performed by the obstetrician or nurse midwife to stimulate labor

2. Performed if the fetus is at 0 or a plus station

3. Increases the risk of prolapsed cord and infection

4. Monitor the FHR before and after amniotomy.

5. Record the time of amniotomy, FHR, and characteristics of the fluid.

6. Meconium-stained amniotic fluid may be associated with fetal distress.

7. Bloody amniotic fluid may indicate abruptio placentae or fetal trauma.

8. An unpleasant odor to the amniotic fluid is associated with infection.

9. Polyhydramnios is associated with maternal diabetes and certain congenital disorders.

10. Oligohydramnios is associated with intrauterine growth restriction and congenital disorders.

11. More variable decelerations are likely to occur after the rupture of the membranes as a result of possible cord compression during contractions.

12. Limit client activity, if prescribed.

D. External version

1. External manipulation of the fetus from an unfavorable presentation into a favorable presentation for birth

2. Indicated for an abnormal presentation that exists after 34 weeks' gestation

3. Monitor vital signs.

4. If the mother is Rh-negative, ensure that Rho(D) immune globulin was given at 28 weeks' gestation.

5. Prepare for a nonstress test to evaluate fetal well-being.

6. IV fluids and tocolytic therapy may be administered to relax the uterus and permit easier manipulation of the fetus.

7. Ultrasound is used during the procedure to evaluate fetal position and placental placement and guide direction of the fetus.

8. The abdominal wall is manipulated to direct the fetus into a cephalic presentation if possible.

9. Monitor blood pressure to identify vena cava compression.

10. Monitor for unusual pain.

11. After the procedure, the following is performed:

  a. A nonstress test to evaluate fetal well-being

  b. Monitoring for uterine activity, bleeding, ruptured membranes, and decreased fetal activity

  c. With Rh-negative clients, a Kleihauer-Betke test is performed as prescribed to detect the presence and amount of fetal blood in the maternal circulation and to identify clients who need additional $Rh_o(D)$ immune globulin.

E. Episiotomy

1. Incision made into the perineum to enlarge the vaginal outlet and facilitate birth; the use of this procedure has declined dramatically in recent years.

2. Check episiotomy site.

3. Institute measures to relieve pain.

4. Provide an ice pack during the first 24 hours.

5. Instruct the client in the use of an ice pack for the first 24 hours, and then sitz baths thereafter.

6. Apply analgesic spray or ointment, as prescribed.

7. Provide perineal care, using clean technique.

8. Instruct the client regarding the proper care of the incision.

9. Instruct the client to dry the perineal area from front to back and to blot the area rather than wipe it.

10. Instruct the client to shower rather than bathe in a tub.

11. Apply a perineal pad without touching the inside surface of the pad.

12. Report any bleeding or discharge from the episiotomy site to the RN.

F. Forceps delivery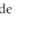

1. Two double-crossed, spoon-like articulated blades are used to assist in the delivery of the fetal head.

2. Reassure the mother and explain the need for the forceps.

3. Monitor the mother and fetus during delivery.

4. Check the neonate and mother after delivery for any possible injury.

5. Assist with the repair of any lacerations.

G. Vacuum extraction

1. A cap-like suction device is applied to the fetal head to facilitate extraction.

2. Suction is used to assist with the delivery of the fetal head.

3. Traction is applied during uterine contractions until the descent of the fetal head is achieved.

4. The suction device would not be kept in place any longer than 25 minutes.

5. Monitor the FHR frequently; fetal monitoring would be used.

6. Check the newborn at birth and monitor him or her throughout the postpartum period for signs of cerebral trauma.

7. Monitor for developing cephalohematoma.
8. Caput succedaneum is normal and will resolve in 24 hours.

▲ **H.** Cesarean delivery
   1. Birth of the fetus usually through a transabdominal, low-segment incision of the uterus
   2. Preoperative
      a. If planned, prepare the mother and partner.
      b. If an emergency, quickly explain the need and procedure to the mother and partner.
      c. Obtain informed consent.
      d. Make sure that the preoperative diagnostic tests are done, including Rh factor determination.
      e. Prepare the mother for the insertion of an IV line and an indwelling urinary catheter.
      f. Prepare the abdomen, as prescribed.
      g. Monitor the mother and fetus continuously.
      h. Provide emotional support.
      i. Administer preoperative medications, as prescribed.
   3. Postoperative
      a. Monitor vital signs.
      b. Perform a fundal assessment; evaluate incision.
      c. Provide pain relief.
      d. Encourage turning, coughing, and deep breathing.
      e. Encourage ambulation.
      f. Encourage bonding/attachment with newborn.
      g. Provide psychological support.
      h. Monitor for signs of infection and bleeding.
      i. Burning and pain during urination may indicate a bladder infection.
      j. A tender uterus and foul-smelling lochia may indicate endometritis.
      k. A productive cough or chills may indicate pneumonia.
      l. Pain, redness, or edema of an extremity may indicate thrombophlebitis.

IX. Premature Rupture of the Membranes ▲

A. Description
   1. The spontaneous rupture of the amniotic membrane before the onset of labor
   2. Gestational age usually determines the plan and intervention.
   3. When the rupture of membranes is before term and birth will be delayed, infection becomes a risk.

B. Data collection ▲
   1. Evidence of fluid pooling in the vaginal vault. The Nitrazine test is positive.
   2. Amount, color, consistency, and odor of fluid need to be assessed.
   3. Vital signs are monitored; elevated temperature may indicate the presence of infection.
   4. Fetal monitoring is necessary; tachycardia in the fetus may indicate infection.

C. Interventions
   1. Assist with tests to assess gestational age.
   2. Avoid vaginal examinations because of the risk of infection.
   3. Monitor maternal and fetal status for signs of compromise or infection.
   4. Assist to administer antibiotics, as prescribed.

X. Prolapsed Umbilical Cord (Fig. 24.3) ▲

A. Description: The umbilical cord is displaced between the presenting part and the amnion, or it is protruding through the cervix, causing compression of the cord and compromising fetal circulation.

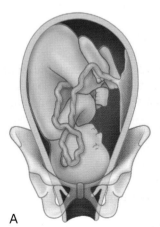 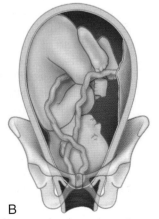 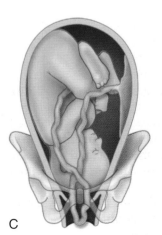 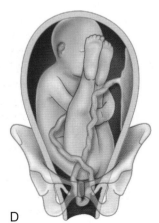

A B C D

FIGURE 24.3 Prolapse of the umbilical cord. Note the pressure of the presenting part on the umbilical cord; this endangers fetal circulation. (A) Occult (hidden) prolapse of the cord. (B) Complete prolapse of the cord. (C) Cord presenting in front of the fetal head may be seen in the vagina. (D) Frank breech presentation with prolapsed cord.

B. Data collection
   1. The client has a feeling that something is coming through the vagina.
   2. The umbilical cord is visible or palpable.
   3. The FHR is irregular and slow.
   4. The fetal heart monitor will show variable deceleration or bradycardia after the rupture of the membranes.
   5. If fetal hypoxia is severe, violent fetal activity may occur and then cease.

C. Interventions (see **Priority Nursing Actions**)
   1. The nurse stays with the client and asks another nurse to call the PHCP immediately.
   2. The goal is to relieve cord pressure immediately so that the fetus receives adequate oxygenation.
   3. The nurse never attempts to push the cord into the uterus.
   4. If the umbilical cord is protruding from the vagina, the cord is wrapped loosely in a sterile towel saturated with warm sterile saline.
   5. This situation is an emergency and delivery must occur usually via a cesarean section.

⚡ PRIORITY NURSING ACTIONS

Umbilical Cord Prolapse

1. Call the RN and stay with the client.
2. Elevate the fetal presenting part that is lying on the cord by applying finger pressure on the fetal part with a gloved hand.
3. Place the client into extreme Trendelenburg's or modified Sims' position, or a knee-chest position.
4. Administer oxygen, 8 to 10 L/min, by face mask to the client.
5. Monitor the FHR and assess the fetus for hypoxia.
6. Prepare to assist with appropriate intravenous fluids or increase the rate of an existing solution.
7. Prepare for immediate birth.
8. Document the event, actions taken, and the client's response.

XI. Supine Hypotension (Vena Cava Syndrome)

A. Description
   1. Occurs when the venous return to the heart is impaired by the weight of the uterus on the vena cava
   2. Results from the partial occlusion of the vena cava and the descending aorta and causes reduced cardiac return, cardiac output, and blood pressure
B. Data collection
   1. Faintness, dizziness, and breathlessness
   2. Pallor, clammy (damp, cool) skin, and sweating
   3. Hypotension and tachycardia
   4. Fetal distress

C. Interventions
   1. Position the client on her side to shift the weight of the fetus off the vena cava until signs and symptoms subside and vital signs stabilize.
   2. Monitor the vital signs and the FHR.

⚠️ To prevent supine hypotension, avoid the supine position; position the client by placing a pillow or wedge under the client's hip to displace the gravid uterus off the vena cava.

XII. Preterm Labor

A. Description
   1. Preterm labor occurs after week 20, but before week 37 of gestation.
   2. Risk factors include a history of medical conditions; present and past obstetrical problems; infection; and social and environmental factors, including substance abuse.
   3. Additional risk factors include a multifetal pregnancy, which contributes to overdistention of uterus; anemia, which decreases oxygen supply to uterus; and age younger than 18 years, or first pregnancy and older than 40 years.
B. Data collection
   1. Uterine contractions (painful or painless)
   2. Abdominal cramping (may be accompanied by diarrhea)
   3. Low back pain
   4. Pelvic pressure or heaviness
   5. Change in the character and amount of usual discharge; may be thicker or thinner, bloody, brown or colorless, odorous
   6. Rupture of amniotic membranes
   7. Presence of fetal fibronectin in cervical canal
   8. Shortening of cervical length
C. Interventions
   1. Focus is on stopping the labor: identify and treat infection, restrict activity, and ensure hydration.
   2. Maintain bed rest if prescribed by the PHCP and a lateral position.
   3. Monitor the fetal status.
   4. Administer fluids as prescribed.
   5. Administer medications as prescribed and monitor for side effects of tocolytics. See Table 27.1 for a description of medications used to treat preterm labor.
   6. Use of 17 alpha-hydroxyprogesterone caproate known as 17P injection to decrease risk of preterm delivery.

XIII. Precipitous Labor and Delivery

A. Description: Labor that lasts less than 3 hours
B. Interventions
   1. Have a precipitous delivery tray available (hemostats, scissors, and cord clamp).
   2. Stay with the client at all times.

3. Provide emotional support and keep the client calm.
4. Encourage the client to pant between contractions.
5. Prepare for the rupturing of the membranes when the head crowns, if they are not already ruptured.
6. Do not try to prevent the fetus from being delivered.
7. If delivery is necessary before the arrival of the PHCP, assist with the following:
   a. Apply gentle pressure to the fetal head upward toward the vagina to prevent damage to the fetal head and vaginal lacerations; support the perineal area. Both actions will constitute the Ritgen maneuver.
   b. Support the infant's body during delivery.
   c. Deliver the infant between contractions, checking for the cord around the neck.
   d. Restitution is used to deliver the posterior shoulder.
   e. Gentle downward pressure is used to move the anterior shoulder under the pubic symphysis.
   f. Bulb suction the newborn's mouth first and then suction each naris.
   g. Dry and cover the newborn to keep the body warm.
   h. Allow the placenta to separate naturally.
   i. Place the newborn on the mother's abdomen or breast to induce uterine contractions.

XIV. Dystocia

A. Description
   1. Difficult labor that is prolonged or more painful
   2. Occurs as a result of problems caused by uterine contractions, the fetus, or the bones and tissues of the maternal pelvis
   3. The fetus may be excessively large, mispositioned, or in an abnormal position.
   4. Contractions may be hypotonic or hypertonic.
   5. Hypotonic contractions are short, irregular, and weak. Amniotomy and oxytocin infusion may be treatment measures.
   6. Hypertonic contractions are painful, occur frequently (6 or more in a 10-minute time period) and are uncoordinated. Treatment depends on cause and includes pain relief measures and rest.
   7. Dystocia can result in maternal dehydration, infection, fetal injury, or death.
B. Data collection
   1. Excessive abdominal pain
   2. Abnormal contraction pattern
   3. Fetal distress
   4. Maternal or fetal tachycardia
   5. Lack of progress of labor
C. Interventions
   1. Check FHR; monitor for fetal distress.
   2. Monitor uterine contractions.
   3. Monitor maternal temperature and heart rate.

4. Assist with pelvic examination, measurements, ultrasound, and other procedures.
5. Prophylactic antibiotics may be prescribed to prevent infection.
6. IV fluids may be prescribed.
7. Monitor intake and output.
8. Monitor for dehydration.
9. Instruct the client in breathing techniques and relaxation exercises.
10. Fetal monitoring is performed if oxytocin is prescribed for hypotonic uterine contractions (oxytocin is not prescribed for hypertonic uterine contractions); refer to Chapter 27 for information on oxytocin.
11. Monitor the color of the amniotic fluid.
12. Provide rest and comfort as with a normal delivery, such as back rubs and position changes.
13. Assess the client's fatigue and pain. Administer sedatives and pain medications, as prescribed.
14. Monitor for prolapse of the cord after the rupture of the membranes.

XV. Amniotic Fluid Embolism

A. Description
   1. Amniotic fluid embolism is the escape of amniotic fluid into the maternal circulation.
   2. The debris-containing amniotic fluid deposits in the pulmonary arterioles and is usually fatal to the mother.
B. Data collection
   1. Abrupt onset of respiratory distress and chest pain
   2. Cyanosis
   3. Fetal bradycardia and distress if delivery has not occurred at the time of the embolism
C. Interventions
   1. Institute emergency measures to maintain life.
   2. Administer oxygen at 8 to 10 L/min by face mask or resuscitation bag delivering 100% oxygen, as prescribed.
   3. Prepare the client for intubation and mechanical ventilation.
   4. Position the client on her side.
   5. IV fluids, blood products, and medications may be prescribed to correct coagulation failure.
   6. Monitor the fetal status.
   7. Prepare for emergency delivery after the client is stabilized.
   8. Provide emotional support to the client, her partner, and the family.

XVI. Fetal Distress

A. Data collection
   1. FHR of less than 110 or more than 160 beats per minute
   2. Meconium-stained amniotic fluid
   3. Fetal hypoactivity or hyperactivity
   4. Progressive decrease in baseline variability
   5. Severe variable decelerations

6. Late decelerations

B. Interventions

1. Place the client in a lateral position.
2. Administer oxygen at 8 to 10 L/min via face mask, as prescribed.
3. Oxytocin, if infusing, is discontinued.
4. IV fluids may be administered as prescribed (usually as a bolus).
5. Monitor the maternal and fetal status.

⚠️ In the event of fetal distress, prepare the client for emergency cesarean delivery.

XVII. Intrauterine Fetal Demise

A. Data collection

1. Loss of fetal movement
2. Absence of fetal heart tones
3. Disseminated intravascular coagulation (DIC) screen: Monitor for coagulation abnormalities, because DIC is a complication that is related to intrauterine fetal demise.
4. Low hemoglobin and hematocrit levels; low platelet count; prolonged bleeding and clotting times
5. Bleeding from puncture sites (which could be indicative of DIC

B. Interventions

1. Encourage the client and her family to verbalize their feelings; provide emotional support.
2. Incorporate religious, spiritual, and cultural health care beliefs and practices into the plan of care.
3. Allow the client choices related to labor and delivery.
4. Assist to administer intravenous fluids, medications, and blood products as prescribed if DIC occurs.

XVIII. Rupture of the Uterus

A. Description

1. Complete or incomplete separation of the uterine tissue as a result of a tear in the wall of the uterus from the stress of labor
2. Complete: Direct communication between the uterine and peritoneal cavities
3. Incomplete: Rupture into the peritoneum covering the uterus, but not into the peritoneal cavity
4. Manifestations vary with the extent of the rupture.
5. Risk factors: Labor after previous cesarean section, overdistended uterus (e.g., multiple fetuses or hydramnios) after cesarean section, abdominal trauma

B. Data Collection

1. Abdominal pain or tenderness
2. Chest pain
3. Contractions may stop or fail to progress
4. Rigid abdomen

5. Absent FHR
6. Signs of maternal shock
7. Fetus palpated outside of the uterus (complete rupture)

C. Interventions

1. Monitor for and assist with treating signs of shock (oxygen, IV fluids, and blood products may be prescribed).
2. Prepare the client for cesarean section (hysterectomy may be necessary).
3. Provide emotional support for the client and partner.

XIX. Uterine Inversion

A. Description

1. Uterus completely or partly turns inside out.
2. This can occur during delivery or after delivery of the placenta.
3. Risk factors: Fundal implantation of the placenta, manual extraction of the placenta, short umbilical cord, uterine atony, leiomyomas, and abnormally adherent placental tissue

B. Data collection

1. A depression in the fundal area of the uterus is noted.
2. Interior of the uterus may be seen through the cervix or protruding through the vagina.
3. Severe pain
4. Hemorrhage
5. Signs of shock

C. Interventions

1. Monitor for hemorrhage and signs of shock, and treat shock.
2. Prepare the client for a return of the uterus to the correct position via the vagina. If unsuccessful, laparotomy with replacement to the correct position is done.

WHAT WOULD YOU DO?

Answer: Near or at term, the normal fetal heart rate is 110 to 160 beats per minute. If fetal tachycardia or bradycardia occurs, the nurse must change the position of the mother, administer oxygen, and check the mother's vital signs including temperature. In addition, the nurse would notify the RN immediately so that further assessment can be done regarding the cause of the tachycardia. The primary health care provider (PHCP) is also notified.

PRACTICE QUESTIONS

1. The nurse is assigned to care for a client who is in early labor. When collecting data from the client, which would the nurse check **first**?

1. Baseline fetal heart rate
2. Intensity of contractions

3. Maternal blood pressure
4. Frequency of contractions

2. Leopold's maneuvers will be performed on a pregnant client. The client asks the nurse about the procedure. Which information would the nurse provide to the client about Leopold's maneuvers?
   1. The maneuvers measure the height of the maternal fundus.
   2. The maneuvers determine the "lie" and "attitude" of the fetus.
   3. The maneuvers are a systematic method for palpating the fetus through the maternal back.
   4. The maneuvers are a systematic method for palpating the fetus through the maternal abdominal wall.

3. The nurse is caring for a client who is in labor. The nurse rechecks the client's blood pressure and notes that it has dropped. To decrease the incidence of supine hypotension, the nurse would encourage the client to remain in which position?
   1. Squatting
   2. Side-lying
   3. Tailor sitting
   4. Semi-Fowler's

4. After a precipitous delivery, the nurse notes that the new mother is passive and only touches her newborn briefly with her fingertips. The nurse would do which to help the woman process what has happened?
   1. Support the mother in her reaction to the newborn.
   2. Encourage the mother to breast-feed soon after birth.
   3. Tell the mother that it is important to hold the newborn.
   4. Document a complete account of the mother's reaction in the birth record.

5. A primigravida's membranes rupture spontaneously. Which action must the nurse take **first**?
   1. Determine the fetal heart rate.
   2. Prepare for immediate delivery.
   3. Monitor the contraction pattern.
   4. Note the amount, color, and odor of the amniotic fluid.

6. The nurse is assigned to assist with caring for a client who has been admitted to the labor unit. The client is 9 cm dilated and is experiencing precipitous labor. Which is the **priority** nursing action?
   1. Prepare for an oxytocin infusion.
   2. Keep the client in a side-lying position.
   3. Prepare the client for epidural anesthesia.
   4. Encourage the client to start pushing with the contractions.

7. The client who is being prepared for a cesarean delivery is brought to the delivery room. To maintain the optimal perfusion of oxygenated blood to the fetus, the nurse would place the client in which position?
   1. Prone position
   2. Semi-Fowler's position
   3. Trendelenburg's position
   4. Supine position with a wedge under the right hip

8. A woman in active labor has contractions every 2 to 3 minutes that last for 45 seconds. The fetal heart rate between contractions is 100 beats per minute. On the basis of these findings which is the **priority** nursing action?
   1. Monitor the maternal vital signs.
   2. Notify the registered nurse (RN) immediately.
   3. Continue monitoring labor and the fetal heart rate.
   4. Encourage relaxation and breathing techniques between contractions.

9. The nurse is assigned to assist with caring for a client who is being admitted to the birthing center in early labor. During admission, which action would the nurse take **initially**?
   1. Estimate the fetal size.
   2. Check pelvic adequacy.
   3. Administer an analgesic.
   4. Determine the maternal vital signs and fetal heart rate.

10. The nurse is assigned to work in the delivery room and is assisting with caring for a client who has just delivered a newborn. The nurse is monitoring for signs of placental separation knowing that which of the following indicates that the placenta has separated?
   1. A change in the uterine contour
   2. Sudden and sharp abdominal pain
   3. A shortening of the umbilical cord
   4. A decrease in blood loss from the introitus

ANSWERS

1. 1

Rationale: The nurse needs to first determine the baseline fetal heart rate. Although options 2, 3, and 4 are components of the data collection process, the fetal heart rate is the priority.

Test-Taking Strategy: Note the strategic word, *first*. Use the ABCs—airway, breathing, and circulation—when selecting an answer. Fetal heart rate reflects the use of the ABCs.

2. 4

Rationale: Leopold's maneuvers comprise a systematic method for palpating the fetus through the maternal abdominal wall. Options 1, 2, and 3 are incorrect descriptions.

Test-Taking Strategy: Note the subject, the purpose of and procedure for Leopold's maneuvers. Visualizing this procedure will assist with directing you to the correct option.

3. 2

Rationale: Pressure from the enlarged uterus on the aorta and the vena cava when the woman is supine can result in hypotension. This can be relieved by having the woman lie on her side. Squatting, tailor sitting, and semi-Fowler's position are incorrect because they would not prevent hypotension.

Test-Taking Strategy: Focus on the subject, measures to decrease the incidence of supine hypotension. Think about the anatomy of the pregnant uterus and the physiological response caused by pressure on the large abdominal vessels. Note that squatting, tailor sitting, and semi-Fowler's position are all comparable or alike in that the client would be in an upright position.

4. 1

Rationale: Women who have experienced precipitous labor and delivery often describe feelings of disbelief that their labor has progressed so rapidly. To assist the woman with understanding what has happened, it is best to support the mother in her reaction to the newborn. Encouraging the mother to breast-feed, telling the mother the importance of holding her newborn, and documenting the maternal reaction to the birth do not acknowledge the mother's feelings.

Test-Taking Strategy: Use therapeutic communication techniques. Supporting the maternal reaction to the newborn is the only choice that acknowledges the mother's feelings.

5. 1

Rationale: When the membranes rupture, the nurse immediately assesses the fetal heart rate to detect changes associated with prolapse or the compression of the umbilical cord. Monitoring the contraction pattern and noting the amount, color, and odor of the amniotic fluid may be performed, but these would not be the first actions. There is no information in the question that indicates the need to prepare the client for immediate delivery.

Test-Taking Strategy: Note the strategic word, *first*. Use the ABCs—airway, breathing, and circulation. Fetal heart rate is associated with fetal circulation.

6. 2

Rationale: Precipitous labor progresses quickly, with frequent contractions and short periods of relaxation between them. This does not allow for the maximal reperfusion of the placenta with oxygenated blood. Priority care of this client includes the promotion of fetal oxygenation. A side-lying position can assist with providing blood flow to the uterus by preventing vena cava and abdominal aorta compression. Further stimulation with oxytocin is contraindicated. There may not be enough time to administer epidural anesthesia before delivery with such quick progression. Pushing with contractions is not indicated, especially with this type of labor. The controlled delivery of the fetus is essential to prevent maternal and fetal injury.

Test-Taking Strategy: Note the strategic word, *priority*. Use the ABCs—airway, breathing, and circulation—and consider the baby's as well as the mother's needs. Maintaining a side lying position will promote fetal oxygenation.

7. 4

Rationale: Vena cava and descending aorta compression by the pregnant uterus impede blood return from the lower trunk and extremities, thereby decreasing cardiac return, cardiac output, and blood flow to the uterus and subsequently to the fetus. The best position to prevent this would be side-lying, with the uterus displaced off of the abdominal vessels. Positioning for abdominal surgery necessitates a supine position; however, a wedge placed under the right hip provides for the displacement of the uterus. A prone or semi-Fowler's position is not practical for this type of abdominal surgery. Trendelenburg's position places pressure from the pregnant uterus on the diaphragm and lungs, thus decreasing respiratory capacity and oxygenation.

Test-Taking Strategy: Note the subject, maintaining optimal perfusion to the fetus. Visualize each of the positions in the options and think about their effect on the fetus.

8. 2

Rationale: Fetal bradycardia between contractions may indicate the need for immediate medical management. The nurse must immediately contact the RN, who then contacts the primary health care provider. Monitoring maternal vital signs and labor progress, and encouraging relaxation and breathing techniques will delay necessary and immediate interventions.

Test-Taking Strategy: Note the strategic word, *priority*. Use the ABCs—airway, breathing, and circulation. Note that the woman is in active labor and the fetal heart rate is below normal. It is imperative that the circulation in the fetus be restored to normal limits.

9. 4

Rationale: To evaluate a woman's physical well-being, her temperature, pulse, respirations, and blood pressure (as well as the fetal heartbeat) are checked. Administering an analgesic is incorrect because it would be too premature for an analgesic; medication given too early tends to slow or stop labor contractions. Estimating fetal size and pelvic adequacy would have been previously performed by the PHCP during prenatal visits.

Maternity Nursing

Test-Taking Strategy: Note the strategic word, *initially,* and use the ABCs—airway, breathing, and circulation; this will direct you to the correct option. Remember, measuring the vital signs is the priority.

10. 1
Rationale: Signs of placental separation include the lengthening of the umbilical cord, a sudden gush of dark blood from the introitus, a firmly contracted uterus, and the uterus changing from a discoid to a globular shape. The client may experience vaginal fullness, but not sudden and sharp abdominal pain.

Test-Taking Strategy: Focus on the subject, indications that the placenta has separated. Thinking about what one would expect to occur when the placenta separates will assist you to eliminate shortening of the umbilical cord and a decrease in blood flow from the introitus. Option 2 is eliminated because of the words *sudden and sharp.*

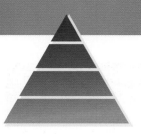
CHAPTER **25**

The Postpartum Period and Associated Complications

PRIORITY CONCEPTS Caregiving; Reproduction

WHAT WOULD YOU DO?

The nurse is caring for a postpartum client and is preparing to measure the amount of lochial flow. What would the nurse do to obtain an accurate assessment?
Answer is located on p. 316.

I. Postpartum

A. Description: Period when the reproductive tract returns to the normal, nonpregnant state

B. Postpartum period: Starts immediately after birth and is usually completed by week 6 following birth

II. Physiological Maternal Changes

A. Involution (Fig. 25.1)
   1. Description
      a. The rapid decrease in the size of the uterus as it returns to the nonpregnant state
      b. Clients who breast-feed may experience a more rapid involution as a result of the release of oxytocin during breast-feeding.
   2. Data collection
      a. Weight of the uterus decreases from 2 lb (900 g) to 2 oz (57 g) in 6 weeks.
      b. Endometrium regenerates.
      c. Fundus steadily descends into the pelvis. The fundal height decreases about 1 cm/day.
      d. By 10 days postpartum, the uterus cannot be palpated abdominally.
      e. A flaccid fundus indicates uterine atony and needs to be massaged until firm.
      f. A tender fundus indicates an infection.
      g. Afterpains decrease in frequency after the first few days.

B. Lochia
   1. Description: Discharge from the uterus that consists of blood from the vessels of the placental site and debris from the decidua

   2. Data collection (Box 25.1)
      a. Rubra: Bright red discharge that occurs from day of birth to day 3 postpartum
      b. Serosa: Brownish-pink discharge that occurs from days 4 to 10 postpartum
      c. Alba: White discharge that occurs from days 11 to 14 postpartum
      d. Normally the discharge smells like normal menstrual flow.
      e. Discharge decreases daily in amount.
      f. Discharge increases with ambulation.

C. Cervix: Cervical involution occurs. After 1 week, the muscle begins to regenerate.

D. Vagina: Vaginal distention decreases, although muscle tone is never restored completely to the pregravid state.

E. Ovarian function and menstruation
   1. Ovarian function depends on the rapidity with which pituitary function is restored.
   2. Menstrual flow resumes within 1 to 2 months in non-breast-feeding mothers.
   3. Menstrual flow usually resumes within 3 to 6 months in breast-feeding mothers.
   4. Breast-feeding mothers may experience amenorrhea during the entire period of lactation so long as they are exclusively breast-feeding.

⚠️ Women may ovulate without menstruating, so breast-feeding would not be considered a form of birth control.

F. Breasts
   1. Breasts continue to secrete colostrum for the first 48 to 72 hours after birth.
   2. A decrease of estrogen and progesterone levels after birth stimulates increased prolactin levels, which promote breast milk production.
   3. Breasts become distended with milk on the third day.
   4. Engorgement occurs on approximately day 4 in both breast-feeding and non-breast-feeding

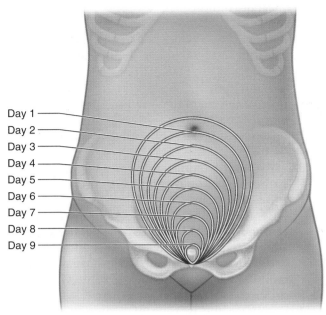

Day 1
Day 2
Day 3
Day 4
Day 5
Day 6
Day 7
Day 8
Day 9

FIGURE 25.1 Involution of the uterus. The height of uterine fundus decreases by approximately 1 cm/day.

BOX 25.1 Amount of Lochia

Scant
Less than 2.5 cm (<1 inch) on menstrual pad in 1 hour

Light
Less than 10 cm (<4 inches) on menstrual pad in 1 hour

Moderate
Less than 15 cm (<6 inches) on menstrual pad in 1 hour

Heavy
Saturated menstrual pad in 1 hour

Excessive
Menstrual pad saturated in 15 minutes

Adapted from Murray S, McKinney E: *Foundations of maternal-newborn and women's health nursing*, ed 5, Philadelphia, 2010, Saunders.

---

mothers. Box 25.2 summarizes care of breasts for non-breast-feeding mothers.
5. Breast-feeding relieves engorgement.
G. Urinary tract
1. May have urinary retention because of a loss of elasticity, tone, and loss of sensation in the bladder from trauma, medications, anesthesia, and lack of privacy
2. Diuresis usually begins within the first 12 hours after birth.
H. Gastrointestinal tract
1. Clients are usually hungry after birth.
2. Constipation can occur, with bowel movement (soft, formed stool) by the second or third postpartum day.
3. Hemorrhoids are common.
I. Vital signs (Table 25.1)

BOX 25.2 Breast Care for Non-Breast-Feeding Mothers

- Avoid nipple stimulation.
- Apply a breast binder, wear a snug-fitting bra, apply ice packs, or take a mild analgesic for engorgement.
- Engorgement usually resolves within 24–36 hours after it begins.

TABLE 25.1 Normal Postpartum Vital Signs

Vital Sign	Description
Temperature	May increase to 100.4°F (38.0°C) during the first 24 hours postpartum as a result of the dehydrating effects of labor; any higher elevation may be caused by infection and must be reported.
Pulse	May decrease to 50 beats per minute (normal puerperal bradycardia); a pulse rate of >100 beats per minute may indicate excessive blood loss or infection.
Blood pressure	Should be normal; suspect hypovolemia if it decreases.
Respirations	Rarely changes; if respirations increase significantly, suspect pulmonary embolism, uterine atony, or hemorrhage.

III. **Postpartum Interventions**
A. Data collection
1. Monitor vital signs.
2. Monitor pain level.
3. Monitor the height, consistency, and location of the fundus (have the client empty the bladder before fundal assessment) (Fig. 25.2).
4. Monitor the color, amount, and odor of the lochia.
5. Check breasts for engorgement.
6. Monitor perineum for swelling or discoloration.
7. Monitor for perineal lacerations or episiotomy for healing.
8. Check incisions or dressings of the client who had a cesarean birth.
9. Monitor intake and output (I&O).
10. Encourage frequent voiding.
11. Monitor bowel status.
12. Encourage ambulation.
13. Check extremities for thrombophlebitis (redness, tenderness, or warmth of legs).
14. $Rh_o(D)$ immune globulin is prescribed to be administered within 72 hours postpartum to the Rh-negative client who has given birth to a Rh-positive newborn.
15. Rubella immunity will be evaluated; if not immune, rubella immunization will be administered.
16. Monitor parent–newborn bonding.
17. Monitor the mother's emotional status.

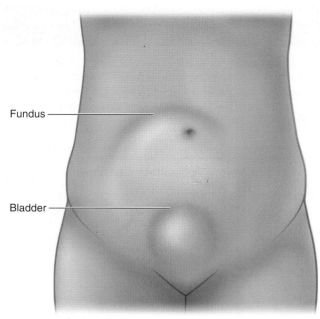

Fundus

Bladder

FIGURE 25.2 A full bladder displaces and prevents contraction of the uterus.

B. Client teaching
1. Demonstrate newborn care skills as necessary.
2. Provide the opportunity for the mother to bathe the newborn.
3. Reinforce instructions to the mother regarding feeding technique.
4. Reinforce instructions to the mother to avoid heavy lifting for at least 3 weeks.
5. Reinforce instructions to the mother to plan at least one rest period per day.
6. Reinforce instructions to the mother that contraception must begin after birth or with the initiation of intercourse (intercourse would be postponed at least until lochia ceases). With rubella immunization, avoid conception for 1 to 3 months based on the primary health care provider's (PHCP) or obstetrician/gynecologist's (OB/GYN) recommendation.
7. Reinforce instructions to the mother regarding the importance of follow-up care, which would be scheduled at 4 to 6 weeks postpartum.
8. Reinforce instructions to the mother to report immediately any signs of chills, fever, increased lochia, or depressed feelings to the PHCP.

IV. Postpartum Discomforts
A. Afterbirth pains
1. Occur as a result of uterine contractions
2. Are more common among multiparas, breast-feeding mothers, clients treated with oxytocin, and clients who had an overdistended uterus during pregnancy (e.g., those who carried twins)

⚠ The nurse would consult with the RN and check the PHCP's prescriptions regarding treatment measures for postpartum discomforts.

B. Perineal discomfort
1. Apply ice packs to the perineum, as prescribed, during the first 24 hours to reduce swelling.
2. After the first 24 hours, apply warmth by sitz baths.
C. Episiotomy
1. Instruct the client to administer perineal care after each voiding.
2. Encourage the use of analgesic spray as prescribed.
3. Assist with administration of analgesics as prescribed if comfort measures are unsuccessful.
D. Perineal lacerations
1. Care as for an episiotomy. Administer perineal care and assist with the use of analgesic spray and administration of analgesics for comfort.
2. Rectal suppositories and enemas may be contraindicated (to avoid injury to sutures).
E. Breast discomfort from engorgement
1. Encourage the wearing of a support bra at all times, even while sleeping.
2. Encourage the use of ice packs between feedings if the client is breastfeeding. Use of ice packs could diminish milk supply in the breast-feeding mother.
3. Encourage the use of warm soaks or a warm shower before feeding for the breast-feeding mother.
4. Assist to administer analgesics as prescribed if comfort measures are unsuccessful.
F. Constipation
1. Encourage adequate intake of fluids (2000 mL/day).
2. Encourage a diet high in fiber.
3. Encourage ambulation.
4. Administer stool softener, laxative, enema, or suppository if needed and prescribed.
G. Postpartum emotional changes (Box 25.3)
1. Acknowledge the client's feelings and demonstrate a caring attitude.
2. Determine availability of family support and other support systems and resources as needed.
3. Encourage and assist the client to verbalize feelings.
4. Monitor the newborn for appropriate growth and development expectations.
5. Assist significant other and other appropriate family members to discuss feelings and identify ways to assist client.

⚠ All clients must be assessed for depression during pregnancy and in the postpartum period.

V. Nutritional Counseling
A. Discuss caloric intake for breast-feeding and non-breast-feeding mothers.
B. Nutritional needs depend on prepregnancy weight, ideal weight for height, and whether the mother is breast-feeding.

BOX 25.3	**Signs and Symptoms of Emotional Changes**

Postpartum Blues
- Anger
- Anxiety
- Cries easily for no apparent reason
- Emotionally labile
- Expresses a let-down feeling
- Fatigue
- Headache
- Insomnia
- Restlessness
- Sadness

Postpartum Depression
- Anxiety
- Appetite changes
- Crying, sadness
- Difficulty concentrating or making decisions
- Fatigue, unable to sleep
- Feelings of guilt
- Irritability and agitation
- Lack of energy
- Less responsive to the infant
- Loss of pleasure in normal activities
- Suicidal thoughts

Postpartum Psychosis
- Break with reality
- Confusion
- Delirium
- Delusions
- Hallucinations
- Panic

Data from Lowdermilk D, Cashion MC, Perry S: *Maternity & women's health care,* ed 9, St. Louis, 2011, Mosby; Lowdermilk D, Cashion MC, Perry S: *Maternity & women's health care,* ed 10, St. Louis, 2012, Mosby; Perry S, Hockenberry M, Lowdermilk D, Wilson D: *Maternal-child nursing care,* ed 4, St. Louis, 2013.

BOX 25.4	**Breast-Feeding Procedure for the Mother**

1. Wash hands and assume a comfortable position.
2. Start with the breast with which the last feeding ended.
3. Brush the newborn's lower lip with nipple.
4. Tickle the lips to have the newborn open the mouth wide.
5. Guide the nipple and surrounding areola into the newborn's mouth.
6. Encourage the newborn to nurse on each breast for 15–20 minutes.
7. After the newborn has nursed, release suction by depressing the newborn's chin or inserting a clean finger into the newborn's mouth.
8. Burp the newborn after the first breast.
9. Repeat the procedure on the second breast until the newborn stops nursing.
10. Burp the newborn again.
11. Listen for audible sucking and swallowing.

C. If the mother is breast-feeding, calorie needs increase by approximately 200 to 500 cal/day, and the mother may require increased fluids and the continuance of prenatal vitamins and minerals.

VI. Breast-Feeding

A. Interventions
1. Put the newborn to the mother's breast as soon as the mother's and newborn's conditions are stable (on the delivery table, if possible).
2. Stay with the mother each time she nurses until she feels secure and confident with the newborn and her feelings.
3. Monitor LATCH (L = latch achieved by newborn; A = audible swallowing; T = type of nipple; C = comfort of mother; H = hold or position of the newborn).
4. Uterine cramping may occur during the first day after birth while the mother is nursing, when oxytocin stimulation causes the uterus to contract.

5. Instruct the client in general hygiene and to wash the breasts once daily.
6. The mother should not use soap on the breasts because it tends to remove natural oils, which increases the chance of cracked nipples.
7. If engorgement occurs, have the mother breast-feed frequently, apply warm packs before feeding, apply ice packs between feedings, and massage the breasts.
8. If cracked nipples develop, expose the nipples to air for 10 to 20 minutes after feeding, rotate the position of the baby for each feeding, and be sure that the baby is latched onto the areola and not just the nipple. Colostrum can also be expressed after the feeding as a moisturizer for the nipple to prevent cracked, dry skin.
9. Bra should be well fitted and supportive; avoid an underwire bra.
10. Breasts may leak between feedings or during coitus. Place a breast pad in the bra.
11. Calories should be increased by 200 to 500 cal/day, and the diet needs to include additional fluids. Prenatal vitamins would be taken, as prescribed.
12. Newborn's stools are usually light yellow, seedy, watery, and frequent.
13. Medications, including over-the-counter medications, need to be avoided unless prescribed, because they may be unsafe when breast-feeding.
14. Gas-producing foods and caffeine would be avoided.
15. Oral contraceptives that contain estrogen are not recommended for breast-feeding mothers. Progestin-only birth control pills are less likely to interfere with the milk supply.
16. The baby will develop his or her own feeding schedule.

B. Breast-feeding procedure for mother (Box 25.4)

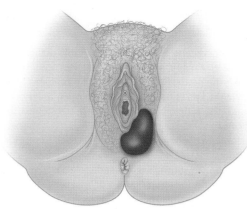

FIGURE 25.3 A vulvar hematoma is caused by rapid bleeding into soft tissue. It causes severe pain and feelings of pressure.

VII. Cystitis

A. Description: Infection of the bladder can occur in the postpartum period, and the postpartum woman would be encouraged to consume adequate fluids and void frequently to avoid bladder distension.

B. Data collection and interventions: Refer to Chapter 51 for information.

⚠ If cystitis is suspected, a urine specimen for culture and sensitivity needs to be obtained before initiating antibiotic therapy.

VIII. Hematoma

A. Description
  1. Localized collection of blood into the tissues; can occur internally, involving the vaginal sulcus or other organs. Vulvar hematomas are the most common (Fig. 25.3).
  2. Predisposing conditions include operative delivery with forceps or injury to a blood vessel.
  3. Can result in shock and be life-threatening

B. Data collection
  1. Abnormal severe pain not relieved with treatment or comfort measures
  2. Pressure in the perineal area
  3. Sensitive, bulging mass in the perineal area with discolored skin
  4. Inability to void
  5. Decreased hemoglobin and hematocrit levels
  6. Restlessness; changes in vital signs indicating shock, such as tachycardia and hypotension

C. Interventions
  1. Monitor vital signs and look for signs of shock.
  2. Monitor the client for abnormal pain or perineal pressure, especially when a forceps delivery has occurred.
  3. Place ice on the hematoma site as prescribed.
  4. Assist with the administration of analgesics as prescribed.

The other hand is cupped to massage and gently compress the fundus toward the lower uterine segment.

One hand remains cupped against the uterus at the level of the symphysis pubis to support the uterus.

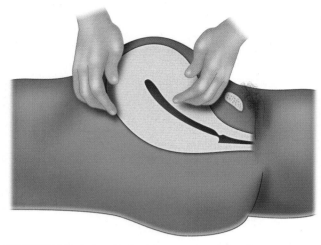

FIGURE 25.4 Technique for fundal massage. One hand remains cupped against the uterus at the level of the symphysis pubis to support the uterus. The other hand is cupped to massage and compress the fundus gently toward the lower uterine segment. (From McKinney E, James S, Murray S, Ashwill J: *Maternal-child nursing,* ed 4, St. Louis, 2013, Saunders.)

  5. Prepare for urinary catheterization if the client is unable to void.
  6. Assist with the administration of blood products as prescribed.
  7. Monitor for signs of infection, such as increased temperature, pulse rate, and white blood cell (WBC) count.
  8. Assist to administer antibiotics as prescribed because infection is common after hematoma formation.
  9. Prepare the client for the incision and evacuation of the hematoma, if necessary.

IX. Uterine Atony

A. Description: A poorly contracted uterus that does not adequately compress large open vessels at the placental site; this can result in hemorrhage. This can involve the anterior, posterior, or both areas of the uterus.

B. Data collection: A soft (boggy) uterus noted on palpation of the uterine fundus.

C. Interventions
  1. Massage the uterus until firm (Fig. 25.4).
  2. Empty the woman's bladder (by voiding or catheterization) if that is contributing to the uterine atony.
  3. The PHCP is notified if interventions do not resolve the atony, because this could be an indication of hemorrhage.

X. Hemorrhage and Shock

A. Description
  1. Bleeding of greater than 1000 mL or more after delivery or a 10% drop in hemoglobin and hematocrit from admission to postdelivery with signs/symptoms of hemorrhage

2. Can occur early, during the first 24 hours after delivery, or later, after the first 24 hours after delivery
3. Early postpartum hemorrhage is within the first 4 hours postpartum.
4. Late postpartum hemorrhage is anything beyond 4 hours postpartum.
5. While postpartum hemorrhage can occur anytime during the postpartum period, the greatest risk is during the 4 hours immediately after delivery.
6. Causes and predisposing factors (Box 25.5)

B. Data collection
1. Persistent significant bleeding: perineal pad is soaked within 15 minutes.
2. Restlessness and increased pulse rate (earlier signs), decrease in blood pressure, cool and clammy skin, ashen or grayish color
3. Complaints of weakness, lightheadedness, dyspnea

C. Interventions: (See Priority Nursing Actions)

⚡ PRIORITY NURSING ACTIONS

Hemorrhage and Shock in the Postpartum Client

1. Notify the RN immediately (stay with the client); the RN will contact the primary health care provider (PHCP).
2. If uterus is atonic, massage gently but firmly to cause it to contract.
3. Elevate client's legs to a 30-degree angle.
4. Administer oxygen by nonrebreather face mask at 8 to 10 L/min.
5. Monitor vital signs and empty bladder by catheterization if prescribed.
6. Assist with the administration of uterotonic medications (e.g., oxytocin, prostaglandins) as prescribed to increase uterine tone.
7. Assist with providing additional or maintaining the existing intravenous (IV) infusion of lactated Ringer's solution or normal saline solution to restore circulatory volume (woman needs to have 2 patent IV lines; a second IV line using 16- to 18-gauge IV catheter may need to be inserted by the RN).
8. Assist the RN with the administration of blood or blood products as prescribed.
9. Insert an indwelling urinary catheter to monitor perfusion of kidneys.
10. Assist the RN to administer emergency medications as prescribed.
11. Prepare for possible surgery or other emergency treatments or procedures.
12. Record event, interventions instituted, and woman's response to interventions.

BOX 25.5 Postpartum Hemorrhage

Causes
- Uterine atony
- Laceration of the cervix or vagina
- Hematoma development in the cervix, perineum, or labia
- Retained placental fragments

Predisposing Factors
- Previous history of postpartum hemorrhage
- Placenta previa
- Abruptio placentae
- Overdistention of the uterus—polyhydramnios, multiple gestation, large neonate
- Infection
- Multiparity
- Dystocia or labor that is prolonged
- Operative delivery—cesarean or forceps delivery, intrauterine manipulation

---

XI. Infection

A. Description: Any infection of the reproductive organs that occurs within 28 days of delivery or abortion; endometritis is inflammation/infection of the inner lining of the uterus.

B. Data collection
1. Fever
2. Chills
3. Anorexia
4. Pelvic discomfort or pain
5. Vaginal discharge that is malodorous. Normal vaginal discharge has a fleshy odor, or an odor similar to a menstrual period.
6. Elevated WBC count

⚠ A temperature up to 100.4°F (38°C) is normal during the first 24 hours postpartum because of dehydration; a temperature of 100.4°F (38°C) or greater after 24 hours postpartum indicates infection.

C. Interventions
1. Monitor vital signs and temperature every 2 to 4 hours.
2. Make the mother as comfortable as possible. Position her for comfort and to promote vaginal drainage.
3. Keep the mother warmed if she is chilled.
4. Isolate the newborn from the mother only if the mother can infect the newborn, such as with an airborne illness.
5. Provide a nutritious, high-calorie, high-protein diet.
6. Encourage fluids to 3000 to 4000 mL/day, if not contraindicated.
7. Encourage frequent voiding; monitor intake and output.
8. Monitor culture results if cultures were prescribed.
9. Assist to administer antibiotics, according to identified organism as prescribed.

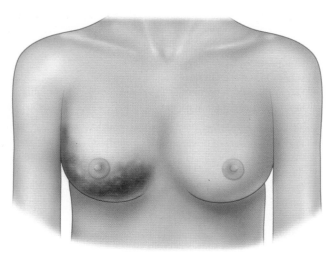

FIGURE 25.5 Mastitis.

XII. Mastitis

A. Description
1. Inflammation of the breast as a result of a blocked duct and infection
2. Primarily occurs in breast-feeding mothers 2 to 3 weeks after delivery, but may occur at any time during lactation

B. Data collection (Fig. 25.5)
1. Localized heat and swelling
2. Pain; tender axillary lymph nodes
3. Elevated temperature
4. Complaints of flu-like symptoms

C. Interventions
1. Instruct the mother in good hand-washing and breast hygiene techniques.
2. Promote comfort.
3. Apply heat to the site, as prescribed.
4. Maintain lactation in breast-feeding mothers.
5. Encourage the manual expression of breast milk or the use of a breast pump every 4 hours.
6. Encourage the mother to support the breasts with a supportive, no underwire bra.
7. Assist to administer analgesics or antibiotics, as prescribed.

XIII. Endometritis

A. Description
1. Infection of the lining of the uterus occurring in the postpartum period; caused by bacteria that invade the uterus at the placental site
2. The infection may spread, involve the entire endometrium, and cause peritonitis or pelvic thrombophlebitis.

B. Data collection
1. Chills and fever
2. Increased pulse
3. Decreased appetite
4. Headache
5. Backache
6. Prolonged, severe afterpains
7. Tender, large uterus
8. Foul odor to lochia or reddish-brown lochia
9. Ileus
10. Elevated WBC count

C. Interventions
1. Monitor vital signs.
2. Place the mother in Fowler's position to facilitate the drainage of lochia.
3. Provide a private room for the mother.
4. Inform the mother that it is not necessary to isolate the newborn from the mother.
5. Instruct the mother in proper hand-washing techniques.
6. Initiate contact precautions, as necessary.
7. Monitor I&O and encourage fluid intake.
8. Intravenous antibiotics may be prescribed.
9. Administer comfort measures, such as back rubs, position changes, and pain medications, as prescribed, and provide emotional support.
10. Oxytocic medications may be prescribed to improve uterine tone.

XIV. Pulmonary Embolism

A. Description: Passage of a thrombus, often originating in a uterine or other pelvic vein, into the lungs, where it disrupts the circulation of the blood

B. Data collection
1. Sudden dyspnea and chest pain
2. Tachypnea and tachycardia
3. Cough and lung crackles
4. Hemoptysis
5. Feeling of impending doom

C. Interventions
1. Administer oxygen.
2. Position the client with the head of the bed elevated.
3. Monitor vital signs frequently, especially respiratory and heart rate and breath sounds.
4. Monitor for signs of respiratory distress and for signs of increasing hypoxemia.
5. Assist to administer intravenous fluids and anticoagulants as prescribed.
6. Prepare to assist the RN and PHCP to administer medications to dissolve the clot if prescribed.

XV. Subinvolution

A. Description: Incomplete involution or the failure of the uterus to return to its normal size and condition

B. Data collection
1. Uterine pain during palpation
2. Uterus is larger than expected
3. More than normal vaginal bleeding

C. Interventions
1. Monitor vital signs.
2. Check the uterus and fundus.
3. Monitor for uterine pain and vaginal bleeding.

BOX 25.6	Data Collection: Types of Thrombophlebitis

Superficial
- Palpable thrombus that feels bumpy and hard
- Tenderness and pain in the affected lower extremity
- Warm and pinkish-red color over the thrombus area

Femoral
- Malaise
- Chills and fever
- Diminished peripheral pulses
- Shiny, white skin over the affected area
- Pain, stiffness, and swelling of the affected leg

Pelvic
- Severe chills
- Dramatic body temperature changes
- Occurrence of pulmonary embolism may be the first sign

BOX 25.7	Client Education for Thrombophlebitis

- Never massage the leg.
- Avoid crossing the legs.
- Avoid prolonged sitting.
- Avoid constrictive clothing.
- Avoid pressure behind the knees.
- Know how to apply elastic stockings (support hose), if prescribed.
- Understand the importance of compliance with anticoagulant therapy, if prescribed.
- Understand the importance of follow-up with the primary health care provider.

---

4. Elevate the legs to promote venous return.
5. Encourage frequent voiding.
6. Monitor the hemoglobin and hematocrit levels.
7. Prepare to assist with the administration of methylergonovine maleate, which provides sustained contraction of the uterus, as prescribed.

XVI. Thrombophlebitis

A. Description
   1. A condition in which a clot forms in a vessel wall as a result of the inflammation of the vessel wall.
   2. A partial obstruction of the vessel can occur.
   3. Increased blood-clotting factors during the postpartum period place the client at risk.
   4. Early ambulation in the postoperative period after cesarean section is a preventive action.

B. Types
   1. Superficial thrombophlebitis
   2. Femoral thrombophlebitis
   3. Pelvic thrombophlebitis

C. Data collection (Box 25.6)

D. Interventions
   1. Specific therapies may depend on the location of the thrombophlebitis.
   2. Check the lower extremities for edema, tenderness, varices, and increased skin temperature.
   3. Maintain bed rest.
   4. Elevate the affected leg.
   5. Apply a bed cradle and keep bedclothes off of the affected leg.
   6. Never massage the leg.
   7. Monitor for manifestations of pulmonary embolism.
   8. Apply hot packs or moist heat to the affected site as prescribed to alleviate discomfort.
   9. Apply elastic stockings (support hose), if prescribed.
   10. Assist to administer analgesics and antibiotics as prescribed.
   11. Intravenous heparin sodium may be prescribed for femoral or pelvic thrombophlebitis to prevent further thrombus formation.

E. Reinforcement of client teaching (Box 25.7).

XVII. Perinatal Loss

A. Description
   1. Perinatal loss is associated with miscarriage, neonatal death, stillbirth, and therapeutic abortion.
   2. Loss and grief may also occur with the birth of a preterm baby, a newborn who has suffered complications with birth, or a newborn with congenital anomalies. It may also occur within a family who is placing a child for adoption.

B. Interventions

⚠ Not all interventions are appropriate for every woman and her family who have experienced perinatal loss. It is crucial to consider religious, spiritual, and cultural health care practices and beliefs when planning care for a woman and her family who have experienced perinatal loss.

   1. Communicate therapeutically and actively listen, providing parents with time to grieve.
   2. Notify the hospital chaplain or other religious person as appropriate.
   3. Discuss with the parents about options such as seeing, holding, bathing, and/or dressing the deceased infant; visitation by other family members or friends; religious, spiritual, or cultural rituals; and funeral arrangements.
   4. Prepare a special memories box with keepsakes such as footprints, handprints, locks of hair, and pictures, if appropriate.
   5. Admit the mother to a private room if possible. Mark the door to the room with a special card (per agency procedure and maintaining confidentiality) that denotes to hospital staff that this family has experienced a loss.
   6. See Chapter 24 for additional information on intrauterine fetal demise.

WHAT WOULD YOU DO?

Answer: To determine most accurately the amount of lochia flow, the nurse would weigh the perineal pad before and after use and identify the amount of time between pad changes. This information is then documented according to agency procedures. The nurse would also note the color, odor, and the presence and characteristics of clots if any are noted.

PRACTICE QUESTIONS

1. The client received epidural anesthesia during labor and had a forceps delivery after pushing for 2 hours. At 6 hours postpartum, the client's systolic blood pressure (BP) dropped 20 points, the diastolic BP dropped 10 points, and her pulse is 120 beats per minute. The client is very anxious and restless. The nurse is told that the client has a vulvar hematoma. Based on this diagnosis, the nurse needs to plan which action?
   1. Reassure the client.
   2. Apply perineal pressure.
   3. Monitor fundal height.
   4. Prepare the client for surgery.

2. The nurse is preparing a list of self-care instructions for a postpartum client who has been diagnosed with mastitis. Which instructions would be included on the list? **Select all that apply.**
   - [ ] 1. Rest during the acute phase.
   - [ ] 2. Wear a supportive, no underwire bra.
   - [ ] 3. Maintain a fluid intake of at least 3000 mL.
   - [ ] 4. Continue to breast-feed if the breasts are not too sore.
   - [ ] 5. Take prescribed antibiotics until the soreness subsides.
   - [ ] 6. Avoid decompression of the breasts by breast-feeding or breast pumping.

3. A postpartum client is getting ready for discharge. The nurse suspects that the client **needs further teaching** related to breast-feeding when she makes which statement?
   1. "I don't need birth control because I will be breast-feeding."
   2. "I need to increase my caloric intake by 500 calories a day."
   3. "I wouldn't use soap to wash my breasts because I will be breast-feeding."
   4. "I need to be sure that I increase my fluid intake and take my prenatal vitamins while breast-feeding."

4. The nurse is caring for a postpartum client with a diagnosis of thrombophlebitis. The client suddenly complains of chest pain and dyspnea. The nurse would **initially** check which item?
   1. Vital signs
   2. Fundal height
   3. Presence of calf pain
   4. Level of consciousness (LOC)

5. The nurse suspects that the client has a pulmonary embolism. Which is the **most important** nursing action?
   1. Monitor the vital signs.
   2. Elevate the head of the bed.
   3. Increase the intravenous flow rate.
   4. Administer oxygen by face mask, as prescribed.

6. The nurse notes that the 4-hour postpartum client has cool, clammy skin and that she is restless and excessively thirsty. The nurse **immediately** notifies the registered nurse and then performs which action?
   1. Checks the vital signs
   2. Begins fundal massage
   3. Encourages ambulation
   4. Encourages the client to drink fluids

7. The nurse is assisting with caring for a postpartum client who is experiencing uterine hemorrhage. When planning to meet the psychosocial needs of the client, the nurse would plan which action?
   1. Maintain strict bed rest
   2. Monitor the vital signs every 2 hours
   3. Perform firm fundal massage every 2 hours
   4. Keep the client and her family members informed of her progress

8. The nurse palpates the fundus and checks the character of the lochia of a postpartum client who is in the fourth stage of labor. Which lochia characteristic would the nurse expect to note?
   1. Red
   2. Pink
   3. White
   4. Serosanguineous

9. After episiotomy and the delivery of a newborn, the nurse performs a perineal check on the mother. The nurse notes a trickle of bright red blood coming from the perineum. The nurse checks the fundus and notes that it is firm. Which determination would the nurse make?
   1. This is a normal expectation after episiotomy.
   2. The mother would be allowed bathroom privileges only.
   3. The bright red bleeding is abnormal and needs to be reported.
   4. The perineal assessment would be performed more frequently.

10. The nurse is assigned to care for the client during the postpartum period. The client asks the nurse what the term involution means. Which description would the nurse give to the client?
    1. The inverted uterus returning to normal
    2. The gradual reversal of the uterine muscle into the abdominal cavity
    3. The descent of the uterus into the pelvic cavity, which occurs at a rate of 2 cm/day
    4. The progressive descent of the uterus into the pelvic cavity, which occurs at a rate of approximately 1 cm/day

11. A mother is breast-feeding her newborn baby and experiences breast engorgement. The nurse would encourage the mother to do which to provide relief of the engorgement?
    1. Breast-feed only during the daytime hours.
    2. Apply cold compresses to the breast before feeding.
    3. Avoid the use of a bra while the breasts are engorged.
    4. Massage the breasts before feeding to stimulate let-down.

12. After delivery the nurse checks the height of the uterine fundus. Which position of the fundus would the nurse expect to note?
    1. To the right of the abdomen
    2. At the level of the umbilicus
    3. About 4 cm above the level of the umbilicus
    4. One fingerbreadth above the symphysis pubis

13. The nurse is caring for a postpartum client. At 4 hours postpartum, the client's temperature is 102°F (38.9°C). Which is the appropriate nursing action?
    1. Apply cool packs to the abdomen.
    2. Continue to monitor the temperature.
    3. Remove the blanket from the client's bed.
    4. Notify the registered nurse (RN), who will then contact the primary health care provider (PHCP).

14. The nurse is assisting with planning care for a postpartum woman who has small vulvar hematomas. To assist with reducing the swelling, the nurse would perform which action?
    1. Check vital signs every 4 hours.
    2. Measure the fundal height every 4 hours.
    3. Prepare a heat pack for application to the area.
    4. Prepare an ice pack for application to the area.

15. The nurse is assigned to care for the client after a cesarean section. To prevent thrombophlebitis, the nurse would encourage the woman to take which **priority** action?
    1. Ambulate frequently.
    2. Wear support stockings.
    3. Apply warm, moist packs to the legs.
    4. Remain on bed rest, with the legs elevated.

ANSWERS

1. 4
Rationale: The information provided in the question indicates that the client is experiencing blood loss. Surgery would be indicated for this complication to stop the bleeding. Reassuring the client, applying perineal pressure, and monitoring the fundal height do not assist with controlling the bleeding in this emergency situation.
Test-Taking Strategy: Focus on the data in the question to determine that the client has a vulvar hematoma. Note that the signs and symptoms in the question indicate the presence of bleeding; this would direct you to the correct option.

2. 1, 2, 3, 4
Rationale: Mastitis is an infection of the lactating breast. Client instructions include resting during the acute phase, wearing a supportive no underwire bra, maintaining a fluid intake of at least 3000 mL/day, and taking analgesics to relieve discomfort. Antibiotics may be prescribed and are taken until the complete prescribed course is finished. They are not stopped when the soreness subsides. Additional supportive measures include the use of moist heat or ice packs.

Continued decompression of the breast by breast-feeding or breast pump is important to empty the breast and prevent the formation of an abscess.
Test-Taking Strategy: Think about the pathophysiology associated with the subject, mastitis. Recalling that supportive measures include rest, moist heat or ice packs, antibiotics, analgesics, increased fluid intake, breast support, and the decompression of the breasts will assist you with answering the question.

3. 1
Rationale: Amenorrhea may occur during breast-feeding, but the client can still ovulate without menstruating. The caloric intake would be increased by 200 to 500 cal/day (per PHCP's prescription), and the diet would include additional fluids and prenatal vitamins, as prescribed. The use of soap on the breasts is avoided because it tends to remove natural oils, which can lead to cracked nipples.
Test-Taking Strategy: Note the strategic words, *needs further teaching.* These words indicate a negative event query and the need to select the incorrect statement. Recalling the physiology related to amenorrhea and ovulation during breast-feeding will direct you to the correct option.

4. 1

Rationale: Pulmonary embolism is a complication of thrombophlebitis. Changes in the vital signs are one of the first things to occur with pulmonary embolism, because pulmonary blood flow is compromised. Fundal height is unrelated to the information in the question. Calf pain is an indicator of thrombophlebitis. Level of consciousness may change as the condition worsens; worsening would indicate hypoxia.

Test-Taking Strategy: Note the strategic word, *initially*. Use the ABCs—airway, breathing, and circulation—to direct you to the correct option.

5. 4

Rationale: Because pulmonary circulation is compromised in the presence of an embolus, cardiorespiratory support is initiated by oxygen administration. Monitoring vital signs and elevating the head of the bed may be components of the plan of care, but they are not the most important actions from the options provided. The nurse would not increase the intravenous rate without a prescription from the PHCP to do so.

Test-Taking Strategy: Note the strategic words, *most important*, and use the ABCs—airway, breathing, and circulation. This will direct you to the correct option: *oxygen is the priority*.

6. 1

Rationale: Signs/symptoms of hypovolemia include cool, clammy, and pale skin; feelings of anxiety and restlessness; and thirst. The nurse would check the vital signs. The nurse does not ambulate the client or encourage fluids until specific prescriptions are given to do so. There is no information in the question to indicate the need for fundal massage.

Test-Taking Strategy: Note the strategic word, *immediately*. Use the ABCs—airway, breathing, and circulation—and the steps of the nursing process to direct you to the correct option.

7. 4

Rationale: Keeping the client and her family informed about her condition will help minimize fear and apprehension. Maintaining strict bed rest, monitoring vital signs, and performing fundal massage every 2 hours address physiological needs.

Test-Taking Strategy: Focus on the subject, meeting psychosocial needs. The correct option is the only option that addresses psychosocial needs.

8. 1

Rationale: The color of the lochia during the fourth stage of labor is bright red, and this may last from 1 to 3 days. The color of the lochia then changes to a pinkish-brown and occurs from day 4 to 10 postpartum. Finally, the lochia changes to a creamy white color that occurs from day 10 to 14 postpartum.

Test-Taking Strategy: Focus on the subject, fourth stage of labor; this will direct you to the correct option. In the immediate postpartum period, the lochia is red in color.

9. 3

Rationale: Lochial flow must be distinguished from bleeding that originates from a laceration or an episiotomy, which is usually brighter red than lochia and presents as a continuous trickle of bleeding, even though the fundus of the uterus is firm. This bright red bleeding is abnormal and needs to be reported. Therefore, the other options are incorrect interpretations.

Test-Taking Strategy: Note the subject, trickle of bright red blood. This would be an indication that the flow is not normal.

10. 4

Rationale: Involution is the progressive descent of the uterus into the pelvic cavity. After birth, descent occurs at a rate of approximately 1 fingerbreadth or 1 cm per day. The other options do not accurately describe involution.

Test-Taking Strategy: Focus on the subject, a description of involution. Use your knowledge of medical terminology to help you to define *involution*. This will assist with directing you to the correct option.

11. 4

Rationale: Comfort measures for breast engorgement include massaging the breasts before feeding to stimulate let-down, wearing a supportive and well-fitting bra at all times, taking a warm shower or applying warm compresses just before feeding, and alternating breasts during feeding.

Test-Taking Strategy: Focus on the subject, engorgement. Eliminate "breast-feeding only in the daytime hours" because of the closed-ended word, *only*. From the remaining options, recalling the self-care measures that promote the comfort of the mother with breast engorgement will direct you to the correct option.

12. 2

Rationale: After delivery, the uterine fundus would be at the level of the umbilicus or 1 to 3 fingerbreadths below it and in the midline of the abdomen. If the fundus is 4 cm above the umbilicus, this may indicate that there are blood clots in the uterus that need to be expelled by fundal massage. If the fundus is noted to the right of the abdomen, it may indicate a full bladder. By about 10 days postpartum, the uterus will be in the symphysis pubis area.

Test-Taking Strategy: Note the subject, height of the fundus after delivery, and visualize the process of involution. Remember that after delivery, the uterine fundus would be at the level of the umbilicus or 1 to 3 fingerbreadths below it and in the midline of the abdomen.

13. 4

Rationale: During the first 24 hours postpartum, the mother's temperature may be elevated as a result of dehydration. However, if the temperature is more than 2°F above normal, this may indicate infection, and the PHCP will need to be notified. Applying cool packs to the abdomen is an inappropriate action, and, additionally, this action requires a prescription. The remaining options may be a component of care but are not the most appropriate based on the data in the question.

Test-Taking Strategy: Focus on the subject, a temperature of 102°F 4 hours after delivery. Noting that this temperature is extreme compared with the normal temperature will direct you to the correct option.

14. 4

Rationale: The application of ice will reduce the swelling caused by hematoma formation in the vulvar area. Checking the vital signs and performing fundal massage every 4 hours and preparing a heat pack for the perineal area will not reduce swelling.

Test-Taking Strategy: Focus on the subject, the reduction of swelling. This will assist you with eliminating monitoring vital signs and performing fundal massage. Recalling the principles related to heat and cold will direct you to the correct option.

15. 1
Rationale: Stasis is believed to be a major predisposing factor for the development of thrombophlebitis. Because cesarean delivery poses a risk factor, the client needs to ambulate early and frequently to promote circulation and prevent stasis.

Wearing support stockings, applying warm, moist packs to the legs and maintaining bed rest with legs elevated are implemented if thrombophlebitis occurs.

Test-Taking Strategy: Focus on the subject, the prevention of thrombophlebitis, and note the strategic word, *priority*. Applying warm, moist packs to the legs and maintaining bed rest with legs elevated are implemented if thrombophlebitis occurs. Although wearing support stockings may be prescribed in the postoperative period to promote venous return, ambulating frequently is the priority preventive measure.

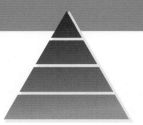

CHAPTER 26

Care of the Newborn

Maternity Nursing

PRIORITY CONCEPTS Development; Health Promotion

WHAT WOULD YOU DO?

The nurse is assisting with collecting initial data on a newborn and notes that the newborn is experiencing tremors. What would the nurse do?
Answer is located on p. 335.

 I. Initial Care of the Newborn

A. Data collection
1. Observe or assist with the initiation of respirations.
2. Determine Apgar score.
3. Note characteristics of cry.
4. Monitor for nasal flaring, grunting, retractions, and abnormal respirations, such as a seesaw respiratory pattern (rise and fall of the chest and abdomen do not occur together).
5. Check for central cyanosis and acrocyanosis.
6. Obtain vital signs.
7. Observe the newborn for signs of hypothermia or hyperthermia.
8. Check for gross anomalies.

B. Interventions
1. Suction the mouth first and then the nares with a bulb syringe.
2. Dry the newborn and stimulate crying by rubbing.
3. Maintain temperature stability; wrap the newborn in warm blankets and place a stockinette cap on the newborn's head.
4. Keep the newborn with the mother to facilitate bonding.
5. Place the newborn at the mother's breast if breastfeeding is planned, or place the newborn on the mother's abdomen.
6. Place the newborn in a radiant warmer.
7. Ensure proper identification.
8. Footprint the newborn and fingerprint the mother on the identification sheet per agency policies and procedures; initiate other agency identification and safety procedures.

9. Place matching identification bracelets on the mother and the newborn.

C. Apgar scoring system
1. Assess each of the five items to be scored and add the points assessed for each item to determine the newborn's total score.
2. Five vital indicators (Table 26.1)
3. Interventions: Apgar score (Table 26.2)

⚠ The newborn's Apgar score is routinely assessed and recorded at 1 minute and 5 minutes after birth and may be repeated later if the score is and remains low.

II. Initial Physical Examination

A. General guidelines
1. Keep the newborn warm during the examination.
2. Begin with general observations; then first perform the assessments that are the least disturbing to the newborn.
3. Initiate nursing interventions for abnormal findings and document findings.
4. The Ballard Scale may be used for gestational age assessment; in this scale, scores are assigned to physical and neurological criteria.

⚠ The phases of newborn instability occur during the first 6 to 8 hours after birth and are known as the transition period between intrauterine and extrauterine existence. These phases include the first period of reactivity, period of decreased responsiveness, and second period of reactivity.

B. Vital signs
1. Heart rate (resting): 120 to 160 beats per minute (apical), 80 to 100 beats per minute (if sleeping), up to 180 beats per minute (if crying); auscultate at the fourth intercostal space for 1 full minute to detect abnormalities.
2. Respirations: 30 to 60 breaths per minute; assess for 1 full minute.

TABLE 26.1   The Five Vital Indicators of the Apgar Score

Indicator	0 Points	1 Point	2 Points
Heart rate	Absent	<100 beats per minute	>100 beats per minute
Respiratory rate/effort	Absent	Slow, irregular breathing, weak cry	Good rate and effort, vigorous cry
Muscle tone	Flaccid, limp	Minimal flexion of the extremities	Good flexion, active motion
Reflex irritability	No response	Minimal response (grimace) to suction or the gentle slap on the soles	Responds promptly with a cry or active movement
Skin color	Pallor or cyanosis	Body skin color normal, extremities blue	Body and extremity skin color normal

TABLE 26.2   Apgar Score Interventions

Score	Intervention
8–10	No intervention except support the newborn's spontaneous efforts
4–7	Stimulate; rub the newborn's back Administer oxygen to the newborn; rescore at specific intervals
0–3	Newborn requires full resuscitation; rescore at specific intervals

Note: The newborn's Apgar score obtained at 5 minutes of age reflects the efficacy of any initial resuscitation efforts.

TABLE 26.3   Fontanels

Location	Characteristics	Closure
Anterior	Soft, flat, and diamond-shaped; 3–4 cm wide by 2–3 cm long	Between the ages of 12 and 18 months
Posterior	Triangular, 0.5–1 cm wide; located between the occipital and parietal bones	Between birth and the age of 2 or 3 months

3. Assess heart rate and respiratory rate first, before assessing other vital signs while the newborn is resting or sleeping.
4. Axillary temperature: 97.7°F (37°C) to 99°F (36.5°C) to <100.3°F (37.9°C)
5. Blood pressure: Usually not done in term newborn unless a cardiac issue is suspected, 80–90/40–50 mm Hg

C. Body measurements (approximate)
  1. Length: 45-55 cm (18 to 22 inches)
  2. Weight: 2500 to 4000 g (5.5–8.75 lb)
  3. Head circumference: 33 to 35 cm (13.2–14 inches)

D. Head
  1. Head would be one-fourth of the body length (cephalocaudal development).
  2. Bones of the skull are not fused.
  3. Sutures (connective tissue between the skull bones) are palpable and may be overlapping because of head molding, but would not be widened.
  4. Fontanels are unossified membranous tissue at the junction of the sutures (Table 26.3)
  5. Molding is asymmetry of the head resulting from pressure in the birth canal; molding disappears in about 72 hours (Fig. 26.1).
  6. Masses from birth trauma
    a. Caput succedaneum is edema of the soft tissue over bone (crosses over the suture line); it subsides within a few days.
    b. Cephalhematoma is swelling caused by bleeding into an area between the bone and its periosteum (does not cross over the suture line); it usually is absorbed within 6 weeks with no treatment.
  7. Head lag
    a. Common when pulling the newborn to a sitting position
    b. When prone, the newborn needs to be able to lift the head slightly and turn the head from side to side.

E. Eyes
  1. Slate gray (light skin), dark blue, or brown-gray (dark skin)
  2. Symmetrical and clear
  3. Pupils equal, round, react to light and accommodation
  4. Blink reflex present
  5. Eyes cross because of weak extraocular muscles.
  6. Ability to track and fixate momentarily
  7. Red reflex is present.
  8. Eyelids often edematous as a result of pressure during the birth process and the effects of eye medication

F. Ears
  1. Symmetrical
  2. Firm cartilage with recoil
  3. Top of pinna on or above line drawn from outer canthus of eye
  4. Low-set ears associated with Down syndrome, renal anomalies, or other genetic or chromosomal syndromes

G. Nose
  1. Flat, broad, in center of face
  2. Obligatory nose breathing
  3. Occasional sneezing to remove obstructions
  4. Nares are patent and would not flare (flaring is an indication of respiratory distress).

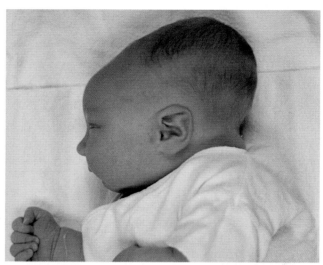

FIGURE 26.1 Molding. (A) Significant molding after vaginal birth. (B) Schematic of bones of skull when molding is present. (A, From Perry S, Hockenberry M, Lowdermilk D, Wilson D: *Maternal-child nursing care*, ed 4, St. Louis, 2010, Mosby. Courtesy Kim Molloy, Knoxville, IA.)

H. Mouth
   1. Pink, moist gums
   2. Soft and hard palates intact
   3. Epstein's pearls (small, white cysts) may be present on the hard palate.
   4. Uvula in midline
   5. Freely moving tongue, symmetrical, has short frenulum
   6. Symmetrical sucking and crying movements
   7. Able to swallow.
   8. Root and gag reflexes present.

⚠ When assessing the newborn's mouth, look for the presence of thrush (Candida albicans), which are white patchy areas on the tongue or gums that cannot be removed with a washcloth; these may be painful.

I. Neck
   1. Short and thick
   2. Head held in midline
   3. Trachea in midline
   4. Good range of motion and ability to flex and extend
   5. Check for torticollis (head inclined to one side as a result of contraction of muscles on that side of the neck).

 J. Chest
   1. Circular appearance because anteroposterior and lateral diameters are about equal (approximately 30–33 cm [12–13.2 inches] at birth)
   2. Diaphragmatic respirations—chest and abdomen would rise and fall in synchrony, not in a *seesaw* pattern.
   3. Bronchial sounds heard during auscultation
   4. Nipples prominent and often edematous; milky secretion (witch's milk) common.

   5. Breast tissue present.
   6. Clavicles need to be palpated to assess for fractures.

K. Skin
   1. Pinkish-red (light-skinned newborn) to pinkish-brown or pinkish-yellow (dark-skinned newborn)
   2. Vernix caseosa is a cheesy white substance on the entire body in preterm newborns, but is more prominent between folds closer to term; may be absent after 42 weeks of gestation.
   3. Lanugo, fine body hair, might be seen, especially on the back.
   4. Milia, small white sebaceous glands, appear on the forehead, nose, and chin.
   5. Dry, peeling skin, increased in postmature newborns
   6. Dark red color (plethoric) common in premature newborns
   7. Cyanosis may be noted with hypothermia, infection, and hypoglycemia, and with cardiac, respiratory, or neurological abnormalities.
   8. Acrocyanosis (peripheral cyanosis of hands and feet) is normal in the first few hours after birth and may be noted intermittently for the next 7 to 10 days (Fig. 26.2).
   9. Check for ecchymosis and petechiae as a result of the trauma of birth.
   10. Check the skin turgor over the abdomen to determine hydration status.
   11. Observe for forceps marks.
   12. Harlequin sign
       a. Deep pink or red color develops over one side of the newborn's body, while the other side remains pale or of normal color.
       b. Harlequin may indicate shunting of blood that occurs with a cardiac problem or may indicate sepsis.
   13. Birthmarks (Table 26.4)

L. Abdomen
   1. Umbilical cord
       a. Umbilical cord would have three vessels—two arteries and one vein; if fewer than three vessels are noted, notify the primary health care provider (PHCP).
       b. Although a two-vessel cord (one artery, one vein) may present no problems or concerns, there is a higher correlation to intrauterine growth restriction (IUGR) and genetic or chromosomal problems.
       c. Small, thin cord may be associated with poor fetal growth.
       d. Check for an intact cord and ensure that the cord clamp is secured.
       e. Cord needs to be clamped for at least the first 24 hours after birth; clamp can be removed

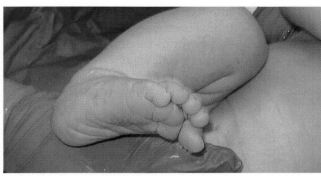

FIGURE 26.2 Acrocyanosis. (From McKinney E, James S, Murray S, Ashwill J: *Maternal-child nursing,* ed 4, St. Louis, 2013, Saunders. Courtesy Todd Shiros, Santa Fe Springs, CA.)

TABLE 26.4   Birthmarks

Birthmark	Characteristics
Telangiectatic nevi (stork bites)	Pale pink or red, flat, dilated capillaries
	On eyelids, nose, lower occipital bone, and nape of neck
	Blanch easily
	More noticeable during crying periods
	Disappear by age 2 years
Nevus flammeus (port-wine stain)	Capillary angioma directly below epidermis
	Nonelevated, sharply demarcated, red to purple, dense areas of capillaries
	Commonly appear on face
	No fading with time
	May require future surgery
Nevus vasculosus (strawberry mark)	Capillary hemangioma
	Raised, clearly delineated, dark red, with rough surface
	Common in head region
	Disappears by age 7–9 years
Mongolian spots	Bluish-black pigmentation
	On lumbar dorsal area and buttocks
	Gradually fade during first and second years of life
	Common in Asian and dark-skinned individuals

when the cord is dried and occluded and no longer bleeding.

   f. Note any bleeding or drainage from the cord.

   g. Cleansing of the cord needs to be done; hospital protocol and PHCP's preference determine the frequency, technique, and skin preparation used for cord care.

   h. If signs of infection, such as moistness, oozing, discharge, and a reddened base occur, antibiotic treatment is prescribed.

2. Gastrointestinal

   a. Monitor cord for meconium staining.

   b. The newborn will be checked for the presence of an umbilical hernia.

   c. Note and report to RN any abdominal depression that may be associated with diaphragmatic hernia.

   d. Note and report to RN any abdominal distention associated with obstruction, mass, or sepsis.

   e. Monitor bowel sounds (present within the first hour after birth).

3. Anus

   a. Ensure that anal opening is present.

   b. First stool meconium would pass within the first 24 hours.

M. Genitals

1. Female

   a. Labia may be swollen; clitoris may be enlarged.

   b. Smegma may be present (thick, white mucus discharge).

   c. Pseudomenstruation, caused by the withdrawal of the maternal hormone estrogen, is possible (blood-tinged mucus).

   d. Hymen tag may be visible.

   e. First voiding would occur within 24 hours.

2. Male

   a. Prepuce (foreskin) covers glans penis.

   b. Scrotum may be edematous.

   c. Verify meatus at tip of penis.

   d. Testes are descended, but may retract if the infant becomes chilled.

   e. The newborn is checked for hernia or hydrocele.

   f. First voiding would occur within 24 hours.

N. Spine

1. Straight

2. Posture flexed

3. Supportive of head momentarily when prone

4. Chin flexed on upper chest

5. Well-coordinated sporadic movements

6. A degree of hypotonicity or hypertonicity may indicate central nervous system damage.

7. Check for hair tufts and dimples along the spinal column (may be indicative of a possible opening).

O. Extremities

1. Flexed

2. Full range of motion; symmetrical movements

3. Fists clenched

4. Ten fingers and ten toes, all separate

5. Legs bowed

6. Major gluteal folds are even.

7. Creases on soles of feet

8. The newborn will be checked for fractures (especially clavicle) or dislocations (hip).
9. The newborn will be checked for developmental dysplasia of the hip; when the thighs are rotated outward, no clicks would be heard. (Ortolani's sign and Barlow's sign are two assessment tools that the PHCP may use to assess for developmental dysplasia of the hip.)
10. Pulses palpable (radial, brachial, and femoral)

 Slight tremors noted in the newborn may be a common finding, but they could also be a sign of hypoglycemia or drug withdrawal.

III. Body Systems: Data Collection and Interventions

 A. Cardiovascular system
1. Keep the newborn warm.
2. Measure the apical heart rate for 1 full minute.
3. The PHCP will listen for murmurs; assess oxygen saturation via pulse oximetry if a murmur is heard.
4. Palpate pulses.
5. Assess for cyanosis; blanch the skin on the trunk and extremities to assess circulation.
6. Observe for cardiac distress when the newborn is feeding.

B. Respiratory system
1. Suction the airway as necessary: Use a bulb syringe for upper airway suctioning (compress bulb before insertion) and a French catheter for deeper suctioning.
2. Observe for respiratory distress and hypoxemia.
   a. Nasal flaring
   b. Increasingly severe retractions
   c. Grunting
   d. Cyanosis
   e. Bradycardia and periods of apnea that last more than 15 seconds
3. Administer oxygen if necessary and as prescribed.

C. Hepatic system
1. Normal or physiological jaundice appears after the first 24 hours in full-term newborns and after the first 48 hours in premature newborns; jaundice occurring before this time (pathological jaundice) may indicate early hemolysis of red blood cells and must be reported to the PHCP.
2. Physiological jaundice peaks about the fifth day of life (indirect bilirubin levels: 6–7 mg/dL).
3. Feed early to stimulate intestinal activity and to keep the bilirubin level low.
4. Prevent chilling, because hypothermia can cause acidosis, which interferes with bilirubin conjugation and excretion.
5. Liver stores the iron passed from the mother for 5 or 6 months.
6. Glycogen storage occurs in the liver.
7. The newborn is at risk for hemorrhagic disorders. Coagulation factors synthesized in the liver depend on vitamin K, which is not synthesized until intestinal bacteria are present.
8. Handle the newborn carefully and monitor for any bruising or bleeding episodes.
9. Watch for meconium stool and subsequent stools.
10. Administer intramuscular phytonadione to the newborn as prescribed to prevent hemorrhagic disorders (usually 0.5–1 mg is prescribed); administer in lateral aspect of the middle third of the vastus lateralis muscle (see Chapter 38).
11. Assess newborn's hemoglobin and blood glucose levels.

D. Renal system
1. The immature kidneys are unable to concentrate urine.
2. A weight loss of approximately 5% to 10% occurs as a result of water loss and limited intake; birth weight would be regained by 10 to 14 days after birth.
3. Weigh the newborn daily.
4. Monitor intake and output; weigh diapers if necessary (1 g of diaper weight equals 1 mL of urine).
5. If the diaper requires weighing, record the weight before putting it on the newborn; after the newborn voids, reweigh the diaper and subtract the prevoided weight.
6. Assess for signs of dehydration (dry mucous membranes, sunken eyeballs, poor skin turgor, sunken fontanels).

E. Immune system
1. Newborn receives passive immunity via the **placenta** (immunoglobulin G).
2. Newborn receives passive immunity from the colostrum (immunoglobulin A).
3. Elevations in immunoglobulin M indicate infection in utero.
4. Use aseptic technique and standard precautions when caring for the newborn.
5. Ensure meticulous hand washing.
6. Ensure that infection-free staff members care for the newborn.
7. Monitor the newborn's temperature.
8. Observe for any cracks or openings in the skin.
9. Administer eye medication within 1 hour after birth to prevent ophthalmia neonatorum (see Chapter 27).
10. Provide cord care.
    a. Umbilical clamp can be removed after 24 hours if cord is dried and occluded and is not bleeding.
    b. Reinforce instructions to the mother how to perform cord care.
    c. Keep the cord clean and dry; alcohol or other solution may be prescribed for cleaning the cord if the cord becomes soiled.
    d. Keep the diaper from covering the cord; fold the diaper below it.

e. Monitor the cord for odor, edema, or discharge.

f. The newborn is typically washed via a sponge bath until the cord falls off (within 7–10 days). Follow alternate instructions if provided by PHCP.

11. Provide circumcision care.

   a. Apply petroleum jelly gauze to the penis, except when a PlastiBell is used.

   b. Remove the petroleum jelly gauze, if applied, after the first voiding following the circumcision.

   c. Observe for edema, infection, or bleeding from the circumcision site.

   d. Reinforce instructions to the mother how to care for the circumcision site.

   e. Clean the penis after each voiding by squeezing warm water over it.

   f. A milky covering over the glans penis is normal and should not be disrupted.

   g. Monitor for urinary retention.

F. Metabolic and gastrointestinal system

1. Newborns are able to digest simple carbohydrates, but are unable to digest fats because of a lack of lipase.

2. Proteins may be broken down only partially, so they may serve as antigens and provoke an allergic reaction.

3. The newborn has a small stomach capacity (less than 10 mL at birth, increasing to about 90 mL by day 10), with rapid intestinal peristalsis (bowel emptying time is 2.5–3 hours).

4. Breast-feeding usually can begin immediately after birth; based on PHCP preference and agency protocols, bottle-fed newborns may be initially offered no more than 30 mL of formula.

5. Observe feeding reflexes, such as rooting, sucking, and swallowing.

6. Assist the mother with breast-feeding or formula feeding; breast-feeding needs to be done every 2 to 3 hours, and formula feeding (minimum of 30 mL, or 1 oz) needs to be done every 3 to 4 hours (or per PHCP preference or agency protocols).

7. Burp the newborn during and after feeding.

8. Monitor for regurgitation or vomiting.

9. Position the newborn on the right side after feeding; however, the side-lying position is not recommended for sleep because this position makes it easy for the newborn to roll to the prone position (prone position is contraindicated because it increases the risk of sudden infant death syndrome).

10. Observe for normal stool and the passage of meconium.

   a. Meconium stool, which is greenish-black with a thick, sticky, tar-like consistency, is usually passed within the first 24 hours of life.

   b. Transitional stool, the second type of stool excreted by the newborn, is greenish-brown and of looser consistency than meconium.

   c. Seedy, yellow stools are usually noted in breast-fed newborns; pale yellow to light brown stools are usually seen in formula-fed newborns.

11. Assist with performing a screening test (including the test for phenylketonuria [PKU]), as prescribed, before discharge and after sufficient protein intake occurs; the newborn should be receiving formula or breast milk for a minimum of 24 hours before screening.

G. Neurological system

1. Newborn head size is proportionally larger than that of an adult because of cephalocaudal development.

2. Myelinization of the nerve fibers is incomplete, so primitive reflexes are present.

3. Fontanels are open to allow for brain growth.

4. Assess for an abnormal head size and a bulging or depressed anterior fontanel.

5. Measure and graph the head circumference in relation to the chest circumference and length.

6. Assess the newborn's movements, noting symmetry, posture, and abnormal movements.

7. Observe for jitteriness, marked tremors, and seizures.

8. The newborn's reflexes will be tested.

9. Assist in assessment for lethargy.

10. Assist in assessment of the pitch of cry.

H. Thermal regulatory system

1. Prevent cold stress (Fig. 26.3).

2. Newborns do not shiver to produce heat.

3. Newborns have brown fat deposits, which produce heat.

4. Prevent heat loss resulting from evaporation by keeping the newborn dry and well wrapped with a blanket.

5. Prevent heat loss resulting from radiation by keeping the newborn away from cold objects and outside walls.

6. Prevent heat loss resulting from convection by shielding the newborn from drafts.

7. Prevent heat loss that results from conduction by performing all treatments on a warm, padded surface.

8. Keep the room temperature warm.

9. Take the newborn's axillary temperature every hour for the first 4 hours of life, every 4 hours for the remainder of the first 24 hours, and then every shift (as per agency protocol).

 Cold stress causes oxygen consumption and energy to be diverted from maintaining normal brain cell function and cardiac function, resulting in serious metabolic and physiological conditions.

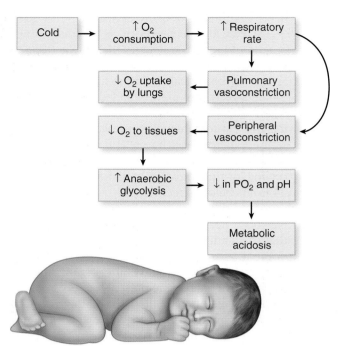

FIGURE 26.3 Effects of cold stress. When a newborn is stressed by cold, oxygen (O₂) consumption increases, and pulmonary and peripheral vasoconstriction occur, decreasing O₂ uptake by the lungs and O₂ delivery to the tissues; anaerobic glycolysis increases; and there is a decrease in partial pressure of oxygen (Po₂) and pH, leading to metabolic acidosis.

I. Reflexes

1. Sucking and rooting
   a. Touch the newborn's lip, cheek, or the corner of the mouth with a nipple.
   b. The newborn turns the head toward the nipple, opens the mouth, takes hold of the nipple, and sucks.
   c. Rooting reflex usually disappears after 3 to 4 months, but may persist for 1 year.
2. Swallowing reflex
   a. Swallowing reflex occurs spontaneously after sucking and obtaining fluids.
   b. Newborn swallows in coordination with sucking without gagging, coughing, or vomiting.
3. Tonic neck or fencing
   a. While the newborn is falling asleep or sleeping, the head is turned gently and quickly to one side.
   b. As the newborn faces the left side, the left arm and leg extend outward, and the right arm and leg flex.
   c. When the head is turned to the right side, the right arm and leg extend outward, and the left arm and leg flex.
   d. Response usually disappears within 3 to 4 months
4. Palmar–plantar grasp
   a. Place a finger in the palm of the newborn's hand and then place a finger at the base of the toes.
   b. The newborn's fingers curl around the examiner's fingers, and the newborn's toes curl downward.
   c. Palmar response lessens within 3 to 4 months.
   d. Plantar response lessens within 8 months.
5. Moro reflex
   a. Hold the newborn in a semi-sitting position and then allow the head and trunk to fall backward to at least a 30-degree angle.
   b. The newborn assumes sharp extension and abduction of the arms with the thumbs and forefingers in a "C" position; this is followed by flexion and adduction to an "embrace" position (legs following a similar pattern).
   c. The Moro reflex is present at birth and is absent by 6 months of age if neurological maturation is not delayed.
   d. A body jerk motion may be the response between 8 to 18 weeks.
   e. A persistent response lasting more than 6 months may indicate neurological abnormality.
6. Startle reflex (often considered the same as the Moro reflex, but the response is different)
   a. The response is best elicited if the newborn is at least 24 hours old.
   b. The examiner makes a loud noise or claps the hands to elicit the response.
   c. The newborn's arms adduct, whereas the elbows flex.
   d. The hands stay clenched.
   e. The reflex would disappear within 4 months.
7. Pull-to-sit response
   a. Pull the newborn up from the wrist while the newborn is in the flat position.
   b. The head lags until the newborn is in an upright position and then the head is level with the chest and shoulders momentarily before falling forward.
   c. The head will then lift for a few minutes.
   d. The response depends on the newborn's general muscle tone and condition and on maturity level.
8. Babinski sign: Plantar reflex
   a. Beginning at the heel of the foot, use a finger to stroke gently upward along the lateral aspect of the sole and then move the finger along the ball of the foot.
   b. The newborn's toes hyperextend, whereas the big toe dorsiflexes.
   c. This reflex disappears after the newborn is 1 year old.
   d. Absence of this reflex indicates the need for a neurological examination.
9. Stepping or walking
   a. Hold the newborn in a vertical position, allowing one foot to touch a table surface.

b. The newborn simulates walking, alternately flexing and extending the feet.

c. The reflex is usually present for 3 to 4 months.

10. Crawling

  a. The newborn is placed on the abdomen.

  b. The newborn begins making crawling movements with the arms and legs.

  c. The reflex usually disappears after about 6 weeks.

IV. Newborn Safety

A. Newborn identification

  1. Information bracelets are applied to the mother and the newborn immediately after birth and before the mother and the newborn are separated; in addition, the newborn's identification pictures and footprints may be obtained before leaving the mother's side in the delivery room.

  2. The bracelets include name, sex, date, time of birth, and identification numbers.

  3. Some agencies use identification bracelets that have radiofrequency transmitters that set off alarms if the newborn is removed from a certain area.

  4. Agencies also conduct unit and hospital-wide drills to prevent newborn abductions.

B. Newborn abduction

  1. The mother is taught to check the identification of any person who comes to remove the baby from her room and is taught other precautions to prevent newborn abduction (nurses must be wearing photo identification or some other security badge) (Box 26.1).

  2. Closed-circuit televisions, code-alert bands, or computer monitoring systems may be used on some units.

  3. The newborn is wheeled in a bassinette rather than carried in a staff member's arms.

BOX 26.1	Precautions to Prevent Infant Abductions

- All personnel must wear identification that is easily visible at all times.
- Teach parents to only allow hospital staff with proper identification to take their newborn from them.
- Question anyone with a newborn near an exit or in an unusual part of the facility.
- Never leave a newborn unattended.
- Teach the parents that the newborn must be observed at all times.
- When the newborn is in the mother's room, position the crib away from the doorway.
- Teach the parents home safety precautions: suggest that the parents do not place announcements in the paper or signs in their yard that may alert an abductor that a new baby is in the home.

V. Reinforce Parent Teaching

A. Formula feeding

  1. Teach sterilization techniques if the water supply is from an area where the purification process of the water is questionable.

  2. Remind the mother not to heat the bottle of formula in a microwave oven.

  3. Inform the mother that formula is a sufficient diet for the first 4 to 6 months.

  4. Assess the mother's ability to burp the newborn.

B. Breast-feeding

  1. Assess the newborn's ability to attach to the mother's breast and suck (Fig. 26.4).

  2. Teach the mother how to pump her breasts and how to store breast milk properly.

  3. Inform the mother that breast milk is a sufficient diet for the first 4 to 6 months.

  4. Give the mother the phone numbers of local organizations that offer support to breast-feeding mothers.

C. Bathing

  1. Bathe the newborn in a warm room before feeding.

  2. Have all equipment for bathing available.

  3. Use a mild soap (not on the face).

  4. Proceed from the cleanest area to the dirtiest area.

  5. Clean eyes from the inner canthus outward.

  6. Special care needs to be taken to clean under the folds of the neck, the underarms, groin, and genital area.

  7. Make bath time enjoyable for both the newborn and the mother.

D. Clothing

  1. Assess diaper and clothing needs for the newborn with the mother.

  2. Instruct the mother that the newborn's head needs to be covered during cold weather to prevent heat loss.

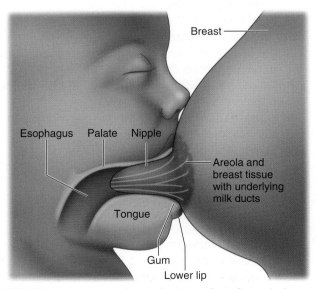

FIGURE 26.4 Correct attachment (latch-on) of an infant at the breast.

3. Instruct the mother to layer the newborn's clothing in cooler weather.

4. To be comfortable, the newborn needs to be dressed in one more layer of clothing than what the parents are wearing.

E. Cord care: See earlier for cord care, "Body Systems Assessment and Interventions."

F. Circumcision: See earlier for circumcision care, "Body Systems: Data Collection and Interventions."

G. Uncircumcised newborn

1. Inform the mother that the foreskin and glans are two similar layers of cells that separate from each other and that the separation process is normally complete by 3 years of age, but can remain adhered until puberty.

2. Instruct the mother not to pull back the foreskin but rather to allow for the natural separation to occur.

3. Inform the mother that as the process of separation occurs, sterile sloughed cells build up between the layers of the foreskin and the glans. When retraction occurs, daily gentle washing of the glans with soap and water is sufficient to maintain adequate cleanliness.

H. Stimulation: Providing stimulation to the newborn such as touching, cuddling, or talking is an important intervention.

VI. Preterm Newborn

A. Description
   1. An **infant** born before 37 weeks of gestation
   2. Primary concern relates to the immaturity of all body systems.

B. Data collection
   1. Respirations are irregular with periods of apnea.
   2. Body temperature is below normal.
   3. The newborn has poor suck and swallow reflexes.
   4. Bowel sounds are diminished.
   5. Urinary output is increased or decreased.
   6. Extremities are thin, with minimal creasing on the soles and palms.
   7. The newborn extends extremities and does not maintain flexion.
   8. Lanugo, on skin and in the hair on the newborn's head, is present in woolly patches.
   9. Skin is thin, with visible blood vessels and minimal subcutaneous fat pads.
   10. Skin may appear jaundiced.
   11. Testes are undescended in boys.
   12. Labia are narrow in girls.

C. Interventions
   1. Monitor vital signs every 2 to 4 hours.
   2. Maintain airway and cardiopulmonary functions.
   3. Administer oxygen and humidification as prescribed.
   4. Monitor intake and output and electrolyte balance.
   5. Monitor weight daily.

6. Maintain the newborn in a warming device.
7. Avoid exposure to infections.

VII. Post-Term Newborn

A. Description: Infant born after 42 weeks of gestation
B. Data collection
   1. Hypoglycemia
   2. Parchment-like skin (dry and cracked) without lanugo
   3. Fingernails long, extended over the ends of the fingers
   4. Profuse scalp hair
   5. Long and thin body
   6. Wasting of fat and muscle in extremities
   7. Meconium staining possible, present on nails and umbilical cord
C. Interventions
   1. Provide normal newborn care.
   2. Monitor for hypoglycemia.
   3. Maintain newborn's temperature.
   4. Monitor for meconium aspiration.

VIII. Small for Gestational Age

A. Description: Newborn who is plotted at or below the 10th percentile on the intrauterine growth curve
B. Data collection
   1. Fetal distress
   2. Decreased or elevated body temperature
   3. Physical abnormalities
   4. Hypoglycemia
   5. Signs of polycythemia
      a. Ruddy appearance
      b. Cyanosis
      c. Jaundice
   6. Signs of infection
   7. Signs of aspiration of meconium
C. Interventions
   1. Maintain airway and cardiopulmonary function.
   2. Maintain body temperature.
   3. Observe for signs of respiratory distress.
   4. Monitor for infection and initiate measures to prevent sepsis.
   5. Monitor for hypoglycemia.
   6. Initiate early feedings and monitor for signs of aspiration.

IX. Large for Gestational Age

A. Description: Newborn who is plotted at or above the 90th percentile on the intrauterine growth curve
B. Data collection
   1. Respiratory distress
   2. Birth trauma or injury
   3. Hypoglycemia
C. Interventions
   1. Monitor vital signs and for respiratory distress.
   2. Monitor for hypoglycemia.

3. Initiate early feedings.
4. Monitor for infection and initiate measures to prevent sepsis.

X. Respiratory Distress Syndrome

A. Description: Serious lung disorder caused by immaturity and the inability to produce surfactant, resulting in hypoxia and acidosis

B. Data collection
   1. Respiratory distress can include tachypnea, nasal flaring, expiratory grunting, retractions, seesaw respirations, decreased breath sounds, apnea.
   2. Pallor and cyanosis
   3. Hypothermia
   4. Poor muscle tone

C. Interventions
   1. Monitor color, respiratory rate, and degree of effort in breathing.
   2. Maintain airway and cardiopulmonary function and support respirations as prescribed.
   3. Monitor arterial blood gases and the oxygen saturation levels as prescribed (arterial blood gases from umbilical artery); ensure that oxygen administered to the newborn is at the lowest possible concentration necessary to maintain adequate arterial oxygenation.
   4. Any premature newborn who requires oxygen support needs to be scheduled for an eye examination before discharge to assess for retinal damage.
   5. Position the newborn on the side or back, with the neck slightly extended.
   6. Administer respiratory therapy (percussion and vibration), as prescribed; use a padded small plastic cup or a small oxygen mask for percussion; use a padded electric toothbrush for vibration.
   7. Provide nutrition.
   8. Support bonding.
   9. Assist to prepare parents for a short-term to long-term period of oxygen dependency, if necessary.
   10. Reinforce encouragement with the mother to pump the breasts for future breast-feeding of her newborn if she so desires.
   11. Encourage as much parental participation in the newborn's care as the condition allows.

⚠ Prepare to assist to administer surfactant replacement (instilled into endotracheal tube) to a newborn with respiratory distress syndrome.

XI. Meconium Aspiration Syndrome

A. Description
   1. Occurs in term or post-term newborns
   2. Exact etiology is unknown, but the release of meconium into the amniotic fluid is thought to be related to a stressful fetal event initiating a biochemical chain of events.
   3. Aspiration can occur in utero or with the first breath.

B. Data collection
   1. Respiratory distress is present at birth; tachypnea, cyanosis, retractions, nasal flaring, grunting, crackles, and rhonchi may be present.
   2. The newborn's nails, skin, and umbilical cord may be stained a yellow-green color.

C. Interventions
   1. If the newborn is delivered in an active crying state with no evidence of respiratory distress, no intervention is necessary.
   2. If the newborn is delivered and exhibits inactivity and lack of cry, endotracheal suctioning is performed. If the newborn also exhibits lack of respiratory effort and a low heart rate, additional interventions will be needed.
   3. Newborns with severe meconium aspiration syndrome may benefit from extracorporeal membrane oxygenation; this therapy uses a modified heart-lung machine and provides oxygen to circulation, allowing the lungs to rest and decreasing pulmonary hypertension and hypoxemia in some conditions, such as meconium aspiration.

XII. Bronchopulmonary Dysplasia (BPD)

A. Description
   1. This chronic pulmonary condition affects newborns who have experienced respiratory failure or have been oxygen dependent for more than 28 days.
   2. X-ray findings are abnormal, indicating areas of over-inflation and atelectasis.

B. Data collection
   1. Tachypnea
   2. Tachycardia
   3. Retraction
   4. Nasal flaring
   5. Labored breathing
   6. Crackles and decreased air movement
   7. Occasional expiratory wheezing

C. Interventions
   1. Monitor airway and cardiopulmonary function; provide oxygen therapy.
   2. Fluid restriction may be prescribed.
   3. Medications include surfactant at birth, bronchodilators, and possibly diuretics, and corticosteroids.

XIII. Transient Tachypnea of the Newborn

A. Description
   1. Respiratory condition that results from the incomplete reabsorption of the fetal lung fluid in full-term newborns
   2. Usually disappears within 24 to 48 hours

B. Data collection
   1. Tachypnea
   2. Expiratory grunting

3. Retractions
4. Nasal flaring
5. Fluid breath sounds per auscultation
6. Cyanosis
C. Interventions
1. Supportive care
2. Oxygen administration

XIV. Intraventricular Hemorrhage

A. Description
1. Bleeding within the ventricles of the brain
2. Risk factors include prematurity, respiratory distress syndrome, trauma, or asphyxia.
B. Data collection: Diminished or absent Moro reflex, lethargy, apnea, poor feeding, high-pitched and shrill cry, seizure activity
C. Interventions: Supportive treatment

XV. Retinopathy of Prematurity

A. Description
1. Vascular disorder involving gradual replacement of retina by fibrous tissue and blood vessels
2. Primarily caused by prematurity and use of supplemental oxygen (>30 days)
B. Data collection: Leukocoria (white tissue on the retrolental space), vitreous hemorrhage, myopia, strabismus, cataracts (check for red reflex)
C. Interventions: Laser photocoagulation surgery

XVI. Necrotizing Enterocolitis (NEC)

A. Description
1. Acute inflammatory disease of the gastrointestinal tract
2. Usually occurs 4 to 10 days after birth and is most frequently seen in preterm newborns
B. Data collection: Increased abdominal girth, decreased or absent bowel sounds, bowel loop distension, vomiting, bile-stained emesis, abdominal tenderness, occult blood in the stools
C. Prevention
1. Withhold feedings for 24 to 48 hours from infants believed to have suffered birth asphyxia. Breast milk is the preferred nutrient after this time period.
2. The use of probiotics with enteral feedings and breast milk has shown evidence of prevention of NEC.
3. Administration of corticosteroids to the mother before birth to promote early gut closure and maturation of the gut mucosa
D. Interventions
1. Hold oral feedings.
2. Insert oral gastric tube to decompress the abdomen.
3. Intravenous antibiotics
4. Intravenous fluids to correct fluid, electrolyte, and acid-base imbalances
5. Surgery if indicated

XVII. Hyperbilirubinemia

A. Description
1. Elevated serum bilirubin level
2. Evaluation is indicated when serum bilirubin levels are more than 12 mg/dL in a term newborn.
3. Therapy is aimed at preventing kernicterus, which results in permanent neurological damage as a result of the deposition of bilirubin in the brain cells.
B. Data collection
1. Jaundice
2. Elevated serum bilirubin level
3. Enlarged liver
4. Poor muscle tone
5. Lethargy
6. Poor sucking reflex
C. Interventions
1. Monitor for the presence of jaundice; assess skin and sclera for jaundice.
   a. Examine the newborn's skin color in natural light.
   b. Press a finger over a bony prominence or the tip of the newborn's nose to press out capillary blood from the tissues.
   c. Note that jaundice starts at the head first and then spreads to the chest, abdomen, arms and legs, and the hands and feet, which are the last to be jaundiced.
2. Keep the newborn well hydrated to maintain blood volume.
3. Facilitate early, frequent feeding to hasten the passage of meconium and to encourage the excretion of bilirubin.
4. Report any signs of jaundice that present during the first 24 hours and any abnormal signs/symptoms to the RN and PHCP.
5. Prepare for phototherapy (bili-light or bili-blanket) and monitor the newborn closely during the treatment.

 At any serum bilirubin level, the appearance of jaundice during the first day of life indicates a pathological process.

D. Phototherapy
1. Description
   a. Phototherapy refers to the use of light to reduce serum bilirubin in the newborn.
   b. Adverse effects from treatment such as eye damage, dehydration, or sensory deprivation, can occur.
2. Interventions
   a. Follow specific instructions for phototherapy and bili-blanket care.
   b. Expose as much of the newborn's skin as possible.

c. Cover the genital area and monitor the genital area for skin irritation or breakdown.

d. Cover the newborn's eyes with shields or patches; make sure the eyelids are closed when shields or patches are applied.

e. Remove the shields or patches at least once per shift (during a feeding time) to inspect the eyes for infection or irritation and to allow for eye contact and bonding with the parents.

f. Measure the lamp energy output to ensure efficacy of the treatment (done with a special device known as a photometer).

g. Monitor skin temperature closely.

h. Increase fluids to compensate for water loss.

i. Expect loose green stools.

j. Monitor the newborn's skin color with the light turned off every 4 to 8 hours.

k. Monitor the skin for bronze baby syndrome, which is a grayish-brown discoloration of the skin, and a complication of phototherapy.

l. Reposition the newborn every 2 hours; monitor the newborn closely.

m. Provide stimulation.

n. If treatment is done at home, teach the parents about care and indications of the need to notify the PHCP.

o. After treatment, continue monitoring for signs of hyperbilirubinemia, because rebound elevations can occur after therapy is discontinued.

p. Turn off phototherapy lights before drawing a blood specimen for serum bilirubin levels and do not leave blood specimen uncovered under the lights (to prevent breakdown of bilirubin in blood specimen).

XVIII. Erythroblastosis Fetalis

A. Description

1. Erythroblastosis fetalis is the destruction of red blood cells that results from an antigen–antibody reaction.

2. The disorder is characterized by hemolytic anemia or hyperbilirubinemia.

3. Exchange of fetal and maternal blood takes place primarily when the placenta separates at birth (Fig. 26.5).

4. Antibodies are harmless to the mother but attach to the erythrocytes in the fetus and cause hemolysis.

5. Sensitization is rare with the first pregnancy.

6. ABO incompatibility is usually less severe.

B. Data collection

1. Anemia

2. Jaundice that develops rapidly after birth and before 24 hours

3. Edema

C. Interventions

1. Rh$_o$(D) immune globulin is administered to the mother during the first 72 hours after delivery if the Rh-negative mother delivers an Rh-positive fetus but remains unsensitized.

2. Assist with exchange transfusion after birth or intrauterine transfusion, as prescribed.

3. The newborn's blood is replaced with Rh-negative blood to stop the destruction of the baby's red blood cells. The Rh-negative blood is gradually replaced with the baby's own blood.

4. Provide support to the parents.

XIX. Sepsis

A. Description: Generalized infection resulting from the presence of bacteria in the blood, such as Group B streptococcal infection

B. Data Collection

1. Pallor

2. Tachypnea, tachycardia

3. Poor feeding

4. Abdominal distention

5. Temperature instability

C. Interventions

1. Assess for periods of apnea or irregular respirations.

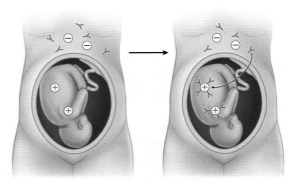

FIRST PREGNANCY

Rh-negative mother   Antibodies

A   Normal Rh-positive infant   Sensitization

SECOND PREGNANCY

B   Sensitized mother   Erythroblastosis fetalis

FIGURE 26.5 Development of maternal sensitization to Rh antigens. (A) Fetal Rh-positive erythrocytes enter the maternal system. Maternal anti-Rh antibodies are formed. (B) Anti-Rh antibodies cross placenta and attack fetal erythrocytes.

2. If apnea is present, stimulate by gently rubbing the chest or foot.

3. Administer oxygen as prescribed.

4. Monitor vital signs; check for fever.

5. Maintain warmth in a radiant warmer.

6. Provide isolation as necessary.

7. Monitor intake and output, and obtain daily weight.

8. Monitor for diarrhea.

9. Check feeding and sucking reflex, which may be poor.

10. Monitor for jaundice.

11. Observe for irritability and lethargy.

12. Assist in preparing for blood cultures and to administer antibiotics as prescribed, and observe carefully for toxicity because a newborn's liver and kidneys are immature.

XX. TORCH Syndrome (See Chapter 23)

XXI. Syphilis

A. Description

1. Syphilis is a sexually transmitted infection.

2. Congenital syphilis can result in premature delivery, skin lesions, and abnormal skeletal development.

3. The organism *Treponema pallidum*, a spirochete, can cross the placenta throughout pregnancy and infect the fetus, usually after 18 weeks' gestation.

4. Risks include preterm birth, stillbirth, and low birth weight.

5. Congenital effects are irreversible and may include central nervous system damage and hearing loss.

B. Data collection

1. Hepatosplenomegaly

2. Joint swelling

3. Palmar rash and lesions

4. Anemia

5. Jaundice

6. Snuffles

7. Ascites

8. Pneumonitis

9. Cerebrospinal fluid changes

C. Interventions

1. Monitor the newborn for signs of syphilis.

2. Prepare the newborn for serological testing, if prescribed.

3. Assist to administer antibiotic therapy as prescribed.

4. Use standard precautions and drainage and secretion (contact) precautions with suspected congenital syphilis.

5. Wear gloves when handling the neonate until antibiotic therapy has been administered for 24 hours.

6. Provide psychological support to the mother, and provide instructions regarding follow-up care of the newborn.

XXII. Addicted Newborn

A. Description

1. A newborn who has become passively addicted to drugs that have passed through the placenta

2. Data collection findings and withdrawal times may vary, depending on specific addicting drugs.

3. See also Fetal Alcohol Spectrum Disorders (FASDs)

B. Data collection

1. Irritability

2. Tremors

3. Hyperactivity and hypertonicity

4. Respiratory distress

5. Vomiting

6. High-pitched cry

7. Sneezing

8. Fever

9. Diarrhea

10. Excessive sweating

11. Poor feeding

12. Extreme sucking of fists

13. Seizures

C. Interventions

1. Monitor respiratory and cardiac status frequently.

2. Monitor temperature and vital signs.

3. Hold newborn firmly and close to the body during feeding and when giving care.

4. Initiate seizure precautions (pad the sides of the crib).

5. Provide small frequent feedings and allow a longer period for feeding.

6. Monitor intake and output.

7. Assist with administering intravenous hydration if prescribed.

8. Protect the newborn's skin from injury that can be caused by constant rubbing from hyperactive jitters.

9. Swaddle the newborn.

10. Place the newborn in a quiet room and reduce stimulation.

11. Allow the mother to express feelings such as anxiety and guilt.

12. Refer the mother for treatment of her substance abuse problem.

XXIII. Fetal Alcohol Spectrum Disorders (FASDs)

A. Description

1. FASDs are a group of conditions caused by maternal alcohol use during pregnancy.

2. The disorders are a result of teratogenesis.

3. FASDs cause cognitive and physical delays.

4. Fetal alcohol syndrome is the most severe of the FASDs. The other disorders included in this category are alcohol-related neurodevelopmental disorder (ARND) and alcohol-related birth defects (ARBDs).

B. Data collection
1. Facial changes
   a. Short palpebral fissures
   b. Hypoplastic philtrum
   c. Short, upturned nose
   d. Flat midface
   e. Thin upper lip
   f. Low nasal bridge
2. Abnormal palmar creases
3. Respiratory distress (apnea, cyanosis)
4. Congenital heart disorders
5. Irritability and hypersensitivity to stimuli
6. Tremors
7. Poor feeding
8. Seizures

C. Interventions
1. Monitor for respiratory distress.
2. Position the newborn on the side to facilitate drainage of secretions; initiate seizure precautions.
3. Keep resuscitation equipment at the bedside.
4. Monitor for hypoglycemia.
5. Assess suck and swallow reflex.
6. Administer small feedings and burp well.
7. Suction as necessary.
8. Monitor intake and output.
9. Monitor weight and head circumference.
10. Decrease environmental stimuli.
11. Make referral to local early intervention system.

 XXIV. Newborn of a Mother With Human Immunodeficiency Virus (HIV)

A. Description
1. The fetus of a mother who is positive for HIV antibody need to be monitored closely throughout the pregnancy.
2. Serial ultrasound screenings need to be done during pregnancy to identify IUGR.
3. Weekly nonstress testing after 32 weeks of gestation and biophysical profiles may be necessary during pregnancy.
4. Neonates born to HIV-positive clients may test positive because the mother's positive antibodies may persist for as long as 18 months after birth.
5. The use of antiviral medication, the reduction of neonate exposure to maternal blood and body fluids, and the early identification of HIV during pregnancy reduce the risk of transmission to the newborn.
6. All neonates born to HIV-positive mothers acquire maternal antibody to HIV infection, but not all acquire the infection.
7. The neonate may be asymptomatic for the first several years of life.

B. Transmission
1. Across placental barrier
2. During labor and birth

3. Breast milk (breast-feeding not done if the mother is HIV-positive; follow PHCP prescription)

C. Data collection
1. Possibly no outward signs at birth
2. Signs of immunodeficiency
3. Hepatomegaly
4. Splenomegaly
5. Lymphadenopathy
6. Impairment in growth and development

D. Interventions
1. Clean the newborn's skin carefully before any invasive procedure, such as the administration of phytonadione, heel sticks, or venipunctures.
2. Circumcisions are not done on newborns with HIV-positive mothers until the newborn's status is determined.
3. Newborn can room with mother.
4. All HIV-exposed newborns need to be treated with medication to prevent infection by *Pneumocystis jiroveci*.
5. Antiretroviral medication may be administered for the first 6 weeks of life or longer if prescribed.
6. Monitor for early signs of immunodeficiency, such as enlarged spleen or liver, lymphadenopathy, and impairment in growth and development.
7. Newborns at risk for HIV infection must be seen by the PHCP at birth and at 1 week, 2 weeks, 1 month, and 2 months of age.
8. Inform the mother that HIV culture is recommended at 1 month and 4 months of age.

E. Immunizations
1. Immunizations with live vaccines, such as measles–mumps–rubella, would not be done until the newborn's, infant's, or child's status is confirmed.
2. If infected, live vaccine will not be given.

 Newborns at risk for HIV infection need to receive all recommended immunizations according to the regular schedule; live vaccines are not administered until HIV status is determined.

XXV. Newborn of a Diabetic Mother

A. Description
1. Infant born to a mother with type 1 or type 2 diabetes or gestational diabetes
2. Hypoglycemia, hyperbilirubinemia, respiratory distress syndrome, hypocalcemia, birth trauma, and congenital anomalies may be present.

B. Data collection
1. Excessive size and weight as a result of excess fat and glycogen in tissues
2. Edema or puffiness in the face and cheeks
3. Signs of hypoglycemia, such as twitching, difficulty feeding, lethargy, apnea, seizure, and cyanosis

4. Hyperbilirubinemia

5. Signs of respiratory distress, such as tachypnea, cyanosis, retractions, grunting, and nasal flaring

C. Interventions

1. Monitor for signs of respiratory distress, birth trauma, and congenital anomalies.

2. Monitor bilirubin and blood glucose levels.

3. Monitor weight.

4. Feed the newborn soon after birth with glucose in water, breast milk, or formula, as prescribed.

5. Prepare to assist in administering intravenous glucose to treat hypoglycemia, if necessary and as prescribed.

6. Monitor for edema.

7. Monitor for respiratory distress, tremor, or seizure.

XXVI. Hypoglycemia

A. Description

1. Hypoglycemia is an abnormally low level of glucose in the blood (<45 mg/dL).

2. Normal blood glucose reference interval is 45 to 60 mg/dL in a 1-day-old newborn and 50 to 90 mg/dL in a newborn older than 1 day (institutional values for normal newborn blood glucose levels vary).

B. Data collection

1. Increased respiratory rate

2. Twitching, nervousness, or tremors

3. Unstable temperature

4. Lethargy, apnea, seizure, cyanosis

C. Interventions

1. Prevent low blood glucose through early feedings.

2. Administer formula orally or assist to administer glucose intravenously, as prescribed.

3. Monitor the blood glucose levels, as prescribed.

4. Monitor for feeding problems.

5. Monitor for apneic periods.

6. Monitor for shrill or intermittent cries.

7. Evaluate lethargy and poor muscle tone.

XXVII. Hypothyroidism

A. Description: Hypothyroidism refers to a decrease in the production of thyroid hormone.

B. Assessment

1. Protruding or thick tongue

2. Dull look

3. Decreased muscle tone

4. Laboratory results reveal low thyroid production.

C. Interventions: Focus on thyroid replacement.

XXVIII. Relief of Choking in an Infant

A. Description: Choking is also known as foreign body airway obstruction (FBAO).

B. Assessment

1. Signs of mild airway obstruction include good air exchange, ability to cough forcefully, and wheezing between coughs.

2. Signs of severe airway obstruction include poor or no air exchange, weak or ineffective cough or no cough, a high-pitched noise while inhaling or no noise, increased respiratory difficulty, cyanosis, and inability to cry.

C. Interventions

1. For mild obstruction, do not interfere with the infant's own attempts to expel the object. Stay with them and continue to monitor. If the obstruction persists, activate the emergency response system and relieve the obstruction.

2. Severe obstruction must be relieved as soon as possible (see Priority Nursing Actions).

PRIORITY NURSING ACTIONS

Choking Infant

1. Sit or kneel with the infant in your lap.
2. Remove clothing from the infant's chest if easily removed.
3. Hold the infant face down with the head lower than the chest while resting on your forearm. The infant's head and jaw must be supported with the hand. The forearm is rested on the thigh to support the infant (Fig. 26.6).
4. Deliver 5 back slaps between the infant's shoulder blades using the heel of the other hand with sufficient force. Place free hand on infant's back while supporting the back of the infant's head with the palm of the hand. Cradle the infant between the two forearms. Turn the infant as a unit while supporting the head and neck.
5. Rest the forearm on the thigh while holding the infant face up. Deliver 5 chest thrusts in the middle of the chest over the lower half of the sternum at a rate of 1 per second with enough force to dislodge the foreign body.
6. Repeat the sequence until the object is removed or the infant becomes unresponsive.
7. If the infant becomes unresponsive, call for help and activate the emergency response system.
8. Begin cardiopulmonary resuscitation (CPR) while checking for a foreign body each time the airway is opened. Do not perform blind finger sweeps.

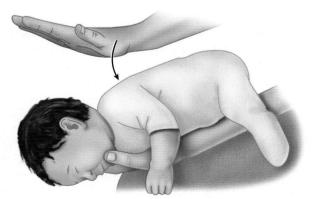

FIGURE 26.6 Relief of choking in the newborn infant.

XXIX. Cardiopulmonary Resuscitation (CPR) Guidelines for Infants

A. Description: Infants include individuals who are 1 year of age or less.

B. The American Heart Association 2020 updated guidelines for CPR can be found in the 2020 *American Heart Association Guidelines for Cardiopulmonary Resuscitation and Emergency Cardiovascular Care* at https://professional.heart.org/en/science-news/2020-aha-guidelines-for-cpr-and-ecc

WHAT WOULD YOU DO?

Answer: Slight tremors noted in the newborn may be a common finding but could also be a sign of hypoglycemia, hypocalcemia, or drug withdrawal. The nurse must notify the registered nurse immediately. Determination of the cause of the tremors is necessary so that treatment can be initiated immediately. This finding must also be immediately reported to the primary health care provider.

PRACTICE QUESTIONS

1. The nurse administers erythromycin ointment (0.5%) to the newborn's eyes and the mother asks the nurse why this is done. The nurse would give which response to the client?
   1. Prevents cataracts in the neonate born to a woman who is susceptible to rubella
   2. Protects the neonate's eyes from possible infections acquired while hospitalized
   3. Minimizes the spread of microorganisms to the neonate from invasive procedures during labor
   4. Prevents ophthalmia neonatorum from occurring after delivery to a neonate born to a woman with an untreated gonococcal infection

2. A client asks the nurse why her newborn baby needs an injection of vitamin K (phytonadione). The nurse would make which statement to the client?
   1. "Your newborn needs vitamin K to develop immunity."
   2. "The vitamin K will protect your newborn from becoming jaundiced."
   3. "Newborns are deficient in vitamin K. This injection prevents your baby from abnormal bleeding."
   4. "Newborns have sterile bowels. The vitamin K will give the bowel the necessary bacteria."

3. The nurse is assigned to assist with caring for a neonate born to a mother who is human immunodeficiency virus (HIV)-positive. The nurse understands that which of these need to be included in the plan of care?
   1. Monitoring the neonate's vital signs routinely
   2. Maintaining standard precautions at all times while caring for the neonate
   3. Instructing breast-feeding mothers regarding the treatment of their nipples with an antifungal cream
   4. Initiating a referral to evaluate for blindness, deafness, learning, or behavioral problems in the neonate

4. The nurse in the newborn nursery receives a telephone call to prepare for the admission of a neonate born at 43 weeks' gestation with Apgar scores of 1 and 4. When planning for the admission of this infant, which is the nurse's **highest priority**?
   1. Turning on the apnea and cardiorespiratory monitor
   2. Connecting the resuscitation bag to the oxygen outlet
   3. Setting up the intravenous line with 5% dextrose in water
   4. Setting the radiant warmer control temperature at 36.5°C (97.6°F)

5. The nurse is assisting in caring for a post-term neonate immediately after admission to the nursery. The **priority** nursing action would be to monitor which clinical parameter?
   1. Urinary output
   2. Blood glucose level
   3. Total bilirubin level
   4. Hemoglobin and hematocrit levels

6. The nurse is reinforcing instructions to a new mother about cord care and how to monitor for the presence of an infection. The nurse would tell the mother that which is a sign of infection?
   1. A darkened drying stump
   2. A moist cord with discharge
   3. A purple stump that shows pinkness around the base
   4. A purple stump that shows some moistness at the base

7. The nurse is reinforcing measures regarding the care of the newborn with a mother. To bathe the newborn, the mother would be taught which intervention?
   1. Begin with the eyes and face.
   2. Start with the dirtiest area first.
   3. Begin with the feet and work upward.
   4. Only wash the diaper area, because this is the only part of the baby that gets soiled.

8. After birth the nurse prevents hypothermia as a result of evaporation by performing which action?
   1. Warming the crib pad
   2. Closing the doors of the room
   3. Drying the baby with a warm blanket
   4. Turning on the overhead radiant warmer

9. The nurse is preparing to care for a newborn who is receiving phototherapy. Which measures need to be implemented? **Select all that apply.**
- ❑ 1. Avoid stimulation.
- ❑ 2. Decrease fluid intake.
- ❑ 3. Expose all of the newborn's skin.
- ❑ 4. Monitor the skin temperature closely.
- ❑ 5. Reposition the newborn every 2 hours.
- ❑ 6. Cover the newborn's eyes with shields or patches.

10. A newborn has just been circumcised and is being discharged home in 2 hours. Which instructions need to be provided by the nurse to the parents? **Select all that apply.**
- ❑ 1. Use only baby wipes to cleanse the penis.
- ❑ 2. Remove the yellow exudate which forms by 24 hours post circumcision.
- ❑ 3. Do not wash penis with soap until the circumcision is healed, which takes 5 to 6 days.
- ❑ 4. Change diaper every 4 hours or more often to inspect the penis for drainage or infection.
- ❑ 5. Monitor the circumcision; penis may appear reddened with small amount of bloody drainage shortly after the procedure.

11. The nurse would monitor for which signs associated with respiratory distress syndrome (RDS) in a preterm newborn?
1. Tachypnea and retractions
2. Acrocyanosis and grunting
3. Hypotension and bradycardia
4. The presence of a barrel chest with acrocyanosis

12. The nurse notes hypotonia, irritability, and a poor sucking reflex in a full-term newborn after admission to the nursery. The nurse suspects fetal alcohol syndrome (FAS) and is aware that which additional sign is consistent with FAS?
1. A length of 19 inches
2. Abnormal palmar creases
3. A birth weight of 6 pounds and 14 ounces
4. A head circumference that is appropriate for gestational age

ANSWERS

1. 4
Rationale: Erythromycin ophthalmic ointment 0.5% is used as a prophylactic treatment for ophthalmia neonatorum, which is caused by the bacteria *Neisseria gonorrhoeae*. The preventive treatment of gonorrhea is required by law. Options 1, 2, and 3 are not the purposes of administering this medication to the newborn.
Test-Taking Strategy: Focus on the subject, the purpose of administering erythromycin ophthalmic ointment to the newborn. Remember that erythromycin ophthalmic ointment 0.5% is used as a prophylactic treatment of ophthalmia neonatorum in newborns.

2. 3
Rationale: Vitamin K is necessary for the body to synthesize coagulation factors, and it is administered to the newborn infant to prevent abnormal bleeding. It promotes the liver's formation of the clotting factors II, VII, IX, and X. Newborn infants are deficient in vitamin K because the bowel does not have the bacteria necessary for synthesizing this fat-soluble vitamin. The normal flora in the intestinal tract produces vitamin K, but the newborn's bowel does not support the normal production of vitamin K until bacteria have adequately colonized it. The bowel becomes colonized by bacteria as food is ingested. Vitamin K does not promote the development of immunity or prevent the infant from becoming jaundiced.
Test-Taking Strategy: Focus on the subject, the purpose of administering vitamin K to a newborn. Because jaundice and immunity are not related to the action of vitamin K, eliminate options 1 and 2. From the remaining options, recall the action of vitamin K to direct you to option 3.

3. 2
Rationale: The neonate born to a mother who is HIV-positive must be cared for with strict attention to standard precautions. This prevents the transmission of the infection from the neonate, if he or she is infected, to others, and it prevents the transmission of other infectious agents to the possibly immunocompromised neonate. The mother would not breast-feed, unless the primary health care provider has specific recommendations about doing so. Monitoring vital signs and referring for sensory/cognitive problems are not care measures specifically associated with the care of a potentially AIDS-infected neonate.
Test-Taking Strategy: Focus on the subject, the care of a neonate infant born to a woman who is HIV-positive. Eliminate options 1 and 4 first because they are not specifically associated with the care of a potentially infected neonate. Recalling that mothers who are HIV-positive would not breast-feed will direct you to the correct option.

4. 2
Rationale: The highest priority during the admission to the nursery of a newborn with low Apgar scores is airway support, which would involve preparing respiratory resuscitation equipment. The remaining options are also important, although they are of lower initial priority. The newborn infant will be placed on a cardiorespiratory monitor. Setting up an intravenous line with 5% dextrose in water would provide circulatory support and may be prescribed. The radiant warmer will provide an external heat source, which is necessary to prevent further respiratory distress.

Test-Taking Strategy: Note the strategic words, *highest priority*. This question asks you to prioritize care on the basis of information about a newborn's condition. Use the ABCs—airway, breathing, and circulation. A method of planning for airway support is to have the resuscitation bag connected to an oxygen source.

5. 2

Rationale: The most common metabolic complication in the post-term newborn is hypoglycemia, which can produce central nervous system abnormalities and cognitive impairment if it is not corrected immediately. Urinary output, although important, is not the highest priority action. The polycythemia contributes to increased bilirubin levels, usually beginning on the second day after delivery. Hemoglobin and hematocrit levels are monitored, because the post-term neonate may exhibit polycythemia; however, this also does not require immediate attention.

Test-Taking Strategy: Note the strategic word, *priority*. Think about the characteristics of a post-term newborn. Recalling that hypoglycemia is a primary concern in the post-term newborn will direct you to the correct option.

6. 2

Rationale: Signs of infection of the umbilical cord are moistness, oozing, discharge, and a reddened base. If signs of infection occur, the primary health care provider is notified. Antibiotic treatment may be necessary.

Test-Taking Strategy: Focus on the subject, signs of infection. Options 1 and 3 identify normal signs and are eliminated first. From the remaining options, noting the word *discharge* will direct you to the correct option.

7. 1

Rationale: Bathing would start at the eyes and face, which are usually the cleanest areas. Next, the external portion of the ears and behind the ears are cleansed. The newborn's neck would be washed, because formula, breast milk, or lint will often accumulate in the folds of the neck. The hands and arms are then washed. The baby's legs are washed, with the diaper area being washed last.

Test-Taking Strategy: Focus on the subject, bathing a newborn. Remember, when bathing an adult or a baby, start with the cleanest part of the body and proceed to the dirtiest part. Therefore, options 2, 3, and 4 are incorrect.

8. 3

Rationale: Evaporation occurs when moisture from the newborn's wet body surface dissipates heat along with moisture. By keeping the newborn dry (and by drying the wet newborn at birth), evaporation is prevented. Conduction occurs when the newborn is on a cold surface, such as a cold pad or mattress. Convection occurs as air moves across the newborn's skin from an open door and heat is transferred to the air. Radiation occurs when heat from the newborn radiates to a colder surface.

Test-Taking Strategy: Recalling the methods of preventing heat loss in a newborn and focusing on the subject, evaporation, and thinking about the definition of evaporation will direct you to the correct option.

9. 4, 5, 6

Rationale: Phototherapy is the use of intense fluorescent lights to reduce serum bilirubin levels in the newborn. Injury from treatment (e.g., eye damage, dehydration, sensory deprivation) can occur. Interventions include exposing as much of the newborn's skin as possible; however, the genital area is covered. The newborn's eyes are also covered with shields or patches to ensure that the eyelids are closed. The shields or patches are removed at least once per shift to inspect the eyes for infection or irritation and to allow for eye contact. The nurse measures the quantity of light every 8 hours, monitors the skin temperature closely, and increases fluids to compensate for water loss. The newborn will have loose green stools and green-colored urine. The newborn's skin color is monitored with the fluorescent light turned off every 4 to 8 hours, and he or she is monitored for bronze baby syndrome, which is a grayish-brown discoloration of the skin. The newborn is repositioned every 2 hours, and stimulation is provided. After treatment, the newborn is monitored for signs of hyperbilirubinemia, because rebound elevations are normal after therapy is discontinued.

Test-Taking Strategy: Focus on the subject, phototherapy. Recalling that injury from treatment and sensory deprivation can occur will assist you with determining the correct interventions.

10. 3, 4, 5

Rationale: The glans penis is normally dark red. Use only water to cleanse the glans penis until complete healing has occurred around day 5 to 6. Diapers need to be changed at least every 4 hours to inspect the glans penis for drainage or signs of infection. After circumcision, a small amount of bloody drainage is expected. Baby wipes may contain alcohol and would not be used to cleanse the glans penis. During the normal healing process, the glans becomes covered with a yellow exudate. This exudate must not be removed. If excessive bleeding is noted from the circumcision, the parent would be instructed to apply gentle pressure to the site of bleeding with a sterile gauze pad. If the bleeding is not controlled, the primary health care provider is notified because a blood vessel may need to be ligated.

Test-Taking Strategy: Focus on the subject, instructions provided to parents following circumcision. Remember that a small amount of bloody drainage and yellow exudate are expected following the procedure.

11. 1

Rationale: The newborn infant with RDS may present with clinical signs of cyanosis, tachypnea, apnea, nasal flaring, chest wall retractions, or audible grunts. Acrocyanosis is a bluish discoloration of the hands and feet that is associated with immature peripheral circulation, and it is not uncommon during the first few hours of life. Options 2, 3, and 4 do not indicate clinical signs of RDS.

Test-Taking Strategy: Focus on the subject, signs of respiratory distress syndrome. Recalling that acrocyanosis may be a normal sign in a newborn infant will assist you with eliminating options 2 and 4. From the remaining options, it is necessary to be familiar with the signs of RDS. In addition, note the relationship between the diagnosis and the signs noted in option 1.

12. 2

Rationale: Features of newborn infants who are diagnosed with FAS include craniofacial abnormalities, IUGR, cardiac abnormalities, abnormal palmar creases, and respiratory distress. Options 1, 3, and 4 are normal findings in the full-term newborn infant.

Test-Taking Strategy: Focus on the subject, signs of fetal alcohol syndrome. Use your knowledge regarding the normal findings in the full-term newborn infant to answer this question. Note that options 1, 3, and 4 are comparable or alike and that they represent normal findings.

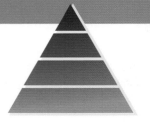

CHAPTER 27

Maternity and Newborn Medications

PRIORITY CONCEPTS **Health Promotion; Safety**

WHAT WOULD YOU DO?

The nurse notes that a pregnant client who has undergone amniocentesis is Rh-negative. What would the nurse do? *Answer is located on p. 346.*

⚠ The Food and Drug Administration initiated the Pregnancy and Lactation Labeling Rule (PLLR). This is a revision to the previous system that used Category A, B, C, D, and X. The PLLR provides more information on the risks and benefits of using medications during pregnancy. The PLLR also provides more information to assist the provider and pregnant mother to make informed decisions together, so as not to deter medication use during pregnancy when it is necessary.

I. Tocolytics

A. Description: Tocolytics are medications that produce uterine relaxation and suppress uterine activity in an attempt to halt uterine contractions and prevent preterm birth (Table 27.1).

B. Uses: To halt uterine contractions and prevent preterm birth

C. Adverse effects and contraindications
  1. See Table 27.1 for a description of adverse effects.
  2. Maternal contraindications include severe preeclampsia and eclampsia, active vaginal bleeding, intrauterine infection, cardiac disease, placental abruption, or poorly controlled diabetes.
  3. Fetal contraindications include estimated gestational age greater than 37 weeks, cervical dilation greater than 4 cm, fetal demise, lethal fetal anomaly, chorioamnionitis, acute fetal distress, and chronic intrauterine growth restriction.

D. Interventions for the client receiving tocolytic therapy
  1. Position the client on her side to enhance placental perfusion and reduce pressure on the cervix.
  2. Monitor maternal vital signs, fetal status, and labor status frequently according to agency protocol.

3. Monitor for signs of adverse effects to the medication.
  4. Monitor daily weight and input and output status, and provide fluid intake as prescribed.
  5. Offer comfort measures and provide psychosocial support to the client and family.
  6. See Table 27.1 for interventions specific to each tocolytic medication.

II. Magnesium Sulfate

A. Description (see Table 27.1)
  1. Magnesium sulfate is a central nervous system depressant and anticonvulsant.
  2. The medication causes smooth muscle relaxation.
  3. The antidote is calcium gluconate.

B. Uses
  1. Stopping preterm labor to prevent preterm birth
  2. Preventing and controlling seizures in preeclamptic and eclamptic clients

C. Adverse effects and contraindications
  1. Magnesium sulfate can cause respiratory depression, depressed reflexes, flushing, hypotension, extreme muscle weakness, decreased urine output, pulmonary edema, and elevated serum magnesium levels.
  2. Continuous intravenous (IV) infusion increases the risk of magnesium toxicity in the newborn.
  3. IV administration would not be used for 2 hours preceding delivery.
  4. Magnesium sulfate may be prescribed for the first 12 to 24 hours postpartum if it is used for preeclampsia.
  5. High doses can cause loss of deep tendon reflexes, heart block, respiratory paralysis, and cardiac arrest.
  6. The medication is contraindicated in clients with heart block, myocardial damage, or kidney failure.
  7. The medication is used with caution in clients with severe kidney impairment.

D. Interventions
  1. Monitor maternal vital signs, especially respirations, every 30 to 60 minutes.

TABLE 27.1 Tocolytics

Medication, Classification, and Actions	Adverse Effects	Nursing Interventions
Terbutaline—selective beta2 agonist that suppresses preterm labor by activating beta2 receptors in the uterus—decreases both frequency and intensity of contractions; primarily used to delay birth for several hours to allow the fetus to mature more before being born	Maternal—pulmonary edema, hypotension, hyperglycemia, and tachycardia Fetus—tachycardia	Assist to administer by injection under the skin Dosing needs to stop after 48 hours and would be interrupted if the maternal heart rate exceeds 120 beats/min
Magnesium sulfate—central nervous system depressant; relaxes smooth muscle, including the uterus; used to halt preterm labor contractions; used for preeclamptic clients to prevent seizure	*Maternal*—depressed respirations, depressed DTRs, hypotension, extreme muscle weakness, flushing, decreased urine output, pulmonary edema, serum magnesium level >7.5 mEq/L	Always use intravenous controller pump for administration
	Newborn—hypotonia and sleepiness	Follow agency protocol for administration
		Discontinue infusion and notify the PHCP if adverse effects occur
		Monitor for respirations <12/min, urine output <100 mL/4 h (25–30 mL/h)
		Monitor DTRs
		Monitor magnesium level and report values outside therapeutic range 4–7.5 mEq/L
		Keep calcium gluconate available (antidote)
Nifedipine—calcium channel blocker; relaxes smooth muscles, including the uterus, by blocking calcium entry	*Maternal*—tachycardia, hypotension, dizziness, headache, nervousness, facial flushing, fatigue, nausea *Newborn*—may cause vascular dilation	Follow agency protocol for administration Avoid use, or use cautiously with magnesium sulfate because severe hypotension can occur Monitor for adverse effects

DTRs, Deep tendon reflexes; *PHCP*, primary health care provider.

2. Assess renal function and electrocardiogram for cardiac function.
3. Monitor magnesium levels—the target range is 4 mEq/L to 7.5 mEq/L; if the magnesium level increases, notify the PHCP.
4. Always administer by IV infusion via an infusion monitoring device such as a controller pump; carefully monitor the dose being administered, and follow agency protocol for administration.
5. Keep calcium gluconate readily accessible in case of a magnesium sulfate overdose because calcium gluconate antagonizes the effect of magnesium sulfate.
6. Monitor deep tendon reflexes hourly for signs of developing toxicity.
7. Test the patellar reflex or knee jerk reflex before administering a repeat parenteral dose (used as an indicator of central nervous system depression; suppressed reflex may be a sign of impending respiratory arrest) (Table 27.2).
8. Patellar reflex must be present and respiratory rate must be greater than 12 breaths/min (or as designated by agency protocol) before each parenteral dose.
9. Monitor intake and output hourly; output needs to be maintained at 25 mL/h to 30 mL/h

TABLE 27.2 Assessing Deep Tendon Reflexes

Grade	Deep Tendon Reflex Response
0	No response
1	Sluggish or diminished
2	Active or expected response
3	Brisker than expected, slightly hyperactive
4	Brisk, hyperactive, with intermittent or transient clonus

Data from Seidel H, Ball J, Dains J, Flynn J, Solomon B, Stewart R: *Mosby's guide to physical examination*, ed 6, St. Louis, 2011, Mosby.

because the medication is eliminated by the kidneys.

⚠ Closely monitor a client receiving IV magnesium sulfate for signs of toxicity. Call the PHCP if respirations are less than 12 breaths/min, indicating respiratory depression, or if any other adverse effects occur.

III. Betamethasone and Dexamethasone

A. Description: Corticosteroids that increase the production of surfactant to accelerate fetal lung maturity and reduce the incidence or severity of respiratory distress syndrome

B. Use: For a client in preterm labor between 28 and 32 weeks' gestation whose labor can be inhibited for 48 hours without jeopardizing the mother or fetus

C. Adverse effects and contraindications
1. May decrease the mother's resistance to infection
2. Pulmonary edema secondary to sodium and fluid retention can occur.
3. Elevated blood glucose levels can occur in a client with diabetes mellitus.

D. Interventions
1. Monitor maternal vital signs, lung sounds, and check for edema.
2. Monitor mother for signs of infection.
3. Monitor white blood cell count.
4. Monitor blood glucose level.
5. Administer by deep intramuscular injection.

IV. Opioid Analgesics

A. Description
1. Used to relieve moderate to severe pain associated with labor
2. Administered by intramuscular or IV route
3. Regular use of opioids during pregnancy may produce withdrawal symptoms in the newborn (irritability, excessive crying, tremors, hyperactive reflexes, fever, vomiting, diarrhea, yawning, sneezing, and seizures).
4. Antidotes for opioids
   a. Naloxone is usually the treatment of choice because it rapidly reverses opioid toxicity; the dose may need to be repeated every few hours until opioid concentrations have decreased to nontoxic levels.
   b. These medications can cause withdrawal in opioid-dependent clients.

B. Hydromorphone hydrochloride
1. Can cause dizziness, nausea, vomiting, sedation, decreased blood pressure, decreased respirations, diaphoresis, flushed face, urinary retention
2. May be prescribed to be administered with an antiemetic such as promethazine to prevent nausea
3. High dosages may result in respiratory depression, skeletal muscle flaccidity, cold clammy skin, cyanosis, and extreme somnolence progressing to seizures, stupor, and coma.
4. Used cautiously in clients delivering preterm newborns
5. Not administered during advanced labor (within 1 hour of expected delivery); if the medication is not adequately removed from the fetal circulation, respiratory depression can occur.

C. Fentanyl: Can cause respiratory depression, dizziness, drowsiness, hypotension, urinary retention, and fetal narcosis and distress

D. Butorphanol tartrate and nalbuphine

BOX 27.1   Prostaglandins

Prostaglandin E₁:
Misoprostol intravaginal tablet

Prostaglandin E₂:
Dinoprostone vaginal gel, insert, suppository

1. Can cause confusion, sedation, sweating, nausea, vomiting, hypotension, sinusoidal-like fetal heart rhythm
2. Use with caution in a client with preexisting opioid dependency because these medications can precipitate withdrawal symptoms in the client and the newborn.

E. Interventions
1. Monitor vital signs, particularly respiratory status; if respirations are 12 breaths/min or less, withhold the medication and contact the PHCP.
2. Monitor the fetal heart rate and characteristics of uterine contractions.
3. Monitor for blood pressure changes (hypotension); maintain the client in a recumbent position (elevate the hip with a wedge pillow or other device).
4. Record the client's response and level of pain relief.
5. Monitor the bladder for distention and retention.
6. Have the antidote naloxone available, especially if delivery is expected to occur during peak drug absorption time.

 Obtain a medication history before the administration of an opioid analgesic. Some medications may be contraindicated if the client has a history of opioid dependency because these medications can precipitate withdrawal symptoms in the client and newborn.

V. Prostaglandins (Box 27.1)

A. Description
1. Ripen the cervix, making it softer and causing it to begin to dilate and efface
2. Stimulate uterine contractions
3. Administered vaginally

B. Uses
1. Preinduction cervical ripening (ripening of the cervix before the induction of labor when the Bishop score is ≤4)
2. Induction of labor
3. Induction of abortion (abortifacient agent)

C. Adverse effects and contraindications
1. Gastrointestinal effects, including diarrhea, nausea, vomiting, and stomach cramps
2. Fever, chills, flushing, headache, hypotension
3. Tachysystole (≥12 uterine contractions in 20 minutes without an alteration in the fetal heart rate pattern)
4. Hyperstimulation of the uterus

> **BOX 27.2** **Contraindications to the Use of Prostaglandins**
>
> - Active cardiac, hepatic, pulmonary, or kidney disease
> - Acute pelvic inflammatory disease
> - Clients in whom vaginal delivery is not indicated
> - Fetal malpresentation
> - History of cesarean section or major uterine surgery
> - History of difficult labor or traumatic labor
> - Hypersensitivity to prostaglandins
> - Maternal fever or infection
> - Nonreassuring fetal heart rate pattern
> - Placenta previa or unexplained vaginal bleeding
> - Regular progressive uterine contractions
> - Significant cephalopelvic disproportion

5. Fetal passage of meconium

6. Contraindications (Box 27.2)

D. Interventions

1. Monitor maternal vital signs, fetal heart rate pattern, and status of pregnancy including indications for cervical ripening or the induction of labor, signs of labor or impending labor, and the Bishop score (see Chapter 24, Table 24.2 for information about the Bishop score).

2. Monitor for contraindications and adverse effects to the medication.

3. Have the client void before administration of medication and then have her maintain a supine with lateral tilt or side-lying position for 30 to 60 minutes (gel) up to 2 hours (insert) after administration, depending on the medication administered.

4. Treatment is discontinued when the Bishop score is 8 or more (cervix ripens) or an effective contraction pattern is established (three or more contractions in a 10-minute period); in addition, signs of adverse effects indicate that the treatment needs to be discontinued.

5. Follow agency protocol for the induction of labor if cervical ripening has occurred and labor has not begun; oxytocin can be initiated if needed 6 to 12 hours after discontinuation of prostaglandin therapy.

VI. Uterine Stimulants (Oxytocics): Oxytocin

A. Description

1. Oxytocin stimulates the smooth muscle of the uterus and increases the force, frequency, and duration of uterine contractions.

2. Oxytocin also promotes milk letdown.

3. For induction of labor, oxytocin is administered by the IV route (other route of administration is intramuscular); if injecting intramuscularly, aspiration is necessary to avoid injection into a blood vessel.

4. Minimal cervical change usually is noted until the active phase of labor is achieved.

B. Uses

1. Induces or augments labor

2. Controls postpartum bleeding

3. Manages an incomplete abortion

C. Adverse effects and contraindications

1. Adverse effects include allergy, dysrhythmia, change in blood pressure, uterine rupture, and water intoxication; intranasal administration may cause nasal vasoconstriction.

2. Oxytocin may produce uterine hypertonicity, resulting in fetal or maternal adverse effects.

3. High doses may cause hypotension, with rebound hypertension.

4. Postpartum hemorrhage can occur and must be monitored for because the uterus may become atonic when the medication wears off.

5. Oxytocin would not be used in a client who cannot deliver vaginally or in a client with hypertonic uterine contractions; it is also contraindicated in a client with active genital herpes.

D. Interventions

1. Monitor maternal vital signs (every 15 minutes), especially the blood pressure and heart rate; weight; intake and output; level of consciousness; and lung sounds.

2. Monitor frequency, duration, and force of contractions and resting uterine tone every 15 minutes.

3. Monitor fetal heart rate every 15 minutes, and notify the PHCP if significant changes occur; use of an internal fetal scalp electrode may be prescribed.

4. Administered by IV infusion via an infusion monitoring device; prescribed additive solution is piggybacked at the port nearest the point of venous insertion (prescribed additive solution may be normal saline, lactated Ringer's, or 5% dextrose in water).

5. Carefully monitor the dose being administered; do not leave the client unattended while the oxytocin is infusing.

6. Administer oxygen if prescribed.

7. Monitor for hypertonic contractions or a nonreassuring fetal heart rate and notify the PHCP if these occur (see **Priority Nursing Actions**).

8. Stop the medication if uterine hyperstimulation or a nonreassuring fetal heart rate occurs; turn the client on her side, increase the IV rate of the prescribed additive solution, and administer oxygen via face mask.

9. Monitor for signs of water intoxication.

10. Have emergency equipment available.

11. Document the dose of the medication and the time it was started, increased, maintained, and discontinued; document the client's response.

12. Keep the client and family informed of the client's progress.

⚡ PRIORITY NURSING ACTIONS

Hypertonic Contractions or a Nonreassuring Fetal Heart Rate Occurrence During Oxytocin Infusion

1. Stop the oxytocin infusion.
2. Turn the client on her side, stay with the client, and ask another nurse to contact the PHCP.
3. Increase the flow rate of the intravenous solution that does not contain the oxytocin.
4. Administer oxygen, 8 L/min to 10 L/min, by snug face mask.
5. Assess maternal vital signs; fetal heart rate and patterns; and frequency, duration, and force of contractions.
6. Document the event, actions taken, and the response.

VII. Medications Used to Manage Postpartum Hemorrhage (Box 27.3)

A. Ergot alkaloids
  1. Description
    a. Methylergonovine maleate is an ergot alkaloid.
    b. Directly stimulate uterine muscle, increase the force and frequency of contractions, and produce a firm tetanic contraction of the uterus
    c. Can produce arterial vasoconstriction and vasospasm of the coronary arteries
    d. Ergot alkaloids are administered postpartum and are not administered before the delivery of the placenta.
  2. Uses
    a. Postpartum hemorrhage
    b. Postabortal hemorrhage resulting from atony or involution
  3. Adverse effects and contraindications
    a. Can cause nausea, uterine cramping, bradycardia, dysrhythmia, myocardial infarction, and severe hypertension
    b. High doses are associated with peripheral vasospasm or vasoconstriction, angina, miosis, confusion, respiratory depression, seizure, or unconsciousness; uterine tetany can occur.
    c. Contraindicated during pregnancy and in clients with significant cardiovascular disease, peripheral vascular disease, or hypertension
  4. Interventions
    a. Monitor maternal vital signs, weight, intake and output, level of consciousness, and lung sounds.

BOX 27.3   **Medications Used to Manage Postpartum Hemorrhage**

- Methylergonovine
- Oxytocin
- Prostaglandin F$_{2\alpha}$: Carboprost tromethamine

---

b. Monitor the blood pressure closely; the medication produces vasoconstriction, and if an increase in blood pressure is noted, withhold the medication and notify the PHCP.
c. Monitor uterine contractions (frequency, strength, and duration).
d. Assess for chest pain, headache, shortness of breath, itching, pale or cold hands or feet, nausea, diarrhea, or dizziness.
e. Assess the extremities for color, warmth, movement, and pain.
f. Assess vaginal bleeding.
g. Notify the PHCP if chest pain or other adverse effects occur.
h. Administer analgesics as prescribed; they may be required because the medication produces painful uterine contractions.

⚠ Check the client's blood pressure before administering an ergot alkaloid. These medications can cause severe hypertension and are contraindicated in a client with hypertension.

B. Prostaglandin F$_{2\alpha}$ (carboprost tromethamine)
  1. Description: Contracts the uterus
  2. Uses: Postpartum hemorrhage
  3. Adverse effects and contraindications
    a. Can cause headache, nausea, vomiting, diarrhea, fever, tachycardia, hypertension
    b. Contraindicated if the client has asthma
  4. Interventions
    a. Monitor vital signs.
    b. Monitor vaginal bleeding and uterine tone.

C. Oxytocin: See Section VI on uterine stimulants.

VIII. Rh$_o$(D) Immune Globulin

A. Description
  1. Prevention of anti-Rh$_o$(D) antibody formation is most successful if the medication is administered twice, at 28 weeks of gestation and again within 72 hours after delivery.
  2. Rh$_o$(D) immune globulin also must be administered within 72 hours after potential or actual exposure to Rh-positive blood and must be given with each subsequent exposure or potential exposure to Rh-positive blood.
B. Use: To prevent isoimmunization in Rh-negative clients who are negative for Rh antibodies and exposed or potentially exposed to Rh-positive red blood cells by amniocentesis, chorionic villus sampling, transfusion, termination of pregnancy, abdominal trauma, or bleeding during pregnancy or the birth process
C. Adverse effects and contraindications
  1. Elevated temperature
  2. Tenderness at the injection site
  3. Contraindicated for Rh-positive clients

4. Contraindicated in clients with a history of systemic allergic reactions to preparations containing human immunoglobulins

5. Not administered to a newborn

D. Interventions

1. Administer to the client by intramuscular injection at 28 weeks' gestation and within 72 hours after delivery.

2. Never administer by the IV route.

3. Monitor for temperature elevation.

4. Monitor injection site for tenderness.

⚠ Rho(D) immune globulin is of no benefit when the client has developed a positive antibody titer to the Rh antigen.

IX. Rubella Vaccine

A. Given subcutaneously before hospital discharge to a nonimmune postpartum client

B. Administered if the rubella titer is less than 1:8

C. Adverse effects: Transient rash, hypersensitivity

D. Contraindicated in a client with a hypersensitivity to eggs

E. Interventions

1. Assess for allergy to duck eggs and notify the PHCP before administration if an allergy exists.

2. Question administration if the client or other family members are immunocompromised.

⚠ The client must avoid pregnancy for 1 to 3 months (or as prescribed) after immunization with rubella vaccine. Inform the client about the need for using a contraception method during this time.

X. Lung Surfactants

A. Description

1. Lung surfactants replenish surfactant and restore surface activity to the lungs to prevent and treat respiratory distress syndrome.

2. Lung surfactants are administered by the intratracheal route.

B. Use: To prevent or treat respiratory distress syndrome in premature newborns

C. Adverse effects and contraindications

1. Adverse effects include transient bradycardia and oxygen desaturation; pulmonary hemorrhage, mucus plugging, and endotracheal tube reflux can also occur.

2. Surfactants are administered with caution in newborns at risk for circulatory overload.

D. Interventions

1. Instill surfactant through the catheter inserted into the newborn's endotracheal tube; avoid suctioning for at least 2 hours after administration.

2. Monitor for bradycardia and decreased oxygen saturation during administration.

3. Monitor respiratory status and lung sounds and for signs of adverse effects.

XI. Eye Prophylaxis for the Newborn

A. Description

1. Preventive eye treatment against ophthalmia neonatorum in the newborn is required by law in the United States.

2. Agent used varies depending on agency protocols, but usually ophthalmic forms of erythromycin are prescribed because they are bacteriostatic and bactericidal, and provide prophylaxis against *Neisseria gonorrhoeae* and *Chlamydia trachomatis*.

B. Use: As a prophylactic measure to protect against *N. gonorrhoeae* and *C. trachomatis*

C. Interventions

1. Clean the newborn's eyes before instilling the medication.

2. Do not flush the eyes after instillation.

⚠ Instillation of eye medication can be delayed for 1 hour after birth to facilitate eye contact and parent-newborn attachment and bonding.

XII. Phytonadione

A. Description

1. The newborn is at risk for hemorrhagic disorders; coagulation factors synthesized in the liver depend on phytonadione (also known as vitamin K), which is not synthesized until intestinal bacteria are present.

2. Newborns are deficient in phytonadione for the first 5 to 8 days of life because of the lack of intestinal bacteria.

B. Use: Prophylaxis and treatment of hemorrhagic disease of the newborn

C. Adverse effect: phytonadione can cause hyperbilirubinemia in the newborn (occurrence is rare).

D. Interventions

1. Protect the medication from light.

2. Administer during the early newborn period.

3. Administer by the intramuscular route in the lateral aspect of the middle third of the vastus lateralis muscle of the thigh.

4. Monitor for bruising at the injection site and for bleeding from the cord.

5. Monitor for jaundice and monitor the bilirubin level, because, although rare, the medication can cause hyperbilirubinemia in the newborn.

XIII. Hepatitis B Vaccine, Recombinant

A. Description: Given intramuscularly to the newborn before discharge

B. Use: Recommended for all newborns to prevent hepatitis B (HBV)

C. Adverse effects: Rash, fever, erythema, and pain at injection site

D. Interventions

1. Parental consent must be obtained.

2. Administer intramuscularly in the lateral aspect of the middle third of the vastus lateralis muscle.

3. If the infant was born to a mother positive for HBV surface antigen, HBV immune globulin must be given within 12 hours of birth in addition to the HBV vaccine. Then follow the regularly scheduled HBV vaccination schedule.

4. Document immunization administration on a vaccination card for the parents to have a record that it was administered.

XIV. Contraceptives

A. Description

1. These medications contain a combination of estrogen and a progestin or a progestin alone.

2. Estrogen-progestin combinations suppress ovulation and change the cervical mucus making it difficult for sperm to enter.

3. Medications that contain only progestins are less effective than the combined medications.

4. Contraceptives usually are taken for 21 consecutive days and stopped for 7 days. The administration cycle is then repeated.

5. Contraceptives provide reversible prevention of pregnancy.

6. Contraceptives are useful in controlling irregular or excessive menstrual cycles.

7. Risk factors associated with the development of complications related to the use of contraceptives include smoking, obesity, and hypertension.

8. Contraceptives are contraindicated in women with hypertension, thromboembolic disease, cerebrovascular or coronary artery disease, estrogen-dependent cancers, and pregnancy.

9. Contraceptives would be avoided with the use of hepatotoxic medications.

10. Contraceptives interfere with the activity of bromocriptine mesylate and anticoagulants and increase the toxicity of tricyclic antidepressants.

11. Contraceptives may alter the blood glucose level.

12. Antibiotics may decrease the absorption and effectiveness of oral contraceptives.

B. Side and adverse effects

1. Breakthrough bleeding
2. Excessive cervical mucus formation
3. Breast tenderness
4. Hypertension
5. Nausea, vomiting

C. Interventions

1. Monitor vital signs and weight.

2. Reinforce instructions to the client in the administration of the medication. (It may take up to 1 week for full contraceptive effect to occur when the medication is begun; the client would be instructed to use a barrier method during this time.)

3. Reinforce instructions to the client with diabetes mellitus to monitor blood glucose levels carefully.

4. The client is instructed to report signs of thromboembolic complications.

5. The client is instructed to notify the PHCP if vaginal bleeding or menstrual irregularities occur or if pregnancy is suspected.

6. The client is instructed to use an alternate method of birth control when taking antibiotics because these may decrease absorption of the oral contraceptive.

7. The client is instructed to perform breast self-examination monthly and about the importance of annual physical examinations.

8. Contraceptive patches

   a. Designed to be worn for 3 weeks and removed for a 1-week period

   b. Applied on clean, dry, intact skin on the buttocks, abdomen, upper outer arm, or upper torso

   c. The client is instructed to peel away half of backing on patch, apply the sticky surface to the skin, remove the other half of the backing, and then press down on the patch with the palm for 10 seconds.

   d. The client is instructed to change the patch weekly, using a new location for each patch.

   e. If the patch falls off and remains off for less than 24 hours (such as when the client is sleeping or is unaware that it has fallen off), it can be reapplied if still sticky, or it can be replaced with a new patch.

   f. If the patch is off for more than 24 hours, a new 4-week cycle must be started immediately.

9. Vaginal ring

   a. Inserted into the vagina by the client, left in place for 3 weeks, and removed for 1 week

   b. The medication is absorbed through mucous membranes of the vagina.

   c. Removed rings need to be wrapped in a foil pouch and discarded, not flushed down the toilet.

10. Implants and depo injections provide long-acting forms of birth control, from 3 months to 5 years in duration.

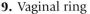 If the client decides to discontinue the contraceptive to become pregnant, recommend that the client use an alternative form of birth control for 2 months after discontinuation to ensure more complete excretion of hormonal agents before conception.

XV. Fertility Medications (Box 27.4)

A. Description

1. Fertility medications act to stimulate follicle development and ovulation in functioning ovaries

Maternity Nursing

- Cetrorelix
- Chorionic gonadotropin
- Clomiphene citrate
- Follitropin alfa
- Follitropin beta
- Ganirelix
- Menotropins
- Urofollitropin alfa

and are combined with human chorionic gonadotropin to maintain the follicles once ovulation has occurred.

2. Fertility medications are contraindicated in the presence of primary ovarian dysfunction, thyroid or adrenal dysfunction, ovarian cysts, pregnancy, or idiopathic uterine bleeding.

3. Fertility medications would be used with caution in clients with thromboembolic or respiratory disease.

B. Side and adverse effects
1. Risk of multiple births and birth defects
2. Ovarian overstimulation (abdominal pain, distention, ascites, pleural effusion)
3. Headache, irritability
4. Fluid retention and bloating
5. Nausea, vomiting
6. Uterine bleeding
7. Ovarian enlargement
8. Gynecomastia
9. Rash
10. Orthostatic hypotension
11. Febrile reactions

C. Interventions
1. The client is instructed regarding administration of the medication.
2. A calendar of treatment days and instructions on when intercourse would occur are provided to increase therapeutic effectiveness of the medication.
3. Information about the risks and hazards of multiple births is provided.
4. The client is instructed to notify the PHCP if signs of ovarian overstimulation occur.
5. The client is instructed about the need for regular follow-up for evaluation.

WHAT WOULD YOU DO?

Answer: The nurse would seek a prescription from the primary health care provider (PHCP) for the administration of Rh_o(D) immune globulin. Rh_o(D) immune globulin is administered to prevent isoimmunization in Rh-negative clients who are negative for Rh antibodies and are exposed or potentially exposed

to Rh-positive red blood cells from the fetus by amniocentesis or chorionic villus sampling, transfusion, termination of pregnancy, abdominal trauma, or bleeding during pregnancy or the birth process. It is administered to the Rh-negative client by intramuscular injection at 28 weeks' gestation and within 72 hours after delivery.

PRACTICE QUESTIONS

❖ **1.** The nurse is monitoring a client who is receiving oxytocin to induce labor. Which assessment findings would indicate to the nurse that the oxytocin infusion needs to be **immediately** discontinued? **Select all that apply.**
- ❏ **1.** Fatigue
- ❏ **2.** Drowsiness
- ❏ **3.** Uterine hyperstimulation
- ❏ **4.** Late decelerations of the fetal heart rate
- ❏ **5.** Early decelerations of the fetal heart rate

❖ **2.** A pregnant client is receiving magnesium sulfate for the management of preeclampsia. The nurse who is assisting in caring for the client determines that the client is experiencing toxicity from the medication if which findings are noted during assessment? **Select all that apply.**
- ❏ **1.** Proteinuria of 3 +
- ❏ **2.** Respirations of 10 breaths/min
- ❏ **3.** Presence of deep tendon reflexes
- ❏ **4.** Urine output of 20 mL in an hour
- ❏ **5.** Serum magnesium level of 6 mEq/L

❖ **3.** The nurse is assisting in monitoring a client in preterm labor who is receiving intravenous magnesium sulfate. The nurse would monitor for which adverse effects of this medication? **Select all that apply.**
- ❏ **1.** Flushing
- ❏ **2.** Hypertension
- ❏ **3.** Increased urine output
- ❏ **4.** Depressed respirations
- ❏ **5.** Extreme muscle weakness
- ❏ **6.** Hyperactive deep tendon reflexes

4. The nursing instructor asks a nursing student to describe the procedure for administering erythromycin ointment to the eyes of a newborn. Which student statement indicates that **further teaching is needed?**
1. "I will flush the eyes after instilling the ointment."
2. "I will clean the newborn's eyes before instilling ointment."
3. "I need to administer the eye ointment within 1 hour after delivery."
4. "I will instill the eye ointment into each of the newborn's conjunctival sacs."

5. A client in preterm labor (31 weeks) who is dilated to 4 cm has been started on magnesium sulfate and her contractions have stopped. If the client's labor can be inhibited for the next 48 hours, the nurse anticipates a prescription for which medication?
1. Nalbuphine
2. Betamethasone
3. $Rh_o(D)$ immune globulin
4. Dinoprostone vaginal insert

6. Methylergonovine is prescribed for a woman to treat postpartum hemorrhage. Before administration of methylergonovine, what is the **priority** nursing assessment?
1. Uterine tone
2. Blood pressure
3. Amount of lochia
4. Deep tendon reflexes

7. The nurse is assisting in caring for a premature infant who needs to receive beractant for respiratory distress syndrome. The nurse plans to assist in administering the medication by which route?
1. Intradermal
2. Intratracheal
3. Subcutaneous
4. Intramuscular

8. An opioid analgesic is administered to a client in labor. The nurse assigned to care for the client ensures that which medication is readily available if respiratory depression occurs?
1. Naloxone
2. Morphine sulfate
3. Betamethasone
4. Meperidine hydrochloride

9. $Rh_o(D)$ immune globulin is prescribed for a client after delivery and the nurse assisting in caring for the client provides information to the client about the purpose of the medication. The nurse determines that the woman understands the purpose if the woman states that it will protect her next baby from which condition?
1. Having Rh-positive blood
2. Developing a rubella infection
3. Developing physiological jaundice
4. Being affected by Rh incompatibility

10. Methylergonovine is prescribed for a client with postpartum hemorrhage. Before administering the medication, the nurse consults with the registered nurse about contacting the primary health care provider (PHCP) who prescribed the medication if which condition is documented in the client's medical history?
1. Hypotension
2. Hypothyroidism
3. Diabetes mellitus
4. Peripheral vascular disease

ANSWERS

 1. 3, 4

Rationale: Oxytocin stimulates uterine contractions and is a common pharmacological method to induce labor. High-dose protocols have been associated with more uterine hyperstimulation and more cesarean births related to fetal stress. Noting late decelerations is a nonreassuring sign, because the health status of the fetus is being compromised. Some PHCPs prescribe the administration of oxytocin in 10-minute pulsed infusions rather than as a continuous infusion. This pulsed method, which is more like endogenous secretion of oxytocin, is reported to be effective for labor induction and requires significantly less oxytocin use. Oxytocin infusion must be stopped when any signs of uterine hyperstimulation are present. Drowsiness and fatigue may be caused by the labor experience. Early decelerations of the fetal heart rate are a reassuring sign and do not indicate fetal distress.

Test-Taking Strategy: Note the strategic word *immediately.* Focus on the subject, an adverse effect of oxytocin. Options 1 and 2 are comparable or alike and can be eliminated first. From the remaining options, recalling that early decelerations of the fetal heart rate are a reassuring sign will direct you to the correct option.

2. 2, 4

Rationale: Magnesium toxicity can occur from magnesium sulfate therapy. Signs of magnesium sulfate toxicity relate to the central nervous system depressant effects of the medication and include respiratory depression, loss of deep tendon reflexes, and a sudden decline in fetal heart rate and maternal heart rate and blood pressure. Urine output must be at least 25 mL to 30 mL per hour. Therapeutic serum levels of magnesium are 4 mEq/L to 7.5 mEq/L. Proteinuria of 3 + is an expected finding in a client with preeclampsia.

Test-Taking Strategy: Focus on the subject, magnesium toxicity. Eliminate option 3 first because it is a normal finding. Next, eliminate option 4, knowing that the therapeutic serum level of magnesium is 4 mEq/L to 7.5 mEq/L. From the remaining options, recalling that proteinuria of 3 + would be noted in a client with preeclampsia will direct you to the correct option.

3. 1,4,5

Rationale: Magnesium sulfate is a central nervous system depressant and relaxes smooth muscle, including the uterus. It is used to halt preterm labor contractions and is used for preeclamptic clients to prevent seizure. Adverse effects include flushing, depressed respirations, depressed deep tendon reflexes, hypotension, extreme muscle weakness, decreased urine output, pulmonary edema, and elevated serum magnesium levels.

Test-Taking Strategy: Focus on the subject, adverse effects of magnesium sulfate. Recalling that this medication is a central nervous system depressant and relaxes smooth muscle will assist you in choosing the correct answer.

4. 1

Rationale: Eye prophylaxis protects the newborn against Neisseria gonorrhoeae and Chlamydia trachomatis. The eyes are not flushed after instillation of the medication because the flush would wash away the administered medication. Options 2, 3, and 4 are correct statements regarding the procedure for administering eye medication to the newborn.

Test-Taking Strategy: Note the strategic words *further teaching is needed*. These words indicate a negative event query and ask you to select an option that is an incorrect statement. Eliminate options 3 and 4 first because they are comparable or alike and relate to instilling the eye medication. From the remaining options, visualize the effect of each. This will direct you to the correct option.

5. 2

Rationale: Betamethasone, a glucocorticoid, is given to increase the production of surfactant to stimulate fetal lung maturation. It is administered to clients in preterm labor at 28 to 32 weeks of gestation if the labor can be inhibited for 48 hours. Nalbuphine is an opioid analgesic. $Rh_o(D)$ immune globulin is given to Rh-negative clients to prevent sensitization. Dinoprostone vaginal insert is a prostaglandin given to ripen and soften the cervix and to stimulate uterine contractions.

Test-Taking Strategy: Focus on the subject, a client at 31 weeks' gestation. Recall that the preterm infant is at risk for respiratory distress syndrome because of immaturity and the inability to produce surfactant. Next, recalling the actions of the medications in the options and that betamethasone is used to increase the production of surfactant will direct you to the correct option.

6. 2

Rationale: Methylergonovine, an ergot alkaloid, is used to prevent or control postpartum hemorrhage by contracting the uterus. Methylergonovine causes continuous uterine contractions and may elevate the blood pressure. A priority assessment before the administration of the medication is to check the blood pressure. The PHCP must be notified if hypertension is present. Although options 1, 3, and 4 may be components of the postpartum assessment, the correct option, blood pressure, is related specifically to the administration of this medication.

Test-Taking Strategy: Note the strategic word, *priority*. Eliminate options 1 and 3 first because they are comparable or alike and related to one another. To choose from the remaining options, use the ABCs—airway, breathing, and circulation. Blood pressure is a method of assessing circulation.

7. 2

Rationale: Respiratory distress syndrome is a serious lung disorder caused by immaturity and the inability to produce surfactant, resulting in hypoxia and acidosis. It is common in premature infants and may occur as a result of lung immaturity caused by surfactant deficiency. The mainstay of treatment is the administration of exogenous surfactant, which is administered by the intratracheal route. Options 1, 3, and 4 are not routes of administration for this medication.

Test-Taking Strategy: Focus on the subject, route of administration for beractant. Note the relationship between the diagnosis *respiratory distress syndrome* and the correct option, *intratracheal*.

8. 1

Rationale: Opioid analgesics may be prescribed to relieve moderate to severe pain associated with labor. Opioid toxicity can occur and cause respiratory depression. Naloxone is an opioid antagonist, which reverses the effects of opioids and is given for respiratory depression. Morphine sulfate and meperidine hydrochloride are opioid analgesics. Betamethasone is a corticosteroid administered to enhance fetal lung maturity.

Test-Taking Strategy: Focus on the subject of the question, the antidote for respiratory depression. Eliminate options 2 and 4 first because they are comparable or alike and are opioid analgesics. Next, eliminate option 3, knowing that this medication is a corticosteroid.

9. 4

Rationale: Rh incompatibility can occur when an Rh-negative mother becomes sensitized to the Rh antigen. Sensitization may develop when an Rh-negative woman becomes pregnant with a fetus who is Rh positive. During pregnancy and at delivery, some of the fetus's Rh-positive blood can enter the maternal circulation, causing the mother's immune system to form antibodies against Rh-positive blood. Administration of $Rh_o(D)$ immune globulin prevents the mother from developing antibodies against Rh-positive blood by providing passive antibody protection against the Rh antigen.

Test-Taking Strategy: Note the subject of the question, the purpose of $Rh_o(D)$ immune globulin. Noting the relationship between the name of the medication, $Rh_o(D)$ immune globulin, and the word incompatibility in the correct option will direct you to this option.

10. 4

Rationale: Methylergonovine is an ergot alkaloid used to treat postpartum hemorrhage. Ergot alkaloids are contraindicated in clients with significant cardiovascular disease, peripheral vascular disease, hypertension, preeclampsia, or eclampsia. These conditions are worsened by the vasoconstrictive effects of the ergot alkaloids. Options 1, 2, and 3 are not contraindications related to the use of ergot alkaloids.

Test-Taking Strategy: Focus on the subject, the purpose, action, and contraindications of methylergonovine. Recalling that ergot alkaloids produce vasoconstriction will direct you to the correct option.

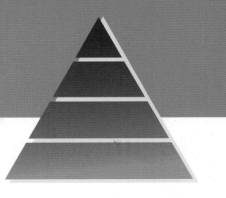

Pediatric Nursing

UNIT VII

Pediatric Nursing

 ## Pyramid to Success

Pyramid Points focus on growth and development, safety, and age-appropriate measures to ensure a safe and hazard-free environment for the child; for protection of the child and the prevention of accidents; and for acute disorders that can occur in children. The focus is on nutrition, specific feeding techniques, positioning techniques, and interventions that will provide and maintain adequate airway, breathing, and circulation patterns for the child. In addition, neglect and/or abuse of the child is a focus. On the NCLEX-PN® examination, be alert to the age of the child, if the age is presented in a question. If an age is presented in the question, think about the specific growth and development characteristics of the age group to answer the question correctly.

 ## Client Needs: Learning Objectives

Safe and Effective Care Environment

Communicating with interprofessional health care team members

Considering issues related to informed consent regarding minors

Delegating care safely as appropriate

Ensuring environmental safety, including home safety and personal safety, related to the developmental age of the child

Establishing priorities

Instituting measures related to the spread and control of infectious agents, particularly communicable diseases

Maintaining confidentiality

Preventing errors and accidents

Protecting the child and other contacts to prevent illness

Providing continuity of care

Providing protective measures

Upholding parent and child rights

Health Promotion and Maintenance

Ensuring that immunization schedules are up to date

Focusing on developmental stages when planning care

Performing physical assessment/data collection techniques specific to the pediatric client

Preventing disease in the pediatric population

Reinforcing instructions to the child and parents regarding care at home

Psychosocial Integrity

Checking the child for neglect and/or abuse

Communicating with the pediatric client

Considering concepts of family dynamics when planning care

Considering cultural, religious, and spiritual beliefs when planning care

Considering end-of-life issues and grief and loss in the pediatric population

Identifying family and support systems for the child

Providing play therapies

Physiological Integrity

Following medication administration procedures

Following nutritional guidelines for the pediatric population

Identifying comfort measures appropriate for the child

Maintaining sensitivity for intrusive procedures needed for the pediatric client

Managing childhood illnesses

Monitoring elimination patterns

Monitoring for age-appropriate normal body structure and function

Monitoring for infectious diseases of the pediatric client

Monitoring for responses to treatments

Providing for consistent rest and sleep patterns

Responding to medical emergencies

Client Needs lists modified from: National Council of State Boards of Nursing, Inc. (NCSBN). *NCLEX-PN Examination: Test Plan for the National Council Licensure Examination for Practical Nurses,* effective April 2020. Chicago: NCSBN.

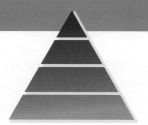

CHAPTER **28**

Integumentary Problems

PRIORITY CONCEPTS Infection; Tissue Integrity

WHAT WOULD YOU DO?

A child being admitted to the pediatric unit is suspected of having impetigo. In order to prevent the spread of this infectious disease, what would the nurse do?

Answer is located on p. 353.

I. Eczema (Dermatitis)

A. Description

1. A superficial inflammatory process that primarily involves the epidermis; there are many types, some of which include atopic dermatitis, and stasis dermatitis.

2. Associated with family history of the disorder, allergies, asthma, or allergic rhinitis

3. The major goals of management are to relieve pruritus, lubricate the skin, reduce inflammation, and prevent or control secondary infections.

B. Forms of eczema (Box 28.1)

C. Data collection

1. Redness

2. Scaliness

3. Itching

4. Minute papules (firm elevated circumscribed lesions smaller than 1 cm in diameter) and vesicles (similar to papules but fluid-filled)

5. Weeping, oozing, and crusting of lesions

6. Adolescent and early adult forms commonly occur in antecubital and popliteal areas.

D. Interventions

1. Avoid exposure to skin irritants such as irritating soaps, detergents, fabric softeners, diaper wipes, and powder.

2. Baths and moisturizers are important; bathing water would be tepid and bath would be limited to 5 to 10 minutes, and the skin should be moisturized immediately after the bath; a thick cream or ointment would be used, such as petroleum jelly.

3. If topical medications are prescribed, they would be applied within 3 minutes after the bath.

4. Antihistamines and topical corticosteroids may be prescribed; corticosteroids are applied in a thin layer and rubbed into the area thoroughly.

5. Antibiotics may be prescribed if secondary infections occur.

6. Cool, wet compresses applied for short periods may help to soothe the skin and alleviate itching; pat the skin dry between cooling treatments.

7. Prevent or minimize scratching. Keep the nails short and clean and place gloves or cotton socks over the hands.

8. Eliminate conditions that increase itching, such as wet diapers, excessive bathing, ambient heat, woolen clothes or blankets, and rough fabrics or furry stuffed animals; exposure to latex should also be avoided.

9. Reinforce instructions to the parents to wash the child's clothing in a mild detergent and rinse it thoroughly. Putting the clothes through a second complete wash cycle without detergent will minimize the amount of residue remaining on the fabric.

10. Reinforce instructions to parents on measures to take to prevent skin infections.

11. Reinforce instructions to parents to monitor the lesions for signs of infection (i.e., honey-colored crusts with surrounding erythema) and to seek immediate medical intervention if such signs are noted.

⚠ A child with an integumentary disorder needs to be monitored for signs of either a skin infection or a systemic infection.

II. Impetigo

A. Description

1. A highly contagious bacterial infection of the skin caused by β-hemolytic streptococci, or *Staphylococcus aureus*, or both.

Infantile
Usually begins at 2–6 months of age and decreases in incidence with age; generally undergoes spontaneous remission by 3 years of age

Childhood
May follow the infantile form; occurs at 2–3 years of age

Preadolescent and Adolescent
Begins at about 12 years of age; may continue into the early adult years or indefinitely

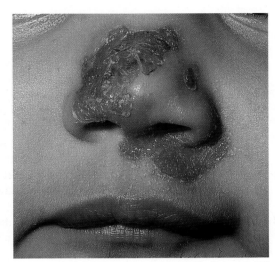

FIGURE 28.1 Impetigo contagiosa. (From Hockenberry M, Wilson D: *Wong's nursing care of infants and children*, ed 9, St. Louis, 2012, Mosby.)

2. Impetigo can occur because of poor hygiene. It can be a primary infection or occur secondarily at a site that has been injured or sustained an insect bite, or at a site that was originally a rash, such as atopic dermatitis, poison ivy, or poison oak.
3. The most common sites of infection are the face, around the mouth, the hands, the neck, and the extremities.
4. The lesions begin as vesicles or pustules surrounded by edema and redness (a pustule is similar to a vesicle except that its fluid content is purulent).
5. The lesions progress to an exudative and crusting stage; after the crusting of the lesions, the initially serous vesicular fluid becomes cloudy, and the vesicle ruptures, leaving a honey-colored crust that covers an ulcerated base.

B. Data collection (Fig. 28.1)
1. Lesions
2. Erythema
3. Pruritus
4. Burning
5. Secondary lymph node involvement

C. Interventions
1. Institute contact isolation, standard precautions and implement agency-specific isolation proce-

dures for the hospitalized child. Strict hygiene practice is important because it is a highly contagious condition.
2. Apply topical antibiotic ointments with a clean/ sterile cotton swab, without touching the tube opening with fingers or skin, and instruct parents in ointment and swab use; the infection is still communicable for 48 hours beyond initiation of antibiotic treatment.
3. Cover lesions with gauze bandages and tape to prevent the spread of infection.
4. Assist the child with daily bathing with antibacterial soap, as prescribed.
5. Apply warm water compresses to the lesions two or three times daily, followed by mild soap and water rinse to soften crusts for removal and to promote healing.
6. Oral antibiotics may be prescribed if there is no response to topical antibiotic treatment. It is extremely important to comply with the prescribed antibiotic regimen because secondary infections such as glomerulonephritis may result if the infectious agent is of a streptococcal type that can affect the nephrons.
7. To prevent skin cracking, apply emollients and reinforce instructions to parents in the use of emollients.
8. Reinforce instructions to the parents in the methods of preventing the spread of the infection, especially careful hand washing.
9. Inform parents that the child needs to use separate towels, linens, and dishes.
10. Inform parents that all linens and clothing used by the child needs to be washed with detergent in hot water separately from linens and clothing of other household members.

III. Pediculosis Capitis (Lice)

A. Description
1. An infestation of the hair and scalp with lice
2. The most common sites of involvement are the occipital area, behind the ears, at the nape of the neck, and, occasionally, the eyebrows and eyelashes.
3. The female louse lays her eggs (nits) on the hair shaft, close to the scalp. The incubation period is 7 to 10 days.
4. Head lice can survive for 48 hours away from the host; nits shed in the environment and can hatch in 7 to 10 days.
5. Head lice live and reproduce only on humans and are transmitted by direct and indirect contact, such as the sharing of brushes, hats, towels, and bedding.
6. All contacts of the infested child need to be examined for lice infestation and referred for treatment as appropriate.

BOX 28.2	Data Collection Findings: Pediculosis Capitis

- Child scratches the scalp excessively.
- Pruritus is caused by the crawling insect and insect saliva on the skin.
- Nits (white eggs) are observable on the hair shaft (it is important to differentiate nits from lint or dandruff, which flakes away easily).
- Adult lice are difficult to see and appear as small tan or grayish specks, which may crawl fast.

B. Data collection (Box 28.2)

C. Interventions

1. Use a pediculicide product as prescribed; follow package instructions for timing the application and for contraindications for their use in children.
2. Daily removal of nits with an extra fine-tooth metal nit comb should be done as a control measure after use of the pediculicide product. Gloves need to be worn for removal of nits. Hairbrushes or combs would be discarded or soaked in boiling water for 10 minutes or in a commercially available lice-killing product for 1 hour.
3. Reinforce instructions to the parents that siblings may also need treatment; grooming items are not to be shared, and a single comb or brush should be used for each individual child.
4. Reinforce instructions to the parents that bedding and clothing used by the child needs to be changed daily, laundered in hot water with detergent, and dried in a hot dryer for 20 minutes; this process would continue for 1 week.
5. Reinforce instructions to the parents that nonessential bedding and clothing can be stored in a tightly sealed bag for 2 weeks and then washed.
6. Reinforce instructions to the parents to seal toys that cannot be washed or dry-cleaned in a plastic bag for 2 weeks.
7. Reinforce instructions to the parents that furniture and carpets need to be vacuumed frequently and that the dust bag from the vacuum needs to be discarded after vacuuming.
8. Reinforce teaching the parents and the child not to share clothing, headwear, brushes, and combs.
9. Lice of the eyelashes or eyebrows may need to be removed manually.

IV. Scabies

A. Description

1. A parasitical skin disorder caused by an infestation of *Sarcoptesscabiei* (itch mite)
2. Endemic among schoolchildren and institutionalized populations as a result of close personal contact
3. Incubation period

BOX 28.3	Data Collection Findings: Scabies

- Pruritic papular rash
- Burrows into the skin (fine grayish-red lines that may be difficult to see)

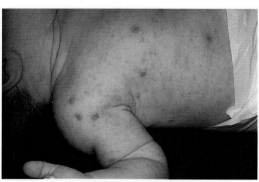

FIGURE 28.2 Scabies rash on an infant. (From Calen JP, Greer KE, Hood AF, Paller AS, Swinyer LJ: *Color atlas of dermatology*, Philadelphia, 1993, Saunders. Courtesy Dr. Steve Estes.)

    a. Female mites burrow into the epidermis, lay eggs, and die in the burrow after 4 to 5 weeks.

    b. The eggs hatch in 3 to 5 days, and the larvae mature and complete their life cycle.

4. Infectious period: During the course of the infestation

B. Data collection (Box 28.3 and Fig. 28.2)

⚠️ Scabies is transmitted by close personal contact with an infected person. Household members and contacts of an infected child need to be treated simultaneously.

C. Interventions

1. Topical application of a scabicide is needed to kill the mites.
2. Various products are available, and a prescription is needed for the product.
3. Lindane shampoo, a product that may be prescribed, is not used in children younger than 2 years because of the risk of neurotoxicity and seizures.
4. Reinforce instructions to the parents in the application of the scabicide.
5. When permethrin is used, it is applied to cool, dry skin at least 30 minutes after bathing; the cream is massaged thoroughly and gently into all skin surfaces (not just the areas that have the rash) from the head to the soles of the feet (avoid contact with the eyes); left on the skin for 8 to 14 hours; and then removed by bathing. A repeat treatment may be necessary.
6. Reinforce instructions to the parents about the importance of frequent hand washing.
7. Reinforce instructions to the parents that all clothing, bedding, and pillowcases used by the child

need to be changed daily; washed in hot water with detergent; dried in a hot dryer; and ironed before reuse; this process would continue for 1 week.

8. Reinforce instructions to the parents that non-washable toys and other items would be sealed in plastic bags for 4 days.

9. Antiitch topical treatment may be necessary, and antibiotics may be prescribed if a secondary infection develops.

V. Burn Injuries (see Priority Nursing Actions)

⚡ PRIORITY NURSING ACTIONS

A Major Burn Injury on the Child

1. Stop the burning process.
2. Assess for patent airway.
3. Begin resuscitation if necessary using CAB—compressions, airway, breathing.
4. Remove burned clothing and jewelry.
5. Cover the wound(s) with a clean cloth at the site of injury (sterile dressings on arrival to the health care facility).
6. Keep the child warm.
7. Transport the child to the emergency department.

A. Pediatric considerations (see Chapter 39 for additional information about burns)

1. Very young children who have been severely burned have a higher mortality rate than older children and adults with comparable burns.

2. Lower burn temperatures and shorter exposure to heat can cause a more severe burn in a child than an adult because a child's skin is thinner.

3. The degree of pain experienced by the child and the ability to communicate it will be different than in an adult with the same exposure.

4. Severely burned children are at increased risk for fluid and heat loss, dehydration, and metabolic acidosis than an adult.

5. The higher proportion of body fluid to body mass in children increases the risk of cardiovascular problems.

6. Burns involving more than 10% of the total body surface area require some form of fluid resuscitation.

7. Infants and children are at increased risk for protein and calorie deficiency because they have smaller muscle mass and less body fat than adults.

8. Scarring is more severe in a child; disturbed body image will be a distinct issue for a child or adolescent, especially as growth continues.

9. An immature immune system presents an increased risk of infection for infants and young children.

10. A delay in **growth** may occur following a burn.

B. Extent of burn injury

1. The rule of nines, used for an adult with a burn injury, gives an inaccurate estimate in children because of the difference in body proportions between children and adults.

2. In the pediatric client, the extent of the burn is expressed as a percentage of the total body surface area (TBSA) using specific age-related charts.

C. Fluid replacement therapy

⚠ To determine adequacy of fluid resuscitation, vital signs (especially heart rate), urine output, adequacy of capillary filling, and sensorium status are assessed.

1. Fluid replacement is necessary during the initial 24-hour period following the burn injury because of the fluid shifts that occur as a result of the injury.

2. Several formulas are available to calculate the child's fluid needs, and the formula used depends on the health care provider's preference.

3. Crystalloid solutions are used during the initial phase of therapy; colloid solutions such as albumin, Plasma-Lyte (combined electrolyte solution), or fresh-frozen plasma are useful in maintaining plasma volume.

4. See Chapter 39 for additional information related to burns and their management.

D. Instructions for parents

1. Keep all matches and lighters out of reach.

2. Check smoke detectors regularly.

3. Turn hot water heater thermostat down to 120°F (48.8°C).

4. Turn pot handles toward back burners on stove when possible.

5. Teach a child about "stop, drop, and roll" as a measure to stop the burning process.

6. Keep children away from outdoor grills and indoor wood burning stoves.

7. Have periodic fire drills.

WHAT WOULD YOU DO?

Answer: For a child suspected of having impetigo, the nurse would institute strict contact precautions and use standard precautions. The nurse would also implement agency-specific isolation procedures for the hospitalized child. Strict hygiene practices are important because impetigo is a highly contagious condition. The nurse would ensure that all health care workers and visitors are aware of the necessary precautions in order to prevent the spread of infection.

PRACTICE QUESTIONS

❖ 1. The school nurse prepares a list of home care instructions for the parents of school children who have been diagnosed with pediculosis capitis (head lice). Which would be included in the list? **Select all that apply.**
   - ❑ 1. Siblings may also need treatment.
   - ❑ 2. Use antilice sprays on all bedding and furniture.
   - ❑ 3. Use a pediculicide shampoo and repeat treatment in 14 days.
   - ❑ 4. Grooming items such as combs and brushes should not be shared.
   - ❑ 5. Launder all the bedding and clothing in hot water and dry on high heat.
   - ❑ 6. Vacuum floors, play areas, and furniture to remove any hairs that may carry live nits.

2. The nurse is reinforcing home-care instructions to the parents of a 3-year-old child with scabies. Which statement by a parent indicates the **need for further teaching?**
   1. "I understand that I need to leave the scabicide on for 4 hours before washing it off."
   2. "I will need to seal up all my child's non-washable toys in a plastic bag for at least 4 days."
   3. "I realize that everyone who has come in contact with my child will need to be treated for scabies."
   4. "I know I need to wash all the clothing and bedding in hot water with detergent and dry in a hot dryer."

❖ 3. The nurse caring for a child who sustained a burn injury plans care based on which pediatric considerations associated with this injury? **Select all that apply.**
   - ❑ 1. Scarring is less severe in a child than in an adult.
   - ❑ 2. A delay in growth may occur after a burn injury.
   - ❑ 3. An immature immune system presents an increased risk of infection for infants and young children.
   - ❑ 4. Fluid resuscitation is unnecessary unless the burned area is more than 25% of the total body surface area.
   - ❑ 5. The lower proportion of body fluid to body mass in a child increases the risk of cardiovascular problems.
   - ❑ 6. Infants and young children are at increased risk for protein and calorie deficiency because they have smaller muscle mass and less body fat than adults.

4. A topical corticosteroid is prescribed by the pediatrician for a child with atopic dermatitis (eczema). Which instruction would the nurse give the parent about applying the cream?
   1. Apply the cream over the entire body.
   2. Apply a thick layer of cream to affected areas only.
   3. Avoid cleansing the area before application of the cream.
   4. Apply a thin layer of cream and rub it into the area thoroughly.

5. The nurse is assisting in performing pediculosis capitis (head lice) checks. Which finding indicates that a child has a "positive" head check?
   1. Maculopapular lesions behind the ears
   2. Lesions in the scalp that extend to the hairline or neck
   3. White flaky particles throughout the entire scalp region
   4. White sacs attached to the hair shafts in the occipital area

ANSWERS

1. 1, 4, 5, 6
Rationale: Bedding and linens need to be washed with hot water and dried on a hot setting. Thorough home cleaning is necessary to remove any remaining lice or nits. Siblings may need to be treated, and combs and brushes may need to be discarded or soaked in boiling water for 10 minutes. Antilice sprays are unnecessary. Additionally, they would never be used on bedding, furniture, or a child. The pediculicide product needs to be used as prescribed, and the parents are instructed to follow package instructions for timing the application and for contraindications for their use in children.
Test-Taking Strategy: Focus on the subject, home care instructions for pediculosis capitis. Eliminate option 2, knowing that antilice sprays should not be used. The pediculicide product needs to be used based on the manufacturer's instructions. All the other choices are acceptable and need to be reiterated to the family.

2. 1
Rationale: The treatment for scabies involves applying a scabicide to cool, dry skin at least 30 minutes after bathing, which needs to be left on the skin for 8 to 14 hours, then washed off. The other statements are correct instructions.
Test-Taking Strategy: Focus on the strategic words, *need for further teaching.* These words indicate a negative event query and ask you to select an option that is an incorrect statement. Recall that the scabicide needs to be left on the skin for 8 to 14 hours before washing it off. The other options are correct instructions.

3. 2, 3, 6
Rationale: Pediatric considerations in the care of a burn victim include the following: Scarring is more severe in a child than in an adult. A delay in growth may occur after a burn injury. An immature immune system presents an increased risk of infection for infants and young children. The higher proportion of body fluid to body mass in a child increases the

risk of cardiovascular problems. Burns involving more than 10% of total body surface area require some form of fluid resuscitation. Infants and young children are at increased risk for protein and calorie deficiencies because they have smaller muscle mass and less body fat than adults.

Test-Taking Strategy: Focus on the subject, pediatric considerations in the care of a child who has sustained a burn injury. To answer correctly, read each option carefully and think about the physiology of a child related to body size.

4. 4

Rationale: Atopic dermatitis is a superficial inflammatory process involving primarily the epidermis. A topical corticosteroid may be prescribed and would be applied sparingly (thin layer) and rubbed into the area thoroughly. The affected area would be cleaned gently before application. A topical corticosteroid would not be applied over extensive areas. Systemic absorption is more likely to occur with extensive application.

Test-Taking Strategy: Focus on the subject, application of a topical corticosteroid. Eliminate option 3 first because it does not make sense not to clean an affected area. Eliminate option 1 because medicated cream would be applied only to areas that are affected. Eliminate option 2 because of the word *thick*.

5. 4

Rationale: Pediculosis capitis is an infestation of the hair and scalp with lice. The nits are visible and attached firmly to the hair shaft near the scalp. The occiput is an area in which nits can be seen. Maculopapular lesions behind the ears or lesions that extend to the hairline or neck are indicative of an infectious process, not pediculosis. White flaky particles are indicative of dandruff.

Test-Taking Strategy: Focus on the subject, the characteristics of pediculosis capitis. Option 3 can be eliminated first because white flaky particles are indicative of dandruff. Recalling that in this infestation nit sacs attach to the hair shaft will direct you to the correct option.

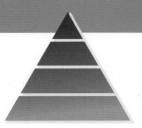

CHAPTER **29**

Hematological and Oncological Problems

PRIORITY CONCEPTS Cellular Regulation; Perfusion

WHAT WOULD YOU DO?

A child with hemophilia who has been in a motor vehicle crash is admitted to the pediatric unit. What would the nurse do in the care of this child?
Answer is located on p. 365.

I. Sickle Cell Anemia

A. Description

1. Sickle cell anemia constitutes a group of diseases termed *hemoglobinopathies*, in which hemoglobin (Hgb) A is partly or completely replaced by abnormal sickle Hgb S.

2. It is caused by the inheritance of a gene for a structurally abnormal portion of the Hgb chain.

3. Risk factors include having parents heterozygous for hemoglobin S or being of African American descent.

4. For screening purposes, the sickle-turbidity test (Sickledex) is frequently used because it can be performed using blood from a finger stick and yields accurate results in 3 minutes. However, if the test result is positive, Hgb electrophoresis is necessary to distinguish between children with the trait and those with the disease.

5. HgbS is sensitive to changes in the oxygen content of the red blood cell (RBC).

6. Insufficient oxygen causes the cells to assume a sickle shape, and the cells become rigid and clumped together, obstructing capillary blood flow (Fig. 29.1).

7. The clinical manifestations occur primarily as a result of obstruction caused by sickled RBCs and increased RBC destruction.

8. Situations that precipitate sickling include fever, dehydration, and emotional or physical stress; any condition that increases the need for oxy-

gen or alters the transport of oxygen can result in sickle cell crisis (acute exacerbation).

9. Sickle cell crises are acute exacerbations of the disease, which vary considerably in severity and frequency; these include vaso-occlusive crisis, splenic sequestration, hyperhemolytic crisis, and aplastic crisis.

10. The sickling response is reversible under conditions of adequate oxygenation and hydration; after repeated sickling, the cell becomes permanently sickled.

11. An interprofessional approach to care is needed, and care focuses on the prevention (preventing exposure to infection and maintaining normal hydration) and treatment (hydration, oxygen, pain management, and bed rest) of the crisis.

B. Sickle cell crisis: Data collection (Box 29.1)

C. Interventions

1. Maintain adequate hydration and blood flow with oral and intravenous (IV) administered fluids. Electrolyte replacement is also provided as needed; without adequate hydration, pain will not be controlled.

2. Administer oxygen, as prescribed, to increase tissue perfusion; blood transfusions may also be prescribed.

3. Assist to administer analgesics as prescribed (around the clock).

4. Assist the child with assuming a comfortable position so that he/she keeps the extremities extended to promote venous return; elevate the head of the bed no more than 30 degrees, avoid putting strain on painful joints, and do not raise the knee gatch of the bed.

5. Encourage the consumption of a high-calorie, high-protein diet with folic acid supplementation.

6. Assist to administer antibiotics, as prescribed, to prevent infection.

7. Monitor for complications, including increasing anemia, decreased perfusion, and shock

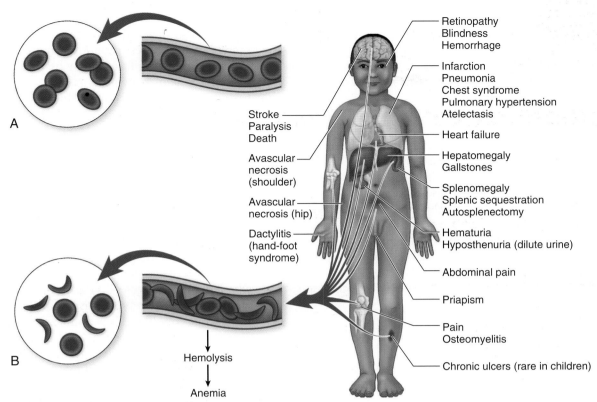

Stroke
Paralysis
Death

Avascular
necrosis
(shoulder)

Avascular
necrosis (hip)

Dactylitis
(hand-foot
syndrome)

Retinopathy
Blindness
Hemorrhage

Infarction
Pneumonia
Chest syndrome
Pulmonary hypertension
Atelectasis

Heart failure

Hepatomegaly
Gallstones

Splenomegaly
Splenic sequestration
Autosplenectomy

Hematuria
Hyposthenuria (dilute urine)

Abdominal pain

Priapism

Pain
Osteomyelitis

Chronic ulcers (rare in children)

A

B

Hemolysis

Anemia

FIGURE 29.1 Differences between (A) normal red blood cells and (B) sickled red blood cells on circulation with related complications.

BOX 29.1 Sickle Cell Crisis

Vaso-Occlusive Crisis
- Caused by stasis of blood with clumping of cells in the microcirculation, ischemia, and infarction
- *Manifestations:* Fever; painful swelling of hands, feet, and joints; and abdominal pain

Splenic Sequestration
- Caused by pooling and clumping of blood in the spleen (hypersplenism)
- *Manifestations:* Profound anemia, hypovolemia, and shock

Hyperhemolytic Crisis
- An accelerated rate of red blood cell destruction
- *Manifestations:* Anemia, jaundice, and reticulocytosis

Aplastic Crisis
- Caused by diminished production and increased destruction of red blood cells, triggered by viral infection or depletion of folic acid
- *Manifestations:* Profound anemia and pallor

(i.e., mental status changes, pallor, and vital sign changes).
8. Reinforce instructions to the child and parents about the early signs and symptoms of crisis and the measures to prevent a crisis.
9. Emphasize the need to maintain strict adherence to immunization schedules; ensure that the child receives pneumococcal and meningococcal vaccines and an annual influenza vaccine be-

cause of the susceptibility to infection from functional asplenia.
10. A splenectomy may be necessary for those who experience recurrent splenic sequestration.
11. Inform the parents of the hereditary aspects of the disorder.

⚠ Administration of meperidine for pain is avoided because of the risk of normeperidine-induced seizures.

II. Iron Deficiency Anemia

A. Description
   1. Iron stores are depleted, which results in a decreased supply of iron for the manufacture of Hgb in RBCs.
   2. Commonly results from blood loss, increased metabolic demand, syndromes of gastrointestinal (GI) malabsorption, and dietary inadequacy
B. Data collection
   1. Pallor
   2. Weakness and fatigue
   3. Low Hgb and hematocrit levels
   4. RBCs that are microcytic and hypochromic
C. Interventions
   1. Increase oral intake of iron; iron-fortified formula will be needed for the infant.
   2. Reinforce instructions to the child and parents regarding food choices that are high in iron. (Refer to Chapter 11 for foods high in iron.)

3. Administer iron supplements as prescribed.

4. Intramuscular injections of iron (using Z-track method) or IV administration of iron may be prescribed in severe cases of anemia.

5. Reinforce teaching the parents about how to administer the iron supplements.

    a. Give them between meals for maximum absorption.

    b. Give them with a multivitamin or fruit juice, because vitamin C increases absorption.

    c. Do not give them with milk or antacids, because these items decrease absorption.

6. Reinforce instructions to the child and parents about the side effects of iron supplements (i.e., black stools, constipation, foul aftertaste).

7. Emphasize the importance of keeping the medication in a safe place out of reach of the child (iron overdose can result if an excess amount is consumed).

    ⚠ Liquid iron preparation stains the teeth. Teach the parents and child that liquid iron would be taken through a straw and that the teeth need to be brushed after administration.

III. Aplastic Anemia

A. Description

1. A deficiency of circulating erythrocytes and all other formed elements of blood, resulting from the arrested development of cells within the bone marrow

2. It can be primary (present at birth) or secondary (acquired).

3. Several possible causes exist, including chronic exposure to myelotoxic agents, viruses, infection, autoimmune disorders, and allergic states.

4. The definitive diagnosis is determined by bone marrow aspiration, which shows the conversion of red bone marrow to yellow fatty bone marrow.

5. Therapeutic management focuses on restoring function to the bone marrow and involves immunosuppressive therapy and bone marrow transplantation (treatment of choice if a suitable donor exists).

6. If the cause is a myelotoxic medication that is being administered for another purpose, the medication may be discontinued to improve bone marrow function.

B. Data collection

1. Pancytopenia (a deficiency of erythrocytes, leukocytes, and thrombocytes)

2. Petechiae, purpura, bleeding, pallor, weakness, tachycardia, and fatigue

C. Interventions

1. Prepare the child for bone marrow transplantation, if planned.

2. Immunosuppressive medications: Antilymphocyte globulin or antithymocyte globulin may be prescribed to suppress the autoimmune response.

3. Colony-stimulating factors may be prescribed to enhance bone marrow production.

4. Corticosteroids and cyclosporine may be prescribed.

5. Blood or platelet transfusions may be prescribed.

6. Advise the parents to obtain a Medic-Alert bracelet for the child.

IV. Hemophilia

A. Description

1. Refers to a group of bleeding disorders resulting from a deficiency of specific coagulation proteins

2. Identifying the specific coagulation deficiency is important so that definitive treatment with the specific replacement agent can be implemented; aggressive replacement therapy is initiated to prevent the chronic crippling effects from joint bleeding.

3. The most common types include factor VIII deficiency (hemophilia A or classic hemophilia) and factor IX deficiency (hemophilia B or Christmas disease).

4. Hemophilia is transmitted as an X-linked recessive disorder (it may also occur as a result of a gene mutation).

5. Carrier females pass on the defect to affected males; female offspring are rarely born with the disorder but may be if they inherit an affected gene from their mother and are offspring of a father with hemophilia.

6. The primary treatment is the replacement of the missing clotting factor; additional medications, such as those to relieve pain or corticosteroids, may be prescribed, depending on the source of bleeding.

B. Data collection

1. Abnormal bleeding in response to trauma or surgery (sometimes is detected after circumcision)

2. Epistaxis (nosebleeds)

3. Joint bleeding that causes pain, tenderness, swelling, and a limited range of motion

4. Tendency to bruise easily

5. Results of tests that measure platelet function are normal; results of tests that measure clotting factor function may be abnormal.

C. Interventions

1. Monitor for bleeding and maintain bleeding precautions.

2. Prepare to assist to administer factor VIII concentrates, either produced through genetic engineering (recombinant) or derived from pooled plasma as prescribed.

3. DDAVP (1-deamino-8-D-arginine vasopressin), a synthetic form of vasopressin, increases plasma factor VIII and may be prescribed to treat mild hemophilia.

4. Monitor for joint pain; immobilize the affected extremity if joint pain occurs.
5. Monitor the neurological status; the child is at risk for intracranial hemorrhage.
6. Monitor the urine for hematuria.
7. Control bleeding by immobilization, elevation, and the application of ice; in addition, apply pressure (15 minutes) for superficial bleeding.
8. Reinforce instructions to the child and parents about the signs of internal bleeding and how to control bleeding if it occurs.
9. Reinforce instructions to the parents regarding activities for the child, emphasizing the avoidance of contact sports and the need for protective devices while learning to walk; assist in developing an appropriate exercise plan.
10. Reinforce instructions to the child to wear protective devices such as helmets and knee and elbow pads when participating in sports such as bicycling and skating.

V. von Willebrand's Disease

A. Description
1. A hereditary bleeding disorder characterized by a deficiency of, or a defect in, the protein called von Willebrand's factor (vWF)
2. The disorder causes platelets to adhere to damaged endothelium; the vWF protein also serves as a carrier protein for factor VIII.
3. It is characterized by an increased tendency to bleed from the mucous membranes.

B. Data collection
1. Epistaxis
2. Gum bleeding
3. Easy bruising
4. Excessive menstrual bleeding

C. Interventions
1. Treatment and care are similar to those measures implemented for hemophilia, including the administration of clotting factors.
2. Provide emotional support to the child and parents, especially if the child is experiencing an episode of bleeding.

⚠️ A child with a bleeding disorder needs to wear a Medic-Alert bracelet.

VI. β-Thalassemia Major (Box 29.2)

A. Description
1. An autosomal-recessive disorder characterized by the reduced production of one of the globin chains in the synthesis of Hgb (both parents must be carriers to produce a child with β-thalassemia major)
2. The incidence is highest in individuals of Mediterranean descent, such as Italians, Greeks, Syrians, and their offspring.

BOX 29.2   Types of β-Thalassemia

- *Thalassemia minor:* Asymptomatic silent carrier case
- *Thalassemia trait:* Produces a mild microcytic anemia
- *Thalassemia intermedia:* Manifested as splenomegaly and moderate to severe anemia
- *Thalassemia major:* Results in severe anemia requiring transfusion support to sustain life (also known as Cooley's anemia)

---

3. Treatment is supportive; the goal of therapy is to maintain normal Hgb levels by the administration of blood transfusions.
4. Bone marrow transplantation may be offered as an alternative therapy.
5. A splenectomy may be performed in a child with severe splenomegaly who requires repeated transfusions (assists in relieving abdominal pressure and may increase the life span of supplemental RBCs).

B. Data collection
1. Frontal bossing
2. Maxillary prominence
3. Wide-set eyes with a flattened nose
4. Greenish-yellow skin tone
5. Hepatosplenomegaly
6. Severe anemia
7. Microcytic, hypochromic RBCs

C. Interventions
1. Blood transfusion may be prescribed.
2. Monitor for iron overload and administer chelation therapy, which may be prescribed to treat iron overload and to prevent organ damage from the elevated levels of iron caused by the multiple transfusion therapy.
3. If the child has had a splenectomy, instruct the parents to report any signs of infection because of the risk of sepsis.
4. Ensure that parents understand the importance of the child receiving pneumococcal and meningococcal vaccines in addition to an annual influenza vaccine and the regularly scheduled vaccines.
5. Provide resources for genetic counseling.

VII. Leukemia

A. Description (also refer to Chapter 41)
1. Malignant increase in the number of leukocytes, usually at an immature stage, in the bone marrow
2. In leukemia, proliferating immature white blood cells (WBCs) depress the bone marrow, causing anemia from decreased erythrocytes, infection from neutropenia, and bleeding from decreased platelet production (thrombocytopenia).
3. The cause is unknown and appears to involve the genetic damage of cells, thus leading to the transformation of cells from a normal state to a malignant state.

4. Risk factors include genetic, viral, immunological, and environmental factors and exposure to radiation, chemicals, and medications.

5. Acute lymphocytic leukemia is the most frequent type of cancer in children.

6. Leukemia is more common among boys than girls after 1 year of age.

7. Prognosis depends on various factors such as age at diagnosis, initial WBC, type of cell involved, and sex of the child.

8. Treatment involves chemotherapy and possibly radiation and hematopoietic stem cell transplantation.

9. The phases of chemotherapy include induction, which achieves a complete remission or disappearance of leukemic cells; intensification or consolidation therapy, which decreases the tumor burden further; central nervous system prophylactic therapy, which prevents leukemic cells from invading the central nervous system; and maintenance, which serves to maintain the remission phase.

B. Data collection

1. Infiltration of the bone marrow causes fever, pallor, fatigue, anorexia, hemorrhage (usually petechiae), and bone and joint pain; pathological fractures can occur as a result of bone marrow invasion with leukemic cells.

2. Signs of infection as a result of neutropenia

3. Hepatosplenomegaly and lymphadenopathy

4. Normal, elevated, or low WBC, depending on the presence of infection or of immature *versus* mature WBCs

5. Decreased Hgb and hematocrit levels

6. Decreased platelet count

7. Positive bone marrow biopsy identifying leukemic blast (immature) phase cells

8. Signs of increased intracranial pressure (ICP) occur as a result of central nervous system involvement (refer to XII. Brain Tumors)

9. Signs of cranial nerve (cranial nerve VII, or the facial nerve, is most commonly affected) or spinal nerve involvement; signs and symptoms relate to the area involved.

10. Signs and symptoms that indicate the invasion of leukemic cells in the kidneys, testes, prostate, ovaries, GI tract, and lungs

C. Infection (Box 29.3)

1. Infection can occur through self- or cross-contamination.

2. Most common sites of infection are the skin (any break in the skin is a potential site of infection), respiratory tract, or GI tract.

D. Bleeding (Box 29.4)

1. Platelet transfusions are generally reserved for active bleeding episodes that do not respond to local treatment and that may occur during induction or relapse therapy.

BOX 29.3   Protecting the Child from Infection

- Initiate protective isolation procedures.
- Maintain frequent and thorough hand washing.
- Maintain the child in a private room with high-efficiency particulate air filtration or laminar airflow system, if possible.
- Be sure that the child's room is cleaned daily.
- Use strict aseptic technique for all nursing procedures.
- Limit the number of caregivers entering the child's room and ensure that anyone entering is wearing a mask.
- Keep supplies for the child separate from supplies for other children.
- Reduce exposure to environmental organisms by eliminating raw fruits and vegetables and fresh flowers and by not leaving standing water in the child's room.
- Assist the child with daily bathing with the use of antimicrobial soap.
- Assist the child with performing oral hygiene frequently.
- Monitor for signs/symptoms of infection.
- Monitor the oral or axillary temperature, pulse, and blood pressure.
- Change wound dressings daily, and inspect wounds for redness, swelling, or drainage.
- Monitor the urine for color and cloudiness.
- Monitor the skin and oral mucous membranes for signs of infection.
- Check the lung sounds.
- Encourage the child to cough and deep breathe.
- Monitor the white blood cell and the neutrophil count.
- Notify the registered nurse if signs of infection are present; prepare to obtain specimens for the culture of open lesions, urine, and sputum.
- Assist with initiation of a bowel program to prevent constipation and rectal trauma.
- Avoid invasive procedures, such as injections, rectal temperatures, and urinary catheterization.
- Assist to administer antibiotic, antifungal, and antiviral medication, as prescribed.
- Assist to administer granulocyte colony-stimulating factor, as prescribed.
- Reinforce instructions to the parents to keep the child away from crowds and those with infections.
- Reinforce instructions to the parents that the child should not receive immunization with a live virus (measles, mumps, rubella, polio) because if the immune system is depressed, the attenuated virus can result in a life-threatening infection; also, the child would not receive the varicella vaccine.
- The inactivated vaccine for poliomyelitis may be administered.
- Reinforce instructions to the parents to inform the teacher that they need to be notified immediately if a case of a communicable disease occurs in another child at school.

---

2. Packed RBCs may be prescribed for a child with severe blood loss.

E. Fatigue and nutrition

1. Assist the child with selecting a well-balanced diet.

2. Provide small meals that require little chewing and will not be irritating to the oral mucosa.

BOX 29.4 **Protecting the Child from Bleeding**

- Examine the child for signs/symptoms of bleeding.
- Handle the child gently.
- Measure the abdominal girth, which can indicate internal hemorrhage.
- Reinforce instructions to the child to use a soft toothbrush and to avoid dental floss.
- Provide soft foods that are cool to warm in temperature.
- Avoid injections, if possible, to prevent trauma to the skin and bleeding.
- Apply firm and gentle pressure to a needle-stick site for at least 10 minutes.
- Pad side rails and sharp corners of the bed and other furniture.
- Discourage the child from engaging in activities that involve the use of objects that can cause injury.
- Reinforce instructions to the child to avoid constrictive or tight clothing.
- Use caution when taking the blood pressure to prevent skin injury.
- Reinforce instructions to the child to avoid blowing his or her nose.
- Avoid rectal suppositories, enemas, and rectal thermometers; initiate a bowel program to prevent constipation and rectal trauma.
- Examine all body fluids and excrement for the presence of blood.
- Count the number of pads or tampons used if the adolescent girl is menstruating.
- Reinforce instructions to the child regarding the signs and symptoms of bleeding.
- Reinforce instructions to the parents to avoid administering nonsteroidal anti-inflammatory drugs and products that contain aspirin to the child.

---

3. If the child cannot take oral feedings, parenteral nutrition or enteral feedings may be prescribed.
4. Assist the child with self-care and mobility activities.
5. Allow for adequate rest periods during care.
6. Avoid performing nursing care activities unless they are essential.

F. Chemotherapy

1. Monitor for severe bone marrow suppression; during the period of greatest bone marrow suppression (the nadir), blood counts will be extremely low.
2. Monitor for infection and bleeding.

3. Protect the child from life-threatening infections.
4. Monitor for nausea, vomiting, and alterations in bowel function.
5. Administer stool softeners as prescribed and if needed to prevent straining and resultant bleeding, if constipation occurs.
6. Provide rectal hygiene gently as needed.
7. Assist to administer antiemetics before beginning chemotherapy as prescribed.

8. Monitor for signs of dehydration.
9. Monitor for signs of hemorrhagic cystitis.
10. Monitor for signs of peripheral neuropathy.
11. Check oral mucous membranes for mucositis; administer frequent mouth rinses per agency procedure and as prescribed to promote healing and/or prevent infection (local oral anesthetics may also be prescribed).
12. Reinforce instructions to the parents regarding the signs/symptoms to monitor after chemotherapy and when to notify the primary health care provider (PHCP).
13. Inform parents that hair loss may occur from chemotherapy; hair will regrow in 3 to 6 months and may be a slightly different color or texture.
14. Reinforce instructions to the parents about the care of a central venous access device, as necessary. (Refer to Chapter 12 for information on central venous access devices.)
15. Listen to the child and family, and encourage them to verbalize their feelings and express their concerns.
16. Introduce the family to other families of children with cancer if appropriate.
17. Consult social services and chaplains, as necessary.

⚠️ Monitor a child receiving chemotherapy closely for signs of infection. Infection is a major cause of death in the immunosuppressed child.

VIII. Hodgkin's Disease

A. Description
1. A type of lymphoma; a malignancy of the lymph nodes that originates in a single lymph node or a single chain of nodes.
2. It predictably metastasizes to nonnodal or extralymphatic sites, especially the spleen, liver, bone marrow, lungs, and mediastinum.
3. Characterized by the presence of Reed-Sternberg cells in the lymph nodes
4. Peak incidence is in mid-adolescence.
5. Possible causes include viral infection and previous exposure to alkylating chemical agents.
6. The prognosis is excellent, with long-term survival rates depending on the stage of the disease.
7. The primary treatment modalities are radiation and chemotherapy; each may be used alone or in combination, depending on the clinical staging of the disease.

B. Data collection

1. Painless enlargement of the lymph nodes
2. Enlarged, firm, nontender, movable nodes in the supraclavicular area; in children, the sentinel node located near the left clavicle may be the first enlarged node.

Pediatric Nursing

3. Nonproductive cough as a result of mediastinal lymphadenopathy
4. Abdominal pain as a result of enlarged retroperitoneal nodes
5. Advanced lymph node and extralymphatic involvement may cause systemic symptoms, such as low-grade and/or intermittent fever, anorexia, nausea, weight loss, night sweats, and pruritus.
6. Positive biopsy of a lymph node (presence of Reed-Sternberg cells) and positive bone marrow biopsy specimen
7. Computed tomography scan of the liver, spleen, and bone marrow may be done to detect metastasis.

C. Interventions
1. For early stages without mediastinal node involvement, the treatment of choice is usually extensive external radiation of the involved lymph node regions.
2. With more extensive disease, radiation in combination with multiagent chemotherapy is used.
3. Monitor for drug-induced pancytopenia and an abnormal depression of all cellular components of the blood, which increases the risk for infection, bleeding, and anemia.
4. Protect the child from infection.
5. Provide a safe, hazard-free environment.
6. Monitor for adverse effects related to chemotherapy or radiation; the most common side effect of extensive irradiation is malaise, which can be difficult for older children and adolescents to tolerate both physically and psychologically (Table 29.1).
7. Monitor for nausea and vomiting; administer antiemetics, as prescribed.

IX. Nephroblastoma (Wilms' Tumor)

A. Description
1. Wilms' tumor is the most common intraabdominal and kidney tumor of childhood; it may present unilaterally and localized, or bilaterally, sometimes with metastasis to other organs.
2. The peak incidence is at 3 years of age.
3. Occurrence is associated with a genetic inheritance and with several congenital anomalies.
4. Therapeutic management includes a combination treatment of surgery (partial to total nephrectomy) and chemotherapy with or without radiation, depending on the clinical stage and histological pattern of the tumor.

B. Data collection
1. A swelling or mass within the abdomen; the mass is characteristically firm, nontender, confined to one side, and deep within the flank.
2. Urinary retention and/or hematuria
3. Anemia caused by hemorrhage within the tumor

TABLE 29.1 Adverse Effects of Radiation Therapy and Nursing Interventions

Body Area and Adverse Effects	Interventions
Gastrointestinal Tract	
Anorexia	Encourage fluids and foods as best tolerated. Provide small, frequent meals. Monitor for weight loss.
Nausea, vomiting	Administer antiemetics around the clock. Monitor for dehydration.
Mucosal ulceration	Provide soothing oral hygiene and prescribed mouth rinses. Topical anesthetic may be prescribed.
Diarrhea	Administer antispasmodics and antidiarrheal preparations as prescribed. Monitor for dehydration.
Skin	
Alopecia (hair loss)	Introduce idea of a wig or head wraps to the child. Provide scalp hygiene. Stress the need for head covering in cold weather.
Dry or moist desquamation	Keep the skin clean. Wash the skin daily, using a mild soap sparingly. Do not remove skin markings for radiation. Avoid exposure to the sun and other extreme temperature changes. For dryness, apply lubricant as prescribed.
Urinary Bladder	
Cystitis	Encourage fluid intake and frequent voiding. Monitor for hematuria.
Bone Marrow	
Myelosuppression	Monitor for fever. Administer antibiotics as prescribed. Avoid the use of suppositories, enemas, and rectal temperatures. Institute neutropenic or bleeding precautions as needed. Monitor for signs of anemia.

Adapted from Hockenberry M, Wilson D: *Wong's nursing care of infants and children*, ed 9, St. Louis, 2013, Mosby; and McKinney E, James S, Murray S, Ashwill J: *Maternal-child nursing*, ed 4, St. Louis, 2013, Saunders.

4. Pallor, anorexia, and lethargy resulting from anemia
5. Hypertension, caused by the secretion of excess amounts of renin by the tumor
6. Weight loss and fever
7. Symptoms of lung involvement, such as dyspnea, shortness of breath, and pain in the chest, if metastasis has occurred

C. Preoperative interventions
1. Monitor vital signs, particularly blood pressure.
2. Avoid palpation of the abdomen; place a sign at the bedside that reads as follows: "Do not palpate abdomen."
3. Measure the abdominal girth at least once daily.

D. Postoperative interventions
1. Monitor temperature and blood pressure closely.
2. Monitor for signs of hemorrhage and infection.
3. Monitor strict intake and output closely.
4. Monitor for abdominal distention, bowel sounds, and other signs of GI activity because of the risk for intestinal obstruction.

⚠️ Avoid palpation of the abdomen in a child with Wilms' tumor and be cautious when bathing, moving, or handling the child. It is important to keep the encapsulated tumor intact. Rupture of the tumor can cause the cancer cells to spread throughout the abdomen, lymph system, and bloodstream.

X. Neuroblastoma

A. Description
1. A tumor that originates from the embryonic neural crest cells that normally give rise to the adrenal medulla and the sympathetic ganglia
2. Most tumors develop in the adrenal gland or the retroperitoneal sympathetic chain; other sites may be within the head, neck, chest, or pelvis.
3. Most children present with the tumor before 10 years of age. Most presenting signs are caused by the tumor compressing adjacent normal tissue and organs.
4. Diagnostic evaluation is aimed at locating the primary site of the tumor.
5. The prognosis is poor because of the frequency of invasiveness of the tumor and because, in most cases, the diagnosis is not made until after metastasis has occurred; the younger the child at diagnosis, the better the survival rate.
6. Therapeutic Management
   a. Surgery is performed to remove as much of the tumor as possible and to obtain samples for biopsy; in early stages, complete surgical removal of the tumor is the treatment of choice.
   b. Surgery is usually limited to biopsy in the later stages because of the extensive metastasis.
   c. Radiation is commonly used with late-stage disease and provides palliation for metastatic lesions in the bones, lungs, liver, or brain.
   d. Chemotherapy is used in the treatment of extensive local or disseminated disease.

B. Data collection: Signs/symptoms depend on the location of the primary tumor.
1. Firm, nontender, irregular mass in the abdomen that crosses the midline
2. Urinary frequency or retention from the compression of the kidney, ureter, or bladder
3. Lymphadenopathy, especially in the cervical and supraclavicular area
4. Bone pain if skeletal involvement occurs
5. Supraorbital ecchymosis (raccoon eyes), periorbital edema, and exophthalmos as a result of the invasion of retrobulbar soft tissue

6. Pallor, weakness, irritability, anorexia, weight loss
7. Signs of respiratory impairment (thoracic lesion)
8. Signs of neurological impairment (intracranial lesion)
9. Paralysis from the compression of the spinal cord

C. Preoperative interventions
1. Monitor for signs and symptoms related to the location of the tumor.
2. Provide emotional support to the child and parents.

D. Postoperative interventions
1. Monitor for postoperative complications related to the location (organ) of the surgery.
2. Monitor for complications related to chemotherapy or radiation, if prescribed.
3. Provide support for the parents, and encourage them to express their feelings; many parents feel guilt for not having recognized signs in the child earlier.
4. Refer the parents to appropriate community services.

XI. Osteosarcoma (Osteogenic Sarcoma)

A. Description
1. The most common bone cancer in children
2. Usually found in the metaphysis of the long bones, especially in the lower extremities, with most tumors occurring in the femur
3. Peak age of incidence is between 10 and 25 years.
4. Symptoms during the earliest stage are almost always attributed to extremity injury or normal growing pains.
5. Treatment may include surgical resection (limb salvage procedure) to save a limb or to remove affected tissue, or amputation.
6. Chemotherapy is used to treat the cancer and may be used before and after surgery.

B. Data collection
1. Localized pain at the affected site (may be severe or dull) that may be attributed to trauma or the vague complaint of "growing pains"; pain is often relieved by a flexed position.
2. Palpable mass
3. Limping if weight-bearing limb is affected
4. Progressively limited range of motion; child curtails physical activity.
5. Child may be unable to hold heavy objects because of their weight and resultant pain in the affected extremity.
6. Pathological fractures at the tumor site

C. Interventions
1. Prepare the child and family for prescribed treatment modalities, which may include surgical resection to remove affected tissue, amputation, and chemotherapy.
2. Communicate honesty and provide support to the child and family.
3. Prepare for prosthetic fitting, as necessary.

4. Assist the child with dealing with self-image problems.

5. Reinforce instructions to the child and parents about the potential development of phantom limb pain that may occur after amputation, characterized by tingling, itching, and a painful sensation in the area where the limb was amputated.

XII. Brain Tumors

A. Description

1. An infratentorial (below the tentorium cerebelli) tumor, the most common brain tumor, is located in the posterior third of the brain (primarily in the cerebellum or brainstem) and accounts for the frequency of symptoms resulting from increased ICP.

2. A supratentorial tumor is located within the anterior two thirds of the brain—mainly the cerebrum.

3. The signs/symptoms of a brain tumor depend on its anatomical location and size, and, to some extent, the age of the child; a number of tests may be used in the neurological evaluation, but the most common diagnostic procedure is magnetic resonance imaging, which determines the location and extent of the tumor.

4. Therapeutic management includes surgery, radiation, and chemotherapy; the treatment of choice is the total removal of the tumor without residual neurological damage.

B. Data collection

1. Headache that is worse when awakening and that improves during the day

2. Vomiting that is unrelated to feeding or eating

3. Change in behavior

4. Clumsiness; awkward gait or difficulty walking

5. Ataxia

6. Facial weakness

7. Diplopia

8. Seizures

9. Signs of increased ICP (Box 29.5)

 Monitor for signs of increased ICP in a child with a brain tumor and after a craniotomy. If signs of increased ICP occur, notify the primary health care provider (PHCP) immediately.

C. Preoperative interventions

1. Monitor neurological status.

2. Institute seizure precautions and safety measures.

3. Monitor the weight and nutritional status.

4. The child's head will be shaved (provide a favorite cap or hat for the child); shaving the head may also be done in the surgical suite.

5. Prepare the child as much as possible; tell the child that he or she will wake up with a large head dressing.

BOX 29.5	Manifestations of Increased Intracranial Pressure in Infants and Children

Infants
- Tense, bulging fontanel
- Separated cranial sutures
- Macewen's sign (cracked pot sound on percussion)
- Irritability
- High-pitched cry
- Increased head circumference
- Distended scalp veins
- Poor feeding
- Crying when disturbed
- Setting sun sign (eyes appear downward, with the sclera seen over the iris, part of the pupil may be covered by the lower eyelid)

Children
- Headache
- Nausea
- Forceful vomiting
- Diplopia; blurred vision
- Seizures

Personality and Behavior Signs
- Irritability, restlessness
- Indifference, drowsiness
- Decline in school performance
- Diminished physical activity and motor performance
- Increased sleeping
- Inability to follow simple commands
- Lethargy

Late Signs
- Bradycardia
- Decreased motor response to command
- Decreased sensory response to painful stimuli
- Alterations in pupil size and reaction
- Decerebrate (extension) or decorticate (flexion) posturing
- Cheyne-Stokes respirations
- Papilledema
- Decreased consciousness
- Coma

From Perry S, Hockenberry M, Lowdermilk D, Wilson D: *Maternal child nursing care*, ed 4, St. Louis, 2010, Elsevier.

D. Postoperative interventions

1. Monitor the neurological and motor function and the level of consciousness.

2. Monitor the temperature closely because it may be elevated as a result of hypothalamus or brainstem involvement during surgery; maintain a cooling blanket by the bedside.

3. Monitor for signs of respiratory infection.

4. Monitor for signs of meningitis (opisthotonos, Kernig's and Brudzinski's signs).

5. Monitor for signs of increased ICP (see Box 29.5) or hemorrhage; check the back of the head dressing for the posterior pooling of blood; notify the

registered nurse immediately if signs of increased ICP or bleeding are noted.

6. Monitor the pupillary response; sluggish, dilated, or unequal pupils are reported immediately, because they may indicate increased ICP and potential brainstem herniation.

7. Monitor for colorless drainage on the dressing or from the ears or nose; this is indicative of cerebrospinal fluid and needs to be reported immediately. Check for the presence of glucose in the drainage (dipstick).

8. Check the surgeon prescription for positioning, including the degree of neck flexion. (Refer to Chapter 55 for additional information on craniotomy.)

9. Monitor IV fluids closely to prevent volume overload.

10. Promote measures that prevent vomiting; vomiting increases ICP and the risk for incisional rupture.

11. Provide a quiet environment.

12. Administer analgesics, as prescribed.

13. Provide emotional support to the child and parents, and promote maximum functioning in the child.

WHAT WOULD YOU DO?

Answer: The child with hemophilia is at risk for bleeding. If the child experienced recent trauma, the nurse would place the child on bleeding precautions and monitor for bleeding. This is the priority intervention. The nurse would monitor vital signs and monitor for joint pain. Joint bleeding would be controlled by immobilization, elevation, and application of ice. Pressure must be applied for 15 minutes for any superficial bleeding. The neurological status must be checked because the child is at risk for intracranial hemorrhage, and the nurse would monitor the urine for hematuria. Blood replacement factors may be prescribed.

PRACTICE QUESTIONS

1. The nurse reinforces instructions to the parents of a child with sickle cell anemia regarding the precipitating factors related to pain crisis. Which, if identified by a parent as a precipitating factor, indicates the **need for further teaching**?
   1. Stress
   2. Trauma
   3. Infection
   4. Fluid overload

❖ 2. The nurse monitors a 5-year-old child admitted to the hospital for a neuroblastoma for signs/symptoms related to the location of the tumor in the adrenal gland. Which descriptions would the nurse expect to be documented in the child's record specific to this tumor? **Select all that apply.**
   ☐ 1. Respiratory impairment
   ☐ 2. Anorexia and weight loss
   ☐ 3. Pallor, weakness, irritability
   ☐ 4. Supraorbital ecchymosis and periorbital edema
   ☐ 5. Firm, nontender, irregular mass in the abdomen
   ☐ 6. Urinary frequency or retention from compression on the bladder

3. The nurse caring for a child with aplastic anemia is reviewing the laboratory results and notes a white blood cell (WBC) count of 6000 mm^3 and a platelet count of 20,000 mm^3. Which nursing intervention would be incorporated into the plan of care?
   1. Encourage naps.
   2. Encourage a diet high in iron.
   3. Encourage quiet play activities.
   4. Maintain strict isolation precautions.

4. The nurse reinforces home care instructions to the parents of a 3-year-old child who has been hospitalized with hemophilia. Which statement by a parent indicates the **need for further teaching**?
   1. "I will supervise my child closely."
   2. "I will pad the corners of the furniture."
   3. "I will remove household items that can easily fall over."
   4. "I will avoid immunizations and dental hygiene treatments for my child."

5. The nurse reinforces instructions to the parents of a child with leukemia regarding measures related to monitoring for infection. Which statement by the parents indicates the **need for further teaching**?
   1. "I need to use proper hand-washing techniques."
   2. "I need to take my child's rectal temperature daily."
   3. "I need to inspect my child's skin daily for redness."
   4. "I need to inspect my child's mouth daily for lesions."

6. The nurse is providing discharge instructions to the parents of a 14-year-old child who is undergoing radiation for Hodgkin's disease. Which statement by a parent indicates the **need for further teaching**?
   1. "I need to watch for diarrhea, so my child does not get dehydrated."
   2. "I think that once my child's hair starts to fall out that I can keep a hat on him."
   3. "I understand that the radiation will cause nausea and vomiting and I need to keep my child hydrated."
   4. "I will need to keep my child's skin from flaking, so we will be allowing showers every 2 or 3 days."

7. A 4-year-old child is hospitalized with a suspected diagnosis of Wilms' tumor. The nurse reviews the plan of care and would question which intervention that is written in the plan?
   1. Palpate the abdomen for a mass.
   2. Check the urine for the presence of hematuria.
   3. Monitor the blood pressure for the presence of hypertension.
   4. Monitor the temperature for the presence of a kidney infection.

8. The nursing instructor asks a student nurse to describe osteogenic sarcoma. Which statement by the student indicates the **need to further research** the disease?
   1. "The femur is the most common site of this sarcoma."
   2. "The child does not experience pain at the primary tumor site."
   3. "If a weight-bearing limb is affected, then limping is a clinical manifestation."
   4. "The symptoms of the disease during the early stage are almost always attributed to normal growing pains."

9. The nurse is monitoring for bleeding in a child after surgery to remove a brain tumor. The nurse checks the head dressing for the presence of blood and notes a colorless drainage on the back of the dressing. Which nursing action is appropriate?
   1. Reinforce the dressing.
   2. Notify the registered nurse (RN).
   3. Document the findings and continue to monitor.
   4. Circle the area of drainage and continue to monitor.

10. The nurse observes a mother giving an oral iron supplement to her 6-year-old child with iron deficiency anemia. Which action by the mother indicates the **need for further teaching**?
    1. The mother administered the iron with milk.
    2. The mother administered the iron with water.
    3. The mother administered the iron with apple juice.
    4. The mother administered the iron with orange juice.

ANSWERS

1. 4
Rationale: Pain crisis may be precipitated by infection, dehydration, hypoxia, trauma, or general stress. The mother of a child with sickle cell disease would encourage a fluid intake of 1.5 to 2 times the daily requirement to prevent dehydration.
Test-Taking Strategy: Note the strategic words, *need for further teaching.* These words indicate a negative event query and ask you to select an option that is an incorrect statement. Recalling that fluid administration is a main component of the treatment of sickle cell anemia to prevent dehydration and pain crisis will direct you to the correct option.

2. 5, 6
Rationale: The signs/symptoms of a neuroblastoma depend on the location of the tumor. When the tumor is found on the adrenal gland, the findings will be consistent with a firm, non-tender, irregular mass in the abdomen. This will likely cause some degree of urinary frequency or retention from compression on the ureter, or kidney. The remaining descriptions are not specific to the location of the tumor on the adrenal gland.
Test-Taking Strategy: Focus on the data in the question, signs and symptoms specific to the tumor in the adrenal gland. Pallor, weakness, irritability, anorexia and weight loss are associated with cancer but are not specific to the location of this tumor. Respiratory impairment would indicate the tumor as located in the thoracic cavity. Supraorbital ecchymosis (raccoon eyes), periorbital edema, and exophthalmos are a result of a tumor around the eye.

3. 3
Rationale: Precautionary measures to prevent bleeding need to be taken when a child has a low platelet count. These

include no injections, no rectal temperatures, the use of a soft toothbrush, quiet activities, and abstinence from contact sports or activities that could cause an injury. Strict isolation would be required if the white blood cell (WBC) count was low. Naps and a diet high in iron are unrelated to the risk of bleeding.
Test-Taking Strategy: Focus on the subject, the intervention that would be incorporated into the plan of care, and note the data in the question. Note that the WBC count is normal and that the platelet count is low. Recall that a low platelet count places the client at risk for bleeding. This will assist you with eliminating the incorrect options.

4. 4
❖ *Rationale:* The nurse needs to stress the importance of immunizations, dental hygiene, and routine well-child care. Options 1, 2, and 3 are appropriate statements. The parents are also provided instructions regarding measures to take in the event of blunt trauma (especially trauma that involves the joints), and they are instructed to apply prolonged pressure to superficial wounds until the bleeding has stopped.
Test-Taking Strategy: Note the strategic words, *need for further teaching.* These words indicate a negative event query and ask you to select an option that is an incorrect statement. Recalling that bleeding is a concern among individuals with this disorder will assist you with eliminating options 1, 2, and 3, because they include measures of protection and safety for the child.

5. 2
Rationale: The risk of injury to the fragile mucous membranes is so great in the child with leukemia that only oral, axillary, or temporal or tympanic temperatures would be taken. Rectal abscesses can easily occur in damaged rectal tissue, so no rectal

temperatures would be taken. In addition, oral temperatures need to be avoided if the child has oral ulcers. Options 1, 3, and 4 are appropriate teaching measures.

Test-Taking Strategy: Note the strategic words, *need for further teaching.* These words indicate a negative event query and ask you to select an option that is an incorrect statement. Options 1, 3, and 4 are reasonable measures and can be easily eliminated. Also, note the word *rectal* in option 2. Recalling that rectal temperatures need to be avoided because of the risk for bleeding and possible infection will direct you to this option.

6. 4

Rationale: The side effects of radiation therapy include dry or moist desquamation (peeling of the skin) and the intervention includes washing the skin daily, using mild soap, applying a lubricant as prescribed. Options 1, 2, and 3 are appropriate statements.

Test-Taking Strategy: Note the, strategic words, *need for further teaching.* These words indicate a negative event query and the need to select the incorrect statement from the parent. Recall that side effects of radiation include anorexia, nausea, vomiting, diarrhea, alopecia, dry or moist desquamation, cystitis, and myelosuppression.

7. 1

Rationale: Wilms' tumor is an intraabdominal and kidney tumor. If Wilms' tumor is suspected, the mass would not be palpated. Excessive manipulation can cause seeding of the tumor and thus cause the spread of the cancerous cells. Hematuria, hypertension, and fever are signs and symptoms that are associated with Wilms' tumor.

Test-Taking Strategy: Focus on the subject, the intervention that the nurse would question. This means that you need to select an option that is an incorrect intervention. Knowledge that Wilms' tumor is an intra-abdominal and kidney tumor will assist you with eliminating options 2, 3, and 4 because of the relationship of these options to renal function.

8. 2

Rationale: Osteogenic sarcoma is the most common bone tumor in children. A clinical manifestation of osteogenic

sarcoma is progressive, insidious, intermittent pain at the tumor site. By the time these children receive medical attention, they may be in considerable pain from the tumor. Options 1, 3, and 4 are accurate regarding osteogenic sarcoma.

Test-Taking Strategy: Focus on the subject, osteogenic sarcoma and note the strategic words, *need to further research.* These words indicate a negative event query and the need to select the incorrect student statement. Recalling that osteogenic sarcoma is a malignant tumor of the bone will direct you to the correct option.

9. 2

Rationale: Colorless drainage on the dressing would indicate the presence of cerebrospinal fluid and needs to be reported to the registered nurse (RN) immediately; the RN would then contact the primary health care provider. The colorless drainage would also be checked for evidence of cerebrospinal fluid; one method is to check for the presence of glucose using a dipstick. Options 1, 3, and 4 are incorrect and delay required immediate interventions.

Test-Taking Strategy: Eliminate options 3 and 4 because they are comparable or alike and indicate to continue to monitor. Also note the subject, colorless drainage following surgery for a brain tumor. This would quickly alert you to the possibility of the presence of cerebrospinal fluid.

10. 1

Rationale: Milk may affect absorption of the iron. Vitamin C increases the absorption of iron by the body. The mother would be instructed to administer the medication with a citrus fruit or a juice that is high in vitamin C. Water will not assist in absorption but will not affect absorption as milk would.

Test-Taking Strategy: Note the strategic word, *need for further teaching.* These words indicate a negative event query and ask you to select an option that is an incorrect action. Recalling that vitamin C increases the absorption of iron will assist you in recognizing that juices contain vitamin C. Also. To select from the remaining options, think about the effect of milk versus water on absorption to answer correctly.

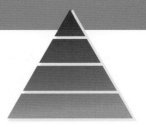

CHAPTER **30**

Pediatric Nursing

Metabolic and Endocrine Problems

PRIORITY CONCEPTS Glucose Regulation; Thermoregulation

WHAT WOULD YOU DO?

A child is diagnosed with phenylketonuria. What interventions would the nurse include in the plan of care?
Answer is located on p.373.

I. Fever
A. Description
1. Fever is an abnormal body temperature elevation.
2. A child's temperature can vary, depending on activity, emotional stress, the type of clothing that the child is wearing, and the temperature of the environment.
3. A fever in an infant less than 1 month old is considered an emergency, and the pediatric specialist needs to be contacted immediately if this occurs.
4. Data collection findings associated with the fever provide important indications of its seriousness.

B. Data collection
1. Temperature elevation: Normal temperature range for a child is 36.4°C to 37°C (97.5°F–98.6°F); 38°C (100.4°F) is considered to be fever.
2. Flushed skin; warm to touch
3. Diaphoresis
4. Chills
5. Restlessness or lethargy

C. Interventions
1. Monitor vital signs. Take the temperature electronically or per agency procedure.
2. Remove excess clothing and blankets, reduce the room temperature, and increase the air circulation. Use other cooling measures, such as the application of a cool compress to the forehead if appropriate.
3. Administer a sponge bath with tepid water for 20 to 30 minutes, and gently squeeze water from a facecloth over the back and chest; recheck the temperature 30 minutes after the bath; do not use alcohol because it can cause peripheral vasoconstriction.
4. Administer antipyretics such as ibuprofen, as prescribed.
5. Aspirin would not be administered, unless specifically prescribed, because of the risk of Reye's syndrome.
6. Retake the temperature 30 to 60 minutes after the antipyretic is administered.
7. Provide adequate fluid intake, as tolerated and prescribed.
8. Monitor for signs and symptoms that indicate dehydration and electrolyte imbalances; monitor laboratory values.
9. Reinforce instructions to the parents regarding how to take the child's temperature, how to safely medicate the child, and when it is necessary to call the primary health care provider (PHCP).

II. Dehydration
A. Description
1. Dehydration is a common fluid and electrolyte imbalance in infants and children.
2. In infants and children, the organs that conserve water are immature, thus placing them at risk for fluid volume deficit.
3. The causes can include decreased fluid intake, diaphoresis, vomiting, diarrhea, diabetic ketoacidosis, and extensive burns or other serious injuries.

⚠ Infants and children are more vulnerable to fluid volume deficit because more of their body water is in the extracellular fluid compartment.

B. Data collection (Table 30.1)
C. Interventions
1. The cause of the dehydration is treated.
2. Monitor vital signs.
3. Monitor weight and for weight changes, including fluid gains and losses.
4. Monitor intake and output and urine for specific gravity.
5. Monitor level of consciousness.

TABLE 30.1 **Evaluating the Extent of Dehydration**

Clinical Signs	Level of Dehydration		
	Mild	Moderate	Severe
Weight loss—infants	3%–5%	6%–9%	≥ 10%
Weight loss—children	3%–4%	6%–8%	10%
Pulse	Normal	Slightly increased	Very increased
Respiratory rate	Normal	Slight tachypnea (rapid)	Hyperpnea (deep and rapid)
Blood pressure	Normal	Normal to orthostatic (>10 mm Hg change)	Orthostatic to shock
Behavior	Normal	Irritable, more thirsty	Hyperirritable to lethargic
Thirst	Slight	Moderate	Intense
Mucous membranes[a]	Normal	Dry	Parched
Tears	Present	Decreased	Absent; sunken eyes
Anterior fontanel	Normal	Normal to sunken	Sunken
External jugular vein	Visible when supine	Not visible except with supra-clavicular pressure	Not visible even with supra-clavicular pressure
Skin[a]	Capillary refill 2 sec	Slowed capillary refill (2–4 sec [decreased turgor])	Very delayed capillary refill (>4 sec) and tenting; skin cool, acrocyanotic or mottled
Urine specific gravity	>1.020	>1.020; oliguria	Oliguria or anuria

[a]These signs are less prominent in the child who has hypernatremia.

Data from Jospe N, Forbes G: Fluids and electrolytes—clinical aspects, *Pediatric Rev* 17:395–403, 1996; and Steiner MJ, DeWalt DA, Byerley JS: Is this child dehydrated? *JAMA* 291:2746–2754, 2004. Table from Perry S, Hockenberry M, Lowdermilk D, Wilson D: *Maternal child nursing care*, ed 4, St. Louis, 2010, Mosby.

6. Monitor skin turgor and mucous membranes for dryness.
7. For mild to moderate dehydration, provide oral rehydration therapy with Pedialyte or a similar rehydration solution as prescribed; avoid carbonated beverages, because they are gas-producing, and fluids that contain high amounts of sugar, such as apple juice.
8. For severe dehydration, maintain NPO (nothing by mouth) status to place the bowel at rest and provide fluid and electrolyte replacement by the intravenous (IV) route as prescribed; if potassium is prescribed for IV administration, before administering ensure that the child has voided and has adequate renal function.
9. Reintroduce a normal diet when rehydration is achieved.
10. Reinforce instructions to the parents about the types and amounts of fluid to encourage, the signs of dehydration, and the indications of the need to notify the PHCP.

III. Phenylketonuria (PKU)

A. Description
   1. A genetic disorder (autosomal recessive disorder) that results in central nervous system damage from toxic levels of phenylalanine (an essential amino acid) in the blood.
   2. Characterized by blood phenylalanine levels greater than 20 mg/dL; normal level is 0 mg/dL to 2 mg/dL.
   3. All 50 states require routine screening of all newborn infants for PKU.
B. Data collection
   1. In all children:
      a. Digestive problems and vomiting
      b. Seizure
      c. Musty odor of the urine
      d. Mental retardation
   2. In older children
      a. Eczema
      b. Hypertonia
      c. Hypopigmentation of the hair, skin, and irises
      d. Hyperactive behavior
C. Interventions
   1. Screening of newborn infants for PKU: The infant would have begun formula or breast milk feeding before specimen collection.
   2. If initial screening is positive, a repeat test is performed and further diagnostic evaluation is required to verify the diagnosis.
   3. Rescreening of infants would be done by 14 days of age if the initial screening was done before 48 hours of age.
   4. If PKU is diagnosed, prepare to implement the following:

a. Restrict phenylalanine intake; high-protein foods (meats and dairy products) and aspartame are avoided because they contain large amounts of phenylalanine.
b. Monitor physical, neurological, and intellectual development.
c. Stress the importance of follow-up treatment.
d. Encourage the parents to express feelings about the diagnosis and the risk of PKU in future children.
e. Reinforce educating the parents about use of special preparation formulas and about the foods that contain phenylalanine.
f. Consult with social care services to assist the parents with financial burdens of specially prepared formulas.

IV. Childhood Obesity

A. Description
  1. A condition where excess body fat negatively impacts the health and well-being of the child.
  2. Body mass index (BMI) is a screening tool that can be used to measure obesity.
  3. BMI is defined as a person's body weight in kilograms divided by the square of a person's height in meters.
  4. As recommended by the Centers for Disease Control and Prevention (CDC), health professionals would use the BMI percentile when measuring children and adolescents aged 2 to 20 years.
  5. Overweight is defined as being above the 85th percentile but less than the 95th percentile.
  6. Obesity is defined as having a BMI greater than the 95th percentile.

B. Effects of obesity
  1. Obesity can lead to problems later in life if diagnosed in childhood, such as physical, social, and emotional health problems.
  2. Asthma, sleep apnea, bone and joint problems, type 2 diabetes, and risk factors leading to heart disease, such as hyperlipidemia can occur.
  3. A child who is obese is more likely to be obese as an adult, which results in the comorbidities associated with obesity later in life, such as type 2 diabetes, heart disease, metabolic syndrome, and cancer.

V. Diabetes Mellitus

A. Description (Fig. 30.1)
  1. Type 1 diabetes mellitus is characterized by the destruction of the pancreatic beta cells, which produce insulin. This results in absolute insulin deficiency.
  2. Type 2 diabetes mellitus usually arises as a result of insulin resistance, in which the body fails to use insulin properly, in combination with relative (rather than absolute) insulin deficiency.

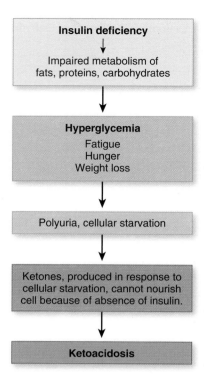

FIGURE 30.1 Insulin deficiency leading to ketoacidosis. (From McKinney E, James S, Murray S, Ashwill J: Maternal-child nursing, ed 4, St. Louis, 2013, Saunders.)

  3. The rate of children and teens being diagnosed with prediabetes and type 2 diabetes is increasing. The number one risk factor for developing type 2 diabetes in childhood is being overweight.
  4. Insulin deficiency requires the use of exogenous insulin to promote appropriate glucose use and prevent complications related to elevated blood glucose levels, such as hyperglycemia, diabetic ketoacidosis, and death.
  5. Diagnosis is based on the presence of classic symptoms and an elevated blood glucose level (a normal blood glucose level is between 70 mg/dL and 99 mg/dL; based on PHCP preference, normal level may be a lower range).
  6. Children may be admitted directly to the pediatric intensive care unit because of the manifestations of diabetic ketoacidosis, which may be the initial occurrence when they are diagnosed with diabetes mellitus.

B. Data collection
  1. Polyuria, polydipsia, and polyphagia
  2. Hyperglycemia
  3. Weight loss
  4. Unexplained fatigue or lethargy
  5. Headache
  6. Occasional enuresis in a previously toilet-trained child
  7. Vaginitis in adolescent girls (caused by *Candida vaginitis*, which thrives in hyperglycemic tissues)

8. Fruity odor to the breath
9. Dehydration
10. Blurred vision
11. Slow wound healing
12. Change in the level of consciousness

C. Long-term effects
1. Failure to grow at a normal rate
2. Delayed maturation
3. Recurrent infections
4. Neuropathy
5. Cardiovascular disease
6. Retinal microvascular disease
7. Renal microvascular disease

D. Complications
1. Hypoglycemia
2. Hyperglycemia
3. Diabetic ketoacidosis
4. Coma
5. Hypokalemia
6. Hyperkalemia
7. Microvascular changes
8. Cardiovascular changes

⚠ For a child with diabetes mellitus, plan to initiate a consultation with the diabetic specialist to plan the child's care.

E. Diet
1. Normal, healthy nutrition is encouraged. The total number of calories is individualized on the basis of the child's age and growth expectations. For type 2 diabetes, the American Diabetes Association recommendation can be found at http://main.diabetes.org/dorg/PDFs/Type-2-Diabetes-in-Youth/Type-2-Diabetes-in-Youth_14-18.pdf.
2. As prescribed by the PHCP, children with diabetes need no special foods or supplements. They need sufficient calories to balance daily expenditure for energy and to satisfy the requirement for growth and development.
3. Dietary intake needs to include three well-balanced meals per day, eaten at regular intervals, plus a midafternoon snack and a bedtime snack; a consistent intake of the prescribed protein, fats, and carbohydrates at each meal and snack is needed (concentrated sweets are discouraged; fat is reduced to 30% or less of the total caloric requirement).
4. Tell the child and parents that the child needs to carry a source of glucose (e.g., glucose tablets) with him/her at all times to treat hypoglycemia if it occurs.
5. Incorporate the diet into the individual child's needs, likes, dislikes, lifestyle, and cultural and socioeconomic patterns.
6. Allow the child to participate in making food choices to provide a sense of control.

F. Exercise
1. Instruct the child regarding dietary adjustments to consider when exercising.
2. Extra food needs to be consumed for increased activity (usually 10–15 g of carbohydrates for every 30–45 minutes of activity).
3. Instruct the child to check the blood glucose level before exercising.
4. Plan an appropriate exercise regimen with the child, and incorporate the child's developmental stage.

G. Insulin
1. Diluted insulin may be required for some infants to provide small enough doses to avoid hypoglycemia. Diluted insulin must be clearly labeled to avoid dosage errors.
2. A laboratory evaluation of the glycosylated hemoglobin level (HgbA1C) would be performed every 3 months. Reference interval for HgbA1C is less than 6%.
3. Illness, infection, and stress increase the need for insulin. Insulin would not be withheld in these situations, because hyperglycemia and ketoacidosis can result.
4. When the child is NPO for a special procedure, verify with the PHCP the need to withhold the morning insulin and when food, fluids, and insulin are to be given.
5. Reinforce instructions to the child and parents regarding the administration of the insulin.
6. Reinforce instructions to the child and parents regarding how to recognize the symptoms of hypoglycemia and hyperglycemia.
7. Reinforce instructions to the parents in the administration of glucagon intramuscularly or subcutaneously if the child has a hypoglycemic reaction and is unable to consume items orally (if semiconscious or unconscious).
8. Reinforce instructions to the child and parents to always have a spare bottle of insulin available.
9. Advise the parents to obtain a Medic-Alert bracelet that indicates the type and daily insulin dosage that has been prescribed for the child.
10. See Chapter 43 for information on insulin pumps and skin sensors.
11. See Chapter 44 for information on insulin types, administration sites, and administration procedure.

H. Blood glucose monitoring
1. Results provide information needed to maintain good glycemic control.
2. Blood glucose monitoring is more accurate than urine testing.
3. Requires that the child prick himself or herself several times a day, as prescribed (Box 30.1)

BOX 30.1 Lessening the Pain of Blood Glucose Monitoring

- Hold the finger under warm water for a few seconds before puncture (enhances blood flow to the finger).
- Use the ring finger or thumb to obtain a blood sample because blood flows more easily to these areas; puncture the finger just to the side of the finger pad because there are more blood vessels in this area and fewer nerve endings.
- Press the lancet device lightly against the skin to prevent a deep puncture.
- Use glucose monitors that require very small blood samples for measurement.

Adapted from Perry S, Hockenberry M, Lowdermilk D, Wilson D: *Maternal child nursing care*, ed 4, St. Louis, 2010, Elsevier.

4. Reinforce instructions to the child and parents about the proper procedure for obtaining the blood glucose level.
5. Inform the child and parents that the procedure must be performed precisely to obtain accurate results.
6. Stress the importance of hand washing before and after performing the procedure to prevent infection.
7. Stress the importance of following the manufacturer's instructions for the blood glucose monitoring device.
8. Reinforce instructions to the child and parents to calibrate the monitor as instructed by the manufacturer.
9. Reinforce instructions to the child and parents to check the expiration date on the test strips used for blood glucose monitoring.
10. Reinforce instructions to the child and parents that if the blood glucose results do not seem reasonable, they need to reread the instructions, reassess the technique, check the expiration date of the test strips, and perform the procedure again to verify the results.

I. Urine testing
1. Reinforce instructions to the parents and child on the procedure for testing the urine for ketones and glucose.
2. Reinforce instructions to the child that the second voided urine specimen is the most accurate.
3. The presence of ketones may indicate impending ketoacidosis.

⚠ Urine glucose testing is an unreliable method of monitoring the glucose level; however, the urine needs to be tested for ketones when the child is ill or when the blood glucose level is consistently greater than 200 mg/dL or as specified by the PHCP.

⚡ PRIORITY NURSING ACTIONS

Hypoglycemia in a Hospitalized Child with Diabetes Mellitus

1. Check the child's blood glucose level.
2. Give the child ½ cup of fruit juice or another acceptable item.
3. Take the child's vital signs.
4. Retest the blood glucose level.
5. Give the child a small snack of carbohydrate and protein.
6. Document the child's signs/symptoms, actions taken, and outcome.

BOX 30.2 Interventions for Hypoglycemia

- If possible, the nurse would confirm the hypoglycemia with a blood glucose reading.
- Administer glucose immediately. The rapid-releasing glucose is followed by a complex carbohydrate and protein, such as a slice of bread or a peanut butter cracker.
- Give an extra snack if the next meal is not planned for more than 30 min or if activity is planned.
- If the child becomes unconscious, squeeze cake frosting or glucose paste onto the gums and retest the blood glucose level if the child does not improve in 15 minutes (monitor the child closely); if the reading remains low, administer additional glucose.
- If the child remains unconscious, it may be necessary to administer glucagon.
- In the hospital, prepare for the administration of intravenous dextrose if the child is unable to consume an oral glucose product.

BOX 30.3 Food Items to Treat Hypoglycemia

- ½ cup orange or other fruit juice or a sugar-sweetened beverage
- 8 oz milk
- 1 small box of raisins
- 3 or 4 hard candies
- 4 sugar cubes (1 tbsp. of sugar)
- 3 or 4 Life Savers
- 1 candy bar
- 1 tsp. honey
- 2 or 3 glucose tablets

J. Hypoglycemia
1. Description
   a. A blood glucose level less than 70 mg/dL (or as specified by the PHCP)
   b. Occurs as a result of too much insulin, not enough food, or excessive activity
   c. Signs include headache, nausea, sweating, tremors, lethargy, hunger, confusion, slurred speech, tingling around the mouth, and anxiety.
2. Interventions (Boxes 30.2 and 30.3) (see Priority Nursing Actions)

BOX 30.4 Interventions for Hyperglycemia

Instruct the parents to notify the primary health care provider when the following occur:
- Blood glucose results remain elevated (usually >200 mg/dL or as specified by the PHCP).
- Moderate or high ketonuria is present.
- The child is unable to take food or fluids.
- The child vomits more than once.
- Illness persists.

BOX 30.5 Sick-Day Rules for the Diabetic Child

- Always give insulin, even if the child does not have an appetite, or contact the primary health care provider (PHCP) for specific instructions.
- Test blood glucose levels at least every 4 hr.
- Test for urinary ketones with each voiding.
- Notify the PHCP if moderate or large amounts of urinary ketones are present.
- Follow the child's usual meal plan.
- Encourage liquids to aid in clearing ketones.
- Encourage rest, especially if urinary ketones are present.
- Notify the PHCP if vomiting, fruity odor to the breath, deep rapid respirations, decreasing level of consciousness, or persistent hyperglycemia occurs.

Adapted from Hockenberry M, Wilson D: *Nursing care of infants and children*, ed 9, St. Louis, 2011, Mosby.

K. Hyperglycemia
  1. Description: Elevated blood glucose level as specified by the PHCP
  2. Signs include polydipsia, polyuria, polyphagia, blurred vision, weakness, weight loss, and syncope.
  3. Interventions (Box 30.4)
  4. Sick-day rules (Box 30.5)

L. Diabetic ketoacidosis (see Fig. 30.1)
  1. Description
    a. A complication of diabetes mellitus that develops when a severe insulin deficiency occurs.
    b. A life-threatening condition
    c. Hyperglycemia that progresses to metabolic acidosis occurs.
    d. Develops over a period of several hours to days
    e. The blood glucose level is more than 300 mg/dL and urine and serum ketones are positive.

⚠ Manifestations of diabetic ketoacidosis include signs of hyperglycemia, Kussmaul's respirations, acetone (fruity) breath odor, increasing lethargy, and decreasing level of consciousness.

  2. Interventions
    a. The goal is to restore the circulating volume and protect against cerebral, coronary, or renal hypoperfusion.
    b. Dehydration is corrected with IV infusions of 0.9% or 0.45% saline, as prescribed.
    c. Hyperglycemia is corrected with IV regular insulin administration, as prescribed.
    d. Monitor vital signs, urine output, and mental status closely.
    e. Correct acidosis and electrolyte imbalances as prescribed.
    f. Administer oxygen, as prescribed.
    g. Monitor blood glucose level frequently.
    h. Monitor potassium level closely because when the child receives insulin to lower the blood glucose level, the serum potassium level will change; if the potassium level decreases, potassium replacement may be required.
    i. The child needs to be voiding adequately before administering potassium; if the child does not have an adequate output, hyperkalemia may result.
    j. Monitor the child closely for signs of fluid overload.
    k. Intravenously administered dextrose is added as prescribed when the blood glucose reaches an appropriate level.
    l. The cause of the hyperglycemia is treated.

WHAT WOULD YOU DO?

Answer: Interventions for phenylketonuria (PKU) include restricting phenylalanine intake. High-protein foods (meats and dairy products) and products that contain aspartame are avoided because they contain large amounts of phenylalanine. Monitoring physical, neurological, and intellectual development is important to detect any abnormalities. The nurse would stress the importance of follow-up treatment with the parents, encourage the parents to express their feelings about the diagnosis and discuss the risk of PKU in future children, educate the parents about the use of special preparation formulas and about the foods that contain phenylalanine, and consult with social care services to assist the parents with any financial burdens.

PRACTICE QUESTIONS

1. A school-age child with type 1 diabetes mellitus has soccer practice three afternoons a week. The nurse reinforces instructions regarding how to prevent hypoglycemia during practice. Which would the nurse tell the child?
   1. Drink a half a cup of orange juice before soccer practice.
   2. Eat twice the amount that is normally eaten at lunchtime.
   3. Take half of the amount of prescribed insulin on practice days.

4. Take the prescribed insulin at noontime rather than in the morning.

2. The nursing instructor asks a nursing student about phenylketonuria (PKU). Which statement made by the student indicates a **need for further teaching**?
   1. "PKU is an autosomal-recessive disorder."
   2. "PKU primarily affects the gastrointestinal system."
   3. "Treatment of PKU includes the dietary restriction of phenylalanine."
   4. "All 50 states require routine screening of all newborns for PKU."

3. The mother of a 6-year-old child who has type 1 diabetes mellitus calls a clinic nurse and tells the nurse that the child has been sick. The mother reports that she checked the child's urine and it was positive for ketones. The nurse would instruct the mother to take which action?
   1. Hold the next dose of insulin.
   2. Come to the clinic immediately.
   3. Encourage the child to drink liquids.
   4. Administer an additional dose of regular insulin.

4. A primary health care provider prescribes an intravenous (IV) solution of 5% dextrose and half-normal saline (0.45%) with 40 mEq of potassium chloride for a child with hypotonic dehydration. The nurse performs which **priority** assessment before this IV prescription is initiated?
   1. Obtains a weight
   2. Takes the temperature
   3. Takes the blood pressure
   4. Checks the amount of urine output

5. An adolescent client with type 1 diabetes mellitus is admitted to the emergency department for treatment of diabetic ketoacidosis. Which assessment findings would the nurse expect to note?
   1. Sweating and tremors
   2. Hunger and hypertension
   3. Cold, clammy skin and irritability
   4. Fruity breath odor and decreasing level of consciousness

6. A mother brings her 3-week-old infant to a clinic for a phenylketonuria (PKU) rescreening blood test. The test indicates a serum phenylalanine level of 0 mg/dL. The nurse reviews this result and makes which interpretation?
   1. It is negative.
   2. It is a concern.
   3. It is inconclusive.
   4. It requires rescreening at age 6 weeks.

7. A child with type 1 diabetes mellitus is brought to the emergency department by the mother, who states that the child has been complaining of abdominal pain and has been lethargic. Diabetic ketoacidosis is diagnosed. Anticipating the plan of care, the nurse prepares to administer which type of IV infusion?
   1. Potassium infusion
   2. NPH insulin infusion
   3. 5% dextrose infusion
   4. Normal saline infusion

8. The nurse has just administered ibuprofen to a child with a temperature of 38.8°C (102°F). The nurse would also take which action?
   1. Withhold oral fluids for 8 hours.
   2. Sponge the child with cold water.
   3. Plan to administer salicylate in 4 hours.
   4. Remove excess clothing and blankets from the child.

9. A child has fluid volume deficit. The nurse collects data and determines that the child is improving and the deficit is resolving if which finding is noted?
   1. The child has no tears.
   2. Urine specific gravity is 1.030.
   3. Capillary refill is less than 2 seconds.
   4. Urine output is less than 1 mL/kg/h.

❖ 10. The nurse would implement which interventions for a child older than 2 years with type 1 diabetes mellitus who has a blood glucose level of 60 mg/dL? **Select all that apply.**
   ❑ 1. Administer regular insulin.
   ❑ 2. Encourage the child to ambulate.
   ❑ 3. Give the child a teaspoon of honey.
   ❑ 4. Provide electrolyte replacement therapy intravenously.
   ❑ 5. Wait 30 minutes and confirm the blood glucose reading.
   ❑ 6. Prepare to administer glucagon subcutaneously if unconsciousness occurs.

ANSWERS

1. 1

Rationale: An extra snack of 10 g to 15 g of carbohydrates eaten before activities and for every 30 to 45 minutes of activity will prevent hypoglycemia. A half cup of orange juice will provide the needed carbohydrates. The child or parents would not be instructed to adjust the amount or time of insulin administration, and meal amounts would not be doubled.

Test-Taking Strategy: Focus on the subject, preventing hypoglycemia during exercise. Options 3 and 4 can be eliminated first using general medication guidelines, because insulin dosages and times would not be adjusted. From the remaining options, recalling the signs/symptoms and treatment associated with hypoglycemia will direct you to the correct option.

2. 2
Rationale: PKU is a genetic disorder that results in central nervous system (CNS) damage from toxic levels of phenylalanine in the blood, not the gastrointestinal system. PKU is an autosomal-recessive disorder and treatment includes the dietary restriction of phenylalanine intake. All 50 states require screening newborns for PKU.
Test-Taking Strategy: Note the strategic words, *need for further teaching*. These words indicate a negative event query and ask you to select an option that is an incorrect statement. Recalling that PKU affects the CNS will direct you to the correct option. Also, recalling that PKU is a recessive disorder and involves the dietary restriction of phenylalanine leads you to eliminate options 1 and 3. Recalling that all 50 states require newborn screening will direct you to the correct option.

3. 3
Rationale: When the child is sick, the mother needs to test for urinary ketones with each voiding. If ketones are present, liquids are essential to aid in clearing the ketones. The child would be encouraged to drink liquids. Bringing the child to the clinic immediately is unnecessary. Insulin doses would not be adjusted or changed.
Test-Taking Strategy: Use general medication guidelines. Eliminate options 1 and 4, noting that they are comparable or alike; insulin doses would not be adjusted or changed. From the remaining options, note the words *positive for ketones*. Recalling that liquids are essential to aid in clearing the ketones will direct you to the correct option.

4. 4
Rationale: In hypotonic dehydration, electrolyte loss exceeds water loss. The priority assessment before administering potassium chloride intravenously would be to assess the status of the urine output. Potassium chloride would not be administered in the presence of oliguria or anuria. If the urine output is less than 1 mL/kg/hr to 2 mL/kg/hr, potassium chloride would not be administered. Although options 1, 2, and 3 are appropriate assessments for a child with dehydration, these assessments are not related specifically to the IV administration of potassium chloride.
Test-Taking Strategy: Note the strategic word, *priority*. Focus on the IV prescription. Recalling that the kidneys play a key role in the excretion and reabsorption of potassium will direct you to the correct option.

5. 4
Rationale: Diabetic ketoacidosis is a complication of diabetes mellitus that develops when a severe insulin deficiency occurs. Hyperglycemia occurs with diabetic ketoacidosis. Signs of hyperglycemia include fruity breath odor and a decreasing level of consciousness. Hunger can be a sign of hypoglycemia or hyperglycemia, but hypertension is not a sign of diabetic ketoacidosis. Hypotension occurs because of a decrease in blood volume related to the dehydrated state that occurs during diabetic ketoacidosis. Cold clammy skin, irritability, sweating, and tremors all are signs of hypoglycemia.

Test-Taking Strategy: Focus on the subject, the signs of diabetic ketoacidosis, and recall that in this condition the blood glucose level is elevated. Eliminate options 1, 2, and 3 because these signs do not occur with hyperglycemia. Recall that fruity breath odor and a change in the level of consciousness can occur during diabetic ketoacidosis.

6. 1
Rationale: Phenylketonuria is a genetic (autosomal recessive) disorder that results in central nervous system damage from toxic levels of phenylalanine (an essential amino acid) in the blood. It is characterized by blood phenylalanine levels greater than 20 mg/dL. The normal level is 0 mg/dL to 2 mg/dL. A result of 0 mg/dL is a negative test result.
Test-Taking Strategy: Eliminate options 3 and 4 first because they are comparable or alike, indicating no definitive finding. Note that the level identified in the question is a low level; this would assist in directing you to the correct option.

7. 4
Rationale: Diabetic ketoacidosis is a complication of diabetes mellitus that develops when a severe insulin deficiency occurs. Hyperglycemia occurs with diabetic ketoacidosis. Rehydration is the initial step in resolving diabetic ketoacidosis. Normal saline is the initial IV rehydration fluid. NPH insulin is never administered by the IV route. Dextrose solutions are added to the treatment when the blood glucose level decreases to an acceptable level. Intravenously administered potassium may be required, depending on the potassium level, but would not be part of the initial treatment.
Test-Taking Strategy: Focus on the subject, treatment for diabetic ketoacidosis. Eliminate option 3, knowing that dextrose would not be administered in a hyperglycemic state. Eliminate option 2 next, knowing that NPH insulin is not administered by the IV route. Recalling that hydration is the initial treatment in diabetic ketoacidosis will direct you to the correct option.

8. 4
Rationale: After administering ibuprofen, excess clothing and blankets need to be removed. The child can be sponged with tepid water, but not cold water because the cold water can cause shivering, which increases metabolic requirements above those already caused by the fever. Aspirin is not administered to a child with fever because of the risk of Reye's syndrome. Fluids would be encouraged to prevent dehydration, so oral fluids would not be withheld.
Test-Taking Strategy: Focus on the subject, interventions for an elevated temperature. Remember that cooling measures such as removing excess clothing and blankets would be done when a child has a fever. Options 1, 2, and 3 are not interventions for a child with a fever.

9. 3
Rationale: Indicators that fluid volume deficit is resolving would be capillary refill less than 2 seconds, specific gravity of 1.002 to 1.025, urine output of at least 1 mL/kg/hr, and adequate tear production. A capillary refill time less than 2 seconds is the only indicator that the child is improving. Urine output of less than 1 mL/kg/hr, a specific gravity of 1.030, and no tears would indicate that the deficit is not resolving.

Test-Taking Strategy: Focus on the subject, assessment findings indicating that fluid volume deficit is resolving. Recall the parameters that indicate adequate hydration status. The only option that indicates an improving fluid balance is option 4. The other options indicate fluid imbalance.

10. 3, 6

Rationale: Hypoglycemia is defined as a blood glucose level less than 70 mg/dL. Hypoglycemia occurs as a result of too much insulin, not enough food, or excessive activity. If possible, the nurse would confirm hypoglycemia with a blood glucose reading. Glucose is administered orally immediately; rapid-releasing glucose is followed by a complex carbohydrate and protein, such as a slice of bread or a peanut butter cracker. An extra snack is given if the next meal is not planned for more than 30 minutes or if activity is planned. If the child becomes unconscious, cake frosting or glucose paste is squeezed onto the gums, and the blood glucose level is retested in 15 minutes; if the reading remains low, additional glucose is administered. If the child remains unconscious, administration of glucagon may be necessary, and the nurse needs to be prepared for this intervention. Encouraging the child to ambulate and administering regular insulin would result in a lowered blood glucose level. Providing electrolyte replacement therapy intravenously is an intervention to treat diabetic ketoacidosis. Waiting 30 minutes to confirm the blood glucose level delays necessary intervention.

Test-Taking Strategy: Focus on the subject, a low blood glucose level, and on the information in the question. Think about the pathophysiology associated with hypoglycemia and how it is treated. Recalling that a blood glucose level of 60 mg/dL indicates hypoglycemia will assist in determining the correct interventions.

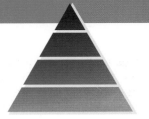

CHAPTER 31

Gastrointestinal Problems

PRIORITY CONCEPTS Elimination; Nutrition

WHAT WOULD YOU DO?

A child suddenly vomits. What would the nurse do to prevent aspiration?
Answer is located on p. 390.

I. Vomiting

A. Description
1. The major concerns when a child is vomiting are the risk of dehydration, the loss of fluid and electrolytes, and the development of metabolic alkalosis.
2. Additional concerns include aspiration, atelectasis, and the development of pneumonia.
3. Causes of vomiting include an acute infectious disease, increased intracranial pressure, toxic ingestion, food intolerance, mechanical obstruction of the gastrointestinal tract, a metabolic disorder, and a psychogenic disorder.

B. Data collection
1. Signs of aspiration
2. Character of vomitus
3. Presence of pain and abdominal cramping
4. Signs of dehydration
5. Signs of fluid and electrolyte imbalances
6. Signs of metabolic alkalosis

C. Interventions
1. Maintain a patent airway.
2. Position the child on his or her side to prevent aspiration.
3. Monitor vital signs.
4. Monitor the character, amount, and frequency of vomiting.
5. Note the force of vomiting, because projectile vomiting is indicative of pyloric **stenosis** or increased intracranial pressure.
6. Monitor the intake and output (I&O) and for signs of dehydration, such as a sunken fontanel (age-appropriate), nonelastic skin turgor, dry mucous membranes, decreased tear production, and oliguria.
7. Monitor the electrolyte levels.
8. Provide oral rehydration therapy, as tolerated and as prescribed. Start feeding slowly, with small amounts of fluid at frequent intervals.
9. Monitor for diarrhea or abdominal pain.
10. Tell the parents to contact the primary health care provider (PHCP) when signs of dehydration, blood in the vomitus, forceful vomiting, or abdominal pain is present.

II. Diarrhea

A. Description
1. Acute diarrhea is a cause of dehydration, particularly in children younger than 5 years of age.
2. Some causes of acute diarrhea include an acute infectious disorder of the gastrointestinal tract, antibiotic therapy, and a parasitic infestation.
3. Some causes of chronic diarrhea include rotavirus, malabsorption syndromes, inflammatory bowel disease, immune deficiencies, food intolerances, and nonspecific factors.
4. Rotavirus is a cause of serious gastroenteritis and is a nosocomial (hospital-acquired) pathogen that is most severe in children ages 3 to 24 months; children younger than 3 months of age have some protection because of maternally acquired antibodies.

B. Data collection
1. Character of stools
2. Pain and abdominal cramping
3. Signs of dehydration and fluid and electrolyte imbalances
4. Signs of metabolic acidosis

C. Interventions
1. Monitor the character, amount, and frequency of diarrhea.
2. Provide enteric isolation as required; instruct the parents in effective hand-washing technique (the child would also be taught this technique).
3. Monitor skin integrity.
4. Monitor strict I&O.

377

5. Monitor electrolyte levels.
6. Monitor for signs/symptoms of dehydration.
7. For mild to moderate dehydration, oral rehydration therapy with Pedialyte or a similar rehydration solution may be prescribed; avoid carbonated beverages because they are gas producing, as well as fluids that contain high amounts of sugar, such as apple juice.
8. For severe dehydration, an NPO (nothing by mouth) status may be prescribed to place the bowel at rest and fluid and electrolyte replacement by the intravenous (IV) route may be prescribed; if potassium is prescribed for IV administration, ensure that the child has voided before administration and has adequate kidney function.
9. Reintroduce a normal diet once rehydration is achieved.

 The major concerns when a child is having diarrhea are the risk of dehydration, the loss of fluid and electrolytes, and the development of metabolic acidosis. Monitoring intake and output is important in assessing hydration status.

III. Cleft Lip and Cleft Palate

A. Description
1. A congenital anomaly that occurs as a result of failure of soft tissue or a bony structure to fuse during embryonic development
2. Involves abnormal openings in the lip or palate that may occur unilaterally or bilaterally and that are readily apparent at birth
3. Causes include hereditary and environmental factors—exposure to radiation or rubella virus, chromosome abnormalities, and teratogenic factors.
4. Prenatal dietary supplementation of folic acid is important to decrease the risk of cleft lip and palate.
5. Closure of cleft lip defect precedes that of the cleft palate and is usually performed by age 3 to 6 months.
6. Cleft palate repair is performed around 1 year of age, following the successful repair of cleft lip if present and to allow for the palatal changes that take place with normal growth; a cleft palate is closed as early as possible to facilitate speech development.
7. The child with cleft palate is at risk for developing frequent otitis media; this can result in hearing loss.
8. A multidisciplinary team approach is taken to address the many needs of the child; some of these professionals include audiologists, orthodontists, plastic surgeons, and occupational and speech therapists.

B. Data collection (Fig. 31.1)
1. Cleft lip can range from a slight notch to a complete separation from the floor of the nose.
2. Cleft palate can include nasal distortion, midline or bilateral cleft, and variable extension from the uvula and the soft and hard palate.

C. Interventions
1. Check the ability to suck, swallow, handle normal secretions, and breathe without distress.
2. Monitor fluid and calorie intake daily, and monitor the weight.
3. Modify feeding techniques; plan to use specialized feeding techniques, obturators, and special nipples and feeders.
4. Hold the child in an upright position, and direct the formula to the side and back of the mouth to prevent aspiration.
5. Feed small amounts gradually and burp frequently.
6. Keep suction equipment and a bulb syringe at the bedside.
7. Reinforce instructions to the parents about special feeding or suctioning techniques.
8. Reinforce instructions to the parents about the *ESSR* method of feeding (enlarge the nipple, stimulate the sucking reflex, swallow, rest to allow the child to finish swallowing what has been placed in the mouth).
9. Encourage parents to express their feelings about the disorder.
10. Encourage parental bonding with the child, including holding and calling the child by name.

D. Postoperative interventions
1. Cleft lip repair
   a. Provide lip protection; a metal appliance or adhesive strips may be taped securely to the cheeks to prevent trauma to the suture line.
   b. Avoid positioning the child on the side of the repair or in the prone position, because these positions can cause rubbing of the surgical site on the mattress (position on the back upright and position to prevent airway obstruction by secretions, blood, or the tongue).
   c. Keep the surgical site clean and dry; after feeding, gently cleanse the suture line of formula or serosanguineous drainage with a solution such as normal saline or as designated by agency procedure.
   d. Apply antibiotic ointment to the site as prescribed.
   e. Elbow restraints would be used to prevent the infant from injuring or traumatizing the surgical site.
   f. Monitor for signs/symptoms of infection at the surgical site.

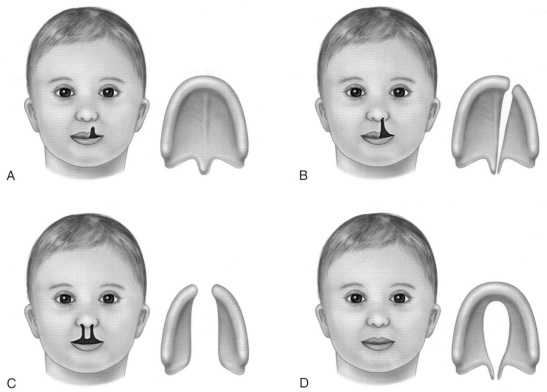

FIGURE 31.1 Variations in clefts of the lip and palate at birth. (**A**) Notch in vermilion border. (**B**) Unilateral cleft lip and palate. (**C**) Bilateral cleft lip and palate. (**D**) Cleft palate.

2. Cleft palate repair
  a. Feedings are resumed by bottle, breast, or cup per surgeon preference; some surgeons prescribe the use of an asepto syringe for feeding or a soft cup such as a Sippy cup.
  b. Oral packing may be secured to the palate (usually removed in 2 to 3 days).
  c. Reinforce instructions to the parents to avoid placing anything in the child's mouth that is harsh and could cause disruption of the surgical site.
3. Soft elbow or jacket restraints may be used (check agency policies and procedures) to keep the child from touching the repair site; remove restraints at least every 1 to 2 hours (or per agency procedure) to check skin integrity and circulation and to allow for exercising the arms.
4. Avoid the use of oral suction or placing objects in the mouth such as a tongue depressor, thermometer, straws, spoons, forks, or pacifiers.
5. Provide analgesics for pain as prescribed.
6. Reinforce instructions to the parents in feeding techniques and in the care of the surgical site.
7. Reinforce instructions to the parents to monitor for signs of infection at the surgical site, such as redness, swelling, or drainage.
8. Encourage the parents to hold the child.
9. Initiate appropriate referrals such as a dental referral and speech therapist referral.

IV. Esophageal Atresia and Tracheoesophageal Fistula (Fig. 31.2)
A. Description
  1. The esophagus terminates before it reaches the stomach, ending in a blind pouch, and/or a fistula is present that forms an unnatural connection with the trachea.
  2. The condition causes oral intake to enter the lungs or a large amount of air to enter the stomach. Choking, coughing, and severe abdominal distention can occur.
  3. Aspiration pneumonia and severe respiratory distress will develop, and death will occur without surgical intervention.
  4. Treatment includes maintenance of a patent airway, prevention of pneumonia, gastric or blind-pouch decompression, supportive therapy, and surgical repair.
B. Data collection
  1. Frothy saliva in the mouth and nose; drooling
  2. The "3 Cs"—coughing and choking during feedings and unexplained cyanosis
  3. Regurgitation and vomiting
  4. Abdominal distention
  5. Increased respiratory distress during and after feeding
C. Preoperative interventions
  1. The infant may be placed in a radiant warmer in which humidified oxygen is administered

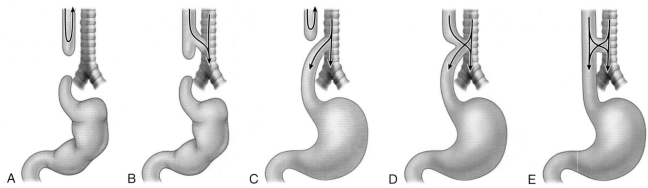

FIGURE 31.2 Congenital atresia of the esophagus and tracheoesophageal fistula. **(A)** Upper and lower segments of the esophagus end in a blind sac (occurring in 5%–8% of such infants). **(B)** Upper segment of the esophagus ends in atresia and connects to the trachea by a fistulous tract (occurring rarely). **(C)** Upper segment of the esophagus ends in a blind pouch; lower segment connects with the trachea by a small fistulous tract (occurring in 80%–95% of such infants). **(D)** Both segments of the esophagus connect by a fistulous tract to the trachea (occurring in less than 1% of such infants). Infant may aspirate with first feeding. **(E)** Esophagus is continuous but connects by a fistulous tract to the trachea; known as H-type.

(intubation and mechanical ventilation may be necessary if respiratory distress occurs).

2. Maintain NPO status.
3. Maintain IV fluids, as prescribed.
4. Monitor respiratory status closely.
5. Suction accumulated secretions from the mouth and pharynx.
6. Maintain in a supine upright position (at least 30 degrees upright) to facilitate drainage and prevent aspiration of gastric secretions.
7. The blind pouch is kept empty of secretions by intermittent or continuous suction as prescribed; monitor its patency closely because clogging from mucus can easily occur.
8. If a gastrostomy tube is inserted, it may be left open so that air entering the stomach through the fistula can escape, minimizing the risk of regurgitation of gastric contents into the trachea.
9. Broad-spectrum antibiotics may be prescribed because of the high risk for aspiration pneumonia.

D. Postoperative interventions

1. Monitor vital signs and respiratory status.
2. Assist in maintaining IV fluids, antibiotics, and parenteral nutrition as prescribed.
3. Monitor strict I&O.
4. Monitor daily weight; monitor for dehydration and possible fluid overload.
5. Monitor for signs of pain.
6. Assist to maintain chest tube patency if present.
7. Inspect the surgical site for signs/symptoms of infection.
8. Monitor for anastomotic leaks as evidenced by purulent drainage from the chest tube, increased temperature, and increased white blood cell count; report these findings to the registered nurse (RN).
9. If a gastrostomy tube is present, it is usually attached to gravity drainage until the infant can tolerate feedings and the anastomosis is healed (usually postoperative day 5 to 7); then feedings are prescribed.

10. Before oral feedings and removal of the chest tube, assist to prepare for an esophagram as prescribed to check the integrity of the esophageal anastomosis.
11. Before feeding, the gastrostomy tube is elevated and secured above the level of the stomach to allow gastric secretions to pass to the duodenum and swallowed air to escape through the open gastrostomy tube.
12. Assist to administer oral feedings with sterile water, followed by frequent small feedings of formula as prescribed.
13. Check the cervical esophagostomy site, if present, for redness, breakdown, or exudate; remove accumulated drainage frequently, and apply protective ointment, a barrier dressing, and/or a collection device as prescribed.
14. Assist to provide nonnutritive sucking using a pacifier for infants who remain NPO for extended periods (a pacifier must not be used if the infant is unable to handle secretions).
15. Reinforce instructions to parents in the techniques of suctioning, gastrostomy tube care and feedings, and skin site care as appropriate.
16. Reinforce instructions to parents to identify behaviors that indicate the need for suctioning, signs of respiratory distress, and signs of a constricted esophagus (e.g., poor feeding, dysphagia, drooling, coughing during feedings, regurgitated undigested food).

V. Gastroesophageal Reflux

A. Description

1. Gastroesophageal reflux is backflow of gastric contents into the esophagus as a result of relaxation or incompetence of the lower esophageal or cardiac sphincter.
2. Most infants with gastroesophageal reflux have a mild problem that improves in approximately 1 year and requires only medical therapy.

3. Gastroesophageal reflux disease (GERD) occurs when gastric contents reflux into the esophagus or oropharynx and produce symptoms.

B. Data collection
1. Passive regurgitation or emesis
2. Poor weight gain
3. Irritability
4. Hematemesis
5. Heartburn (in older children)
6. Anemia from blood loss

C. Interventions
1. Monitor the amount and characteristics of the emesis.
2. Monitor the relationship of the vomiting to the times of feedings and infant activity.
3. Monitor the breath sounds before and after feedings.
4. Monitor for signs of aspiration, such as drooling, coughing, or dyspnea following feeding.
5. Place suction equipment at the bedside.
6. Monitor I&O.
7. Monitor for signs and symptoms of dehydration.
8. Assist to maintain the IV fluids, as prescribed.

⚠️ Complications of GERD include esophagitis, esophageal strictures, aspiration of gastric contents, and aspiration pneumonia.

D. Positioning
1. The infant is placed in the supine position during sleep (to reduce the incidence of sudden infant death syndrome) unless the risk of death from aspiration or other serious complications of GERD greatly outweigh the risks associated with the prone position (check the PHCP's prescription); otherwise, the prone position is only acceptable while the infant is awake and can be monitored.
2. In children older than 1 year, position with the head of the bed elevated.

E. Diet
1. Provide small, frequent feedings with predigested formula to decrease the amount of regurgitation.
2. Nutrition via nasogastric (NG) tube feedings may be prescribed if severe regurgitation and poor growth are present.
3. For infants, formula may be thickened by adding rice cereal to the formula (follow agency procedure); then cross-cut the nipple.
4. Breast-feeding may continue, and the mother may provide more frequent feeding times or express milk for thickening with rice cereal.
5. Burp the infant frequently when feeding, and handle the infant minimally after feedings; monitor for coughing during feeding and other signs of aspiration.
6. For toddlers, feed solids first, followed by liquids.
7. Reinforce instructions to the parents to avoid feeding the child fatty foods, chocolate, tomato

products, carbonated liquids, fruit juices, citrus products, and spicy foods.
8. Reinforce instructions to the parents that the child would avoid vigorous play after feeding, and avoid feeding just before bedtime.

F. Medications
1. Antacids for symptom relief
2. Proton pump inhibitors and histamine 2 (H_2) antagonists to decrease acid secretion

VI. Hypertrophic Pyloric Stenosis

A. Description
1. Hypertrophy of the circular muscles of the pylorus causes the narrowing of the pyloric canal between the stomach and the duodenum.
2. The stenosis usually develops during the first few weeks of life and causes projectile vomiting, dehydration, metabolic alkalosis, and failure to thrive.

B. Data collection
1. Vomiting that progresses from mild regurgitation to forceful and projectile that usually occurs after a feeding
2. Vomitus contains gastric contents, such as milk or formula. It may contain mucus, may be blood-tinged, and does not usually contain bile.
3. Hunger and irritability
4. Peristaltic waves visible from left to right across the epigastrium during or immediately after a feeding
5. Olive-shaped mass in the epigastrium just right of the umbilicus
6. Dehydration and malnutrition
7. Electrolyte imbalance
8. Metabolic alkalosis

C. Interventions
1. Monitor strict I&O.
2. Monitor vomiting episodes and stools.
3. Obtain daily weights.
4. Monitor for signs of dehydration and electrolyte imbalance.
5. Assist to prepare the child and parents for pyloromyotomy, if prescribed.

D. Pyloromyotomy
1. Description: An incision through the muscle fibers of the pylorus, which may be performed by laparoscopy
2. Interventions preoperatively
   a. Monitor the hydration status by checking the daily weight measurements, I&O, and urine for specific gravity.
   b. Correct fluid and electrolyte imbalances; IV fluids may be prescribed for rehydration.
   c. Maintain NPO status.
   d. Monitor the number and character of stools.
   e. Maintain the patency of the NG tube that is placed for stomach decompression.

3. Postoperative interventions
   a. Monitor I&O.
   b. Begin small, frequent feedings postoperatively as prescribed.
   c. Gradually increase amount and interval between feedings until a full feeding schedule has been reinstated.
   d. Feed the infant slowly, burping frequently, and handle the infant minimally after feedings.
   e. Monitor for abdominal distention.
   f. Monitor the surgical wound and for signs of infection.
   g. Reinforce instructions to the parents about wound care and feeding.

VII. Lactose Intolerance

A. Description: The inability to tolerate lactose as a result of an absence or deficiency of lactase, which is an enzyme found in the secretions of the small intestine that is required for the digestion of lactose

B. Data collection
   1. Symptoms occur after the ingestion of milk products.
   2. Abdominal distention
   3. Crampy, abdominal pain; colic
   4. Diarrhea and excessive flatus

C. Interventions
   1. Eliminate the offending dairy product or administer an enzyme replacement.
   2. Provide information to the parents about enzyme tablets that predigest the lactose in milk or supplement the body's own lactase.
   3. Soy-based formula can be substituted for cow's milk formula or human milk.
   4. Allow milk consumption as tolerated.
   5. If milk is consumed, it should be taken when other foods are consumed rather than by itself.
   6. Encourage the consumption of hard cheese, cottage cheese, or yogurt (which contains inactive lactase enzyme) rather than milk.
   7. Encourage the consumption of small amounts of dairy foods daily to help colonic bacteria adapt to ingested lactose.
   8. Reinforce instructions to parents about foods that contain lactose, including hidden sources.

⚠ A child with lactose intolerance can develop calcium and vitamin D deficiency. Instruct parents about the importance of providing these supplements.

VIII. Celiac Disease

A. Description
   1. Celiac disease is also known as gluten enteropathy or celiac sprue.
   2. Intolerance to gluten, the protein component of wheat, barley, rye, and oats, is characteristic.
   3. Celiac disease results in the accumulation of the amino acid glutamine, which is toxic to intestinal mucosal cells.
   4. Intestinal villi atrophy occurs, which affects absorption of ingested nutrients.
   5. Symptoms of the disorder occur most often between the ages of 1 and 5 years.
   6. There is usually an interval of 3 to 6 months between the introduction of gluten in the diet and the onset of symptoms.
   7. Strict dietary avoidance of gluten minimizes the risk of developing malignant lymphoma of the small intestine and other gastrointestinal malignancies.

B. Data collection
   1. Acute or insidious diarrhea. Stools are watery and pale with an offensive odor.
   2. Steatorrhea
   3. Anorexia
   4. Abdominal pain and distention
   5. Muscle wasting, particularly in the buttocks and extremities
   6. Vomiting
   7. Anemia
   8. Irritability

C. Celiac crisis
   1. Precipitated by fasting, infection, or ingestion of gluten
   2. Causes profuse watery diarrhea and vomiting
   3. Can lead to rapid dehydration, electrolyte imbalance, and severe acidosis

D. Interventions
   1. Gluten-free diet and the substitution of corn, rice, and millet as grain sources
   2. Lifelong elimination of gluten sources such as wheat, rye, oats, and barley
   3. Mineral and vitamin supplements, including iron, folic acid, and fat-soluble supplements A, D, E, and K
   4. Reinforce teaching the parents about a gluten-free diet and to read food labels carefully for hidden sources of gluten (Box 31.1).
   5. Reinforce instructions to parents regarding measures to prevent celiac crisis.
   6. Inform the parents about the Celiac Sprue Association.

IX. Appendicitis

A. Description
   1. Inflammation of the appendix
   2. When the appendix becomes inflamed or infected, perforation may occur within a matter of hours, leading to peritonitis, sepsis, septic shock, and potential death.
   3. Treatment is the surgical removal of the appendix before perforation occurs.

BOX 31.1 **Basics of a Gluten-Free Diet**

Foods Allowed

Meat such as beef, pork, poultry, and fish; eggs; milk and dairy products; vegetables; fruits; rice; corn; gluten-free flour; puffed rice; cornflakes; cornmeal; and precooked gluten-free cereals.

Foods Prohibited

Commercially prepared ice cream; malted milk; prepared puddings; and grains, including anything made from wheat, rye, oats, or barley, such as breads, rolls, cookies, cakes, crackers, cereal, spaghetti, macaroni noodles, beer, and ale unless they are prepared gluten free.

B. Data collection
   1. Pain in periumbilical area that descends to the right lower quadrant
   2. Abdominal pain that is most intense at McBurney's point
   3. Referred pain that indicates the presence of peritoneal irritation
   4. Rebound tenderness and abdominal rigidity
   5. Elevated white blood cell count
   6. Side-lying position with abdominal guarding (legs flexed) to relieve pain
   7. Difficulty walking and pain in the right hip
   8. Low-grade fever
   9. Anorexia, nausea, and vomiting after the pain develops
   10. Diarrhea
C. Peritonitis
   1. Description: Results from a perforated appendix.
   2. Data collection
      a. Increased fever
      b. Progressive abdominal distention
      c. Tachycardia and tachypnea
      d. Pallor
      e. Chills
      f. Restlessness and irritability

⚠ An indication of a perforated appendix is the sudden relief of pain and then a subsequent increase in pain accompanied by right guarding of the abdomen.

D. Appendectomy
   1. Description: Surgical removal of the appendix
   2. Preoperative interventions
      a. Maintain NPO status.
      b. IV fluids and electrolytes may be prescribed to prevent dehydration and correct electrolyte imbalances.
      c. Monitor for signs of a ruptured appendix and peritonitis.
      d. Monitor for change in the level of pain; pain medications may be avoided so as to not mask pain changes associated with perforation.

   e. Antibiotics may be prescribed.
   f. Monitor bowel sounds.
   g. Position the child in a right side-lying or low to semi-Fowler's position to promote comfort.
   h. Apply ice packs to the abdomen for 20 to 30 minutes every hour, if prescribed.
   i. Avoid the application of heat to the abdomen and the administration of laxatives or enemas because of the risk of perforation.
   3. Postoperative interventions
      a. Monitor the temperature for signs of infection.
      b. Maintain NPO status until bowel function has returned. Advance the diet gradually, as tolerated and as prescribed, when bowel sounds return.
      c. Monitor the incision for signs of infection, such as redness, swelling, drainage, and pain.
      d. Monitor drainage from the drain which may be inserted if perforation occurred.
      e. Position in a right side-lying or low to semi-Fowler's position with the legs slightly flexed to facilitate drainage.
      f. Change the dressing, as prescribed, and record the type and amount of drainage.
      g. Perform wound irrigations, if prescribed.
      h. Maintain NG tube suction and the patency of the tube, if present.
      i. Administer antibiotics and analgesics, as prescribed.

X. Hirschsprung's Disease

A. Description
   1. Congenital anomaly also known as congenital aganglionosis or aganglionic megacolon
   2. The disease occurs as the result of an absence of ganglion cells in the rectum and other areas of the affected intestine.
   3. The disease results in mechanical obstruction because of inadequate motility in an intestinal segment.
   4. The disease may be a familial congenital defect or may be associated with other anomalies, such as Down syndrome and genitourinary abnormalities.
   5. A rectal biopsy demonstrates histological evidence of the absence of ganglionic cells.
   6. The most serious complication is enterocolitis; signs include fever, severe prostration, gastrointestinal bleeding, and explosive watery diarrhea.
   7. Treatment for mild or moderate disease is based on relieving the chronic constipation with stool softeners and rectal irrigations; however, surgery may be required for severe disease.
   8. Treatment for moderate to severe disease involves a two-step surgical procedure:
      a. Initially, in the neonatal period, a temporary colostomy is created to relieve obstruction and allow the normally innervated, dilated bowel to return to its normal size.

b. When the bowel returns to its normal size, a complete surgical repair is performed via a pull-through procedure to excise portions of the bowel; at this time, the colostomy is closed.

B. Data collection
  1. Newborns
    a. Failure to pass meconium stool
    b. Refusal to suck
    c. Abdominal distention
    d. Bile-stained vomitus
  2. Children
    a. Failure to gain weight and delayed growth
    b. Abdominal distention
    c. Vomiting
    d. Constipation alternating with diarrhea
    e. Ribbon-like and foul-smelling stools
  3. Interventions: Medical management
    a. Maintain low-fiber, high-calorie, high-protein diet; parenteral nutrition may be necessary in extreme situations.
    b. Administer stool softeners as prescribed.
    c. Administer daily rectal irrigations with normal saline to promote adequate elimination and prevent obstruction as prescribed.

C. Surgical management: Preoperative interventions
  1. Monitor the bowel function and administer bowel preparations, as prescribed.
  2. Maintain NPO status.
  3. Monitor hydration and fluid and electrolyte status. IV fluids may be prescribed for hydration.
  4. Administer antibiotics or colonic irrigations with an antibiotic solution as prescribed to clear the bowel of bacteria.
  5. Monitor strict I&O and weight.
  6. Measure the abdominal girth.
  7. Avoid taking rectal temperatures.
  8. Monitor for respiratory distress associated with abdominal distention.

D. Postoperative interventions
  1. Monitor vital signs, avoiding taking the temperature rectally.
  2. Measure abdominal girth daily and as frequently as prescribed.
  3. Check the surgical site for redness, swelling, and drainage.
  4. Check the stoma if present for bleeding or skin breakdown (stoma would be red and moist).
  5. Check the anal area for the presence of stool, redness, or discharge.
  6. Maintain NPO status until bowel sounds return or flatus is passed and as prescribed, usually within 48 to 72 hours.
  7. Maintain the NG tube to allow intermittent suction until peristalsis returns.
  8. Maintain IV fluids until the child tolerates appropriate oral intake, advancing the diet from clear liquids to regular as tolerated and as prescribed.

9. Monitor for dehydration and fluid overload.
10. Monitor strict I&O.
11. Obtain daily weight.
12. Monitor for pain and provide comfort measures as required and as prescribed.
13. Reinforce instructions to the parents regarding colostomy care and skin care.
14. Reinforce teaching the parents about the appropriate diet and the need for adequate fluid intake.

XI. Intussusception (Fig. 31.3)

A. Description
  1. The telescoping of one portion of the bowel into another
  2. Results in an obstruction of the passage of intestinal contents
B. Data collection
  1. Colicky abdominal pain that causes the child to scream and draw his or her knees to the abdomen
  2. Vomiting of gastric contents
  3. Bile-stained fecal emesis
  4. Currant jelly-like stools that contain blood and mucus
  5. Hypoactive or hyperactive bowel sounds
  6. Tender and distended abdomen, possibly with a palpable sausage-shaped mass in the upper right quadrant
C. Interventions
  1. Monitor for signs of perforation and shock as evidenced by fever, increased heart rate, change in the level of consciousness or blood pressure, and respiratory distress, and report immediately.

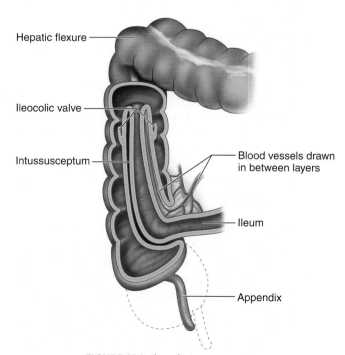

FIGURE 31.3 Ileocolic intussusception.

2. Antibiotics, IV fluids, and decompression via NG tube may be prescribed.

3. Monitor for the passage of normal, brown stool, which indicates that the intussusception has reduced itself.

4. Prepare for hydrostatic reduction as prescribed, if no signs of perforation or shock occur (in hydrostatic reduction, air or fluid is used to exert pressure on the area involved to lessen, diminish, or resolve the prolapse).

5. Posthydrostatic reduction

　a. Monitor for the return of normal bowel sounds, for the passage of barium, and the characteristics of stool.

　b. Administer clear fluids and advance the diet gradually as prescribed.

6. If surgery is required, postoperative care is similar to that following any abdominal surgery.

XII. Abdominal Wall Defects

A. Omphalocele

1. Occurs when there is a herniation of the abdominal contents through the umbilical ring (hernia of the umbilical cord), usually with an intact peritoneal sac

2. The protrusion is covered by a translucent sac that may contain bowel or other abdominal organs.

3. Immediately after birth, the sac is covered with sterile gauze soaked in normal saline to prevent drying of abdominal contents; a layer of plastic wrap is placed over the gauze to provide additional protection against moisture loss.

4. Rupture of the sac results in the evisceration of the abdominal contents. Once the infant is stabilized, synthetic material (Silastic) is used to cover the intestines.

5. Monitor the vital signs every 2 to 4 hours. Temperature is particularly important, because the infant can lose heat through the sac.

6. Preoperatively: Maintain NPO status. IV fluids will be prescribed to maintain hydration and electrolyte balance. Monitor for signs of infection, and handle the infant carefully to prevent the rupture of the sac.

7. Postoperatively: Control pain, prevent infection, maintain fluid and electrolyte balance, and ensure adequate nutrition.

B. Gastroschisis

1. Occurs when the herniation of the intestine is lateral (usually on the right) to the umbilical ring

2. There is no membrane covering the exposed bowel.

3. The exposed bowel is covered loosely in saline-soaked pads, and the abdomen is loosely wrapped in a plastic drape or bowel bag; wrapping directly around the exposed bowel is contraindicated because if the exposed bowel expands, wrapping could cause pressure and necrosis.

4. Preoperatively: Care is similar to that for omphalocele; surgery is performed within several hours after birth because no membrane is covering the sac.

5. Postoperatively: Most infants develop prolonged ileus, require mechanical ventilation, and need parenteral nutrition; otherwise, care is similar to that for omphalocele.

XIII. Umbilical Hernia

A. Description

1. A hernia is a protrusion of the bowel through an abnormal or weakened opening in the abdominal wall.

2. In children, a hernia most commonly occurs at the umbilicus and through the inguinal canal.

3. A hydrocele is the presence of abdominal fluid in the scrotal sac.

B. Data collection

1. Umbilical hernia: A soft swelling or protrusion around the umbilicus that is usually reducible with the finger

2. Inguinal hernia

　a. Painless inguinal swelling that is reducible

　b. Swelling may disappear during periods of rest and is most noticeable when the infant cries or coughs.

3. Incarcerated hernia

　a. Occurs when the descended portion of the bowel becomes tightly caught in the hernial sac, compromising blood supply

　b. Represents a medical emergency requiring surgical repair

　c. Data collection findings—irritability, tenderness at site, anorexia, abdominal distention, difficulty defecating

　d. May lead to complete intestinal obstruction and gangrene

4. Noncommunicating hydrocele

　a. Occurs when residual peritoneal fluid is trapped with no communication with the peritoneal cavity

　b. Usually disappears by the age of 1 year

5. Communicating hydrocele

　a. Associated with a hernia that remains open from the scrotum to the abdominal cavity

　b. Data collection findings include a bulge in the inguinal area of the scrotum that increases with crying or straining and that decreases when the child is at rest.

C. Postoperative interventions (hernia)

1. Monitor vital signs.

2. Monitor for wound infection (redness or drainage).

3. Monitor I&O and hydration status.

4. Advance the diet, as tolerated and as prescribed.

5. Administer analgesics, as prescribed.

D. Postoperative interventions (hydrocele)

1. Provide ice bags and a scrotal support to relieve pain and swelling.
2. Reinforce instructions to the parents that tub bathing needs to be avoided until the incision heals.
3. Reinforce instructions to the parents that strenuous physical activities need to be avoided.
4. Advise parents that the scrotum may not immediately return to normal size.

XIV. Constipation and Encopresis

A. Description

1. Constipation is the infrequent and difficult passage of dry, hard stools.
2. Encopresis is constipation with fecal incontinence; children often complain that soiling is involuntary and occurs without warning.
3. If the child does not have a neurological or anatomical disorder, encopresis is usually the result of fecal impaction and an enlarged rectum caused by chronic constipation.

B. Assessment

1. Constipation
   a. Abdominal pain and cramping without distention
   b. Palpable movable fecal masses
   c. Normal or decreased bowel sounds
   d. Malaise and headache
   e. Anorexia, nausea, and vomiting
2. Encopresis
   a. Evidence of soiling clothing
   b. Scratching or rubbing of the anal area
   c. Fecal odor
   d. Social withdrawal

C. Interventions

1. Maintain a diet high in fiber and fluids to promote bowel elimination (Box 31.2).
2. Monitor treatment regimen for severe encopresis for 3 to 6 months.
3. Decrease sugar and milk intake.
4. Administer enemas as prescribed until impaction is clear.
5. Monitor for hypernatremia and hyperphosphatemia when administering repeated enemas.
   a. Signs of hypernatremia include increased thirst; dry, sticky mucous membranes; flushed skin; increased temperature; nausea and vomiting; oliguria; and lethargy.
   b. Signs of hyperphosphatemia include tetany, muscle weakness, dysrhythmias, and hypotension.
6. Administer stool softeners or laxatives as prescribed.
7. Encourage the child to sit on the toilet for 5 to 10 minutes approximately 20 to 30 minutes after breakfast and dinner, to assist with defecation.

BOX 31.2 **High-Fiber Foods**

Bread and Grains
- Whole-grain bread or rolls
- Whole-grain cereals
- Bran
- Pancakes, waffles, and muffins with fruit or bran
- Unrefined (brown) rice

Vegetables
- Raw vegetables, especially broccoli, cabbage, carrots, cauliflower, celery, lettuce, and spinach
- Cooked vegetables, including those listed above and asparagus, beans, Brussels sprouts, corn, potatoes, rhubarb, squash, string beans, and turnips

Fruits
- Prunes, raisins, or other dried fruits
- Raw fruits, especially those with skins or seeds, other than ripe banana or avocado

Miscellaneous
- Legumes (beans), popcorn, nuts, and seeds
- High-fiber snack bars

XV. Irritable Bowel Syndrome

A. Description

1. Occurs as a result of increased motility, which can lead to spasm and pain
2. Diagnosis is based on the elimination of pathological conditions.
3. Self-limiting, intermittent problem with no definitive treatment
4. Stress and emotional factors may contribute to its occurrence.

B. Data collection

1. Diffuse abdominal pain unrelated to meals or activity
2. Alternating constipation and diarrhea with the presence of undigested food and mucus in the stool

C. Interventions

1. Reassure the parents that the problem is self-limiting and intermittent and that it will resolve.
2. Anticholinergics may be prescribed. (Antidepressants may be needed in severe cases.)
3. Encourage the maintenance of a healthy, well-balanced, moderate-fiber and low-fat diet.
4. Encourage health-promotion activities, such as exercise and school activities.
5. Inform the parents about psychosocial resources, if required.

XVI. Imperforate Anus

A. Description: The incomplete development or absence of the anus in its normal position in the perineum.

B. Types

1. A membrane is noted over the anal opening, with a normal anus just above the membrane.

- Failure to pass meconium stool
- Absence or stenosis of the anal rectal canal
- Presence of an anal membrane
- External fistula to the perineum

2. There is complete absence of the anus (anal agenesis) with a rectal pouch ending some distance above.
3. Rectum ends blindly or has a fistula connection to the perineum, urethra, bladder, or vagina.

C. Data collection (Box 31.3)
D. Preoperative interventions
1. Determine the patency of the anus.
2. Monitor for the presence of stool in the urine and vagina. Report this immediately.
3. Assist to administer IV fluids as prescribed.
4. Prepare the child and parents for the surgical procedures, including the potential for colostomy.

E. Postoperative interventions
1. Monitor the skin for signs of infection.
2. The preferred position is a side-lying prone position with the hips elevated or a supine position with the legs suspended at a 90-degree angle to the trunk to reduce edema and pressure on the surgical site.
3. Keep the anal surgical incision clean and dry, and monitor for redness, swelling, or drainage.
4. Maintain NPO status and the NG tube, if one has been placed.
5. Maintain IV fluids until gastrointestinal motility returns as prescribed.
6. Assist to provide colostomy care, if prescribed.
7. A new colostomy stoma will be red and edematous, but this would decrease with time.
8. Reinforce instructions to parents about the procedure to perform anal dilation, if prescribed, to achieve and maintain bowel patency.
9. Reinforce instructions to use only dilators supplied by the PHCP and a water-soluble lubricant and to insert the dilator no more than 1 cm to 2 cm into the anus to prevent damage to the mucosa.

XVII. Hepatitis

A. This section contains specific information regarding hepatitis as it relates to infants and children. Refer to Chapters 23 and 45 for additional information about hepatitis.
B. Description: An acute or chronic inflammation of the liver that may be caused by a virus, a medication reaction, or another disease process
C. Hepatitis A virus (HAV)
1. Highest incidence occurs among preschool or school-age children who are younger than 15 years old.

2. Many affected children are asymptomatic, but mild nausea, vomiting, and diarrhea may occur.
3. Infected children who are asymptomatic can still spread HAV to others.

D. Hepatitis B virus (HBV)
1. Most HBV in children is acquired perinatally.
2. Newborns are at risk if the mother is infected with HBV or was a carrier of HBV during pregnancy.
3. Possible routes of maternal-fetal (infant) transmission include the leakage of the virus across the placenta late in pregnancy or during labor, the ingestion of amniotic fluid or maternal blood, and breast-feeding, especially if the mother has cracked nipples.
4. The severity in the infant varies from no liver disease to fulminant (severe, acute course) or chronic, active disease.
5. In children and adolescents, HBV occurs in specific high-risk groups, including the following:
   a. Children with hemophilia or other disorders who have received multiple blood transfusions
   b. Children or adolescents who are involved in drug abuse
   c. Institutionalized children
   d. Preschool-age children in endemic areas
   e. Children who may be involved with heterosexual activity or sexual activity with homosexual males
6. HBV infection can cause a carrier state and lead to eventual cirrhosis or hepatocellular carcinoma during adulthood.

E. Hepatitis C virus (HCV)
1. Transmission is primarily by the parenteral route.
2. Some children may be asymptomatic, but HCV often becomes a chronic condition, and it can cause cirrhosis and hepatocellular carcinoma.

F. Hepatitis D virus
1. Infection occurs in children already infected with HBV.
2. Acute and chronic forms tend to be more severe than HBV and can lead to cirrhosis.
3. Children with hemophilia are more likely to be infected, as are those who are IV drug users.

G. Hepatitis E virus
1. Uncommon among children
2. Is not a chronic condition, does not cause chronic liver disease, and has no carrier state

H. Data collection (Box 31.4)
I. Diagnostic evaluation: See Chapter 10 for the laboratory studies that are used to diagnose hepatitis.
J. Prevention
1. Immunoglobulin provides passive immunity and may be effective for preexposure prophylaxis to prevent HAV infection.
2. Hepatitis B immunoglobulin provides passive immunity and may be effective in preventing

infection following a one-time exposure (needs to be given immediately after exposure), such as an accidental needle puncture or other contact of contaminated material with mucous membranes; it needs to also be given to newborns whose mothers are hepatitis B surface antigen (HBsAg)-positive.

3. Hepatitis A and hepatitis B vaccines (see Chapter 37 for information on immunizations)

⚠️ Proper hand washing and standard precautions can prevent the spread of viral hepatitis.

K. Interventions
1. Strict hand washing is required.
2. Hospitalization is required in the event of coagulopathy or fulminant hepatitis.
3. Standard precautions and enteric precautions are followed during hospitalization; provide enteric precautions for at least 1 week after the onset of jaundice with HAV.
4. A hospitalized child is not usually isolated in a separate room unless he or she is fecally incontinent and items are likely to become contaminated with feces.
5. Children are discouraged from sharing toys.
6. Reinforce instructions to the child and parents regarding good hand-washing techniques.
7. Reinforce instructions to parents to thoroughly disinfect diaper-changing surfaces using 1/4 cup of bleach in 1 gallon of water.
8. Maintain comfort and provide adequate rest and sleep.
9. Provide a low-fat, balanced diet.
10. Inform the parents that because HAV is not infectious 1 week after the onset of jaundice, the child may return to school at that time if he or she feels well enough.
11. Inform the parents that jaundice may get worse before it resolves.
12. Caution parents about administering any medications to the child. (Remember that the liver is unable to detoxify and excrete medications.)
13. Reinforce instructions to parents regarding the signs that indicate the worsening of the child's condition, such as a change in the neurological status, bleeding, and fluid retention.

XVIII. Ingestion of Poisons (see Priority Nursing Actions)

> ⚡ **PRIORITY NURSING ACTIONS**
>
> **Poisoning Treatment in the Emergency Department**
>
> 1. Assess the child and intervene accordingly.
> 2. Terminate exposure to the poison.
> 3. Identify the poison.
> 4. Take measures to prevent absorption of the poison.
> 5. Document the occurrence, assessment of findings, poison ingested, treatment measures, and the child's response.

A. Lead poisoning
1. Description: Excessive accumulation of lead in the blood
2. Causes
   a. The pathway for exposure may be food, air, or water.
   b. Dust and soil contaminated with lead may be a source of exposure.
   c. Lead enters the child's body through ingestion or inhalation, or through placental transmission to an unborn child when the mother is exposed; the most common route is hand to mouth from lead containing contaminated objects, such as loose paint chips, pottery, or ceramicware coupled with the inhalation of lead dust in the environment.
   d. When lead enters the body, it affects the erythrocytes, bones, teeth, organs, and tissues, including the brain and nervous system. The most serious consequences are the effects on the central nervous system.
3. Universal screening
   a. Recommended in high-risk areas at the age of 1 to 2 years. Children at high risk must be screened earlier.
   b. Any child between the ages of 3 and 6 years who has not been screened must be tested.
4. Targeted screening
   a. Acceptable in low-risk areas
   b. At the age of 1 to 2 years (or a child between the ages of 3 and 6 years who has not been

TABLE 31.1 Blood Lead Level Test Results and Intervention

Level (mcg/dL)	Intervention
<5	Reassess or rescreen in 1 year or sooner if exposure status changes.
5–14	Provide family lead education, follow-up testing, and social service referral for home assessment if necessary.
15–19	Provide family lead education, follow-up testing, and social service referral if necessary; on follow-up testing, prepare to assist in initiating actions for blood lead level of 20–44 mcg/dL.
20–44	Assist with coordination of care, clinical management, including treatment, environmental investigation, and lead-hazard control.
45–69	Assist with coordination of care and clinical management within 48 hours, including treatment, environmental investigation, and lead hazard control (the child must not remain in a lead-hazardous environment if resolution is necessary).
≥70	Medical treatment is provided immediately, including coordination of care, clinical management, environmental investigation, and lead-hazard control.

Adapted from Perry S, Hockenberry M, Lowdermilk D, Wilson D: *Maternal child nursing care*, ed 4, St. Louis, 2010, Elsevier.

screened) may be targeted for screening if determined to be at risk.

5. Blood lead level test: Used for screening and diagnosis (Table 31.1)
6. Erythrocyte protoporphyrin test
    a. An indicator of anemia
    b. Normal value for a child is 35 mcg/100 mL of whole blood or less
7. Chelation therapy
    a. Removes lead from the circulating blood and from some organs and tissues
    b. Does not counteract any effects of the lead
    c. Medications include calcium disodium edetate and succimer, an oral preparation; British anti-Lewisite is used in conjunction with edetate.
    d. British anti-Lewisite is administered by the IV route or via deep intramuscular route and is contraindicated in children with an allergy to peanuts because the medication is prepared in a peanut oil solution; it is also contraindicated in children with a glucose 6-phosphate dehydrogenase (G6PD) deficiency and would not be administered with iron.
    e. The function of the renal, hepatic, and hematological systems must be monitored closely.
    f. Adequate urinary output is ensured before administering the medication, and it is important to monitor the output and pH of the urine closely during and after therapy.
    g. Provide adequate hydration and monitor kidney function for nephrotoxicity when the medication is given because the medication is excreted via the kidneys.
    h. Follow-up of lead levels needs to be done to monitor progress.
    i. Reinforce instructions to parents about lead hazards and safety, medication administration, and the need for follow-up.
    j. Confirm that the child will be discharged to a home without lead hazards.
B. Acetaminophen poisoning
    1. Description
        a. The seriousness of the ingestion is determined by the amount ingested and the length of time before intervention.
        b. A toxic dose is 150 mg/kg or higher in children.
    2. Data collection
        a. First 2 to 4 hours: Malaise, nausea, vomiting, sweating, pallor, and weakness
        b. Latent period: 24 to 36 hours; child improves.
        c. Hepatic involvement: May last up to 7 days and be permanent; right upper quadrant pain, jaundice, confusion, stupor, elevated liver enzymes and bilirubin levels, and prolonged prothrombin time
    3. Interventions
        a. Administer the antidote: *N*-acetylcysteine.
        b. Antidote is diluted in juice or soda because of its offensive odor.
        c. Loading dose is followed by maintenance doses.
        d. In the unconscious child, prepare to administer gastric lavage with activated charcoal to decrease the absorption of acetaminophen.
        e. If using activated charcoal with lavage, do not also use *N*-acetylcysteine because activated charcoal will inactivate the antidote.
C. Acetylsalicylic acid poisoning
    1. Description
        a. May be caused by acute or chronic ingestion
        b. Acute: Severe toxicity occurs with 300 to 500 mg/kg.
        c. Chronic: More than 100 mg/kg/day for 2 days or more; can be more serious than acute ingestion
    2. Data collection
        a. Gastrointestinal effects: Nausea, vomiting, and thirst from dehydration
        b. Central nervous system effects: Hyperpnea, confusion, tinnitus, seizures, coma, respiratory failure, and circulatory collapse
        c. Renal effects: Oliguria
        d. Hematopoietic effects: Bleeding tendencies
        e. Metabolic effects: Diaphoresis, fever, hyponatremia, hypokalemia, dehydration, and hypoglycemia

3. Interventions
   a. Prepare to administer activated charcoal to decrease the absorption of salicylate.
   b. Emesis or cathartic measures may be prescribed.
   c. Assist to administer IV fluids; sodium bicarbonate may be prescribed to correct metabolic acidosis.
   d. Other interventions may include external cooling, anticonvulsants, vitamin K (if bleeding), and oxygen.
   e. Prepare the child for dialysis as prescribed if the child is unresponsive to the therapy.

D. Corrosives
   1. Description
      a. Items that can cause poisoning include household cleaners, detergents, bleach, paint or paint thinners, or batteries.
      b. Liquid corrosives can cause more damage to the victim than other types of corrosives, such as granular.
   2. Data collection
      a. Severe burning in the mouth, throat, or stomach
      b. Edema of the mucous membranes, lips, tongue, and pharynx
      c. Vomiting
      d. Drooling and inability to clear secretions
   3. Interventions
      a. Dilute corrosive with water or milk as prescribed (usually no more than 4 oz).
      b. Inducing vomiting is contraindicated because vomiting redamages the mucous membranes.
      c. Neutralization of the ingested corrosive is not done because it can cause a reaction producing heat and burns.

⚠ Educate parents to call the poison control center immediately in the event of poisoning. The parents need to be instructed to post the poison control center telephone number near each phone in the house and have it in their mobile phones.

XIX. Intestinal Parasites

A. Description: Common infections in children are giardiasis and pinworms.
   1. Giardiasis is caused by protozoa and it is prevalent among children in crowded environments, such as classrooms and daycare centers.
   2. Pinworms (enterobiasis) are universally present in temperate climate zones and easily transmitted in crowded environments.

B. Data collection
   1. Giardiasis
      a. Diarrhea and vomiting
      b. Anorexia
      c. Failure to thrive
      d. Abdominal cramps with intermittent loose stools and constipation
      e. Steatorrhea
      f. Stool specimens from three or more collections are used for diagnosis
   2. Pinworms
      a. Intense perianal itching
      b. Irritability and restlessness
      c. Poor sleeping
      d. Bed-wetting

C. Interventions
   1. Giardiasis
      a. Medications that may be prescribed include metronidazole, tinidazole, nitazoxanide, or albendazole.
      b. Performance of meticulous hand washing by caregivers
      c. Reinforce education to the family and caregivers regarding sanitary practices.
   2. Pinworms
      a. Perform a visual inspection of the anus with a flashlight 2 to 3 hours after sleep.
      b. The tape test is the most common diagnostic test.
      c. Reinforce educating the family and caregivers regarding the tape test. A loop of transparent tape is placed firmly against the child's perianal area; it is removed in the morning and placed in a glass jar or plastic bag and transported to the primary care provider for analysis.
      d. Medications that may be prescribed include mebendazole, pyrantelpamoate, and albendazole; these medications are not used in children younger than the age of 2 years.
      e. The medication regimen may be repeated in 2 weeks to prevent reinfection.
      f. All members of the family are treated for the infection.
      g. Reinforce teaching the family and caregivers about the importance of meticulous hand washing and about washing all clothes and bed linens in hot water.

WHAT WOULD YOU DO?

Answer: If a child suddenly vomits, the nurse must maintain a patent airway. The child would be positioned upright or on the side to prevent aspiration. Suctioning equipment must be obtained and kept at the bedside. The nurse needs to check the character and amount of vomitus. The force of the vomiting would be assessed because projectile vomiting may indicate pyloric stenosis or increased intracranial pressure. The nurse must also monitor intake and output and for signs of dehydration.

PRACTICE QUESTIONS

❖ **1.** The nurse is reviewing the postoperative surgeon's prescriptions for a 3-week-old infant with Hirschsprung's disease admitted to the hospital for surgery. Which prescriptions documented in the child's record would the nurse question? **Select all that apply.**
   ❑ **1.** Measure abdominal girth daily.
   ❑ **2.** Monitor strict intake and output.
   ❑ **3.** Take temperature measurements rectally.
   ❑ **4.** Start clear liquid diet after 8 hours postoperative.
   ❑ **5.** Maintain intravenous (IV) fluids until the child tolerates oral intake.
   ❑ **6.** Monitor the surgical site for redness, swelling, and drainage.

2. The nurse is monitoring for signs of dehydration in a 1-year-old child who has been hospitalized for diarrhea and prepares to take the child's temperature. Which method of temperature measurement needs to be avoided?
   1. Rectal
   2. Axillary
   3. Electronic
   4. Tympanic

3. A mother of a child with a diagnosis of intussusception calls the nurse into the hospital room because the child is screaming in pain. The nurse quickly assesses the child. Which manifestations of perforation and shock would the nurse report **immediately**? **Select all that apply.**
   ❑ **1.** Fever
   ❑ **2.** Ribbon-like stools
   ❑ **3.** Increased heart rate
   ❑ **4.** Hypoactive bowel sounds
   ❑ **5.** Profuse projectile vomiting
   ❑ **6.** Change in the level of consciousness

4. A child with a diagnosis of a hernia has been scheduled for a surgical repair in 2 weeks. The nurse reinforces instructions to the parents about the signs of possible incarcerated hernia. The nurse tells the parents that which manifestation requires primary health care provider (PHCP) notification by the parents?
   1. Pain
   2. Diarrhea
   3. Constipation
   4. Increased flatus

5. The nurse reinforces home-care instructions to the parents of a child with hepatitis regarding the care of the child and the prevention of the transmission of the virus. Which statement by a parent indicates a **need for further teaching**?

   1. "Frequent hand washing is important."
   2. "I need to provide a well-balanced, high-fat diet to my child."
   3. "I need to clean contaminated household surfaces with bleach."
   4. "Diapers should never be changed near any surfaces that are used to prepare food."

6. The nurse is assigned to care for a child who is scheduled for an appendectomy. Which prescriptions does the nurse anticipate to be prescribed? **Select all that apply.**
   ❑ **1.** Administer a Fleet enema.
   ❑ **2.** Initiate an intravenous line.
   ❑ **3.** Maintain nothing-by-mouth status.
   ❑ **4.** Administer intravenous antibiotics.
   ❑ **5.** Administer preoperative medications.
   ❑ **6.** Place a heating pad on the abdomen to decrease pain.

7. A child is brought to the emergency room and the mother reports that the child accidentally swallowed paint thinner after mistaking it for water. The nurse must perform which action **first**?
   1. Begin resuscitation.
   2. Terminate exposure to the poison.
   3. Take measures to prevent absorption of the poison.
   4. Check the airway, breathing, and circulation status of the child.

8. The nurse is caring for an 18-month-old child who has been vomiting. Which is the appropriate position to place the child during naps and sleep time?
   1. A supine position
   2. A side-lying position
   3. Prone, with the head elevated
   4. Prone, with the face turned to the side

9. An infant returns to the nursing unit after the surgical repair of a cleft lip located on the right side of the lip. Which is the **best** position to place this infant at this time?
   1. A flat position
   2. A prone position
   3. On his or her left side
   4. On his or her right side

10. The nurse reviews the record of an infant who is seen in the clinic. The nurse notes that a diagnosis of esophageal atresia with tracheoesophageal fistula (TEF) is suspected. The nurse expects to note which **most likely** manifestation of this condition in the medical record?
   1. Incessant crying
   2. Coughing at nighttime
   3. Choking with feedings
   4. Severe projectile vomiting

11. The nurse is reviewing the record of a child with a diagnosis of pyloric stenosis. Which data would the nurse expect to note as having been documented in the child's record?
    1. Watery diarrhea
    2. Projectile vomiting
    3. Increased urine output
    4. Vomiting large amounts of bile

12. The nurse reinforces instructions to the mother about dietary measures for a 5-year-old child with lactose intolerance. The nurse would tell the mother that which supplement will be required as a result of the need to avoid lactose in the diet?

1. Fats and vitamin A
2. Zinc and vitamin C
3. Calcium and vitamin D
4. Thiamine and vitamin B

13. The nurse reinforces home-care instructions to the parents of a child with celiac disease. Which food item would the nurse advise the parents to include in the child's diet?
    1. Rice
    2. Oatmeal
    3. Rye toast
    4. Wheat bread

ANSWERS

❖ **1. 3, 4**
Rationale: Postoperative management of Hirschsprung's disease includes taking vital signs but avoiding taking the temperature rectally. The client needs to remain NPO (nothing by mouth) status until bowel sounds return or flatus is passed, usually within 48 to 72 hours. The other options are correct postoperative management.
Test-Taking Strategy: Focus on the subject, postoperative prescriptions that need to be questioned for the management for Hirschsprung's disease. Maintaining NPO status and having a nasogastric tube is important until peristalsis returns. The infant's temperature is not to be taken rectally. Monitoring abdominal girth, dehydration and fluid overload, and pain management are all a part of postoperative management.

2. 1
Rationale: Rectal temperature measurements would be avoided if diarrhea is present. The use of a rectal thermometer can stimulate peristalsis and cause more diarrhea. Axillary or tympanic measurements of temperature would be acceptable. Most measurements are performed via electronic devices.
Test-Taking Strategy: Focus on the subject, the method of temperature measurement that would be avoided. Note that the child has diarrhea. Eliminate option 3 first because most methods of temperature measurement are performed with the use of an electronic device. Next, note the diagnosis stated in the question; this would direct you to the correct option.

3. 1, 3, 6
Rationale: The child with intussusception classically presents with severe abdominal pain that is crampy and intermittent and that causes the child to draw in his or her knees to the chest. The signs of perforation and shock are evidenced by fever, an increased heart rate, a change in the level of consciousness or blood pressure, and respiratory distress and need to be reported immediately. The options for hypoactive bowel sounds, profuse projectile vomiting, and ribbon-like stools are a part of the presentation picture of a child with intussusception but are not signs of shock.

Test-Taking Strategy: Note the strategic word, *immediately*. Knowing the signs of perforation and shock related to intussusception is required to answer this question. Think about the pathophysiology of a perforation. This will assist in eliminating options 2, 4, and 5 because these are symptoms that are used to diagnose intussusception.

4. 1
Rationale: The parents of a child with a hernia need to be instructed about the signs of an incarcerated hernia. These signs include irritability, tenderness and pain at the site of the hernia, anorexia, abdominal distension, and difficulty defecating. The parents need to be instructed to contact the PHCP immediately if an incarcerated hernia is suspected. These signs may lead to a complete intestinal obstruction and gangrene. Diarrhea, increased flatus, and constipation are not associated with an incarcerated hernia.
Test-Taking Strategy: Focus on the subject, signs of a possible incarcerated hernia and the need to notify the PHCP. Use the definition of the word *incarcerated hernia* to help answer this question; this will assist you with eliminating options 2, 3, and 4.

5. 2
Rationale: The child with hepatitis needs to consume a well-balanced, low-fat diet to allow the liver to rest. Options 1, 3, and 4 are components of the homecare instructions to the family of a child with hepatitis.
Test-Taking Strategy: Note the strategic words, *need for further teaching*. These words indicate a negative event query and ask you to select an option that is an incorrect statement. Options 1, 3, and 4 can be eliminated by remembering the basic principles related to standard precautions.

6. 2, 3, 4, 5
Rationale: During the preoperative period, enemas or laxatives must not be administered. In addition, heat must not be applied to the abdomen. Any of these interventions can cause the rupture of the appendix and resultant peritonitis. Intravenous fluids would be started, and the child would not receive anything by mouth while awaiting surgery.

Antibiotics are usually administered because of the risk of perforation. Preoperative medications are administered as prescribed.

Test-Taking Strategy: Consider the anatomical location of the subject, appendicitis, and think about the concern of rupture of the appendix for clients with this disorder. This will assist you with determining the correct interventions. Next, think about the actions that could cause pressure or stress on the appendix and resultant rupture to direct you to the correct options.

❖ **7. 4**
Rationale: Actions to take in the case of a child swallowing poison include assessing the child and treating the child first, not the poison. Airway, breathing, and circulation, and vital signs need to be assessed. Resuscitation measures would be initiated if the assessment indicates a need. The next step is to terminate exposure to the poison, such as emptying the mouth of pills or other materials or flushing the skin with water. Then identify the poison, if possible, and take measures to prevent absorption of the poison, such as administering the antidote if known. Transport the child to an emergency department for further treatment.

Test-Taking Strategy: Note the strategic word, *first* and recall the actions to be taken in an emergency situation. Use the steps of the nursing process and think about the steps to take and which one would be done first. This will assist you in selecting the correct option. Also, use of the ABCs—airway, breathing, and circulation will direct you to the correct option.

8. 2
Rationale: The vomiting child needs to be placed in an upright or side-lying position to prevent aspiration. Options 1, 3, and 4 will place the child at risk for aspiration if vomiting occurs.

Test-Taking Strategy: Eliminate options 3 and 4 first, because they are comparable or alike. In addition, these positions would place the child at risk for aspiration if vomiting occurred. Visualize the remaining two positions. Option 1 is also inappropriate and would cause aspiration.

9. 3
Rationale: After the repair of a cleft lip, the infant would be positioned on the side opposite to the repair to prevent contact of the suture lines with the bed linens. In this case it is best to place the infant on the left side. Additionally, the flat or prone position can result in aspiration if the infant vomits.

Test-Taking Strategy: Note the strategic word, *best*. Consider the anatomical location of the surgical site, *right side*, and think about the risk of aspiration and disruption of the surgical site. You would be easily directed to the correct option with the use of these concepts.

10. 3
Rationale: Any child who exhibits the "3 Cs"—coughing and choking during feedings and unexplained cyanosis—would be suspected of having a tracheoesophageal fistula (TEF). Options 1, 2, and 4 are not specifically associated with TEF.

Test-Taking Strategy: Note the strategic words, *most likely*. Focus on the subject, signs/symptoms of TEF, and think about the pathophysiology associated with this condition. Recalling the "3 Cs" associated with TEF will direct you to the correct option.

11. 2
Rationale: Signs/symptoms of pyloric stenosis include projectile, nonbilious vomiting; irritability; hunger and crying; constipation; and signs of dehydration, including a decrease in urine output.

Test-Taking Strategy: Focus on the subject, signs/symptoms of pyloric stenosis. Considering the anatomical location of this disorder and the definition of the word *stenosis* will assist you with eliminating the incorrect options. Watery diarrhea and increased urine output are not symptoms of pyloric stenosis. Vomiting bile would indicate that the pyloric sphincter is working because bile is produced in the liver and stored in the gallbladder.

12. 3
Rationale: Lactose intolerance is the inability to tolerate lactose, the sugar that is found in dairy products. Removing milk from the diet can provide relief from symptoms. Additional dietary changes may be required to provide adequate sources of calcium and vitamin D.

Test-Taking Strategy: Focus on the subject, adequate nutrition for the child with lactose intolerance. Knowledge that lactose is the sugar that is found in dairy products will easily direct you to the correct option because dairy products are a major source of calcium. Fats, zinc, and thiamine (a B vitamin) are not associated with lactose intolerance.

13. 1
Rationale: Dietary management is the mainstay of treatment for celiac disease. All wheat, rye, barley, and oats would be eliminated from the diet and replaced with corn and rice. Vitamin supplements, especially fat-soluble vitamins and folate, may be required during the early period of treatment to correct deficiencies. These restrictions are likely to be life long, although small amounts of grains may be tolerated after the gastrointestinal ulcerations have healed.

Test-Taking Strategy: Focus on the subject, dietary management for the child with celiac disease. Think about the pathophysiology of this disease. Recalling that corn and rice are substitute food replacements among clients with this disease will direct you to the correct option.

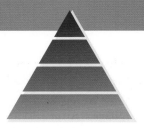
CHAPTER **32**

Eye, Ear, Throat, and Respiratory Problems

PRIORITY CONCEPTS **Gas Exchange; Sensory Perception**

WHAT WOULD YOU DO?

A child with pneumonia complains of pain in the pleural area on the affected side. What would the nurse do?
Answer is located on p. 408.

I. Strabismus

A. Description
1. Called "squint" or "cross-eye"
2. A condition in which the eyes are not aligned as a result of a lack of coordination of the extraocular muscles
3. Most often results from a muscle imbalance or the paralysis of the extraocular muscles, but it may also result from a congenital defect
4. Amblyopia (reduced visual acuity) may occur if not treated early because the brain receives two messages as a result of the nonparallel visual axes.
5. Permanent loss of vision can occur if not treated early.
6. This condition is considered a normal finding in a young infant, but it would not be present after about age 4 months.
7. Treatment of the condition depends on the cause.

B. Data collection
1. Crossed eyes
2. Squinting; tilts the head or closes one eye to see
3. Loss of binocular vision
4. Impairment in depth perception
5. Frequent headache
6. Diplopia; photophobia

C. Interventions
1. Corrective lenses to improve eye alignment
2. Instruct the parents regarding patching (occlusion therapy) of the "good" eye to strengthen the weak eye.
3. Prepare for surgery to realign the weak muscles as prescribed if nonsurgical interventions are unsuccessful.

4. Reinforce instructions to the parents about the need for follow-up visits.

II. Conjunctivitis

A. Description
1. Inflammation of the conjunctiva; frequently known as pinkeye
2. May be caused by allergy, infection, or trauma
3. Bacterial or viral conjunctivitis is extremely contagious.

B. Data collection
1. Itching, burning, or scratchy eyelids
2. Redness of the conjunctiva and sclera
3. Edema
4. Redness

⚠ Chlamydial conjunctivitis is rare among older children; if diagnosed in a child who is not sexually active, he or she needs to be assessed for possible sexual abuse.

C. Interventions
1. Viral Conjunctivitis
   a. The infection will usually resolve in 7 to 14 days; in some cases it can take 2 to 3 weeks or more to resolve.
   b. Antiviral medications may be prescribed to treat more serious forms of conjunctivitis, such as those caused by herpes simplex virus or varicella zoster virus; antibiotics are not effective against viruses.
2. Bacterial conjunctivitis
   a. Mild cases may improve without antibiotic treatment.
   b. An antibiotic, usually prescribed topically as eye drops or ointment, may be prescribed to shorten the length of infection, reduce complications, and reduce the spread to others.
3. Allergic conjunctivitis
   a. Removing the allergen from the environment often improves the condition.

b. Allergy medication and eye drops such as topical antihistamine and vasoconstrictors may be prescribed.

4. General Interventions

   a. The primary health care provider (PHCP) needs to be consulted regarding going to school and contact with others.

   b. Instruct the child and parents about the administration of prescribed medications.

   c. Instruct in infection control measures such as good hand washing and not sharing towels and washcloths.

   d. Instruct the child to avoid rubbing the eyes to prevent injury.

   e. Instruct a child who is wearing contact lenses to discontinue wearing them and to obtain new lenses to eliminate the chance of reinfection that can occur from the use of old lenses.

   f. Instruct an adolescent that eye makeup needs to be discarded and replaced.

   g. For additional information, refer to Centers for Disease Control and Prevention at https://www.CDC.gov/conjunctivitis/index.html.

III. Otitis Media

A. Description

   1. Otitis media is an inflammatory disorder usually caused by an infection of the middle ear occurring as a result of a blocked Eustachian tube, which prevents normal drainage; can be acute or chronic.

   2. Otitis media is a common complication of an acute respiratory infection (most commonly from respiratory syncytial virus [RSV] or influenza).

   3. Infants and children have Eustachian tubes that are shorter, wider, and straighter, which makes them more prone to otitis media.

B. Prevention

   1. Feed infants in upright position to prevent reflux.

   2. Maintain routine immunizations.

   3. Encourage breast-feeding for at least the first 6 months of age.

   4. Avoid exposure to tobacco smoke and allergens.

C. Data collection

   1. Fever

   2. Acute onset of ear pain

   3. Crying, irritability, lethargy

   4. Loss of appetite

   5. Rolling of head from side to side

   6. Pulling on or rubbing the ear

   7. Purulent ear drainage may be present

   8. Red, opaque, bulging, immobile tympanic membrane on otoscopic examination

   9. Signs of hearing loss (indicative of chronic otitis media)

D. Interventions

   1. Encourage fluid intake (may be difficult if the child is in pain).

2. Reinforce instructions to the child to avoid chewing as much as possible during the acute period because chewing increases pain.

3. Provide local heat or cold as prescribed to relieve discomfort and have the child lie with the affected ear down.

4. Reinforce instructions to parents with regard to the appropriate procedure to clean drainage from the external ear canal with sterile swabs or gauze; frequent cleansing and the application of moisture barriers may be prescribed to prevent ear excoriation from the drainage.

5. Reinforce instructions to parents about the administration of analgesics or antipyretics such as acetaminophen or ibuprofen as prescribed to decrease fever and pain.

6. Reinforce instructions to parents about the administration of antibiotics if prescribed, emphasizing that the prescribed period of administration is necessary to eliminate infective organisms.

7. In healthy infants over 6 months and children, careful use of antibiotics is recommended because of concerns about drug-resistant *Streptococcus pneumoniae*; usually, waiting up to 72 hours for spontaneous resolution is a safe and appropriate management of acute otitis media.

8. Reinforce instructions to parents that screening for hearing loss may be necessary.

9. Reinforce instructions to parents about the procedure for administering ear medications such as topical pain relief drops if prescribed.

E. Otitis Externa

   1. Description

      a. Inflammation of the external auditory canal, which can occur with or without infection

      b. Also known as "swimmer's ear"

   2. Data Collection

      a. Rapid onset of symptoms within 48 hours; symptoms include otalgia, pruritus, fullness, drainage, and impaired hearing.

      b. A low-grade fever may be present.

      c. Tenderness on manipulation of the pinna and tragus is noted on physical exam.

      d. May have regional lymphadenopathy

   3. Interventions: Treatment is indicated with topical antibiotics and may include neomycin with or without polymyxin B or fluoroquinolone preparation.

⚠ To administer ear medications in a child younger than age 3, pull the ear lobe down and back. In a child older than 3 years, pull the pinna up and back.

F. Myringotomy

   1. Description

      a. A surgical incision into the tympanic membrane to provide drainage of the purulent middle ear fluid; may be done by a laser-assisted procedure

b. Insertion of tympanoplasty tubes into the middle ear may be done to allow continued drainage and to equalize pressure and allow ventilation of the middle ear.

2. Postoperative interventions

a. Reinforce instructions to parents and child to keep the ears dry.

b. The child would wear earplugs while bathing, shampooing, and swimming (diving and submerging under water are not allowed).

c. Parents can administer an analgesic such as acetaminophen or ibuprofen as prescribed to relieve discomfort following insertion of tympanoplasty tubes.

d. Parents would be taught that the child should not blow his or her nose for 7 to 10 days after surgery.

e. Reinforce instructions to parents that if the tubes fall out, it is not an emergency, but the PHCP needs to be notified; inform the parents of the appearance of the tubes (tiny, white, spool-shaped tubes).

IV. Tonsillitis and Adenoiditis

A. Description

1. *Tonsillitis* refers to inflammation and infection of the tonsils, which is lymphoid tissue located in the pharynx (Fig. 32.1).

2. *Adenoiditis* refers to inflammation and infection of the adenoids (pharyngeal tonsils), located on the posterior wall of the nasopharynx.

3. Enlarged tonsils and adenoids may lead to an obstructive sleep apnea in children, manifested by snoring and periods of sudden waking and fragmented sleep; a polysomnography and referral to ear, nose, and throat specialist may be needed.

4. Can be the result of a viral, bacterial, or fungal infection. Group A streptococcus ("strep throat") is a common bacterial infection of the oropharynx, particularly in children, which can result in streptococcal toxic shock syndrome. Mononucleosis is another possible cause of tonsillitis and adenoiditis.

5. Tonsillectomy (surgical removal of the tonsils) and adenoidectomy (surgical removal of the adenoids) may be necessary depending on the number of infections per year as well as signs of obstructive respiratory disturbance.

B. Data collection

1. Persistent or recurrent sore throat

2. Enlarged bright red tonsils that may be covered with white exudate

3. Difficulty swallowing

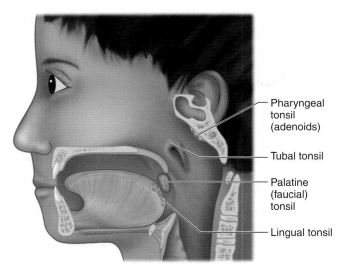

FIGURE 32.1 Location of various tonsillar masses.

Pharyngeal tonsil (adenoids)
Tubal tonsil
Palatine (faucial) tonsil
Lingual tonsil

4. Mouth breathing and an unpleasant mouth odor

5. Fever

6. Cough

7. Enlarged adenoids may cause a nasal quality of speech, mouth breathing, hearing difficulty, snoring, or obstructive sleep apnea.

C. Interventions preoperatively

1. Monitor for signs of active infection.

2. Monitor bleeding and clotting studies, because the throat is very vascular.

3. Prepare the child for a sore throat postoperatively and inform him or her that they will need to drink liquids.

4. Check for any loose teeth to decrease the risk of aspiration during surgery.

D. Interventions postoperatively

1. Position the child prone or side-lying to facilitate drainage.

2. Have suction equipment available, but do not suction unless there is an airway obstruction.

3. Monitor for signs of bleeding (frequent swallowing may indicate bleeding). If bleeding occurs, turn the child to the side and notify the registered nurse (RN) immediately.

4. Discourage coughing, clearing of the throat, or nose blowing to prevent bleeding.

5. Provide an ice collar or analgesics (rectally or intravenously) for discomfort, as prescribed.

6. Administer antiemetics, as prescribed, to prevent vomiting.

7. Provide clear, cool, non-citrus, and noncarbonated fluids (crushed ice, ice pops).

8. Avoid red, purple, or brown liquids, which will simulate the appearance of blood if the child vomits.

9. Avoid milk products such as milk, ice cream, and pudding initially, because they will coat the throat, causing the child to clear the throat.

10. Soft foods may be prescribed 1 to 2 days postoperatively.

11. Do not give the child any straws, forks, or sharp objects that can be put into the mouth.

12. Mouth odor, slight ear pain, and a low-grade fever may occur for a few days postoperatively, but the parents would be instructed to notify the PHCP if bleeding, a persistent earache, or fever occurs.

13. Reinforce instructions to the parents to keep the child away from crowds until healing has occurred; usually the child is able to resume normal activities after 1 to 2 weeks postoperatively.

14. Reinforce instructions to the parents to monitor the child for postoperative bleeding both within the first 24 hours and again 7 to 10 days after surgery.

V. Epistaxis (Nosebleeds)

A. Description

   1. The nose, especially the septum, is a highly vascular structure, and bleeding usually results from direct trauma, foreign bodies, nose picking, and mucosal inflammation.

   2. Recurrent epistaxis and severe bleeding may indicate underlying disease.

B. Interventions

   1. See Priority Nursing Actions.

   2. If bleeding cannot be controlled, packing or cauterization of the bleeding vessel may be prescribed.

⚡ PRIORITY NURSING ACTIONS

Nosebleed in a Child

1. Remain calm and keep the child calm and quiet.
2. Have the child sit up and lean forward (not lying down).
3. Apply continuous pressure to the nose with the thumb and forefinger for at least 10 minutes.
4. Insert cotton or wadded tissue into each nostril and apply ice or a cold cloth to the bridge of the nose if bleeding persists.

VI. Epiglottitis

A. Description

   1. A bacterial form of croup

   2. An inflammation of the epiglottis occurs, which may be caused by *Haemophilus influenzae* type B or *Streptococcus pneumonia*; children immunized with *H. influenza* type b (Hib vaccine) are at less risk for epiglottitis.

   3. Occurs most frequently among children who are 2 to 8 years of age, but can occur from infancy to adulthood

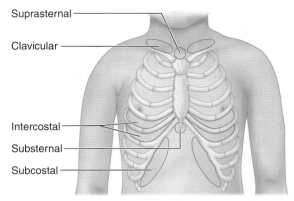

Suprasternal —
Clavicular —
Intercostal —
Substernal —
Subcostal —

FIGURE 32.2 Location of retractions.

   4. Onset is abrupt; occurs most often in the winter.

   5. Considered an emergency situation because it can progress rapidly to severe respiratory distress

B. Data collection

   1. High fever

   2. Sore, red, and inflamed throat (large, cherry red, edematous epiglottis) and pain during swallowing

   3. Absence of spontaneous cough

   4. Dysphonia (muffled voice), dysphagia, dyspnea, and drooling

   5. Agitation

   6. Retractions and the child struggles to breathe (Fig. 32.2)

   7. Inspiratory stridor aggravated by the supine position

   8. Tachycardia

   9. Tachypnea progressing to more severe respiratory distress (hypoxia, hypercapnia, respiratory acidosis, decreased level of consciousness)

  10. Tripod positioning: while supporting the body with the hands, the child leans forward, thrusts the chin forward, and opens the mouth in an attempt to widen the airway.

  11. A fiberoptic nasal laryngectomy may be necessary to assist in diagnosis.

C. Interventions

   1. Maintain a patent airway.

   2. Monitor respiratory status and breath sounds, noting nasal flaring, the use of accessory muscles, retractions, and the presence of stridor.

   3. Do not measure the temperature by the oral route.

   4. Monitor pulse oximetry.

   5. Prepare the child for lateral neck films to confirm the diagnosis (accompany the child to the radiology department).

   6. Maintain an NPO (nothing by mouth) status.

   7. Do not leave the child unattended.

   8. Avoid placing the child in a supine position because this position will further affect the respiratory status.

9. Do not restrain the child or take any other measure that may agitate the child.

10. Assist to administer intravenous (IV) fluids as prescribed; insertion of an IV may need to be delayed until an adequate airway is established because this procedure may agitate the child.

11. IV antibiotics may be prescribed; these are usually followed by oral antibiotics (blood cultures may be necessary to identify the organism).

12. Administer analgesics and antipyretics (acetaminophen or ibuprofen) to reduce fever and throat pain as prescribed.

13. Administer corticosteroids to decrease inflammation and reduce throat edema as prescribed.

14. Heliox (mixture of helium and oxygen) may be prescribed; this medication reduces the work of breathing, reduces airway turbulence, and helps relieve airway obstruction.

15. Medications that promote mucosal vasoconstriction and reduce edema may be prescribed.

16. Provide cool-mist oxygen therapy as prescribed; high humidification cools the airway and decreases swelling.

17. Have resuscitation equipment available and prepare for endotracheal intubation or tracheotomy for severe respiratory distress.

18. Ensure that the child is up to date with immunizations, including Hib conjugate vaccine. (See Chapter 37)

⚠ If epiglottitis is suspected, no attempts would be made to visualize the posterior pharynx, obtain a throat culture, or take an oral temperature. Otherwise, spasm of the epiglottis can occur, leading to complete airway occlusion.

VII. Laryngotracheobronchitis (Croup)

A. Description

  1. Inflammation of the larynx, trachea, and bronchi

  2. Most common type of croup; may be viral or bacterial and most frequently occurs in children younger than 5 years

  3. Common causative organisms include parainfluenzae virus types 2 and 3, RSV, *Mycoplasma pneumoniae*, and influenza A and B.

  4. Characterized by gradual onset that may be preceded by an upper respiratory infection

 B. Data collection (Box 32.1)

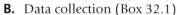 **C.** Interventions

  1. Maintain a patent airway.

  2. Monitor the respiratory status and pulse oximetry; check for nasal flaring, sternal retraction, and inspiratory stridor (see Fig. 32.2).

  3. Monitor for adequate respiratory exchange; monitor for pallor or cyanosis.

BOX 32.1 Progression of Symptoms in Laryngotracheobronchitis

Stage I
- Low-grade fever
- Hoarseness
- Seal bark and brassy cough (croup cough)
- Inspiratory stridor
- Fear
- Irritability and restlessness

Stage II
- Continuous respiratory stridor
- Retractions
- Use of accessory muscles
- Crackles and wheezing
- Labored respirations

Stage III
- Continued restlessness
- Anxiety
- Pallor
- Diaphoresis
- Tachypnea
- Signs of anoxia and hypercapnia

Stage IV
- Intermittent cyanosis that progresses to consistent cyanosis
- Apneic episodes that progress to cessation of breathing

Adapted from Perry S, Hockenberry M, Lowdermilk D, Wilson D: *Maternal child nursing care*, ed 4, St. Louis, 2010, Mosby.

4. Elevate the head of the bed and provide rest.

5. Provide humidified oxygen via a cool-mist tent for the hospitalized child (Table 32.1).

6. Reinforce instructions to the parents to use a cool-air vaporizer or humidifier at home. Other measures include having the child breathe in the cool night air or the air from an open freezer and taking the child to a cool basement or garage.

7. Provide and encourage fluid intake. IV fluids may be prescribed to maintain hydration status if the child is unable to take oral fluids.

8. Administer analgesics as prescribed to reduce fever.

9. Reinforce teaching the parents to avoid administering cough syrups and cold medicines, which may dry and thicken secretions.

10. Assist to administer corticosteroids, if prescribed, to reduce inflammation and edema.

11. Assist to administer antibiotics, as prescribed, noting that they are not indicated unless a bacterial infection is present.

12. Heliox (mixture of helium and oxygen) may be prescribed; this medication reduces the work of breathing, reduces airway turbulence, and helps to relieve airway obstruction.

TABLE 32.1 Advantages and Disadvantages of Various Oxygen-Delivery Systems.

Systems	Advantages	Disadvantages
Oxygen mask	Various sizes available Delivers higher O_2 concentration than cannula Able to provide a predictable concentration of oxygen if Venturi mask is used, whether child breathes through nose or mouth	Skin irritation Fear of suffocation Accumulation of moisture on face Possibility of aspiration of vomitus Difficulty with controlling O_2 concentrations (except with Venturi mask)
Nasal cannula	Provides low to moderate O_2 concentration (22%–40%) Child is able to eat and talk while receiving O_2 Possibility of more complete observation of child because nose and mouth remain unobstructed	Must have patent nasal passages May cause abdominal distention, discomfort, or vomiting Difficulty controlling O_2 concentration if child breathes through mouth Inability to provide mist, if desired
Oxygen tent	Provides lower O_2 concentrations (FIO_2 up to 0.3–0.5) Child is able to receive desired inspired O_2 concentrations, even while eating	Necessity for tight fit around bed to prevent leakage of oxygen Cool and wet tent environment Poor access to child; inspired O_2 levels fall when the tent is entered
Oxygen hood, face tent	Provides high O_2 concentrations (FIO_2 up to 1.00) Free access to child's chest for assessment	High-humidity environment Need to remove child for feeding and care

FIO$_2$, Fraction of inspired oxygen; *O$_2$*, oxygen.
Data from Hockenberry M, Wilson D: *Wong's nursing care of infants and children*, ed 9, St. Louis, 2013, Mosby.

13. Have resuscitation equipment available.
14. Provide appropriate reassurance and education to the parents or caregivers.

⚠ Isolation precautions need to be implemented for a hospitalized child with an upper respiratory infection until the cause of the infection is known.

VIII. Bronchitis

A. Description
1. Inflammation of the trachea and bronchi; may be referred to as *tracheobronchitis*
2. Usually occurs in association with an upper respiratory infection
3. Is usually a mild disorder; causative agent is most often viral.

B. Data collection
1. Fever
2. Dry, hacking, and nonproductive cough that is worse at night and becomes productive in 2 to 3 days

C. Interventions

1. Treat the symptoms as necessary.
2. Monitor for respiratory distress.
3. Provide cool, humidified air for the child.
4. Encourage increased fluid intake; child may drink beverages that he or she likes as long as respiratory status is stable.
5. Administer antipyretics for fever as prescribed.
6. Cough suppressant may be prescribed to promote rest but are used cautiously because they dry secretions.

IX. Bronchiolitis and Respiratory Syncytial Virus (RSV)

A. Description
1. An inflammation of the bronchioles that causes a thick production of mucus, which occludes the bronchiole tubes and the small bronchi

2. RSV is an acute viral infection and a common cause of bronchiolitis (other organisms that cause bronchiolitis include adenoviruses, parainfluenza viruses, and human metapneumovirus).

3. RSV is highly communicable and is usually transferred via droplets or by direct contact with respiratory secretions.
4. RSV occurs primarily in the fall, winter, and spring.
5. RSV is rarer in children older than 2 years, with a peak incidence at approximately 6 months of age.
6. At-risk children include children who have a chronic or disabling condition and those who are immunocompromised.
7. Identification of the virus is done via testing of nasal or nasopharyngeal secretions.
8. Prevention measures include encouraging breastfeeding, avoiding tobacco smoke exposure, and using good hand-washing technique.
9. Administering palivizumab, a monoclonal antibody, to high-risk infants; see American Academy of Pediatrics for further information about palivizumab at http://www.aappublications.org/news/2017/10/19/RSV101917.

B. Data collection (Box 32.2)
C. Interventions

1. For the child with bronchiolitis, interventions are aimed at treating symptoms and include airway maintenance, cool humidified air and oxygen, adequate fluid intake, and medications.
2. For a hospitalized child with RSV, place the child in a single room.
3. Ensure that nurses caring for the child with RSV do not care for other high-risk children.
4. Use standard precautions during care including contact and droplet precautions; using good hand-washing techniques is necessary.

BOX 32.2 Data Collection: Respiratory Syncytial Virus

Initial Manifestations
- Rhinorrhea
- Eye or ear drainage
- Pharyngitis
- Coughing
- Sneezing
- Wheezing
- Intermittent fever

Manifestations as the Disease Progresses
- Increased coughing and wheezing
- Signs of air hunger
- Tachypnea and retractions
- Periods of cyanosis

Manifestations in Severe Illness
- Tachypnea greater than 70 breaths per minute
- Decreased breath sounds and poor air exchange
- Listlessness
- Apneic episodes

Adapted from Perry S, Hockenberry M, Lowdermilk D, Wilson D: *Maternal child nursing care*, ed 4, St. Louis, 2010, Mosby.

---

5. Monitor airway status and maintain a patent airway.
6. For most effective airway maintenance, position the child at a 30- to 40-degree angle with the neck slightly extended to maintain an open airway and decrease pressure on the diaphragm.
7. Provide cool, humidified oxygen as prescribed.
8. Monitor pulse oximetry levels.
9. Encourage fluids; IV fluids may be necessary until the acute stage has passed.
10. Periodic suctioning may be necessary if nasal secretions are copious; use of a bulb syringe for suctioning may be effective and would be done before feeding to promote comfort and adequate intake.
11. Antiviral medication may be prescribed.

⚠ Cough suppressants are administered with caution because they can dry secretions and interfere with the clearance of respiratory secretions.

X. Pneumonia

A. Description
1. Inflammation of the pulmonary parenchyma and/ or alveoli caused by a virus, mycoplasmal agents, bacteria, or aspiration of foreign substances
2. The causative agent is usually introduced into the lungs through inhalation or from the bloodstream.
3. Viral pneumonia occurs more frequently than bacterial pneumonia, is seen in children of all ages, and is often associated with a viral upper respiratory infection.
4. Primary atypical pneumonia, usually caused by *Mycoplasma pneumoniae* or *Chlamydia pneumoniae*,

occurs most often in the fall and winter months and is more common in crowded living conditions; most often seen in children between the ages of 5 and 12 years.
5. Bacterial pneumonia is often a serious infection requiring hospitalization when pleural effusion or empyema accompanies the disease; hospitalization is also necessary for children with staphylococcal pneumonia (*Streptococcus pneumoniae* is a common cause).
6. Aspiration pneumonia occurs when food, secretions, liquids, or other materials enter the lung and cause inflammation and a chemical pneumonitis. Classic symptoms include an increasing cough or fever with foul-smelling sputum, deteriorating results as seen by chest x-ray films, and other signs of airway involvement.
7. Prevention of viral and bacterial pneumonia includes immunization of infants and children with the pneumococcal vaccine. (See Chapter 37)

B. Viral pneumonia
1. Data collection
   a. Acute or insidious onset
   b. Mild fever, slight cough, and malaise to high fever, severe cough, and diaphoresis
   c. Nonproductive or productive cough of small amounts of whitish sputum
   d. Wheezes or fine crackles
2. Interventions
   a. Treatment is symptomatic.
   b. Administer oxygen with cool humidified air as prescribed.
   c. Increase fluid intake.
   d. Administer antipyretics for fever as prescribed.
   e. Administer chest physiotherapy and postural drainage as prescribed.

C. Primary atypical pneumonia
1. Data collection
   a. Acute or insidious onset
   b. Fever, chills, anorexia, headache, malaise, and muscle pain
   c. Rhinitis, sore throat, and dry, hacking cough
   d. Cough is nonproductive initially and then produces seromucoid sputum, which becomes mucopurulent or blood streaked.
2. Interventions:
   a. Treatment is symptomatic.
   b. Recovery generally occurs in 7 to 10 days.

D. Bacterial pneumonia
1. Data collection
   a. Infant: Acute onset, irritability, lethargy, poor feeding, abrupt fever (may be accompanied by seizure), and respiratory distress (air hunger, tachypnea, and circumoral cyanosis)
   b. Older child: Headache, chills, abdominal pain, chest pain, and meningeal symptoms (meningism)
   c. Hacking, nonproductive cough

d. Diminished breath sounds or scattered crackles

e. With consolidation, decreased breath sounds are more pronounced.

f. As the infection resolves, the cough becomes productive and the child expectorates purulent sputum; coarse crackles and wheezing are noted.

2. Interventions

a. Blood cultures are taken and antibiotic therapy is initiated as soon as the diagnosis is suspected; in a hospitalized infant or child, IV antibiotics are usually prescribed.

b. Administer oxygen for respiratory distress as prescribed, and monitor oxygen saturation via pulse oximetry.

c. Place the child in a cool mist tent as prescribed; cool humidification moistens the airways and assists in temperature reduction.

d. Suction mucus from the infant, using a bulb syringe to maintain a patent airway if the infant is unable to handle secretions.

e. Administer chest physiotherapy and postural drainage every 4 hours as prescribed.

f. Promote bed rest to conserve energy.

g. Encourage the child to lie on the affected side (if pneumonia is unilateral) to splint the chest and reduce the discomfort caused by pleural rubbing.

h. Encourage fluid intake (administer cautiously to prevent aspiration); intravenously administered fluids may be necessary.

i. Administer antipyretics for fever and bronchodilators as prescribed.

j. Monitor temperature frequently because of the risk for febrile seizures.

k. Institute isolation precautions with pneumococcal or staphylococcal pneumonia (according to agency policy).

l. Cough suppressant may be prescribed before rest times and meals if the cough is disturbing (administered with caution because they can interfere with the clearance of respiratory secretions).

m. Continuous closed-chest drainage may be necessary if purulent fluid is present (usually noted in *Staphylococcus* infections).

n. Fluid accumulation in the pleural cavity may be removed by thoracentesis; thoracentesis also provides a means for obtaining fluid for culture and for instilling antibiotics directly into the pleural cavity.

⚠ Children with a respiratory disorder would be monitored for weight loss and for signs of dehydration. Signs of dehydration include a sunken fontanel (infants), nonelastic skin turgor, decreased and concentrated urinary output, dry mucous membranes, and decreased tear production.

BOX 32.3	Laboratory Tests to Assist with the Diagnosis of Asthma

- *Pulmonary function tests (PFTs):* Spirometry testing assesses the presence and degree of disease and can determine the response to treatment.
- *Peak expiratory flow rate (PEFR) measurement:* Measures the maximum flow of air that can be forcefully exhaled in 1 second; the child uses a peak expiratory flow meter (PEFM) to determine a "personal best value" that can be used for comparison at other times, such as during and after an asthma attack.
- *Bronchoprovocation testing:* Testing done to identify inhaled allergens; the mucous membranes are directly exposed to the suspected allergen in increasing amounts.
- *Skin testing:* Done to identify specific allergens.
- *Exercise challenges:* Exercise is used to identify the occurrence of exercise-induced bronchospasm.
- *Radioallergosorbent test (RAST):* A blood test used to identify a specific allergen.
- *Chest radiograph:* May show hyperexpansion of the airways.

Note: Some tests place the child at risk for an asthma attack; therefore, testing would be done under close supervision.

XI. Asthma

A. Description

1. Asthma is a chronic inflammatory disease of the airways.

2. Asthma is classified on the basis of disease severity; management includes medications, environmental control of allergens, and child/family education.

3. The allergic reaction in the airways caused by the precipitant can result in an immediate reaction with obstruction occurring, and it can result in a late bronchial obstructive reaction several hours after the initial exposure to the precipitant.

4. Mast cell release of histamine leads to a bronchoconstrictive process, bronchospasm, and obstruction.

5. Diagnosis is made on the basis of the child's symptoms, history and physical examination, chest radiograph, and laboratory tests (Box 32.3). See Table 32.2 for a classification system for asthma severity.

6. Precipitants triggering an asthma attack (Box 32.4)

7. Status asthmaticus refers to an acute asthma attack; the child displays respiratory distress despite vigorous treatment measures; this is a medical emergency that can result in respiratory failure and death if not treated.

B. Data collection

1. Child has episodes of dyspnea, wheezing, breathlessness, chest tightness, and cough, particularly at night and/or in the early morning.

TABLE 32.2   **Asthma Severity Classification System.**

Severity	Characteristics	Treatment
Mild intermittent	Intermittent symptoms less than once per week Nighttime symptoms less than twice a month Asymptomatic and normal between exacerbations FEV1 > 80% predicted, PFT > 20% variability	Inhaled SABA or cromolyn before exercise or allergen exposure No daily medications needed
Mild persistent	Symptoms more than 2 times/week but less than once/day May affect activity and sleep Nighttime symptoms more than twice a month FEV1 > 80% predicted, PFT 20%–30% variability	One daily controlled medication, low-dose inhaled corticosteroid; cromolyn/nedocromil, leukotriene modifiers Inhaled SABA as needed
Moderate persistent	Daily symptoms, but not continual, nighttime symptoms more than once a week but not every night Affect activity and sleep Daily use of SABA FEV1 60%–80% predicted, PFT >30% variability	Daily controller medications; combined inhaled medium-dose corticosteroid and LABA, especially for nighttime symptoms, cromolyn/nedocromil, leukotriene modifiers Inhaled SABA as needed
Severe persistent	Continuous daily symptoms Frequent nighttime symptoms Frequent exacerbations Physical activity limited by asthma FEV1 less than or equal to 60% predicted, PFT variability >30%	Inhaled SABA as needed Multiple daily controller medications, high-dose inhaled corticosteroid, LABA, cromolyn/nedocromil, leukotriene modifiers, may need long-term corticosteroids

FEV1, Forced expiratory volume in 1 second; *LABA,* long-acting beta-adrenergic agonists; *PFT,* pulmonary function test; *SABA,* short-acting beta adrenergic.
Adapted from National Asthma Education and Prevention Program (NAEPP). Expert Panel 3 Summary Report 2007: Guidelines for the Diagnosis and Management of Asthma. NIH publication no. 08-5846. U.S. Department of Health & Human Services, Public Health Service, National Institutes of Health (NIH), National Heart, Lung, and Blood Institute (NHLBI), Bethesda, MD.

2. Acute asthma attacks

  a. Episodes of progressively worsening shortness of breath, cough, wheezing, chest tightness, decrease in expiratory airflow secondary to bronchospasm, mucosal edema, and mucus plugging; air is trapped behind occluded or narrow airways and hypoxemia can occur.

  b. The attack begins with irritability, restlessness, headache, feeling tired, and/or chest tightness; just before the attack, the child may present with itching localized at the front of the neck or over the upper part of the back.

  c. Respiratory symptoms include a hacking, irritable, nonproductive cough caused by bronchial edema.

  d. Accumulated secretions stimulate the cough; the cough becomes rattling, and there is production of frothy, clear, gelatinous sputum.

  e. The child experiences retractions.

  f. Hyperresonance on percussion of the chest is noted.

  g. Breath sounds are coarse and loud, with crackles, coarse rhonchi, and inspiratory and expiratory wheezing; expiration is prolonged.

  h. Child may be pale or flushed, and the lips may have a deep, dark red color that may progress to cyanosis (also observed in the nail beds and skin, especially around the mouth).

  i. Restlessness, apprehension, and diaphoresis occur.

  j. Child speaks in short, broken phrases.

  k. Younger children assume the tripod sitting position; older children sit upright, with the shoulders in a hunched-over position, the hands on the bed or a chair, and the arms braced to facilitate the use of the accessory muscles of breathing (child refuses to lie down).

  l. Exercise-induced attack: A cough, shortness of breath, chest pain or tightness, wheezing, and endurance problems occur during exercise.

  m. Severe spasm or obstruction: Breath sounds and wheezing cannot be heard (silent chest), and the cough is ineffective (represents a lack of air movement).

  n. Ventilatory failure and asphyxia: Shortness of breath, with air movement in the chest restricted to the point of absent breath sounds is noted; this is accompanied by a sudden rise in the respiratory rate.

C. Interventions: Acute episode (see Priority Nursing Actions)

⚡ **PRIORITY NURSING ACTIONS**

Acute Asthma Attack

1. Check airway patency and respiratory status.
2. Assist to administer humidified oxygen by nasal cannula or face mask.
3. Assist to administer quick-relief (rescue) medications.
4. Assist to initiate an intravenous (IV) line.
5. Prepare the child for a chest radiograph if prescribed.
6. Prepare to obtain a blood sample for determining arterial blood gas levels, if prescribed.

BOX 32.4	Examples of Precipitants Triggering an Asthma Attack

Allergens
Outdoor: Trees, shrubs, weeds, grasses, molds, pollen, air pollution, sand dust, spores
Indoor: Dust, dust mites, mold, cockroach antigen

Irritants
Tobacco smoke, wood smoke, odors, sprays
Exposure to occupational irritants
Exercise
Cold air
Changes in weather or temperature

Environmental Change
Moving to a new home, starting a new school
Colds and infections

Animals
Cats, dogs, rodents, horses

Medications
Aspirin, nonsteroidal anti-inflammatory drugs, antibiotics, β-blockers

Strong Emotions
Fear, anger, laughing, crying

Conditions
Gastroesophageal reflux disease, tracheoesophageal fistula

Food Additives
Sulfite preservatives

Foods
Nuts, milk, and other dairy products

Endocrine Factors
Menses, pregnancy, thyroid disease

Data from Perry S, Hockenberry M, Lowdermilk D, Wilson D: *Maternal child nursing care*, ed 4, St. Louis, 2010, Mosby.

BOX 32.5	Quick-Relief (Rescue) Medications

Short-acting β₂-agonists (for bronchodilation)
Anticholinergics (for the relief of acute bronchospasm)
Systemic corticosteroids (for their anti-inflammatory action to treat reversible airflow obstruction)

 D. Medications
  1. Quick-relief (rescue medications): Used to treat symptoms and exacerbations (Box 32.5)
  2. Long-term control (preventer medications): Used to achieve and maintain control of inflammation (Box 32.6)
  3. Nebulizer, metered-dose inhaler (MDI): May be used to administer medications; if the child has difficulty using the MDI, medication can be administered by nebulization (medication is mixed with saline and then nebulized with compressed air by a machine).

BOX 32.6	Long-Term Control (Medications to Prevent Attacks)

Inhaled corticosteroids (for anti-inflammatory action)
Antiallergy medications (to prevent an adverse response upon exposure to an allergen)
Nonsteroidal anti-inflammatory drugs (for anti-inflammatory action)
Long-acting β₂ agonists (for long-acting bronchodilation)
Leukotriene modifiers (to prevent bronchospasm and inflammatory cell infiltration)
Monoclonal antibody (blocks the binding of immunoglobulin E [IgE] to mast cells to inhibit inflammation)

---

  4. If the MDI is used to administer a corticosteroid, a spacer would be used to prevent yeast infections in the child's mouth.
  5. The child's growth patterns need to be monitored when corticosteroids are prescribed.
E. Chest physiotherapy
  1. Includes breathing exercises and physical training
  2. Chest physiotherapy will strengthen the respiratory musculature and produce more efficient breathing patterns.
  3. Chest physiotherapy is not recommended during an acute exacerbation.
F. Allergen control
  1. Testing may be done to identify allergens.
  2. Reinforce teaching the child and parents about measures to prevent and reduce exposure to allergens (see Box 32.4).
G. Homecare measures
  1. Reinforce instructions to the family in measures to eliminate environmental allergens.
  2. Avoid extremes of environmental temperature; in cold temperatures, instruct the child to breathe through the nose, not the mouth, and to cover the nose and mouth with a scarf.
  3. Avoid exposure to individuals with a respiratory infection.
  4. Reinforce instructions to the child and family with regard to recognizing early symptoms of an asthma attack.
  5. Reinforce instructions to the child and family about medications.
  6. Reinforce instructions to the child and family how to use a nebulizer, MDI, or peak expiratory flowmeter (PEF). The PEF measures how fast air comes out of the lungs after exhaling forcefully following a full inhalation.
  7. Reinforce instructions to the child and family about the importance of home monitoring of the peak expiratory flow rate; a decrease in the expiratory flow rate may indicate impending infection or exacerbation.

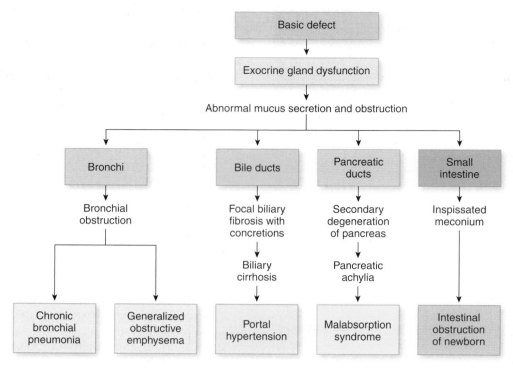

FIGURE 32.3 Various effects of exocrine gland dysfunction in cystic fibrosis.

8. Reinforce instructions to the child in the cleaning of devices used for inhaled medications (yeast infections can occur with the use of aerosolized corticosteroids).
9. Encourage adequate rest, sleep, and a well-balanced diet.
10. Reinforce instructions to the child in the importance of adequate fluid intake to liquefy secretions.
11. Assist in developing an exercise program.
12. Reinforce instructions to the child in the procedure for respiratory treatments and exercises as prescribed.
13. Encourage the child to cough effectively.
14. Encourage the parents to keep immunizations up to date; annual influenza vaccinations are recommended for children 6 months of age and older.
15. Inform other healthcare providers and school personnel of the asthma condition.
16. Allow the child to take control of self-care measures based on age appropriateness.

XII. Cystic Fibrosis (CF) (Fig. 32.3)

A. Description
1. A chronic multisystem disorder and autosomal-recessive trait disorder that is characterized by exocrine gland dysfunction
2. The mucus produced by the exocrine glands is abnormally thick and copious, which causes obstruction of the small passageways of the affected organs, particularly in the respiratory, gastrointestinal, and reproductive systems.

BOX 32.7 Quantitative Sweat Chloride Test

- The production of sweat is stimulated (pilocarpine iontophoresis), the sweat is collected, and the sweat electrolytes are measured (75 mg of sweat is needed).
- Normally, the sweat chloride concentration is lower than 40 mEq/L.
- A chloride concentration higher than 60 mEq/L is a positive test result (higher than 40 mEq/L is diagnostic in infants younger than 3 months of age).
- Chloride concentrations between 40 and 60 mEq/L are highly suggestive of cystic fibrosis and require a repeat test.

---

3. Common symptoms are associated with pancreatic enzyme deficiency and pancreatic fibrosis, caused by duct blockage, progressive chronic lung disease as a result of infection, and sweat gland dysfunction, resulting in increased sodium and chloride sweat concentrations.
4. An increase in sodium and chloride in sweat and saliva forms the basis for one diagnostic test, the sweat chloride test (Box 32.7).
5. CF is a progressive and incurable disorder, and respiratory failure is a common cause of death; organ transplantation may be an option to increase survival rate.

B. Respiratory system
1. Symptoms are produced by the stagnation of mucus in the airway, which leads to bacterial colonization and the destruction of lung tissue.

2. Emphysema and atelectasis occur as the airways become increasingly obstructed.

3. Chronic hypoxemia causes the contraction and hypertrophy of the muscle fibers in the pulmonary arteries and arterioles, thus leading to pulmonary hypertension and eventual cor pulmonale.

4. Pneumothorax from ruptured bullae and hemoptysis from the erosion of the bronchial wall occur as the disease progresses.

5. Other respiratory symptoms
   a. Wheezing and cough
   b. Dyspnea
   c. Cyanosis
   d. Clubbing of the fingers and toes
   e. Barrel chest
   f. Repeated episodes of bronchitis and pneumonia

C. Gastrointestinal system
   1. Meconium ileus in the newborn is the earliest manifestation.
   2. Intestinal obstruction (distal intestinal obstructive syndrome) caused by thick intestinal secretions. Signs include pain, abdominal distention, nausea, and vomiting.
   3. Steatorrhea (frothy, foul-smelling stools)
   4. Deficiency of the fat-soluble vitamins A, D, E, and K, which causes easy bruising, bleeding, and anemia
   5. Malnutrition and failure to thrive
   6. Hypoalbuminemia from the diminished absorption of protein occurs and results in generalized edema.
   7. Rectal prolapse can result from the large, bulky stools and increased intraabdominal pressure.
   8. Pancreatic fibrosis can occur and places the child at risk for diabetes mellitus.

D. Integumentary system
   1. Abnormally high concentrations of sodium and chloride in the sweat
   2. Parents report that the infant tastes "salty" when kissed.
   3. Dehydration and electrolyte imbalance, especially during hyperthermic conditions

E. Reproductive system
   1. Can delay puberty in females
   2. Fertility can be inhibited by highly viscous cervical secretions, which act as a plug and block sperm entry.
   3. Males are usually sterile (but not impotent) as a result of the blockage of the vas deferens by abnormal secretions or the failure of the normal development of duct structures.

F. Diagnostic tests
   1. Quantitative sweat chloride test is positive (see Box 32.7).
   2. Newborn screening may be done in some states and may consist of immunoreactive trypsino-

gen analysis and direct DNA analysis for mutant genes.
   3. Chest x-ray reveals atelectasis and obstructive emphysema.
   4. Pulmonary function tests provide evidence of abnormal small airway function.
   5. Stool fat and/or enzyme analysis: A 72-hour stool sample is collected to check the fat and/or enzyme (trypsin) content, or both (food intake is recorded during the collection).

G. Interventions: Respiratory system
   1. Goals of treatment include preventing and treating pulmonary infection by improving aeration, removing secretions, and administering antibiotic medications.
   2. Monitor respiratory status, including lung sounds and the presence and characteristics of a cough.
   3. Chest physiotherapy (via percussion and postural drainage) when awakening and in the evening (more frequently during pulmonary infection) needs to be done every day to maintain pulmonary hygiene; it would not be performed before or immediately after a meal.
   4. A Flutter Mucus Clearance Device (a small, handheld plastic pipe with a stainless-steel ball on the inside) facilitates the removal of mucus and may be prescribed; store away from small children because if the device separates, the steel ball poses a choking hazard.
   5. Handheld percussors or a special vest device that provides high-frequency chest wall oscillation may be prescribed to help loosen secretions.
   6. A positive expiratory pressure mask may be prescribed; use of this mask forces secretions to the upper airway for expectoration.
   7. The child needs to be taught the forced expiratory technique (huffing) to mobilize secretions for expectoration.
   8. Bronchodilator medication by aerosol may be prescribed, and the medication opens the bronchi for easier expectoration (administered before the chest physiotherapy when the child has reactive airway disease or is wheezing). Medications that decrease the viscosity of mucus may also be prescribed.
   9. A physical exercise program with the aim of stimulating mucus expectoration and establishing an effective breathing pattern needs to be instituted.
   10. Aerosolized antibiotics may be prescribed, or IV antibiotics may be prescribed and administered at home through a central venous access device.
   11. Oxygen may be prescribed during acute episodes; monitor closely for oxygen narcosis (signs include nausea and vomiting, malaise, fatigue, numbness and tingling of extremities, substernal distress) because the child with CF may have chronic carbon dioxide retention.
   12. Lung transplantation may be an option.

H. Interventions: Gastrointestinal system

1. The child with CF requires a high-calorie, high-protein, and well-balanced diet to meet energy and growth needs; multivitamins and vitamins A, D, E, and K are also administered.
2. Monitor weight and for failure to thrive.
3. Monitor stool patterns and for signs of intestinal obstruction.
4. The goal of treatment for pancreatic insufficiency is to replace pancreatic enzymes; pancreatic enzymes are administered within 30 minutes of eating and administered with all meals and all snacks (not given if the child is NPO).
5. The amount of pancreatic enzymes administered depends on the PHCP's preference and usually is adjusted to achieve normal growth and a decrease in the number of stools to two or three daily (additional enzymes are needed if the child is consuming high-fat foods).
6. Enteric-coated pancreatic enzymes are not to be crushed or chewed; capsules can be taken apart and the contents can be sprinkled on a small amount of food for administration.
7. Monitor for constipation, intestinal obstruction, and rectal prolapse.
8. Monitor for signs of gastroesophageal reflux; place the infant in an upright position after eating, and teach the child to sit upright after eating.

I. Additional interventions

1. Monitor blood glucose level and for signs of diabetes mellitus.
2. Ensure adequate salt intake and fluids that provide an adequate supply of electrolytes during extremely hot weather and when the child has a fever.
3. Monitor bone growth in the child.
4. Monitor for signs of retinopathy or nephropathy.
5. Provide emotional support to the parents, particularly when the child is diagnosed; parents will be fearful and uncertain about the disorder and the care involved.
6. Provide support to the child as he or she transitions through the stages of growth.
7. Reinforce teaching to the child and parents about the care involved and encourage independence in the child to care for self, as it is age-appropriate.

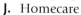

J. Homecare

1. Homecare involves educating the parents and the child about all of the aspects of care for the disorder.
2. Inform the parents and child about the signs of complications, actions to take, and the importance of follow-up as critical.
3. Reinforce instructions to the parents to be sure that the child receives the recommended immunizations on schedule; in addition, annual influ-

enza vaccinations are recommended for children 6 months of age and older.
4. Inform the child and parents about the CF Foundation.

 An alteration in respiratory status can create a frightening experience for both the child and parents. A calm and reassuring nursing approach will assist in reducing fear.

XIII. Sudden Infant Death Syndrome (SIDS)

A. Description

1. SIDS refers to the unexpected death of an apparently healthy infant younger than 1 year for whom an investigation of the death and a thorough autopsy fails to demonstrate an adequate cause of death.
2. Several theories are proposed as to the cause, but the exact cause is unknown.
3. Most frequently occurs during winter months
4. Death usually occurs during sleep periods, but not necessarily at night.
5. Most frequently affects infants from 2 to 3 months of age
6. Incidence is higher in boys.
7. Incidence is higher in Native Americans, African Americans, and Hispanics, and in lower socioeconomic groups.
8. Incidence has been found to be lower in breast-fed infants and infants sleeping with a pacifier.
9. High-risk conditions for SIDS
   a. Prone position
   b. Use of soft bedding or sleeping in a noninfant bed such as a sofa
   c. Overheating (thermal stress)
   d. Cosleeping
   e. Mother who is cigarette smoking or partakes in substance abuse during pregnancy
   f. Exposure to tobacco smoke after birth

B. Data collection

1. Child is apneic, blue, and lifeless.
2. Frothy blood-tinged fluid is in the nose and mouth.
3. Child may be found in any position, but typically is found in a disheveled bed, with blankets over the head, and huddled in a corner.
4. Child may appear to have been clutching bedding.
5. Diaper may be wet and full of stool.

C. Prevention and interventions

1. Infants need to be placed in the supine position for sleep.
2. Mother needs to be taught about the risk factors: cigarette smoking and substance abuse during pregnancy; use of soft bedding; sleeping in a noninfant bed such as a sofa; overheating (thermal stress); cosleeping; exposure to tobacco

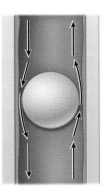
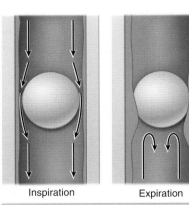
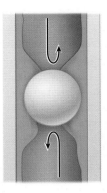

Inspiration   Expiration

FIRST-DEGREE OBSTRUCTION	SECOND-DEGREE OBSTRUCTION	COMPLETE OBSTRUCTION
Obstruction allows passage of air in both directions	Air able to move past the obstruction in one direction only. Air passages enlarge during inspiration and diminish during expiration.	Air unable to move in either direction. FB and edematous mucosa obliterate passage.

FIGURE 32.4 Manifestations of airway obstruction by foreign body (FB).

smoke after birth; stuffed animals or other toys need to be removed from the crib while the infant is sleeping.

3. Reinforce teaching to parents about monitoring for positional plagiocephaly caused by the supine sleeping position; signs include flattened posterior occiput and development of a bald spot in the posterior occiput area.

4. To assist in preventing positional plagiocephaly, teach the parents to alter head position during sleep, avoid excessive time in infant seats and bouncers, and place the infant in a prone position while awake (monitor the infant when in the prone position).

5. If SIDS occurs, the parents need a great deal of support as they grieve and mourn, especially because the event was sudden, unexpected, and unexplained.

 XIV. Foreign-Body Aspiration

A. Description (Fig. 32.4)
1. Swallowing and aspirating a foreign body (or bodies) into the air passages
2. Most inhaled foreign bodies lodge in the mainstem or lobar bronchus.
3. The most common offending foods are round in shape and include hot dogs, candy, peanuts, popcorn, and grapes.

B. Data collection
1. Initially, choking, gagging, coughing, and retractions are general findings.
2. If the condition worsens, cyanosis may occur.
3. Laryngotracheal obstruction leads to dyspnea, stridor, cough, and hoarseness.
4. Bronchial obstruction produces paroxysmal cough, wheezing, asymmetrical breath sounds, and dyspnea.

5. If any obstruction progresses, unconsciousness and asphyxiation may occur.
6. Partial obstructions may occur without symptoms.
7. The distressed child cannot speak, becomes cyanotic, and collapses.

C. Interventions
1. Emergency care: Abdominal thrust maneuver is used for the removal of a foreign body (or relief of choking) in a child; refer to the American Heart Association document at https://hinman.org/Clinicians/Handouts/2017/Th113-Th114-Fr141-Fr142.pdf.
2. After initiating emergency care measures, removal by endoscopy may be necessary.
    a. Postprocedure, the child receives high-humidity air.
    b. Observe for signs and symptoms of airway edema.
3. Prevention
    a. Keep any small object out of reach of small children.
    b. Avoid giving small children small, round food items.
4. Parent, daycare provider, babysitter education
    a. Reinforce teaching about the hazards of aspiration.
    b. Discuss potential situations in which small items may be aspirated.
    c. Reinforce teaching about the symptoms of aspiration.
    d. Reinforce teaching about how to perform emergency care measures.

XV. Tuberculosis

A. Description (see Chapter 47)
1. A contagious disease caused by *Mycobacterium tuberculosis*, which is an acid-fast bacillus

Pediatric Nursing

BOX 32.8 **Tuberculin Skin Test or Mantoux Test Interpretation**

Induration that measures 15 mm or more is considered to be a positive reaction in children 4 years old or older who do not have any risk factors.

Induration that measures 10 mm or more is considered to be a positive reaction in children younger than 4 years old and in those with chronic illness or who are at high risk for exposure to tuberculosis.

Induration that measures 5 mm or more is considered to be positive for those in the highest-risk groups, such as children with immunosuppressive conditions or human immunodeficiency virus (HIV) infection.

---

2. Multidrug-resistant strains of *M. tuberculosis* occur as a result of client or family noncompliance with therapeutic regimens.

3. The route of transmission of *M. tuberculosis* is via the inhalation of droplets from an individual with active tuberculosis (TB).

4. There is an increased incidence in urban low-income areas, nonwhite racial or ethnic groups, and first-generation immigrants from endemic countries.

5. Most children are infected by a family member or another individual with whom they have frequent contact (e.g., a babysitter).

 B. Data collection

1. May be asymptomatic or develop symptoms such as malaise, fever, cough, weight loss, anorexia, and lymphadenopathy

2. Specific symptoms related to the site of infection, such as the lungs, brain, or bone, may be present.

3. With increased time, asymmetrical expansion of the lungs, decreased breath sounds, crackles, and dullness to percussion develop.

 C. Tuberculin skin test (TST) or Mantoux test (Box 32.8)

1. Will produce a positive reaction 2 to 10 weeks after the initial infection

2. Determines whether the child has been infected and has developed a sensitivity to the protein of the tubercle bacillus. A positive reaction does not confirm the presence of active disease (exposure *versus* presence).

3. After the child reacts positively, he or she will always react positively. A positive reaction in a previously negative child indicates that the child has been infected since their last test.

 4. TB testing would not be done at the same time as measles immunization (viral interference from the measles vaccine may cause a false-negative result).

 D. Sputum culture

1. A definitive diagnosis is made by demonstrating the presence of mycobacteria in a culture.

2. Chest x-rays are supplemental to sputum cultures and are not definitive alone.

3. Because an infant or young child often swallows sputum rather than expectorates it, gastric washings (aspiration of lavaged contents from the fasting stomach) may be done to obtain a specimen; the specimen is obtained in the early morning before breakfast.

E. Interventions

1. Medications

   a. A 9-month course of isoniazid may be prescribed to prevent a latent infection from progressing to clinically active TB and to prevent initial infection in children in high-risk situations; a 12-month course may be prescribed for the child infected with human immunodeficiency virus (HIV).

   b. Recommendation for the child with clinically active TB may include combination administration of isoniazid, rifampin, and pyrazinamide daily for 2 months, and then isoniazid and rifampin twice weekly for 4 months.

   c. Inform the parents and child that bodily fluids, including urine, may turn an orange-red color with some TB medications.

   d. Direct observed therapy may be necessary for some children.

2. Place children with active disease who are contagious on respiratory isolation until medications have been initiated, sputum cultures demonstrate a diminished number of organisms, and cough is improving; this includes use of a personally fitted air-purifying N95 or N100 respirator (mask) by the nurse caring for the child.

3. Stress the importance of adequate rest and adequate diet.

4. Reinforce instructions to the child and family about measures to prevent the transmission of TB.

5. Case finding and follow-up with known contacts is critical to decrease the number of cases of individuals with active TB.

WHAT WOULD YOU DO?

Answer: For the child with pneumonia, to reduce the discomfort in the pleural area, the nurse would encourage the child to lie on the affected side (if pneumonia is unilateral) to splint the chest. This position reduces the discomfort associated with pleural rubbing. The primary health care provider's prescription for positioning is always followed. In addition, a mild analgesic may be administered if it is prescribed.

PRACTICE QUESTIONS

❖ 1. The nurse is preparing for the admission of an infant with a diagnosis of bronchiolitis caused by the respiratory syncytial virus (RSV). Which interventions would be included in the plan of care? **Select all that apply.**
   ❑ 1. Place the infant in a private room.
   ❑ 2. Place the infant in a room near the nurses' station.
   ❑ 3. Ensure that the infant's head is in a flexed position.
   ❑ 4. Wear a mask at all times when in contact with the infant.
   ❑ 5. Place the child in a tent that delivers warm, humidified air.
   ❑ 6. Position the infant side-lying, with the head lower than the chest.

2. After a tonsillectomy, the child begins to vomit bright red blood. Which is the **initial** nursing action?
   1. Turn the child to the side.
   2. Notify the registered nurse (RN).
   3. Administer the prescribed antiemetic.
   4. Maintain NPO (nothing by mouth) status.

3. The nurse reinforces instructions to the mother of a child with croup about the measures to take if an acute spasmodic episode occurs. Which statement by the mother indicates the **need for further teaching**?
   1. "I will take my child out into the humid night air."
   2. "I will place a steam vaporizer in my child's bedroom."
   3. "I will place a cool-mist humidifier in my child's bedroom."
   4. "I will place my child in a closed bathroom and allow my child to inhale steam from the running water."

4. The nurse reinforces instructions to the mother of a child who has been hospitalized with croup. Which statement made by the mother would indicate the **need for further teaching**?
   1. "I will give my child cough syrup if a cough develops."
   2. "During an attack, I will take my child to a cool location."
   3. "I can give acetaminophen if my child develops a fever."
   4. "I will be sure that my child drinks at least three to four glasses of fluids every day."

5. The nurse is working in the emergency department and is caring for a child who has been diagnosed with epiglottitis. Which is an indication that the child may be experiencing airway obstruction?
   1. Retractions and coughing
   2. Nasal flaring and bradycardia
   3. Tripod positioning and dyspnea
   4. A low-grade fever and complaints of a sore throat

6. The nurse has provided instructions to the mother of an infant with viral pneumonia. Which statement by the mother would indicate the **need for further teaching**?
   1. "I understand I will need to have my baby on antibiotics for this pneumonia."
   2. "I will need to give a cough suppressant before meals if his cough gets too bad."
   3. "I will be careful and allow my baby to sleep, so he can conserve energy and fight this infection."
   4. "I understand that my baby has viral pneumonia and I need to monitor his temperature because of the risk for febrile seizures."

7. The nurse is instructing the mother of a child with cystic fibrosis (CF) about the appropriate dietary measures. Which meal **best** illustrates the **most appropriate** diet for a client with CF?
   1. Veggie salad and a caramel apple
   2. Strawberry jelly sandwich and pretzels
   3. Plate of nachos and cheese and a cupcake
   4. Chicken tenders and a baked potato with butter

8. The nursing instructor asks a nursing student about sudden infant death syndrome (SIDS). Which statement by the student indicates **further teaching is needed**?
   1. "Some of the interventions that are used to prevent SIDS include having infants sleep in the supine position."
   2. "The incidence of SIDS has been found to be higher in breast-fed infants and infants that use a pacifier."
   3. "Infants exposed to cigarette smoking during pregnancy and after birth are considered at risk for SIDS."
   4. "SIDS refers to sudden infant death syndrome that can occur in healthy infants under 1 year of age, and no exact cause is known."

9. Isoniazid is prescribed for a 2-year-old child with a positive tuberculin skin test. The mother of the child asks the nurse how long the child will need to take the medication. Which time frame is the appropriate response to the mother?
   1. 4 months
   2. 9 months
   3. 12 months
   4. 18 months

10. The nurse is instructing a mother of a 1-year-old child with strabismus about the treatment options. Which statement by the mother would indicate the **need for further teaching**?
    1. "My child will outgrow this by the time he is 2 years old and be able to see just fine."
    2. "I will have my child wear an eye patch over the good eye to help strengthen the weak eye."
    3. "If this eye patch does not work I know that we will have to do surgery to correct my child's crossed eyes."
    4. "There are a few causes of this condition and they tell me my child has crossed eyes because of a muscle imbalance."

11. The nurse has provided instructions to the mother of a child who has been diagnosed with bacterial conjunctivitis. Which statement by the mother would indicate the **need for further teaching**?
    1. "I need to wash my hands frequently."
    2. "I need to clean the eye, as prescribed."
    3. "I need to give the eye drops, as prescribed."
    4. "I need to use hot compresses to relieve the eye irritation."

12. The nurse is assigned to care for a child after a myringotomy with the insertion of tympanostomy tubes. The nurse notes a small amount of reddish drainage from the child's ear after the surgery. On the basis of this finding, which action would the nurse take?
    1. Document the findings.
    2. Notify the RN immediately.
    3. Change the ear tubes so that they do not become blocked.
    4. Check the ear drainage for the presence of cerebrospinal fluid.

13. The nurse assists to prepare a teaching plan regarding the administration of eardrops for the parents of a 2-year-old child with otitis media. Which would be included in the plan?
    1. Wear gloves when administering the eardrops.
    2. Pull the ear up and back before instilling the eardrops.
    3. Pull the earlobe down and back before instilling the eardrops.
    4. Hold the child in a sitting position when administering the eardrops.

ANSWERS

❖ **1. 1, 2, 4**
Rationale: The hospitalized infant with RSV needs to be isolated in a private room. The infant needs to be placed in a room near the nurses' station for close observation of respiratory status. The infant would be positioned with the head and chest elevated at a 30- to 40-degree angle and the neck slightly extended to maintain an open airway and to decrease pressure on the diaphragm. Cool, humidified oxygen is delivered to relieve dyspnea, hypoxemia, and insensible water loss from tachypnea. Contact, droplet, and standard precautions are necessary to reduce the nosocomial transmission of RSV.
Test-Taking Strategy: Focus on the subject, care of the child with RSV. Recalling the mode of transmission of RSV will assist you with determining that the infant needs to be placed in a private room and that droplet, contact, and standard precautions need to be maintained. Recalling the reasons to maintain a patent airway (edema and the accumulation of mucus obstruct the bronchioles) will assist you with determining that the infant needs to be observed closely, that the infant's head needs to be elevated, and that the infant would receive cool, humidified oxygen.

2. 1
Rationale: After a tonsillectomy, if bleeding occurs, the child is turned to the side and the RN or PHCP is notified. An NPO status would be maintained, and an antiemetic may be prescribed; however, the initial nursing action would be to turn the child to the side.

Test-Taking Strategy: Note the strategic word, *initial*. Although all of the options may be appropriate to maintain physiological integrity, the initial action is to turn the child to the side.

3. 2
Rationale: Steam from warm running water in a closed bathroom and cool mist from a bedside humidifier are effective for reducing mucosal edema. Cool-mist humidifiers are recommended compared with steam vaporizers, which present a danger of scalding burns. Taking the child out into the humid night air may also relieve mucosal swelling. Remember, however, that a cold mist may precipitate bronchospasm.
Test-Taking Strategy: Note the strategic words, *need for further teaching*. These words indicate a negative event query and the need to select the incorrect statement. Recall the goals of reducing mucosal edema and providing a safe environment. Note the word *steam* in option 2. Option 2 would provide an unsafe environment for the child.

4. 1
Rationale: Cough syrups should not be given unless specifically prescribed because they may dry and thicken secretions. During a croup attack, the child can be taken to a cool basement or garage. Acetaminophen is used if a fever develops. Adequate hydration of 500 to 1000 mL of fluids daily is important for thinning secretions.
Test-Taking Strategy: Note the strategic words, *need for further teaching*. These words indicate a negative event query and ask you to select an option that is an incorrect statement.

Knowledge of the pathophysiology related to croup will assist you with eliminating options 3 and 4 first. Recalling that taking the child to a cool location during an attack is appropriate will direct you to the correct option from the remaining options.

5. 3
Rationale: Clinical manifestations that are suggestive of airway obstruction include tripod positioning (leaning forward supported by the hands and arms with the chin thrust out and the mouth open), nasal flaring, tachycardia, retractions, and dyspnea. Epiglottitis is the bacterial form of croup with symptoms of a high fever, sore throat, and an absence of spontaneous cough.
Test-Taking Strategy: Focus on the subject, signs/symptoms of airway obstruction. Eliminate option 2 first because tachycardia rather than bradycardia will occur in a child who is experiencing respiratory distress. Eliminate option 4 next, knowing that a high fever occurs with epiglottitis. From the remaining options, recall that tripod positioning and dyspnea are present in airway obstruction and no spontaneous cough is evident.

6. 1
Rationale: The child with viral pneumonia will not be prescribed antibiotics; it is bacterial pneumonia that requires antibiotics for treatment. It is important to monitor the infant for fever spikes because of the risk for febrile seizures. Use of a cough suppressant may be prescribed before rest times and meals if the cough is disturbing and unproductive. Promoting bed rest to conserve energy, encouraging fluid intake and the administration of antipyretics for fever, and bronchodilators are typical interventions for pneumonia.
Test-Taking Strategy: Note the strategic words, *need for further teaching*. These words indicate a negative event query and ask you to select an option that is an incorrect statement. Knowledge of pneumonia will assist you with eliminating options 2 and 4 as these are correct interventions. Recalling that bacterial pneumonia requires antibiotics will direct you to the correct option.

7. 4
Rationale: Children with CF are managed with a high-calorie, high-protein diet. Pancreatic enzyme replacement therapy is undertaken, and fat-soluble vitamin supplements are administered. Fats are not restricted unless steatorrhea cannot be controlled by increased levels of pancreatic enzymes. Chicken tenders and a baked potato with butter provide a high-calorie and high-protein meal that includes fat.
Test-Taking Strategy: Focus on the subject, dietary measures for a child with CF. Note the strategic words, *best* and *most appropriate*. Eliminate options 1, 2, and 3 because they are not high in protein or calories. From the remaining options, recalling the appropriate diet for the child with CF will direct you to the correct option.

8. 2
Rationale: The incidence of SIDS has been found to be lower in breast-fed infants and infants who sleep with a pacifier. Options 1, 3 and 4 are correct statements about SIDS.

Test-Taking Strategy: Note the strategic words, *further teaching is needed*. These words indicate a negative event query and ask you to select an option that is an incorrect statement. Knowledge of SIDS will assist you in eliminating options 3 and 4. Recalling prevention and interventions for SIDS will direct you to the correct option.

9. 2
Rationale: Isoniazid is given to prevent TB infection from progressing to active disease. A chest x-ray film is obtained before the initiation of preventive therapy. In infants and children, the recommended duration of isoniazid therapy is 9 months. For children with human immunodeficiency virus infection, a minimum of 12 months is recommended.
Test-Taking Strategy: Focus on the subject, treatment for TB. Knowledge regarding treatment with isoniazid in a 2-year-old child is required to answer this question. Remember that in infants and children, the recommended duration of isoniazid therapy is 9 months.

10. 1
Rationale: Although strabismus is considered a normal finding in young infants, it would not be present after 4 months of age, so the 1 year old will likely not outgrow the condition. The use of an eye patch helps to strengthen the weak eye and surgery may be required for the condition. A muscle imbalance or the paralysis of the extraocular muscles may be the cause or strabismus could be congenital.
Test-Taking Strategy: Note the strategic words, *need for further teaching*. These words indicate a negative event query and ask you to select an option that is an incorrect statement. Knowledge of the interventions and descriptions for strabismus will assist you to eliminate options 2, 3, and 4. Recalling that this condition needs to be treated will direct you to the correct option.

11. 4
Rationale: Parents are to be instructed to use cool compresses to lessen eye irritation and wear dark glasses for photophobia. Options 1, 2, and 3 are correct measures.
Test-Taking Strategy: Note the strategic words, *need for further teaching*. These words indicate a negative event query and ask you to select an option that is an incorrect statement. Recall that instructions to the parents include infection control measures, use of cool compresses, administration of eye drops, and to avoid rubbing the eye. Also, noting the word *hot* in option 4 will direct you to this option.

12. 1
Rationale: After a myringotomy with the insertion of tympanostomy tubes, the child is monitored for ear drainage. A small amount of reddish drainage is normal during the first few days after surgery. However, any heavy bleeding or bleeding that occurs after 3 days needs to be reported. The nurse would document the findings. Options 2, 3, and 4 are not necessary.
Test-Taking Strategy: Note the subject, a small amount of reddish drainage. Considering both the anatomical location of the surgery and the subject of the question will direct you to the correct option.

13. 3

Rationale: When administering eardrops to a child who is younger than 3 years old, the ear needs to be pulled down and back. For children who are older than 3 years old, the ear is pulled up and back. Gloves do not need to be worn by the parents, but hand washing needs to be performed before and after the procedure. The child needs to be in a side-lying position with the affected ear facing upward to facilitate the flow of medication down the ear canal by gravity.

Test-Taking Strategy: Focus on the subject, administering eardrops to a 2-year-old child. Visualizing this procedure will assist you with eliminating options 1 and 4 first. From the remaining options, recalling the anatomy of the 2-year-old's ear canal will direct you to the correct option.

CHAPTER 33

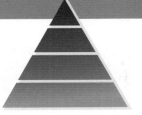

Cardiovascular Problems

PRIORITY CONCEPTS Gas Exchange; Perfusion

WHAT WOULD YOU DO?

A child diagnosed with a congenital heart defect suddenly develops difficulty breathing. What would the nurse do? *Answer is located on p. 420.*

I. Hyperlipidemia

A. Description
1. A condition in which there are high levels of lipids circulating in the blood, which can predispose a child to heart disease
2. Laboratory values for lipids for individuals aged 2 to 19 years are as follows:
   a. Total cholesterol: Less than 170 mg/dL is acceptable, 170 to 199 mg/dL is borderline, 200 mg/dL or greater is high.
   b. Low-density lipoprotein cholesterol: Less than 110 mg/dL is acceptable, 110 to 129 mg/dL is borderline, 130 mg/dL or greater is high.
   c. High-density lipoprotein cholesterol: Greater than 45 mg/dL is acceptable, 40 to 45 mg/dL is borderline, less than 40 mg/dL is low.
   d. Triglycerides: Less than 100 mg/dL for 9 years and younger is acceptable; less than 130 mg/dL for 10 years and older is acceptable.
   e. Any person with hyperlipidemia as a child is likely to have the condition later in life, and it predisposes them to cardiac events.

B. Interventions
   a. Referral to a specialist (cardiology) would be made if there is an elevation in any of the above values.
   b. Treatment focuses on lifestyle modifications and behavior changes.

II. Heart Failure (HF)

A. Description
1. The inability of the heart to pump a sufficient amount of blood to meet the metabolic and oxygen needs of the body

2. In infants and children, inadequate cardiac output is most commonly caused by congenital heart defects (**shunt**, obstruction, or a combination of both) that produce an excessive volume or pressure load on the myocardium.
3. In infants and children, a combination of both left- and right-sided heart failure is usually present (Box 33.1).
4. The goals of treatment are to improve cardiac function, remove accumulated fluid and sodium, decrease cardiac demands, improve tissue oxygenation, and decrease oxygen consumption.

B. Data collection of early signs
1. Tachycardia, especially during rest and slight exertion
2. Tachypnea
3. Profuse scalp diaphoresis, especially in infants
4. Fatigue and irritability
5. Sudden weight gain related to excess fluid retention
6. Respiratory distress

C. Interventions
1. Monitor for early signs of HF.
2. Monitor for respiratory distress (count respirations for 1 minute).
3. Monitor apical pulse (count apical pulse for 1 minute) and monitor for abnormal rhythms.
4. Monitor temperature for hyperthermia and for other signs of infection, particularly respiratory infection.
5. Monitor strict intake and output (I&O); weigh diapers as appropriate for most accurate output.
6. Monitor daily weight to check for fluid retention; a weight gain of 0.5 kg (1 lb) in 1 day is caused by the accumulation of fluid.
7. Monitor for facial or peripheral-dependent edema, listen to lung sounds, and report abnormal findings indicating excessive fluid in the body.
8. Elevate the head of the bed in a semi-Fowler's position.
9. Maintain a neutral thermal environment to prevent cold stress in infants.

413

BOX 33.1	Signs/Symptoms of Heart Failure in Infants and Children

Left-Sided Failure
- Crackles and wheezes
- Cough
- Dyspnea
- Grunting (infants)
- Head bobbing (infants)
- Nasal flaring
- Orthopnea
- Periods of cyanosis
- Retractions
- Tachypnea

Right-Sided Failure
- Ascites
- Hepatosplenomegaly
- Jugular vein distention
- Oliguria
- Peripheral edema, especially dependent edema and periorbital edema
- Weight gain

10. Provide rest and decrease environmental stimuli.
11. Administer cool humidified oxygen as prescribed, using an oxygen hood for young infants and a nasal cannula or face mask for older infants and children.
12. Organize nursing activities to allow for uninterrupted sleep.
13. Maintain adequate nutritional status.
14. Feed when hungry and soon after awakening, conserving energy and oxygen supply.
15. Provide small, frequent feedings, conserving energy and oxygen supply.
16. Administer medications as prescribed, which may include digoxin, diuretics, and afterload reducers such as angiotensin-converting enzyme (ACE) inhibitors.
17. Administer digoxin as prescribed.
    a. Check apical heart rate for 1 minute before administration.
    b. Withhold digoxin if the apical pulse is less than 90 to 110 beats/min in infants and young children and less than 70 beats/min in older children, as prescribed.
    c. Check the prescribed dose carefully to ensure it is a safe, age-appropriate dose; follow agency policy and question any unclear prescription.
18. Monitor digoxin levels and for signs of digoxin toxicity, including anorexia, poor feeding, nausea, vomiting, bradycardia, dysrhythmias; report any signs to the registered nurse (RN) immediately.
19. The optimal therapeutic digoxin level range is 0.8 to 2 ng/mL; toxicity is usually seen at greater than 2 ng/mL level.

20. Administer ACE inhibitors as prescribed.
    a. Monitor for hypotension, renal dysfunction, and cough when ACE inhibitors are administered.
    b. The blood pressure; serum protein, albumin, blood urea nitrogen, creatinine levels, and white blood cell count; urine output; urinary specific gravity, and urinary protein level are monitored.
21. Administer diuretics such as furosemide as prescribed.
    a. Monitor for signs and symptoms of hypokalemia (serum potassium level less than 3.5 mEq/L, including muscle weakness and cramping and confusion, irritability, restlessness, and inverted T wave or prominent U waves on the electrocardiogram (ECG).
    b. If signs/symptoms of hypokalemia are present and the child is also being administered digoxin, then monitor closely for digoxin toxicity because hypokalemia potentiates digoxin toxicity.
22. Administer potassium supplements and provide dietary sources of potassium as prescribed.
    a. Supplemental potassium is prescribed if the need is indicated by low serum potassium levels and if adequate kidney function is evident; supplemental potassium is usually necessary when administering a potassium-losing diuretic such as furosemide.
    b. Encourage foods that the child will eat that are high in potassium, as appropriate, such as bananas, baked potato skins, and peanut butter.
23. Monitor serum electrolyte levels, particularly the potassium level (normal level is 3.5–5.0 mEq/L).
24. Limit fluid intake as prescribed in the acute stage.
25. Monitor for signs/symptoms of dehydration, including sunken fontanel (infant), nonelastic skin turgor, dry mucous membranes, decreased tear production, decreased urine output, and concentrated urine.
26. Monitor sodium level as prescribed.
    a. Normal level is 135 mEq/L to 145 mEq/L.
    b. Many infant formulas have slightly more sodium than breast milk.
27. Reinforce instructions to parents regarding administration of digoxin (Box 33.2).
28. Reinforce instructions to parents in cardiopulmonary resuscitation (CPR). The guidelines for CPR for the child older than 1 year of age are the same as they are for an adult. For American Heart Association current CPR guidelines refer to https://eccguidelines.heart.org/circulation/cpr-ecc-guidelines/.

⚠ The parents would be provided with a medication guide for any medication prescribed for the infant or child. In addition, the nurse needs to review the instructions in the guide and provide an opportunity for the parents to demonstrate medication administration procedures.

BOX 33.2 **Homecare Instructions for Administering Digoxin**

- Administer the medication as prescribed.
- Use an accurate measuring device as provided by the pharmacist.
- Administer the medication 1 hour before or 2 hours after feedings.
- Use a calendar to mark off the dose that has been administered.
- Do not mix the medication with food or fluid.
- If a dose is missed and 4 or more hours have elapsed, withhold the dose and give the next dose at the scheduled time. If less than 4 hours have elapsed, administer the missed dose.
- If the child vomits, do not administer a second dose (follow primary health care provider's [PHCP's] prescription).
- If more than two consecutive doses have been missed, notify the PHCP. Do not increase or double the dose to make up for missed doses.
- If the child has teeth, give water after the medication. If possible, brush the child's teeth to prevent tooth decay from the sweetened liquid.
- Monitor for signs of toxicity such as poor feeding or vomiting.
- If the child becomes ill, notify the PHCP.
- Keep the medication in a locked cabinet.
- Call the poison control center immediately if accidental overdose occurs.

BOX 33.3 **Signs/Symptoms of Decreased Cardiac Output**

- Decreased peripheral pulses
- Activity intolerance
- Feeding difficulties
- Hypotension
- Irritability, restlessness, and lethargy
- Oliguria
- Pale, cool extremities
- Tachycardia

III. Defects with Increased Pulmonary Blood Flow

A. Description
1. Intracardiac communication along the septum or an abnormal connection between the great arteries allows for the blood to flow from the high-pressure left side of the heart to the low-pressure right side of the heart.
2. The infant typically demonstrates signs and symptoms of HF.

B. Atrial septal defect (ASD)
1. An abnormal opening between the atria that causes an increased flow of oxygenated blood into the right side of the heart
2. Right atrial and ventricular enlargement occurs.
3. Infant may be asymptomatic or may develop HF.
4. Signs/symptoms of decreased cardiac output may be present (Box 33.3).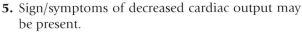
5. Management
   a. May be closed with the use of devices during a cardiac catheterization
   b. Open repair with cardiopulmonary bypass is usually performed before the child reaches school age.

C. Atrioventricular canal defect
1. Results from incomplete fusion of the endocardial cushions
2. Most common cardiac defect in children with Down syndrome
3. A characteristic murmur is present.

4. The infant usually has mild to moderate HF. Cyanosis increases with crying.
5. Sign/symptoms of decreased cardiac output may be present.
6. Management can include either pulmonary artery banding for infants with severe symptoms (palliative) or complete repair via cardiopulmonary bypass.

D. Patent ductus arteriosus (PDA)
1. Failure of the fetal ductus arteriosus (shunt that connects the aorta and the pulmonary artery) to close within the first weeks of life
2. A characteristic machinery-like murmur is present. The infant may be asymptomatic or he or she may show signs of HF.
3. A widened pulse pressure and bounding pulses are present.
4. Signs/symptoms of decreased cardiac output may be present.
5. Management
   a. Indomethacin (prostaglandin inhibitor) may be administered to close a patent ductus in premature infants and some newborns.
   b. The defect may be closed during cardiac catheterization or may require surgical management.

E. Ventricular septal defect (VSD)
1. An abnormal opening between the right and left ventricles
2. Many VSDs close spontaneously during the first year of life in children who have small or moderate defects.
3. A characteristic murmur is present; HF is common.
4. Signs/symptoms of HF and of decreased cardiac output may be present.
5. Management
   a. Device closure during cardiac catheterization may be possible.
   b. Open repair with cardiopulmonary bypass may be done.

IV. Obstructive Defects

A. Description
1. Blood exiting the heart meets an area of anatomical narrowing (stenosis), thus causing obstruction of blood flow.

2. The location of narrowing is usually near the valve of the obstructive defect.

3. Infants and children exhibit signs of HF.

4. Children with mild obstruction may be asymptomatic.

B. Aortic stenosis

1. Aortic stenosis is a narrowing or stricture of the aortic valve, causing resistance to blood flow from the left ventricle into the aorta, resulting in decreased cardiac output, left ventricular hypertrophy, and pulmonary vascular congestion.

2. Valvular stenosis is the most common type and is usually caused by malformed cusps, resulting in a bicuspid rather than a tricuspid valve, or fusion of the cusps.

3. A characteristic murmur is present.

4. Infants with severe defects demonstrate signs of decreased cardiac output.

5. Children show signs of activity intolerance, chest pain, and dizziness when standing for long periods of time.

6. Management

 a. Dilation of the narrowed valve may be done during cardiac catheterization.

 b. Surgical aortic valvotomy (palliative) may be done; a valve replacement may be required at a second procedure.

C. Coarctation of the aorta

1. Coarctation of the aorta refers to the localized narrowing near the insertion of the ductus arteriosus.

2. Signs of HF may occur in infants.

3. Signs/symptoms of decreased cardiac output may be present.

4. Children may experience headaches, dizziness, fainting, and epistaxis resulting from hypertension.

5. Management of the defect may be done via balloon angioplasty in children; restenosis can occur. Surgical management may be necessary.

> ⚠ With coarctation of the aorta, the blood pressure is higher in the upper extremities than the lower extremities. In addition, bounding pulses in the arms, weak or absent femoral pulses, and cool lower extremities may be present.

D. Pulmonary stenosis

1. Narrowing at the entrance to the pulmonary artery

2. Resistance to blood flow causes right ventricular hypertrophy and decreased pulmonary blood flow. The right ventricle may be hypoplastic.

3. Pulmonary atresia is the extreme form of pulmonary stenosis in that there is total fusion of the commissures and no blood flows to the lungs.

4. A characteristic murmur is present.

5. May be asymptomatic

6. Newborns with severe narrowing will be cyanotic.

7. If pulmonary stenosis is severe, HF occurs.

8. Signs and symptoms of decreased cardiac output may occur.

9. Management: Dilation of the narrowed valve may be done during cardiac catheterization. Surgical intervention may be necessary.

V. Defects Associated with Decreased Pulmonary Blood Flow

A. Description

1. Obstructed pulmonary blood flow and an anatomical defect (ASD or VSD) between the right and left sides of the heart

2. Pressure in the right side of the heart increases as a result of obstructed blood flow, exceeding pressure in the left side, which allows desaturated blood to shunt right to left, causing desaturation in the left side of the heart and in the systemic circulation.

3. Typically, hypoxemia and cyanosis appear.

B. Tetralogy of Fallot

1. Includes four defects: VSD, pulmonary stenosis, overriding aorta, and right ventricular hypertrophy

2. If pulmonary vascular resistance is higher than systemic resistance, the shunt is from right to left. If systemic resistance is higher than pulmonary resistance, the shunt is from left to right.

3. Infants

 a. May be acutely cyanotic at birth or may have mild cyanosis that progresses over the first year of life as the pulmonic stenosis worsens

 b. A characteristic murmur is present.

 c. Acute episodes of cyanosis and hypoxia (hypercyanotic spells), called *blue spells* or *tet spells*, occur when the infant's oxygen requirements exceed the blood supply (usually during crying, feeding, or defecating).

4. Children: With increasing cyanosis, squatting, clubbing of the fingers, and poor growth may occur.

 a. Squatting is a compensatory mechanism to facilitate increased return of blood flow to the heart for oxygenation.

 b. Clubbing is an abnormal enlargement in the distal phalanges; seen in the fingers.

5. Surgical management: Palliative shunt

 a. The shunt increases pulmonary blood flow and increases oxygen saturation in infants who cannot undergo primary repair.

 b. The shunt provides blood flow to the pulmonary arteries from the left or right subclavian artery.

6. Surgical management: Complete repair, if necessary, is usually performed in the first year of life. The repair requires a median sternotomy and cardiopulmonary bypass.

C. Tricuspid atresia
1. Failure of the tricuspid valve to develop
2. There is no communication from the right atrium to the right ventricle.
3. Blood flows through an ASD or a patent foramen ovale to the left side of the heart and through a VSD to the right ventricle and out to the lungs.
4. Often associated with pulmonic stenosis and the transposition of the great arteries.
5. A complete mixing of unoxygenated and oxygenated blood in the left side of the heart occurs, which results in systemic desaturation, pulmonary obstruction, and decreased pulmonary blood flow.
6. Cyanosis, tachycardia, and dyspnea are seen in the newborn.
7. Older children exhibit signs of chronic hypoxemia and clubbing.
8. Management: If the ASD is small, the defect may be closed during cardiac catheterization; otherwise, surgery is needed.

⚠ Clubbing is symptomatic of chronic hypoxia. Peripheral circulation is diminished and oxygenation of vital organs and tissues is compromised.

VI. Mixed Defects

A. Description
1. Fully saturated systemic blood flow mixes with the desaturated blood flow, which causes a desaturation of the systemic blood flow.
2. Pulmonary congestion occurs, and cardiac output decreases.
3. Signs of HF are present; symptoms depend on the degree of desaturation.

B. Hypoplastic left heart syndrome
1. The underdevelopment of the left side of the heart that results in a hypoplastic left ventricle and aortic atresia
2. Mild cyanosis and signs of HF occur until the ductus arteriosus closes. Progressive deterioration with cyanosis and decreased cardiac output then occur, which lead to cardiovascular collapse.
3. Without intervention, this is fatal during the first few months of life.
4. Surgical treatment is necessary.

C. Transposition of the great arteries or transposition of the great vessels
1. The pulmonary artery leaves the left ventricle, and the aorta exits from the right ventricle.
2. No communication exists between the systemic and pulmonary circulations.
3. Infants with minimal communication are severely cyanotic at birth.
4. Infants with large septal defects or a PDA may be less severely cyanotic but may have symptoms of HF.

5. Cardiomegaly is evident a few weeks after birth.
6. Surgery is usually required.

D. Total anomalous pulmonary venous connection
1. Failure of the pulmonary veins to join the left atrium
2. Results in mixed blood being returned to the right atrium and shunted from the right to the left through an ASD
3. The right side of the heart hypertrophies, whereas the left side may remain small.
4. Signs/symptoms of HF develop.
5. Cyanosis worsens with pulmonary vein obstruction. After obstruction occurs, the infant's condition deteriorates rapidly.
6. Surgical treatment is necessary.

E. Truncus arteriosus
1. The failure of normal septation and the division of the embryonic bulbar trunk into the pulmonary artery and the aorta, which results in a single vessel that overrides both ventricles
2. Blood from both ventricles mixes in the common great artery, thus causing desaturation and hypoxemia.
3. A characteristic murmur is present.
4. The infant exhibits moderate to severe HF, variable cyanosis, poor growth, and activity intolerance.
5. Surgical treatment is necessary.

VII. Interventions: Cardiovascular Defects

A. Monitor for signs of a defect in the infant or child (see previous descriptions of defects).
B. Monitor the vital signs closely.
C. Monitor the respiratory status for the presence of nasal flaring and the use of accessory muscles. The RN is notified immediately if any changes occur.
D. Breath sounds are auscultated for crackles, wheezes, or rhonchi.
E. If respiratory effort is increased, place the child in reverse Trendelenburg position (elevate the head and upper body) to decrease the work of breathing.
F. Administer humidified oxygen, as prescribed.
G. Endotracheal tube and ventilator care may be necessary.
H. Monitor for hypercyanotic spells and intervene immediately if they occur (see **Priority Nursing Actions**).

⚡ PRIORITY NURSING ACTIONS

Hypercyanotic Spell Occurring in an Infant

1. Place the infant in a knee-chest position.
2. Prepare to administer 100% oxygen.
3. Assist to administer morphine sulfate.
4. Assist to administer fluids intravenously.
5. Document occurrence, actions taken, and the infant's response.

I. Monitor for signs of HF, such as fluid retention in the hands, feet, chest, and around the eyes.

J. Monitor the peripheral pulses.

K. Monitor the I&O and notify the RN immediately if a decrease in urine output occurs (weigh diapers as necessary).

L. Obtain daily weight.

M. Provide adequate nutrition (high-calorie requirements), as prescribed.

N. Assist to administer medications, as prescribed.

O. Plan interventions to allow maximal rest for the child; keep the child as stress-free as possible.

P. Prepare the child and parents for cardiac catheterization, if appropriate.

VIII. Cardiac Catheterization

A. Description (see Chapter 49)
   1. An invasive diagnostic procedure used to determine cardiac defects
   2. Provides information about the oxygenation saturation of the blood in the great vessels and heart chambers
   3. May be carried out on an outpatient basis
   4. May be diagnostic, interventional, or electrophysiological in purpose
   5. Risks include hemorrhage from the entry site, clot formation and subsequent blockage distally, and transient dysrhythmias.
   6. General anesthesia is usually unnecessary.

B. Preprocedural nursing interventions
   1. Check the accurate height and weight, because this assists with the selection of the correct catheter size.
   2. Obtain a history of the presence of allergic reactions to iodine.
   3. Check for symptoms of infection, including diaper rash.
   4. Check and mark bilateral pulses (e.g., dorsalis pedis, posterior tibial).
   5. Check the baseline oxygen saturation.
   6. Familiarize the parents and child with hospital procedures and equipment.
   7. Reinforce educating the parents and child, if age appropriate, about the procedure.
   8. Allow the parents and child to verbalize their feelings and concerns regarding the procedure and the disorder.

C. Postprocedural nursing interventions
   1. Monitor findings on the cardiac monitor and the oxygen saturation for 4 hours after the procedure.
   2. Check the pulses below the catheter site for equality and symmetry.
   3. Check the temperature and color of the affected extremity, and report coolness immediately, which may indicate arterial obstruction.
   4. Monitor vital signs frequently, per the primary health care provider's (PHCP's) orders.
   5. Check the pressure dressing for intactness and signs of hemorrhage.
   6. Check the bedsheets under the extremity for blood, which indicates bleeding from the entry site.
   7. If bleeding is present, apply continuous direct pressure above the entry site and report it immediately.
   8. Immobilize the affected extremity for at least 4 to 6 hours for a venous entry site and for 6 to 8 hours for an arterial entry site, as prescribed.
   9. Hydrate the child via the oral route, the intravenous route, or both, as prescribed.
   10. Administer acetaminophen or ibuprofen for pain or discomfort, as prescribed.
   11. Prepare the parents and child, if appropriate, for surgery.

D. Discharge teaching for the child and parents
   1. Remove the dressing on the day after the procedure and cover it with a bandage for 2 to 3 days.
   2. Keep the site clean and dry.
   3. Have the child avoid tub baths for 2 to 3 days.
   4. Observe for redness, edema, drainage, bleeding, and fever, and report any of these signs immediately.
   5. Avoid strenuous activity, if applicable (the child may return to school, if appropriate).
   6. Provide a diet as tolerated.
   7. Administer acetaminophen or ibuprofen for pain, discomfort, or fever.
   8. Stress the importance of keeping follow-up appointments with the PHCP.

IX. Cardiac Surgery

A. Postoperative interventions
   1. Monitor vital signs frequently, especially temperature, and notify the RN immediately if fever occurs.
   2. Monitor for signs of sepsis, such as fever, chills, diaphoresis, lethargy, and altered levels of consciousness. Notify the RN immediately if any signs occur.
   3. Maintain strict aseptic technique.
   4. Assist with monitoring lines, tubes, or catheters that are in place and monitor for signs and symptoms of infection.
   5. Monitor for signs of discomfort, such as irritability or restlessness, and any changes in heart rate, respiratory rate, and blood pressure.
   6. Assist to administer pain medications, as prescribed, and note their effectiveness.
   7. Assist to administer antibiotics and antipyretics, as prescribed.
   8. Encourage rest and sleep periods.
   9. Facilitate parent–child contact as soon as possible.

B. Postoperative homecare (Box 33.4)

BOX 33.4 Homecare After Cardiac Surgery (Based upon Surgeon's Prescriptions)

- Omit play outside for several weeks.
- Avoid activities in which the child could fall and injure themselves, such as bike riding, for 2–4 weeks.
- Avoid crowds for 2 weeks after discharge.
- Follow a no-added-salt diet if prescribed.
- Do not add any new foods to the infant's diet (if an allergy exists to the new food, the manifestations may be interpreted as a postoperative complication).
- Do not place creams, lotions, or powders on the incision until completely healed.
- The child may return to school usually the third week after discharge, starting with half-days.
- The child is not to participate in physical education for 2 months.
- Reinforce instructions to the parents to discipline the child normally.
- Reinforce instructions to the parents about the importance of the 2-week follow-up.
- Avoid immunizations, invasive procedures, and dental visits for 2 months; following this time period, the immunization schedule and dental visits need to be resumed.
- Advise the parents regarding the importance of a dental visit every 6 months after age 3 years and to inform the dentist of the cardiac problem so that antibiotics can be prescribed if necessary.
- Reinforce instructions to the parents to call the primary health care provider if coughing, tachypnea, cyanosis, vomiting, diarrhea, anorexia, pain, or fever occur, or any swelling, redness, or drainage occurs at the site of the incision.

BOX 33.5 Jones Criteria for Diagnosis of Rheumatic Fever

Major Criteria
- Carditis
- Arthralgia
- Chorea
- Erythema marginatum
- Subcutaneous nodules

Minor Criteria
- Fever
- Arthralgia
- Elevated erythrocyte sedimentation rate or positive C-reactive protein level
- Prolonged PR interval on electrocardiogram

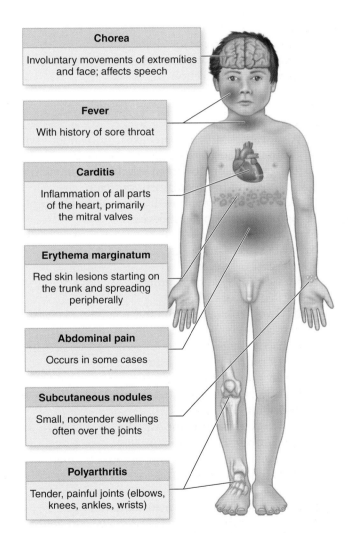

Chorea
Involuntary movements of extremities and face; affects speech

Fever
With history of sore throat

Carditis
Inflammation of all parts of the heart, primarily the mitral valves

Erythema marginatum
Red skin lesions starting on the trunk and spreading peripherally

Abdominal pain
Occurs in some cases

Subcutaneous nodules
Small, nontender swellings often over the joints

Polyarthritis
Tender, painful joints (elbows, knees, ankles, wrists)

FIGURE 33.1 Clinical manifestations of rheumatic fever.

X. Rheumatic Fever

A. Description
1. An inflammatory autoimmune disease that affects the connective tissues of the heart, joints, skin (subcutaneous tissues), blood vessels, and central nervous system
2. The most serious complication is rheumatic heart disease, which affects the cardiac valves, particularly the mitral valve.
3. Manifests 2 to 6 weeks after an untreated or partially treated group A β-hemolytic streptococcal infection of the upper respiratory tract
4. Jones criteria are used to determine the diagnosis (Box 33.5).

B. Data collection (Fig. 33.1)
1. Low-grade fever that spikes in the late afternoon
2. Elevated antistreptolysin O titer
3. Elevated erythrocyte sedimentation rate
4. Elevated C-reactive protein
5. Aschoff's bodies (lesions) in the heart, blood vessels, brain, and serous surfaces of the joints and pleurae
6. A macular erythematous rash, primarily on the trunk and extremities

⚠ Data collection of a child with suspected rheumatic fever includes inquiring about a recent sore throat because rheumatic fever manifests 2 to 6 weeks after an untreated or partially treated group A β-hemolytic streptococcal infection of the upper respiratory tract.

C. Interventions
1. Monitor vital signs.
2. Control joint pain and inflammation with massage and alternating hot and cold applications, as prescribed.
3. Provide bed rest during the acute febrile phase.
4. Limit physical exercise for the child with carditis.
5. Assist to administer antibiotics, as prescribed.
6. Assist to administer salicylates and antiinflammatory agents, as prescribed. (These medications would not be instituted before the diagnosis is confirmed, because they mask polyarthritis.)
7. Initiate seizure precautions if the child is experiencing chorea.
8. Reinforce instructions to the parents about the importance of follow-up and the need for antibiotic prophylaxis for dental work, infection, and invasive procedures.
9. Inform the parents to ask the school nurse to notify them if anyone in school develops a streptococcal throat infection.

XI. Kawasaki Disease

A. Description
1. Also called mucocutaneous lymph node syndrome. It is an acute systemic inflammatory illness.
2. The cause is unknown but may be associated with an infection by an organism or toxin.
 3. Cardiac involvement is the most serious complication. Aneurysms can develop.

B. Data collection
1. Acute stage
   a. Fever
   b. Conjunctival hyperemia
   c. Red throat
   d. Swollen hands, rash, and enlargement of the cervical lymph nodes
2. Subacute stage
   a. Cracking lips and fissures
   b. Desquamation of the skin on the tips of the fingers and toes
   c. Joint pain
   d. Cardiac manifestations
   e. Thrombocytosis
3. Convalescent stage: Child appears normal, but signs of inflammation may be present.

C. Interventions
1. Monitor temperature frequently.
2. Check heart sounds and the heart rate and rhythm.
3. Check extremities for edema, redness, and desquamation.
4. Examine eyes for conjunctivitis.
5. Monitor mucous membranes for inflammation.
6. Monitor strict I&O.
7. Administer soft foods and liquids that are neither too hot nor too cold.
8. Weigh the child daily.

9. Provide passive range-of-motion exercises to facilitate joint movement.
10. Administer acetylsalicylic acid as prescribed for its antipyretic and antiplatelet effects (additional anticoagulation may be necessary if aneurysms are present).
11. Intravenous immunoglobulin may be prescribed to reduce the duration of the fever and the incidence of coronary artery lesions and aneurysms; intravenous immunoglobulin is a blood product, so blood precautions when administering it are warranted.
12. Reinforce parent education (see Box 33.6).

BOX 33.6 **Parent Education for Kawasaki Disease**

- Follow-up care is essential to recovery.
- The signs/symptoms of Kawasaki disease include the following:
  - Irritability that may last for up to 2 months after the onset of symptoms.
  - Peeling of the hands and feet.
  - Pain in the joints that may persist for several weeks.
  - Stiffness in the morning, after naps, and in cold temperatures.
- Record the temperature (because fever is expected) until child has been afebrile for several days.
- Notify the primary health care provider (PHCP) if the temperature is 101°F (38.3°C) or higher.
- Salicylates such as acetylsalicylic acid may be prescribed.
- Signs of aspirin toxicity include tinnitus, headache, vertigo, bruising; do not administer aspirin or aspirin-containing products if child has been exposed to chickenpox or the flu.
- Signs/symptoms of bleeding include epistaxis (nosebleeds), hemoptysis (coughing up blood), hematemesis (vomiting up blood), hematuria (blood in urine), melena (blood in stool), and bruises on body.
- Signs/symptoms of cardiac complications include chest pain or tightness (older children), cool and pale extremities, abdominal pain, nausea and vomiting, irritability, restlessness, and uncontrollable crying.
- Child would avoid contact sports, if age appropriate, if taking aspirin or anticoagulants.
- Avoid administration of measles, mumps, and rubella (MMR) or varicella vaccine to the child for 11 months after intravenous immunoglobulin therapy, if appropriate.
- Notify the PHCP if any signs of complication occur.

WHAT WOULD YOU DO?

Answer: The nurse would monitor respiratory status closely in a child who has a congenital heart defect. If respiratory effort is increased, the nurse needs to place the child in a reverse Trendelenburg position, elevating the head and upper body, to decrease the work of breathing. In addition, the child needs to sleep with the head elevated on several pillows and would remain in a semi- or high Fowler's position during waking hours.

PRACTICE QUESTIONS

1. The nurse reviews the record of a child who was just seen by the primary health care provider (PHCP). The PHCP has documented a diagnosis of suspected aortic stenosis. Which specific sign/symptom of aortic stenosis would the nurse anticipate?
   1. Pallor
   2. Hyperactivity
   3. Activity intolerance
   4. Gastrointestinal disturbances

2. The nurse has reinforced homecare instructions to the parent of a child who is being discharged after cardiac surgery. Which statement by the parent indicates the **need for further teaching**?
   1. "A balance of rest and exercise is important."
   2. "I can apply lotion or powder to the incision if it is itchy."
   3. "Activities during which the child could fall need to be avoided for 2 to 4 weeks."
   4. "Large crowds of people need to be avoided for at least 2 weeks after this surgery."

3. The nurse is told that a child with rheumatic fever (RF) will be arriving to the nursing unit for admission. Which question would the nurse ask the family to elicit information specific to the development of RF?
   1. "Has the child complained of back pain?"
   2. "Has the child complained of headaches?"
   3. "Has the child had any nausea or vomiting?"
   4. "Has the child had a sore throat or a fever within the past 2 months?"

4. The nurse is providing instructions to a parent of a child with patent ductus arteriosus (PDA). Which statement by the parent would indicate a **need for further teaching**?
   1. "I know that my child will outgrow this problem, just give him time."
   2. "I know that I need to be alert for signs of heart failure with this defect until it is repaired."
   3. "The doctors tell me that my child has a heart murmur caused by the ductus not closing after birth."
   4. "As I understand it, my child may have to have his defect closed, either during a catheterization or by surgery."

5. The nurse assists with admitting a child with a diagnosis of acute stage Kawasaki disease. When obtaining the child's medical history, which manifestation is likely to be noted?
   1. Cracked lips
   2. A normal appearance
   3. Conjunctival hyperemia
   4. Desquamation of the skin

❖ 6. The nurse caring for an infant with congenital heart disease is monitoring the infant closely for signs of heart failure (HF). The nurse would observe for which **early** signs of HF? **Select all that apply.**
   - ☐ 1. Cough
   - ☐ 2. Irritability
   - ☐ 3. Scalp diaphoresis
   - ☐ 4. Tachypnea, tachycardia
   - ☐ 5. Slow and shallow breathing

7. The nurse was caring for an infant who had come to the nursing unit for observation and treatment of tetralogy of Fallot. The child suddenly becomes cyanotic and the oxygen saturation reading drops to 60%. The nurse would perform which action **first**?
   1. Assist to administer morphine sulfate.
   2. Place the child in a knee-chest position.
   3. Administer 100% oxygen by face mask.
   4. Prepare to administer intravenous fluids.

8. The nurse is monitoring the daily weight of an infant with heart failure (HF). Which finding alerts the nurse to suspect fluid accumulation and thus the need to notify the registered nurse?
   1. Bradypnea
   2. Diaphoresis
   3. Decreased blood pressure (BP)
   4. A weight gain of 1 lb in 1 day

9. The nurse provides homecare instructions to the parents of a child with heart failure regarding the procedure for the administration of digoxin. Which statement by a parent indicates the **need for further teaching**?
   1. "I will not mix the medication with food."
   2. "If more than one dose is missed, I will call the doctor."
   3. "I will take my child's pulse before administering the medication."
   4. "If my child vomits after medication administration, I will repeat the dose."

10. A primary health care provider has prescribed oxygen as needed for a 10-month-old infant with heart failure (HF). In which situation would the nurse administer the oxygen to the child?
    1. When the child is sleeping
    2. When changing the child's diapers
    3. When the mother is holding the child
    4. When drawing blood for electrolyte levels

Pediatric Nursing

ANSWERS

1. 3

Rationale: The child with aortic stenosis shows signs of activity intolerance, chest pain, and dizziness when standing for long periods. Pallor may be noted, but it is not specific to this type of disorder alone. Options 2 and 4 are not related to this disorder.

Test-Taking Strategy: Focus on the subject, a sign/symptom of aortic stenosis. It is necessary to know that activity intolerance is characteristic of aortic stenosis. Options 2 and 4 can be eliminated first because they are not associated with a cardiac disorder. To select from the remaining options, think about the pathophysiology of the disorder to direct you to the correct option.

2. 2

Rationale: The mother would be instructed that lotions and powders should not be applied to the incision site because these items can affect the skin integrity and the healing process. Options 1, 3, and 4 are accurate instructions regarding home care after cardiac surgery.

Test-Taking Strategy: Note the strategic words, *need for further teaching*. These words indicate a negative event query and ask you to select an option that is an incorrect statement. Using the general principles related to postoperative incisional site care will direct you to the correct option.

3. 4

Rationale: Rheumatic fever (RF) characteristically presents 2 to 6 weeks after an untreated or partially treated group A β-hemolytic streptococcal infection of the upper respiratory tract. Initially, the nurse determines whether the child has had a sore throat or an unexplained fever within the past 2 months. Options 1, 2, and 3 are unrelated to RF.

Test-Taking Strategy: Focus on the subject, the etiology associated with RF. Note the similarity between rheumatic "fever" in the question and the word *fever* in the correct option.

4. 1

Rationale: A patent ductus arteriosus (PDA) is caused by a failure of the ductus to close within the first weeks of life. The infant may be asymptomatic or show signs of heart failure. The defect may be closed during cardiac catheterization or may require surgery. A characteristic machine-like murmur is present with PDA.

Test-Taking Strategy: Note the strategic words, *need for further teaching*. These words indicate a negative event query and the need to select the incorrect statement by the parent. Think about the pathophysiology associated with PDA to assist in answering correctly.

5. 3

Rationale: During the acute stage of Kawasaki disease, the child presents with fever, conjunctival hyperemia, a red throat, swollen hands, a rash, and enlargement of the cervical lymph nodes. During the subacute stage, cracking lips and fissures, desquamation of the skin on the tips of the fingers and toes, joint pain, cardiac manifestations, and thrombocytosis occur. During the convalescent stage, the child appears normal, but signs of inflammation may be present.

Test-Taking Strategy: Focus on the subject, acute stage of Kawasaki disease. Think about the pathophysiology associated with this disorder. It is necessary to know the manifestations that occur in each stage to answer correctly.

❖ **6. 2, 3, 4**

Rationale: The early signs of HF include tachycardia, tachypnea, profuse scalp sweating, fatigue, irritability, sudden weight gain, and respiratory distress. A cough may occur with HF as a result of mucosal swelling and irritation, but it is not an early sign. Slow and shallow breathing is not associated with heart failure.

Test-Taking Strategy: Note the strategic word, *early*. Think about the physiology and the effects on the heart when fluid overload occurs. These concepts will assist with directing you to the correct option.

7. 2

Rationale: The child who is cyanotic with oxygen saturations dropping to 60% is having a hypercyanotic episode. Hypercyanotic episodes often occur among infants with tetralogy of Fallot. If a hypercyanotic episode occurs, the infant is placed in a knee-chest position immediately. The knee-chest position improves systemic arterial oxygen saturation by decreasing venous return so that smaller amounts of highly saturated blood reach the heart. Additional interventions include administering 100% oxygen by face mask, morphine sulfate, and intravenous fluids, as prescribed.

Test-Taking Strategy: Note the strategic word, *first*. Recall the priority nursing actions to take if a hypercyanotic spell occurs in an infant. Read each option carefully. Think about the steps to take and which one needs to be done first; this will assist you in selecting the correct first action.

8. 4

Rationale: A weight gain of 0.5 kg (1 lb) in 1 day is a result of the accumulation of fluid. The nurse would monitor the urine output, monitor for evidence of facial or peripheral edema, check the lung sounds, and report the weight gain. Tachypnea and an increased BP would occur with fluid accumulation. Diaphoresis is a sign of HF, but it is not specific to fluid accumulation and it usually occurs with exertional activities.

Test-Taking Strategy: Focus on the subject, fluid accumulation. Note the relationship between fluid accumulation in the question and weight gain in the correct option.

9. 4

Rationale: The parents need to be instructed that if the child vomits after the digoxin is administered, they are not to repeat the dose. Options 1, 2, and 3 are accurate instructions regarding the administration of this medication. Additionally, the parents need to be instructed that if a dose is missed and it is not noticed until 4 hours or more later, the dose should not be administered.

Test-Taking Strategy: Note the strategic words, *need for further teaching*. These words indicate a negative event query and ask you to select an option that is an incorrect statement. Principles related to the administration of medication to children will assist you with eliminating option 1. General knowledge regarding digoxin administration will assist you with eliminating option 3. From the remaining options, select option 4 over option 2 because if the child vomits, it would be difficult to determine whether the medication was absorbed by the body.

10. 4
Rationale: Oxygen administration may be prescribed for the infant with HF for stressful periods, especially during bouts of crying or invasive procedures. Drawing blood is an invasive procedure that would likely cause the child to cry.
Test-Taking Strategy: Focus on the subject, care of the infant with heart failure. Read the options and recall the situations that would place stress and an increased workload on the heart. This concept will direct you to the correct option.

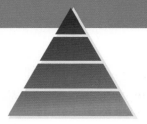

Pediatric Nursing

CHAPTER **34**

Renal and Urinary Problems

PRIORITY CONCEPTS Elimination; Inflammation

WHAT WOULD YOU DO?

The nurse notes that there has been no urinary output for 1 hour in an infant who underwent surgical repair of hypospadias. What would the nurse do?
Answer is located on p. 428.

I. Urinary Tract Infection (UTI)
A. Bacterial invasion of the urinary tract from flora from the skin or gastrointestinal tract
B. Uncircumcised infants are more likely to develop a UTI than circumcised infants.
C. Hygiene (wiping from front to back) is important in children to prevent this problem.
D. Children may experience asymptomatic bacteriuria, so if there is a suspicion of infection in the urinary tract they should be screened and treated accordingly.
E. See Chapter 51 for additional information.

II. Glomerulonephritis
A. Description
  1. Glomerulonephritis is a term that refers to a group of kidney disorders characterized by inflammatory injuries in the glomerulus, most of which are caused by an immunological reaction.
  2. Results in proliferative and inflammatory changes within the glomerular structure
  3. Destruction, inflammation, and sclerosis of the glomeruli of the kidneys may occur.
  4. Inflammation of the glomeruli results from an antigen–antibody reaction produced by an infection elsewhere in the body.
  5. Loss of kidney function develops.
B. Causes
  1. Immunological disease
  2. Autoimmune disease
  3. Antecedent group A β-hemolytic streptococcal infection of the pharynx or skin

  4. History of pharyngitis or tonsillitis 2 to 3 weeks before the onset of symptoms
C. Types
  1. Acute: Occurs 2 to 3 weeks after a streptococcal infection
  2. Chronic: May occur after the acute phase or slowly over time
D. Complications
  1. Kidney failure
  2. Hypertensive encephalopathy
  3. Seizure
  4. Pulmonary edema
  5. Heart failure
E. Data collection
  1. Periorbital and facial edema that is more prominent in the morning
  2. Anorexia
  3. Decreased urinary output
  4. Cloudy, smoky, brown-colored urine (hematuria)
  5. Pallor, irritability, and lethargy
  6. In the older child, headaches, abdominal or flank pain, and dysuria
  7. Hypertension
  8. Proteinuria that produces a persistent and excessive foam in the urine
  9. Azotemia
  10. Increased blood urea nitrogen and creatinine levels
  11. Increased antistreptolysin O titer (used to diagnose disorders caused by streptococcal infections)
F. Interventions (see **Priority Nursing Actions**)
  1. Monitor vital signs, daily weight, intake and output (I&O), and characteristics of urine.
  2. Measure daily weight at the same time of the day, using the same scale, and wearing the same clothing.
  3. Limit activity; provide safety measures.
  4. Diet restrictions of sodium depend on the stage and severity of the disease, especially the extent of the edema; in addition, potassium may be restricted during periods of oliguria.

⚡ PRIORITY NURSING ACTIONS

Fluid Volume Overload in a Child with Glomerulonephritis

1. Check airway patency, vital signs, and weight.
2. Check for dyspnea, bounding rapid pulse, dysrhythmias, and hypertension.
3. Check for distended hand and neck veins.
4. Assess level of generalized edema (anasarca) and check amount of urinary output.
5. Notify the primary health care provider (PHCP) as directed by the registered nurse and assist with carrying out prescriptions, including water and sodium restriction and the administration of diuretics.

5. Monitor for complications (i.e., kidney failure, hypertensive encephalopathy, seizure, pulmonary edema, and heart failure).
6. Assist with the administration of diuretics (if significant edema and fluid overload are present), antihypertensives (for hypertension), and antibiotics (to the child with evidence of persistent streptococcal infection), as prescribed.
7. Initiate seizure precautions and assist with the administration of anticonvulsants, as prescribed, for seizures associated with hypertensive encephalopathy.

8. Reinforce instructions to the parents to report signs of bloody urine, headache, or edema.

9. Reinforce instructions to the parents that the child needs to obtain appropriate and adequate treatment for infections, specifically for a sore throat, upper respiratory infection, and skin infection.

⚠️ Measuring the daily weight and monitoring for weight changes are the most useful and effective methods for determining fluid balance.

III. Nephrotic Syndrome

A. Description
   1. A kidney disorder characterized by massive proteinuria, hypoalbuminemia (hypoproteinemia), and edema (Fig. 34.1)
   2. The primary objectives of therapeutic management are to reduce the excretion of urinary protein, maintain protein-free urine, reduce edema, prevent infection, and minimize complications.
B. Data collection (Box 34.1)

⚠️ The classic manifestations of nephrotic syndrome are massive proteinuria, hypoalbuminemia, and edema.

C. Interventions
   1. Monitor the vital signs, I&O, and daily weights.
   2. Monitor the urine for specific gravity and protein.
   3. Monitor for edema.
   4. Nutrition: A regular diet without added salt is prescribed if the child is in remission. Sodium is restricted during periods of massive edema (fluids may also be restricted).
   5. Corticosteroid therapy is prescribed as soon as the diagnosis has been determined; monitor the child closely for signs of infection and other adverse effects of corticosteroids (see Chapter 44).
   6. Immunosuppressant therapy may be prescribed to reduce the relapse rate and to induce long-term remission, or if the child is unresponsive to corticosteroid therapy, immunosuppressant therapy may be administered in conjunction with the corticosteroid.
   7. Diuretics may be prescribed to reduce edema.
   8. Plasma expanders such as salt-poor human albumin may be prescribed for the severely edematous child.
   9. Reinforce instructions to the parents about testing the urine for protein, medication administration, the side and adverse effects of the medication(s), and the general care of the child.
   10. Reinforce instructions to the parents regarding the signs of infection and the need to avoid contact with other children who may be infectious.

IV. Hemolytic-Uremic Syndrome

A. Description
   1. Thought to be associated with bacterial toxins, chemicals, and viruses that cause acute kidney injury in children
   2. Occurs primarily among infants and small children between the ages of 6 months and 5 years
   3. Clinical features include acquired hemolytic anemia, thrombocytopenia, kidney injury, and central nervous system symptoms.
B. Data collection
   1. Triad of anemia, thrombocytopenia, and renal failure (Box 34.2)
   2. Proteinuria, hematuria, and the presence of urinary casts
   3. Blood urea nitrogen and serum creatinine levels are elevated; hemoglobin and hematocrit levels are decreased.
C. Interventions
   1. Hemodialysis or peritoneal dialysis may be prescribed if the child is anuric (dialysate solution is prescribed to meet the child's electrolyte needs).
   2. Strict monitoring of fluid balance is necessary. Fluid restrictions may be prescribed if the child is anuric.
   3. Institute measures to prevent infection.
   4. Provide adequate nutrition.
   5. Other treatments may include medications to treat manifestations and the administration of blood products to treat severe anemia (administered with caution to prevent fluid overload).

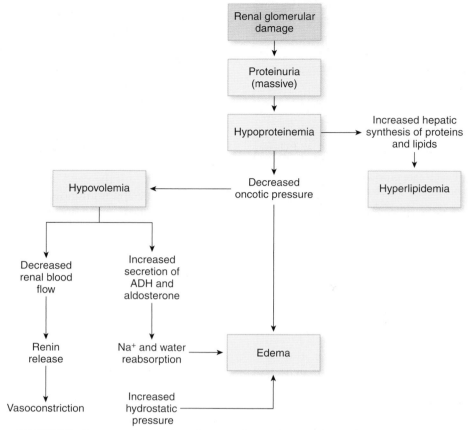

FIGURE 34.1 Sequence of events in nephrotic syndrome. *ADH*, antidiuretic hormone; *Na+*, sodium.

| BOX 34.1 | **Findings in Nephrotic Syndrome** |

- The child gains weight.
- Periorbital and facial edema are most prominent in the morning.
- Leg, ankle, labial, or scrotal edema occur.
- Urine output decreases, and the urine is dark and frothy.
- Ascites (fluid in the abdominal cavity)
- Blood pressure is normal or slightly decreased.
- Lethargy, anorexia, and pallor occur.
- Massive proteinuria
- Decreased serum protein (hypoproteinemia) and elevated serum lipid levels

---

| BOX 34.2 | **Manifestations of Hemolytic-Uremic Syndrome** |

- Vomiting
- Irritability
- Lethargy
- Marked pallor
- Hemorrhagic manifestations: bruising, petechiae, jaundice, bloody diarrhea
- Oliguria or anuria
- Central nervous system involvement: seizures, stupor, and coma

---

V. Enuresis

A. Description

  1. Enuresis refers to a condition in which a child is unable to control bladder function, even though the child has reached an age at which control of voiding is expected or the child has successfully completed a bladder control program.

  2. A child does not have control over this condition.

B. Primary enuresis: Wetting that occurs in a child that has not fully mastered toilet training

C. Nighttime (nocturnal) enuresis

  1. Nighttime (nocturnal) enuresis is bedwetting in a child who has never been dry for extended periods.

  2. Most children eventually outgrow bedwetting without therapeutic intervention.

  3. The child is unable to sense a full bladder and does not awaken to void.

  4. The child may have delayed maturation of the central nervous system.

  5. The child should be evaluated for any pathological causes before the diagnosis of nighttime (nocturnal) enuresis is made.

D. Daytime (diurnal) enuresis: Bedwetting that occurs during the day

E. Secondary enuresis

  1. The onset of wetting occurs after a period of established urinary continence.

2. If the child complains of dysuria, urgency, or frequency, the child needs to be assessed for a UTI.

F. Interventions

1. A urinalysis and urine culture may be prescribed to rule out infection or an existing disorder.
2. Assist the family with identifying a treatment plan that best fits the needs of the child.
3. Limit fluid intake at night and encourage the child to void just before going to bed.
4. Provide reward systems for dryness as appropriate for the child.
5. Incorporate behavioral conditioning techniques such as timed voiding program every two hours.
6. Medications may be prescribed to treat enuresis.
7. Encourage follow-up to determine the effectiveness of the treatment.

VI. Cryptorchidism

A. Description: Occurs when one or both testes fail to descend through the inguinal canal and into the scrotal sac

B. Data collection: Testes not palpable or easily guided into the scrotum

C. Interventions

1. Monitor during the first 6 months of life to determine whether spontaneous descent occurs.
2. Surgical correction is commonly done at 6 months of age and before 12 months of age depending on the pediatric surgeon preference (if the testes do not descend spontaneously).
3. Monitor for bleeding and infection postoperatively.
4. Reinforce instructions to the parents regarding postoperative homecare measures, including preventing infection, pain control, and activity restrictions.
5. Provide an opportunity for parental counseling if the parents are concerned about the future fertility of the child.

VII. Epispadias and Hypospadias (Fig. 34.2)

A. Description: Congenital defects that involve the abnormal placement of the urethral orifice of the penis; these anatomical defects can lead to the easy entry of bacteria into the urine.

B. Data collection

1. Epispadias: Urethral orifice is located on the dorsal surface of the penis; often occurs with exstrophy of the bladder (see VIII. Bladder Exstrophy).
2. Hypospadias: Urethral orifice is located along the ventral surface of the penis, anywhere from the scrotum to the glans.

C. Surgical interventions: Performed before the age of toilet training, preferably between 6 and 12 months of age

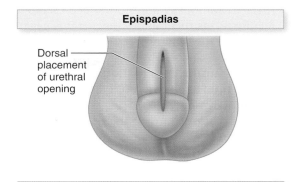

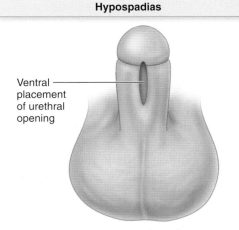

FIGURE 34.2 Epispadias and hypospadias are genital anomalies in which the urethral opening is above or below its normal location on the glans of the penis.

 Circumcision is not performed on a newborn with epispadias or hypospadias. Although there are other surgical techniques used to repair these defects, the pediatric surgeon may prefer using the foreskin for surgical reconstruction of the defect.

D. Postoperative interventions for hypospadias

1. The child will have a dressing and may have some type of urinary diversion, stent (used to maintain the patency of the urethral opening), or catheter while the meatus is healing (dressing changes are not done unless specifically prescribed; check surgeon's orders).
2. Monitor vital signs.
3. Encourage fluid intake to maintain adequate urine output and to maintain the patency of the stent if present.
4. Monitor I&O and urine for cloudiness or a foul odor.
5. Notify the registered nurse (RN) if there is no urinary drainage for 1 hour, because this may indicate kinks in the system or obstruction by sediment.
6. Assist to provide pain medication or medication to relieve bladder spasms (anticholinergic), as prescribed.

7. Assist to administer antibiotics, as prescribed.

8. Reinforce instructions to the parents regarding the care of the urinary diversion, stent, or catheter if present.

9. Reinforce instructions to the parents to avoid giving the child a tub bath until the stent, if present, is removed.

10. Reinforce instructions to the parents about fluid intake, medication administration, signs and symptoms of infection, and the need to follow-up with the surgeon for dressing removal approximately 4 days after surgery.

VIII. Bladder Exstrophy

A. Description

1. A congenital anomaly characterized by the extrusion of the urinary bladder to the outside of the body through a defect in the lower abdominal wall

2. Cause is unknown; it is possibly a combination of genetic and environmental risk factors during pregnancy.

3. The condition can include specific defects of the abdominal wall, bladder, genitals, pelvic bones, rectum, and anus.

4. Children with bladder exstrophy will also experience vesicoureteral reflux, a condition in which urine flows backwards into the ureters to the kidney; epispadias is also noted in males.

5. Treatment requires surgical management and occurs in a series of staged reconstructions to repair the affected organs, muscles, and bones.

6. Initial surgery for the closure of the abdominal defect is normally planned within the first few days of life.

7. Goals of subsequent surgeries are to reconstruct the bladder and genitalia and enable the child to achieve urinary continence.

B. Data collection

1. Exposed bladder mucosa and epispadias in males
2. Defects of the abdominal wall
3. Vesicoureteral reflux
4. Defects of the rectum and anus

C. Interventions

1. Monitor urinary output.
2. Monitor for signs of urinary tract or wound infection.
3. Maintain the integrity of the exposed bladder mucosa.

4. Prevent the bladder tissue from drying while allowing for the drainage of urine until surgical closure is performed. Immediately after birth, as prescribed, the exposed bladder is covered with a sterile, nonadherent dressing to protect it until closure can be performed.

5. Laboratory values and urinalysis are monitored to assess for kidney function.

6. Assist to administer antibiotics, as prescribed.

7. Provide emotional support to the parents and encourage the verbalization of their fears and concerns.

⚠ Applying petroleum jelly to the bladder mucosa is avoided because it tends to dry out, adhere to the bladder mucosa, and damage the delicate tissues when the dressing is removed.

IX. Sexually Transmitted Infections (STIs)

A. Screening for certain STIs should be done for certain children and adolescents. See http://www.aap.org/en-us/advocacy-and-policy/aap-health-initiatives/adolescent-sexual-health/Pages/Sexually-Transmitted-Infections.aspx for specific recommendations.

B. Refer to Chapter 23 for more detailed information on STIs.

WHAT WOULD YOU DO?

Answer: Following surgical repair for hypospadias, the urinary output is monitored closely. The nurse would notify the registered nurse (RN) if there is no urinary output for 1 hour because this may indicate kinks in the urinary diversion or stent placed during the surgical procedure or an obstruction caused by sediment. The RN will perform an assessment and contact the surgeon if necessary.

PRACTICE QUESTIONS

❖ **1.** The nurse is assigned to care for a child who is suspected of having glomerulonephritis. The nurse reviews the child's record and notes that which findings are associated with the diagnosis of glomerulonephritis? **Select all that apply.**

- ❑ 1. Headache
- ❑ 2. Hypotension
- ❑ 3. Red-brown urine
- ❑ 4. Periorbital edema
- ❑ 5. Increased urine output
- ❑ 6. A low blood urea nitrogen (BUN) level

❖ **2.** A child is admitted to the hospital with a probable diagnosis of nephrotic syndrome. Which findings would the nurse expect to observe? **Select all that apply.**

- ❑ 1. Ascites
- ❑ 2. Anorexia
- ❑ 3. Weight loss
- ❑ 4. Proteinuria
- ❑ 5. Decreased serum lipids
- ❑ 6. Periorbital and facial edema

❖ **3.** The nurse is planning care for a child with hemolytic-uremic syndrome (HUS). The child has been anuric and will be receiving peritoneal dialysis treatment. The nurse would plan to include which interventions in the care of the child? **Select all that apply.**
   ❑ 1. Provide adequate nutrition.
   ❑ 2. Restriction of fluids, as prescribed
   ❑ 3. Institute measures to prevent infection.
   ❑ 4. Monitoring the arteriovenous (AV) fistula
   ❑ 5. Administer blood products to treat severe anemia.
   ❑ 6. Anticipate the child will have central nervous system involvement.

4. The nurse is assisting with gathering admission assessment data on a 2-year-old child who has been diagnosed with nephrotic syndrome. The nurse collects data knowing that which is a common characteristic associated with nephrotic syndrome?
   1. Hypotension
   2. Generalized edema
   3. Increased urinary output
   4. Frank, bright red blood in the urine

5. The child with cryptorchidism is being discharged after orchiopexy, which was performed on an outpatient basis. The nurse would reinforce instructions to the parents about which **priority** care measure?
   1. Measuring intake and output
   2. Administering anticholinergics
   3. Preventing infection at the surgical site
   4. Applying cold, wet compresses to the surgical site

6. The nurse is reinforcing discharge instructions to the parent of a 2-year-old child who has had an orchiopexy to correct cryptorchidism. Which statement by the parent indicates a **need for further teaching**?
   1. "I'll check his temperature."
   2. "I'll give him medication so he'll be comfortable."
   3. "I'll let him decide when to return to his play activities."
   4. "I'll check his voiding to be sure there are no problems."

7. The nurse collects a urine specimen preoperatively from a child with epispadias who is scheduled for surgical repair. The nurse reviews the child's record for the laboratory results of the urine test and would **most likely** expect to note which finding?
   1. Hematuria
   2. Bacteriuria
   3. Glucosuria
   4. Proteinuria

8. An 18-month-old child is being discharged after surgical repair of hypospadias. Which postoperative nursing care measure would the nurse stress to the parents as they prepare to take this child home?
   1. Leave diapers off to allow the site to heal.
   2. Avoid tub baths until the stent has been removed.
   3. Encourage toilet training to ensure that the flow of urine is normal.
   4. Restrict the fluid intake to reduce urinary output for the first few days.

9. The parents of a newborn have been told that their child was born with bladder exstrophy and the parents ask the nurse about this condition. Which response would the nurse give to the parents about bladder exstrophy?
   1. "It is a hereditary disorder that occurs in every other generation."
   2. "It is caused by the use of medications taken by the mother during pregnancy."
   3. "It is a condition in which the urinary bladder is abnormally located in the pelvic cavity."
   4. "It is an extrusion of the urinary bladder to the outside of the body through a defect in the lower abdominal wall."

10. A parent with a 6 year-old-child diagnosed with enuresis discusses with the nurse the measures that are being taken to help her child. Which statement by the parent indicates a **need for further teaching**?
   1. "I make sure that my child goes potty before going to bed."
   2. "I will praise my child and think of a reward for him for staying dry."
   3. "I take away privileges such as TV time when the bed is wet in the morning."
   4. "I make sure that my child does not have anything to drink 2 hours before bedtime."

ANSWERS

❖ 1. 1, 3, 4

Rationale: Signs of glomerulonephritis include headache; abdominal or flank pain; gross hematuria resulting in dark, smoky, cola-colored or red-brown urine; and periorbital edema or facial edema. Clients are hypertensive and have decreased urine output. BUN levels may be elevated.

Test-Taking Strategy: Focus on the subject, the manifestations of glomerulonephritis. Eliminate option 2 first because hypertension, not hypotension, is a classic symptom of glomerulonephritis. Recalling that decreased urine output and elevated BUN levels are associated with this condition will assist with directing you to the correct options.

❖ 2. 1, 2, 4, 6

Rationale: Nephrotic syndrome is a kidney disorder that is characterized by massive proteinuria, hypoalbuminemia, periorbital and facial edema, ascites, elevated serum lipids, and anorexia. The urine volume is decreased and the urine is dark and frothy in appearance. The child with this condition gains weight.

Test-Taking Strategy: Note the child's diagnosis and think about the subject, nephrotic syndrome and its associated characteristics, to answer the question. Think about the pathophysiology associated with this disorder to answer correctly. Remember it is characterized by massive proteinuria, hypoalbuminemia, periorbital and facial edema, weight gain, ascites, elevated serum lipids, anorexia, and pallor.

❖ 3. 1, 2, 3, 5, 6

Rationale: HUS is thought to be associated with bacterial toxins, chemicals, and viruses that cause acute kidney injury in children. A child with HUS who is undergoing peritoneal dialysis for the treatment of anuria will be prescribed fluid restrictions. The treatment also involves providing adequate nutrition, preventing infection, and anticipating central nervous system (CNS) involvement which may include seizure, stupor, and coma. Blood products may be prescribed to treat severe anemia but is administered with caution to prevent fluid overload. Peritoneal dialysis does not require an AV fistula (only hemodialysis does).

Test-Taking Strategy: Focus on the subject, hemolytic-uremic syndrome, and recall your knowledge of the care of a client with this diagnosis. Also focus on the data in the question. Noting the word *peritoneal* will assist you with eliminating option 4. From the remaining options, remember that because the child is anuric, fluids will be restricted.

4. 2

Rationale: Nephrotic syndrome is defined as massive proteinuria, hypoalbuminemia, and edema. The urine is dark, foamy, and frothy, but microscopic hematuria may be present. Frank, bright red blood in the urine does not occur. Urine output is decreased and the blood pressure is normal or slightly decreased.

Test-Taking Strategy: Focus on the subject, the characteristics of nephrotic syndrome. Eliminate option 3 first because urine output is likely to be decreased in a client with a renal disorder. From the remaining options, associate edema with nephrotic syndrome, because this will be helpful to you if you encounter a similar question.

5. 3

Rationale: The most common complications associated with orchiopexy are bleeding and infection. The parents are instructed in postoperative homecare measures, including the prevention of infection, pain control, and activity restrictions. The measurement of intake and output is not required. Anticholinergics are prescribed for the relief of bladder spasms; they are not necessary after orchiopexy. Cold, wet compresses are not prescribed. The moisture from a wet compress presents a potential for infection.

Test-Taking Strategy: Note the strategic word, *priority*. Use Maslow's Hierarchy of Needs theory to answer the question. Of the options presented, the potential for infection is the physiological priority.

6. 3

Rationale: All vigorous activities need to be restricted for 2 weeks after surgery to promote healing and prevent injury. This will prevent dislodging of the suture, which is internal. Normally, 2-year-old children will want to be very active. Therefore, allowing the child to decide when to return to his play activities may prevent healing and cause injury. The parents would be taught to monitor the child's temperature; provide analgesics, as needed; and monitor the urine output.

Test-Taking Strategy: Note the strategic words, *need for further teaching*. These words indicate a negative event query and ask you to select an option that is an incorrect statement. Option 1 is an important action for recognizing signs of infection. Option 2 is appropriate for keeping pain to a minimum. Option 4 monitors the voiding pattern, which is also important after this type of surgery.

7. 2

Rationale: Epispadias is a congenital defect that involves the abnormal placement of the urethral orifice of the penis. In clients with this condition, the urethral opening is located anywhere on the dorsum of the penis. This anatomical characteristic leads to the easy access of bacterial entry into the urine. Options 1, 3, and 4 are not characteristically noted with this condition.

Test-Taking Strategy: Note the strategic words, *most likely*. Use your knowledge regarding the anatomical characteristics of epispadias to answer the question. Options 1, 3, and 4 do not relate to the potential for infection, which can be present with this condition.

8. 2

Rationale: After hypospadias repair, the parents are instructed to avoid giving the child a tub bath until the stent has been removed to prevent infection. Rather, sponge baths are given. Diapers are placed on the child to prevent the contamination of the surgical site. Toilet training would not be an issue during this stressful period. Fluids need to be encouraged to maintain hydration.

Test-Taking Strategy: Focus on the subject, homecare instructions following surgical repair of hypospadias. Option 3 is eliminated first because toilet training should not be initiated during times of stress, such as after surgery. Eliminate option 1 because this action can cause the contamination of the surgical site. Option 4 is inappropriate because fluids need to be encouraged rather than restricted.

9. 4

Rationale: Bladder exstrophy is a congenital anomaly that is characterized by the extrusion of the urinary bladder to the outside of the body through a defect in the lower abdominal wall. The cause is unknown and there is a higher incidence among males. Options 1, 2, and 3 are not characteristics of this disorder.

Test-Taking Strategy: Focus on the subject, the characteristics of bladder exstrophy. If you are unfamiliar with this condition, note the relationship of the word *exstrophy* in the name of the disorder to the word *extrusion* in the correct option; this would remind you that this condition is located *external* to the body.

10. 3

Rationale: Praising the child and providing a reward system suited for the child is appropriate and is not a punitive system to treat enuresis. Taking privileges away such as TV time is inappropriate and a punitive action. Limiting fluid intake at night and encouraging the child to void just before going to bed are effective interventions.

Test-Taking Strategy: Note the strategic words, *need for further teaching*. These words indicate a negative event query and ask you to select an option that is an incorrect statement. Options 1, 2, and 4 can be eliminated by remembering the interventions used to treat enuresis.

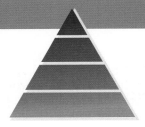

CHAPTER **35**

Neurological and Cognitive Problems

PRIORITY CONCEPTS Intracranial Regulation; Safety

WHAT WOULD YOU DO?

The nurse notes signs of increased intracranial pressure (ICP) in a child who has undergone insertion of a ventriculoperitoneal shunt for the treatment of hydrocephalus. What would the nurse do?
Answer is located on p. 439.

I. Cerebral Palsy

A. Description
1. A disorder characterized by impaired movement and posture resulting from an abnormality in the extrapyramidal or pyramidal motor system
2. The most common clinical type is spastic cerebral palsy, which represents an upper motor neuron type of muscle weakness.
3. Less common types of cerebral palsy are athetoid, ataxic, and mixed.

B. Data collection
1. Extreme irritability and crying
2. Feeding difficulties
3. Abnormal motor performance
4. Alterations of muscle tone; stiff and rigid arms or legs
5. Delayed developmental milestones
6. Persistence of primitive infantile reflexes (e.g., Moro, tonic neck) after 6 months (most primitive reflexes disappear by 3–4 months of age)
7. Abnormal posturing (e.g., opisthotonic [exaggerated arching of the back]) (Fig. 35.1)
8. Seizure may occur.

C. Interventions
1. The goals of management are early recognition and intervention to maximize the child's abilities.
2. A multidisciplinary team approach is implemented to meet the many needs of the child.
3. Therapeutic management includes physical therapy, occupational therapy, speech therapy, education, and recreation.

4. Determine the child's developmental level and intelligence.
5. Encourage early intervention and participation in school programs is encouraged.
6. Prepare for using mobilizing devices to help prevent or reduce deformities.
7. Encourage communication and interaction with the child on his or her developmental age rather than his or her chronological age level.
8. Provide a safe environment by removing sharp objects, using a protective helmet if the child falls frequently, and implementing seizure precautions, if necessary.
9. Provide safe, appropriate toys for the child's age and developmental level.
10. Position the child upright after meals.
11. Medications may be prescribed to relieve muscle spasms, which cause intense pain; antiseizure medications may also be prescribed.
12. Provide the parents with information about the disorder and treatment plan; encourage support groups for parents.

II. Head Injury

A. Description
1. Head injury is the pathological result of any mechanical force to the skull, scalp, meninges, or brain (Fig. 35.2).
   a. Open head injury occurs when there is a fracture of the skull or a penetration of the skull by an object.
   b. Closed head injury is the result of blunt trauma. It is more serious because of the chance of increased intracranial pressure (ICP) in a "closed" vault. This type of injury can also be caused by shaken baby syndrome.
2. Manifestations depend on the type of injury and the subsequent amount of increased ICP.

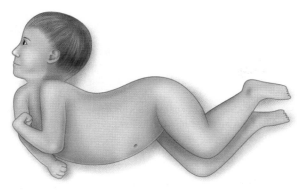

FIGURE 35.1 Abnormal posturing: Opisthotonos.

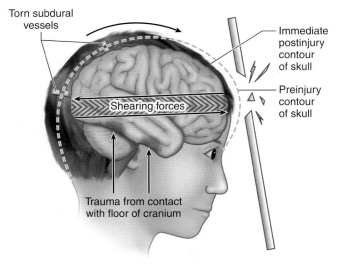

FIGURE 35.2 Mechanical distortion of cranium during closed head injury.

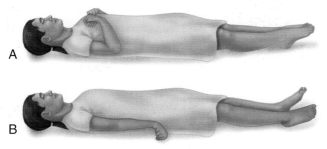

FIGURE 35.3 (A) Decorticate (flexion) posturing. (B) Decerebrate (extension) posturing.

fisted, and the lower extremities are extended and adducted; seen with severe dysfunction of the cerebral cortex (Fig. 35.3).

 f. Decerebrate (extension) posturing: Rigid extension and pronation of the arms and the legs; a sign of dysfunction at the level of the midbrain (see Fig. 35.3)

 g. Cheyne-Stokes respirations

 h. Coma

C. Interventions

  Immobilize the neck and spine after a head injury if a cervical or other spinal injury is suspected. When a spinal cord injury is ruled out, elevate the head of the bed 15 to 30 degrees, if not contraindicated and as prescribed, to facilitate venous drainage.

 1. Monitor the airway and administer oxygen as prescribed.

 2. Check injuries. (Refer to Chapter 55 for information on spinal cord injuries.)

 3. Position the child so that the head is maintained midline to avoid jugular vein compression, which can increase ICP.

 4. Monitor vital signs and neurological function (monitor level of consciousness closely).

 5. Notify the primary health care provider (PHCP) if signs of increased ICP occur.

 6. Keep stimuli to a minimum; attempt to minimize crying in the infant.

 7. Sedating medications are withheld during the acute phase of the injury so that any change in level of consciousness can be assessed.

 8. Initiate seizure precautions (Box 35.1).

 9. Monitor for decreased responsiveness to pain (a significant sign of altered level of consciousness).

 10. Maintain an NPO (nothing by mouth) status or provide clear liquids, if prescribed, until it is determined that vomiting will not occur.

 11. Assist with monitoring prescribed intravenous fluids carefully to avoid increasing any cerebral edema and to minimize the possibility of overhydration.

 12. Monitor for a fluid or electrolyte alteration (could indicate injury to the hypothalamus or posterior pituitary).

 B. Data collection: Increased ICP

  The child's level of consciousness provides the earliest indication of an improvement or deterioration of the neurological condition.

 1. Early signs

  a. Slight change in vital signs

  b. Slight change in level of consciousness

  c. Infant: Irritable, high-pitched cry, bulging fontanel, increased head circumference, dilated scalp veins, Macewen sign (cracked-pot sound on percussion of the head), setting-sun sign (sclera visible above the iris)

  d. Child: Headache, nausea, vomiting, visual disturbance (diplopia), seizure

 2. Late signs

  a. Decrease in level of consciousness

  b. Bradycardia

  c. Decreased motor and sensory responses

  d. Alteration in pupil size and reactivity

  e. Decorticate (flexion) posturing: Adduction of the arms at the shoulders; arms are flexed on the chest with the wrists flexed and the hands

- Raise the side rails when the child is sleeping or resting.
- Pad the side rails and other hard objects.
- Place a waterproof mattress or pad on the bed or crib.
- Instruct the child to wear or carry medical identification.
- Instruct the child regarding precautions to take during potentially hazardous activities.
- Instruct the child to swim with a companion.
- Instruct the child to use a protective helmet and padding during bicycle riding, skateboarding, and inline skating.
- Alert caregivers to the need for any special precautions.

- Deep, rapid, or intermittent and gasping respirations
- Wide fluctuations or noticeable slowing of the pulse
- Widening pulse pressure or extreme fluctuations in blood pressure
- Sluggish, dilated, or unequal pupils
  Notify the registered nurse (RN) or primary health care provider (PHCP) immediately if these signs develop!

13. Check wounds and dressings for the presence of drainage and monitor for nose or ear drainage, which could indicate leakage of cerebrospinal fluid (CSF); if this is noted, notify the registered nurse (RN) immediately.
14. Assist to administer tepid sponge baths or place on a hypothermia blanket as prescribed if hyperthermia occurs.
15. Avoid suctioning through the nares because of the possibility of the catheter entering the brain through a fracture, which places the child at high risk for a secondary infection.
16. As prescribed, assist with the administration of medications such as acetaminophen for headache, anticonvulsants for seizures, and antibiotics if a laceration is present; prepare to administer prophylactic tetanus toxoid.
17. A corticosteroid or osmotic diuretic may be prescribed to reduce cerebral edema.
18. Monitor for signs of brainstem involvement (Box 35.2).
19. Monitor for signs of epidural hematoma: Asymmetrical pupils (one dilated, nonreactive pupil) may indicate a neurosurgical emergency that requires evacuation of the hematoma. Notify the RN immediately if this is noted.

⚠ Drainage from the nose or ear needs to be tested for the presence of glucose. Drainage that is positive for glucose (as tested with reagent strips) indicates leakage of CSF. The RN and PHCP would be notified immediately if the drainage tests positive for glucose.

III. Hydrocephalus

A. Description
   1. An imbalance of CSF absorption and production may be caused by a malformation, tumor, hemorrhage, an infection, or trauma.
   2. Results in head enlargement and increased ICP
B. Types
   1. Communicating
      a. Hydrocephalus occurs as a result of impaired absorption within the subarachnoid space.
      b. Obstruction of the CSF flow in the ventricular system does not occur.
   2. Noncommunicating: Obstruction of CSF flow in the ventricular system does occur.
C. Data collection
   1. Infant
      a. Increased head circumference
      b. Thin, widely separated bones of the head that produce a cracked-pot sound (Macewen's sign) on percussion
      c. Anterior fontanel that is tense, bulging, and nonpulsating; sutures will separate before fontanel bulging.
      d. Dilated scalp veins
      e. Frontal bossing
      f. "Setting sun" eyes
   2. Child
      a. Behavior changes (e.g., irritability, lethargy)
      b. Headache when awakening
      c. Nausea and vomiting
      d. Ataxia
      e. Nystagmus
   3. Late signs: A high, shrill cry and seizure
D. Surgical interventions
   1. The goal of surgery is to prevent further CSF accumulation by bypassing the blockage and draining the fluid from the ventricles to a location where it may be reabsorbed.
   2. In a ventriculoperitoneal shunt, the CSF drains into the peritoneal cavity from the lateral ventricle (Fig. 35.4).
   3. In a ventriculoatrial shunt, the CSF drains into the right atrium of the heart from the lateral ventricle, bypassing the obstruction. This is used for older children and those with pathological conditions of the abdomen.
   4. Shunt revision may be necessary as the child grows.
   5. An alternative to shunt placement is endoscopic third ventriculostomy, in which a small opening in the floor of the third ventricle is made that allows CSF to bypass the fourth ventricle and return to the circulation to be absorbed. This treatment may not be appropriate for some types of hydrocephalus.

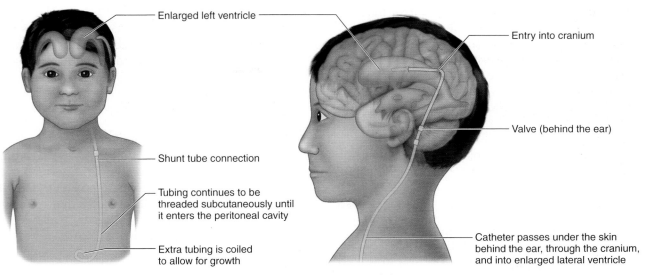

FIGURE 35.4 Ventriculoperitoneal shunt.

E. Preoperative interventions
  1. Monitor intake and output (I&O). Administer small frequent feedings as tolerated until a preoperative NPO status is prescribed.
  2. Reposition the head frequently and use special devices such as an egg crate mattress under the head to prevent pressure sores.
  3. Prepare the child and family for diagnostic procedures and surgery.

F. Postoperative interventions
  1. Monitor vital signs and neurological signs.
  2. Position the child on the unoperated side to prevent pressure on the shunt valve.
  3. Keep the child flat, as prescribed, to avoid the rapid reduction of intracranial fluid.
  4. Observe for increased ICP. If increased ICP occurs, elevate the head of the bed to 15 to 30 degrees to enhance gravity flow through the shunt and report the observations to the RN.
  5. Measure head circumference.
  6. Monitor for signs of infection. Check dressings for drainage.
  7. Monitor intake and output.
  8. Provide comfort measures. Assist with the administration of medications, as prescribed.
  9. Reinforce instructions to the parents regarding how to recognize shunt infection or malfunction.
  10. In an infant, irritability, a high shrill cry, lethargy, and feeding poorly may indicate shunt malfunction or infection.
  11. In a toddler, headache and a lack of appetite are the earliest common signs of shunt malfunction.
  12. In older children, the most valuable indicator of shunt malfunction is an alteration in the child's level of consciousness.

⚠ A high shrill cry in an infant can be a sign of increased ICP.

IV. Meningitis

A. Description
  1. Meningitis is an infectious process of the central nervous system that is caused by bacteria and viruses that may be acquired as a primary disease or as a result of complications of neurosurgery, trauma, infection of the sinuses or ears, or systemic infections.
  2. The diagnosis of bacterial meningitis is made by testing CSF obtained by lumbar puncture. The fluid of a child with meningitis is cloudy with increased pressure, increased white blood cell count, elevated protein, and decreased glucose levels.
  3. Bacterial meningitis can be caused by a variety of organisms, most commonly *Haemophilus influenza* type B, *Streptococcus pneumoniae*, or *Neisseria meningitides*; meningococcal meningitis occurs in epidemic form and can be transmitted by droplets from nasopharyngeal secretions.
  4. Viral meningitis is associated with viruses such as mumps, paramyxovirus, herpesvirus, and enterovirus.

B. Data collection
  1. Signs/symptoms vary, depending on the type, the age of the child, and the duration of the preceding illness.
  2. Fever, chills, and headache
  3. Vomiting and diarrhea
  4. Poor feeding or anorexia
  5. Nuchal rigidity
  6. Poor or high-shrill cry
  7. Altered level of consciousness (e.g., lethargy, irritability)
  8. Bulging anterior fontanel in the infant
  9. Positive Kernig's sign (the inability to extend the leg when the thigh is flexed anteriorly at the hip) and Brudzinski's sign (neck flexion causes

adduction and flexion movements of the lower extremities) in children and adolescents

10. Muscle or joint pain (meningococcal infection and *Haemophilus influenzae* infection)
11. Petechial or purpuric rashes (meningococcal infection)
12. Ear that chronically drains (pneumococcal meningitis)

C. Interventions
1. Provide respiratory isolation precautions and maintain them for at least 24 hours after antibiotics are initiated.
2. Assist to administer antibiotics and antipyretics as prescribed. (Antibiotics are administered as soon as they are prescribed after lumbar puncture.) Antiseizure medications may also be prescribed.
3. Assist with performing a neurological assessment and monitor for seizures. Monitor for the complication of inappropriate antidiuretic hormone secretion, which causes fluid retention (cerebral edema) and dilutional hyponatremia.
4. Monitor for any change in the level of consciousness and irritability.
5. Monitor for a purpuric or petechial rash and for signs of thromboemboli.
6. Monitor nutritional status; monitor I&O.
7. Monitor for hearing loss.
8. Determine close contacts of the child with meningitis, because the contacts will need prophylactic treatment.
9. Pneumococcal conjugate vaccine is recommended for all children beginning at age 2 months to protect against meningitis; streptococcal pneumococci can cause many bacterial infections, including meningitis (see Chapter 37 for information on vaccines).

V. Submersion Injury

A. Description
1. Survival of at least 24 hours after submersion in a fluid medium
2. Hypoxia and asphyxiation are the primary problems because they result in extensive cell damage. Cerebral cells sustain irreversible damage after 4 to 6 minutes of submersion.
3. Additional problems include aspiration and hypothermia.
4. The outcome is predicted based on the length of submersion in non-icy water. The outcome may be good if submersion was for less than 5 minutes and the child exhibits neurological responsiveness, reactive pupils, and a normal cardiac rhythm.
5. A child who was submerged for more than 10 minutes and does not respond to cardiopulmonary life support measures within 25 minutes has an extremely poor prognosis (severe neurological impairment or death).

B. Interventions
1. Provide ventilatory and circulatory support; if child has had a severe cerebral insult, endotracheal intubation and mechanical ventilation may be required.
2. Monitor respiratory status because respiratory compromise and cerebral edema may occur 24 hours after the incident.
3. Monitor for aspiration pneumonia.
4. Monitor neurological status closely; if spontaneous purposeful movement and normal brainstem function are not apparent 24 hours after the event, the child most likely suffered severe neurological deficits.
5. Reinforce teaching to the parents to provide adequate supervision of infants and small children around water to prevent accidents.

VI. Reye's Syndrome

A. Description
1. An acute encephalopathy that follows a viral illness. It is characterized pathologically by cerebral edema and fatty changes in the liver; laboratory studies will assist in making a diagnosis; a definitive diagnosis is made by liver biopsy.
2. The exact cause is not clear; most commonly follows a viral illness such as influenza or varicella.
3. Administration of aspirin and aspirin-containing products is not recommended for children with a febrile illness or children with varicella or influenza because of its association with Reye's syndrome.
4. Acetaminophen or ibuprofen is usually prescribed for pediatric clients.
5. Early diagnosis and aggressive treatment is important; the goal of treatment is to maintain effective cerebral perfusion and control increasing ICP.

B. Data collection
1. History of systemic viral illness 4 to 7 days before the onset of symptoms
2. Malaise
3. Nausea and vomiting
4. Signs of altered hepatic function such as lethargy
5. Progressive neurological deterioration
6. Increased blood ammonia levels

C. Interventions
1. Provide rest and decrease stimulation in the environment.
2. Monitor neurological status.
3. Monitor for altered level of consciousness and signs of increased ICP.
4. Monitor for signs of altered hepatic function and the results of liver function studies.
5. Monitor I&O.
6. Monitor for signs of bleeding and signs of impaired coagulation, such as a prolonged bleeding time.

BOX 35.3   Interventions for Seizures

- Ensure airway patency.
- Have suction equipment and oxygen available.
- Time the seizure episode.
- If the child is standing or sitting, ease the child down to the floor and place him or her in a side-lying position.
- Place a pillow or folded blanket under the child's head. If no bedding is available, place your own hands under the child's head, or place the child's head in your own lap.
- Loosen restrictive clothing.
- Remove eyeglasses from the child, if present.
- Clear the area of any hazards or hard objects.
- Allow the seizure to proceed and end without interference.
- If vomiting occurs, turn the child to one side as a unit.
- Do not restrain the child, place anything in the child's mouth, or give any food or liquids to the child.
- Prepare to assist with the administration of medications, as prescribed.
- Remain with the child until he or she fully recovers.
- Observe for incontinence, which may have occurred during the seizure.
- Document the occurrence.

VII. Seizure Disorders

A. Description (see Chapter 55 for additional information on seizures)
1. Excessive and unorganized neuronal discharges in the brain that activate associated motor and sensory organs
2. Classified as generalized, partial, or unclassified, depending on the area of the brain involved
3. Types of generalized seizures include tonic-clonic, absence, myoclonic, and atonic.
4. Partial seizures arise from a specific area in the brain and cause limited symptoms; types include simple partial and complex partial.

B. Data collection
1. Obtain information from the parents about the time of onset, precipitating events, and behavior before and after the seizure.
2. Determine the child's history related to seizures.
3. Ask the child about the presence of an aura (a warning sign of impending seizure).
4. Monitor for apnea and cyanosis.
5. Post seizure: The child is disoriented and sleepy.

C. Seizure precautions (see Box 35.1)

D. Interventions (Box 35.3)

E. Anticonvulsant medications (see Chapter 56 for information about medications)

⚠ Never place anything, including an airway device or padded tongue blade, into the mouth of a child during a seizure.

VIII. Neural Tube Defects

A. Description
1. Central nervous system defect that results from the failure of the neural tube to close during embryonic development
2. Folic acid is recommended before and during pregnancy to reduce the occurrence of these conditions.
3. Associated deficits may include sensorimotor disturbance, dislocated hips, talipes equinovarus (clubfoot), and hydrocephalus.
4. Defect closure is performed immediately after birth.

B. Types
1. Spina bifida occulta
   a. Posterior vertebral arches fail to close in the lumbosacral area; there is a small gap in the spine but no opening or sac on the back.
   b. The nerves and spinal cord remains intact and the defect usually does not cause any disability.
2. Closed neural tube defects
   a. The spinal column is affected by malformations of fat, bone, or meninges.
   b. A dimple or tuft of hair may be an indication of a closed neural tube deficit.
   c. Usually there are few or no symptoms; but in some situations the malformation causes partial paralysis or other problems such as with urinary and bowel dysfunction.
3. Meningocele
   a. The protrusion involves meninges and a sac-like cyst that contains fluid in the midline of the back, usually in the lumbosacral area.
   b. The spinal cord is not involved or damaged.
   c. Neurological deficits are usually not present; some people with meningocele will have no symptoms, while others may have problems.
4. Myelomeningocele
   a. The bones of the spinal column do not form completely.
   b. Some of the spinal cord and tissues covering the spinal cord protrude out of an opening in the back.
   b. The sac (defect) is covered by a thin membrane that is prone to leakage or rupture.
   c. Partial or complete paralysis in the parts of the body below the spinal column are evident; bowel and urinary problems are common.
   d. The child may develop hydrocephalus, which can lead to learning and intellectual disabilities.

C. Data collection
1. Depends on the spinal cord involvement
2. Visible spinal defect
3. Flaccid paralysis of the legs
4. Altered bladder and bowel function

Pediatric Nursing

5. Hip and joint deformities

6. Hydrocephalus

D. Interventions

1. Evaluate the sac and measure the lesion.

2. Assist with performing a neurological assessment.

3. Monitor for increased ICP, which may indicate developing hydrocephalus.

4. Measure the head circumference. Check the anterior fontanel for fullness.

5. Protect the sac as prescribed. Cover with a sterile, moist (normal saline), nonadherent dressing to maintain its moisture and contents.

6. Change the dressing that covers the sac on a regular schedule, as prescribed, or whenever it becomes soiled to reduce the risk of infection. Diapering may be contraindicated until the defect has been repaired.

7. Use aseptic technique to prevent infection.

8. Check the sac for redness, clear or purulent drainage, abrasions, irritation, and signs of infection.

9. Early signs of infection include elevated temperature, irritability, lethargy, and nuchal rigidity.

10. Place the child in a prone position to minimize tension on the sac and the risk of trauma; the head is turned to one side for feeding.

11. Check for physical impairments such as hip and joint deformities.

12. Assist with preparing the child and family for surgery.

13. Assist with the administration of antibiotics preoperatively and postoperatively, as prescribed, to prevent infection.

14. Reinforce teaching to the parents and eventually the child about long-term homecare.

    a. Positioning, feeding, skin care, and range-of-motion exercises

    b. Instituting a bladder elimination program and performing clean intermittent catheterization

    c. Administering antispasmodics (these act on the smooth muscle of the bladder) as prescribed to increase bladder capacity and improve continence

    d. Implementing a bowel program as appropriate and as needed, including a high-fiber diet, increased fluids, and suppositories

    e. The child is at high risk for allergy to latex and rubber products because of the frequent exposure to latex during implementation of care measures.

IX. Attention Deficit Hyperactivity Disorder

A. Description

1. A behavior disorder that is characterized by inappropriate degrees of inattention, overactivity, and impulsivity

2. Childhood problems include lowered intellectual development, some minor physical abnormalities, sleep disturbances, behavioral or emotional disorders, and difficulty with social relationships.

3. Early diagnosis is important to prevent impaired emotional and psychological development.

4. Diagnosis is established on the basis of self-reports, parent and teacher reports, and the use of assessment tools.

B. Data collection

1. Fidgets with hands or feet or squirms in a seat

2. Easily distracted by external or internal stimuli

3. Difficulty with following through on instructions

4. Poor attention span

5. Shifts from one uncompleted activity to another

6. Talks excessively

7. Interrupts or intrudes on others

8. Engages in physically dangerous activities without considering the possible consequences

C. Interventions

1. Provide parents with information about the disorder and treatment plan; encourage support groups for the parents.

2. Treatment includes behavioral therapy, medication, maintaining a consistent environment, and appropriate classroom placement.

3. Behavioral therapy focuses on preventing undesirable behavior.

4. Maintaining a consistent home and classroom environment, providing environmental and physical safety measures is important.

5. Promote self-esteem.

6. Stimulant medications may be prescribed; possible side/adverse effects include appetite suppression and weight loss, nervousness, tics, insomnia, and increased blood pressure.

7. Reinforce instructions to the child and parents regarding medication administration and the need for regular follow-up.

X. Autism Spectrum Disorders

A. Description

1. Autism spectrum disorders (ASDs) are complex neurodevelopmental disorders of unknown etiology composed of qualitative alterations in social interaction and verbal impairment with repetitive, restricted, and stereotyped behavioral patterns.

2. ASD impairments range from mild to severe; types include autism, Asperger syndrome, and Rett syndrome.

3. Symptoms are usually noted by the parents by 3 years of age.

4. The cause of the disorder is not specifically known; however, it has been linked to a wide range of antepartum, intrapartum, and postpartum conditions and exposure to hazardous chemicals. Genetic predisposition is also linked to the disorder.

5. The disorder is accompanied by intellectual and social behavioral deficits, and the child exhibits peculiar and bizarre characteristics with social interaction, communication, and behavior.

6. Despite their relatively moderate to severe disability, some children with autism (known as savants) excel in particular areas, such as art, music, memory, mathematics, or perceptual skills such as puzzle building.

7. Diagnosis is established on the basis of symptoms and with the use of several screening tools.

B. Data collection

1. Social
   a. Abnormal lack of comfort-seeking behaviors
   b. Abnormal or lack of social play
   c. Impairment in peer relationships
   d. Lack of awareness of the existence or feelings of others
   e. Abnormal imitation of others

2. Communication
   a. Lack of, impaired, or abnormal speech such as producing a monotone voice or echolalia
   b. Abnormal nonverbal communication (does not use gestures to communicate)

3. Behavior
   a. Persistent preoccupation or attachment to objects; range of interests restricted
   b. Self-injurious behaviors
   c. Must maintain routine; any environmental change produces marked distress.
   d. Produces repetitive body movements such as rocking or head banging
   e. Lack of imaginative play

C. Interventions

1. Determine the child's routines, habits, and preferences, and maintain consistency as much as possible.

2. Determine the specific ways in which the child communicates and use these methods.

3. Avoid placing demands on the child.

4. Implement safety precautions, as necessary, for self-injurious behaviors such as head banging.

5. Assist to initiate referrals to special programs, as required.

6. Provide support to the parents.

7. The Modified Checklist for Autism in Toddlers, Revised with Follow-up (M-CHAT-R/F™) is used to screen toddlers for this disorder. https://www.cpqcc.org/sites/default/files/M-CHAT-R_F_1.pdf.

 Ensuring a safe environment for a child with autism is a priority.

XI. Intellectual Disability

A. Description

1. In intellectual disability, a child manifests subaverage intellectual functioning along with deficits in adaptive skills.

2. Down syndrome is a congenital condition that results in moderate to severe retardation and has been linked to an extra group G chromosome, chromosome 21 (trisomy 21).

B. Data collection

1. Deficits in cognitive skills and level of adaptive functioning
2. Delays in fine and gross motor skills
3. Speech delays
4. Decreased spontaneous activity
5. Nonresponsiveness
6. Irritability
7. Poor eye contact during feeding

C. Interventions

1. Medical strategies are focused on correcting structural deformities and treating associated behaviors.
2. Assist to implement community and educational services using a multidisciplinary approach.
3. Promote care skills as much as possible.
4. Assist with communication and socialization skills.
5. Facilitate appropriate playtimes.
6. Initiate safety precautions as necessary.
7. Assist the family with decisions regarding care.
8. Provide information regarding support services and community agencies.

WHAT WOULD YOU DO?

Answer: Following insertion of a ventriculoperitoneal shunt for the treatment of hydrocephalus, the nurse would monitor the child for signs of increased ICP. In the child, early signs include a change in the level of consciousness, headache, nausea, vomiting, visual disturbance (diplopia), and seizure. Normally, the surgeon prescribes that the child be kept flat to avoid rapid reduction of intracranial fluid. If increased ICP occurs, the nurse needs to elevate the head of the bed to 15–30 degrees to enhance gravity flow through the shunt. The nurse would also notify the registered nurse (RN) immediately. The RN will assess the child and contact the surgeon immediately.

PRACTICE QUESTIONS

1. The nurse instructs a mother of a child who has seizures regarding seizure precautions. Which statement by the mother indicates a **need for further teaching**?

   1. "I will make my child wear a medical identification alert bracelet."
   2. "I know that my child will need to have a companion when swimming."
   3. "I will need to give antiseizure medications when my child has a seizure."
   4. "I will have my child wear a bike helmet when riding a bike or skateboarding."

2. A child has a basilar skull fracture. Which primary health care provider's prescription would the nurse question?
1. Restrict fluid intake.
2. Insert an indwelling urinary catheter.
3. Keep an intravenous (IV) line patent.
4. Suction via the nasotracheal route as needed.

3. Which laboratory result would verify the diagnosis of bacterial meningitis?
1. Clear cerebrospinal fluid with high protein and low glucose levels
2. Cloudy cerebrospinal fluid with low protein and low glucose levels
3. Cloudy cerebrospinal fluid with high protein and low glucose levels
4. Decreased pressure and cloudy cerebrospinal fluid with a high protein level

4. The nurse reinforces instructions to the parent of a child with meningococcal meningitis. Which statement by the parent indicates a **need for further teaching**?
1. "I can give my child acetaminophen for fever."
2. "I will watch for any hearing loss that may occur."
3. "I know that I will need to watch for any rash that my child may develop."
4. "I will need to get my other children the pneumococcal vaccine, but not the baby yet, he is only 3 months."

5. The parents of a child recently diagnosed with cerebral palsy ask the nurse about the disorder. The nurse bases the response on the understanding that cerebral palsy is which type of condition?
1. An infectious disease of the central nervous system
2. An inflammation of the brain as a result of a viral illness
3. A congenital condition that results in moderate to severe retardation
4. A chronic disability characterized by impaired muscle movement and posture

6. The nurse is reviewing the postoperative prescriptions for an infant with hydrocephalus, who came back from surgery with a ventriculoperitoneal shunt. Which of the surgeon's prescriptions does the nurse question?
1. Position the infant on the nonoperative side.
2. Keep the head of the bed elevated 45 degrees.
3. Monitor for signs of infection and check dressings for drainage.
4. Observe for irritability, a high shrill cry, lethargy, and poor feeding.

7. The nurse is reviewing the record of a child with increased intracranial pressure and notes that the child has exhibited signs of decerebrate posturing. During data collection about the child, the nurse expects to note which characteristic of this type of posturing?
1. Flaccid paralysis of all extremities
2. Adduction of the arms at the shoulders
3. Rigid extension and pronation of the arms and legs
4. Abnormal flexion of the upper extremities and extension and adduction of the lower extremities

8. A child is diagnosed with Reye's syndrome. The nurse assists with developing a nursing care plan for the child and would include which intervention in the plan?
1. Assess hearing loss
2. Monitor urine output
3. Change body position every 2 hours
4. Provide a quiet atmosphere with dimmed lighting

9. The nurse provides homecare instructions to the parent of a child with attention deficit hyperactivity disorder regarding behavioral therapy interventions. Which statement by the parent indicates a **need for further teaching**?
1. "I hear that the side effects of the medication that my child will be on can cause overeating."
2. "I know that consistent medication and regular follow-up visits are a part of the plan for my child."
3. "I know I need to maintain a consistent home environment because my child is easily distracted."
4. "I understand that I will need to learn some behavioral modification techniques to help my child's impulsivity."

ANSWERS

1. 3

Rationale: Antiseizure medications are given on a routine basis to prevent a seizure; they are not rescue medications given at the time of a seizure. Padding the side rails, having a child wear a medical alert bracelet, swimming with a companion, and wearing a protective helmet while riding a bike or skateboarding are just a few of the precautions that are discussed with families.

Test-Taking Strategy: Note the strategic words, *need for further teaching*. These words indicate a negative event query and ask you to select an option that is an incorrect statement. Recalling that antiseizure medications are administered on a daily routine basis and the seizure precautions taught to parents will direct you to the correct option.

2. 4

Rationale: Nasotracheal suctioning is contraindicated in a child with a basilar skull fracture. Because of the location of the injury, the suction catheter may be introduced into the brain. Fluids are restricted to prevent fluid overload. The child may require a urinary catheter for the accurate monitoring of I&O. An IV line is maintained to administer fluids or medications, if necessary.

Test-Taking Strategy: Focus on the subject, the prescription that the nurse would question. Note that options 1, 2, and 3 are comparable or alike in that they all address the subject of fluid intake or output.

3. 3

Rationale: A diagnosis of meningitis is made by testing the cerebrospinal fluid (CSF) obtained by lumbar puncture. In the case of bacterial meningitis, findings usually include increased pressure, cloudy cerebrospinal fluid, a high protein level, and a low glucose level.

Test-Taking Strategy: Focus on the subject, verifying the diagnosis of meningitis. Eliminate options 1 and 4 first because clear CSF and decreased pressure are not likely to be found if an infectious process such as meningitis is suspected. From this point, recalling that a high protein level indicates a possible diagnosis of meningitis will direct you to the correct option.

4. 4

Rationale: Pneumococcal conjugate vaccine is recommended for all children beginning at age 2 months to protect against meningitis; streptococcal pneumococci can cause many bacterial infections, including meningitis. Options 1, 2, and 3 are correct statements.

Test-Taking Strategy: Note the strategic words, *need for further teaching*. These words indicate a negative event query and ask you to select an option that is an incorrect statement. Recalling that vaccines would be given to children beginning at age 2 months will direct you to the correct option.

5. 4

Rationale: Cerebral palsy is a chronic disability characterized by impaired movement and posture resulting from an abnormality in the extrapyramidal or pyramidal motor system. Meningitis is an infectious process of the central nervous system. Encephalitis is an inflammation of the brain that occurs as a result of viral illness or central nervous system infection. Down syndrome is an example of a congenital condition that results in moderate to severe retardation.

Test-Taking Strategy: Eliminate options 1 and 2 first, noting that they are comparable or alike. Next, note the relationship between the words *palsy* in the question and *impaired muscle movement* in the correct option.

6. 2

Rationale: Postoperative management for positioning of infants with hydrocephalus who have undergone ventriculoperitoneal shunt is flat in bed to avoid the rapid reduction of intracranial fluid. The nurse observes for increased ICP; if it occurs the nurse would elevate the head of the bed to 15 to 30 degrees to enhance gravity flow through the shunt and notify the registered nurse. The nurse would position the infant on the non-operative side to prevent pressure on the shunt valve. The nurse would monitor for signs of infection and check dressings for drainage. A high shrill cry in an infant can be a sign of increased ICP.

Test-Taking Strategy: Focus on the subject, postoperative interventions for ventriculoperitoneal shunt and the prescription that the nurse would question. Think about the purpose of this shunt and why it is needed to assist in answering. Remember that the head of the bed would be flat to avoid the rapid reduction of intracranial fluid. All other options are correct interventions.

7. 3

Rationale: Decerebrate (extension) posturing is characterized by the rigid extension and pronation of the arms and legs. Option 1 is incorrect. Options 2 and 4 describe decorticate (flexion) posturing.

Test-Taking Strategy: Focus on the subject, characteristics of decerebrate (extension) posturing. Recalling the clinical manifestations associated with decerebrate posturing will direct you to the correct option. Remember that decerebrate posturing is characterized by the rigid extension and pronation of the arms and legs.

8. 4

Rationale: Reye's syndrome is an acute encephalopathy that follows a viral illness and is characterized pathologically by cerebral edema and fatty changes in the liver. A definitive diagnosis is made by liver biopsy. In Reye's syndrome, supportive care is directed toward monitoring and managing cerebral edema. Decreasing stimuli in the environment by providing a quiet environment with dimmed lighting would decrease the stress on the cerebral tissue and neuron responses. Hearing loss and urine output are not affected. Changing the body position every 2 hours would not affect the cerebral edema directly. The child needs to be positioned with the head elevated to decrease the progression of the cerebral edema and promote drainage of cerebrospinal fluid.

Test-Taking Strategy: Focus on the subject, nursing care for the child with Reye's syndrome. Think about the pathophysiology associated with Reye's syndrome. Recalling that cerebral edema is a concern for a child with Reye's cyndrome will direct you to the correct option.

9. 1

Rationale: The treatment plan for children with attention deficit hyperactivity disorder includes stimulant medications that may have the adverse effect of appetite suppression and weight loss, not overeating. Treatment for these children includes behavioral therapy, maintaining a consistent environment, and appropriate classroom placement. Regular medication administration and regular follow-up visits are also important instructions for the parents.

Test-Taking Strategy: Note the strategic words, *need for further teaching*. These words indicate a negative event query and ask you to select an option that is an incorrect statement. Think about the pathophysiology of the disorder and recall the treatment plan for children with attention deficit hyperactivity disorder includes stimulant medications. This will assist you in answering correctly.

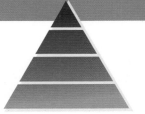

CHAPTER **36**

Musculoskeletal Problems

PRIORITY CONCEPTS Development; Mobility

WHAT WOULD YOU DO?

The nurse is assessing an infant with clubfoot who is in a cast. The nurse notes that the tissue distal to the cast is pale and edematous and the infant shows signs of pain with passive movement. What would the nurse do?
Answer is located on p. 448.

I. Developmental Dysplasia of the Hip

A. Description
   1. Disorders related to abnormal development of the hip that may develop during fetal life, infancy, or childhood; in these disorders, the head of the femur is seated improperly in the acetabulum or hip socket of the pelvis.
   2. Degrees of developmental dysplasia of the hip (Box 36.1)

BOX 36.1 Degrees of Developmental Dysplasia of the Hip

Acetabular Dysplasia (Preluxation)
- Mildest form
- Neither subluxation nor dislocation
- Delay in acetabular development occurs
- Femoral head remains in the acetabulum

Subluxation
- Incomplete dislocation of the hip
- Femoral head remains in the acetabulum
- Stretched capsule and ligamentum teres causes head of the femur to be partially displaced

Dislocation
- Femoral head loses contact with acetabulum and is displaced posteriorly and superiorly over the fibrocartilaginous rim
- Ligamentum teres—elongated and taut

B. Data collection (Fig. 36.1)
   1. Neonates: Laxity of the ligaments around the hip
   2. Infants
      a. Shortening of the limb on the affected side (Galeazzi sign, Allis's sign)
      b. Restricted abduction of the hip on the affected side when the child is placed supine with the knees and hips flexed (limited range of motion in the affected hip)
      c. Unequal gluteal folds when the infant is prone and the legs are extended against the examining table
      d. Positive Ortolani's test: The Ortolani maneuver is a test to assess for hip instability. In the Ortolani maneuver, the examiner abducts the thigh and applies gentle pressure forward over the greater trochanter. A "clicking" sensation indicates a dislocated femoral head moving into the acetabulum.
      e. Positive Barlow's test: The examiner adducts the hips and applies gentle pressure down and back with the thumbs. In hip dysplasia, the examiner can feel the femoral head move out of the acetabulum.
   3. Older infant and child
      a. Affected leg is shorter than the other.
      b. The head of the femur can be felt to move up and down in the buttock when the extended thigh is pushed first toward the child's head and then pulled distally.
      c. Positive Trendelenburg's sign: The child stands on one foot and then the other foot, holding onto a support and bearing weight on the affected hip; the pelvis tilts downward on the normal side, instead of upward, as it would be with normal stability.
      d. Greater trochanter is prominent.
      e. Marked lordosis or waddling gait is noted in bilateral dislocations.

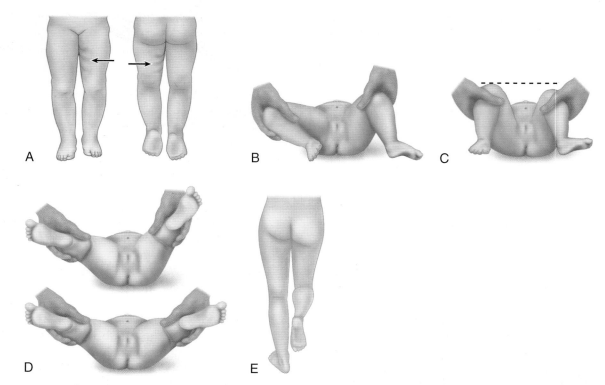

FIGURE 36.1 Signs of developmental dysplasia of the hip. (A) Asymmetry of gluteal and thigh folds. (B) Limited hip abduction, as seen during flexion. (C) Apparent shortening of the femur, as indicated by the level of the knees in flexion. (D) Ortolani click (if infant is under 4 weeks of age). (E) Positive Trendelenburg's sign of gait (if child is weight bearing).

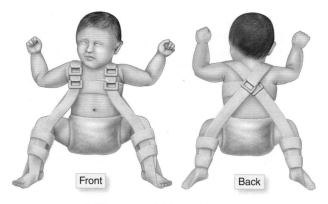

Front   Back

FIGURE 36.2 Child in Pavlik harness.

C. Interventions
  1. Birth to 6 months of age: Splinting of the hips with a Pavlik harness to maintain flexion, abduction, and external rotation; worn continuously until the hip is stable, in about 3 to 6 months (Fig. 36.2).
  2. Age 6 to 18 months: Gradual reduction by traction followed by closed reduction or open reduction (if necessary) under general anesthesia. The child is then placed in a hip spica cast for 2 to 4 months until the hip is stable, and then a flexion-abduction brace is applied for approximately 3 months.
  3. Older child: Operative reduction and reconstruction may be required.

4. Reinforce instructions to the parents regarding the proper care of a Pavlik harness, spica cast, or abduction brace.

II. Congenital Clubfoot

A. Description
  1. Complex deformity of the ankle and foot that includes forefoot adduction, midfoot supination, hindfoot varus, and ankle equinus. The defect may be unilateral or bilateral.
  2. The goal of treatment is to achieve a painless plantigrade (able to walk on the sole of the foot with the heel on the ground) and stable foot.
  3. Long-term interval follow-up is required until the child reaches skeletal maturity.

B. Data collection: Deformities are described on the basis of the position of the ankle and foot.
  1. Talipes varus: An inversion or bending inward
  2. Talipes valgus: An eversion or bending outward
  3. Talipes equinus: Plantar flexion in which the toes are lower than the heel
  4. Talipes calcaneus: Dorsiflexion in which the toes are higher than the heel

C. Interventions
  1. Treatment begins as soon after birth as possible.
  2. Manipulation and casting are performed weekly for about 8 to 12 weeks because of the rapid growth during early infancy; a splint is then applied if casting and manipulation are successful.

3. Surgical intervention may be necessary if normal alignment is not achieved by about 6 to 12 weeks of age.
4. Monitor for pain and monitor the neurovascular status of the toes.

⚠ Contact the registered nurse (RN) or primary health care provider (PHCP) immediately if signs of neurovascular impairment are noted in a child with a cast or brace.

III. Idiopathic Scoliosis

A. Description
1. A three-dimensional spinal deformity that usually involves lateral curvature, spinal rotation that results in rib asymmetry, and hypokyphosis of the thorax
2. Usually diagnosed during the preadolescent growth spurt. Screenings are important at times when growth spurts occur.
3. Surgical (spinal fusion, which may be done by thoracoscopic surgery, placement of an instrumentation system, or use of metallic staples placed into vertebral bodies) and nonsurgical (bracing) interventions are used; the type of treatment depends on the location and degree of the curvatures, the age of the child, the amount of growth that is yet anticipated, and any underlying disease processes.
4. Long-term monitoring is essential to detect any progression of the curve.

B. Data collection
1. Asymmetry of the ribs and flanks is noted when the child bends forward at the waist and hangs the arms down toward the feet (Adam's test).
2. Hip height, rib positioning, and shoulder height are asymmetrical. (This can be noted when standing behind the undressed child.) A leg-length discrepancy is also apparent.
3. Radiographs are performed to confirm the diagnosis.

C. Interventions
1. Monitor the progression of the curvatures.
2. Prepare the child and parents for the use of a brace, if prescribed.
3. Prepare the child and parents for surgery (spinal fusion and the placement of internal instrumentation systems), if prescribed.

⚠ The potential for altered role performance, body image disturbance, fear, anger, and isolation exist for a child with a disabling condition and a condition that requires wearing a body brace.

D. Braces
1. Braces are not curative, but they may slow the progression of the curvature to allow for skeletal growth and maturity.

2. Braces usually are prescribed to be worn from 16 to 23 hours a day.
3. Inspect the skin for signs of redness or breakdown.
4. Keep the skin clean and dry, and avoid lotions and powders because these cake and lead to skin breakdown.
5. Advise the child to wear soft, nonirritating clothing under the brace.
6. Reinforce instructions to the child and parents regarding the prescribed exercises, which help to maintain and strengthen the spinal and abdominal muscles during treatment.
7. Encourage verbalization about body image and other psychosocial issues.

E. Postoperative interventions
1. Maintain proper alignment. Avoid twisting movements.
2. Logroll the child when turning him or her to maintain alignment.
3. Monitor the neurovascular status of the extremities.
4. Encourage coughing, deep breathing, and the use of incentive spirometry.
5. Check for pain and assist with the administration of analgesics, as prescribed.
6. Monitor for incontinence.
7. Monitor for signs/symptoms of infection.
8. Monitor for superior mesenteric artery syndrome, which is caused by mechanical changes in the position of the child's abdominal contents during surgery, and notify the RN immediately if it occurs. Symptoms include emesis and abdominal distention similar to that which occurs during intestinal obstruction or paralytic ileus.
9. Reinforce instructions to the child and parents regarding activity restrictions.
10. Reinforce instructions to the child how to logroll from a side-lying position to a sitting position, and assist the child with ambulation.
11. Be alert to signs of a potential body image problem.

IV. Juvenile Idiopathic Arthritis

A. Description
1. An autoimmune, inflammatory disease affecting the joints and other tissues, such as the articular cartilage, which occurs most often in girls
2. Treatment is supportive (there is no cure) and directed toward preserving joint function, controlling inflammation, minimizing deformity, and reducing the effect that the disease may have on the development of the child.

3. Treatment includes medication, physical and occupational therapy, and child and family education.
4. A pediatric rheumatology team can manage the complex needs of the child and family most effec-

Pediatric Nursing

BOX 36.2 **Data Collection: Juvenile Idiopathic Arthritis**

- Stiffness, swelling, and limited motion occur in the affected joints.
- The affected joints are warm to the touch, tender, and painful.
- Joint stiffness is present when arising in the morning and after inactivity.
- Uveitis (the inflammation of structures in the uveal tract) can occur and cause blindness.

BOX 36.3 **Medications Used for the Treatment of Juvenile Idiopathic Arthritis**

Corticosteroid injections: Prescribed when only a few joints are involved. Usually they do not have any significant side effects.

Oral Corticosteroids: These may be prescribed but only for as short a time and at the lowest dose possible. Long-term use is associated with side effects such as weight gain, poor growth, osteoporosis, cataracts, avascular necrosis, hypertension, and risk of infection.

Disease-Modifying Anti-Rheumatic drugs (DMARDs): These are prescribed when many joints are involved or the child does not respond to corticosteroid joint injections. Biologics also may be prescribed, and these include antitumor necrosis factor agents. All of these medications cause side effects that need to be discussed with the child and/or parents.

---

tively; the team may consist of a pediatric rheumatologist, physical and occupational therapist, social worker, and nurse specialist.

    5. Surgical intervention may be implemented if the child has problems with joint contractures and unequal growth of extremities.

 B. Data collection (Box 36.2)

    1. There are no definitive tests to diagnose the condition.

    2. Certain laboratory tests (e.g., an elevated erythrocyte sedimentation rate, the presence of leukocytosis) may support evidence of the disease.

    3. Radiographs may show soft tissue swelling and joint space widening as a result of increased synovial fluid in the joint.

C. Interventions

    1. Facilitate social and emotional development.

    2. Reinforce instructions to the parents and child in the administration of medications. Medications may be given alone or in combination and are prescribed in a step-like fashion that is dependent on the disease's response to each level (Box 36.3).

    3. Assist the child with range-of-motion exercises. Instruct the child and parents with regard to prescribed exercises.

    4. Encourage the normal performance of activities of daily living.

    5. Reinforce instructions to the parents and child in the use of hot and cold packs, splinting, and positioning the affected joint in a neutral position during painful episodes. Begin simple isometric exercises as soon as the child is able.

    6. Encourage and support prescribed physical and occupational therapy.

    7. Reinforce instructions to the child and parents about the importance of preventive eyecare and the reporting of visual disturbances.

    8. Assess the child's and family's perceptions regarding the chronic illness. Plan to discuss the nature of a chronic illness and the grief associated with the new recognition of life alterations

that result from the chronic progression of the disorder.

V. Marfan Syndrome

A. Description

    1. A disorder of connective tissue that affects the skeletal system, cardiovascular system, eyes, and skin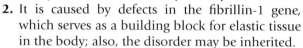

    2. It is caused by defects in the fibrillin-1 gene, which serves as a building block for elastic tissue in the body; also, the disorder may be inherited.

    3. There is no cure for the disorder.

B. Data collection

    1. Tall and thin body structure; slender fingers, long arms and legs, curvature of the spine

    2. Presence of visual problems

    3. Presence of cardiac problems

C. Interventions

    1. Monitor for vision problems and obtain visual examinations on a regular schedule.

    2. Monitor for curvature of the spine, especially during adolescence.

    3. Cardiac medications may be prescribed to slow the heart rate, which will decrease stress on the aorta.

    4. Reinforce instructions to the parents that the child needs to avoid participating in competitive athletics and contact sports to avoid injuring the heart.

    5. Reinforce instructions to the parents to inform the dentist of the condition; antibiotics need to be taken before dental procedures to prevent endocarditis.

    6. Surgical replacement of the aortic root and valve may be necessary.

VI. Legg-Calve-Perthes Disease

A. Description

    1. A condition affecting the hip where the femur and pelvis meet in the joint

2. Blood supply is temporarily interrupted to the head of the femur and the bone dies and stops growing.

B. Assessment

    1. Limping

    2. Pain or stiffness in the hip, groin, thigh, or knee

    3. Limited range of motion in the affected joint

C. Interventions

    1. Physical therapy, particularly stretching exercises

    2. Use of crutches to avoid bearing weight on the affected hip

    3. Bed rest and traction if pain is severe

    4. Casting to keep the femoral head within its socket

    5. Use of a nighttime brace

    6. Hip replacement surgery

VII. Fractures (see also Chapter 57)

A. Description

    1. A break in the continuity of the bone as a result of trauma, twisting, or bone decalcification

    2. Fractures in children usually occur as a result of increased mobility and inadequate or immature motor and cognitive skills; they may result from trauma or bone diseases such as a congenital bone disease or bone tumors.

> ⚠ Fractures during infancy are generally rare and warrant further investigation to rule out the possibility of child abuse and to recognize bone structure defects.

B. Data collection

    1. Pain or tenderness over the involved area

    2. Obvious deformity

    3. Edema

    4. Ecchymosis

    5. Muscle spasm

⚡ PRIORITY NURSING ACTIONS

Extremity Fracture in a Child

1. Check the extent of the injury and immobilize the affected extremity.
2. If a compound fracture exists, cover the wound with a sterile dressing (apply a clean dressing if a sterile dressing is unavailable).
3. Elevate the injured extremity.
4. Apply cold packs to the injured area.
5. Continue to monitor neurovascular status.
6. Transport to the nearest emergency department.

---

    6. Loss of function

    7. Crepitation

C. Initial care of a fracture (see **Priority Nursing Actions**)

D. Interventions

    1. Reduction

        a. Restoring the bone to proper alignment

        b. Closed reduction: Accomplished by the manual alignment of the fragments, followed by immobilization

        c. Open reduction: Requires the surgical insertion of internal fixation devices (e.g., rods, wires, pins) that help maintain alignment until healed

    2. Retention: The application of traction or a cast to maintain alignment until healing occurs

E. Traction (see Chapter 57)

    1. Russell skin traction

        a. Used to stabilize a fractured femur before surgery

        b. Similar to Buck's traction but provides a double pull using a knee sling that pulls at the knee and foot

    2. Balanced suspension

        a. Used with skin or skeletal traction to approximate fractures of the femur, tibia, or fibula

        b. Traction is produced by a counterforce other than the child.

        c. Provide pin care if pins are used with the skeletal traction.

    3. 90-degree–90-degree traction

        a. The lower leg is supported by a boot cast or a calf sling.

        b. A skeletal Steinmann pin or Kirschner wire is placed in the distal fragment of the femur, allowing a 90-degree angle at both the hip and the knee.

    4. Interventions

        a. Maintain the correct amount of weight, as prescribed.

        b. Ensure that the weights hang freely. They should not be resting on the floor or bed.

        c. Check all ropes for fraying and all knots for tightness; be sure that the ropes are appropriately tracking in the grooves of the pulley wheels.

        d. Monitor the neurovascular status of the involved extremity.

        e. Protect the skin from breakdown.

        f. Monitor for signs/symptoms of complications of immobilization, such as constipation, skin breakdown, lung congestion, renal complications, and disuse syndrome of unaffected extremities.

        g. Monitor for sensory deprivation. Provide therapeutic and diversional play.

F. Casts (see Chapter 57)

    1. Description

        a. Made of plaster or fiberglass to provide for the immobilization of bones and joints after a fracture or injury

        b. Fractures of the hip or the knee may require a spica cast.

Pediatric Nursing

2. Interventions

  a. Examine the cast for pressure areas.

  b. Ensure that no rough casting material remains in contact with the skin; assist with petaling the cast edges with waterproof adhesive tape as necessary to ensure a smooth cast edge.

  c. If a hip spica cast is placed, the cast edges are around the perineum and buttocks and may need to be taped with waterproof tape.

  d. Monitor the extremity for circulatory impairment, such as more pain than would be expected for the type of injury, edema, rubor, pallor, numbness and tingling, coolness, decreased sensation or mobility, or diminished pulse.

  e. Notify the RN immediately if circulatory impairment occurs.

  f. Prepare to assist with bivalving or cutting of the cast if circulatory impairment occurs; prepare for emergency fasciotomy if cast removal does not improve the neurocirculatory compromise.

  g. Reinforce instructions to the family and the child not to stick objects down the cast.

  h. Reinforce teaching the family and the child to keep the cast clean and dry.

  i. Reinforce instructions to the family and the child with regard to isometric exercises to prevent muscle atrophy.

WHAT WOULD YOU DO?

Answer: Compartment syndrome is a condition in which pressure increases in a confined anatomical space, leading to decreased blood flow, ischemia, and dysfunction of these tissues. This complication can occur with casts. Signs of this complication include unrelieved or increased pain in the limb; pale, dusky, or edematous tissue distal to the involved area; pain with passive movement; loss of sensation (paresthesia); and pulselessness (a late sign). The nurse should notify the registered nurse (RN) immediately. The RN will assess the child and then contact the primary health care provider (PHCP) immediately because of the risk of tissue ischemia and necrosis if neurovascular impairment is noted.

PRACTICE QUESTIONS

1. The nurse is reinforcing instructions to the parents of a child with scoliosis regarding the use of a brace. Which statement by a parent indicates the **need for further teaching**?

  1. "I need to have my child wear a soft fabric under the brace."

  2. "I will apply lotion under the brace to prevent skin breakdown."

  3. "I need to encourage my child to perform the prescribed exercises."

  4. "I need to avoid applying powder under the brace, because it will cake."

2. The mother of a child with juvenile idiopathic arthritis calls the nurse because the child is experiencing a painful exacerbation of the disease. The mother asks the nurse if the child should perform range-of-motion (ROM) exercises at this time. The nurse would make which response to the mother?

  1. "Avoid all exercise during painful periods."

  2. "The ROM exercises must be performed every day."

  3. "Have the child perform simple isometric exercises during this time."

  4. "Administer additional pain medication before performing the ROM exercises."

3. A 4-year-old child sustains a fall at home injuring the right arm and is brought to the emergency department by the mother. The nurse would perform which emergency actions in the care of the child? **Select all that apply.**

  ❑ **1.** Elevate the right arm.

  ❑ **2.** Apply warm packs to the right arm.

  ❑ **3.** Check the neurovascular status of the right extremity.

  ❑ **4.** Check the range of motion (ROM) of the right arm and shoulder.

  ❑ **5.** Determine the level of pain using a pediatric pain assessment tool.

4. The nurse assists to create a nursing care plan for the child with an arm cast and would include which interventions in the plan? **Select all that apply.**

  ❑ **1.** Instruct parents to keep the cast clean and dry.

  ❑ **2.** Monitor the extremity for circulatory impairment.

  ❑ **3.** Instruct the child not to stick objects down the cast.

  ❑ **4.** Ensure that rough cast materials are cut off to keep the edges smooth.

  ❑ **5.** Notify the registered nurse (RN) immediately if circulatory impairment occurs.

5. The mother of a child with Marfan syndrome asks the nurse what can be done to help her child. Which are the **best** responses by the nurse? **Select all that apply.**

  ❑ **1.** "You will need to keep your child indoors and avoid sports."

  ❑ **2.** "You will need to consider surgery in the future if recommended."

  ❑ **3.** "You will need to make regular pediatric appointments for your child."

❏ 4. "You will need to make regular eye examination appointments for your child."

❏ 5. "You will need to be sure your child takes prescribed cardiac medication(s) to decrease stress on the aorta."

❏ 6. "You will need to let the dentist know so antibiotics can be prescribed before any procedure."

6. The nurse is assisting a primary health care provider (PHCP) during an examination of an infant with hip dysplasia. The PHCP performs the Ortolani maneuver. Which data would the nurse expect to note during the examination?

1. Full range of motion (ROM) of the legs
2. Marked asymmetry on the affected side
3. The unstable femoral head pops out of the acetabulum.
4. The dislocated femoral head pops back into the acetabulum.

7. The nurse provides information to the parent of a 2-week-old infant who was diagnosed with clubfoot at the time of birth. Which statement by the parent indicates the **need for further teaching** regarding this disorder?

1. "I understand treatment needs to be started as soon as possible."
2. "I realize my child will require follow-up care until fully grown."
3. "I need to bring my child back to the clinic in 2 months for a new cast."
4. "I need to come to the clinic every week with my child for the casting."

8. The nurse reinforces home care instructions to the parents of a child with a brace for scoliosis. Which statement by a parent indicates a **need for further teaching**?

1. "I will inspect the skin under the brace for redness or breakdown."
2. "I will encourage my child to do their exercises to maintain strength."
3. "I understand that my child needs to wear this brace for 12 hours a day."
4. "I understand that this brace is not a cure for scoliosis; it only slows the progression of the curvature."

9. The nurse is assigned to care for a child who is in skeletal traction. The nurse needs to avoid which action when caring for the child?

1. Keeping the weights hanging freely
2. Ensuring that the ropes are in the pulleys
3. Placing the bed linens on the traction ropes
4. Ensuring that the weights are out of the child's reach

10. The nurse is performing a neurovascular check on a hospitalized child who had a cast applied to the lower leg. The child complains of tingling in the toes distal to the fracture site. Which action would the nurse take?

1. Elevate the extremity.
2. Document the findings.
3. Notify the registered nurse (RN).
4. Ambulate the child with crutches.

ANSWERS

1. 2

Rationale: The use of either lotions or powders needs to be avoided because they can become sticky or cake under the brace, thus causing irritation. Options 1, 3, and 4 are appropriate statements regarding the care of a child with a brace.

Test-Taking Strategy: Note the strategic words, *need for further teaching*. These words indicate a negative event query and ask you to select an option that is an incorrect statement. Recalling that lotions and powders need to be avoided because of the irritation they can cause will direct you to the correct option.

2. 3

Rationale: During painful episodes, hot or cold packs, splinting, and positioning the affected joint in a neutral position help to reduce the pain. Although resting the extremity is appropriate, it is important to begin simple isometric or tensing exercises as soon as the child is able. These exercises do not involve joint movement.

Test-Taking Strategy: Use general medication guidelines to assist in eliminating option 4. Additional medication would not be given. Eliminate options 1 and 2 because of the closed-ended words, *all* and *must,* in these options.

❖ **3. 1, 3, 5**

Rationale: Emergency nursing actions to take for a child sustaining an extremity fracture include elevating the injured extremity, checking the extent of the injury including pain level, immobilizing the affected extremity, applying cold packs to the injured area, and monitoring the neurovascular status of the extremity.

Test-Taking Strategy: Focus on the subject, emergency actions to take when a child sustains an extremity fracture. Recall that heat will increase circulation to the extremity causing further swelling and increasing the pain; this will assist in eliminating option 2. Next, eliminate option 4 because range of motion can cause further injury; determining the extent of the injury is necessary before any movement is done.

❖ **4. 1, 2, 3, 5**

Rationale: Cutting the cast is not appropriate; cast material can drop into the cast and cause skin irritation and skin breaks. The edges can be covered with waterproof adhesive tape to ensure a smooth cast edge. Instruct the parents and the child to keep the cast clean and dry, and not to stick objects down the cast. Monitoring for circulatory impairment is important and immediately reporting signs of impairment to the RN is necessary.

Test-Taking Strategy: Focus on the subject, cast care. Read each option carefully thinking about the principles related to case care and the complications. Recall that maintaining skin integrity is a priority concern to answer correctly.

❖ **5. 2, 3, 4, 5, 6**
Rationale: Parents of the child with Marfan syndrome need to be instructed to monitor for vision problems and get regular eye examinations, and avoid participation in contact sports; however, it is not necessary for the child to stay indoors. The nurse needs to monitor the curvature of the spine as the child grows. Antibiotics need to be taken before any dental procedure to prevent endocarditis. Cardiac medications need to be taken to decrease stress on the aorta, and surgical replacement of the aortic root and valve may be necessary. Making regular pediatric appointments is important for monitoring the child.
Test-Taking Strategy: Note the strategic word, *best*. This indicates that all the answers may be correct, but you will need to select the ones that are better than the others. Focus on the subject, Marfan syndrome. Think about the interventions that are taken to decrease stress on the aorta and to prevent endocarditis. This will assist you with answering the question.

6. 4
Rationale: With the Ortolani maneuver, the examiner reduces the dislocated femoral head back into the acetabulum. A positive Ortolani maneuver is a palpable clunk as the femoral head moves over the acetabular ring. Options 1 and 2 are data collection techniques for the identification of the clinical manifestations of hip dysplasia, but they do not describe the Ortolani maneuver. When performing the Barlow maneuver, the examiner pushes the unstable femoral head out of the acetabulum.
Test-Taking Strategy: Focus on the subject, the expected finding when performing the Ortolani maneuver. Eliminate options 1 and 2 first, because they are data collection techniques. From the remaining options, it is necessary to know the action/purpose of the Ortolani maneuver.

7. 3
Rationale: Treatment for clubfoot is started as soon as possible after birth. Serial manipulation and casting are performed at least weekly. If sufficient correction is not achieved within 3 to 6 months, surgery is usually indicated. Because clubfoot can recur, all children with the condition require long-term interval follow-up until they reach skeletal maturity to ensure an optimal outcome.

Test-Taking Strategy: Focus on the subject, the treatment plan for clubfoot. Note the strategic words, *need for further teaching*. These words indicate a negative event query and the need to select the incorrect statement. This will assist you with eliminating options 1 and 2. Recalling that serial manipulations and casting are required weekly will direct you to the correct option.

8. 3
Rationale: The brace needs to be worn from 16 to 23 hours a day. Braces are not curative; they slow the progression of the curvature. The skin under the brace needs to be inspected for any redness or breakdown. The child would continue to perform prescribed exercise to help maintain and strengthen the spinal and abdominal muscles.
Test-Taking Strategy: Focus on the subject, the treatment plan for scoliosis. Note the strategic words, *need for further teaching*. These words indicate a negative event query and the need to select the incorrect statement. Recall that the brace needs to be worn from 16 to 23 hours a day. The other options are correct.

9. 3
Rationale: Bed linens would not be placed on the traction ropes because of the risk of disrupting the traction apparatus. Options 1, 2, and 4 are appropriate measures when caring for a child who is in skeletal traction.
Test-Taking Strategy: Focus on the subject, the action that the nurse avoids. This tells you that you need to select an option that is an incorrect intervention. Use knowledge regarding the care of the child in traction to direct you to the correct option.

10. 3
Rationale: Reduced sensation to touch or complaints of numbness or tingling at a site distal to the fracture may indicate poor tissue perfusion. This finding needs to be reported to the registered nurse or PHCP. Options 1, 2, and 4 are inappropriate and would delay the required and immediate interventions.
Test-Taking Strategy: Focus on the subject, the action that the nurse would take. Note the data in the question and recall the signs of circulatory compromise. Noting the child's complaint will assist with directing you to the correct option.

CHAPTER **37**

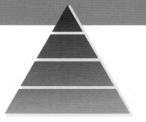

Immune Problems and Infectious Diseases

PRIORITY CONCEPTS Infection; Safety

WHAT WOULD YOU DO?

The nurse is assisting with the admission of a child with a diagnosis of mumps to the pediatric unit. What would the nurse include in the plan of care for the child?
Answer is located on p. 460

I. **Immune Disorders:** For information on the function of the immune system, the immune response, immunodeficiency, and other immune disorders, hypersensitivity and allergies, and skin testing, see Chapter 59.

⚠ Standard precautions are instituted in the care of all children. Additional transmission based precautions such as airborne, droplet, and contact may also need to be instituted depending on the child's disease and method of transmission, and other conditions present in the child. For example, in addition to standard precautions, the nurse may need to institute droplet precautions for a child with influenza but if that same child has a wound infection or scabies then contact precautions are also necessary.

II. **Human Immunodeficiency Virus (HIV) Infection and Acquired Immunodeficiency Syndrome (AIDS)**
A. Description
   1. AIDS is a disorder caused by HIV and characterized by generalized dysfunction of the immune system (see Fig. 59.1 – systemic anaphylactic reaction).
   2. The diagnosis of AIDS is associated with certain illnesses or conditions.
   3. HIV infects CD4+ T cells; a gradual decrease in CD4+ T-cell count occurs, and this results in a progressive immunodeficiency; the risk for opportunistic infections is present (see Box 37.1 for AIDS-Defining Conditions in Children).
   4. HIV is transmitted through blood, semen, vaginal secretions, and breast milk; the incubation period is months to years.

5. Horizontal transmission occurs through intimate sexual contact or parenteral exposure to blood or body fluids that contain the virus.
6. Vertical (perinatal) transmission occurs from an HIV-infected pregnant woman to her fetus (see Chapter 23).
7. The most common opportunistic infection that occurs in children infected with HIV is *Pneumocystis jiroveci* pneumonia; *P. jiroveci* pneumonia most frequently occurs between the ages of 3 and 6 months.

⚠ An infant or child infected with HIV is at risk for developing a life-threatening opportunistic infection. Monitor the infant or child closely for signs of infection and report these signs immediately if they occur.

B. Data collection (see Boxes 37.1 and 37.2)
C. Diagnostic tests: Before testing, counseling would be provided to parents; issues that would be addressed include the causes of HIV, reasons for testing, implications of positive test results, confidentiality issues, and beneficial effects of early intervention (Table 37.1).

III. **Care of the Child with HIV Infection or AIDS**
A. An interprofessional health care approach is taken; primary goals are to decelerate the replication of the virus, prevent opportunistic infections, provide nutritional support, treat symptoms, and treat opportunistic infections.
B. Prophylaxis (*P. jiroveci* pneumonia and other opportunistic infections)
   1. Provide prophylaxis as prescribed against *P. jiroveci* pneumonia and other opportunistic infections, particularly during the first year of life of an infant born to an HIV-infected mother.
   2. After 1 year of age, the need for prophylaxis is determined on the basis of the presence and severity of immunosuppression or a history of *P. jiroveci* pneumonia.

451

BOX 37.1 Common Acquired Immunodeficiency Syndrome (AIDS)-Defining Conditions in Children

- Candidal esophagitis
- Cryptosporidiosis
- Cytomegalovirus disease
- Herpes simplex disease
- Human immunodeficiency virus encephalopathy
- Lymphoid interstitial pneumonitis
- *Mycobacterium avium-intracellulare* infection
- *Pneumocystis jiroveci* pneumonia
- Pulmonary candidiasis
- Recurrent bacterial infections
- Wasting syndrome

Data from Perry S, Hockenberry M, Lowdermilk D, Wilson D: *Maternal-child nursing care*, ed 4, St. Louis, 2010, Mosby.

BOX 37.2 Common Findings in Children with Human Immunodeficiency Virus Infection

- Chronic cough
- Chronic or recurrent diarrhea
- Developmental delay or regression of developmental milestones
- Failure to thrive
- Hepatosplenomegaly
- Lymphadenopathy
- Malaise and fatigue
- Night sweats
- Oral candidiasis
- Parotitis
- Weight loss

Adapted from Perry S, Hockenberry M, Lowdermilk D, Wilson D: *Maternal-child nursing care*, ed 4, St. Louis, 2010, Mosby.

3. Continuing prophylaxis is based on the child's HIV status, history of opportunistic infections, and CD4+ counts.

C. Antiretroviral medications (Refer to Chapter 60)

⚠ Before an antiretroviral medication is administered, the medication is checked to be sure it is safe for pediatric administration. The contraindications for use and the adverse effects are also checked before administration.

1. The goal of antiretroviral medication is to suppress viral replication to slow the decline in the number of CD4+ cells, preserve immune function, reduce the incidence and severity of opportunistic infections, and delay disease progression.
2. The medications affect different stages of the HIV life cycle to prevent reproduction of new virus particles.

3. Combination therapy may be prescribed and includes the use of more than one antiretroviral medication.

D. Immunizations

⚠ Immunization against childhood diseases is recommended for all children exposed to and infected with HIV.

1. If a child has symptomatic HIV infection or has severe immunosuppression, guidelines are as follows:
   a. Only the inactivated influenza vaccine that is given intramuscularly would be used (influenza vaccine should be given yearly).
   b. Measles vaccine would not be given; immunoglobulin may be prescribed after measles exposure.
   c. Only the inactivated polio vaccine that is given intramuscularly would be used.
   d. Rotavirus vaccine should not be given.
   e. Varicella-zoster (VCZ) virus vaccine should not be given; VCZ immunoglobulin may be prescribed after chickenpox exposure.
   f. Tetanus immunoglobulin may be prescribed for tetanus-prone wounds.

E. Caregiver instructions
   1. Wash hands frequently.
   2. Monitor the child for fever, malaise, fatigue, weight loss, vomiting, diarrhea, altered activity level, and oral lesions; notify the primary health care provider (PHCP) if any of these occur.
   3. Monitor the child for signs/symptoms of opportunistic infections, such as pneumonia.
   4. Antiretroviral medications and other medications are administered to the child as prescribed.
   5. The child needs to be restricted from having contact with persons who have infections or other contagious or potentially contagious illnesses.
   6. Keep the child's immunizations up to date.
   7. Keep the child home when sick.
   8. Avoid direct unprotected contact with the child's body fluids.
   9. Monitor the child's weight.
   10. Provide a high-calorie and high-protein diet for the child.
   11. Administer appetite stimulants to the child, as prescribed and as needed.
   12. Do not share eating utensils with the child.
   13. Wash all eating utensils in the dishwasher.
   14. Cover any of the child's unused food and formula and refrigerate (discard unused refrigerated formula and food after 24 hours).
   15. Do not allow the child to eat fresh fruits or vegetables or raw meat or fish (neutropenic diet if immunosuppressed).

TABLE 37.1 Diagnostic Tests for Human Immunodeficiency Virus

Test	Age-Appropriate Use	Test Determines	Special Considerations
Enzyme-linked immuno-sorbent assay (ELISA)	18 months or older	Response of antibodies to HIV	If used and found to be positive in infants younger than 18 months, indicates only that the mother is infected because maternal antibodies are transmitted transplacentally; another diagnostic test is used.
Western blot	18 months or older	Presence of HIV antibodies	Same as above
Polymerase chain reaction (PCR)	Younger than 18 months	Presence of proviral deoxyribonucleic acid (DNA)	Very accurate for diagnosing infants 1–4 months of age
p24 antigen	Younger than 18 months	HIV antigen specific	Very accurate for diagnosing infants 1–4 months of age
CD4+ lymphocyte count, T-lymphocyte count	Infant up to 13 years	Immune system status related specifically to suppression	Age adjustment is essential, because normal counts are relatively high in infants and steadily decline until 6 years of age. Severe suppression in all age groups is <15% total lymphocytes (less than 750 cells/L in an infant younger than 12 months, less than 500 cells/L in a child 1–5 years, less than 200 cells/L in a child 6–12 years).

HIV, Human immunodeficiency virus.
Adapted from Branson BM, Handsfield HH, Lampe MA, et al.: Centers for Disease Control and Prevention: Revised recommendations for HIV testing of adults, adolescents, and pregnant women in health-care settings. *MMWR Recomm Rep* 55(RR14):1–17, 2006. Available from: http://www.cdc.gov/mmwr/preview/mmwrhtml/rr5514a1.htm.

16. Wear gloves when caring for the child, especially when in contact with body fluids and changing diapers.
17. Change the child's diapers frequently, away from food areas.
18. Fold the child's soiled disposable diapers inward, close with the tabs, and dispose in a tightly covered plastic-lined container.
19. Dispose of trash daily.
20. Clean up any of the child's body fluid spills with a bleach solution (10:1 ratio of water to bleach).

F. Education for an adolescent infected with HIV
1. High-risk behaviors and the importance of avoiding high-risk behaviors
2. Methods of HIV transmission
3. The importance of abstinence from sexual contact, such as intercourse
4. The importance of using safe condoms if intercourse is planned
5. Resources available for support and other issues
6. For specific information about transmission based precautions needed for each communicable disease, refer to Chapter 14.

IV. Rubeola (Measles)

A. Description
1. Agent: Paramyxovirus virus
2. Incubation period: 10 to 20 days
3. Communicable period: From 4 days before to 5 days after the rash appears; mainly during the prodromal stage (this pertains to early symptoms that may mark the onset of disease)
4. Source: Respiratory tract secretions, blood, or urine of an infected person

5. Transmission: Airborne particles, direct contact with infectious droplets, or transplacental transmission

B. Data collection (Fig. 37.1)
1. Fever
2. Malaise
3. The "3 Cs": Coryza, cough, and conjunctivitis
4. Rash appears as red, erythematous maculopapular eruption starting on the face and spreading downward to the feet; blanches easily with pressure and gradually turns a brownish color (lasts 6–7 days); may have desquamation.
5. Koplik spots: Small, red spots with a bluish-white center and a red base. They are located on the buccal mucosa and last for approximately 3 days.

C. Interventions
1. Use airborne and contact precautions if the child is hospitalized.
2. Restrict the child to quiet activities and bed rest.
3. Use a cool-mist vaporizer for cough and coryza.
4. Dim the lights if photophobia is present.
5. Administer antipyretics for fever, as prescribed.
6. Administer vitamin A supplementation as prescribed.

V. Roseola (Exanthema Subitum)

A. Description
1. Agent: Human herpesvirus type 6
2. Incubation period: 5 to 15 days
3. Communicable period: Unknown but thought to extend from the febrile stage to the time that the rash first appears
4. Source and transmission: Unknown; institute standard precautions and other precautions based on child's symptoms and disease.

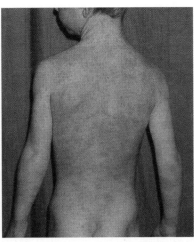

FIGURE 37.1 Rubeola (measles). (From Hockenberry, Wilson, 2012.)

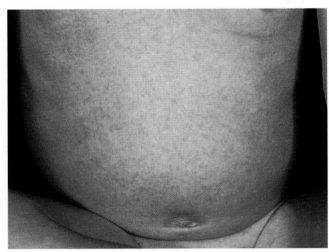

FIGURE 37.2 Roseola (exanthema subitum). (From Habif, 2004.)

 B. Data collection (Fig. 37.2)
1. Sudden high fever (greater than 102°F [38.8°C]) of 3 to 5 days' duration in a child who appears well, followed by a rash (rose-pink macules that blanch with pressure)
2. The rash appears several hours to 2 days after the fever subsides and lasts 1 to 2 days.

C. Interventions: Supportive

VI. Rubella (German Measles)

A. Description
1. Agent: Rubella virus
2. Incubation period: 14 to 21 days
3. Communicable period: 7 days before to about 5 days after the rash appears
4. Source: Nasopharyngeal secretions. The virus is also present in the blood, stool, and urine.
5. Transmission
   a. Airborne or direct contact with infectious droplets
   b. Indirectly via articles freshly contaminated with nasopharyngeal secretions, feces, or urine
   c. Transplacental

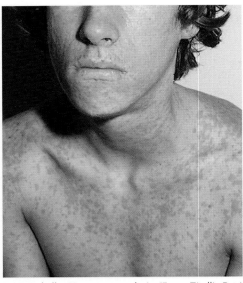

FIGURE 37.3 Rubella (German measles). (From Zitelli, Davis, 2007.) Courtesy Dr. Michael Sherlock, Lutherville, MD.)

B. Data collection (Fig. 37.3)
1. Low-grade fever
2. Malaise
3. Pinkish-red maculopapular rash that begins on the face and spreads to the entire body within 1 to 3 days
4. Petechiae red, pinpoint spots may occur on the soft palate.

C. Interventions
1. Use airborne and contact precautions if the child is hospitalized; provide supportive treatment.
2. Isolate the infected child from pregnant women.

VII. Mumps

A. Description
1. Agent: Paramyxovirus
2. Incubation period: 14 to 21 days
3. Communicable period: Immediately before and after parotid gland swelling begins
4. Source: The saliva of an infected person and possibly the urine
5. Transmission: Direct contact or droplet spread from an infected person

B. Data collection
1. Fever
2. Headache and malaise
3. Anorexia
4. Jaw or ear pain aggravated by chewing, followed by parotid glandular swelling
5. Orchitis or oophoritis may occur.
6. Aseptic meningitis may occur.
7. Deafness may occur.

C. Interventions
1. Institute droplet, and contact precautions.
2. Provide bed rest until the parotid gland swelling subsides.
3. Avoid foods that require chewing.

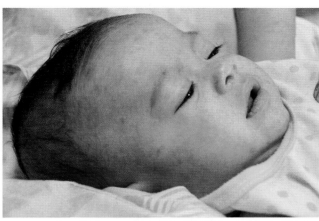

FIGURE 37.4 Chickenpox (varicella). (CDC/Rebecca Martin, PhD.)

4. Apply hot or cold compresses to the neck, as prescribed.

5. Apply warmth and local support with snug-fitting underpants to relieve orchitis.

6. Monitor closely for signs of aseptic meningitis, a complication of mumps (see Chapters 35 and 55 for information on meningitis).

VIII. Chickenpox (Varicella)

A. Description

1. Agent: VCZ virus

2. Incubation period: 13 to 17 days

3. Communicable period: 1 to 2 days before the onset of the rash to 6 days after the first crop of vesicles, when crusts have formed

4. Source: Respiratory tract secretions of an infected person; skin lesions

 5. Transmission: Direct contact, droplet, airborne spread, and contaminated objects

B. Data collection (Fig. 37.4)

1. Slight fever, malaise, and anorexia are followed by a macular rash that first appears on the trunk and scalp and then moves to the face and extremities.

2. Lesions become pustules, begin to dry, and develop a crust.

3. Lesions may appear on the mucous membranes of the mouth, the genital area, and the rectal area.

C. Interventions

 1. In the hospital setting, ensure airborne and droplet precautions.

 2. In the home setting, isolate the infected child until the vesicles have dried.

3. An antiviral agent may be used to treat varicella infections in susceptible immunocompromised persons to decrease the number of lesions; shorten the duration of fever; and decrease itching, lethargy, and anorexia.

4. The use of VCZ immune globulin or intravenous immune globulin (IVIG) is recommended for children who are immunocompromised, who

have no previous history of varicella, and who are likely to contract the disease and have complications as a result.

5. Provide supportive care.

⚠ Isolate high-risk children, such as children who have immunosuppressive disorders, from a child with a communicable disease.

IX. Pertussis (Whooping Cough)

A. Description

1. Agent: Bordetella pertussis

2. Incubation period: 5 to 21 days (usually 10 days)

3. Communicable period: Greatest during the catarrhal stage (i.e., when discharge from respiratory secretions occurs)

4. Source: Discharge from the respiratory tract of the infected person

 5. Transmission: Direct contact or droplet spread from the infected person; indirect contact with freshly contaminated articles

B. Data collection

 1. Symptoms of respiratory infection followed by increased severity of cough with a loud whooping inspiration

2. May experience cyanosis, respiratory distress, and tongue protrusion

3. Listlessness, irritability, and anorexia

C. Interventions

 1. Isolate the child during the catarrhal stage. If the child is hospitalized, institute droplet and contact precautions.

2. Antimicrobial therapy may be prescribed.

 3. Reduce environmental factors that cause coughing spasms, such as dust, smoke, and sudden changes in temperature.

4. Ensure adequate hydration and nutrition.

5. Provide suction and humidified oxygen, if needed.

6. Monitor the cardiopulmonary status (via a monitor as prescribed) and pulse oximetry.

 7. Infants do not receive maternal immunity to pertussis; the tetanus-diphtheria–acellular pertussis (Tdap) vaccine would be administered to women in the postpartum period and those in close contact with the infant to prevent the spread of pertussis to infants.

X. Diphtheria

A. Description

1. Agent: Corynebacterium diphtheriae

2. Incubation period: 2 to 5 days

3. Communicable period: Variable; until virulent bacilli are no longer present (3 negative cultures of discharge from the nose, nasopharynx, skin, and other lesions); usually 2 weeks, but can be as long as 4 weeks

Pediatric Nursing

4. Source: Discharge from the mucous membrane of the nose, nasopharynx, skin, and other lesions of the infected person
5. Transmission: Direct contact with an infected person, carrier, or contaminated articles

B. Data collection
1. Low-grade fever, malaise, and sore throat
2. Foul-smelling and mucopurulent nasal discharge
3. Dense pseudomembrane formation in the throat that may interfere with eating, drinking, and breathing
4. Lymphadenitis, neck edema, and "bull neck"

C. Interventions
1. Institute airborne and contact precautions for the hospitalized child.
2. Assist to administer diphtheria antitoxin, as prescribed (after a skin or conjunctival test to rule out sensitivity to horse serum).
3. Provide bed rest.
4. Assist to administer antibiotics, as prescribed.
5. Provide suction and humidified oxygen, as needed.
6. Provide tracheostomy care if a tracheostomy is necessary.

XI. Poliomyelitis

A. Description
1. Agent: Enteroviruses
2. Incubation period: 7 to 14 days
3. Communicable period: Unknown. The virus is present in the throat and feces shortly after infection and persists for approximately 1 week in the throat and 4 to 6 weeks in the feces.
4. Source: The oropharyngeal secretions and feces of an infected person
5. Transmission: Direct contact with an infected person; fecal-oral and oropharyngeal routes

B. Data collection
1. Fever, malaise, anorexia, nausea, headache, and sore throat
2. Abdominal pain followed by soreness and stiffness of the trunk, neck, and limbs that may progress to central nervous system paralysis

C. Interventions
1. Enteric and contact precautions
2. Supportive treatment
3. Bed rest
4. Monitoring for signs of respiratory paralysis
5. Physical therapy

XII Scarlet Fever

A. Description
1. Agent: Group A β-hemolytic streptococci
2. Incubation period: 1 to 7 days
3. Communicable period: Approximately 10 days during the incubation period and clinical illness; during the first 2 weeks of the carrier stage, although this stage may persist for months

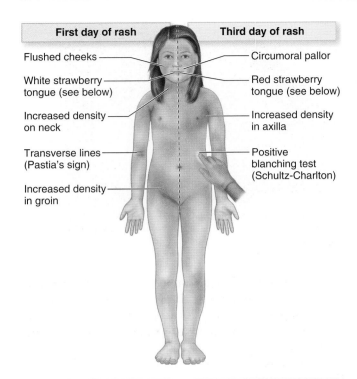

First day of rash	Third day of rash

Flushed cheeks — Circumoral pallor
White strawberry tongue (see below) — Red strawberry tongue (see below)
Increased density on neck — Increased density in axilla
Transverse lines (Pastia's sign) — Positive blanching test (Schultz-Charlton)
Increased density in groin

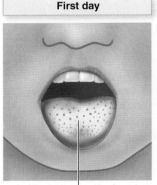 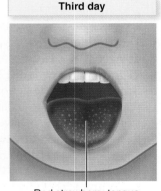

First day	Third day

White strawberry tongue   Red strawberry tongue

FIGURE 37.5 Scarlet fever.

4. Source: Nasopharyngeal secretions of an infected person or carriers
5. Transmission: Direct contact with an infected person or droplet spread; indirectly by contact with contaminated articles or the ingestion of contaminated milk or other foods

B. Data collection (Fig. 37.5)
1. Abrupt high fever, flushed cheeks, vomiting, headache, enlarged lymph nodes in the neck, malaise, and abdominal pain
2. A red, fine, sandpaper-like rash develops in the axilla, groin, and neck and spreads to cover the entire body, except the face.
3. The rash blanches with pressure (Schultz-Charlton): pink or red lines of petechiae are noted in areas of deep creases and folds of the joints (Pastia's sign).
4. Desquamation, a sheet-like sloughing of the skin of the palms and soles, appears by week 1 to week 3.
5. The tongue is initially coated with a white, furry covering with red projecting papillae (white

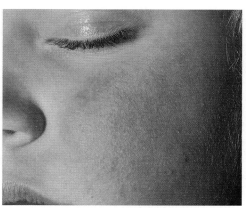

FIGURE 37.6 Erythema infectiosum (fifth disease): Slapped-face appearance. (From Habif, 2004.)

strawberry tongue). By the third to fifth day, the white coat sloughs off, leaving a red, swollen tongue (red strawberry tongue).

6. Tonsils are reddened, edematous, and covered with exudate.
7. Pharynx is edematous and beefy red.

C. Interventions

1. Institute droplet and contact precautions until 24 hours after the initiation of antibiotic therapy.
2. Provide supportive therapy.
3. Provide bed rest.
4. Encourage fluid intake.

XIII. Erythema Infectiosum (Fifth Disease)

A. Description

1. Agent: Human parvovirus B19
2. Incubation period: 4 to 14 days; may be as long as 20 days
3. Communicable period: Uncertain, but before the onset of symptoms in most children
4. Source: Infected person
5. Transmission: Unknown; possibly respiratory secretions and blood

B. Data collection

1. Before rash, asymptomatic or mild fever, malaise, headache, and runny nose
2. Stages of the rash
   a. Erythema of the face (slapped-cheek appearance) develops, chiefly on the cheeks, and disappears by 1 to 4 days (Fig. 37.6).
   b. Approximately 1 day after the rash appears on the face, maculopapular red spots appear and are symmetrically distributed on the extremities. The rash progresses from the proximal to distal surfaces and may last a week or more.
   c. The rash subsides but may reappear if the skin is irritated or traumatized by factors such as the sun, heat, cold, exercise, or friction.

C. Interventions

1. The child is not usually hospitalized.
2. Pregnant women need to avoid the infected individual.

3. Provide supportive care.
4. Assist with the administration of antipyretics, analgesics, and anti-inflammatory medications, as prescribed.

XIV. Infectious Mononucleosis

A. Description

1. Agent: Epstein-Barr virus
2. Incubation period: 4 to 6 weeks
3. Communicable period: Unknown
4. Source: Oral secretions
5. Transmission: Direct intimate contact

B. Data collection

1. Fever, sore throat, malaise, headache, fatigue, nausea, abdominal pain, and enlarged, red tonsils
2. Lymphadenopathy and hepatosplenomegaly
3. A discrete macular rash that is most prominent over the trunk may occur.

C. Interventions

1. Provide supportive care.
2. Monitor for signs of splenic rupture.

 Teach the parents of a child with mononucleosis to monitor for signs of splenic rupture, which include abdominal pain, left upper quadrant pain, and left shoulder pain.

XV. Rocky Mountain Spotted Fever

A. Description

1. Agent: Rickettsia rickettsii
2. Incubation period: 2 to 14 days
3. Source: Tick from a mammal source, most often from wild rodents and dogs
4. Transmission: The bite of an infected tick

B. Data collection

1. Fever, malaise, anorexia, vomiting, headache, and myalgia
2. A maculopapular or petechial rash primarily on the extremities (ankles and wrists) but that may spread to other areas; characteristically on the palms and soles

C. Interventions

1. Provide vigorous supportive care.
2. Assist to administer antibiotics, as prescribed.
3. Reinforce teaching to the child and parents about protection from tick bites (Box 37.3).

XVI. Community-Associated Methicillin-Resistant *Staphylococcus aureus* (CA-MRSA)

A. Description

1. *S. aureus* is a bacterium that is normally located on the skin or in the nose of healthy people. When present without symptoms, it is called *colonization*, and when symptoms are present, it is called an *infection*.
2. MRSA is a strain of *S. aureus* that is resistant to methicillin and most often occurs in people who

were hospitalized or treated at a health care facility (hospital-acquired MRSA).

3. CA-MRSA is a MRSA infection that occurs in a healthy person who has not been hospitalized or had a medical procedure done within the past year.

4. Persons at risk for CA-MRSA include athletes, prisoners, daycare attendees, military recruits, persons who abuse intravenous drugs, persons living in crowded settings, persons with poor hygiene practices, persons who use contaminated items, persons who get tattoos, and persons with a compromised immune system.

5. CA-MRSA is spread through person-to-person contact, contact with contaminated items, or infection of a preexisting cut or wound that is not protected by a dressing.

6. The bacteria can enter the bloodstream through the cut or wound and cause sepsis, cellulitis, endocarditis, osteomyelitis, septic arthritis, toxic shock syndrome, pneumonia, organ failure, and death.

B. Prevention measures

1. Frequent hand washing and strict aseptic technique in health care facilities
2. Hand washing and practicing good personal hygiene
3. Avoiding sharing of personal items
4. Regular cleaning of shared equipment such as athletic equipment, whirlpools, or saunas

5. Cleaning a cut or wound thoroughly
6. Ensure tattoo or body piercing facilities adhere to strict guidelines regarding preventing infection.

C. Data collection

1. Appearance of a skin infection: Red, swollen area, warmth around the area, drainage of pus, pain at the site, fever
2. Symptoms of a more serious infection: Chest pain, cough, fatigue, chills, fever, malaise, headache, muscle aches, shortness of breath, rash

D. Interventions

1. Institute contact precautions.
2. Check skin lesions.
3. Prepare to drain an infected skin site and culture the wound and wound drainage.
4. Prepare to obtain blood cultures, sputum cultures, and urine cultures.
5. Prepare to administer antibiotics as prescribed.
6. Reinforce educating the parent and family about the causes and modes of transmission, signs/symptoms, and importance of treatment prescribed.

XVII. Influenza

A. Description

1. Various strains of influenza can occur.
2. It is a viral infection that affects the respiratory system and is highly contagious.
3. Children, pregnant women, persons with pre- existing health conditions, and persons with a compromised immune system are at high risk for developing complications.
4. It is caused by contact with an infected person or by touching something such as a toy or tissue that the infected person has touched.

B. Prevention

1. Flu vaccine
2. Wash the child's hands frequently and teach hand-washing techniques.
3. Avoid children who are ill.
4. Keep the child home from school or away from others until the child has been fever-free (without the use of antipyretics) for at least 24 hours.
5. For additional information on influenza, refer to Centers for Disease Control and Prevention (CDC) website: https://www.cdc.gov/vaccines/hcp/vis/vis-statements/hib.html.

⚠ The signs/symptoms of flu usually last a week. If they last longer, the presence of complications would be suspected.

C. Data collection

1. Fever that occurs suddenly and is high
2. Headache, body aches, fatigue, chills, cough, congestion, sore throat, loss of appetite, vomiting, diarrhea

D. Interventions
 1. Institute droplet precautions.
 2. Antiviral medications if prescribed, fluids, rest, pain relievers such as acetaminophen or ibuprofen
 3. Reinforce family and child teaching about prevention measures.

XVIII. COVID-19 (Coronavirus)

A. The SARS-CoV-2 is the coronavirus that causes COVID-19.

B. At the current time, it is noted that the disease causes much milder symptoms in babies and children than in adults.

C. As with adults, existing underlying conditions such as asthma or diabetes mellitus place the child at greater risk for more severe symptoms. Parents should be taught to seek immediate medical care if the child experiences difficulty breathing, vomiting and the inability to hold in fluids, confusion, inability to arouse, or develops cyanosis.

D. Transmission is via contact with the virus via respiratory droplets; droplet precautions and possibly contact precautions are necessary.

E. Most common symptoms are fever and cough; children can also experience sore throat, excessive fatigue, or diarrhea.

F. Prevention includes avoiding crowds, maintaining 6 feet of social distancing especially from sick people, handwashing, use of hand sanitizer, wearing masks, coughing and sneezing into the elbow, keeping the hands away from the face, and keeping things clean such as toys or surfaces frequently touched.

G. A concern is the development of pediatric inflammatory multisystem syndrome (PIMS) and although this is a rare condition, it is thought that it might be related to exposure to the coronavirus.

H. PIMS can cause inflammation of the blood vessels throughout the body and this inflammation can limit blood flow, damaging the heart and other organs. It has characteristics similar to toxic shock syndrome and Kawasaki disease (see Chapter 33 for information on Kawasaki disease).

I. Symptoms of PIMS include fever, abdominal pain, vomiting, diarrhea, red rash, red cracked lips, red eyes, swollen glands in the neck, swollen hands and feet.
 From: Milstone, A. (2020). Coronavirus in babies and kids. *Health*. The John Hopkins University, https://www.hopkinsmedicine.org/health/conditions-and-diseases/coronavirus/coronavirus-in-babies-and-children.

XIX. Immunizations

A. Guidelines (see **Priority Nursing Actions**)
 1. In the United States the recommended age for beginning primary immunizations of infants is at birth.

⚡ PRIORITY NURSING ACTIONS

Administering a Parenteral Vaccine

1. Verify the prescription for the vaccine.
2. Obtain an immunization history from the parents and ask about allergies.
3. Provide information to the parents about the vaccine.
4. Obtain parental consent.
5. Check the lot number and expiration date and prepare the injection.
6. Select the appropriate site for administration.
7. Administer the vaccine.
8. Document the administration, site of administration, lot number, and expiration date of the vaccine.
9. Provide a vaccination record to the parents.

---

 2. Children who began primary immunizations at the recommended age but failed to receive all of the required doses do not need to begin the series again. Rather, they need to receive only the missed doses.
 3. If there is a suspicion that the parent will not bring the child to the pediatrician or health care clinic for follow-up immunizations according to the optimal immunization schedule, any of the recommended vaccines can be administered simultaneously.

B. General contraindications and precautions
 1. A vaccine is contraindicated if the child experienced an anaphylactic reaction to a previously administered vaccine or a component in the vaccine.
 2. Live virus vaccines generally are not administered to individuals with severely deficient immune systems, those with a severe sensitivity to gelatin, or pregnant women.
 3. A vaccine is administered with caution to an individual with a moderate or severe acute illness, with or without fever.

C. Guidelines for administration (Box 37.4)

 ⚠️ Children born preterm need to receive the full dose of each vaccine at the appropriate chronological age.

D. Recommended immunization schedules (Box 37.5): For the most up-to-date information about schedules and specific information for each type of vaccine, refer to Immunization Schedules at Centers for Disease Control and Prevention (CDC) website: https://www.cdc.gov/vaccines/schedules/.

E. Reactions to a vaccine
 1. Local reactions
   a. Tenderness, erythema, and swelling at the injection site
   b. Low-grade fever
   c. Behavioral changes, such as drowsiness, unusual crying, and eating less

BOX 37.4 Guidelines for the Administration of Vaccines

- Follow the manufacturer's recommendations for the route of administration, storage, and the reconstitution of the vaccine.
- If refrigeration is necessary, store the vaccine on a center shelf and not on the door. Frequent temperature changes from opening the refrigerator door can alter the potency of the vaccine.
- A vaccine information statement needs to be given to the parents or the individual, and informed consent for administration needs to be obtained.
- Check the expiration date on the vaccine bottle.
- Parenteral vaccines are given in separate syringes in different injection sites.
- Vaccines that are administered intramuscularly are given in the vastus lateralis muscle (best site) or the ventrogluteal muscle. The deltoid can be used for children 36 months and older.
- Vaccines that are administered subcutaneously are given into the fatty areas in the lateral upper arms and the anterior thighs.
- Adequate needle length and gauge are as follows: intramuscular, 1 inch, 23–25 gauge; subcutaneous, $\frac{5}{8}$ inch, 25 gauge (needle length may vary, depending on the child's size).
- Mild side effects may include fever, soreness, swelling, or redness at the injection site.
- A topical anesthetic may be applied to the injection site before the injection.
- For painful or red injection sites, advise the parent to apply cool compresses for the first 24 hours and to then use warm or cool compresses as long as needed.
- An age-appropriate dose of acetaminophen or ibuprofen, per health care provider's preference, may be administered every 4–6 hours for vaccine-associated discomfort.
- Maintain an immunization record: document the day, month, and year of administration; the manufacturer and lot number of vaccine; the name, address, and title of the person who administered the vaccine; and the site and route of administration.
- A vaccine adverse event report needs to be filed, and the health department needs to be notified if an adverse reaction to an immunization occurs.

BOX 37.5 Recommended Childhood and Adolescent Immunizations: 2020

Birth: Hepatitis B vaccine (HepB)
1 month: HepB
2 months: Inactivated poliovirus vaccine (IPV); diphtheria, tetanus, acellular pertussis (DTaP) vaccine; *Haemophilus influenzae* type b conjugate vaccine (Hib); pneumococcal conjugate vaccine (PCV), rotavirus (RV)
4 months: DTaP, Hib, IPV, PCV, RV
6 months: DTaP, Hib, HepB, IPV, PCV, RV (dose may be needed depending on type of vaccine used for first and second doses)
12–15 months: Hib; PCV; measles, mumps, rubella (MMR) vaccine; hepatitis A, first dose (second dose is given 6–18 months after the first dose); varicella vaccine
15–18 months: DTaP
18–33 months: Hepatitis A (second dose given 6–18 months after the first dose)
4–6 years: DTaP, IPV, MMR, varicella vaccine
11–12 years: MMR (if not administered at 4–6 years); diphtheria, tetanus, acellular pertussis adolescent preparation (Tdap); meningococcal vaccine (MCV4) with a booster at age 16; human papillomavirus (HPV) (first dose to girls at age 11–12 years, second dose 2 months after first dose, and third dose 6 months after first dose)

Centers for Disease Control and Prevention (CDC), (2020). *Recommended Child and Adolescent Immunization Schedule for ages 18 years or younger, United States, 2020.* https://www.cdc.gov/vaccines/schedules/hcp/imz/child-adolescent.html. Note: Influenza vaccine is recommended annually for children beginning at age 6 months.

subcutaneous injection of an antihistamine such as diphenhydramine and epinephrine may be prescribed.

   c. For moderate or severe distress, establish an airway; provide cardiopulmonary resuscitation to the child if necessary; elevate the head; epinephrine, fluids, and vasopressors may be prescribed; monitor vital signs and urine output.

  2. Minimizing local reactions
   a. Select a needle of adequate length to deposit the vaccine deep into the muscle or subcutaneous mass.
   b. Inject the vaccine into the appropriate, recommended site.
  3. Anaphylactic reactions
   a. The goals of treatment are to secure and protect the airway, restore adequate circulation, and prevent further exposure to the antigen.
   b. For a mild reaction with no evidence of respiratory distress or cardiovascular compromise,

WHAT WOULD YOU DO?

Answer: Droplet and contact precautions would be instituted for the child with mumps to prevent its transmission. It is transmitted by direct contact or droplet spread from an infected person. The nurse would also plan to provide bed rest until the parotid gland swelling subsides. If prescribed, hot or cold compresses would be applied to the neck to alleviate discomfort. Foods that require chewing would be avoided. If orchitis occurs, warmth and local support with snug-fitting underpants will relieve discomfort. The nurse would also monitor the child closely for signs of aseptic meningitis, a complication of mumps.

PRACTICE QUESTIONS

❖ **1.** A child with rubeola (measles) is being admitted to the hospital. When preparing for the admission of the child, which precautions would be implemented? **Select all that apply.**
 ❑ **1.** Enteric
 ❑ **2.** Contact
 ❑ **3.** Airborne
 ❑ **4.** Protective
 ❑ **5.** Neutropenic

2. The mother of a toddler with mumps asks the nurse what she needs to watch for in her child with this disease. The nurse bases the response on the understanding that mumps is which type of communicable disease?
 1. Skin rash caused by a virus
 2. Skin rash caused by a bacteria
 3. Respiratory disease caused by virus involving the lymph nodes
 4. Respiratory disease caused by a virus involving the parotid gland

3. A 6-month-old infant receives a diphtheria, tetanus, and acellular pertussis (DTaP) immunization at the well-baby clinic. The parent returns home and calls the clinic to report that the infant has developed swelling and redness at the site of injection. Which instruction by the nurse is appropriate?
 1. Monitor the infant for a fever.
 2. Bring the infant back to the clinic.
 3. Apply an ice pack to the injection site.
 4. Leave the injection site alone, because this always occurs.

4. A child is diagnosed with scarlet fever. The nurse collects data regarding the child. Which is characteristic of scarlet fever?
 1. Pastia's sign
 2. Abdominal pain and flaccid paralysis
 3. Dense pseudoformation membrane in the throat
 4. Foul-smelling and mucopurulent nasal drainage

5. A child is diagnosed with infectious mononucleosis. The nurse reinforces homecare instructions to parents about the care of the child. Which instruction would the nurse provide to the parents?
 1. Maintain the child on bed rest for 2 weeks.
 2. Maintain respiratory precautions for 1 week.
 3. Notify the pediatrician if the child develops a fever.
 4. Notify the pediatrician if the child develops abdominal or left shoulder pain.

6. A child is diagnosed with chicken pox. The nurse collects data regarding the child. Which finding is characteristic of chicken pox?
 1. Macular rash on the trunk and scalp
 2. Pseudomembrane formation in the throat
 3. Maculopapular or petechial rash on the extremities
 4. Small, red spots with a bluish-white center and red base

7. The nurse is reviewing instructions to a parent of a 6-year-old on how to prevent influenza. Which statement by the parent indicates a **need for further teaching**?
 1. "I will get a flu shot and I will have my child get a flu shot too."
 2. "I will avoid having my child come into contact with sick children."
 3. "I will have my child wash her hands frequently during the flu season."
 4. "I will not let my child play with other children who have the flu unless they are taking acetaminophen."

8. The nurse reviews measures to prevent tick bites with a parent of a child with Rocky Mountain spotted fever. Which statement by the parent indicates a **need for further teaching**?
 1. "I will have my child wear long sleeves and long pants to keep covered up."
 2. "I will have my child stay on well-worn paths and not stray into tall grass."
 3. "I will check my child for ticks after being exposed to a high-risk tick-infected area."
 4. "I will have my child wear dark colored clothing so the tick will not be attracted to the colors."

❖ **9.** Which home care instructions would the nurse plan to reinforce to the mother of a child with acquired immunodeficiency syndrome (AIDS)? **Select all that apply.**
 ❑ **1.** Frequent hand washing is important.
 ❑ **2.** The child needs to avoid exposure to other illnesses.
 ❑ **3.** The child's immunization schedule will need revision.
 ❑ **4.** Kissing the child on the mouth will never transmit the virus.
 ❑ **5.** Clean up body fluid spills with bleach solution (10:1 ratio of water to bleach).
 ❑ **6.** Fever, malaise, fatigue, weight loss, vomiting, and diarrhea are expected to occur and do not require special intervention.

10. The nurse reviews the home care instructions with a parent of a 3-year-old with pertussis. Which statement by the parent indicates a **need for further teaching**?
 1. "I know that my child will make a loud whooping sound."
 2. "I understand this whooping cough is viral and I have to let it run its course."
 3. "I understand that I need to watch for respiratory distress signs with pertussis."
 4. "I can reduce the environmental factors that can trigger coughing, like dust and smoke."

Pediatric Nursing

ANSWERS

❖ **1.** 2, 3

Rationale: Rubeola is transmitted via airborne particles or direct contact with infectious droplets. Airborne precautions and contact precautions are required; a mask and gloves are worn by those who come in contact with the child. Gowns and gloves are not indicated. Articles that are contaminated need to be bagged and labeled. Options 1, 4, and 5 are not indicated for rubeola.

Test-Taking Strategy: Focus on the subject, precautions needed for a child with rubeola. Recalling that rubeola is transmitted via airborne particles and direct contact with infectious droplets will direct you to the correct option. Also note that option 4 and 5 are comparable or alike and can be eliminated.

2. 4

Rationale: Mumps is caused by a paramyxovirus that causes swelling from the parotid gland, causing jaw and ear pain. It is transmitted via direct contact or droplets spread from an infected person, from infected saliva, and possibly by contact with urine. Droplet and contact precautions are indicated during the period of communicability. Options 1, 2, and 3 are incorrect.

Test-Taking Strategy: Options 1 and 2 can be eliminated first, because they are comparable or alike and address a skin rash. Recall the cause of mumps as a virus causing swelling from the parotid gland, causing jaw and ear pain. Involvement of lymph nodes would cause neck swelling.

3. 3

Rationale: Occasionally tenderness, redness, or swelling may occur at the site of the injection. This can be relieved with cool packs for the first 24 hours and followed by warm or cool compresses if the inflammation persists. It is not necessary to bring the infant back to the clinic. Option 1 may be an appropriate intervention, but it is not specific to the question.

Test-Taking Strategy: Option 4 can be eliminated first because of the closed-ended word, *always.* Eliminate option 1 next because it does not relate specifically to the subject, swelling and redness at the injection site. Next, eliminate option 2 as an unnecessary intervention.

4. 1

Rationale: Pastia's sign is a rash seen among children with scarlet fever that will blanch with pressure, except in areas of deep creases and in the folds of joints. The tongue is initially coated with a white furry covering with red projecting papillae (white strawberry tongue). By the fourth to fifth day, the white strawberry tongue sloughs off and leaves a red, swollen tongue (strawberry tongue). The pharynx is edematous and beefy red in color. Option 2 is associated with poliomyelitis. Options 3 and 4 are characteristics of diphtheria.

Test-Taking Strategy: Focus on the subject, the characteristic associated with scarlet fever. Remember that Pastia's sign describes the rash noted with scarlet fever. Recalling this knowledge will assist in answering correctly.

5. 4

Rationale: The parents need to be instructed to notify the pediatrician if abdominal pain (especially in the left upper quadrant) or left shoulder pain occurs, because this may indicate splenic rupture. Children with enlarged spleens are also instructed to avoid contact sports until the splenomegaly resolves. Bed rest is not necessary and children usually self-limit their activity. Respiratory precautions are not required, although transmission can occur via direct intimate contact or contact with infected blood. Fever is treated with acetaminophen.

Test-Taking Strategy: Focus on the subject, home care instructions for infectious mononucleosis. Use knowledge regarding the organs that are affected in clients with infectious mononucleosis. Options 1 and 2 can be eliminated first because they are unnecessary interventions for this disease. From the remaining options, knowledge that splenic rupture is a concern will direct you to the correct option.

6. 1

Rationale: A macular rash that first appears on the trunk and scalp and then moves to the face and the extremities is a characteristic of chicken pox. Pseudomembrane formation in the throat is characteristic of diphtheria. A maculopapular or petechial rash primarily on the extremities is characteristic of Rocky Mountain spotted fever. Small red spots with a bluish-white center and red base are known as Koplik spots and are characteristic of measles.

Test-Taking Strategy: Note the subject, the characteristics of chicken pox. Eliminate option 2 because it does not refer to a rash. Of the remaining options, eliminate 4 because that does not identify a location for the rash. Recall that the rash for chicken pox occurs on the trunk and scalp and not the extremities.

7. 4

Rationale: Children who have influenza need to be kept home and away from other children until they are fever-free without the use of antipyretics. Influenza may be prevented with the annual vaccine, by avoiding other children who are sick, and with frequent hand washing.

Test-Taking Strategy: Note the strategic words, *need for further teaching.* These words indicate a negative event query and ask you to select an option that is an incorrect statement. Recalling that influenza can be prevented by the flu vaccine, avoiding children who are sick, frequent hand washing, and not letting others play with a child until fever-free are all correct ways to prevent influenza.

8. 4

Rationale: Protection from tick bites includes wearing light-colored clothing to make the ticks more visible if they get on the child. Prevention of Rocky Mountain spotted fever includes measures to take to protect getting tick bites and includes wearing long-sleeved shirts, long pants tucked into socks, and a hat. Checking for ticks on children after they have been exposed to a high-risk area and using insect repellents containing diethyltoluamide and permethrins are also measures to take.

Test-Taking Strategy: Note the strategic words, *need for further teaching.* These words indicate a negative event query and ask you to select an option that is an incorrect statement. Recalling the measures used to protect from ticks will direct you in selecting the correct option.

❖ **9. 1, 2, 5**

Rationale: AIDS is a disorder that is caused by the human immunodeficiency virus (HIV) and is characterized by a generalized dysfunction of the immune system. Homecare instructions include the following: frequent hand washing; monitoring for fever, malaise, fatigue, weight loss, vomiting, diarrhea, altered activity level, and oral lesions and notifying the primary health care provider if these occur; monitoring for signs and symptoms of opportunistic infections; administering antiretroviral medications, as prescribed; avoiding exposure to other illnesses; keeping immunizations up to date; avoiding kissing the child on the mouth; monitoring the weight and providing a high-calorie, high-protein diet; washing eating utensils in the dishwasher; and avoiding the sharing of eating utensils. Gloves are worn for care, especially when in contact with body fluids or changing diapers. Diapers are changed frequently and away from food areas, and soiled disposable diapers are folded inward, closed with their tabs, and disposed of in a tightly covered plastic-lined container. Any body fluid spills are cleaned with a bleach solution made up of a 10:1 ratio of water to bleach.

Test-Taking Strategy: Focus on the subject, home care of the child with AIDS. Recalling that this disorder is characterized by a generalized dysfunction of the immune system and recalling the modes of transmission will assist you with selecting the homecare instructions.

10. 2

Rationale: Pertussis is caused by the bacteria *Bordetella pertussis,* and treatment requires antimicrobial therapy. Symptoms of pertussis consist of a respiratory infection followed by increased severity of cough with a loud whooping on inspiration. The child may experience respiratory distress, and the parents need to be instructed on reducing environmental factors that cause coughing spasms, such as dust, smoke, and sudden changes in temperature.

Test-Taking Strategy: Note the strategic words, *need for further teaching.* These words indicate a negative event query and ask you to select an option that is an incorrect statement. Recalling that pertussis is caused by a bacteria, not a virus, will direct you to the correct option.

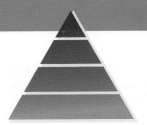

CHAPTER 38

Pediatric Medication Administration and Calculations

Pediatric Nursing

PRIORITY CONCEPTS Development; Safety

WHAT WOULD YOU DO?

The nurse is preparing to administer a medication that has an unpleasant taste to an infant. What would the nurse do to minimize this unpleasant effect?
Answer is located on p. 468.

I. Oral Medications

A. Most oral pediatric medications are in liquid or suspension form because children usually cannot swallow a tablet.

B. Solutions may be measured by using an oral plastic syringe or other acceptable measurement or administration device; the device used depends on the developmental age of the child (Fig. 38.1).

C. Medications in suspension settle to the bottom of the bottle between uses, so thorough mixing is required before the pouring of the medication.

D. Suspensions need to be administered immediately after measurement to prevent settling and thus the administration of an incomplete dose.

E. Administer oral medications with the child sitting in an upright position with the head elevated to prevent aspiration if the child cries or resists.

F. Place the small child sideways on the adult's lap; the child's closest arm would be placed under the adult's arm and behind the adult's back; cradle the child's head, hold his or her hand, and administer the medication slowly with a plastic spoon, small plastic cup, or a syringe without needle.

G. If a tablet or capsule has been administered, check the child's mouth to ensure that it has been swallowed; if swallowing is a problem, some tablets can be crushed and given in small amounts of puréed food or flavored syrup (enteric-coated tablets, timed-release tablets, and capsules cannot be crushed).

H. Follow generally accepted medication administration guidelines for children (Box 38.1).

⚠ Newborns and infants have an immature liver and immature kidneys, so metabolism and elimination of medications are delayed.

II. Parenteral Medications

A. Subcutaneous and intramuscularly administered medications

1. Medications usually given via the subcutaneous route are insulin and some immunizations.

2. Any site with sufficient subcutaneous tissue may be used for subcutaneous injections; common sites include the central third of the lateral aspect of the upper arm, the abdomen, and the center third of the anterior thigh.

3. The safe use of all injection sites is based on normal muscle development and the size of the child; the preferred site for intramuscular injections in infants is the vastus lateralis, but agency policies and procedures need to be followed (Table 38.1 and Fig. 38.2).

4. For pediatric clients, the usual needle length is ½ inch to 1 inch, and the usual needle gauge is 22 to 25; needle length also can be estimated by grasping the muscle between the thumb and forefinger, from which half the resulting distance would be the needle length.

5. Pediatric dosages for subcutaneous and intramuscular administration are calculated to the nearest hundredth and measured with the use of a tuberculin syringe; always follow agency guidelines.

6. Place a plain or decorated adhesive bandage over the puncture site to help the child view the experience in a somewhat pleasant way.

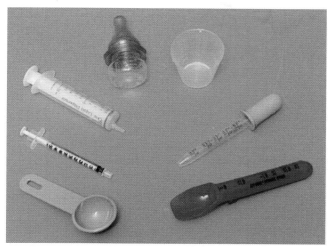

FIGURE 38.1 Acceptable devices for measuring and administering oral medication to children (*clockwise from bottom left*): Measuring spoon, plastic syringes, calibrated nipple, plastic medicine cup, calibrated dropper, hollow-handed medicine spoon. (From Hockenberry, Wilson, 2005.)

⚠ The role of a licensed practical/vocational nurse (LPN/LVN) is to monitor intravenous (IV) solutions and notify the registered nurse if any unexpected event occurs. It is important for the LPN/LVN to understand the guidelines related to IV administration and the various types of administration even though the primary role is monitoring.

III. Guidelines for Intravenous Medication Administration

A. Intravenous medications (IV) are diluted for administration.

B. When an infant or a child is receiving an IV medication, the IV site needs to be monitored closely for signs of infiltration and inflammation immediately before, during, and after the completion of the administration of each medication.

C. IV medications may be prescribed in a manner that requires a continuous infusion through a primary infusion line.

D. IV medications may be prescribed intermittently; several doses may be administered in a 24-hour period.

E. Medications for IV administration are diluted according to the directions accompanying the medication and according to the pediatrician's prescriptions and agency procedures.

F. Infusion time for IV medications is determined on the basis of the directions accompanying the medication, the pediatrician's order, and agency procedures.

G. Note that agency procedures related to the volume of flush (normal saline) for peripheral IV lines and for central lines will be followed. This may differ in children based on age and weight.

H. The flush volume (3–20 mL) is included in the child's intake; the flush is usually administered before administering an IV medication and after the IV medication is completed and is infused at the same rate as the medication.

BOX 38.1 Medication Administration Guidelines for Children

- Two identifiers are required before medication administration, such as name, medical record number, and birth date.
- Obtain information from the parents about successful methods for administering medications to their children.
- Ask the parents about any known allergies.
- To avoid aspiration, liquid forms of medication are safer to swallow than other forms.
- Straws often help older children swallow pills.
- Avoid putting medications in foods, such as milk, cereal, or baby food, because it may cause an unpleasant taste to the food and the child may refuse to accept that same food in the future. In addition, the child may not consume the entire serving and will not receive the required medication dosage.
- If the taste of the medication is unpleasant, have the child drink the medication through a straw.
- Offer juice, a soft drink, or a frozen juice bar after the child swallows a medication.
- Always read the pharmacological indications for administration. Some items such as fruit syrups can be acidic and would not be used with medications that react negatively in an acid medium.
- Record the most successful method of administering medications and pertinent nursing prescriptions on the child's care plan for other nursing staff to follow; this notation also saves the child frustration, fear, and anxiety.

Data from Potter P, Perry A, Stockert P, Hall A: *Fundamentals of nursing*, ed 8, St. Louis, 2013, Mosby; and Perry S, Hockenberry M, Lowdermilk D, Wilson D: *Maternal-child nursing care*, ed 4, St. Louis, 2010, Mosby.

I. Intermittent IV medication administration
   1. Children receiving IV medications intermittently may or may not have a primary IV solution infusing.
   2. If a primary IV solution is infusing, the medication may be administered by IV piggyback via a secondary line.
   3. If a primary IV solution does not exist, an indwelling infusion catheter is used for medication administration, and the medication may be administered by push or piggyback; medication administration instructions need to be checked for dilution and infusion time procedures.
   4. All intermittent medication administrations are preceded and followed by a normal saline flush to ensure that the medication has cleared the IV tubing and the total dose has been administered.
   5. Electronic devices such as controllers or pumps are used to regulate and administer IV fluids and intermittent IV medications.
J. Special IV administration sets
   1. Special IV administration sets, such as a burette, may be used for medication preparation and administration via piggyback.
   2. These special sets are all microdrip sets calibrated to deliver 60 drops (gtt)/mL.

TABLE 38.1 **Intramuscular Injections: Amount of Milliliters (mL) by Muscle Group**

Muscle	Neonate	Infants 1–12 Months	Toddlers 1–2 Years	Preschool to Child 3–12 Years	Adolescent 12–18 Years
Vastus lateralis	0.5	0.5–1	0.5–1	1–1.5	1.5–2
Rectus femoris	Not safe	Not safe	0.5–1	1–1.5	1.5–2
Ventrogluteal	Not safe	Not safe	Not safe	0.5–3	2–3
Deltoid	Not safe	Not safe	0.5–1	0.5–1	1–1.5

Modified from Kee J, Marshall S: *Clinical calculations: With applications to general and specialty areas*, ed 7, St. Louis, 2013, Saunders.

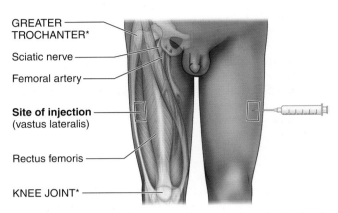

GREATER TROCHANTER*

Sciatic nerve

Femoral artery

Site of injection (vastus lateralis)

Rectus femoris

KNEE JOINT*

FIGURE 38.2 Intramuscular injection site—vastus lateralis. Landmarks are indicated by asterisks and boxes.

BOX 38.3 **Common Measurement Abbreviations**

Abbreviation	Meaning
BSA	body surface area
g	gram(s)
gr	grain(s)
kg	kilogram(s)
lb	pound(s)
m²	square meters
mcg	microgram(s)
mg	milligram(s)
mL	milliliter(s)
SA	surface area

BOX 38.2 **Conversion of Body Weight**

Measurements
- 1 lb = 16 oz
- 1 kg = 2.2 lb

Pounds to Kilograms
- 2.2 lbs = 1 kg
- To convert pounds to kilograms, divide by 2.2.
- Kilograms are expressed to the nearest tenth.

Kilograms to Pounds
- 1 kg = 2.2 lbs
- To convert kilograms to pounds, multiply by 2.2.
- Pounds are expressed to the nearest tenth.

3. The total capacity of these special IV administration sets is 100 mL to 150 mL, calibrated in 1-mL increments so that exact measurements of small volumes are possible.
4. The medication is mixed with the appropriate amount of a diluent, added to the special IV administration set, and allowed to infuse at the prescribed rate.
5. The special IV administration set needs to be labeled clearly to identify the medication and fluid dosage added.
6. During medication infusion time, a label is attached that indicates that the medication is infusing.
7. During the flush infusion time, a label is attached indicating that the flush is infusing.

K. Syringe pump for IV medication administration
1. A syringe containing the medication is fitted into a pump that is connected to the IV tubing through a Y connector.
2. The medication is administered over the prescribed time.

⚠ The 24-hour fluid intake and all IV fluid amounts need to be monitored closely, including the amount of flush volume, which all need to be documented accurately to prevent overhydration. For children, the maximum amount of IV fluid administered in a 24-hour period varies and is usually based on body weight and other factors. The prescription and agency guidelines for the procedures related to the administration of IV fluids and medications are always followed.

IV. Calculation of Medication Dosage by Body Weight
A. Conversion of body weight
1. There are many mobile application devices available to assist with calculating dosages, but it is important to know how to do these calculations without the use of a mobile device.
2. See Box 38.2 for body weight conversions.
B. Calculating daily dosages based on weight
1. Abbreviations (Box 38.3)

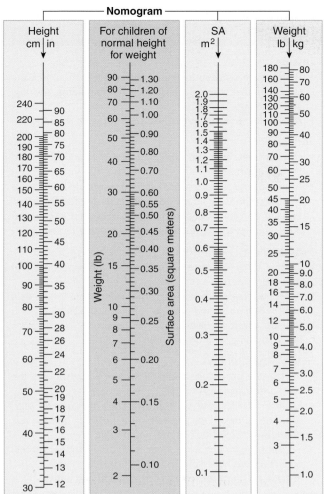

┌──────── Nomogram ────────┐

| Height cm \| in | For children of normal height for weight | SA m² | Weight lb \| kg |

FIG. 38.3 West nomogram for estimation of surface areas in infants and children. First, find height; next, find weight; finally, draw a straight line connecting the height and weight. The body surface area (in square meters [m²]) is indicated where a straight line connecting the height and weight intersects the surface area *(SA)* column or, if the child is approximately of normal proportion, from weight alone *(beige area)*.

2. Dosages are expressed in terms of milligrams per kilogram per day, milligrams per pound per day, or milligrams per kilogram per dose.
3. The total daily dosage is usually administered in divided (more than one) doses per day as prescribed.
4. Express the child's body weight in kilograms or pounds to correlate with the dosage specifications.
5. Calculate the total daily dosage.
6. Divide the total daily dosage by the number of doses to be administered in 1 day.

V. Calculation of Body Surface Area

A. The body surface area (BSA) is determined by comparing body weight and height with averages or norms on a graph called a *nomogram.*
B. Not all children are the same size at the same age; therefore, the nomogram chart can be used to determine the BSA of the child. BSA calculators may be available in some facilities to determine the BSA.

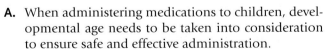

BOX 38.4   How to Use the Nomogram

1. *Example:* Use the nomogram to estimate the body surface area (BSA) of a child whose height is 58 inches and whose weight is 12 kg. Look at Fig. 38.3 and note that the height is on the left-hand side of the chart and the weight is on the right-hand side of the chart.
2. Place a ruler on the chart and line up the left side of the ruler on the height and the right side of the ruler on the weight. Read the BSA at the point where the straight edge of the ruler intersects the surface area (SA) column.
3. The estimated SA is given in square meters (m²).
   Answer: This child's BSA is 0.66 m².

BOX 38.5   Calculating Medication Dosage

Example: The dosage recommendation is 4 mg/m². The child has a body surface area of 1.1 m². What is the dosage to be administered?
   Answer: 1.1 × 4 mg = 4.4 mg

C. Look at the nomogram chart (Fig. 38.3); note that the height is on the left-hand side of the chart, and the weight is on the right-hand side.
D. Place a ruler across the chart.
E. Line up the left side of the ruler on the height and the right side of the ruler on the weight; read the BSA at the point where the straight edge of the ruler intersects the surface area (SA) column.
F. The estimated SA is given in square meters (m²).
G. Box 38.4 gives a sample practice question using the nomogram .

VI. Calculations Based on BSA

A. When dosage recommendations for children are in milligrams, micrograms, or units per square meter, calculating the dosage is simple multiplication (Box 38.5).
B. When dosages are specified only for adults, a formula is used to calculate the child's dosage (Box 38.6).

VII. Developmental Considerations for Administering Medications

A. When administering medications to children, developmental age needs to be taken into consideration to ensure safe and effective administration.
B. General interventions
   1. Always be prepared for the procedure with all necessary equipment and assistance.
   2. For the hospitalized child, ask the parent or child or both if the parent would like to remain for the procedure.
   3. Determine appropriate pre- and post administration comfort measures.
   4. Try to make the event as pleasant as is possible.
C. Box 38.7 lists developmental considerations when giving medications.

BOX 38.6   Calculating a Child's Dosage From the Adult Dosage

When dosages are specified only for adults, a formula is used to calculate a child's dosage from the adult dosage. The adult dosage is based on a standardized body surface area (BSA) of 1.73 m².

Example: A primary health care provider has prescribed an antibiotic for a child. The average adult dose is 250 mg. The child has a BSA of 0.41 m². What is the dose for the child?

Answer: 59.24 mg
Formula:

$$\frac{\text{BSA of a child (m}^2)}{1.73 \text{ m}^2} \times \text{Adult dose} = \text{Child's dose}$$

$$\frac{0.41}{1.73} \times 250 \text{ mg} = 59.24 \text{ mg}$$

WHAT WOULD YOU DO?

Answer: When administering a medication with an unpleasant taste to an infant, the nurse would draw the required dose into a syringe without the needle and place the syringe into the side and toward the back of the infant's mouth; the medication needs to be administered slowly, allowing the infant to swallow.

PRACTICE QUESTIONS

1. Morphine sulfate, 2.5 mg, is prescribed for a child. The safe pediatric dose is 0.05 mg/kg/dose to 0.1 mg/kg/dose. The child weighs 50 kg. Which statement accurately describes the prescribed dosage for this child?
   1. The dose is too low.
   2. The dose is too high.
   3. The dose is within the safe dosage range.
   4. There is not enough information to determine the safe dosage range.

❖ 2. The primary health care provider's (PHCP's) prescription reads acetaminophen 240 mg orally every 6 hours as needed for relief of pain, for a 5-year-old child. The medication label reads "acetaminophen 160 mg per 5 mL." The nurse has determined that the dose prescribed is safe. How many mL per dose would the nurse administer to the child?
   Fill in the blank.
   *Answer:*_____ mL

❖ 3. The PHCP has prescribed phenobarbital sodium, 25 mg orally twice daily, for a child with febrile seizures. The medication label reads as follows: "Phenobarbital sodium, 20 mg/5 mL." The nurse has determined that the dose prescribed is a safe dose for the child. How many milliliters per dose would the nurse administer to the child?
   Fill in the blank.
   *Answer:*_____ mL

BOX 38.7   Developmental Considerations for Administering Medications

Infants
- Perform the procedure quickly, allowing the infant to swallow; then offer comfort measures, such as holding, rocking, and cuddling.
- Allow self-comforting measures, such as the use of a pacifier.

Toddlers
- Offer a brief, concrete explanation of the procedure, and then perform it.
- Accept aggressive behavior, within reasonable limits, as a healthy response, and provide outlets for the toddler.
- Provide comfort measures immediately after the procedure, such as touch, holding, cuddling, and a favorite toy.

Preschoolers
- Offer a brief, concrete explanation of the procedure and then perform it.
- Accept aggressive behavior, within reasonable limits, as a healthy response, and provide outlets for the child.
- Provide comfort measures after the procedure, such as touch, holding, or a favorite toy.

School-Age Children
- Explain the procedure, allowing for some control over the body and situation.
- Explore feelings and concepts through therapeutic play, drawings of own body and self in the hospital, and the use of books and realistic hospital equipment.
- Set appropriate behavior limits; such as, it is alright to cry or scream but not to bite.
- Provide activities for releasing aggression and anger.
- Use the opportunity to teach about how medication helps the disorder.

Adolescents
- Explain the procedure, allowing for some control over the body and situation.
- Explore concepts of self, hospitalization, and illness, and correct any misconceptions.
- Encourage self-expression, individuality, and self-care needs.
- Encourage participation in the procedure.

Data from McKenry L, Salerno E: *Mosby's pharmacology in nursing,* St. Louis, 2003, Mosby.

4. Sulfisoxazole 1 g orally four times daily is prescribed for an adolescent with a urinary tract infection. The medication label reads, "250-mg tablets." The nurse has determined that the prescribed dose is safe. How many tablets per dose would the nurse administer to the adolescent?
   Fill in the blank.
   *Answer:*_____ tablets

5. The pediatrician has prescribed an antibiotic for a child. The average adult dose is 500 mg. The child has a body surface area (BSA) of 0.63 m². What is the dose for the child?
   Fill in the blank.
   Answer: _____ mg

ANSWERS

1. 3

Rationale: Use the formula for calculating a safe dosage range.
Dosage parameters:

$$0.05 \text{ mg/kg/dose} \times 50 \text{ kg} = 2.5 \text{ mg/dose}$$

$$0.1 \text{ mg/kg/dose} \times 50 \text{ kg} = 5 \text{ mg/dose}$$

The dose is within the safe dosage range.
Test-Taking Strategy: Focus on the subject, the safe dosage range of the medication. Calculate the dosage parameters with the use of the safe dosage range identified in the question and the child's weight in kilograms. Verify the answer with the use of a calculator.

❖ **2. 7.5**
Rationale: Use the medication calculation formula.
Formula:

$$\frac{\text{Desired}}{\text{Available}} \times \text{Volume} = \frac{240 \text{ mg}}{160 \text{ mg}} \times 5 \text{ mL} = 7.5 \text{ mL/dose}$$

Test-Taking Strategy: Focus on the subject, milliliters per dose. Next, use the formula to determine the correct dosage, knowing that 160 mg = 5 mL. Verify the answer with the use of a calculator.

❖ **3. 6.25**
Rationale: Use the medication calculation formula.
Formula:

$$\frac{\text{Desired}}{\text{Available}} \times \text{Volume} = \frac{25 \text{ mg}}{20 \text{ mg}} \times 5 \text{ mL} = 6.25 \text{ mL/dose}$$

Test-Taking Strategy: Focus on the subject, milliliters per dose. Use the formula to determine the correct dosage, and use a calculator to verify the answer.

4. 4
Rationale: Change grams to milligrams, knowing that 1000 mg = 1 g. When converting from grams to milligrams (larger to smaller), move the decimal point three places to the right; thus, 1.0 g = 1000 mg. Then, use the medication calculation formula.
Formula:

$$\frac{\text{Desired}}{\text{Available}} \times \text{Tablet} = \frac{1000 \text{ mg}}{250 \text{ mg}} \times 1 \text{ tablet} = 4 \text{ Tablets}$$

Test-Taking Strategy: Focus on the subject, tablets per dose. Change grams to milligrams first. Then, use the formula to determine the correct dosage. Remember to verify the answer with the use of a calculator.

5. 182
Rationale: When calculating pediatric dosages that are specified for adults, calculate the child's dose using the formula that incorporates body surface area (BSA) values. Standard adult BSA value is 1.73 m², the child's BSA is 0.63 m².
Formula:

$$\frac{\text{BSA of child } (\text{m}^2)}{1.73 \text{ m}^2} \times \text{Adult dose} = \text{Child's dose}$$

$$\frac{0.63}{1.73} \times 500 \text{ mg} = 182 \text{ mg}$$

Test-Taking Strategy: Focus on the subject, child's dose based on the adult dose. Focus on the data in the question. Use BSA in the formula to determine the correct dose, and use a calculator to verify your answer.

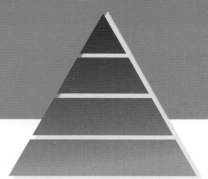

UNIT VIII

Integumentary Problems of the Adult Client

 Pyramid to Success

The Pyramid to Success focuses on the concept that the integumentary system provides the first line of defense against infections. Focus is on the protective measures necessary to prevent infection, including infection from colonization with a multidrug resistant organism, such as methicillin-resistant *Staphylococcus aureus* (MRSA). Pyramid Points address the risk factors related to the development of integumentary disorders, and the preventive measures related to skin cancer. Also described are the emergency measures related to bites and stings, and for a client who sustained a burn injury. Psychosocial issues related to the body image disturbances that can occur as the result of an integumentary disorder are addressed.

 Client Needs: Learning Objectives

Safe and Effective Care Environment

Consulting with interprofessional health care team members regarding treatments

Ensuring that informed consent has been obtained for treatments and procedures

Establishing priorities of care

Handling of hazardous and infectious materials

Instituting standard and other precautions

Client Needs lists modified from: National Council of State Boards of Nursing, Inc. (NCSBN). *NCLEX-PN Examination: Test Plan for the National Council Licensure Examination for Practical Nurses,* effective April 2020. Chicago: NCSBN.

Maintaining confidentiality related to the disorder

Making referrals to appropriate health care providers

Practicing asepsis techniques and preventing infection

Health Promotion and Maintenance

Implementing disease prevention measures

Performing physical assessment/data collection techniques for the integumentary system

Promoting health screening and health promotion programs to prevent skin disorders

Providing instructions to the client regarding prevention measures and care for an integumentary disorder

Psychosocial Integrity

Addressing end-of-life issues

Discussing unexpected body image changes

Identifying coping mechanisms

Identifying situational role changes

Identifying support systems

Physiological integrity

Monitoring for alterations in body systems

Providing adequate nutrition for healing

Providing basic care and comfort

Providing emergency care

Monitoring for expected effects of treatments

Monitoring for fluid and electrolyte imbalances and other complications

Monitoring laboratory reference intervals

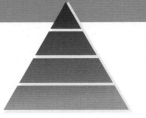

CHAPTER 39

Integumentary Problems

PRIORITY CONCEPTS Infection; Tissue Integrity

WHAT WOULD YOU DO?

A burn client undergoes an autograft to the lower right leg. What would the nurse do when caring for the graft site? *Answer is located on p. 487.*

I. Anatomy and Physiology

A. The skin is the largest sensory organ of the body, with a surface area of 15 to 20 square feet (1.4–1.9 square meters) and a weight of approximately 9 lb (4 kg).

B. Functions
1 Acts as the first line of defense against infection
2. Protects underlying tissues and organs from injury
3. Receives stimuli from the external environment; detects touch, pressure, pain, and temperature stimuli; relays information to the nervous system
4. Regulates normal body temperature
5. Excretes salts, water, and organic wastes
6. Protects the body from excessive water loss
7. Synthesizes vitamin D_3, which converts to calcitriol, for normal calcium metabolism.
8. Stores nutrients

C. Layers
1. Epidermis
2. Dermis
3. Hypodermis (subcutaneous fat)

D. Epidermal appendages
1. Nails
2. Hair
3. Glands
   a. Sebaceous
   b. Sweat

E. Normal bacterial flora
1. Types of normal bacterial flora include the following:
   a. Gram-positive and gram-negative staphylococci
   b. *Pseudomonas* sp.
   c. *Streptococcus* sp.

2. Organisms are shed with normal exfoliation.
3. A pH of 4.2 to 5.6 halts the growth of bacteria.

II Risk Factors for Integumentary Disorders

A. Exposure to chemical and environmental pollutants
B. Exposure to radiation
C. Race and age
D. Exposure to the sun or use of indoor tanning
E. Lack of personal hygiene habits
F. Use of harsh soaps or other harsh products
G. Some medications, such as long-term glucocorticoid use or herbal preparations
H. Nutritional deficiencies
I. Moderate to severe emotional stress
J. Infection, with injured areas as the potential entry points for infection
K. Repeated injury or irritation
L. Genetic predisposition
M. Systemic illnesses
N. Immunocompromised client
O. Prolonged pressure or immobility
P. Impaired sensory perception
Q. Excess skin moisture

III Psychosocial Impact

A. Change in body image, decreased general well-being, and decreased self-esteem
B. Social isolation and fear of rejection (because of embarrassment about changes in skin appearance)
C. Restrictions in physical activity
D. Pain
E. Disruption or loss of employment
F. Cost of medication, hospitalization, and follow-up care, including dressing supplies

IV. Phases of Wound Healing

A. Phases
1. Inflammatory: Begins at the time of injury and lasts 3 to 5 days; manifestations include local edema, pain, redness, and warmth.

471

2. Proliferation: Begins the fourth day after injury and lasts 2 to 4 weeks; scar tissue forms and granulation tissue forms in the tissue bed.

3. Maturation: Begins as early as 3 weeks after the injury and may last for 1 year; scar tissue becomes thinner and is firm and inelastic during palpation.

B. Healing by intention

  1. First intention: Wound edges are approximated and held in place (i.e., with sutures) until healing occurs; wound is easily closed and dead space is eliminated.

  2. Second intention: This type of healing occurs with injuries or wounds that have tissue loss and require gradual filling in of the dead space with connective tissue.

  3. Third intention: This type of healing involves delayed primary closure and occurs with wounds that are intentionally left open for several days for irrigation or removal of debris and exudates; once debris has been removed and inflammation resolves, the wound is closed by first intention.

C. Types of exudate from wounds: Refer to Box 39.1.

V. Diagnostic Tests

A. Skin biopsy

  1. Description

    a. Skin biopsy is the collection of a small piece of skin tissue for histopathological study.

    b. Methods include punch, excisional, and shave.

  2. Preprocedure interventions

    a. Verify informed consent has been obtained.

    b. Cleanse site as prescribed.

  3. Postprocedure interventions

    a. Place specimen in the appropriate container and send to pathology laboratory for analysis.

    b. Use surgically aseptic technique for biopsy site dressings.

    c. Monitor the biopsy site for bleeding and infection.

    d. Reinforce instructions to the client to keep the dressing dry and in place for at least 8 hours and to then clean the area daily and use antibiotic ointment, as prescribed (sutures are usually removed in 7–10 days).

    e. Reinforce instructions to the client to report signs of excessive drainage, redness, or other signs of infection.

B. Skin/wound cultures

  1. A small skin culture sample is obtained with the use of a sterile applicator and the appropriate type of culture tube (e.g., bacterial or viral). Methods include scraping, punch biopsy, and collecting fluid. Local anesthesia may be used.

  2. Wound cleansing with nonantimicrobial cleanser or noncytotoxic solution such as normal saline would be done prior to obtaining a swab culture.

BOX 39.1	Types of Exudate from Wounds

Serous
- Clear or straw-colored
- Occurs as a normal part of the healing process

Serosanguineous
- Pink-colored as a result of the presence of a small amount of blood cells mixed with serous drainage
- Occurs as a normal part of the healing process

Sanguineous
- Red drainage from trauma to a blood vessel
- May occur with wound cleansing or other trauma to the wound bed
- Sanguineous drainage is uncommon in wounds

Hemorrhaging
- Frank blood from a leaking blood vessel
- May require emergency treatment to control bleeding
- Hemorrhage is an abnormal wound exudate

Purulent
- Yellow, gray, or green drainage as a result of infection in the wound

---

  3. A nasal swab is also commonly done to determine exposure to certain types of bacteria and viruses.

  4. Postprocedure intervention

    a. Viral culture is immediately placed on ice.

    b. Sample is sent to the laboratory to identify an existing organism.

⚠ Obtain skin culture samples or any other type of culture specimens before instituting antibiotic therapy.

C. Diascopy

  1. Technique allows clearer inspection of lesions by eliminating the erythema caused by increased blood flow to the area.

  2. A glass slide is pressed over the lesion, causing blanching and revealing the lesion more clearly.

D. Data collection of the skin (see Chapter 13)

VI. *Candida albicans*

A. Description

  1. A superficial fungal infection of the skin and mucous membranes

  2. Also known as a yeast infection (oral candidiasis) or thrush when it occurs in the mouth

  3. Risk factors include local environment of moisture and maceration, immunosuppression, chemotherapy, long-term antibiotic therapy, diabetes mellitus, and obesity.

  4. Common areas of occurrence include skin folds, perineum, vagina, axilla, and under the breasts.

B. Data collection

  1. Skin: red and irritated appearance that itches and stings

2. Mucous membranes of the mouth: red and whitish patches

C. Interventions

1. Reinforce instructions to the client to keep skinfold areas clean and dry.

2. For the hospitalized client, inspect skinfold areas frequently, turn and reposition the client frequently, and keep the skin and bed linens clean and dry.

3. Provide frequent mouth care as prescribed and avoid irritating products.

4. Provide food and fluids that are tepid in temperature and nonirritating to mucous membranes.

5. Antifungal medications may be prescribed.

VII Herpes Zoster (Shingles)

A. Description

1. With a history of chickenpox, shingles is caused by the reactivation of the varicella-zoster virus; shingles can occur during any immunocompromised state in a client with a history of chickenpox.

2. The dormant virus is located in the dorsal nerve root ganglia of the sensory cranial and spinal nerves.

3. Herpes zoster eruptions occur in a segmental distribution on the skin area along the infected nerve and show up after several days of discomfort in the area.

4. Diagnosis is determined by visual examination and by Tzanck smear to verify a herpes infection and viral culture to identify the organism.

5. Postherpetic neuralgia (severe pain) can remain after the lesions resolve.

6. It is contagious to individuals who never had chickenpox and have not been vaccinated against the disease.

7. Herpes simplex virus is another type of virus; type 1 infection causes a cold sore (usually on the lip), and type 2 causes genital herpes typically below the waist (both types are contagious and may be present together).

B. Data collection

1. Unilaterally clustered skin vesicles along peripheral sensory nerves on the trunk, thorax, or face

2. Fever, malaise

3. Burning and pain

4. Pruritus

5. Paresthesia

C. Interventions

1. Isolate the client until lesions are crusted over and dry because exudate from the lesions contains the virus (maintain standard and other precautions as appropriate, such as contact and/or airborne precautions as long as vesicles are present).

2. Assess for signs and symptoms of infection, including skin infections and eye infections; skin necrosis can also occur.

3. Assess neurovascular status and seventh cranial nerve function; Bell's palsy is a complication.

4. Use an air mattress and bed cradle on the client's bed if hospitalized, and keep the environment cool; warmth and touch aggravate the pain.

5. Prevent the client from scratching and rubbing the affected area.

6. Reinforce instructions to the client to wear lightweight, loose cotton clothing and to avoid wool and synthetic clothing.

7. Reinforce teaching the client about the prescribed therapies; astringent compresses may be prescribed to relieve irritation and pain and to promote crust formation and healing.

8. Reinforce teaching the client about measures to keep the skin clean to prevent infection.

9. Reinforce teaching the client about topical treatment or antiviral therapies; antiviral therapies begun within 3 days of the rash reduce pain and lessen the likelihood of postherpetic neuralgia.

10. The zoster vaccine (live), the vaccination for shingles, is recommended for adults 60 years of age and older to reduce the risk of occurrence and the long-term pain.

11. Antiviral medications may be prescribed; refer to Chapter 60 for information on antiviral medications.

VIII. Methicillin-Resistant *Staphylococcus aureus* (MRSA)

A. Description

1. Skin or wound infected with MRSA can be community acquired, such as through sports when skin-to-skin contact and sharing of equipment occurs. It can also be hospital acquired, such as in the case of a surgical site infection (SSI). See Chapter 14 for additional types of health care–associated infections.

2. An MRSA screening with a nasal swab may be done for clients who are having surgery, who have been previously hospitalized, or who live in group settings. Clients with positive cultures or with a history of a positive culture are isolated.

3. Infection can range from mild to severe and can present as folliculitis or furuncles.

4. Folliculitis is a superficial infection of the follicle caused by *Staphylococcus* and presents as a raised, red rash with pustules; furuncles are also caused by *Staphylococcus* and occur deep in the follicle and present as large raised bumps that may or may not have a pustule and are very painful.

5. If MRSA infects the blood, sepsis, organ damage, and death can occur.

⚠ MRSA is contagious and is spread to others by direct contact with infected skin or infected articles; for the client with MRSA, the infection can also be spread to other parts of the body.

B. Data collection: A culture and sensitivity of the skin or wound confirms the presence of MRSA and leads to the choice of appropriate antibiotic therapy.

C. Interventions
1. Maintain standard precautions and contact precautions as appropriate to prevent spread of infection to others.
2. Monitor the client closely for signs of further infection, which may result in systemic illness or organ damage.
3. Administer antibiotic therapy as prescribed.
4. For additional information on MRSA, refer to Chapter 37.

IX. Erysipelas and Cellulitis

A. Description
1. Erysipelas is an acute, superficial, rapidly spreading inflammation of the dermis and lymphatics caused by group A *Streptococcus*, which enters the tissue via an abrasion, bite, trauma, or wound.
2. Cellulitis is an infection of the dermis and underlying hypodermis; the causative organism is usually group A *Streptococcus* or *S. aureus*.

B. Data collection
1. Pain and tenderness
2. Erythema and warmth
3. Edema
4. Fever

C. Interventions
1. Promote rest of the affected area.
2. Apply warm compresses as prescribed to promote circulation and to decrease discomfort, erythema, and edema.
3. Apply antibacterial dressings, ointments, or gels as prescribed.
4. Administer antibiotics as prescribed for an infection; obtain a culture of the area before initiating the antibiotics.

X. Poison Ivy, Poison Oak, and Poison Sumac

A. Description: Dermatitis that develops from contact with urushiol from poison ivy, oak, or sumac plants

B. Data collection
1. Papulovesicular lesions
2. Severe pruritus

C. Interventions
1. Cleanse the oil from the plant off of the skin immediately.
2. Apply cool, wet compresses to relieve the itching.
3. Apply topical products to relieve the itching and discomfort.
4. Topical or oral glucocorticoids may be prescribed for severe reactions.

XI. Bites and Stings

A. Spider bites
1. Almost all types of spider bites are venomous, and most are not harmful, but bites or stings from brown recluse spiders, black widow spiders, tarantulas (as well as from scorpions, bees, and wasps) can produce toxic reactions in humans. Tetanus prophylaxis needs to be current because spider bites can be contaminated with tetanus spores.
2. Brown recluse spider
   a. Bite can cause a skin lesion, a necrotic wound, or systemic effects from the toxin (loxoscelism).
   b. Application of ice to decrease enzyme activity of the venom and to limit tissue necrosis must be done immediately and intermittently for up to 4 days after the bite.
   c. Topical antiseptics and antibiotics may be necessary if the site becomes infected.
3. Black widow spider
   a. Bite causes a small red papule.
   b. Venom causes neurotoxicity.
   c. Ice is applied immediately to inhibit the action of the neurotoxin.
   d. Systemic toxicity can occur and the victim may require supportive therapy in the hospital.
4. Tarantulas
   a. Bite causes swelling, redness, numbness, lymph inflammation, and pain at the bite site.
   b. The tarantula launches its barbed hairs, which penetrate the skin and eyes of the victim, producing a severe inflammatory reaction.
   c. Tarantula hairs are removed as soon as possible using sticky tape to pull hairs from the skin, and the skin is thoroughly irrigated; saline irrigations are done for eye exposure.
   d. The involved extremity is elevated and immobilized to reduce the pain and swelling.
   e. Antihistamines and topical or systemic corticosteroids may be prescribed; tetanus prophylaxis is necessary.

B. Scorpion stings
1. Scorpions inject venom into the victim through a stinging apparatus on their tail.
2. Most stings cause local pain, inflammation, and mild systemic reactions that are treated with analgesics, wound care, and supportive treatment.
3. The bark scorpion can inflict a severe and potentially fatal systemic response, especially in children and elderly; the venom is neurotoxic; the victim must be taken to the emergency department immediately (an antivenom is administered for bark scorpion bites).

C. Bees and wasps
1. Stings usually cause a wheal and flare reaction.

2. Emergency care involves quick removal of the stinger and application of an ice pack.

3. The stinger is removed by gently scraping or brushing it off with the edge of a needle or similar object; tweezers are not used because of the risk of pinching the venom sac.

4. If the victim is allergic to the venom of a bee or wasp, a severe allergic response can occur (hives, pruritus, swelling of the lips and tongue) that can progress to life-threatening anaphylaxis; immediate emergency care is required.

5. Individuals who are allergic need to carry an epinephrine autoinjector for self-administration of intramuscular epinephrine if a bee or wasp sting occurs. After use of the epinephrine auto injector, the individual must seek emergency medical attention. Persons need to have two injectors available and obtain a replacement as soon as possible.

D. Snake bites

1. Some snakes are venomous and can cause a serious systemic reaction in the victim.

2. The victim must be immediately moved to a safe area away from the snake and would rest to decrease venom circulation; the extremity is immobilized and kept below the level of the heart.

3. Constricting clothing and jewelry are removed before swelling occurs.

4. The victim is kept warm and is not allowed to consume caffeinated or alcoholic beverages, which may speed absorption of the venom.

5. If unable to seek emergency medical attention promptly, a constricting band may be applied proximal to the wound to slow the venom circulation; monitor the circulation frequently and loosen the band if edema occurs.

6. The wound is not incised or sucked to remove the venom; ice is not applied to the wound.

7. Emergency care in a hospital is required as soon as possible; an antivenom may be administered along with supportive care. The snake would not be transported with the victim for identification purposes unless it can be safely placed in a sealed container during transportation.

⚠ For spider bites, scorpion bites, or other stings or bites, the Poison Control Center must be contacted as soon as possible to determine the best initial management.

XII. Frostbite

A. Description

1. Frostbite is damage to tissues and blood vessels as a result of prolonged exposure to cold.

2. Fingers, toes, face, nose, and ears often are affected.

B. Data collection

1. First degree: Involves white plaque surrounded by a ring of hyperemia and edema

2. Second degree: Large, clear fluid-filled blisters with partial-thickness skin necrosis

3. Third degree: Involves the formation of small hemorrhagic blisters, usually followed by eschar formation involving the hypodermis, requiring débridement

4. Fourth degree: No blisters or edema noted; full-thickness necrosis with visible tissue loss extending into muscle and bone, which may result in gangrene. Amputation may be required.

C. Interventions

1. Rewarm the affected part rapidly and continuously with a warm water bath or towels at 104°F to 107.6°F (40°C–42°C) to thaw the frozen part.

2. Handle the affected area gently and immobilize.

3. Avoid the use of dry heat, and never rub or massage the part, which may result in further tissue damage.

4. The rewarming process may be painful; analgesics may be necessary.

5. Avoid compression of the injured tissues and apply only loose and nonadherent sterile dressings.

6. Monitor for signs of compartment syndrome.

7. Tetanus prophylaxis is necessary, and topical and systemic antibiotics may be prescribed.

8. Débridement of necrotic tissue may be necessary; amputation may be necessary if gangrene develops.

XIII. Actinic Keratoses

A. Actinic keratoses are caused by chronic exposure to the sun and appear as rough, scaly, red or brown lesions; usually found on the face, scalp, arms, and back of the hands.

B. Lesions are considered premalignant, and there is a risk for slow progression to squamous cell carcinoma.

C. Treatment includes medications and therapies such as excision, cryotherapy, curettage, and laser therapy. (See Chapter 40 for information on medications.)

XIV Skin Cancer

A. Description

1. Skin cancer is a malignant lesion of the skin, which may or may not metastasize.

2. Overexposure to the sun is a primary cause; other causes and conditions that place the individual at risk include chronic skin damage from repeated injury and irritation such as tanning and use of tanning beds, genetic predisposition, ionizing radiation, light-skinned race, age older than 60 years, an outdoor occupation, and exposure to chemical carcinogens.

Adult—Integumentary

3. Diagnosis is confirmed by a skin biopsy.

B. Types

1. Basal cell: Basal cell cancer arises from the basal cells contained in the epidermis; metastasis is rare, but underlying tissue destruction can progress to organ tissue.
2. Squamous cell: Squamous cell cancer is a tumor of the epidermal keratinocytes and can infiltrate surrounding structures and metastasize to lymph nodes.
3. Melanoma: Melanoma may occur any place on the body, especially where birthmarks or new moles are apparent; it is highly metastatic to the brain, lungs, bone, and liver, with survival depending on early diagnosis and treatment.

 C Data collection (Table 39.1)

1. Change in color, size, or shape of preexisting lesion
2. Pruritus
3. Local soreness

 The client needs to be informed about the risks associated with overexposure to the sun and taught about the importance of performing monthly self-skin assessments.

D Interventions

1. Reinforce instructions to the client regarding risk factors and preventive measures.
2. Reinforce instructions to the client to perform monthly self-skin assessments and to monitor for lesions that do not heal or that change characteristics.
3. Reinforce instructions to the client to have moles or lesions removed that are subject to chronic irritation.
4. Reinforce instructions to the client to avoid contact with chemical irritants.
5. Reinforce instructions to the client to wear layered clothing and use sunscreen lotions with an appropriate skin protection factor when outdoors.
6. Reinforce instructions to the client to avoid sun exposure between 10:00 a.m. and 4:00 p.m.
7. Management may include surgical or nonsurgical interventions; if medication is prescribed, provide instructions about its use.
8. Assist with surgical management, which may include cryosurgery, curettage and electrodessication, or surgical excision of the lesion.

XV. Psoriasis

A. Description

1. Psoriasis is a chronic, noninfectious skin inflammation occurring with remissions and exacerbations involving keratin synthesis that results in psoriatic patches; it may lead to an infection in the affected area.
2. Various forms exist, with psoriasis vulgaris being the most common.

TABLE 39.1   Appearance of Skin Cancer Lesions

Basal Cell Carcinoma

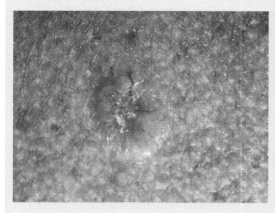

Waxy nodule with pearly borders
Papule, red, central crater
Metastasis is rare

Squamous Cell Carcinoma

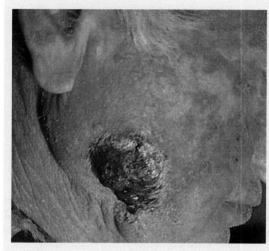

Oozing, bleeding, crusting lesion
Potentially metastatic
Larger tumors associated with a higher risk for metastasis

Melanoma

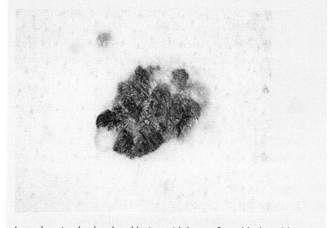

Irregular, circular, bordered lesion with hues of tan, black, or blue
Rapid infiltration into tissue, highly metastatic

Figures from Ignatavicius D, Workman ML: *Medical-surgical nursing: Patient centered collaborative care*, ed 8, Philadelphia, 2016, Saunders.

3. Possible causes of the disorder include stress, trauma, infection, hormonal changes, obesity, an autoimmune reaction, and climate changes; a genetic predisposition may also be a cause.

4. The disorder may also be exacerbated by the use of certain medications.

5. Koebner phenomenon is the development of psoriatic lesions at a site of injury, such as a scratched or sunburned area. Frequent cleansing of the area may prevent or lessen this phenomenon.

6. In some individuals with psoriasis, arthritis develops, which leads to joint changes similar to those seen in rheumatoid arthritis.

7. The goal of therapy is to reduce cell proliferation and inflammation, and the type of therapy prescribed depends on the extent of the disease and the client's response to treatment.

B. Data collection
   1. Pruritus
   2. Shedding, silvery-white scales on a raised, reddened, round plaque that usually affects the scalp, knees, elbows, extensor surfaces of arms and legs, and sacral regions
   3. A yellow discoloration, pitting, and thickening of the nails are noted, if they are affected
   4. Joint inflammation with psoriatic arthritis

C. Pharmacological therapy: Refer to Chapter 40 for medications used to treat psoriasis.

D. Interventions and client education
   1. Provide emotional support to the client with associated altered body image and decreased self-esteem.
   2. Reinforce instructions to the client in the use of prescribed therapies and to avoid over-the-counter medications.
   3. Reinforce instructions to the client not to scratch the affected areas and to keep the skin lubricated as prescribed to minimize itching.
   4. Monitor for and reinforce instructions to the client to recognize and report the signs/symptoms of secondary skin problems, such as infection.
   5. Reinforce instructions to the client to wear light cotton clothing over affected areas.
   6. Assist the client with identifying ways to reduce stress if stress is a predisposing factor.

XVI. Acne Vulgaris

A. Description
   1. Acne is a chronic skin disorder that usually begins during puberty. The incidence is the same for males and females; however, severe conditions affect males more often; lesions develop on the face, neck, chest, shoulders, and back.
   2. Acne requires active treatment for control until it resolves.
   3. The types of lesions include comedones (open and closed), pustules, papules, and nodules.

4. The exact cause is unknown but may include androgenic influence on the sebaceous glands, increased sebum production, and proliferation of *Propionibacterium acnes* (the organism that converts sebum into irritant fatty acids).

5. Exacerbations coincide with the menstrual cycle because of hormonal activity; oily skin and a genetic predisposition may be contributing factors.

B. Data collection
   1. Closed comedones are whiteheads and non-inflamed lesions that develop as follicles and enlarge with the retention of horny cells.
   2. Open comedones are blackheads that result from continuing accumulation of horny cells and sebum, which dilates the follicles.
   3. Pustules and papules result as the inflammatory process progresses.
   4. Nodules result from total disintegration of a comedone and subsequent collapse of the follicle.
   5. Deep scarring can result from nodules.

C. Interventions
   1. Reinforce instructions to the client with regard to prescribed skin-cleansing methods, with an emphasis on not scrubbing the face and using only the prescribed topical agents.
   2. Reinforce instructions to the client about the administration of topical or oral medications as prescribed.
   3. Reinforce instructions to the client not to squeeze, prick, or pick at lesions.
   4. Reinforce instructions to the client to use products labeled noncomedogenic and cosmetics that are water-based and to avoid contact with excessively oil-based products.
   5. Reinforce instructions to the client on the importance of follow-up treatment.
   6. Refer to Chapter 40 for information on the medications used to treat acne.

XVII. Stevens-Johnson Syndrome

A. A medication-induced skin reaction that occurs through an immunological response; common medications causing the reaction include antibiotics (especially sulfonamides), antiseizure medications, and nonsteroidal antiinflammatory drugs (NSAIDs).

B. Similar to toxic epidermal necrolysis (TEN), another medication-induced skin reaction that results in diffuse erythema and large blister formation on the skin and mucous membranes

C. May be mild or severe and cause vesicles, erosions, and crusts on the skin; if severe, systemic reactions occur that involve the respiratory system, renal system, and eyes, resulting in blindness, and it can be fatal. Initial clinical manifestations include flulike symptoms and erythema of the skin and mucous membranes. Serious systemic symptoms and complications occur when the ulcerations involve the larynx, bronchi, and esophagus.

D. Most commonly occurs in clients who have an impaired immune system

E. Treatment includes immediate discontinuation of the medication causing the syndrome; antibiotics, corticosteroids, and supportive therapy may be necessary.

XVIII. Pressure Injury

A. Description

1. A pressure injury is an impairment of skin integrity.

2. A pressure injury can occur anywhere on the body; tissue damage results when the skin and underlying tissue are compressed between a bony prominence and an external surface for an extended period of time.

3. The tissue compression restricts blood flow to the skin, which can result in tissue ischemia, inflammation, and necrosis; once a pressure injury develops, it is difficult to heal.

 4. Prevention of skin breakdown in any part of the body is a major role for the nurse.

 B. Risk factors

1. Skin pressure

2. Skin shearing and friction

3. Immobility

4. Malnutrition

5. Incontinence

6. Decreased sensory perception

C. Data collection and staging (Table 39.2)

 D. Interventions

> Avoid direct massage to a reddened skin area because massage can damage the capillary beds and cause tissue necrosis.

1. Identify clients at risk for developing a pressure injury.

2. Institute measures to prevent pressure injuries such as appropriate positioning, using pressure relief devices, ensuring adequate nutrition, and developing a plan for skin cleansing and care.

3. Check the skin frequently and monitor for an alteration in skin integrity.

4. Keep the client's skin dry and the sheets wrinkle free; if the client is incontinent, check him or her frequently and change pads or any items placed under the client immediately after they are soiled.

5. Use creams and lotions to lubricate the skin and a barrier protection ointment for the incontinent client.

6. Turn and reposition the immobile client every 2 hours, or more frequently if necessary; provide active and passive range-of-motion exercises at least every 8 hours.

7. If a pressure injury is present, record the location and size of the wound (length, width, depth), monitor and record the type and amount of exudates (a culture of the exudate may be prescribed), and check for undermining and tunneling.

8. Serosanguineous exudate (blood-tinged amber fluid) is expected for the first 48 hours; purulent exudates indicate colonization of the wound with bacteria.

9. Use agency protocols for skin assessment and management of a wound; depending on agency policy, it may be required to have picture documentation on file of a pressure injury or other disruption in skin integrity that may include a client identifier, measuring device, and a label indicating wound laterality and location.

10. Treatment may include wound dressings and débridement procedures; skin grafting may be necessary (Tables 39.3 and 39.4).

11. Other treatments may include electrical stimulation to the wound area (increases blood vessel growth and stimulates granulation), vacuum-assisted wound closure (removes infectious material from the wound and promotes granulation), hyperbaric oxygen therapy (administration of oxygen under high pressure raises tissue oxygen concentration), and the use of topical growth factors (biologically active substances that stimulate cell growth).

⚡ PRIORITY NURSING ACTIONS

Burn Injury: Care in the Emergency Department

1. Assess for airway patency.
2. Administer oxygen as prescribed.
3. Obtain vital signs.
4. Assist to initiate an intravenous (IV) line and begin fluid replacement as prescribed.
5. Elevate the extremities if no fractures are obvious.
6. Keep the client warm, and maintain an NPO (nothing by mouth) status.

XIX. Burn Injuries (See Priority Nursing Actions)

A. Description: Cell destruction of the layers of the skin caused by heat, friction, electricity, radiation, or chemicals

B. Burn size

1. Small burns: The response of the body to injury is localized to the injured area.

2. Large or extensive burns

  a. Major or extensive burns consist of 25% or more of the total body surface area for an adult and 10% or more of the total body surface area for a child.

  b. The response of the body to the injury is systemic.

  c. The burn affects all the major systems of the body.

TABLE 39.2 Stages of Pressure Injuries

Stage I

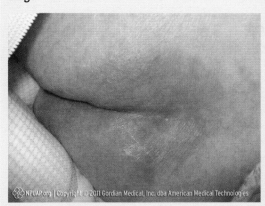

Skin is intact
Area is red and does not blanch with external pressure
Area may be painful, firm, soft, warmer or cooler compared with adjacent tissue

Stage II

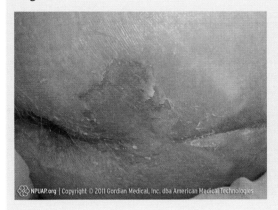

Skin is not intact
Partial-thickness skin loss of the dermis occurs
Presents as a shallow open ulcer with a red-pink wound bed or as intact or open/ruptured serum-filled blister

Stage III

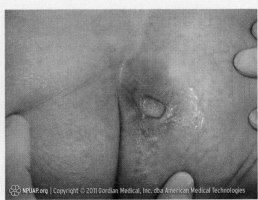

Full-thickness skin loss extends into the dermis and subcutaneous tissues, and slough may be present
Subcutaneous tissue may be visible
Undermining and tunneling may or may not be present

Stage IV

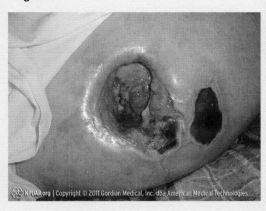

Full-thickness skin loss is present with exposed bone, tendon, or muscle
Slough or eschar may be present
Undermining and tunneling may develop

Suspected Deep-Tissue Injury

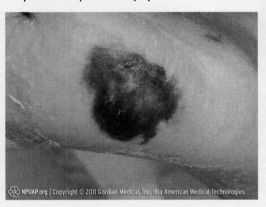

Ischemic subcutaneous tissue injury under intact skin
Appears purple or maroon colored
May be painful, firm, or boggy

Unstageable

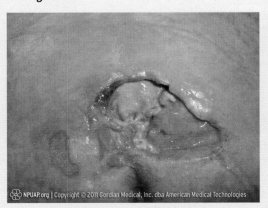

Full-thickness tissue loss in which the wound bed is covered by slough and/or eschar
The true depth, and therefore stage, of the wound cannot be determined until the slough and/or eschar is removed to visualize the wound bed

Figures from National Pressure Ulcer Advisory Panel (NPUAP). All photographs displayed are reprinted with permission of the copyright holder, Gordian Medical, Inc. dba American Medical Technologies.
Adapted from Ignatavicius D, Workman ML: *Medical-surgical nursing: Patient centered collaborative care*, ed 8, Philadelphia, 2016, Saunders.

TABLE 39.3   Types of Dressings and Mechanism of Action for Pressure Injuries

Pressure Injury Stage	Dressing Type	Mechanism of Action
I	None Transparent dressing Hydrocolloid dressing	Slow resolution within 7–10 days
II	Composite film Hydrocolloid dressing Hydrogel	Heals through reepithelialization
III	Hydrocolloid Hydrogel covered with foam dressing Gauze Growth factors	Heals through granulation and reepithelialization
IV	Hydrogel covered with foam dressing Calcium alginate Gauze	Heals through granulation, reepithelialization, and scar tissue development
Unstageable	Adherent film Gauze with a prescribed solution Enzymes None	Eschar loosens and lifts at edges as healing occurs; surgical débridement may be necessary

Data from Perry AG, Potter PA, Ostendorf, W: *Clinical nursing skills & techniques,* ed 8, St. Louis, 2014, Mosby.

TABLE 39.4   Types of Dressing Materials

Type	Indications, Uses, Considerations	Frequency of Dressing Changes
Alginate	Provides hemostasis, débridement, absorption, and protection Can be used as packing for deep wounds and for infected wounds	When dressing is saturated (every 3–5 days) or more frequently
	Requires a secondary dressing for securing	
Biological	Provides protection and débridement after eschar removal	Topical growth factors: Changed daily
	May be used for dormant and nonhealing wounds that do not respond to other topical therapies	Skin substitutes: The need for dressing change varies
	May be used for burns or before pigskin and cadaver skin grafts	
	Conforms to uneven wound surfaces; reduces pain	
	Requires a secondary dressing for securing	
Cotton gauze	Continuous dry dressing provides absorption and protection	Clean base: Every 12–24 hours
	Continuous wet dressing provides protection, a means for the delivery of topical treatment, and débridement	Necrotic base: Every 4–6 hours
	Wet to damp dressing provides atraumatic mechanical débridement	
	May be painful during removal	
Foam	Provides absorption, protection, insulation, and débridement Conforms to uneven wound surfaces	When dressing is saturated or more frequently
	Requires a secondary dressing for securing	
Hydrocolloidal	Provides absorption, protection, and débridement	Clean base: On leakage of exudates
	Is waterproof and is painless on removal	Necrotic base: Every 24 hours
Hydrogel	Provides absorption, protection, and débridement	Clean base: Every 24 hours
	Conducive to use with topical agents	Necrotic base: Every 6–8 hours
	Conforms to uneven wound surfaces but allows only partial wound visualization	
	Requires a secondary dressing for securing	
	Can promote the growth of *Pseudomonas* and other microorganisms	

Adult—Integumentary

TABLE 39.4 **Types of Dressing Materials—cont'd**

Type	Indications, Uses, Considerations	Frequency of Dressing Changes
Adhesive transparent film	Provides protection for partial-thickness lesions, débridement, and serves as a secondary (cover) dressing	Clean base: On leakage of exudates Necrotic base: every 24 hours
	Provides good wound visualization	
	Is waterproof and reduces pain	
	Use is limited to superficial lesions	
	Is nonabsorbent, adheres to normal and healing tissue	
	Dressing may be difficult to apply	

From Ignatavicius D, Workman ML: *Medical-surgical nursing: Patient-centered collaborative care*, ed 7, Philadelphia, 2013, Saunders.

C. Estimating the extent of injury (Fig. 39.1)

D. Burn depth

  1. Superficial-thickness burn

   a. Involves injury to the epidermis; the blood supply to the dermis is still intact.

   b. Mild to severe erythema (pink to red) is present, but no blisters.

   c. The skin blanches with pressure.

   d. Burn is painful, with a tingling sensation, and the pain is eased by cooling.

   e. Discomfort lasts about 48 hours; healing occurs in approximately 3 to 6 days.

   f. No scarring occurs and skin grafts are not required.

  2. Superficial partial-thickness burn

   a. Involves injury deeper into the dermis; the blood supply is reduced.

   b. Large blisters may cover an extensive area.

   c. Edema is present.

   d. Mottled pink to red base and a broken epidermis, with a wet, shiny, and weeping surface is characteristic.

   e. Burn is painful and sensitive to cold air.

   f. Heals in 10 to 21 days with no scarring, but some minor pigment changes may occur.

   g. Grafts may be used if the healing process is prolonged.

  3. Deep partial-thickness burn

   a. Extends deeper into the skin dermis

   b. Blister formation usually does not occur because the dead tissue layer is thick and sticks to underlying viable dermis.

   c. Wound surface is red and dry with white areas in deeper parts.

   d. May or may not blanch, and edema is moderate.

   e. Can convert to a full-thickness burn when tissue damage increases with infection, hypoxia, or ischemia

   f. Generally heals in 3 to 6 weeks, but scar formation results, and skin grafting may be necessary.

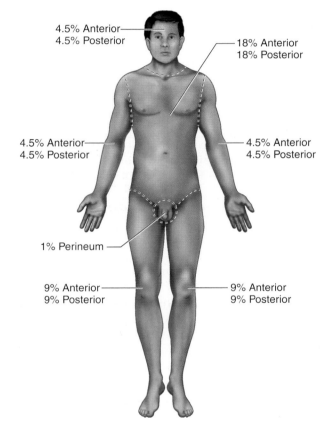

FIGURE 39.1 The rule of nines for estimating burn percentage.

  4. Full-thickness burn

   a. Involves injury and destruction of the epidermis and the dermis; the wound will not heal by reepithelialization and grafting may be required.

   b. Appears as a dry, hard, leathery eschar (burn crust or dead tissue must slough off or be removed from the wound before healing can occur).

   c. Appears waxy white, deep red, yellow, brown, or black.

   d. Injured surface appears dry.

   e. Edema is present under the eschar.

   f. Sensation is reduced or absent because of nerve ending destruction.

Adult—Integumentary

g. Healing may take weeks to months and depends on establishing an adequate blood supply.

h. Scarring and wound contractures are likely to develop.

5. Deep full-thickness burn

a. Injury extends beyond the skin into underlying fascia and tissues, and muscle, bone, and tendons are damaged.

b. Injured area appears black and sensation is completely absent.

c. Eschar is hard and inelastic.

d. Healing takes months and grafts are required.

E. Age and general health

1. Mortality rate is higher for children younger than 4 years old, particularly for children from birth to 1 year of age, and for clients older than 65 years.

2. Debilitating disorders, such as cardiac, respiratory, endocrine, and renal disorders, negatively influence the client's response to injury and treatment.

3. Mortality rate is higher when the client has a preexisting disorder at the time of the burn injury.

F. Burn location

1. Burns of the head, neck, and chest are associated with pulmonary complications.

2. Burns of the face are associated with corneal abrasion.

3. Burns of the ear are associated with auricular chondritis.

4. Hands and joints require intensive therapy to prevent disability.

5. The perineal area is prone to autocontamination by urine and feces.

6. Circumferential burns of the extremities can produce a tourniquet-like effect and lead to vascular compromise (compartment syndrome).

7. Circumferential thorax burns lead to inadequate chest wall expansion and pulmonary insufficiency.

XX. Inhalation Injuries

A. Smoke inhalation injury

1. Description: Respiratory injury that occurs when the victim inhales products of combustion during a fire

⚠ Airway is a priority concern in an inhalation injury.

2. Data collection

a. Facial burns

b. Erythema

c. Swelling of the oropharynx and nasopharynx

d. Singed nasal hairs

e. Flaring nostrils

f. Stridor, wheezing, and dyspnea

g. Hoarse voice

h. Sooty (carbonaceous) sputum and cough

i. Tachycardia

j. Agitation and anxiety

B. Carbon monoxide poisoning

1. Description

a. Carbon monoxide is a colorless, odorless, and tasteless gas that has an affinity for hemoglobin 200 times greater than that of oxygen.

b. Oxygen molecules are displaced and carbon monoxide reversibly binds to hemoglobin to form carboxyhemoglobin.

c. Tissue hypoxia occurs.

2. Data collection (Table 39.5)

C. Direct thermal heat injury

1. Description

a. Thermal heat injury can occur to the lower airways by the inhalation of steam or explosive gases, or the aspiration of scalding liquids.

b. Injury can occur to the upper airways, which appear erythematous and edematous, with mucosal blisters and ulcerations.

c. Mucosal edema can lead to upper airway obstruction, especially during the first 24 to 48 hours.

d. All clients with head or neck burns need to be monitored closely for the development of airway obstruction and are considered immediately for endotracheal intubation if obstruction occurs.

2. Data collection

a. Erythema and edema of the upper airways

b. Mucosal blisters and ulcerations

TABLE 39.5   Carbon Monoxide Poisoning

Blood Level (%)	Clinical Manifestations
1–10	Normal level
11–20 (mild poisoning)	Headache
	Flushing
	Decreased visual acuity
	Decreased cerebral functioning
	Slight breathlessness
21–40 (moderate poisoning)	Headache
	Nausea and vomiting
	Drowsiness
	Tinnitus and vertigo
	Confusion and stupor
	Pale to reddish-purple skin
	Decreased blood pressure
	Increased and irregular heart rate
41–60 (severe poisoning)	Coma
	Seizures
61–80 (fatal poisoning)	Death

Modified from Ignatavicius D, Workman ML: *Medical-surgical nursing: Patient-centered collaborative care*, ed 7, Philadelphia, 2013, Saunders.

XXI. Pathophysiology of Burns

A. Following a burn, vasoactive substances are released from the injured tissue and cause an increase in the capillary permeability, allowing the plasma to seep into the surrounding tissues.

B. The direct injury to the vessels increases capillary permeability (capillary permeability decreases 18–26 hours after the burn, but it does not normalize until 2–3 weeks after the injury).

C. Extensive burns result in generalized body edema and a decrease in circulating intravascular blood volume.

D. The fluid losses result in a decrease in organ perfusion.

E. The heart rate increases, cardiac output decreases, and the blood pressure drops.

F. Initially, hyponatremia and hyperkalemia occur.

G. The hematocrit level increases as a result of plasma loss; this initial increase falls to less than normal on the third to fourth day after the burn as a result of red blood cell damage and loss at the time of injury.

H. Initially, the body shunts blood from the kidneys, causing oliguria; then the body begins to reabsorb fluid and diuresis of the excess fluid occurs over the next days to weeks.

I. Blood flow to the gastrointestinal tract is diminished, which leads to intestinal ileus and gastrointestinal dysfunction.

J. Immune system function is depressed, which results in immunosuppression and thus increases the risk of infection and sepsis.

K. Pulmonary hypertension can develop, resulting in a decrease in the arterial oxygen tension level and a decrease in lung compliance.

L. Evaporative fluid losses through the burn wound are greater than normal, and the losses continue until complete wound closure occurs.

M. If the intravascular space is not replenished with intravenously administered fluids, hypovolemic shock and ultimately death may occur.

XXII. Management of the Burn Injury

A Resuscitation/emergent phase (Table 39.6)
  1. Prehospital care
    a. Begins at the scene of the accident and ends when emergency care is obtained
    b. Remove the victim from the source of the burn.
    c. Check the ABCs—airway, breathing, and circulation.
    d. Check for associated trauma, including inhalation injury.
    e. Conserve body heat.
    f. Cover burns with sterile or clean cloths.
    g. Remove constrictive jewelry and clothing.
    h. Insert IV access.
    i. Transport to the emergency department.

TABLE 39.6   Phases of Management of Burn Injury

Phase	Goal
Resuscitation/Emergent Phase Begins at the time of injury Ends with the restoration of normal capillary permeability	The primary goal is to maintain the client's airway, administer intravenous fluids to prevent hypovolemic shock, and preserve vital organ functioning
Duration usually 48–72 hours	
Includes prehospital care and emergency department care	
Resuscitative Phase Begins with the initiation of fluids Ends when capillary integrity returns to near-normal levels and large fluid shifts have decreased	The goal is to prevent shock by maintaining adequate circulating blood volume and maintaining vital organ perfusion
Amount of fluid administered is based on client's weight and extent of injury	
(Most fluid replacement formulas are calculated from the time of injury and not from the time of arrival at the hospital)	
Acute Phase Begins when the client is hemodynamically stable, capillary permeability is restored, and diuresis has begun	The emphasis during this phase is placed on restorative therapy, and the phase continues until wound closure is achieved
Usually begins 48–72 hours after time of injury	
Focus on infection control, wound care, wound closure, nutritional support, pain management, physical therapy	
Rehabilitative Phase Overlaps acute phase of care Extends beyond hospitalization	The goals of this phase are designed so that the client can gain independence and achieve maximal function

  2. Emergency department care is a continuation of the care administered at the scene of the injury.
  3. Major burns
    a. Evaluate the degree and extent of the burn, and treat life-threatening conditions.
    b. Ensure a patent airway, and administer 100% oxygen as prescribed.
    c. Monitor for respiratory distress and determine the need for intubation.
    d. Check the oropharynx for blisters and erythema.
    e. Monitor arterial blood gases and carboxyhemoglobin level.
    f. For an inhalation injury, administer 100% oxygen via a tight-fitting nonrebreather face mask, as prescribed until the carboxyhemoglobin level decreases to less than 15%.

g. Initiate peripheral IV access to nonburned skin proximal to any extremity burn, or prepare for the insertion of a central venous line as prescribed.

h. Monitor for hypovolemia and prepare to administer fluids intravenously to maintain the fluid balance.

i. Monitor the vital signs closely.

j. Insert a Foley catheter as prescribed and maintain urine output at 30 to 50 mL/hour.

k. Maintain NPO (nothing by mouth) status.

l. Insert a nasogastric tube as prescribed to remove gastric secretions and prevent aspiration.

m. Administer tetanus prophylaxis as prescribed.

n. Administer pain medication, as prescribed, via the IV route.

o. Administer pain medication before dressings changes and procedures.

p. Prepare the client for an escharotomy or fasciotomy as prescribed.

4. Minor burns

a. Administer pain medication as prescribed.

b. Instruct the client regarding the use of oral analgesics as prescribed.

c. Administer tetanus prophylaxis as prescribed.

d. Administer wound care as prescribed, which may include cleansing, debriding loose tissue, removing any damaging agents, followed by the application of topical antimicrobial cream and a sterile dressing.

e. Reinforce instructions to the client regarding follow-up care, including active range-of-motion exercises and wound care treatments.

 B. Resuscitative phase (see Table 39.6)

1. Fluid resuscitation

a. The amount of fluid administered depends on how much IV fluid per hour is required to maintain a urinary output of 30 to 50 mL/hour.

b. Successful fluid resuscitation is evaluated by stable vital signs, an adequate urine output, palpable peripheral pulses, and intact level of consciousness and thought processes.

c. IV fluid replacement may be titrated (adjusted) on the basis of urinary output plus serum electrolyte levels to meet the perfusion needs of the client with burns.

d. If the hemoglobin and hematocrit levels decrease or if the urinary output exceeds 50 mL/hour, the rate of IV fluid administration may be decreased.

⚠ Urinary output is the most reliable and most sensitive noninvasive assessment parameter for cardiac output and tissue perfusion.

2. Interventions

a. Monitor for tracheal or laryngeal edema and administer respiratory treatments as prescribed.

b. Monitor the pulse oximetry and prepare for arterial blood gas and carboxyhemoglobin levels if inhalation injury is suspected.

c. Elevate the head of the bed to 30 degrees or more for burns of the face and head.

d. Monitor for fluid overload and pulmonary edema.

e. Initiate electrocardiographic monitoring.

f. Monitor the temperature, and check for infection.

g. Initiate protective isolation techniques; maintain strict hand washing; use sterile sheets and linens when caring for the client; and use gloves, cap, masks, shoe covers, scrub clothes, and plastic aprons.

h. Clip body hair around wound margins.

i. Monitor daily weights, expecting a weight gain of 15 to 20 lbs during the first 72 hours.

j. Monitor gastric output and pH levels and for gastric discomfort and bleeding, indicating a stress ulcer.

k. Administer antacids, H_2-receptor antagonists, and antiulcer medications such as prescribed to prevent a stress ulcer.

l. Auscultate the bowel sounds for ileus and monitor for abdominal distention and gastrointestinal dysfunction.

m. Monitor stools for occult blood.

n. Obtain a urine specimen for myoglobin and hemoglobin levels.

o. Monitor IV fluids and hourly intake and output to determine the adequacy of fluid replacement therapy; notify the primary health care provider (PHCP) if urine output is less than 30 mL/hour or greater than 50 mL/hour.

p. Elevate circumferential burns of the extremities on pillows above the level of the heart to reduce dependent edema if no obvious fractures are present; diuretics increase the risk of hypovolemia and are generally avoided as a means of decreasing edema.

q. Monitor pulses and capillary refill of the affected extremities, and check the perfusion of the distal extremity with a circumferential burn.

r. Prepare for chest and other radiographs to rule out fractures or associated trauma.

s. Keep the room temperature warm.

t. Place the client on an air-fluidized bed or other special mattress, and use a bed cradle to keep the sheets off the client's skin.

3. Pain: Depending on the extent of the injury, opioid analgesics may be needed.

⚠ Avoid the intramuscular or subcutaneous medication routes for medication administration because absorption through the soft tissue is unreliable when hypovolemia and large fluid shifts occur.

4. Nutrition
   a. Proper nutrition is essential to promote wound healing and prevent infection.
   b. The basal metabolic rate is 40 to 100 times higher than normal with a burn injury.
   c. Maintain NPO status until bowel sounds are heard, and then advance to clear liquids, as prescribed.
   d. Nutrition may be provided via enteral tube feedings or parenteral nutrition through a central line.
   e. Provide a diet high in protein, carbohydrates, fats, and vitamins.
   f. Monitor calorie intake and daily weights.

5. Escharotomy
   a. A lengthwise incision is made through the burn eschar to relieve constriction and pressure and to improve circulation.
   b. Escharotomy is performed for circulatory compromise caused by circumferential burns.
   c. Escharotomy is performed at the bedside without anesthesia because nerve endings have been destroyed by the burn injury.
   d. Escharotomy can be performed on the thorax to improve ventilation.
   e. Following escharotomy, check pulses, color, movement, and sensation of affected extremity, and control any bleeding with pressure.
   f. Pack the incision gently with fine-mesh gauze as prescribed after escharotomy.
   g. Apply topical antimicrobial agents to the area as prescribed.

6. Fasciotomy
   a. An incision is made that extends through the subcutaneous tissue and fascia.
   b. The procedure is performed if adequate tissue perfusion does not return following an escharotomy.
   c. Fasciotomy is performed in the operating room with the client under general anesthesia.
   d. After the procedure, check the pulse, color, movement, and sensation of the affected extremity, and control any bleeding with pressure.
   e. Apply topical antimicrobial agents and dressings to the area, as prescribed.

C. Acute phase (see Table 39.6)
   1. Continue with protective isolation techniques.
   2. Provide wound care as prescribed, and prepare for wound closure.
   3. Provide pain management.
   4. Provide adequate nutrition as prescribed.
   5. Prepare the client for rehabilitation.

D. Wound care
   1. Description: The cleansing, débridement, and dressing of the burn wounds
   2. Hydrotherapy
      a. Wounds are cleansed by immersion, showering, or spraying.
      b. Hydrotherapy occurs for 30 minutes or less to prevent increased sodium loss through the burn wound, heat loss, pain, and stress.
      c. Client would be medicated before the procedure.
      d. Hydrotherapy is generally not used for clients who are hemodynamically unstable or those with new skin grafts.
      e. Care is taken to minimize bleeding and to maintain body temperature during the procedure.
      f. If hydrotherapy is not used, wounds are washed and rinsed while the client is in bed before the application of antimicrobial agents.
   3. Débridement (Box 39.2)
      a. Débridement is the removal of eschar or necrotic tissue to prevent bacterial proliferation under the eschar and to promote wound healing.
      b. Débridement may be mechanical, enzymatic, or surgical.
      c. Deep partial or full-thickness burns: Wound is cleansed and débrided, and topical antimicrobial agents are applied once or twice daily.

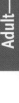

BOX 39.2 **Débridement**

Mechanical
- Performed during hydrotherapy; involves use of washcloths or sponges to cleanse and débride eschar and the use of scissors and forceps to lift and trim away loose eschar
- May include wet-to-dry or wet-to-wet dressing changes
- Painful procedure; may cause bleeding

Enzymatic
- Application of topical enzyme agents directly to the wound; the agent digests collagen necrotic tissue.

Surgical
- Excision of eschar or necrotic tissue via a surgical procedure in the operating room

Tangential Technique
- Very thin layers of the necrotic burn surface are excised until bleeding occurs (bleeding indicates that a healthy dermis or subcutaneous fat has been reached).

Fascial Technique
- The burn wound is excised to the level of superficial fascia; this technique is usually reserved for very deep and extensive burns.

Adult—Integumentary

E. Wound closure
  1. Description
    a. Wound closure prevents infection and loss of fluid.
    b. Closure promotes healing.
    c. Closure prevents contractures.
    d Wound closure is performed on day 5 to 21 following the injury, depending on the extent of the burn.
  2. Wound coverings (Box 39.3)
  3. Autografting
    a. Autografting provides permanent wound coverage.
    b. Autografting is the surgical removal of a thin layer of the client's own unburned skin, which is then applied to the excised burn wound.
    c. Autografting is performed in the operating room with the client under anesthesia.
    d. Monitor for bleeding after the graft because bleeding beneath an autograft can prevent adherence.
    e. If prescribed, small amounts of blood or serum can be removed by gently rolling the fluid from the center of the graft to the periphery with a sterile gauze pad, where it can be absorbed.
    f. For large accumulations of blood, the PHCP will aspirate the blood with the use of a small-gauge needle and syringe.
    g. Autografts are immobilized after surgery for 3 to 7 days to allow time for the graft to adhere and attach to the wound bed.
    h. Position the client for the immobilization and elevation of the graft site to prevent the movement and shearing of the graft.
  4. Care of the graft site
    a. Elevate and immobilize the graft site.
    b. Keep the site free from pressure.
    c. Avoid weight bearing.
    d. When the graft takes, if prescribed, roll a cotton-tipped applicator over the graft to remove exudate, because exudate can lead to infection and prevent graft adherence.

BOX 39.3   Wound Coverings

Biological
Amniotic Membranes
- Amniotic membranes from human placentas are used to adhere to the wound.
- This is effective as a dressing until epithelial cell regrowth occurs.
- Frequent changes are required, because amnion does not develop a blood supply, and it disintegrates in approximately 48 hours.

Allograft or Homograft (Human Tissue)
- Donated human cadaver skin is provided through a skin bank.
- Monitor for wound exudate and signs of infection.
- Rejection can occur within 24 hours.
- The risk of transmitting a blood-borne infection exists with the use of this covering.

Xenograft or Heterograft (Animal Tissue)
- Pigskin is harvested after slaughter and preserved for storage.
- Monitor for infection and wound adherence.
- Rejection can occur within 24–72 hours.
- This tissue is placed over granulation tissue and replaced every 2–5 days until the wound heals naturally or until closure with an autograft is complete.

Cultured Skin
- Cultured skin is grown in a laboratory from a small specimen of epidermal cells from an unburned portion of the client's body.
- Cell sheets are grafted onto the client to generate a permanent skin surface.
- Cell sheets are not durable; care must be taken when applying them to ensure adherence and prevent sloughing.

Autograft
- Skin is taken from a remote, unburned area of the client's own body and transplanted to cover the burn wound.
- The graft is placed either on a clean granulated bed or over a surgically excised area of the burn.
- Autograft provides for permanent skin coverage.

Nonbiological
Artificial Skin
- Artificial skin consists of two layers: a Silastic epidermis and a porous dermis made from bovine hide collagen and shark cartilage.
- After application, fibroblasts move into the collagen part of the artificial skin and create a structure that is similar to that of normal dermis.
- The artificial dermis then dissolves and is replaced with normal blood vessels and connective tissue called neodermis.
- The neodermis supports a standard autograft that is placed over it when the Silastic layer is removed.

Biosynthetic
- This type of covering is made of a combination of biosynthetic and synthetic materials.
- It is placed in contact with the wound surface, and it forms an adherent bond until epithelialization has occurred.
- Its porous substance allows exudate to pass through it.
- Monitor for wound exudate and signs of infection.

Synthetic
- Synthetic coverings are applied directly to the surface of a clean or surgically prepared wound, and they remain in place until they fall off or are removed.
- The covering is transparent or translucent; therefore, the wound can be inspected without removing the dressing.
- Pain at the wound site is reduced because the covering prevents the contact of the wound with air.

e. Monitor for foul-smelling drainage, increased temperature, increased white blood cell count, hematoma formation, and fluid accumulation.

f. Reinforce instructions to the client to avoid using fabric softeners and harsh detergents in the laundry.

g. Reinforce instructions to the client to lubricate the healing skin with prescribed agents.

h. Reinforce instructions to the client to protect the affected area from sunlight.

i. Reinforce instructions to the client to use splints and support garments as prescribed.

5. Care of the donor site

a. Method of care varies, depending on the PHCP's preference.

b. A nonadherent gauze dressing may be applied at the time of surgery to maintain pressure and to stop any oozing; always check surgeon's orders.

c. The PHCP may prescribe site treatment with gauze impregnated with petrolatum or with a biosynthetic dressing.

d. Keep the donor site clean, dry, and free from pressure.

e. Prevent the client from scratching the donor site.

f. Apply lubricating lotions to soften the area and to reduce the itching after the donor site is healed.

g. Donor site can be reused after healing has occurred (heals spontaneously within 7–14 days with proper care).

F. Physical therapy

1. An individualized program of splinting, positioning, exercises, ambulation, and activities of daily living is implemented early during the acute phase of recovery to maximize the functional and cosmetic outcomes.

2. Perform range-of-motion exercises as prescribed to reduce edema and to maintain strength and joint function.

3. Ambulate the client as prescribed to maintain the strength of the lower extremities.

4. Apply splints as prescribed to maintain proper joint position and prevent contractures.

a. Static splints immobilize the joint and are applied for periods of immobilization, during sleeping, and for clients who cannot maintain proper positioning.

b. Dynamic splints exercise the affected joint.

c. Avoid pressure to skin areas when applying splints, which could lead to further tissue and nerve damage.

5. Scarring is controlled by elastic wraps and bandages that apply continuous pressure to the healing skin during the period of time when the skin is vulnerable to shearing.

6. Antiburn scar support garments are usually worn 23 hours a day until the burn scar tissue has matured, which takes 18 months to 2 years.

G. Rehabilitative phase (see Table 39.6)

1. Description

a. Rehabilitation is the final phase of burn care.

2. Goals

a. Promote wound healing.

b. Minimize deformities.

c. Increase strength and function.

d. Provide emotional support.

WHAT WOULD YOU DO?

Answer: The nurse would elevate and immobilize the graft site, keep the site free from pressure, and not allow the client to bear weight on the extremity. When the graft takes, if prescribed, the nurse would roll a cotton-tipped applicator over it to remove exudate, because exudate can lead to infection and prevent graft adherence. The nurse needs to monitor for signs of infection such as foul-smelling drainage, increased temperature, and increased white blood cell count; and monitor for hematoma formation, or fluid accumulation.

PRACTICE QUESTIONS

❖ 1. An adult client was burned as a result of an explosion. The burn initially affected the client's entire face (the anterior half of the head) and the upper half of the anterior torso, and there were circumferential burns to the lower half of both arms. The client's clothes caught on fire and the client ran, which caused subsequent burn injuries of the posterior surface of the head and the upper half of the posterior torso. According to the rule of nines, what is the extent of this client's burn injury? **Fill in the blank.**
Answer: _____%

2. The nurse, employed in a long-term care facility, is planning the clinical assignments for the day. The nurse prepares the assignment and would not assign which staff member to the client with a diagnosis of herpes zoster?

1. A staff member who has never had roseola
2. A staff member who has never had mumps
3. An unlicensed assistive personnel who has never had chickenpox
4. An unlicensed assistive personnel who has never had German measles

❖ 3. A client returns to the clinic for follow-up treatment after a skin biopsy of a suspicious lesion that was performed 1 week ago. The biopsy report indicates that the lesion is a melanoma. The nurse under-

stands that which characteristics describe this type of a lesion? **Select all that apply.**
- ❑ 1. Metastasis is rare.
- ❑ 2. It is encapsulated.
- ❑ 3. It is highly metastatic.
- ❑ 4. It is characterized by local invasion.
- ❑ 5. Lesion is a nevus that has changed in color.

❖ **4.** The nurse is reviewing the health care record of a client with a lesion that has been diagnosed as basal cell carcinoma. The nurse would expect which characteristics of this type of lesion to be documented in the client's record? **Select all that apply.**
- ❑ 1. Lesion has a waxy border
- ❑ 2. An irregularly shaped lesion
- ❑ 3. Pearly papule, with a central crater
- ❑ 4. A small papule with a dry, rough scale
- ❑ 5. A firm nodular lesion topped with a crust

5. The nurse reinforces instructions to a group of clients regarding measures that will assist with the prevention of skin cancer. Which statement by a client indicates the **need for further teaching**?
1. "I need to wear sunscreen when participating in outdoor activities."
2. "I need to avoid sun exposure before 10:00 AM and after 4:00 PM."
3. "I need to wear a hat, opaque clothing, and sunglasses when in the sun."
4. "I need to examine my body monthly for any lesions that may be suspicious."

6. A client arrives at the emergency department and has experienced frostbite to the right hand. What would the nurse expect to find when inspecting the client's hand?
1. A pink, edematous hand
2. Fiery red skin with edema in the nail beds
3. Black fingertips surrounded by an erythematous rash
4. A white color of the skin which is insensitive to touch

7. The evening nurse reviews the nursing documentation in the client's chart and notes that the day nurse has documented that the client has a stage 2 pressure injury in the sacral area. What would the nurse expect to find when checking the client's sacral area?
1. Intact skin
2. The presence of tunneling
3. A deep, crater-like appearance
4. Partial-thickness skin loss of the epidermis

8. The nurse inspects the skin of a client who is suspected of having psoriasis. Which finding would the nurse note if this disorder is present?
1. Oily skin
2. Silvery-white scaly lesions
3. Patchy hair loss and round, red macules with scales
4. The presence of wheal patches scattered about the trunk

9. The nurse is told that an assigned client is suspected of having methicillin-resistant Staphylococcus aureus (MRSA). Which precautions must the nurse institute during the care of the client?
1. Wear gloves only.
2. Wear a mask and gloves.
3. Wear a gown and gloves.
4. Wear a mask and a faceshield.

10. The client arrives at the emergency department after a burn injury that occurred in their home basement and an inhalation injury is suspected. Which would the nurse anticipate as being prescribed for the client?
1. Oxygen via nasal cannula at 10 L
2. Oxygen via nasal cannula at 15 L
3. 100% oxygen via an aerosol mask
4. 100% oxygen via a tight-fitting, nonrebreather face mask

11. The nurse is caring for a client who has just been admitted to the nursing unit after receiving flame burns to the face and chest. The nurse notes a hoarse cough, and the client is expectorating sputum with black flecks. The client suddenly becomes restless, and his color is becoming dusky. Based on this data, which interpretation would the nurse make?
1. The client is hypotensive.
2. Pain is present from the burn injury.
3. The burn has probably caused laryngeal edema, which has occluded the airway.
4. The client is afraid and is having a panic attack as a result of the unfamiliar surroundings.

12. Which would be the anticipated therapeutic outcome of an escharotomy procedure performed for a circumferential arm burn?
1. The return of distal pulses
2. Decreasing edema formation
3. Brisk bleeding from the injury site
4. The formation of granulation tissue

13. The nurse is caring for a client with circumferential burns of both legs. Which leg position is appropriate for this type of a burn?
1. A dependent position
2. Elevation of the knees
3. Flat, without elevation
4. Elevation above the level of the heart

14. The nurse is assisting with caring for a client who is receiving intravenous fluids and who has sustained full-thickness burn injuries of the back and legs. The nurse understands that which would provide the **most** reliable indicator for determining the adequacy of the fluid resuscitation?
1. Vital signs
2. Urine output
3. Mental status
4. Peripheral pulses

15. The nurse is assigned to care for a client with herpes zoster. Based on an understanding of the cause of this disorder, the nurse determines that this definitive diagnosis was made by which diagnostic test?
1. Positive patch test
2. Positive culture results
3. Abnormal biopsy results
4. Wood's light examination indicative of infection

ANSWERS

1. 36%

Rationale: According to the rule of nines, with the initial burn, the anterior half of the head equals 4.5%, the upper half of the anterior torso equals 9%, and the lower halves of both arms equal 9%. The subsequent burn included the posterior half of the head, which equals 4.5%, and the upper half of the posterior torso, which equals 9%. This totals 36%.

Test-Taking Strategy: Focus on the subject, the rule of nines. Knowledge of this rule is necessary in order to answer this question. According to the rule, the entire head equals 9%, each arm equals 9% (both arms, 18%), the anterior and posterior torsos each equal 18% (entire torso, 36%), each leg equals 18% (both legs, 36%), and the perineum equals 1%. Remember the following: 9% (head) + 18% (arms) + 36% (torsos) + 36% (legs) + 1% (perineum) = 100%.

2. 3

Rationale: Herpes zoster is caused by a reactivation of the varicella zoster virus, which is the causative virus of chickenpox. Individuals who have not been exposed to the varicella zoster virus are susceptible to chickenpox. Options 1, 2, and 4 are not associated with the herpes zoster virus.

Test-Taking Strategy: Note the subject, safe assignment-making. Recalling that herpes zoster is caused by a reactivation of the varicella zoster virus will assist you with answering the question.

3. 3, 5

Rationale: Melanomas are pigmented malignant lesions that originate in the melanin-producing cells of the epidermis. The lesion is a nevus that changes in color. This skin cancer is highly metastatic and a person's survival depends on early diagnosis and treatment. Basal cell carcinomas arise in the basal cell layer of the epidermis. Early malignant basal cell lesions often go unnoticed, and although metastasis is rare, underlying tissue destruction can progress to include vital structures. Squamous cell carcinomas are malignant neoplasms of the epidermis. They are characterized by local invasion and the potential for metastasis.

Test-Taking Strategy: Focus on the subject, a melanoma, and use knowledge regarding the various types of skin cancers. Recalling that melanomas are highly metastatic will direct you to the correct option.

4. 1, 3

Rationale: Basal cell carcinoma appears as a pearly papule with a central crater and a rolled, waxy border. A melanoma is an irregularly shaped pigmented papule or plaque with a red, white, or blue color. Squamous cell carcinoma is a firm nodular lesion that is topped with a crust or a central area of ulceration. Actinic keratosis, which is a premalignant lesion, appears as a small macule or papule with a dry, rough, adherent yellow or brown scale.

Test-Taking Strategy: Focus on the subject, basal cell carcinoma. Recall characteristics and etiology of basal cell cancer to direct you to the correct option. Remember that it appears as a pearly papule with a central crater and a rolled, waxy border.

5. 2

Rationale: The client would be instructed to avoid sun exposure between the hours of approximately 10:00 a.m. and 4:00 p.m. Sunscreen, a hat, opaque clothing, and sunglasses would be worn for outdoor activities. The client would be instructed to examine the body monthly for the appearance of any possible cancerous or precancerous lesions.

Test-Taking Strategy: Note the strategic words, *need for further teaching*. These words indicate a negative event query and ask you to select an option that is an incorrect statement. A careful reading of the question and each of the options and thinking about the causes of skin cancer will direct you to the correct option.

6. 4

Rationale: The findings related to frostbite include a white or blue skin color and skin that is hard, cold, and insensitive to touch. As thawing occurs, so does flushing of the skin, the development of blisters or blebs, or tissue edema. Gangrene can develop in 9 to 15 days.

Test-Taking Strategy: Focus on the subject, diagnosis of frostbite. The words, *insensitive to touch*, would assist with directing you to the correct option.

7. 4

Rationale: With a stage 2 pressure injury, the skin is not intact. There is partial-thickness skin loss of the epidermis or dermis. The ulcer is superficial and it may look like an abrasion, blister, or shallow crater. The skin is intact with a stage 1 pressure injury. A deep, craterlike appearance occurs during stage 3 and tunneling develops during stage 4.

Test-Taking Strategy: Focus on the subject, findings associated with a stage 2 pressure injury. Use your knowledge of the characteristics associated with each stage of pressure injuries. Remember, with a stage 2 pressure injury, the skin is not intact and there is partial-thickness skin loss

8. 2
Rationale: Psoriatic patches are covered with silvery-white scales. There is no patchy hair loss or round, red macules with scales. The skin is dry and there is no presence of wheal patches scattered about the trunk.
Test-Taking Strategy: Focus on the subject, psoriasis. Think about the appearance of this skin condition. Recall that psoriasis is associated with the presence of silvery white scaly patches. This will direct you to the correct option.

9. 3
Rationale: MRSA is contagious and is spread to others by direct contact with infected skin or infected articles. The Centers for Disease Control and Prevention recommends the wearing of gowns and gloves when in close contact with a person who has MRSA. Masks are not necessary unless the client has a coexisting condition that presents a risk of airborne or droplet transmission of disease. Face shields are not necessary unless the client has a coexisting condition; for example, a draining wound that presents the risk of splashing during wound cleansing.
Test-Taking Strategy: Focus on the subject, precautions for a client with MRSA. Eliminate option 1 because of the closed-ended word, *only*. Consider the mode of transmission of MRSA. This will assist to eliminate options 1, 2, and 4.

10. 4
Rationale: If an inhalation injury is suspected, the administration of 100% oxygen via a tight-fitting, nonrebreather face mask is prescribed until the carboxyhemoglobin level decreases to less than 15%. With inhalation injuries, the oropharynx is inspected for evidence of erythema, blisters, or ulcerations. The need for endotracheal intubation is also determined. Options 1, 2, and 3 are incorrect.
Test-Taking Strategy: Focus on the subject, inhalation injury. Recalling that 100% oxygen is required after an inhalation injury will assist you with eliminating options 1 and 2. From the remaining options, recall that a tight-fitting nonrebreather mask is preferred so that the client will not rebreathe exhaled air.

11. 3
Rationale: The client exhibits several warning signs of an inhalation injury: a history of a flame burn to the face, hoarseness, cough, carbonaceous sputum, singed facial hair, facial edema, and color change. Additionally, one of the cardinal signs of hypoxia is restlessness.
Test-Taking Strategy: Use the ABCs—airway, breathing, and circulation—to answer the question. The only option that addresses the airway is option 3.

12. 1
Rationale: Escharotomies are performed to alleviate the compartment syndrome that can occur when edema forms under nondistensible eschar in a circumferential burn. Escharotomies are performed through avascular eschar to subcutaneous fat. Although bleeding may occur from the site, it is considered a complication rather than an anticipated therapeutic outcome. The formation of granulation tissue is not the intent of an escharotomy, and escharotomy will not affect the formation of edema.
Test-Taking Strategy: Note the subject, a therapeutic outcome. Use the ABCs—airway, breathing, and circulation—to answer the question. The only option that addresses circulation is the correct option.

13. 4
Rationale: Circumferential burns of the extremities may compromise circulation. Elevating injured extremities above the level of the heart and performing active exercise help to reduce dependent edema formation. Options 1, 2, and 3 are incorrect.
Test-Taking Strategy: Focus on the subject, circumferential burns. Remember that when an injury such as a burn occurs, edema occurs. Option 4 addresses a position that will reduce edema.

14. 2
Rationale: Successful or adequate fluid resuscitation in the adult is signaled by stable vital signs, adequate urine output, palpable peripheral pulses, and a clear sensorium. The most reliable indicator for determining the adequacy of fluid resuscitation is the urine output. For an adult, the hourly urine volume needs to be 30 to 50 mL.
Test-Taking Strategy: Note the subject, fluid resuscitation. Also note the strategic word, *most*. Note the relationship between urine output and the subject of administering fluids.

15. 2
Rationale: With the classic presentation of herpes zoster, the clinical examination is diagnostic. However, a viral culture of the lesion provides the definitive diagnosis. Herpes zoster (shingles) is caused by a reactivation of the varicella-zoster virus, the virus that causes chickenpox. A patch test is a skin test that involves the administration of an allergen to the surface of the skin to identify specific allergies. A biopsy would provide a cytological examination of tissue. In a Wood's light examination, the skin is viewed under ultraviolet light to identify superficial infections of the skin.
Test-Taking Strategy: Focus on the subject, diagnosing herpes zoster. Recalling that herpes zoster is caused by a virus will assist in directing you to the correct option. Also remember that a biopsy will determine tissue type, whereas a culture will identify an organism.

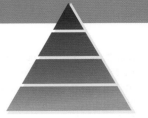

CHAPTER **40**

Integumentary Medications

PRIORITY CONCEPTS Clinical Judgment; Safety

WHAT WOULD YOU DO?

A topical glucocorticoid is prescribed for a hospitalized client to treat an inflammatory skin condition on the neck. What would the nurse do when administering the medication? *Answer is located on p. 497.*

I. Poison Ivy Treatment (Box 40.1)

A. Treatment of lesions includes calamine lotion and commercial products that soothe lesions, compresses and solutions that are astringent and antiseptic, and/or colloidal oatmeal baths to relieve discomfort.

B. Topical corticosteroids are effective to prevent or relieve inflammation, especially when used before blisters form.

C. Oral corticosteroids may be prescribed for severe reactions and an antihistamine such as diphenhydramine may be prescribed.

II. Medications to Treat Dermatitis (Box 40.2)

A. Description

  1. Superficial inflammatory process involving primarily epidermis; there are many types, some of which include atopic dermatitis, contact dermatitis, and stasis dermatitis.

  2. May be treated with moisturizer and topical glucocorticoids; systemic immunosuppressants may also be prescribed if topical treatment is ineffective.

B. Topical immunosuppressants

  1. Tacrolimus and pimecrolimus creams.

  2. Side and adverse effects include redness, burning, and itching; causes sensitization of the skin to sunlight. Treated areas need to be protected from direct sunlight.

  3. Tacrolimus may increase the risk of varicella-zoster infection in children.

  4. Tacrolimus may increase risk of developing skin cancer and lymphoma.

⚠️ When administering any topical medication or patches, the nurse and family caregivers need to always wear gloves to protect themselves from absorption of the medication. Caregivers would also be taught to wash hands thoroughly before and after administration.

III. Topical Glucocorticoids

A. Description

  1. Anti-inflammatory, antipruritic, and vasoconstrictive actions

  2. Preparations vary in potency and depend on the concentration and type of preparation, and method of application (occlusive dressings enhance absorption, increasing the effects).

  3. Systemic effects are more likely to occur with prolonged therapy and when extensive skin surfaces are treated.

⚠️ Topical glucocorticoids can be absorbed into the systemic circulation; absorption is greater in permeable skin areas (scalp, axilla, face and neck, eyelids, perineum) and less in areas where permeability is poor (palms, soles, back).

B. Contraindications

  1. Clients demonstrating previous sensitivity to corticosteroids

  2. Clients with current systemic fungal, viral, or bacterial infections

  3. Clients with current complications related to glucocorticoid therapy

C. Local adverse effects

  1. Burning, dryness, irritation, itching

  2. Skin atrophy

  3. Thinning of the skin, striae, purpura, telangiectasia (causes threadlike red line on the skin)

| BOX 40.1 | **Poison Ivy Treatment Products** |

| BOX 40.1 | **Poison Ivy Treatment Products** |

- Calamine lotion
- Hydrocortisone
- Pramoxine
- Zinc acetate; isopropanol; benzyl alcohol

| BOX 40.3 | **Medications to Treat Actinic Keratosis** |

- Diclofenac sodium 3% gel
- Fluorouracil
- Imiquimod 5% cream
- Ingenol mebutate

| BOX 40.2 | **Medications to Treat Atopic Dermatitis** |

Systemic Immunosuppressants
- Azathioprine
- Cyclosporine
- Methotrexate
- Oral glucocorticoids

Topical Immunosuppressants
- Pimecrolimus 1% cream
- Tacrolimus

4. Acneiform eruptions
5. Hypopigmentation
6. Overgrowth of bacteria, fungi, and viruses
D. Systemic adverse effects
1. Growth retardation in children
2. Adrenal suppression
3. Cushing's syndrome
4. Ocular effects (glaucoma and cataracts)
E. Interventions
1. Monitoring plasma cortisol levels may be prescribed if prolonged therapy is necessary.
2. Wear gloves, wash the area just before application to increase medication penetration.
3. Apply sparingly in a thin film, rubbing gently.
4. Avoid use of a dry occlusive dressing unless specifically prescribed by the primary health care provider (PHCP).
5. Instruct client to report signs of adverse effects to the PHCP.

⚠ In the adult, intact skin is generally impermeable to most topical medications. However, medications would not be applied to open areas unless prescribed because undesired absorption can occur.

IV. **Medications to Treat Actinic Keratosis (Box 40.3)**
A. Description
1. Actinic keratoses are caused by prolonged exposure to the sun and appear as rough, scaly, red or brown lesions usually found on the face, scalp, arms, and back of the hands.
2. Lesions can progress to squamous cell carcinoma.
3. Treatment includes medications and therapies such as excision, cryotherapy, curettage, and laser therapy.

B. Medications include fluorouracil, diclofenac sodium, imiquimod 5% cream, aminolevulinic acid, and ingenol mebutate.
1. Fluorouracil
a. A topical medication that affects DNA and RNA synthesis and causes a sequence of responses that result in healing; results are usually seen in 2 to 6 weeks but may take 1 to 2 months longer for complete healing.
b. Side and adverse effects include itching, burning, inflammation, rash, and increased sensitivity to sunlight.
2. Diclofenac sodium
a. A nonsteroidal anti-inflammatory topical medication; it may take 3 months to be effective.
b. Adverse effects include dry skin, itching, redness, and rash.
3. Imiquimod 5% cream
a. In addition to treating actinic keratoses, this topical medication has been used to treat venereal warts; it may take up to 4 months to be effective.
b. Side and adverse effects include redness, skin swelling, itching, burning, sores, blisters, scabbing, and crusting of the skin.
4. Aminolevulinic acid
a. A topical medication used in conjunction photodynamic therapy; the medication is applied and 14 to 18 hours later the medication is activated by exposing the lesions to special blue light.
b. Side and adverse effects include burning, stinging, redness, and swelling of the skin; treated areas need to be protected from sunlight and bright indoor lights.
5. Ingenol mebutate
a. Indicated for the topical treatment of actinic keratosis; application recommendations need to be followed closely because of the risk of allergic reaction and development of herpes zoster.
b. Side and adverse effects include skin reactions, erythema, flaking/scaling, crusting, swelling, postulation, and erosion/ulceration; allergic reactions; herpes zoster.

V. Sunscreens

A. Ultraviolet (UV) light can damage the skin and cause premalignant actinic keratoses and some types of skin cancer.

B. Sunscreens prevent the penetration of UV light and protect the skin.

C. Organic (chemical) sunscreens absorb UV light; inorganic (physical) sunscreens reflect and scatter UV light.

D. A sunscreen that protects against both UVB and UVA rays and one that has a sun protection factor (SPF) of at least 15 needs to be used.

E. Sunscreens are most effective when applied at least 30 minutes before exposure to the sun (sunscreens containing *para*-aminobenzoic acid or padimate O require application 2 hours before sun exposure).

F. Sunscreen needs to be reapplied every 2 to 3 hours and after swimming or sweating; otherwise, the duration of protection is reduced.

G. Products containing *para*-aminobenzoic acid need to be avoided by individuals allergic to benzocaine, sulfonamides, or thiazides.

H. Sunscreens can cause contact dermatitis and photosensitivity reactions.

> ⚠ The client would be informed that UV light is greatest between the hours of 10:00 a.m. and 4:00 p.m., and that sunglasses, protective clothing, and a hat needs to be worn to reduce the risk of skin damage from the sun.

VI. Medications to Treat Psoriasis (Box 40.4)

A. Description
   1. Psoriasis is a chronic inflammatory disorder that has varying degrees of severity.
   2. Treatment is based on the severity of symptoms and aims to suppress the proliferation of keratinocytes or suppress the activity of inflammatory cells.

B. Topical medications
   1. Glucocorticoids
      a. Used for mild psoriasis
      b. Would not be applied to the face, groin, axilla, or genitalia because the medication is readily absorbable, making the skin vulnerable to glucocorticoid-induced atrophy
   2. Tazarotene
      a. Is a vitamin A derivative
      b. Local reactions include itching, burning, stinging, dry skin, and redness; other, less common effects include rash, desquamation, contact dermatitis, inflammation, fissuring, and bleeding.
      c. Sensitization to sunlight can occur and the client would be instructed to use sunscreen and wear protective clothing.
      d. Medication is usually applied once daily in the evening to dry skin.

BOX 40.4 Medications and Treatments for Psoriasis

Topical Medications
- Calcipotriene
- Coal tar
- Corticosteroids
- Keratolytics (topical salicylic acid; sulfur)
- Tazarotene

Systemic Medications
- Acitretin
- Cyclosporine
- Glucocorticoids
- Methotrexate

Systemic Biological Medications
- Adalimumab
- Brodalumab
- Etanercept
- Guselkumab
- Infliximab
- Ixekizumab
- Ustekinumab
- Risankizumab
- Secukinumab

Phototherapy
- Coal tar and ultraviolet B irradiation
- Photochemotherapy (psoralen and ultraviolet A therapy)

---

   3. Calcipotriene
      a. Is an analog of vitamin D
      b. May take up to 1 to 3 weeks to produce a desired effect
      c. Can cause local irritation; high-dose applications have rarely caused hypercalcemia.
   4. Coal tar
      a. Suppresses DNA synthesis, miotic activity, and cell proliferation
      b. Has an unpleasant odor and may cause irritation, burning, and stinging; can also stain the skin and hair and increase sensitivity to sun
      c. May increase risk for cancer development in high doses
   5. Keratolytics
      a. Soften scales and loosen the horny layer of the skin, resulting in minimal peeling to extensive desquamation
      b. Salicylic acid: Can be absorbed systemically and can cause salicylism, which is characterized by dizziness and tinnitus, hyperpnea, and psychological disturbances; salicylic acid is not applied to large surface areas or open wounds because of the risk of systemic effects.
      c. Sulfur: Promotes peeling and drying and is used to treat acne, dandruff, seborrheic dermatitis, and psoriasis

C. Systemic medications
   1. Methotrexate

a. Reduces proliferation of epidermal cells

b. Can be toxic; causes gastrointestinal effects such as diarrhea, ulcerative stomatitis, and bone marrow depression leading to blood dyscrasias

c. Can be hepatotoxic; hepatic function needs to be monitored during therapy.

d. This medication is teratogenic; women of child-bearing age would wait 3 months after discontinuation of the medication before becoming pregnant.

2. Acitretin

a. Inhibits keratinization, proliferation, and differentiation of cells; has anti-inflammatory and immunomodulatory actions; used for severe psoriasis and reserved for use in those who have not responded to safer medications.

b. Is embryotoxic and teratogenic: Medication is contraindicated during pregnancy; pregnancy must be ruled out and two reliable forms of contraception need to be implemented before the medication is started (contraception must be implemented at least 1 month before treatment begins and be continued for at least 3 years after treatment is discontinued).

c. If pregnancy occurs during treatment with the medication, the medication is discontinued immediately and possible termination of the pregnancy is discussed.

d. Dermatological effects include hair loss, skin peeling, dry skin, rash, pruritus, and nail disorders; other effects include rhinitis from mucous membrane irritation, inflammation of the lips, dry mouth, dry eyes, nosebleed, gingivitis, stomatitis, bone and joint pain, and spinal disorders.

e. Can be hepatotoxic; can elevate triglyceride levels and reduce levels of high-density lipoprotein cholesterol

f. Must not be taken with alcohol, vitamin A supplementation, or tetracycline

3. Cyclosporine

a. An immunosuppressant that inhibits proliferation of B and T cells

b. Can be toxic and cause kidney damage

c. Used for severe psoriasis and reserved for use in those who have not responded to a safer medication

D. Systemic biological medications (clients need to be tested for tuberculosis or other infections before initiation of medications)

1. Tumor necrosis factor (TNF) antagonists

a. Lower amount of TNF-α and interrupt inflammatory process of psoriasis

b. Adalimumab: Administered by subcutaneous injection, usually every other week. Injection sites would be rotated.

c. Etanercept: Administered by subcutaneous injection twice weekly for 3 months, then weekly

d. Infliximab: Administered by intravenous route 3 times over 6 weeks and then every 8 weeks

e. Adverse effects, which are generally not severe, include upper respiratory infections, abdominal pain, headache, rash, injection site reactions, and urinary tract infections; may promote serious infections, including bacterial sepsis, invasive fungal infections, tuberculosis, and reactivation of hepatitis B.

f. Contraindicated for persons with a history of certain cancers, severe or recurrent infection, heart failure, or demyelinating neurological diseases; given with caution to persons with numbness or tingling

g. Increases risk of developing lymphoma

2. Ustekinumab

a. A human monoclonal antibody administered by subcutaneous route

b. Can decrease the activity of the immune system and increase the risk for certain types of cancer

c. Adverse effects of the medication include upper respiratory infections, headache, tiredness, redness at injection site, back pain, and fatigue.

d. Contraindicated in clients who have a history of cancer; also contraindicated in clients with infection or reversible posterior leukoencephalopathy syndrome (rare condition that affects the brain and can cause death)

e. The client would not receive any live virus vaccines because the viruses used in some types of vaccines can cause infection in those with a weakened immune system; in addition, the PHCP needs to be informed if anyone in the household needs a vaccine.

f. The client would not receive the bacillus Calmette-Guérin (BCG) vaccine during the 1 year before, or 1 year after, taking the medication.

g. The client needs to inform the PHCP if he or she is receiving phototherapy, has any other medical condition, is pregnant or plans to become pregnant, or is breast-feeding or plans to breast-feed.

3. Secukinumab

a. Human interlukin-17A antagonist

b. Blocks cytokines to interrupt inflammatory cycle of psoriasis

c. Administered by subcutaneous route

d. Adverse effects include cold symptoms, diarrhea, and upper respiratory infections.

e. Safety with pregnancy has not been established.

E. Phototherapy

1. Coal tar and ultraviolet B (UVB) irradiation: Treatment that involves the application of coal tar

for 8 to 10 hours; coal tar is washed off and the area is exposed to short-wave UVB.

2. Photochemotherapy (psoralen and ultraviolet A [UVA] therapy)

a. Combines the use of long-wave radiation (UVA) with oral methoxsalen (used in very specific cases; photosensitive medication).

b. Can cause pruritus, nausea, and erythema; may accelerate the aging process of the skin; may increase the risk of skin cancer.

VII. Acne Products (Box 40.5; Fig. 40.1)

A. Description

1. Acne lesions that are mild may be treated with nonpharmacological measures, such as gentle cleansing 2 or 3 times daily (oil-based moisturizing products need to be avoided), dermabrasion, or comedo extraction.

2. Mild acne is usually treated pharmacologically with topical agents (antimicrobials and retinoids).

3. Moderate acne is usually treated with oral antibiotics and comedolytics.

4. Severe acne is usually treated with isotretinoin.

5. Hormonal medications may be prescribed to treat acne in female clients.

6. Combination therapy may be prescribed to treat acne.

7. Actions of the medications may include suppressing the growth of *Propionibacterium acnes*, reducing inflammation, promoting keratolysis, unplugging existing comedones and preventing their development, and normalizing hyperproliferation of epithelial cells within the hair follicles; some medications cause thinning of the skin, which facilitates penetration of other medications.

8. For topical applications: Site would be washed and allowed to dry completely before application; hands would be washed after application.

9. All topical products are kept away from the eyes, inside the nose, lips, mucous membranes, hair, and inflamed or denuded skin.

B. Topical antibiotic products

1. Benzoyl peroxide

a. Can produce drying and peeling

b. Severe local irritation (burning, blistering, scaling, swelling) may require reducing the frequency of application.

c. Some products may contain sulfites; monitor for serious allergic reactions.

2. Clindamycin and erythromycin

a. Both products are antibiotics that suppress the growth of *P. acnes.*

b. Combination therapy with benzoyl peroxide prevents the emergence of resistant bacteria; fixed-dose combinations include clindamycin/benzoyl peroxide and erythromycin/benzoyl peroxide.

BOX 40.5 **Acne Products**

Topical Antibiotics
- Benzoyl peroxide
- Clindamycin and erythromycin
- Clindamycin/tretinoin combination gel
- Dapsone
- *Fixed dose combinations:* Clindamycin/benzoyl peroxide and erythromycin/benzoyl peroxide

Topical Retinoids
- Adapalene
- Azelaic acid
- Tazarotene
- Tretinoin

Oral Medications
- Doxycycline
- Erythromycin
- Isotretinoin
- Minocycline
- Tetracycline

Hormonal Medications
- Oral contraceptives
- Spironolactone

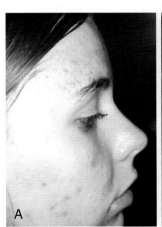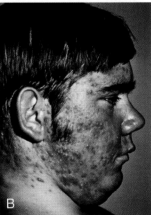

FIGURE 40.1 Acne vulgaris. (A) Comedones with a few inflammatory pustules. (B) Papulopustular acne. (From Perry et al., 2010.)

3. Dapsone: Side and adverse effects include oiliness, peeling, dryness, and erythema of the skin (oral form of medication is used to treat leprosy).

C. Topical retinoids

1. Tretinoin

a. A derivative of vitamin A (vitamin A supplements need to be discontinued during therapy).

b. In addition to treating acne, it may be prescribed to reduce fine wrinkles, skin roughness, and mottled hyperpigmentation as with age spots.

c. Can cause localized adverse effects such as blistering, peeling, crusting, burning, and swelling of the skin.

d. Abrasive products and keratolytic products are discontinued before using tretinoin to decrease localized adverse effects.

e. Instruct the client to apply a sunscreen with an SPF of 15 or greater and to wear protective clothing when outdoors due to sensitivity to UV light.

2. Adapalene: Similar to tretinoin and sensitizes the skin to UV light; adverse effects include burning and itching after application, redness, dryness, and scaling of the skin. Initially may worsen acne; benefits seen in 8 to 12 weeks.

3. Tazarotene

a. Is a derivative of vitamin A (vitamin A supplements need to be discontinued during therapy)

b. In addition to acne, it is used to treat wrinkles and psoriasis.

c. Can cause itching, burning, and dry skin and sensitizes the skin to UV light.

4. Azelaic acid can cause burning, itching, stinging, and redness of the skin; it can also cause hypopigmentation of the skin in clients with a dark complexion.

D. Oral antibiotics

1. Includes doxycycline, minocycline, tetracycline, erythromycin, trimethoprim-sulfamethoxazole, cephalosporines, and penicillins.

2. Improvement develops slowly with the use of oral antibiotics and may take 3 to 6 months for some improvement to be noted; following control of symptoms, the client is usually switched to a topical antibiotic.

E. Isotretinoin

1. Derivative of vitamin A (vitamin A supplements need to be discontinued during therapy); in addition, the use of tetracyclines can increase the risk of adverse effects and need to be discontinued before use of isotretinoin.

2. Used to treat severe cystic acne; reserved for persons who have not responded to other therapies, including systemic antibiotics

3. Side and adverse effects include nosebleeds; inflammation of the lips or eyes; dryness or itching of the skin, nose, or mouth; pain, tenderness, or stiffness in the joints, bones, or muscles; and back pain.

4. Less common adverse effects include rash, hair loss, peeling of the skin, headache, and reduction in night vision.

5. Causes sensitization of the skin to UV light

6. The medication elevates triglyceride levels, which would be measured before and during therapy; alcohol consumption needs to be eliminated during therapy because alcohol could potentiate elevation of serum triglyceride levels.

7. The medication may cause depression in some clients; if depression occurs, the medication would be discontinued.

BOX 40.6	**Burn Products**

- Mafenide acetate
- Silver sulfadiazine
- Bacitracin topical ointment (first-degree burns only)
- Povidone-iodine

⚠ Isotretinoin is highly teratogenic and can cause fetal abnormalities. If prescribed, the client needs to follow strict rules of the iPLEDGE program. It must not be used if the client is pregnant.

F. iPLEDGE program

1. A risk management program that ensures no woman starting an isotretinoin prescription is pregnant and that no woman taking this medication becomes pregnant

2. Access to the medication is controlled through a central automated system.

3. Strict rules must be followed by the client, the PHCP prescribing the medication, pharmacist dispensing the medication, and wholesaler of the medication to ensure safety and to ensure that the woman is not pregnant when therapy is initiated, and that she does not become pregnant while taking the medication.

4. Information on the iPLEDGE program can be found on the US Food and Drug Administration web site: https://www.fda.gov/media/80023/download.

G. Hormonal medications

1. Hormonal medications such as oral contraceptives and spironolactone may be prescribed to treat acne in female clients.

2. These medications decrease androgen activity, resulting in decreased production of sebum.

3. Spironolactone is teratogenic; therefore, contraception during its use is necessary.

4. Side and adverse effects of spironolactone include breast tenderness, menstrual irregularities, and hyperkalemia.

VIII. Burn Products (Box 40.6)

A. Silver sulfadiazine

1. Has broad spectrum of activity against gram-negative bacteria, gram-positive bacteria, and yeast

2. Silver is released slowly from the cream, which is selectively toxic to bacteria.

3. Used primarily to prevent sepsis in clients with burns

4. Not a carbonic anhydrase inhibitor; does not cause acidosis

5. Apply 1/16-inch film (keep burn covered at all times with silver sulfadiazine).

6. Side and adverse effects include rash and itching, blue-green or gray skin discoloration, leukopenia, and interstitial nephritis.

7. Monitor complete blood cell count, particularly the white blood cells, frequently; if leukopenia develops, the PHCP is notified (medication is usually discontinued).

B. Mafenide acetate

    1. Water-soluble cream that is bacteriostatic for gram-negative and gram-positive organisms

    2. Used to treat burns to reduce bacteria present in avascular tissues

    3. Diffuses through the devascularized areas of the skin and may precipitate metabolic acidosis with the client displaying hyperventilation; monitor blood gases and electrolytes.

    4. Apply 1/16-inch film directly to the burn.

    5. Side and adverse effects can include local pain and rash. Medicate for pain before application.

    6. Side and adverse effects include bone marrow depression, hemolytic anemia, and metabolic acidosis.

    7. Keep burn covered with mafenide acetate at all times.

    8. Notify the PHCP if hyperventilation occurs; if acidosis develops, mafenide acetate is washed off the skin and usually discontinued for 1 to 2 days.

WHAT WOULD YOU DO?

Answer: Topical glucocorticoids can be absorbed into the systemic circulation; absorption is greater in permeable skin areas (scalp, axilla, face and neck, eyelids, perineum). The nurse would wash the area just before application and apply the medication sparingly in a thin film, rubbing the area gently. The nurse would also monitor the client for signs of systemic absorption.

PRACTICE QUESTIONS

1. Salicylic acid is prescribed for a client with a diagnosis of psoriasis. The nurse monitors the client, knowing that which finding indicates the presence of systemic toxicity from this medication?

    1. Tinnitus

    2. Diarrhea

    3. Constipation

    4. Decreased respirations

2. The health education nurse provides instructions to a group of clients regarding measures that will assist with preventing skin cancer. Which instructions would the nurse provide? **Select all that apply.**

    ❏ **1.** Sunscreen needs to be applied every 8 hours.

    ❏ **2.** Use sunscreen when participating in outdoor activities.

    ❏ **3.** Wear a hat, opaque clothing, and sunglasses when in the sun.

    ❏ **4.** Avoid sun exposure in the late afternoon and early evening hours.

    ❏ **5.** Examine your body monthly for any lesions that may be suspicious.

3. Silver sulfadiazine is prescribed for a client with a burn injury. Which laboratory finding requires the **need for monitoring** by the nurse?

    1. Glucose level of 99 mg/dL

    2. Platelet level of 300,000 mm^3

    3. Magnesium level of 1.5 mEq/L

    4. White blood cell count of 3000 mm^3

4. A burn client is receiving treatments of topical mafenide acetate to the site of injury. The nurse monitors the client, knowing that which finding indicates the occurrence of a systemic effect?

    1. Hyperventilation

    2. Elevated blood pressure

    3. Local rash at the burn site

    4. Local pain at the burn site

5. Isotretinoin is prescribed for a client with severe acne. Before the administration of this medication, the nurse anticipates that which laboratory test will be prescribed?

    1. Potassium level

    2. Triglyceride level

    3. Hemoglobin A1C

    4. Total cholesterol level

6. A client with severe acne is seen in the clinic and the primary health care provider (PHCP) prescribes isotretinoin. The nurse reviews the client's medication record and would contact the PHCP if the client is also taking which medication?

    1. Digoxin

    2. Phenytoin

    3. Vitamin A

    4. Furosemide

7. The nurse is applying a topical corticosteroid to a client with eczema. The nurse would apply the medication to which body area to decrease the potential for systemic absorption? **Select all that apply.**

    ❏ **1.** Back

    ❏ **2.** Axilla

    ❏ **3.** Eyelids

    ❏ **4.** Soles of the feet

    ❏ **5.** Palms of the hands

8. The clinic nurse is performing an admission assessment on a client and notes that the client is taking azelaic acid. The nurse determines that which client complaint may be associated with the use of this medication?

    1. Itching

    2. Euphoria

3. Drowsiness

4. Frequent urination

9. Silver sulfadiazine is prescribed for a client with a partial-thickness burn and the nurse provides teaching about the medication. Which statement made by the client indicates a **need for further teaching** about the treatments?
   1. "The medication is an antibacterial."
   2. "The medication will help heal the burn."
   3. "The medication is likely to cause stinging initially."

4. "The medication needs to be applied directly to the wound."

10. The camp nurse asks the children preparing to swim in the lake if they have applied sunscreen. The nurse reminds the children that chemical sunscreens are **most effective** when applied at which times?
    1. Immediately before swimming
    2. 5 minutes before exposure to the sun
    3. Immediately before exposure to the sun
    4. At least 30 minutes before exposure to the sun

ANSWERS

1. 1
Rationale: Salicylic acid is absorbed readily through the skin and systemic toxicity (salicylism) can result. Symptoms include tinnitus, dizziness, hyperpnea, and psychological disturbances. Constipation and diarrhea are not associated with salicylism.
Test-Taking Strategy: Focus on the subject, systemic toxicity. Noting the name of the medication will assist in directing you to the correct option if you can recall the toxic effects that occur with acetylsalicylic acid. These medications cause tinnitus if systemic toxicity occurs.

2. 2, 3, 5
Rationale: The client needs to be instructed to avoid sun exposure between the hours of brightest sunlight: 10 a.m. to 4 p.m. Sunscreen, a hat, opaque clothing, and sunglasses needs to be worn for outdoor activities. The client would be instructed to examine the body monthly for the appearance of any cancerous or precancerous lesions. Sunscreen would be reapplied every 2 to 3 hours and after swimming or sweating; otherwise, the duration of protection is reduced.
Test-Taking Strategy: Focus on the subject, measures to prevent skin cancer. Read each option carefully. Noting the time frames in options 1 and 4 will assist in eliminating these options.

3. 4
Rationale: Silver sulfadiazine is used for the treatment of burn injuries. Adverse effects of this medication include rash and itching, blue-green or gray skin discoloration, leukopenia, and interstitial nephritis. The nurse needs to monitor a complete blood count, particularly the white blood cells, frequently for the client taking this medication. If leukopenia develops, the primary health care provider (PHCP) is notified and the medication is usually discontinued. The white blood cell count noted in option 4 is indicative of leukopenia. The other laboratory values are not specific to this medication, and are also within normal limits.
Test-Taking Strategy: Note the strategic words, need for monitoring. Eliminate options 1, 2, and 3 because they are comparable or alike and are within normal limits. In addition, recall that leukopenia is an adverse effect requiring discontinuation of the medication.

4. 1
Rationale: Mafenide acetate is a carbonic anhydrase inhibitor and can suppress renal excretion of acid, thereby causing acidosis. Clients receiving this treatment need to be monitored for signs of an acid-base imbalance (hyperventilation). If this occurs, the medication will probably be discontinued for 1 to 2 days. Options 3 and 4 describe local rather than systemic effects. An elevated blood pressure may be expected from the pain that occurs with a burn injury.
Test-Taking Strategy: Note the subject, *a systemic effect*. Options 3 and 4 can be eliminated because they are comparable or alike and are local rather than systemic effects. From the remaining options, recall that the client in pain would likely have an elevated blood pressure. This would direct you to the correct option.

5. 2
Rationale: Isotretinoin can elevate triglyceride levels. Blood triglyceride levels need to be measured before treatment and periodically thereafter until the effect on triglycerides has been evaluated. There is no indication that isotretinoin affects potassium, hemoglobin A1C, or total cholesterol levels.
Test-Taking Strategy: Note the subject, laboratory values that need to be monitored specifically for the client taking isotretinoin. It is necessary to recall that the medication can affect triglyceride levels in the client.

6. 3
Rationale: Isotretinoin is a metabolite of vitamin A and can produce generalized intensification of isotretinoin toxicity. Because of the potential for increased toxicity, vitamin A supplements would be discontinued before isotretinoin therapy. There are no contraindications associated with digoxin, phenytoin, or furosemide.
Test-Taking Strategy: Focus on the subject, the need to contact the PHCP to ensure client safety. Recall that isotretinoin is a metabolite of vitamin A. Vitamin A is a fat-soluble vitamin; therefore, it is possible to develop toxic levels. This will direct you to the correct option.

7. 1, 4, 5
Rationale: Topical corticosteroids can be absorbed into the systemic circulation. Absorption is higher from regions where the skin is especially permeable (scalp, axilla, face, eyelids, neck, perineum, genitalia), and lower from regions where

permeability is poor (back, palms, soles). The nurse needs to avoid areas of higher absorption to prevent systemic absorption.

Test-Taking Strategy: Focus on the subject, permeability and the potential for increased systemic absorption. Eliminate options 2 and 3 because these body areas are comparable or alike in terms of skin substance. From the remaining options, think about permeability of the skin area. This would direct you to the correct options.

8. 1

Rationale: Azelaic acid is a topical medication used to treat mild to moderate acne. Adverse effects include burning, itching, stinging, redness of the skin, and hypopigmentation of the skin in clients with a dark complexion. The effects noted in the other options are not specifically associated with this medication.

Test-Taking Strategy: Focus on the subject, the purpose and use of azelaic acid. Focusing on the name of the medication and recalling that acne medications commonly cause local irritation will direct you to the correct option.

9. 3

Rationale: Silver sulfadiazine is an antibacterial that has a broad spectrum of activity against gram-negative bacteria, gram-positive bacteria, and yeast. It is applied directly to the wound to assist in healing. It does not cause stinging when applied.

Test-Taking Strategy: Note the strategic words, *need for further teaching*. These words indicate a negative event query and ask you to select an option that is an incorrect statement. Recall the characteristics of this medication and think about the principles associated with the topical application of medications to a burn wound.

10. 4

Rationale: Sunscreens are most effective when applied at least 30 minutes before exposure to the sun so that they can penetrate the skin. All sunscreens need to be reapplied after swimming or sweating.

Test-Taking Strategy: Knowledge that sunscreens need to penetrate the skin will assist in eliminating options 2 and 3. Next, noting the strategic words, *most effective*, will assist in directing you to the correct option.

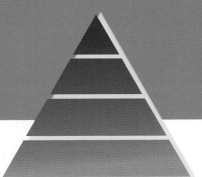

UNIT IX

Oncological and Hematological Problems of the Adult Client

 ## Pyramid to Success

Pyramid Points focus on treatment modalities related to an oncological problem, such as pain management, internal and external radiation, and chemotherapy. In preparation for the NCLEX®, focus on the following oncological problems: skin cancer; leukemia; breast cancer; testicular cancer; stomach, bowel, and pancreatic cancers; bladder cancer; prostate cancer; and lung cancer. Particular attention is given to the nursing care related to these conditions and treatment modalities, client adaptation to acceptance of diagnosis and associated lifestyle changes, and the effect of the treatment for the condition on daily life. Also, concentrate on the complications related to chemotherapy and the nursing measures required to monitor for these complications and to prevent life-threatening conditions, such as infection and bleeding.

 ## Client Needs: Learning Objectives

Safe and Effective Care Environment

Discussing oncology-related consultations and referrals with the interprofessional health care team

Ensuring that advance directives are in the client's medical record

Ensuring that informed consent for treatments and procedures has been obtained

Ensuring advocacy related to the client's decisions

Establishing priorities

Handling hazardous and infectious materials related to radiation and chemotherapy safely

Implementing protective, standard, and other precautions

Maintaining medical and surgical asepsis and preventing infection

Providing confidentiality regarding diagnosis

Upholding client rights

Health Promotion and Maintenance

Discussing expected body image changes related to chemotherapy and treatment

Providing client and family instructions regarding home care

Providing instructions regarding regular breast or testicular self-examinations

Respecting the client's lifestyle choices

Teaching about health promotion programs regarding risks for cancer

Teaching about health screening measures for cancer

Psychosocial Integrity

Assessing the client's ability to cope, adapt, and/or solve problems during illness or stressful events

Assessing the concerns of the client who survived cancer

Assisting the client and family to cope with the alteration in body image

Discussing end-of-life and grief and loss issues related to death and the dying process

Mobilizing appropriate support and resource systems

Promoting a positive environment to maintain optimal quality of life

Respecting religious and cultural preferences

Physiological Integrity

Assisting to administer blood and blood products

Assisting with care to central venous access devices and implanted ports

Caring for the client receiving chemotherapy or radiation therapy

Managing pain

Monitoring diagnostic tests and laboratory values, such as white blood cell and platelet counts

Monitoring for expected and unexpected responses to radiation and chemotherapy

Protecting the client from the life-threatening adverse effects of treatments

Providing basic care and comfort

Providing nutrition

Client Needs lists modified from: National Council of State Boards of Nursing, Inc. (NCSBN). *NCLEX-PN Examination: Test Plan for the National Council Licensure Examination for Practical Nurses,* effective April 2020. Chicago: NCSBN.

CHAPTER **41**

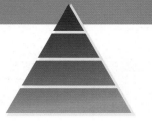

Oncological and Hematological Problems

PRIORITY CONCEPTS Cellular Regulation; Safety

WHAT WOULD YOU DO?

The laboratory reports that a client with leukemia has a platelet count of 19,000 mm³. What would the nurse do?
Answer is located on p. 527.

I. Cancer

A. Description
1. Cancer is a malignant neoplastic disorder that can involve all body organs with manifestations that vary according to the body system affected and type of tumor cells.
2. Cells lose their normal growth-controlling mechanism, and the growth of cells is uncontrolled.
3. Cancer produces serious health problems such as impaired immune and hematopoietic (blood-producing) function; altered gastrointestinal (GI) tract structure and function; motor and sensory deficits; and decreased respiratory function.

B. Metastasis (Box 41.1)
1. Cancer cells move from their original location to other sites.
2. Routes of metastasis
   a. Local seeding: Distribution of shed cancer cells occurs in the local area of the primary tumor.
   b. Blood-borne metastasis: Tumor cells enter the blood, which is the most common cause of cancer spread.
   c. Lymphatic spread: Primary sites rich in lymphatics are more susceptible to early metastatic spread.

C. Cancer classification
1. Solid tumors: Associated with the organs from which they develop, such as breast cancer or lung cancer
2. Hematologic cancers: Originate from blood cell-forming tissues, such as the leukemias, lymphomas, and multiple myeloma

D. Grading and staging (Box 41.2)

1. Grading and staging are methods used to describe the tumor.
2. These methods describe the extent of the tumor, the extent to which malignancy has increased in size, the involvement of regional nodes, and metastatic development.
3. Grading a tumor classifies the cellular aspects of the cancer and is an indicator of tumor growth rate and spread.
4. Staging classifies the severity and clinical aspects of the cancer and degree of metastasis at diagnosis.

E. Factors that influence cancer development
1. Environmental factors
   a. Chemical carcinogens: Factors include industrial chemicals, drugs, and tobacco.
   b. Physical carcinogens: Factors include ionizing radiation (diagnostic and therapeutic x-rays) and ultraviolet radiation (sun, tanning beds, and germicidal lights), chronic irritation, and tissue trauma.
   c. Viral carcinogens: Viruses capable of causing cancer are known as oncoviruses (e.g., Epstein-Barr virus, hepatitis B virus, human papillomavirus [HPV]).
   d. *Helicobacter pylori* infection is associated with an increased risk of gastric cancer.
2. Obesity and dietary factors including preservatives, contaminants, additives, alcohol, and nitrates
3. Genetic predisposition: Factors include an inherited predisposition to specific cancers, inherited conditions associated with cancer, familial clustering, and chromosomal aberrations.
4. Age: Advancing age is a significant risk factor for the development of cancer.
5. Immune function: The incidence of cancer is higher in immunosuppressed individuals, such as those with acquired immunodeficiency syndrome and organ transplant recipients who are taking immunosuppressive medications.

501

BOX 41.1　Common Sites of Metastasis

Bladder Cancer
- Lung
- Bone
- Liver
- Pelvic, retroperitoneal structures

Brain Tumors
- Central nervous system

Breast Cancer
- Bone
- Lung
- Brain
- Liver

Colorectal Cancer
- Liver

Lung Cancer
- Brain
- Liver

Prostate Cancer
- Bone
- Lung
- Liver
- Kidneys

Testicular Cancer
- Lung
- Bone
- Liver
- Adrenal glands
- Retroperitoneal lymph nodes

BOX 41.3　From WebMD: Understanding Cancer—Symptoms

Warning Signs of Cancer—Caution
- **C**hange in bowel or bladder habits
- **A**ny sore that does not heal
- **U**nusual bleeding or discharge
- **T**hickening or lump in breast or elsewhere
- **I**ndigestion
- **O**bvious change in wart or mole
- **N**agging cough or hoarseness

Data from WebMD: Understanding cancer—symptoms (web site): www.webmd.com/cancer/understanding-cancer-symptoms. Ignatavicius et al. (2021), p. 371.

BOX 41.4　Diagnostic Tests

- Biopsy
- Bone marrow examination (particularly if a hematolymphoid malignancy is suspected)
- Chest radiograph
- Complete blood count (CBC)
- Computed tomography (CT) scan
- Cytology studies (Papanicolaou smear)
- Evaluation of serum tumor markers (e.g., carcinoembryonic antigen and alpha-fetoprotein)
- Liver function studies
- Magnetic resonance imaging (MRI)
- Positron emission tomography (PET) scan
- Proctoscopic examination (including guaiac test for occult blood)
- Radiographic studies (mammography)
- Radioisotope scanning (liver, brain, bone, lung)

BOX 41.2　Grading and Staging

Grading
- Grade I: Cells differ slightly from normal cells and are well differentiated (mild dysplasia).
- Grade II: Cells are more abnormal and are moderately differentiated (moderate dysplasia).
- Grade III: Cells are very abnormal and are poorly differentiated (severe dysplasia).
- Grade IV: Cells are immature (anaplasia) and undifferentiated; cell of origin is difficult to determine.

Staging
- Stage 0: Carcinoma in situ
- Stage I: Tumor limited to the tissue of origin; localized tumor growth
- Stage II: Limited local spread
- Stage III: Extensive local and regional spread
- Stage IV: Distant metastasis

F. Prevention: Avoidance of known or potential carcinogens and avoidance or modification of the factors associated with the development of cancer cells

G. Early detection (Box 41.3)
  1. Mammography
  2. Papanicolaou (Pap) test
  3. Rectal exams and stools for occult blood
  4. Sigmoidoscopy, colonoscopy
  5. Breast self-examination (BSE) and clinical breast examination
  6. Testicular self-examination
  7. Skin inspection

II. Diagnostic Tests

A. Diagnostic tests to be performed depend on the suspected primary or metastatic sites of the cancer; invasive procedures require informed consent (Box 41.4).

B. Biopsy
  1. Description
     a. Biopsy is the definitive means of diagnosing cancer and provides histological proof of malignancy.
     b. Biopsy involves the surgical incision of a small piece of tissue for microscopic examination.

2. Types

   a. Needle: Aspiration of cells

   b. Incisional: A wedge of suspected tissue is removed from a larger mass

   c. Excisional: Complete removal of the entire lesion

   d. Staging: Multiple needle or incisional biopsies in tissues in which metastasis is suspected or likely (see Boxes 41.1 and 41.2)

3. Tissue examination

   a. Following excision, a frozen section or a permanent paraffin section is prepared to examine the specimen.

   b. The advantage of the frozen section is the speed with which the section can be prepared and the preliminary diagnosis made; only minutes are required for this test.

   c. Permanent paraffin section takes approximately 24 hours; however, it provides clearer details than the frozen section.

4. Interventions

   a. The procedure is usually performed in an outpatient surgical setting.

   b. Prepare the client for the diagnostic procedure in accordance with the primary health care provider's (PHCP's) instructions and provide postprocedural instructions.

   c. Ensure that informed consent has been obtained.

 III. Pain Control

 Assess the client's pain; pain is what the client describes or says it is. Do not under medicate the cancer client who is in pain.

A. Causes of pain

   1. Bone destruction

   2. Obstruction of an organ

   3. Compression of peripheral nerves

   4. Infiltration and distention of tissue

   5. Inflammation and necrosis

   6. Psychological factors, such as fear or anxiety; a distress screening tool may be used to assess emotional health (see http://www.cancer.org /treatment/treatmentsandsideeffects/emotion alsideeffects/distressinpeoplewithcancer/dist ress-in-people-with-cancer-tools-to-measure-distress).

B. Interventions

   1. Collaborate with other members of the health care team to develop a pain management program.

   2. Administer oral preparations if possible and if they provide adequate relief of pain; the transdermal or transmucosal route may also be prescribed.

   3. Mild or moderate pain may be treated with salicylates, acetaminophen, and nonsteroidal anti-inflammatory drugs (NSAIDs).

   4. Severe pain is treated with opioids, such as codeine sulfate, morphine sulfate, methadone, and hydromorphone hydrochloride; neuropathic pain is treated with a variety of anticonvulsants and antidepressants, as well as opioids.

   5. Subcutaneous injections and continuous intravenous (IV) infusions of opioids provide rapid pain control; equianalgesic comparison charts would be used when switching opioid route of administration.

   6. Monitor vital signs and for side/adverse effects of medications; notify the registered nurse (RN) if side/adverse effects occur.

   7. Monitor for effectiveness of medications.

   8. Provide nonpharmacological techniques of pain control, such as distraction, relaxation, guided imagery, biofeedback, massage, and heat-cold application. Holistic care, such as aromatherapy, may also be beneficial.

IV. Surgery

A. Description: Surgery is indicated to diagnose, stage, and treat certain types of cancer.

B. Prophylactic surgery

   1. Prophylactic surgery is performed in clients with an existing premalignant condition or a known family history or genetic mutation that strongly predisposes the person to the development of cancer.

   2. An attempt is made to remove the tissue or organ at risk and thus prevent the development of cancer.

C. Curative surgery: All gross and microscopic tumor is either removed or destroyed.

D. Control (cytoreductive or "debulking") surgery

   1. Control surgery is a debulking procedure that consists of removing a large part of a locally invasive tumor, such as advanced ovarian cancer.

   2. Surgery decreases the number of cancer cells and increases the chance that other therapies will be successful.

E. Palliative surgery

   1. Palliative surgery is performed to improve the quality of life during the survival time.

   2. Palliative surgery is performed to reduce pain, relieve airway obstruction, relieve obstructions in the GI and urinary tracts, relieve pressure on the brain or spinal cord, prevent hemorrhage, remove infected or ulcerated tumors, or drain abscesses.

F. Reconstructive or rehabilitative surgery is performed to improve the quality of life by restoring maximal function and appearance (e.g., breast reconstruction after mastectomy).

G. Adverse effects of surgery

   1. Loss or loss of function of a specific body part

   2. Reduced function as a result of organ loss

   3. Scarring or disfigurement

4. Grieving about an altered body image or an imposed change in lifestyle
5. Pain, infection, bleeding thromboembolism

 V. Chemotherapy

A. Description
  1. Chemotherapy kills or inhibits the reproduction of neoplastic cells and kills normal cells
  2. The effects are systemic because chemotherapy is usually administered systemically.
  3. Normal cells most profoundly affected include those of the skin, hair, lining of the GI tract; spermatocytes; and hematopoietic cells.
  4. Usually several chemotherapy and biotherapy agents are used in combination (combination therapy) to increase the therapeutic response.
  5. Combination chemotherapy is planned by the PHCP or the oncologist so that medications with overlapping toxicities and nadirs (the time during which bone marrow activity and white blood cell [WBC] counts are at their lowest) are not administered at or near the same time; this will minimize immunosuppression.
  6. Chemotherapy may be combined with other treatments, such as surgery and radiation.

B. Common side/adverse effects include fatigue, alopecia, nausea and vomiting, mucositis, skin changes, and myelosuppression (neutropenia, anemia, and thrombocytopenia).

C. See Chapter 42 for information about the care of the client receiving chemotherapy.

VI. Radiation Therapy

A. Description
  1. Radiation therapy destroys cancer cells with minimal exposure of normal cells to the damaging effects of radiation; the cells that are damaged die or become unable to divide.
  2. Radiation therapy is effective on tissues directly within the path of the radiation beam.
  3. Side effects include local skin changes and irritation, alopecia (hair loss), fatigue (most common side effect of radiation), and altered taste sensation; the effects vary according to the site of treatment.
  4. External-beam radiation (also called teletherapy) and internal radiation (also called brachytherapy) are the types of radiation therapy that are most commonly used to treat cancer.

 B. External-beam radiation (teletherapy): The actual radiation source is external to the client.
  1. Instruct the client regarding skin care (Box 41.5).
  2. The client does not emit radiation and does not pose a hazard to anyone else.

C. Internal radiation (brachytherapy)
  1. The radiation source comes into direct, continuous contact with tumor tissues for a specific time.

BOX 41.5   Client Education Guide: Radiation Therapy for Cancer

- Wash the irradiated area gently each day with either water alone or with a mild soap and water.
- Use the hand rather than a washcloth to wash the area.
- Rinse the soap thoroughly from the skin.
- Take care not to remove the markings that indicate exactly where the beam of radiation is to be focused.
- Dry the irradiated area with patting motions rather than rubbing motions; use a clean, soft towel or cloth.
- Do not use powders, ointments, lotions, or creams on the skin at the radiation site unless they are prescribed by the radiologist.
- Wear soft clothing over the skin at the radiation site.
- Avoid wearing belts, buckles, straps, or any type of clothing that binds or rubs the skin at the radiation site.
- Avoid exposure of the irradiated area to the sun.
- Avoid heat exposure.

---

  2. The radiation source is within the client; for a period of time, the client emits radiation and can pose a hazard to others.
  3. Brachytherapy includes a sealed or unsealed source of radiation.
  4. Unsealed radiation source
    a. Administration is via the oral or IV route or by instillation into the body cavities.
    b. The source is not confined completely to one body area and it enters body fluids and eventually is eliminated via various excreta, which are radioactive and harmful to others. Most of the source is eliminated from the body within 48 hours, at which point neither the client nor the excreta are radioactive or harmful.
  5. Sealed radiation source (**Priority Nursing Actions;** Box 41.6)

⚡ PRIORITY NURSING ACTIONS

Sealed Radiation Implant Becomes Dislodged

1. Encourage the client to lie still.
2. Use long-handled forceps to retrieve the radioactive source.
3. Deposit the radioactive source in a lead container.
4. Contact the registered nurse (RN) and radiation oncologist.
5. Document the occurrence and actions taken.

---

  6. Sealed radiation source
    a. A sealed temporary or permanent radiation source (solid implant) is implanted within the tumor target tissues.

BOX 41.6 Care of the Client with a Sealed Radiation Implant

- Place the client in a private room with a private bath.
- Place a caution sign on the client's door.
- Organize nursing tasks to minimize exposure to the radiation source.
- Nursing assignments to a client with a radiation implant need to rotated.
- Limit exposure time to 30 minutes per care provider per 8-hour shift.
- Wear a dosimeter film badge to measure radiation exposure.
- Wear a lead shield to reduce the transmission of radiation.
- The nurse would not care for more than one client with a radiation implant at one time.
- Do not allow a pregnant nurse to care for the client.
- Do not allow children who are younger than 16 years of age or pregnant women to visit the client.
- Limit visitors to 30 minutes per day; visitors must be at least 6 feet from the source.
- Save the bed linens and dressings until the source is removed, and then dispose of the linens and dressings in the usual manner.
- Other equipment can be removed from the room at any time.

    b. The client emits radiation while the implant is in place, but the excreta are not radioactive.

  7. Removal of sealed radiation sources

    a. The client is not radioactive after removal.

    b. Inform the client that cancer is not contagious.

    c. Inform the client to follow PHCP's prescription regarding resumption of sexual intercourse if the implant was cervical or vaginal.

    d. Advise the client who had a cervical or vaginal implant to notify the PHCP if any of the following occur: severe diarrhea, frequent urination, urethral burning for more than 24 hours, hematuria, heavy vaginal bleeding, extreme fatigue, abdominal pain, fever greater than 100°F (38°C), or other signs of infection.

VII. Hematopoietic Stem Cell Transplantation

A. Description

  1. Bone marrow transplantation (BMT) and peripheral blood stem cell transplantation (PBSCT) are procedures that replace stem cells that have been destroyed by high doses of chemotherapy and/or radiation therapy.

  2. BMT and PBSCT are most commonly used in the treatment of leukemia and lymphoma but are also used to treat other cancers, such as neuroblastoma and multiple myeloma.

  3. The goal of treatment is to rid the client of all leukemic or other **malignant** cells through treatment with high doses of chemotherapy and whole-body irradiation.

  4. Because these treatments are damaging to bone marrow cells, without the replacement of blood-forming stem cell function through transplantation, the client would die of infection or hemorrhage.

B. Types of donor stem cells

  1. Allogeneic: Stem cell donor is usually a sibling, a parent with a similar tissue type, or a person who is not related to the client (unrelated donor).

  2. Syngeneic: Stem cells are from an identical twin.

  3. Autologous

    a. Autologous donation is the most common type.

    b. The client receives his or her own stem cells.

    c. Stem cells are harvested during disease remission and are stored frozen to be reinfused later.

C. Procedure

  1. Harvest

    a. The stem cells used in PBSCT come from the bloodstream in a 4- to 6-hour process called *apheresis* or *leukapheresis* (the blood is removed through a central venous catheter and an apheresis machine removes the stem cells and returns the remainder of the blood to the donor).

    b. In BMT, marrow is harvested through multiple aspirations from the iliac crest to retrieve sufficient bone marrow for the transplant.

    c. Marrow from the client is filtered for residual cancer cells.

    d. Allogenic marrow is transfused immediately; autologous marrow is frozen for later use (cryopreservation).

    e. Harvesting is done before the initiation of the conditioning regimen.

  2. *Conditioning* refers to an immunosuppression therapy regimen used to eradicate all malignant cells, provide a state of immunosuppression, and create space in the bone marrow for the engraftment of the new marrow.

  3. Transplantation

    a. Stem cells are administered through the client's central line in a manner similar to that of a blood transfusion.

    b. Stem cells may be administered by IV infusion or by IV push directly into the central line.

  4. Engraftment

    a. The transfused stem cells move to the marrow-forming sites of the recipient's bones.

    b. Engraftment occurs when the WBC, erythrocyte, and platelet counts begin to rise.

    c. When successful, the engraftment process takes 2 to 5 weeks.

D. Posttransplantation period: Infection, bleeding, or neutropenia and thrombocytopenia are major concerns until engraftment occurs.

Adult—Oncological and Hematological

BOX 41.7 Classification of Leukemia

Acute Lymphocytic Leukemia
- Mostly lymphoblasts present in the bone marrow
- Age of onset is usually younger than 15 years

Acute Myelogenous Leukemia
- Mostly myeloblasts present in the bone marrow
- Age of onset is usually between 15 and 39 years

Chronic Myelogenous Leukemia
- Mostly granulocytes present in the bone marrow
- Age of onset is usually in the fourth decade

Chronic Lymphocytic Leukemia
- Mostly lymphocytes present in the bone marrow
- Age of onset is usually older than 50 years

⚠ During the posttransplantation period, the client remains without any natural immunity until the donor stem cells begin to proliferate and engraftment occurs.

 E. Complications
  1. Failure to engraft: If the transplanted stem cells fail to engraft, the client will die unless another transplantation is attempted and is successful.
  2. Graft-*versus*-host disease in allogeneic transplants
     a. Although the recipient cannot recognize donated cells as foreign or nonself because of total immunosuppression, the immune-competent cells of the donor recognize the recipient's cells as foreign and mount an immune offense against them.
     b. Graft-*versus*-host disease is managed cautiously with immunosuppressive agents to avoid suppressing the new immune system to such an extent that the client becomes more susceptible to infection, or the transplanted cells stop engrafting.
  3. Hepatic venoocclusive disease
     a. The disease involves occlusion of the hepatic venules by thrombosis or phlebitis.
     b. Signs include right upper quadrant abdominal pain, jaundice, ascites, weight gain, and hepatomegaly.
     c. Early detection is critical because there is no known way to open the hepatic vessels.
     d. The client will be treated with fluids and supportive therapy.

VIII. Skin Cancer (See Chapter 39)

 IX. Leukemia (Box 41.7)
  A. Description
     1. Leukemia refers to a group of hematological malignancies involving abnormal overproduction of leukocytes, usually at an immature stage, in the bone marrow.

  2. The two major types of leukemia are lymphocytic (involving abnormal cells from the lymphoid pathway) and myelocytic or myelogenous (involving abnormal cells from the myeloid pathways).
  3. Leukemia may be acute, with a sudden onset, or chronic, with a slow onset and persistent symptoms over a period of years.
  4. Leukemia affects the bone marrow, causing anemia, leukopenia, the production of immature cells, thrombocytopenia, and a decline in immunity.
  5. The cause is unknown and appears to involve genetically damaged cells, leading to the transformation of cells from a normal state to a malignant state.
  6. Risk factors include genetic, viral, immunological, and environmental factors and exposure to radiation, chemicals, and medications, such as previous chemotherapy.

  B. Data collection
  1. Anorexia, fatigue, weakness, weight loss
  2. Anemia
  3. Overt bleeding (nosebleeds, gum bleeding, rectal bleeding, hematuria, increased menstrual flow) and occult bleeding (e.g., as detected in a fecal occult blood test)
  4. Ecchymoses, petechiae
  5. Prolonged bleeding after minor abrasions or lacerations
  6. Elevated temperature
  7. Enlarged lymph nodes, spleen, and liver
  8. Palpitations, tachycardia, orthostatic hypotension
  9. Pallor and dyspnea on exertion
  10. Headache
  11. Bone pain and joint swelling
  12. Normal, elevated, or reduced WBC count
  13. Decreased hemoglobin and hematocrit levels
  14. Decreased platelet count
  15. Positive bone marrow biopsy identifying leukemic blast-phase cells

  C. Infection
  1. Infection can occur through autocontamination or cross-contamination. The WBC count may be extremely low during the period of greatest bone marrow depression, known as the nadir.
  2. Common sites of infection are the skin, respiratory tract, and GI tract.
  3. Initiate protective isolation procedures.
  4. Ensure frequent and thorough hand washing by the client, family, and PHCPs.
  5. Staff and visitors with known infections or exposure to communicable diseases must avoid contact with the client until risk of infectious spread has passed.
  6. Use strict aseptic technique for all procedures.
  7. Keep supplies for the client separate from supplies for other clients; keep frequently used equipment in the room for the client's use only.
  8. Limit the number of staff entering the client's room to reduce the risk of cross-infection.

BOX 41.8   Mouth Care for the Client with Mucositis

- Inspect the mouth daily.
- Offer complete mouth care before and after every meal and at bedtime.
- Brush the teeth and tongue with a soft-bristled toothbrush or sponge.
- Provide mouth rinses every 12 hours with the prescribed solution.
- Administer topical anesthetic agents to mouth sores, as prescribed.
- Avoid the use of alcohol- or glycerin-based mouthwashes or swabs because they are irritating to the mucosa.
- Offer soft foods that are cool to warm in temperature rather than foods that are hard or spicy.

---

9. Maintain the client in a private room with the door closed.
10. Place the client in a room with a high-efficiency particulate air filtration or a laminar airflow system, if possible.
11. Reduce exposure to environmental organisms by eliminating raw fruits and vegetables (low-bacteria diet) from the diet, eliminate fresh flowers and live plants, and avoid leaving standing water in the client's room.
12. Be sure that the client's room is cleaned daily.
13. Assist the client with daily bathing with the use of an antimicrobial soap.
14. Assist the client with performing oral hygiene frequently.
15. Initiate a bowel program to prevent constipation and rectal trauma.
16. Avoid invasive procedures, such as injections, insertion of rectal thermometers, enemas, and urinary catheterization.
17. Change wound dressings daily and inspect the wounds for redness, swelling, or drainage.
18. Monitor the urine for cloudiness and other signs of infection.
19. Monitor the skin and oral mucous membranes for signs of infection (Box 41.8).
20. Encourage the client to cough and deep breathe; check breath sounds.
21. Monitor temperature, pulse, respirations, blood pressure, and for pain.
22. Monitor the WBC and neutrophil counts.
23. Notify the PHCP if signs of infection are present and the nurse would prepare to obtain specimens for the culture of the blood, open lesions, urine, and sputum; chest radiograph may be prescribed.
24. Administer prescribed antibiotic, antifungal, and antiviral medications.
25. Reinforce homecare instructions.
    a. To avoid crowds and those with infections
    b. To maintain a low-bacteria diet and to avoid drinking water that has been standing for longer than 15 minutes

c. To avoid activities that expose him or her to infection, such as changing a pet's litter box, working with houseplants, or gardening
d. That neither they nor their household contacts would receive immunization with a live virus such as measles, mumps, rubella, polio, varicella, shingles, and some influenza vaccines including the H1N1 vaccine

⚠️ Infection is a major cause of death in the immuno-suppressed client.

D. Bleeding
1. During the period of greatest bone marrow suppression (the nadir), the platelet count may be extremely low.
2. The client is at risk for bleeding when the platelet count decreases to less than 50,000 mm³, and spontaneous bleeding frequently occurs when the platelet count is less than 20,000 mm³.
3. Clients with platelet counts less than 20,000 mm³ may need a platelet transfusion.
4. For clients with anemia and fatigue, packed red blood cells may be prescribed.
5. Monitor the laboratory values, as appropriate.
6. Examine the client for signs/symptoms of bleeding, such as petechiae; examine all body fluids and excrement for the presence of blood.
7. Handle the client gently; use caution when obtaining blood pressure measurements to prevent skin injury.
8. Monitor for signs of internal hemorrhage (e.g., pain, rapid and weak pulse, increased abdominal girth, abdomen guarding, and change in mental status).
9. Provide soft foods that are cool to warm to avoid oral mucosa damage.
10. Avoid injections, if possible, to prevent trauma to the skin and bleeding; apply firm and gentle pressure to a needle-stick site for at least 5 minutes, or longer if needed.
11. Pad the side rails and sharp corners of the bed and furniture.
12. Avoid rectal suppositories, enemas, and thermometers.
13. If the female client is menstruating, count the number of pads or tampons used.
14. Assist with administration of blood products as prescribed.
15. Reinforce instructions to the client to use a soft toothbrush and to avoid dental floss.
16. Reinforce instructions to the client to use only an electric razor for shaving.
17. Reinforce instructions to the client to avoid blowing the nose.
18. Discourage the client from engaging in activities that involve the use of sharp objects; contact sports also need to be avoided.
19. Reinforce instructions to the client to avoid using NSAIDs and products that contain aspirin.

E. Fatigue and nutrition
1. Assist the client with selecting a well-balanced diet.

2. Provide small, frequent meals (high calorie, high protein, high carbohydrate) that require little chewing to reduce energy expenditure at mealtimes.

3. Assist the client with self-care and mobility activities.

4. Allow for adequate rest periods during care.

5. Do not perform activities unless they are essential; assist the client with scheduling important or pleasurable activities during periods of highest energy.

6. Blood products may be prescribed for anemia.

F. Additional interventions

   1. Chemotherapy

     a. Induction therapy is aimed at achieving a rapid, complete remission of all manifestations of the disease.

     b. Consolidation therapy is administered early in remission with the aim of curing.

     c. Maintenance therapy may be prescribed for months or years following successful induction and consolidation therapy; the aim is to maintain remission.

   2. Administer antibiotic, antibacterial, antiviral, and antifungal medications as prescribed.

   3. Administer colony-stimulating factors as prescribed.

   4. Blood replacements may be prescribed.

   5. Maintain infection and bleeding precautions.

   6. BMT may be indicated.

   7. Reinforce instructions to the client about appropriate homecare measures.

   8. Provide psychosocial support and support services for home care.

X. Lymphoma: Hodgkin's Disease

A. Description

   1. Lymphomas, classified as Hodgkin's and non-Hodgkin's, depending on the cell type, are characterized by abnormal proliferation of lymphocytes.

   2. Hodgkin's disease is a malignancy of the lymph nodes that originates in a single lymph node or a chain of nodes.

   3. Metastasis occurs to other, adjacent lymph structures and eventually invades nonlymphoid tissue.

   4. The disease usually involves the lymph nodes, tonsils, spleen, and bone marrow; it is characterized by the presence of Reed-Sternberg cells in the nodes.

   5. Possible causes include viral infections; clients treated with combination chemotherapy for Hodgkin's disease have a greater risk of developing acute leukemia and non-Hodgkin's lymphoma, among other secondary malignancies.

   6. Prognosis depends on the stage of the disease.

B. Data collection

   1. Fever

   2. Malaise, fatigue, weakness

   3. Night sweats

   4. Loss of appetite, significant weight loss

   5. Anemia, thrombocytopenia

   6. Enlarged lymph nodes, spleen, and liver

   7. Positive biopsy of lymph nodes, with cervical nodes most often affected first

   8. Presence of Reed-Sternberg cells in nodes

   9. Positive computed tomography (CT) scan of the liver and spleen

C. Interventions

   1. For earlier stages (I and II), without mediastinal node involvement, the treatment of choice is extensive external radiation of the involved lymph node regions.

   2. With more extensive disease, radiation along with multiagent chemotherapy is used.

   3. Monitor for side effects related to chemotherapy or radiation.

   4. Monitor for signs of infection and bleeding.

   5. Maintain infection and bleeding precautions.

   6. Discuss the possibility of sterility with the client receiving radiation and/or chemotherapy and inform the male client of fertility options such as sperm banking.

XI. Multiple Myeloma

A. Description

   1. A malignant proliferation of plasma cells and tumors within the bone

   2. Excessive number of abnormal plasma cells invade the bone marrow, develop into tumors, and ultimately destroy the bone; invasion of the lymph nodes, spleen, and liver occurs.

   3. The abnormal plasma cells produce an abnormal antibody (myeloma protein or the Bence Jones protein) found in the blood and urine.

   4. Multiple myeloma causes decreased production of immunoglobulin and antibodies and increased levels of uric acid and calcium, which can lead to kidney failure.

   5. The disease typically develops slowly and the cause is unknown.

B. Data collection

   1. Bone (skeletal) pain, especially in the pelvis, spine, and ribs

   2. Weakness and fatigue

   3. Recurrent infection

   4. Anemia

   5. Urinalysis shows Bence Jones proteinuria and elevated total serum protein level

   6. Osteoporosis (bone loss and the development of pathological fractures)

   7. Thrombocytopenia and leukopenia

   8. Elevated calcium and uric acid levels

   9. Kidney failure

10. Spinal cord compression and paraplegia
11. Bone marrow aspiration shows an abnormal number of immature plasma cells.

⚠️ The client with multiple myeloma is at risk for pathological fractures. Therefore, provide skeletal support during moving, turning, and ambulating, and provide a hazard-free environment.

C. Interventions
1. Assist with administration of chemotherapy as prescribed.
2. Provide supportive care to control symptoms and prevent complications, especially bleeding, bone fractures, hypercalcemia, kidney failure, and infections.
3. Maintain neutropenic and bleeding precautions, as necessary.
4. Monitor for signs of bleeding, infection, and skeletal fractures.
5. Encourage the consumption of at least 2 L of fluid per day to offset potential problems associated with hypercalcemia, hyperuricemia, and proteinuria, and encourage additional fluid intake as indicated and tolerated.
6. Monitor for signs of kidney failure. Collect 24-hour urine as prescribed.
7. Encourage ambulation to prevent renal problems and slow down bone resorption.
8. IV fluids and diuretics may be prescribed to increase the renal excretion of calcium.
9. Blood transfusions may be prescribed for anemia.
10. Administer analgesics, as prescribed, and provide nonpharmacological therapies to control pain.
11. Administer antibiotics for infection, as prescribed.
12. Bisphosphonate medications may be prescribed to slow bone damage and reduce pain and risk of fractures.
13. Prepare the client for local radiation therapy, if prescribed.
14. Reinforce instructions to the client regarding homecare measures and the signs and symptoms of infection.

XII. Testicular Cancer

A. Description
1. Testicular cancer arises from germinal epithelium from the sperm-producing germ cells or from nongerminal epithelium from other structures in the testicles.
2. The average age at the time of diagnosis is 33 years.
3. The cause of testicular cancer is unknown, but a history of undescended testicle (cryptorchidism) and genetic predisposition have been associated with testicular tumor development.
4. Metastasis occurs to the lung, liver, bone, and adrenal glands via the blood, and to the retroperitoneal lymph nodes via lymphatic channels.

B. Early detection: Perform monthly testicular self-examination (Fig. 41.1).

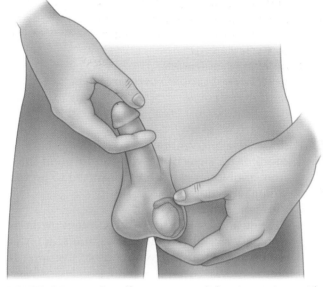

FIGURE 41.1 Testicular self-examination and client instructions. 1. The best time to perform this examination is right after a shower when your scrotal skin is moist and relaxed, thus making the testicles easy to feel. 2. Gently lift each testicle. Each one should feel like an egg; it needs to feel firm but not hard, and smooth with no lumps. 3. Using both hands, place your middle fingers on the underside of each testicle and your thumbs on top. 4. Gently roll each testicle between the thumb and fingers to feel for any lumps, swellings, or masses. 5. If you notice any changes from one month to the next, notify your primary health care provider.

1. Performing testicular self-examination: Perform monthly; a day of the month is selected and the examination is performed on the same day each month.
2. Client instructions (see Fig. 41.1).

C. Data Collection
1. Painless testicular swelling occurs.
2. "Dragging" or "pulling" sensation is experienced in the scrotum.
3. Palpable lymphadenopathy, abdominal masses, and gynecomastia may indicate metastasis.
4. Late signs include back or bone pain and respiratory symptoms.

D. Interventions
1. Chemotherapy may be prescribed.
2. Prepare the client for radiation therapy as prescribed.
3. Prepare the client for unilateral orchiectomy, if prescribed, for diagnosis and primary surgical management or radical orchiectomy (surgical removal of the affected testis, spermatic cord, and regional lymph nodes).
4. Prepare the client for retroperitoneal lymph node dissection, if prescribed, to stage the disease and reduce tumor volume so that chemotherapy and radiation therapy are more effective.
5. Discuss reproduction, sexuality, and fertility information and options with the client.
6. Identify reproductive options such as sperm storage, donor insemination, and adoption.

BOX 41.9   Premalignant Cancers: Stages of Cervical Intraepithelial Neoplasia

- **Stage I:** Mild dysplasia
- **Stage II:** Moderate dysplasia
- **Stage III:** Severe dysplasia to carcinoma in situ

BOX 41.10   Treatment for Cervical Cancer

Nonsurgical
- Chemotherapy
- Cryosurgery
- External radiation
- Internal radiation implants (intracavitary)
- Laser therapy

Surgical
- Conization
- Hysterectomy
- Pelvic exenteration

E. Postoperative interventions
1. Monitor for signs of bleeding and wound infection; antibiotics may be administered to prevent wound infection.
2. Monitor intake and output.
3. Provide and explain pain management methods; to reduce swelling in the first 48 hours, apply an ice pack with an intervening protective layer of cloth.
4. Notify the RN if chills, fever, increasing pain or tenderness at the incision site, or drainage from the incision occurs.
5. After the orchiectomy, the client will be instructed to avoid heavy lifting and strenuous activity for the length of time prescribed by the PHCP.
6. Instruct the client to perform a monthly testicular self-examination on the remaining testicle (see Fig. 41.1).
7. Inform the client that sutures will be removed approximately 7 to 10 days after surgery.

XIII. Cervical Cancer

A. Description
1. Preinvasive cancer is limited to the cervix (Box 41.9).
2. Invasive cancer is in the cervix and other pelvic structures.
3. Metastasis is usually confined to the pelvis, but distant metastasis occurs through lymphatic spread.
4. Premalignant changes are described on a continuum from dysplasia, which is the earliest premalignancy change, to carcinoma in situ, which is the most advanced premalignant change.

B. Risk factors
1. HPV infection (vaccination against HPV is effective to avoid HPV infection and thus cervical cancer)
2. Cigarette smoking, both active and passive
3. Reproductive behavior, including early first intercourse (before the age of 17 years), multiple sex partners, or male partners with multiple sex partners
4. Screening via regular gynecological examinations and Pap test, with treatment of precancerous abnormalities, decreases the incidence and mortality of cervical cancer.

C. Data collection
1. Painless vaginal postmenstrual and postcoital (after sexual intercourse) bleeding
2. Foul-smelling or serosanguineous vaginal discharge
3. Pelvic, lower back, leg, or groin pain
4. Anorexia and weight loss
5. Leakage of urine and feces from the vagina
6. Dysuria (painful urination)
7. Hematuria
8. Cytological changes on Pap test

D. Interventions (Box 41.10)

E. Cryosurgery
1. Involves freezing of the tissues using a probe with subsequent necrosis and sloughing
2. No anesthesia is required, although cramping may occur during the procedure.
3. A heavy, watery discharge will occur for several weeks after the procedure.
4. Reinforce instructions to the client to avoid intercourse and the use of tampons while the discharge is present.

F. Laser therapy
1. Used when all boundaries of the lesion are visible during colposcopic examination
2. Energy from the beam is absorbed by fluid in the tissues, which causes them to vaporize.
3. Minimal bleeding is associated with the procedure.
4. Slight vaginal discharge is expected after the procedure; healing occurs in 6 to 12 weeks.

G. Conization
1. A cone-shaped area of the cervix is removed.
2. Conization allows the woman to retain reproductive capacity.
3. Long-term follow-up care is needed, because new lesions can develop.
4. The risks of the procedure include hemorrhage, uterine perforation, incompetent cervix, cervical stenosis, and preterm labor in future pregnancies.

H. Hysterectomy
1. Description
   a. Hysterectomy is performed for microinvasive cancer if childbearing is not desired.

> ## BOX 41.11 Types of Pelvic Exenteration
>
> **Anterior**
> - Removal of the uterus, ovaries, fallopian tubes, vagina, bladder, urethra, and pelvic lymph nodes
>
> **Posterior**
> - Removal of the uterus, ovaries, fallopian tubes, descending colon, rectum, and anal canal
>
> **Total**
> - Combination of anterior and posterior

  b. A vaginal approach is most commonly performed.

  c. A radical hysterectomy and bilateral lymph node dissection may be performed for cancer that has spread beyond the cervix but not to the pelvic wall.

2. Postoperative interventions

  a. Monitor vital signs.

  b. Assist with coughing and deep-breathing exercises.

  c. Assist with range-of-motion (ROM) exercises and provide early ambulation.

  d. Apply antiembolism stockings or sequential compression devices as prescribed.

  e. Monitor intake and output, urinary catheter drainage, and hydration status.

  f. Monitor bowel sounds.

  g. Monitor the incision site for signs of infection.

  h. Administer pain medication, as prescribed.

  i. Reinforce postoperative instructions to the client to limit stair climbing for 1 month as prescribed and to avoid tub baths and sitting for long periods.

  j. Avoid strenuous activity or lifting anything weighing more than 20 pounds (9 kg).

  k. Instruct the client to consume foods that aid in tissue healing, including protein, fruits, and vegetables.

  l. Instruct the client to avoid sexual intercourse for 3 to 6 weeks as prescribed.

  m. Instruct the client about the signs/symptoms associated with complications.

Monitor vaginal bleeding following hysterectomy. More than 1 saturated pad per hour may indicate excessive bleeding; report this occurrence to the RN.

XIV. Pelvic exenteration (Box 41.11)

A. Description

1. Pelvic exenteration, the removal of pelvic contents, is a radical surgical procedure performed for recurrent cancer if no evidence of tumor outside the pelvis and no lymph node involvement exist.

2. When the bladder is removed, an ileal conduit is created and located on the right side of the abdomen to divert urine.

3. A colostomy may need to be created on the left side of the abdomen for the passage of feces.

B. Postoperative interventions

1. Similar to postoperative interventions following hysterectomy

2. Monitor for signs of altered respiratory status.

3. Monitor incision site for infection.

4. Monitor intake and output and for signs of dehydration.

5. Monitor for hemorrhage, shock, and deep vein thrombosis.

6. Apply antiembolism stockings or sequential compression devices as prescribed.

7. Administer prophylactic heparin as prescribed.

8. Administer perineal irrigations and sitz baths as prescribed.

9. Instruct the client to avoid strenuous activity for 6 months.

10. Instruct the client that the perineal opening, if present, may drain for several months.

11. Reinforce instructions to the client in the care of the ileal conduit and colostomy, if created.

12. Provide sexual counseling because vaginal intercourse is not possible after anterior and total pelvic exenteration.

13. Internal radiation therapy is used for clients for whom surgery is not an option.

XV. Ovarian Cancer

A. Description

1. Ovarian cancer grows rapidly, spreads quickly, and is often bilateral.

2. Metastasis occurs by direct spread to the organs in the pelvis, by distal spread through lymphatic drainage, or by peritoneal seeding.

3. In its early stages, ovarian cancer is often asymptomatic; because most women are diagnosed in advanced stages, ovarian cancer has a higher mortality rate than any other cancer of the female reproductive system.

4. An exploratory laparotomy is performed to diagnose and stage the tumor.

5. A transvaginal ultrasound can also be used; however, this screening does not decrease mortality.

B. Data collection

1. Abdominal discomfort or swelling

2. GI disturbances

3. Dysfunctional vaginal bleeding

4. Abdominal mass

5. Elevated tumor marker (i.e., CA 125)

C. Interventions

1. External radiation may be used if the tumor has invaded other organs; intraperitoneal radioisotopes may be instilled for stage 1 disease.

2. Chemotherapy is used postoperatively for most stages of ovarian cancer.

3. Intraperitoneal chemotherapy, which involves the instillation of chemotherapy into the abdominal cavity, may be prescribed.

4. Total abdominal hysterectomy and bilateral salpingo-oophorectomy with tumor debulking may be necessary.

XVI. Endometrial (Uterine) Cancer

A. Description
1. Endometrial cancer is a slow-growing tumor arising from the endometrial mucosa of the uterus, associated with the menopausal years.
2. Metastasis occurs through the lymphatic system to the ovaries and pelvis and via the blood to the lungs, liver, and bone, or intra-abdominally to the peritoneal cavity.

B. Risk factors
1. Use of estrogen replacement therapy (ERT)
2. Nulliparity
3. Polycystic ovary disease
4. Increased age
5. Late menopause
6. Family history of uterine cancer or hereditary nonpolyposis colorectal cancer
7. Obesity
8. Hypertension
9. Diabetes mellitus

C. Data collection
1. Abnormal bleeding, especially in postmenopausal women
2. Vaginal discharge
3. Low back, pelvic, or abdominal pain (pain occurs late in the disease process)
4. Enlarged uterus (in advanced stages)

D. Nonsurgical interventions
1. External or internal radiation (intracavitary radiation) is used alone or in combination with surgery, depending on the stage of cancer.
2. Chemotherapy is used to treat advanced or recurrent disease.
3. Progesterone therapy with medication for estrogen-dependent tumors may be prescribed.
4. Tamoxifen, an antiestrogen medication may also be prescribed.

E. Surgical interventions: Total abdominal hysterectomy and bilateral salpingo-oophorectomy

XVII. Breast Cancer

A. Description
1. Breast cancer is classified as invasive when it penetrates the tissue surrounding the mammary duct and grows in an irregular pattern.
2. Metastasis occurs via lymph nodes.
3. Common sites of metastasis are the bone and lungs; metastasis may also occur to the brain and liver.
4. Diagnosis is made by breast biopsy through a needle aspiration or by the surgical removal of the tumor with a microscopic examination for malignant cells.

B. Risk factors
1. Family history of breast cancer due to genetic predisposition
2. Early menarche and late menopause
3. Previous cancer of the breast, uterus, or ovaries
4. Nulliparity, late first birth
5. Obesity
6. High-dose radiation exposure of the chest

C. Data collection
1. Mass felt during BSE (usually felt in the upper outer quadrant, beneath the nipple, or in axilla)
2. Presence of the lesion on mammography
3. A fixed, irregular nonencapsulated mass; typically painless except in the late stages
4. Asymmetry, with the affected breast being higher
5. Nipple retraction or elevation
6. Bloody or clear nipple discharge
7. Skin dimpling, retraction, or ulceration
8. Skin edema or peau d'orange skin, which may indicate lymphatic involvement (blocked skin drainage causes skin edema and an "orange peel" appearance)
9. Axillary lymphadenopathy
10. Lymphedema of the affected arm
11. Symptoms of bone or lung metastasis in late stage

D. Early Detection: Regular BSE
1. Perform regularly 7 to 10 days after menses
2. Postmenopausal clients or clients who have had a hysterectomy need to also perform a BSE regularly.

E. Reinforce client instructions (Fig. 41.2)

F. Nonsurgical interventions
1. Chemotherapy
2. Radiation therapy
3. Hormonal manipulation via the use of medication in postmenopausal women or other medications for estrogen receptor–positive tumors
4. Monoclonal antibodies such as trastuzumab for human epidermal growth factor receptor 2–positive (HER-2+) breast cancer

G. Surgical interventions: Surgical breast procedures with possible breast reconstruction (Box 41.12)

H. Postoperative interventions
1. Monitor vital signs.
2. Position the client in a semi-Fowler's position; turn her from the back to the unaffected side, with the affected arm elevated above the level of the heart to promote drainage and prevent lymphedema.
3. Encourage coughing and deep breathing.
4. If a suction type of drain (such as a Jackson-Pratt) is in place, maintain suction and record the amount of drainage and the drainage characteristics; reinforce instructions to the client about home management of the drain (Fig. 41.3).
5. Monitor operative site for infection, swelling, or the presence of fluid collection under the skin flaps or in the arm.
6. Monitor incision site for restriction of dressing, impaired sensation, or color changes of the skin.

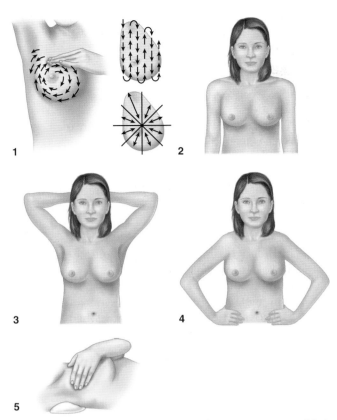

FIGURE 41.2 Breast self-examination and client instructions. 1. While in the shower or bath, when the skin is slippery with soap and water, examine your breasts. Use the pads of your second, third, and fourth fingers to firmly press every part of the breast. Use your right hand to examine your left breast and your left hand to examine your right breast. Using the pads of the fingers on your left hand, examine the entire breast with the use of small circular motions in a spiral or in an up-and-down motion so that the entire breast area is examined. Repeat the procedure using your right hand to examine your left breast. Repeat the pattern of palpation under the arm. Check for any lump, hard knot, or thickening of the tissue. 2. Look at your breasts in a mirror. Stand with your arms at your side. 3. Raise your arms overhead, and check for any changes in the shape of your breasts, any dimpling of the skin, or any changes in the nipple. 4. Place your hands on your hips and press down firmly, tightening the pectoral muscles. Observe for asymmetry or changes, keeping in mind that your breasts probably do not match exactly. 5. While lying down, feel your breasts as described in step 1. When examining your right breast, place a folded towel under your right shoulder, and put your right hand behind your head. Repeat the procedure when examining your left breast. Mark on your calendar that you have completed your breast self-examination; note any changes or unique characteristics that you want to discuss with your primary health care provider.

7. If breast reconstruction was performed, the client will return from surgery with a surgical support garment and the temporary prosthesis in place.
8. Provide the use of a pressure sleeve, as prescribed, if edema is severe.
9. Maintain fluid and electrolyte balance; administer diuretics and provide a low-salt diet, as prescribed, for severe lymphedema.
10. Consult with the RN and the physical therapist regarding the appropriate exercise program, and assist the client with prescribed exercise.
11. Reinforce instructions regarding homecare measures (Box 41.13).

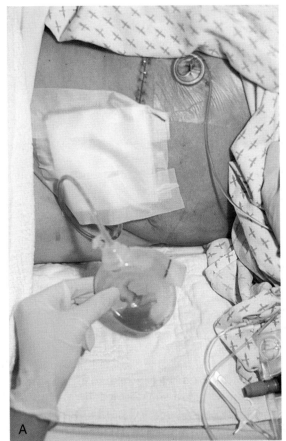

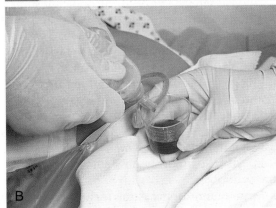

FIGURE 41.3 Jackson-Pratt device. (A) Drainage tubes and reservoir. (B) Emptying drainage reservoir. (From Potter, P. A., & Perry, A. G., Stocker, P. A., Hall, A. M. (2013). *Fundamentals of Nursing* (8th ed., p. 1211). St. Louis: Elsevier Mosby.)

BOX 41.13   Client Instructions After Mastectomy

- Avoid overuse of the arm during the first few months.
- To prevent lymphedema, keep the affected arm elevated; consultation with lymphedema specialist may be prescribed.
- Provide incision care with an emollient, as prescribed, to soften and prevent wound contracture.
- Encourage use of Reach to Recovery volunteers.
- Encourage the client to perform breast self-examination on the remaining breast.
- Protect the affected hand and arm.
- Avoid strong sunlight on the affected arm.
- Do not let the affected arm hang dependent.
- Do not carry a pocketbook or anything heavy over the affected arm.
- Avoid trauma, cuts, bruises, or burns to the affected side.
- Avoid wearing constricting clothing or jewelry on the affected side.
- Wear gloves when gardening.
- Use thick oven mitts when cooking.
- Use a thimble when sewing.
- Apply hand cream several times daily.
- Use cream cuticle remover.
- Call the primary health care provider if signs of inflammation occur in the affected arm.
- Wear a Medic-Alert bracelet stating which arm is lymphedematous.

⚠ No IVs lines, no injections, no blood pressure measurements, and no venipunctures would be done on the arm on the side of the mastectomy. The arm on the side of the mastectomy is protected, and any intervention that could traumatize the affected arm is avoided because of the risk for lymphedema.

XVIII. Esophageal Cancer

A. Description
  1. Esophageal cancer is a malignancy found in the esophageal mucosa, formed by squamous cell carcinoma (SCC) or adenocarcinoma.
  2. The cause is unknown, but major risk factors include cigarette smoking, alcohol consumption, chronic reflux, Barrett's esophagus, and vitamin deficiencies.
  3. Complications include dysphagia, painful swallowing, loss of appetite, and malaise.
  4. The goal of treatment is to inhibit tumor growth and maintain nutrition.

B. Data Collection
  1. Dysphagia
  2. Odynophagia (painful swallowing)
  3. Epigastric pain or sternal pain

C. Interventions
  1. Monitor nutritional status, including daily weight, intake and output, and calories consumed.
  2. Inform the client about diet changes that make eating easier.

  3. Prepare the client for chemotherapy and radiation as prescribed.
  4. Prepare the client for surgical resection of the tumor as prescribed.

XIX. Gastric Cancer

A. Description
  1. Gastric cancer is a malignant growth of the mucosal cells in the inner lining of the stomach, with invasion to the muscle and beyond in advanced disease.
  2. No single causative agent has been identified, but it is believed that *H. pylori* infection and a diet of smoked, highly salted, processed, or spiced foods have carcinogenic effects; other risk factors include smoking, alcohol and nitrate ingestion, and a history of gastric ulcers.
  3. Complications include GI hemorrhage, obstruction, metastasis, and dumping syndrome.
  4. The goal of treatment is to remove the tumor and provide a nutritional program.

B. Data collection
  1. Early
     a. Indigestion
     b. Abdominal discomfort
     c. Full feeling
     d. Epigastric, back, or retrosternal pain
  2. Late
     a. Weakness and fatigue
     b. Anorexia and weight loss
     c. Nausea and vomiting
     d. A sensation of pressure in the stomach
     e. Dysphagia and obstructive symptoms
     f. Iron deficiency anemia
     g. Ascites
     h. Palpable epigastric mass

C. Interventions
  1. Monitor vital signs.
  2. Monitor hemoglobin and hematocrit levels; blood transfusions as prescribed.
  3. Monitor weight.
  4. Monitor nutritional status; encourage small, bland, easily digestible meals with vitamin and mineral supplements.
  5. Administer pain medication, as prescribed.
  6. Prepare the client for chemotherapy or radiation therapy, as prescribed.
  7. Prepare the client for surgical resection of the tumor, as prescribed (Box 41.14).

D. Postoperative interventions
  1. Monitor vital signs.
  2. Place in Fowler's position for comfort.
  3. Administer analgesics and antiemetics, as prescribed.
  4. Monitor intake and output; administer fluids and electrolyte replacement by IV as prescribed; administer parenteral nutrition as indicated.

BOX 41.14 **Surgical Interventions for Gastric Cancer**

Subtotal Gastrectomy

Billroth I
- Also called gastroduodenostomy
- Partial gastrectomy; the remaining segment is anastomosed to the duodenum

Billroth II
- Also called gastrojejunostomy
- Partial gastrectomy; the remaining segment is anastomosed to the jejunum

Total Gastrectomy
- Also called esophagojejunostomy
- Removal of the stomach, with the attachment of the esophagus to the jejunum or the duodenum

---

5. Maintain NPO (nothing by mouth) status, as prescribed, for 1 to 3 days until peristalsis returns; monitor bowel sounds.
6. Monitor nasogastric suction. Following gastrectomy, drainage from the nasogastric tube is normally bloody for 24 hours postoperatively, changes to brown-tinged, and is then yellow or clear.
7. Do not irrigate or remove the nasogastric tube (follow agency procedures); assist the PHCP with irrigation or removal.
8. Advance the diet from NPO to sips of clear water to six small bland meals a day, as prescribed.
9. Monitor for complications such as hemorrhage, dumping syndrome, diarrhea, hypoglycemia, and vitamin B_{12} deficiency.

XX. Pancreatic Cancer

A. Description
1. Most pancreatic tumors are highly malignant, rapidly growing adenocarcinomas originating from the epithelium of the ductal system.
2. Pancreatic cancer is associated with increased age, a history of diabetes mellitus, alcohol use, a history of previous pancreatitis, smoking, the ingestion of a high-fat diet, and exposure to environmental chemicals.
3. Symptoms usually do not occur until the tumor is large; therefore, the prognosis is poor.
4. Endoscopic retrograde cholangiopancreatography for visualization of the pancreatic duct and biliary system and collection of tissue and secretions may be done.

B. Data collection
1. Nausea and vomiting
2. Jaundice
3. Unexplained weight loss
4. Clay-colored stools
5. Glucose intolerance
6. Abdominal pain

C. Interventions
1. Radiation
2. Chemotherapy
3. Whipple procedure, which involves a pancreaticoduodenectomy with the removal of the distal third of the stomach, a pancreaticojejunostomy, a gastrojejunostomy, and a choledochojejunostomy
4. Postoperative care measures are similar to those for the care of a client with pancreatitis and for a client after gastric surgery; monitor the blood glucose levels for transient hyperglycemia or hypoglycemia resulting from the surgical manipulation of the pancreas.

XXI. Intestinal Tumors

A. Description
1. Intestinal tumors are malignant lesions that develop in the cells lining the bowel wall or that develop as adenomatous polyps in the colon or rectum.
2. Tumor spread is by direct invasion and through the circulatory or lymphatic systems.
3. Complications include bowel perforation with peritonitis, abscess and/or fistula formation, hemorrhage, and complete intestinal obstruction.

B. Risk factors for colorectal cancer
1. Age older than 50 years
2. Familial polyposis, family history of colorectal cancer
3. Previous colorectal polyps, history of colorectal cancer
4. History of chronic inflammatory bowel disease
5. History of ovarian or breast, endometrial, and stomach cancers

C. Data collection
1. Blood in the stool (most common manifestation) detected by fecal occult blood testing, sigmoidoscopy, and colonoscopy
2. Anorexia, vomiting, and weight loss
3. Anemia
4. Abnormal stools
   a. Ascending colon tumor: Diarrhea
   b. Descending colon tumor: Constipation, some diarrhea, or flat, ribbon-like stool caused by partial obstruction
   c. Rectal tumor: Alternating constipation and diarrhea
5. Guarding or abdominal distention, abdominal mass (late sign)
6. Cachexia (late sign)
7. Masses noted on barium enema, colonoscopy, CT scan, sigmoidoscopy

D. General interventions
1. Monitor for signs of complications, which include bowel perforation with peritonitis, abscess and/or fistula formation (fever associated with pain), hemorrhage (signs of shock), and complete intestinal obstruction.
2. Monitor for signs of bowel perforation, which include low blood pressure, rapid and weak pulse, distended abdomen, and elevated temperature.
3. Monitor for signs of intestinal obstruction, which include vomiting (may be fecal contents), pain, constipation, and abdominal distention; provide comfort measures.
4. Note that an early sign of intestinal obstruction is increased peristaltic activity, which produces an increase in bowel sounds; as the obstruction progresses, hypoactive sounds may be heard.
5. Prepare for radiation preoperatively if prescribed to facilitate surgical resection and postoperatively to decrease the risk of recurrence or to reduce pain, hemorrhage, bowel obstruction, or metastasis.

E. Nonsurgical interventions
1. Preoperative radiation for local control and postoperative radiation for palliation may be prescribed.
2. Postoperative chemotherapy to control symptoms and the spread of disease

F. Surgical interventions: Bowel, local lymph node resection, and creation of a colostomy or ileostomy

G. Colostomy, ileostomy
1. Preoperative interventions
   a. Consultation with the enterostomal therapist may be necessary to assist with identifying the optimal placement of the ostomy.
   b. Instruct the client in prescribed preoperative diet; bowel preparation (laxatives and enemas) may be prescribed.

   c. Intestinal antiseptics and antibiotics may be prescribed to decrease the bacterial content of the colon and to reduce the risk of infection from the surgical procedure.
2. Postoperative: Colostomy
   a. If a pouch system is not in place, apply a petroleum jelly gauze over the stoma to keep it moist, and keep it covered by a dry sterile dressing; place a pouch system on the stoma as soon as possible.
   b. Monitor the pouch system for proper fit and signs of leakage; empty the pouch when one-third full.
   c. Monitor the stoma for size, color changes, unusual bleeding, and necrotic tissue.
   d. Note that the normal stoma color is red or pink, which indicates high vascularity.
   e. Note that a pale pink stoma indicates low hemoglobin and hematocrit levels.
   f. Monitor the functioning of the colostomy.
   g. Expect that stool will be liquid postoperatively but will become more solid, depending on the area of the colostomy.
   h. Expect liquid stool from an ascending colon colostomy, loose to semiformed stool from a transverse colon colostomy, or close to normal stool from a descending colon colostomy.
   i. Fecal matter should not be allowed to remain on the skin.
   j. Administer analgesics and antibiotics, as prescribed.
   k. Irrigate the perineal wound, if present and if prescribed, and monitor for signs of infection.
   l. Inform the client to avoid foods that cause excessive gas formation and odor.
   m. Reinforce instructions about stoma care and irrigations, as prescribed.
   n. The client is instructed on how to resume normal activities, including work, travel, and sexual intercourse, as prescribed; provide psychosocial support.
3. Postoperative: Ileostomy
   a. Healthy stoma is red in color.
   b. Postoperative drainage will be dark green and progress to yellow as the client begins to eat.
   c. Stool is liquid.
   d. The risk for dehydration and electrolyte imbalance exists.

 Monitor stoma color. A dark blue, purple, or black stoma indicates compromised circulation, requiring RN and PHCP notification.

XXII. Lung Cancer

A. Description
1. Lung cancer is a malignant tumor of the bronchi and peripheral lung tissue.
2. The lungs are a common target for metastasis from other organs.
3. Bronchogenic cancer (tumors originate in the epithelium of the bronchus) spreads through direct extension and lymphatic dissemination.
4. Classified according to histological cell type; types include small cell lung cancer (SCLC) and non–small cell lung cancer (NSCLC); epidermal (squamous cell), adenocarcinoma, and large cell anaplastic carcinoma are classified as NSCLC because of their similar responses to treatment.
5. Diagnosis is made by a chest x-ray, CT scan, or magnetic resonance imaging (MRI), which shows a lesion or mass, and by bronchoscopy and sputum studies, which demonstrate a positive cytological study for cancer cells.

B. Causes
1. Cigarette smoking; also exposure to "passive" tobacco smoke, or second-hand smoke

2. Exposure to environmental and occupational pollutants

C. Data collection
1. Cough
2. Wheezing, dyspnea
3. Hoarseness
4. Hemoptysis, blood-tinged or purulent sputum
5. Chest pain
6. Anorexia and weight loss
7. Weakness
8. Diminished or absent breath sounds, respiratory changes

D. Interventions
1. Monitor vital signs.
2. Monitor breathing patterns and breath sounds and for signs of respiratory impairment; monitor for hemoptysis.
3. Monitor for tracheal deviation.
4. Administer analgesics, as prescribed, for pain management.
5. Place the client in Fowler's position for ease of breathing.
6. Administer oxygen, as prescribed, and humidification to moisten and loosen secretions.
7. Monitor the pulse oximetry.
8. Provide respiratory treatments, as prescribed.
9. Administer bronchodilators and corticosteroids, as prescribed, to decrease bronchospasm, inflammation, and edema.
10. Provide a high-calorie, high-protein, high-vitamin diet.
11. Provide activity (as tolerated), rest periods, and active and passive ROM exercises.

E. Nonsurgical interventions
1. Radiation therapy for localized intrathoracic lung cancers and for the palliation of hemoptysis, obstructions, dysphagia, superior vena cava (SVC) syndrome, and pain
2. Chemotherapy may be prescribed for the treatment of nonresectable tumors or as adjuvant therapy.

F. Surgical interventions
1. Laser therapy: To relieve endobronchial obstruction
2. Thoracentesis and pleurodesis: To remove pleural fluid and relieve hypoxia
3. Thoracotomy (opening into the thoracic cavity) with pneumonectomy: Surgical removal of one entire lung
4. Thoracotomy with lobectomy: Surgical removal of one lobe of the lung for tumors confined to a single lobe
5. Thoracotomy with segmental resection: Surgical removal of a lobe segment

G. Preoperative interventions
1. Explain the potential postoperative need for chest tubes.
2. Note that closed-chest drainage is not usually used for a pneumonectomy and that the serous fluid that accumulates in the empty thoracic cavity eventually consolidates, thus preventing shifts of the mediastinum, heart, and remaining lung.

H. Postoperative interventions
1. Monitor vital signs.
2. Monitor cardiac and respiratory statuses; monitor lung sounds.
3. Monitor the chest tube drainage system, which drains air and blood that accumulates in the pleural space; monitor for *excess* bleeding. (See Chapter 18 for care of the client with a chest tube.)
4. Administer oxygen as prescribed.
5. Check the PHCP's prescriptions regarding client positioning; avoid complete lateral turning.
6. Monitor the pulse oximetry.
7. Provide activity as tolerated.
8. Encourage active ROM exercises of the operative shoulder as prescribed.

 The airway is the priority for a client with lung or laryngeal cancer.

XXIII. Laryngeal Cancer

A. Description
1. Laryngeal cancer is a malignant tumor of the larynx.
2. Laryngeal cancer presents as malignant ulcerations with underlying infiltration and is spread by local extension to adjacent structures in the throat and neck and by the lymphatic system.
3. Diagnosis is made by laryngoscopy and biopsy showing a positive cytological study for cancer cells.
4. Laryngoscopy allows for evaluation of the throat and biopsy of tissues; chest radiography, CT, and MRI are used for staging.

B. Risk factors
1. Cigarette smoking
2. Heavy alcohol use and the combined use of tobacco and alcohol
3. Exposure to environmental pollutants (e.g., asbestos, wood dust)
4. Exposure to radiation

C. Data collection
1. Persistent hoarseness and sore throat
2. Painless neck mass
3. The feeling of a lump in the throat
4. Burning sensation in the throat
5. Dysphagia
6. Change in voice quality
7. Dyspnea
8. Weakness and weight loss
9. Hemoptysis
10. Foul breath odor

D. Interventions
1. Place the client in Fowler's position to promote optimal air exchange.
2. Monitor the respiratory status.

Adult—Oncological and Hematological

3. Monitor for signs of food and fluid aspiration.
4. Administer oxygen, as prescribed.
5. Provide respiratory treatments, as prescribed.
6. Provide activity, as tolerated.
7. Provide a high-calorie, high-protein diet.
8. Prepare to provide nutritional support via parenteral nutrition, nasogastric tube feedings, or gastrostomy or jejunostomy tube, as prescribed.
9. Administer analgesics for pain as prescribed.
10. Encourage clients to stop smoking and drinking alcohol to increase effectiveness of treatments.

E. Nonsurgical interventions
1. Radiation therapy if the cancer is limited to a small area in one vocal cord
2. Chemotherapy, which may be performed in combination with radiation and surgery

F. Surgical interventions
1. The goal is to remove the cancer while preserving as much normal function as possible.
2. Surgical intervention depends on the tumor size, location, and the amount of tissue to be resected.
3. Types of resection include cordal stripping, cordectomy, partial laryngectomy, and total laryngectomy.
4. A tracheostomy is performed with a total laryngectomy; this airway opening is permanent and is referred to as a laryngectomy stoma.

G. Preoperative interventions
1. Discuss self-care of the airway, alternative methods of communication, suctioning, pain-control methods, the critical care environment, and nutritional support.
2. Encourage the client to express feelings about changes in body image and the loss of voice.
3. Describe the rehabilitation program and provide information about the tracheostomy and suctioning.

H. Postoperative interventions
1. Monitor vital signs.
2. Monitor respiratory status and airway patency, and provide frequent suctioning to remove bloody secretions.
3. Place the client in high Fowler's position.
4. Maintain mechanical ventilator support or a tracheostomy collar with humidification, as prescribed.
5. Monitor the pulse oximetry.
6. Maintain surgical drains in the neck area, if present.
7. Observe for hemorrhage and edema in the neck.
8. Monitor IV fluids or parenteral nutrition, if prescribed, until nutrition is administered via a nasogastric, gastrostomy, or jejunostomy tube.
9. Provide oral hygiene.
10. Monitor the gag and cough reflexes and the ability to swallow.
11. Increase activity, as tolerated.
12. Monitor the color, amount, and consistency of the sputum.
13. Provide stoma and laryngectomy care (Box 41.15).

BOX 41.15 Stoma Care after Laryngectomy

- Protect the neck from injury.
- Provide instructions in how to clean the incision and provide stoma care.
- Provide instructions to wear a stoma guard and/or loose-fitting, high-collared clothing to cover the stoma and for shielding and preventing debris from entering the stoma.
- Avoid swimming, showering, and using aerosol sprays.
- Reinforce teaching the client clean suctioning technique.
- Advise the client to increase humidity in the home.
- Increase fluid intake as prescribed.
- Avoid exposure to persons with infections.
- Alternate rest periods with activity.
- Demonstrate how to perform range-of-motion exercises for the arms, shoulders, and neck as prescribed.
- Advise the client to wear a Medic-Alert bracelet.

---

14. Provide consultation with a speech and language pathologist, as prescribed (Box 41.16).
15. Reinforce the method of communication that is established preoperatively.

XXIV. Prostate Cancer

A. Description
1. Prostate cancer, a slow-growing malignancy of the prostate gland, is a common cancer in American men; most prostate tumors are adenocarcinomas arising from androgen-dependent epithelial cells.
2. The risk increases in men with each decade after the age of 50 years.
3. Prostate cancer can spread via direct invasion of surrounding tissues or by metastasis, through the bloodstream and lymphatics, to the bony pelvis and spine.
4. Bone metastasis is a concern; it may also spread to the lungs, liver, and kidneys.
5. The cause of prostate cancer is unclear, but advancing age, heavy metal exposure, smoking, and history of sexually transmitted infection are contributing factors.

B. Data collection
1. Asymptomatic during the early stages
2. Hard, pea-sized nodule or irregularities palpated on rectal examination
3. Gross, painless hematuria
4. Late symptoms include weight loss, urinary obstruction, and pain radiating from the lumbosacral area down the leg.
5. Prostate-specific antigen (PSA) level is elevated in various noncancerous conditions and therefore would not be used as a screening test without a digital rectal examination (DRE); it is routinely used to monitor response to therapy.
6. Diagnosis is made through biopsy of the prostate gland.

BOX 41.16 **Speech Rehabilitation after Laryngectomy**

Esophageal Speech
Client produces esophageal speech by "burping" the air that is swallowed.
Voice produced is monotone; it cannot be raised or lowered, and it carries no pitch.
Client needs to have adequate hearing because he or she uses the mouth to shape words as they are heard.

Mechanical Devices
One device, the *electrolarynx*, is placed against the side of the neck; the air inside the neck and pharynx is vibrated, and the client articulates.
Another device consists of a plastic tube that is placed inside the client's mouth and vibrates during articulation.

Tracheoesophageal Fistula
A fistula is surgically created between the trachea and the esophagus, with the eventual placement of a prosthesis that is used to produce speech.
Prosthesis provides the client with a means for diverting the air from the lungs through the trachea, into the esophagus, and out of the mouth.
Speech is produced by lip and tongue movements.

C. Nonsurgical interventions
   1. Prepare the client for hormone manipulation therapy (androgen suppression therapy) as prescribed or active surveillance with PSA and DRE.
   2. Luteinizing hormone may be prescribed to slow the rate of growth of the tumor.
   3. Medication adverse effects include reduced libido, hot flashes, breast tenderness, osteoporosis, loss of muscle mass, and weight gain. The client needs to be informed of these effects.
   4. Pain medication, radiation therapy, corticosteroids, and bisphosphonates may be prescribed for palliation of advanced prostate cancer.
   5. Prepare the client for external beam radiation or brachytherapy, which may be prescribed alone or with surgery, preoperatively or postoperatively, to reduce the lesion and limit metastasis.
   6. Prepare the client for the administration of chemotherapy in cases of hormone-resistant tumors.
D. Surgical interventions
   1. Prepare the client for orchiectomy (palliative), if prescribed, which will limit the production of testosterone.
   2. Prepare the client for prostatectomy, if prescribed.
   3. The radical prostatectomy can be performed via a retropubic, perineal, or suprapubic approach.
   4. Cryosurgical ablation is a minimally invasive procedure that may be an alternative to radical prostatectomy; liquid nitrogen freezes the gland, and the dead cells are absorbed by the body.

E. Transurethral resection of the prostate (TURP) may be performed for palliation in prostate cancer clients.
   1. The procedure involves insertion of a scope into the urethra to excise prostatic tissue.
   2. Monitor for hemorrhage; bleeding is common following TURP.
   3. Postoperative continuous bladder irrigation (CBI) may be prescribed, which prevents catheter obstruction from clots.
   4. Monitor for signs of transurethral resection syndrome, which include signs of cerebral edema and increased intracranial pressure, such as increased blood pressure, bradycardia, confusion, disorientation, muscle twitching, visual disturbances, and nausea and vomiting; notify the RN immediately.
   5. Antispasmodics may be prescribed for bladder spasm.
   6. Inform the client to monitor and report dribbling or incontinence postoperatively, and teach perineal exercises.
   7. Sterility is possible following the surgical procedure.
F. Suprapubic prostatectomy
   1. Suprapubic prostatectomy is removal of the prostate gland by an abdominal incision with a bladder incision.
   2. The client will have an abdominal dressing that may drain copious amounts of urine, and the abdominal dressing will need to be changed frequently.
   3. Severe hemorrhage is possible, and monitoring for blood loss is an important nursing intervention.
   4. Antispasmodics may be prescribed for bladder spasms.
   5. CBI is prescribed and carried out to maintain pink-colored urine (Box 41.17).
   6. Sterility occurs with this procedure.
G. Retropubic prostatectomy
   1. Retropubic prostatectomy refers to the removal of the prostate gland by a low abdominal incision without opening the bladder.
   2. Less bleeding occurs with this procedure compared with the suprapubic procedure, and the client experiences fewer bladder spasms.
   3. Abdominal drainage is minimal.
   4. CBI may be used.
   5. Sterility occurs with this procedure.
H. Perineal prostatectomy
   1. The prostate gland is removed through an incision made between the scrotum and anus.
   2. Minimal bleeding occurs with this procedure.
   3. The client needs to be monitored closely for infection because the risk of infection is increased with this type of prostatectomy.
   4. Urinary incontinence is common.
   5. The procedure causes sterility.

BOX 41.17   Continuous Bladder Irrigation

Description

A three-way (lumen) irrigation is used to decrease bleeding and to keep the bladder free from clots. One lumen is for inflating the balloon (30 mL), one is for instillation (inflow), and one lumen is for outflow.

Interventions

- Maintain traction on the catheter, if applied, to prevent bleeding by pulling the catheter taut and taping it to the abdomen or thigh.
- Instruct the client to keep the leg straight if traction is applied to the catheter and it is taped to the thigh.
- Catheter traction is not released without a primary health care provider's (PHCP's) prescription; it is usually released after any bright red drainage has diminished.
- Use only sterile bladder irrigation solution or prescribed solution, to prevent water intoxication.
- Run the solution at a rate, as prescribed, to keep the urine pink. Run the solution rapidly if bright red drainage or clots are present; monitor output closely. Run the solution at approximately 40 drops (gtt)/minute when the bright red drainage clears.
- If the urinary catheter becomes obstructed, notify the registered nurse (RN); turn off the continuous bladder irrigation, and assist to irrigate the catheter with 30–50 mL of normal saline, if prescribed; notify the PHCP if the obstruction does not resolve.
- Discontinue continuous bladder irrigation and indwelling urinary catheter as prescribed, usually 24–48 hours after surgery.
- Monitor for continence and urinary retention when the catheter is removed; inform the client that some burning, frequency, and dribbling may occur after catheter removal.
- Inform the client that he would be voiding 150–200 mL of clear yellow urine every 3–4 hours by 3 days after surgery.
- Inform the client that he may pass small clots and tissue debris for several days.
- Instruct the client, as prescribed, to avoid heavy lifting, stressful exercise, driving, the Valsalva maneuver, and sexual intercourse for 2–6 weeks to prevent strain.
- Instruct the client to call the PHCP if bleeding occurs or if there is a decrease in the urinary stream.
- Encourage the client to drink 2400–3000 mL of fluid each day, preferably before 8:00 p.m. to prevent nocturia.
- Instruct the client to avoid alcohol, caffeinated beverages, and spicy foods to prevent the overstimulation of the bladder.
- Reinforce instructions to the client that, if the urine becomes bloody, he needs to rest and increase the fluid intake; if the bleeding does not subside, he must notify the PHCP.

---

4. Monitor for arterial bleeding as evidenced by bright red urine with numerous clots; if it occurs, increase CBI and notify the RN immediately.
5. Monitor for venous bleeding as evidenced by burgundy-colored urine output; if it occurs, notify the RN; the surgeon may apply traction on the catheter.
6. Monitor hemoglobin and hematocrit levels.
7. Expect red to light pink urine for 24 hours, turning to amber in 3 days.
8. Ambulate the client as early as possible and as soon as urine begins to clear in color.
9. Inform the client that a continuous feeling of an urge to void is normal.
10. Reinforce instructions to the client to avoid attempts to void around the catheter because this will cause bladder spasms.
11. Administer antibiotics, analgesics, stool softeners, and antispasmodics as prescribed.
12. Monitor the three-way indwelling urinary catheter, which usually has a 30- to 45-mL retention balloon.
13. Maintain CBI with sterile bladder irrigation solution as prescribed to keep the catheter free of obstruction and maintain the urine pink in color (see Box 41.17).

⚠ Following TURP, monitor for transurethral resection syndrome or severe hyponatremia (water intoxication) caused by the excessive absorption of bladder irrigation during surgery (signs include altered mental status, bradycardia, increased blood pressure, and confusion).

J. Postoperative interventions: Suprapubic prostatectomy
1. Monitor suprapubic and indwelling urinary catheter drainage.
2. Monitor CBI if prescribed.
3. Note that the indwelling urinary catheter will be removed 2 to 4 days postoperatively if the client has a suprapubic catheter.
4. If prescribed, clamp the suprapubic catheter after the indwelling urinary catheter is removed, and instruct the client to attempt to void; after the client has voided, assess the residual urine in the bladder by unclamping the suprapubic catheter and measuring the output.
5. Prepare for removal of the suprapubic catheter when the client consistently empties the bladder and residual urine is 75 mL or less.
6. Monitor the suprapubic incision dressing, which may become saturated with urine, until the incision heals; dressing may need to be changed frequently.

K. Postoperative interventions: Retropubic prostatectomy
1. Note that because the bladder is not entered, there is no urinary drainage on the abdominal dressing; if urinary or purulent drainage is noted on the dressing, notify the RN.

---

6. Reinforce teaching to the client on how to perform perineal exercises.

I. Postoperative interventions
1. Monitor vital signs.
2. Monitor urinary output and urine for hemorrhage or clots.
3. Increase fluids to 2400 to 3000 mL/day, unless contraindicated.

2. Monitor for fever and increased pain, which may indicate an infection.

L. Postoperative interventions: Perineal prostatectomy
   1. Note that the client will have an incision, which may or may not have a drain.
   2. Avoid the use of rectal thermometers, rectal tubes, and enemas because they may cause trauma and bleeding.

XXV. Bladder Cancer

A. Description
   1. Bladder cancer is a papillomatous growth in the bladder urothelium that undergoes malignant changes and that may infiltrate the bladder wall.
   2. Predisposing factors include cigarette smoking, exposure to industrial chemicals, and exposure to radiation.
   3. Common sites of metastasis include the liver, bones, and lungs.
   4. As the tumor progresses, it can extend into the rectum, vagina, other pelvic soft tissues, and retroperitoneal structures.

B. Data collection
   1. Gross or microscopic, painless hematuria (most common sign)
   2. Frequency, urgency, and dysuria
   3. Clot-induced obstruction
   4. Bladder wash specimens and biopsy confirm the diagnosis.

C. Radiation
   1. Radiation therapy is indicated for advanced disease that cannot be eradicated by surgery; palliative radiation may be used to relieve pain and bowel obstruction and control potential hemorrhage and leg edema caused by venous or lymphatic obstruction.
   2. Intracavitary radiation may be prescribed, which protects adjacent tissue.
   3. External beam radiation combined with chemotherapy or surgery may be prescribed to improve survival.
   4. Complications of radiation
      a. Abacterial cystitis
      b. Proctitis
      c. Fistula formation
      d. Ileitis or colitis
      e. Bladder ulceration and hemorrhage

D. Chemotherapy
   1. Intravesical instillation
      a. An alkylating chemotherapeutic agent is instilled into the bladder.
      b. This method provides a concentrated topical treatment with little systemic absorption.
      c. The medication is injected into a urethral catheter and retained for 2 hours.
      d. Following instillation, the client's position is rotated every 15 to 30 minutes, starting in the supine position, to avoid lying on a full bladder.
      e. After 2 hours, the client voids in a sitting position and is instructed to increase fluids to flush the bladder.
      f. Treat the urine as a biohazard, and send it to the radioisotope laboratory for monitoring.
      g. For 6 hours following intravesical chemotherapy, disinfect the toilet with household bleach after the client has voided.
   2. Systemic chemotherapy: Used to treat inoperable tumors or distant metastasis.
   3. Complications of chemotherapy
      a. Bladder irritation
      b. Hemorrhagic cystitis

E. Surgical interventions
   1. Transurethral resection of the bladder tumor
      a. Local resection and fulguration (destruction of tissue by electrical current through electrodes placed in direct contact with the tissue)
      b. Performed for very early tumors for cure or for inoperable tumors for palliation
   2. Partial cystectomy
      a. The removal of up to half of the bladder
      b. Performed for early stage tumors and for clients who cannot tolerate a radical cystectomy
      c. During the initial postoperative period, the bladder capacity is markedly reduced to approximately 60 mL; however, as the bladder tissue expands, the capacity increases to 200 to 400 mL.
      d. Maintenance of a continuous output of urine after surgery is critical to prevent bladder distention and stress on the suture line.
      e. A urethral catheter and a suprapubic catheter may be in place, and the suprapubic catheter may be left in place for 2 weeks until healing occurs.
   3. Cystectomy and urinary diversion (Fig. 41.4)
      a. Various surgical procedures are performed to create alternative pathways for urine collection and excretion.
      b. Urinary diversion may be performed with or without cystectomy (bladder removal).
      c. The surgery may be performed in two stages if the tumor is extensive, with the creation of the urinary diversion first and the cystectomy several weeks later.
      d. If a radical cystectomy is performed, lower-extremity lymphedema may occur as a result of lymph node dissection, and male impotence may occur.
   4. Ileal conduit
      a. The ileal conduit is also called ureteroileostomy or Bricker's procedure.
      b. Ureters are implanted into a segment of the ileum, with the formation of an abdominal stoma.

Ureterostomy
Diverts urine directly to the skin surface through a ureteral-skin opening (stoma).
After ureterostomy the client must wear a pouch.

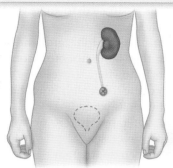

Cutaneous ureterostomy

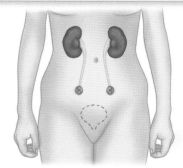

Bilateral cutaneous ureterosigmoidostomy

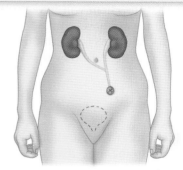

Cutaneous ureteroureterostomy

Ileal reservoir
Diverts urine into a surgically created pouch or pocket that functions as a bladder. The stoma is continent and the client removes urine by regular self-catheterization.

Catheter —

Continent internal ileal reservoir (Kock pouch)

Sigmoidostomy
Diverts urine to the large intestine so no stoma is required. The client excretes urine with bowel movements and bowel incontinence may result.

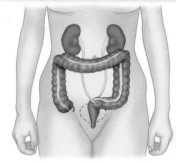

Ureterosigmoidostomy

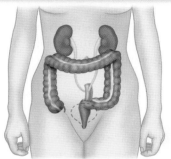

Ureteroileosigmoidostomy

Conduit
Collects urine in a portion of the intestine which is then opened onto the skin surface as a stoma. After the creation of a conduit the client must wear a pouch.

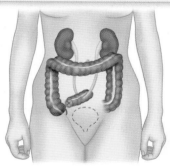

Colon conduit

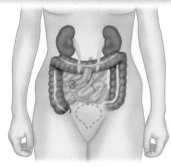

Ileal (Bricker's) conduit

FIGURE 41.4 Urinary diversion procedures used in the treatment of bladder cancer.

c. The urine flows into the conduit and is continually propelled out through the stoma by peristalsis.

d. The client is required to wear an appliance over the stoma to collect the urine (Box 41.18).

e. Complications include obstruction, pyelonephritis, leakage at the anastomosis site, stenosis, hydronephrosis, calculi, skin irritation and ulceration, and stomal defects.

5. Kock pouch

a. The Kock pouch is a continent internal ileal reservoir created from a segment of the ileum and the ascending colon.

b. The ureters are implanted into the side of the reservoir, and a special nipple valve is constructed to attach the reservoir to the skin.

c. Postoperatively, the client will have an indwelling urinary catheter in place to drain urine continuously until the pouch has healed.

d. The catheter is irrigated gently with normal saline to prevent obstruction caused by mucus or clots.

e. Following removal of the urinary catheter, the client is instructed in how to self-catheterize and to drain the reservoir at 4- to 6-hour intervals (Box 41.19).

BOX 41.18 Urinary Stoma Care

- Instruct the client in how to change the appliance in the morning when urinary production is slowest.
- Collect equipment, remove collection bag, and use water or commercial solvent to loosen adhesive.
- Cleanse the skin around the stoma and under the drainage bag with mild nonresidue soap and water.
- Inspect the skin for excoriation, and instruct the client to prevent urine from coming into contact with the skin.
- After the skin is dry, apply skin adhesive around the appliance.
- Instruct the client to cut the stoma opening of the skin barrier just large enough to fit over the stoma (no more than 3 mm larger than the stoma).
- Instruct the client that the stoma will begin to shrink, requiring a smaller stoma opening on the skin barrier.
- Apply the skin barrier before attaching the pouch or face plate.
- Place the appliance over the stoma and secure in place.
- Encourage self-care; teach the client to use a mirror.
- Instruct the client that the pouch may be drained by a bedside bag or leg bag, especially at night.
- Instruct the client to empty the urinary collection bag when it is one-third full to prevent pulling of the appliance and leakage.
- Instruct the client to check the appliance seal if perspiring occurs.
- Instruct the client to leave the urinary pouch in place as long as it is not leaking and to change it every 5–7 days.
- Use a nonkaraya gum product, because urine erodes karaya gum.
- To control odor, instruct the client to drink adequate fluids, wash the appliance thoroughly with soap and lukewarm water, and soak the collection pouch in dilute white vinegar for 20–30 minutes; a special deodorant tablet can also be placed into the pouch while it is being worn.
- Instruct the client who takes baths to keep the level of the water below the stoma and to avoid oily soaps.
- If the client plans to shower, instruct the client to direct the flow of water away from the stoma.

BOX 41.19 Self-Irrigation and Catheterization of Stoma

Irrigation
- Instruct the client to wash hands and use clean technique.
- Instruct the client to use a catheter and syringe, instill 60 mL of normal saline or water into the reservoir, and aspirate gently or allow to drain.
- Instruct the client to irrigate until the drainage remains free of mucus but to be careful not to overirrigate.

Catheterization
- Instruct the client to wash hands and use clean technique.
- Initially, instruct the client to insert a catheter every 2–3 hours to drain the reservoir; during each week thereafter, increase the interval by 1 hour until catheterization is done every 4–6 hours.
- Lubricate the catheter well with water-soluble lubricant, and instruct the client never to force the catheter into the reservoir.
- If resistance is met, instruct the client to pause, rotate the catheter, and apply gentle pressure to insert.
- Instruct the client to notify the primary health care provider (PHCP) if the client is unable to insert the catheter.
- When urine has stopped, instruct the client to take several deep breaths and move the catheter in and out 2–3 inches (5–7.5 cm) to ensure that the pouch is empty.
- Instruct the client to withdraw the catheter slowly and pinch the catheter when withdrawn so that it does not leak urine.
- Instruct the client to carry catheterization supplies with him or her.

6. Indiana pouch
   a. A continent reservoir is created from the ascending colon and the terminal ileum, thus making a pouch larger than the Kock pouch.
   b. Postoperatively, care is similar as with the Kock pouch.
7. Creation of a neobladder
   a. Similar to the creation of an internal reservoir but different because instead of emptying through an abdominal stoma, it empties through a pelvic outlet into the urethra.
   b. The client empties the neobladder by relaxing the external sphincter and creating abdominal pressure or by intermittent self-catheterization.
8. Percutaneous nephrostomy or pyelostomy
   a. These procedures are used when the cancer is inoperable to prevent or treat obstruction.
   b. Involves a percutaneous or surgical insertion of a nephrostomy tube into the kidney for drainage
   c. Nursing interventions involve stabilizing the tube to prevent dislodgment and monitoring output.
9. Ureterostomy
   a. Ureterostomy may be performed as a palliative procedure if the ureters are obstructed by the tumor.
   b. The ureters are attached to the surface of the abdomen, where the urine flows directly into a drainage appliance without a conduit.
   c. Potential problems include infection, skin irritation, and the obstruction of urinary flow as a result of strictures at the opening.
10. Vesicostomy
    a. The bladder is sutured to the abdomen, and a stoma is created in the bladder wall.
    b. The bladder empties through the stoma.
F. Preoperative interventions
   1. Reinforce instructions about preoperative, operative, and postoperative management, including diet, medications, nasogastric tube placement, IV lines, NPO status, pain control, coughing and

deep breathing, leg exercises, and postoperative activity.

2. Assist the RN to demonstrate appliance application and use for those clients who will have a stoma.

3. Arrange an enterostomal nurse consult and for a visit with a person who has had urinary diversion.

4. Antimicrobials for bowel preparation are administered as prescribed.

5. Encourage discussion of feelings, including the effects on sexual activities.

G. Postoperative interventions

 Monitor urinary output closely following bladder surgery. Assist the RN with gentle irrigation of the ureteral catheter (if present and prescribed) to prevent obstruction. Follow the PHCP's prescriptions and agency policy regarding irrigation.

1. Monitor vital signs.

2. Monitor incision site.

3. Check the stoma (it needs to be red and moist) every hour for the first 24 hours.

4. Monitor for edema in the stoma, which may be present during the immediate postoperative period.

5. If the stoma appears dark and dusky, notify the RN and the PHCP immediately, because this indicates necrosis.

6. Monitor for the prolapse or retraction of the stoma; notify the RN.

7. Monitor for the return of bowel function; monitor for expected return of peristalsis in 3 to 4 days.

8. Maintain NPO status, as prescribed, until bowel sounds return.

9. Monitor for continuous urine flow (30 to 60 mL/hr).

10. The RN is notified if the urine output is less than 30 mL/hr or if there is no urine output for more than 15 minutes.

11. Ureteral stents or catheters may be in place for 2 to 3 weeks or until healing occurs; maintain stability of catheters to prevent dislodgment.

12. Monitor for hematuria.

13. Monitor for signs of peritonitis.

14. Monitor for bladder distention after a partial cystectomy.

15. Monitor for shock, hemorrhage, thrombophlebitis, and lower-extremity lymphedema after a radical cystectomy.

16. Monitor the urinary drainage pouch for leaks and check the skin integrity (see Box 41.18).

17. Monitor urine pH (do not place the dipstick into the stoma), because highly alkaline or acidic urine can cause skin irritation and facilitate crystal formation.

18. Reinforce instructions to the client regarding the potential for urinary tract infection or the development of calculi.

19. Reinforce instructions to the client to check the skin for irritation and to monitor the urinary drainage pouch for any leakage.

20. Encourage the client to express feelings about changes in body image and sexual function, as well as embarrassment.

XXVI. Oncological Emergencies

A. Sepsis and disseminated intravascular coagulation (DIC)

1. Description: The client with cancer is at increased risk for infection, particularly gram-negative organisms, in the bloodstream (sepsis or septicemia) and DIC, a life-threatening problem frequently associated with sepsis.

2. Interventions

   a. Prevent the complication through early identification of clients at high risk for sepsis and DIC.

   b. Maintain strict aseptic technique with the immunocompromised client and monitor closely for infection and signs of bleeding.

   c. IV antibiotics may be prescribed.

   d. Anticoagulants may be prescribed during the early phase of DIC.

   e. Cryoprecipitated clotting factors may be prescribed when DIC progresses and hemorrhage is the primary problem.

 Notify the RN and PHCP immediately if signs of an oncological emergency occur.

B. Syndrome of inappropriate antidiuretic hormone (SIADH)

1. Description

   a. Tumors can produce, secrete, or stimulate substances that mimic antidiuretic hormone (ADH).

   b. Mild symptoms include weakness, muscle cramps, loss of appetite, and fatigue; serum sodium levels range from 115 mEq/L to 120 mEq/L.

   c. More serious signs/symptoms relate to water intoxication and include weight gain, personality changes, confusion, and extreme muscle weakness.

   d. As the serum sodium level approaches 110 mEq/L, seizures, coma, and eventually death may occur unless the condition is rapidly treated.

2. Interventions

   a. Initiate fluid restriction and increased sodium intake, as prescribed.

   b. As prescribed, assist with the administration of an antagonist to ADH.

   c. Monitor the serum sodium levels.

   d. Treat the underlying cause with chemotherapy or radiation to reduce the tumor.

C. Spinal cord compression
  1. Description
      a. Spinal cord compression occurs when a tumor directly enters the spinal cord or when the vertebral column collapses from tumor entry, impinging on the spinal cord.
      b. Spinal cord compression causes back pain, usually before neurological deficits occur.
      c. Neurological deficits relate to the spinal level of compression and include numbness and tingling; the loss of urethral, vaginal, and rectal sensation; and muscle weakness.
  2. Interventions
      a. Early recognition: Monitor for back pain and neurological deficits.
      b. Administer high-dose corticosteroids to reduce swelling around the spinal cord and relieve symptoms.
      c. Prepare the client for immediate radiation and/or chemotherapy to reduce the size of the tumor and relieve compression.
      d. Surgery may need to be performed to remove the tumor and relieve the pressure on the spinal cord.
      e. Reinforce instructions to the client regarding the use of neck or back braces, if prescribed.

D. Hypercalcemia
  1. Description
      a. Hypercalcemia is a late manifestation of extensive malignancy that occurs most often in clients with bone metastasis, when the bone releases calcium into the bloodstream.
      b. Decreased physical mobility contributes to or worsens hypercalcemia.
      c. Early signs include fatigue, anorexia, nausea, vomiting, constipation, confusion, and polyuria.
      d. More serious signs/symptoms include severe muscle weakness, diminished deep tendon reflexes, paralytic ileus, dehydration, and electrocardiography changes.
  2. Interventions
      a. Monitor the serum calcium level and electrocardiographic changes.
      b. Oral or parenteral (normal saline) fluids may be prescribed.
      c. Medications to lower the calcium level and control nausea and vomiting may be prescribed.
      d. Prepare the client for dialysis if the condition becomes life-threatening or is accompanied by renal impairment.
      e. Encourage walking to prevent breakdown of bone.

E. Superior vena cava (SVC) syndrome
  1. Description
      a. Occurs when the SVC is compressed or obstructed by tumor growth (commonly associated with lung cancer and lymphoma)
      b. Signs/symptoms result from the blockage of blood flow in the venous system of the head, neck, and upper trunk.
      c. Early signs/symptoms generally occur in the morning and include edema of the face (especially around the eyes) and tightness of the shirt or blouse collar (Stokes sign).
      d. As the condition worsens, edema in the arms and hands, dyspnea, erythema of the upper body, swelling of the veins in the chest and neck, and epistaxis (nosebleed) occur.
      e. Life-threatening signs and symptoms include airway obstruction, hemorrhage, cyanosis, mental status changes, decreased cardiac output, and hypotension.
  2. Interventions
      a. Monitor for early signs/symptoms of SVC syndrome.
      b. Place the client in semi-Fowler's position, and corticosteroids and diuretics are administered as prescribed.
      c. Prepare the client for high-dose radiation therapy to the mediastinal area and possible surgery to insert a metal stent in the vena cava.

F. Tumor lysis syndrome
  1. Description
      a. Tumor lysis syndrome occurs when large quantities of tumor cells are destroyed rapidly and intracellular components such as potassium and uric acid are released into the bloodstream faster than the body can eliminate them.
      b. Tumor lysis syndrome can indicate that cancer treatment is destroying tumor cells; however, if left untreated, it can cause severe tissue damage and death.
      c. Hyperkalemia, hyperphosphatemia with resultant hypocalcemia, and hyperuricemia occur; hyperuricemia can lead to acute kidney injury.
  2. Interventions
      a. Encourage oral hydration; IV hydration may be prescribed for the client experiencing nausea; monitor renal function and intake and output and ensure that the client is on a renal diet low in potassium and phosphorus.
      b. Diuretics may be prescribed to increase the urine flow through the kidneys.
      c. Medications that increase the excretion of purines, such as allopurinol may be prescribed.
      d. The IV infusion of glucose and insulin may be prescribed to treat hyperkalemia.
      e. Prepare the client for dialysis if hyperkalemia and hyperuricemia persist despite treatment.

XXVII. Anemia

A. Description

1. Condition in which the blood lacks adequate healthy red blood cells or hemoglobin, with most common causes being acute blood loss, decreased or faulty red blood cell production, or the destruction of red blood cells

2. There are several types of anemia, with the main types being anemia related to acute and chronic blood loss, anemia of chronic diseases (including cancers, immunodeficiency syndrome, renal disease, liver diseases, and autoimmune conditions), anemias caused by nutritional deficiencies (such as iron, folate, or vitamin B12 deficiency), and hereditary anemias (including sickle cell anemia and thalassemia).

3. Treatment of anemia focuses on treating the cause of the condition and varies based on the type of anemia.

4. Acute blood loss anemia is characterized by normal red blood cell size, shape, color, and hemoglobin saturation. Hemoglobin, hematocrit, or red blood cell levels can be low. Red blood cell indices are unremarkable.

5. Clients at risk include postoperative clients, clients with an active bleeding problem, or immunocompromised clients with a reduction in blood components.

B. Assessment

1. Fatigue
2. Weakness
3. Pallor or slight jaundice due to the destruction of red blood cells
4. Shortness of breath
5. Dysrhythmias
6. Chest pain
7. Tachycardia
8. Cool extremities

C. Interventions

1. Administer blood products and hematopoietic medications as prescribed, which are used to treat anemia related to acute and chronic conditions.

2. Encourage a diet rich in the deficient nutrient if the anemia is caused by malnutrition, such as iron, folate, or vitamin B12 supplementation.

3. Control and address the source of bleeding if anemia is caused by acute blood loss and assess client for sources of frank and occult bleeding. Contact the PCHP and prepare for replacement therapy.

4. Plasmapheresis, immune globulin administration, or corticosteroid therapy may be necessary if the anemia is related to an autoimmune response.

XXVIII. Iron Deficiency Anemia

A. Description

1. Iron stores are depleted, resulting in a decreased iron supply for the manufacture of hemoglobin in red blood cells.

2. Commonly results from blood loss, increased metabolic demands, syndromes of gastrointestinal malabsorption, and dietary inadequacy

B. Assessment

1. Pallor
2. Weakness and fatigue
3. Low hemoglobin, hematocrit, and mean cellular volume (MCV) levels
4. Red blood cells that are microcytic and hypochromic

C. Interventions

1. Increase oral intake of iron and instruct client in food choices that are high in iron (see Box 11.2 in Chapter 11 for iron-rich foods).

2. Administer iron supplements as prescribed.

3. Intramuscular injections of iron (using Z-track method) or IV administration of iron may be prescribed in severe cases of anemia.

4. Teach clients how to administer the iron supplements.

   a. Take between meals for maximum absorption.

   b. Take with a multivitamin or fruit juice, because vitamin C increases absorption.

   c. Do not take with milk or antacids, because these items decrease absorption.

   d. Instruct the client about the side effects of iron supplements (black stools, constipation, and foul aftertaste). Liquid iron preparations stain the teeth. Teach the client that liquid iron should be taken through a straw and that the teeth should be brushed after administration.

XXIX. Vitamin B12 Deficiency Anemia

A. Description

1. A macrocytic anemia that results from an inadequate intake of vitamin B12 or lack of absorption of ingested vitamin B12 from the intestinal tract

2. Pernicious anemia results from a deficiency of intrinsic factor (normally secreted by the gastric mucosa), necessary for intestinal absorption of vitamin B12; gastric disease or surgery can result in a lack of intrinsic factor.

B. Assessment

1. Severe pallor
2. Fatigue
3. Weight loss
4. Smooth, beefy red tongue
5. Slight jaundice
6. Paresthesias of the hands and feet
7. Disturbances with gait and balance

C. Interventions

1. Increase dietary intake of foods rich in vitamin B12 such as meats, poultry, fish, shellfish, eggs, dairy products, citrus fruits, dried beans, green leafy vegetables, liver, nuts, and brewer's yeast.

2. Administer vitamin B12 injections as prescribed, weekly initially and then monthly for maintenance (lifelong) if the anemia is the result of a deficiency of intrinsic factor or disease or surgery of the ileum.

XXX. Folate Deficiency Anemia

A. Description
   1. A macrocytic anemia in which red blood cells are larger than normal and are oval-shaped rather than round-shaped due to the lack of inadequate intake of folate (vitamin B9)
   2. Folic acid is required for DNA synthesis required for red blood cell formation and maturation.
   3. Common causes include dietary deficiency; malabsorption syndromes such as celiac disease, Crohn's disease, or small bowel resection; medications (such as antiseizure medications) that decrease the absorption of folic acid; a condition (including pregnancy) that increases the requirement of folic acid; chronic alcoholism; and chronic hemodialysis.
B. Assessment
   1. Dyspepsia
   2. Smooth, beefy red tongue
   3. Pallor, fatigue and weakness
   4. Tinnitus
   5. Tachycardia
C. Interventions
   1. Encourage the client to eat foods rich in folic acid, such as green leafy vegetables, beef, liver, fish, legumes.
   2. Administer folic acid as prescribed.

XXXI. Aplastic Anemia

A. Description
   1. Aplastic anemia is a deficiency of circulating erythrocytes and all other formed elements of blood, resulting from the arrested development of cells within the bone marrow.
   2. It can be primary (present at birth) or secondary (acquired).
   3. Several possible causes exist, including chronic exposure to myelotoxic agents, viruses and infections such as hepatitis, Epstein-Barr virus, autoimmune disorders such as human immunodeficiency virus, and allergic states.
   4. The definitive diagnosis is determined by bone marrow aspiration (shows conversion of red bone marrow to fatty bone marrow).
   5. Therapeutic management focuses on restoring function to the bone marrow and involves immunosuppressive therapy and bone marrow transplantation (treatment of choice if a suitable donor exists).

   6. If the cause is a myelotoxic medication that is being administered for another purpose, the medication may be discontinued to improve bone marrow function.
B. Assessment
   1. Pancytopenia (deficiency of erythrocytes, leukocytes, and thrombocytes)
   2. Petechiae, purpura, bleeding, pallor, weakness, tachycardia, and fatigue
C. Interventions
   1. Prepare the client for bone marrow transplantation if planned.
   2. Administer immunosuppressive medications as prescribed; antilymphocyte globulin or antithymocyte globulin may be prescribed to suppress the autoimmune response.
   3. Colony-stimulating factors may be prescribed to enhance bone marrow production.
   4. Corticosteroids and cyclosporine may be prescribed.
   5. Administer blood transfusions if prescribed and monitor for transfusion reactions.

XXXII. Sickle Cell Anemia: See Chapter 29 for more information regarding sickle cell anemia

XXXIII. Thalassemia: See Chapter 29 for more information regarding thalassemia

WHAT WOULD YOU DO?

Answer: The normal platelet count is 150,000–400,000 mm³. If the count is low, the client would be placed on bleeding precautions. The registered nurse (RN) and primary health care provider (PHCP) need to be notified of the laboratory result. The nurse needs to examine the client for signs of bleeding, including checking all body fluids and excrement and monitoring for signs of internal hemorrhage (e.g., pain; rapid and weak pulse, drop in blood pressure, and other signs of shock; increased abdominal girth; and abdomen guarding. The nurse needs to handle the client gently and use caution when taking blood pressure to prevent skin injury. Other interventions include soft foods that are cool to warm to avoid oral mucosa damage; avoiding injections to prevent trauma to the skin and bleeding; applying firm and gentle pressure to a needle-stick site for at least 5 minutes, or longer if needed; padding corners of the bed and furniture; and avoiding rectal suppositories, enemas, and thermometers. The client needs to use a soft toothbrush and avoid dental floss, use only an electric razor for shaving, and avoid blowing the nose.

PRACTICE QUESTIONS

❖ **1.** The nurse is assisting with creating a plan of care for the client with multiple myeloma. Which nursing intervention needs to be included to assess for and prevent renal failure for this client? **Select all that apply.**
- ❑ 1. Encouraging fluids
- ❑ 2. Providing frequent oral care
- ❑ 3. Coughing and deep breathing
- ❑ 4. Monitoring the red blood cell count
- ❑ 5. Monitoring serum calcium and uric acid levels

❖ **2.** The nurse is assisting with conducting a health-promotion program to community members regarding testicular cancer. The nurse determines that **further teaching is needed** if a community member states that which is a sign/symptom of testicular cancer? **Select all that apply.**
- ❑ 1. Alopecia
- ❑ 2. Back pain
- ❑ 3. Painless testicular swelling
- ❑ 4. A heavy sensation in the scrotum
- ❑ 5. Elevation in prostate-specific antigen (PSA) levels

3. The nurse is reviewing the laboratory results of a client with leukemia who has received a regimen of chemotherapy. Which laboratory finding is indicative of the massive cell destruction that occurs with the chemotherapy?
- 1. Anemia
- 2. Decreased platelets
- 3. Increased uric acid level
- 4. Decreased leukocyte count

❖ **4.** The client is receiving external radiation to the neck for cancer of the larynx. The nurse monitors the client knowing that which are side/adverse effects of the external radiation? **Select all that apply.**
- ❑ 1. Dyspnea
- ❑ 2. Diarrhea
- ❑ 3. Sore throat
- ❑ 4. Constipation
- ❑ 5. Red and dry skin over neck

❖ **5.** The nurse is reinforcing instructions to a client receiving external radiation therapy. The nurse determines that the client **needs further teaching** if the client states an intention to take which action? **Select all that apply.**
- ❑ 1. Eat a high-protein diet.
- ❑ 2. Avoid exposure to sunlight.
- ❑ 3. Wash the skin with a mild soap, and pat it dry.
- ❑ 4. Apply pressure on the radiated area to prevent bleeding.
- ❑ 5. Avoid standing within 6 feet of persons younger than the age of 18 years.

❖ **6.** The nurse is caring for a client with an internal radiation implant. The nurse needs to observe which principle(s)? **Select all that apply.**
- ❑ 1. Pregnant women are not allowed into the client's room.
- ❑ 2. Limit the time with the client to 1 hour per 8-hour shift.
- ❑ 3. Wear a lead apron while delivering bedside care to the client.
- ❑ 4. Remove the dosimeter badge when entering the client's room.
- ❑ 5. Individuals younger than 16 years old are allowed in the room if they stay 6 feet away from the client.

❖ **7.** The nurse provides skin care instructions to the client who is receiving external radiation therapy. Which statement(s) by the client indicates the **need for further teaching?** **Select all that apply.**
- ❑ 1. "I will handle the area gently."
- ❑ 2. "I will wear loose-fitting clothing."
- ❑ 3. "I will avoid the use of deodorants."
- ❑ 4. "I will limit sun exposure to 1 hour daily."
- ❑ 5. "I will apply moisturizer with a cotton tipped applicator for itching."

8. The client is hospitalized for the insertion of an internal cervical radiation implant. While giving care, the nurse finds the radiation implant in the bed. Which is the **immediate** nursing action?
- 1. Reinsert the implant into the vagina.
- 2. Call the primary health care provider (PHCP).
- 3. Pick up the implant with gloved hands and flush it down the toilet.
- 4. Pick up the implant with long-handled forceps and place into a lead container.

❖ **9.** The nurse is assisting with creating a plan of care for a client with pancytopenia as a result of chemotherapy. The nurse would suggest including which in the plan of care? **Select all that apply.**
- ❑ 1. Restricting all visitors
- ❑ 2. Restricting fluid intake
- ❑ 3. Restricting fresh fruits and vegetables in the diet
- ❑ 4. Applying a face mask to the client if outside the client room
- ❑ 5. Inserting an indwelling urinary catheter to prevent skin breakdown

❖ **10.** The client with carcinoma of the lung develops syndrome of inappropriate antidiuretic hormone (SIADH) as a complication of the cancer. Besides treatment of the lung cancer, the nurse anticipates that which intervention(s) may be prescribed to treat the SIADH? **Select all that apply.**
- ❑ 1. Increase fluid intake
- ❑ 2. Decreased sodium intake

❏ **3.** Institute safety measures

❏ **4.** Frequent monitoring of sodium blood levels

❏ **5.** Gather data about the neurological status frequently

❏ **6.** Medication that is antagonistic to antidiuretic hormone (ADH)

❖ **11.** The client is admitted to the hospital with a diagnosis of suspected Hodgkin's disease. Which sign(s)/(symptom(s) of the client are associated with Hodgkin's disease? **Select all that apply.**

❏ **1.** Fatigue

❏ **2.** Joint pain

❏ **3.** Weakness

❏ **4.** Weight gain

❏ **5.** Night sweats

❏ **6.** Enlarged lymph nodes

❖ **12.** When reinforcing teaching about signs/symptoms of ovarian cancer with a community group of women, the nurse emphasizes which as being a **most** typical manifestation of the disease?

1. Pelvic cramping

2. Sharp abdominal pain

3. Abdominal distention or fullness

4. Postmenopausal vaginal bleeding

❖ **13.** The nurse is caring for a client after a mastectomy. Which finding would indicate that the client is experiencing a complication that may become a chronic problem related to the surgery?

1. Pain at the incisional site

2. Arm edema on the operative side

3. Sanguineous drainage in the Jackson-Pratt drain

4. Complaints of decreased sensation near the operative site

❖ **14.** The nurse is reinforcing discharge instructions to a client with cancer of the prostate after a suprapubic prostatectomy. The nurse would reinforce which discharge instruction(s)? **Select all that apply.**

❏ **1.** Avoid driving a car for 1 week.

❏ **2.** Restrict fluid intake to prevent incontinence.

❏ **3.** Take the prescribed stool softener every day.

❏ **4.** Avoid lifting objects heavier than 20 pounds for 6 weeks.

❏ **5.** Inspect the incision on the scrotum every day for any redness.

❏ **6.** Notify the primary health care provider (PHCP) if small blood clots are noticed during urination.

❖ **15.** The nurse is reviewing the laboratory results of a client who is receiving chemotherapy and notes that the platelet count is 10,000 mm^3. On the basis of this laboratory value, the nurse would perform which intervention(s)? **Select all that apply.**

❏ **1.** Monitor stools for occult blood.

❏ **2.** Keep away from persons who have colds or feel ill.

❏ **3.** Instruct the client not to bend over at the waist or lift.

❏ **4.** Floss teeth and rinse mouth with mouthwash after every meal.

❏ **5.** Instruct the client to blow nose very gently without blocking either nostril.

ANSWERS

❖ **1. 1, 5**

Rationale: To prevent renal failure in the client with multiple myeloma, the nurse would encourage fluids and monitor serum calcium and uric acid levels. Hypercalcemia secondary to bone destruction is a priority concern in the client with multiple myeloma. The nurse needs to encourage fluids in adequate amounts to maintain an output of 1.5 to 2 L a day. Clients require approximately 3 L of fluid per day. The fluid is needed not only to dilute the calcium and uric acid but also to prevent protein from precipitating in the renal tubules. Oral care, encouraging coughing and deep breathing, and monitoring the red blood cell count are important for clients with cancer, but these interventions are not specific to prevention or assessment of renal failure.

Test-Taking Strategy: Focus on the subject, decreasing the risk for renal failure in clients with multiple myeloma. Think about the pathophysiology associated with multiple myeloma. Recall that hypercalcemia and high levels of uric acid can lead to urinary stone formation and renal impairment. Encouraging fluids is specific to the care of a client and decreasing the likelihood of urinary stone formation. This will direct you to the correct option.

❖ **2. 1, 5**

Rationale: Alopecia is not a sign/symptom of testicular cancer. However, it may occur as a result of radiation or chemotherapy. Elevated PSA levels are associated with prostate problems. Testicular swelling without pain and a feeling of heaviness in the scrotum occur with testicular cancer as a result of the tumor growing. Back pain may indicate metastasis to the retroperitoneal lymph nodes.

Test-Taking Strategy: Note the strategic words, *further teaching is needed.* These words indicate a negative event query and ask you to select an option that is incorrect. Also focus on the subject, sign/symptom of testicular cancer. Remember that alopecia occurs as a result of chemotherapy rather than of the disease. Elevated PSA levels are related to prostate problems.

3. 3

Rationale: Hyperuricemia, elevated levels of uric acid, is especially common after treatment for leukemias and lymphomas, because the therapy results in massive cell destruction and the release of uric acid. Anemia (low red blood cell count), low platelet levels, and low white blood cell counts are associated with the bone marrow abnormalities that are a part of the leukemias and lymphoma disease process.

Test-Taking Strategy: Focus on the subject, the effects associated with massive cell destruction. Note that the incorrect options are comparable or alike options because these laboratory tests all reflect bone marrow production. Recalling the cell response to destruction will assist with directing you to the correct option.

❖**4. 3, 5**

Rationale: External radiation is used to treat cancer in a specific area by emission of ionizing radiation beams that destroy cancer cells and have minimal damage to the surrounding normal cells. The client receiving external radiation experiences both general side/adverse effects such as fatigue, nausea, and anorexia and localized side/adverse effects in the specific area receiving radiation. A client who is receiving radiation to the larynx is most likely to experience a sore throat and dry, reddened skin in the throat area. Diarrhea or constipation occur with radiation to the gastrointestinal (GI) tract. Dyspnea may occur with lung involvement.

Test-Taking Strategy: Eliminate diarrhea and constipation first because they are comparable or alike, and both are GI related. Consider the anatomical location of the radiation therapy to direct you to the correct option.

❖**5. 4, 5**

Rationale: The client would avoid pressure on the radiated area and wear loose-fitting clothing to prevent a disruption in the skin integrity. A client receiving external radiation is not radioactive and does not need to avoid other persons, including young people. A diet high in protein assists in the healing process. Avoiding sunlight and washing the skin with gentle soap and patting dry will assist with preventing skin disruption.

Test-Taking Strategy: Note the strategic words, *needs further teaching.* These words indicate a negative event query and ask you to select an option that is an incorrect statement. The word *pressure* in option 4 would be an indication that this is an inappropriate measure. Recall that the radiation is from an external source so the client does not emit any radiation.

❖**6. 1, 3**

Rationale: A client receiving treatment for cancer with internal radioactive implant is emitting radioactive beams, and others in the environment must take precautions to avoid injury. Pregnant persons are not allowed in the room. Nurses delivering bedside care must wear a lead apron which will stop the radioactive beams. The time that the nurse spends in the room of a client with an internal radiation implant is 30 minutes per 8-hour shift. The dosimeter badge must be worn when in the client's room. Children younger than 16 years old and pregnant women are not allowed in the client's room. These guidelines protect individuals from radiation exposure.

Test-Taking Strategy: Focus on the subject, principles to observe for the client with an internal radiation implant. Understand that the client is emitting radiation and persons in the environment must take precautionary actions. Persons who are actively growing are at increased risk for injury, so

know that pregnant women and persons younger than 16 are not allowed in the room. Recall the designated limits of exposure to assist in selecting the correct answers.

❖**7. 4, 5**

Rationale: The client needs to be instructed to avoid exposure to the sun because of the risk of burns, resulting in altered tissue integrity. No lotions, ointments, deodorants, or medications would be applied to the skin area unless prescribed by the radiologist.

Test-Taking Strategy: Note the strategic words, *need for further teaching.* These words indicate a negative event query and ask you to select an option that is an incorrect statement. Eliminate option 1 because of the word *gently* and option 2 because of the word *loose.* From the remaining options, recalling that sun exposure is to be avoided will assist you with answering the question.

❖**8. 4**

Rationale: A lead container and long-handled forceps must be kept in the client's room at all times during internal radiation therapy. Lead is an element that has a high density and high atomic number and is used to shield persons from radiation. If dislodged, the implant must be handled carefully to limit radiation exposure to the client and all persons in the environment. If the implant becomes dislodged, the nurse would pick up the implant with long-handled forceps and place it into the lead container. The radiation safety officer of the institution must be notified. Although the PHCP needs to be notified, this is not the immediate action. The nurse cannot reinsert the implant. A radioactive implant is specifically placed inside the client to kill the cancer while limiting damage to adjacent tissues and organs. Touching the implant with gloves and flushing this down the toilet exposes the nurse and the environment to unsafe levels of radiation.

Test-Taking Strategy: Note the strategic word, *immediate,* which indicates a priority nursing action. Evaluate each option to determine whether it is consistent with safe action of radioactive devices and whether it is a priority. Also think about the roles of the nurse. Option 4 is the safe immediate action.

❖**9. 3, 4**

Rationale: A client who is experiencing pancytopenia (decrease in all blood cells types: red, white, and platelets) is at high risk for infection because of significantly low immunity. The client should not eat fresh fruits and vegetables because of the risk for ingesting bacteria. All foods need to be cooked thoroughly. The client would wear a mask when outside of the room, to avoid potential infection spread from persons in the hallways. Not all visitors are restricted, but the client is protected from people with known infections. Fluids need to be encouraged because dehydration increases the risk for infection. Invasive measures such as an indwelling urinary catheter would be avoided to prevent infection.

Test-Taking Strategy: Note the subject, pancytopenia and care of the immunocompromised client. Eliminate option 1 because of the word *all.* Next, evaluate each option regarding the potential for risk for infection; this will assist in selecting the correct answers.

❖ 10. 3, 4, 5, 6
Rationale: Syndrome of inappropriate antidiuretic hormone (SIADH) is a condition in which excessive amounts of water are reabsorbed by the kidney and put into the systemic circulation. The increased water causes hyponatremia (decreased serum sodium levels) and some degree of fluid retention. SIADH is a potential complication associated with cancer, especially small cell lung cancer. SIADH is managed by treating the condition and its cause. The SIADH induces low sodium blood levels and results in altered neurological states, including confusion and unresponsiveness. Treatment of SIADH includes fluid restriction, increased sodium intake, and a medication with a mechanism of action that is antagonistic to antidiuretic hormone (ADH), such as demeclocycline. Sodium blood levels and neurological status are monitored closely and safety interventions need to be instituted. The client would not be treated with an increase in fluid intake or a decrease in the sodium intake.
Test-Taking Strategy: Focus on the subject, the client's complication SIADH, and recall that in clients with SIADH excessive amounts of water are reabsorbed by the kidney and put into the systemic circulation. It is the opposite of diabetes insipidus. Understand that there is fluid retention resulting in low sodium levels severe enough to cause neurological signs/symptoms. Select options which do not increase fluid or decrease sodium. Select options that involve gathering data about sodium levels and neurological status. An altered neurological status often requires safety interventions to prevent injury in a client who is unable to maintain safety.

❖ 11. 1, 3, 5, 6
Rationale: Hodgkin's disease (lymphoma) is a chronic, progressive neoplastic disorder of the lymphoid tissue that is characterized by the painless enlargement of lymph nodes with progression to extralymphatic sites, such as the spleen and liver. Other signs and symptoms include fatigue, weakness, weight loss, and night sweats. Weight gain and joint pain are not associated with Hodgkin's disease.
Test-Taking Strategy: Focus on the subject, signs/symptoms associated with Hodgkin's disease (lymphoma). Recall that Hodgkin's disease specifically affects the lymph nodes. Clients often experience night sweats and alterations in blood cells, so select signs/symptoms related to anemia and altered immunity.

12. 3
Rationale: Ovarian cancer is a leading cause of death from gynecological cancers and symptoms are usually vague. A common sign/symptom of ovarian cancer is abdominal distention or fullness. Less common are symptoms of urinary frequency and urgency, and gastrointestinal symptoms such as a change in bowel habits. Pelvic cramping, sharp abdominal pain, or postmenopausal vaginal bleeding are not the most typical signs/symptoms.
Test-Taking Strategy: Note the strategic word, *most.* Focus on the subject, most typical sign/symptom of ovarian cancer. Read each option and think about the manifestation. Recalling that the signs/symptoms are vague will assist you to the correct answer.

13. 2
Rationale: Clients who undergo mastectomy for breast cancer, especially those with axillary node resection, may develop chronic lymphedema or excessive swelling in the arm and hand. Lymphedema is a complication that may develop immediately after mastectomy, months, or even years after surgery. Slight edema may occur in the immediate postoperative period but would decrease especially if the client rests with the arm supported on a pillow. Women need to avoid injury to the arm on the affected side and not allow venipunctures or blood pressures to be taken in that arm. Pain and numbness near the incision and drainage from the surgical site are expected occurrences after mastectomy and are not indicative of a complication.
Test-Taking Strategy: Note the subject, a complication of a mastectomy, and consider the normal and expected occurrences after a mastectomy. This will assist in answering. Also, determine whether any finding in the options could develop into a long-term complication.

❖ 14. 3, 4
Rationale: A suprapubic approach involves a lower abdominal incision to remove the prostate to treat prostate cancer. The nurse will reinforce instructions about the incision activity, medications, and when to contact the urologist. The client would take the prescribed stool softener because constipation will lead to straining and cause pain and tension on the surgical site. The client needs to avoid lifting more than 20 pounds for 6 weeks to avoid tension on the surgical site. Driving a car and sitting for long periods of time are restricted for at least 3 weeks. A daily fluid intake of 2 to 2.5 L/day (unless contraindicated) would be maintained to limit clot formation and prevent infection. The incision is not on the scrotum but in the lower abdominal area. Small pieces of tissue or blood clots can be passed during urination for up to 2 weeks after surgery and do not need to be reported.
Test-Taking Strategy: Focus on the subject, postprostatectomy discharge instructions. Eliminate option 1 because of the short time frame. Eliminate option 2 because of the words, *restrict fluid intake.* Thinking about the anatomical location of this surgery will eliminate option 5. Recall that small blood clots are expected after this type of surgery, so option 6 can be eliminated.

❖ 15. 1, 3, 5
Rationale: Platelets or thrombocytes are necessary for a client to clot. A high risk of hemorrhage exists when the platelet count decreases to less than 20,000 mm^3. Fatal central nervous system hemorrhage or massive gastrointestinal hemorrhage can occur when the platelet count is less than 10,000 mm^3. The client may be treated with medications or platelet or blood transfusions to improve the platelet count. The nurse needs to monitor the client's stools for blood, both obvious and occult. The client would be very gentle if blowing the nose and not cause any pressure to build up in the head. The client would not bend over at the waist because this action would increase the pressure within the head and increase the risk for an intracerebral bleed. Clients with decreased immunity, which is not the focus of the question, need to avoid ill persons. The client would not floss the teeth and only use a soft toothbrush to avoid bleeding in the mouth.
Test-Taking Strategy: Focus on the subject, precautions for clients at risk for bleeding. Recall the normal platelet count and determine that a low count places the client at risk for bleeding. Evaluate each option in light of avoiding serious bleeding, especially intracranially. This will assist in answering correctly.

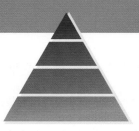

CHAPTER **42**

Oncological and Hematological Medications

PRIORITY CONCEPTS Cellular Regulation; Safety

WHAT WOULD YOU DO?

The nurse notes that a client who needs to receive a scheduled antineoplastic medication has a segmented neutrophil count of 10%. What would the nurse do?
Answer is located on p. 538.

I. Antineoplastic Medications

A. Description
   1. Antineoplastic medications kill or inhibit the reproduction of neoplastic cells.
   2. Antineoplastic medications are used to cure, increase survival time, and decrease life-threatening complications.
   3. The effect of antineoplastic medications may not be limited to neoplastic cells; normal cells also are affected by the medication.
   4. Cell cycle phase-specific medications affect cells only during a certain phase of the reproductive cycle (Fig. 42.1).
   5. Cell cycle phase-nonspecific medications affect cells in any phase of the reproductive cycle (see Fig. 42.1).
   6. Usually, several medications are used in combination to increase the therapeutic response.
   7. Antineoplastic medications may be combined with other treatments, such as surgery and radiation.
   8. Although the intravenous (IV) route is most common for administration, antineoplastic medication may be given by the oral, intraarterial, isolated limb perfusion, or intracavitary route; dosing is usually based on the client's body surface area (BSA) and type of cancer.
   9. Chemotherapy dosing is usually based on total BSA, which requires a current, accurate height and weight for BSA calculation (before each medication administration) to ensure that the client receives optimal doses of chemotherapy medications.

 Side and adverse effects from chemotherapy result from the effects of the antineoplastic medication on normal cells.

B. Side/adverse effects
   1. Mucositis
   2. Alopecia
   3. Anorexia, nausea, vomiting
   4. Diarrhea
   5. Anemia
   6. Low white blood cell count (neutropenia)
   7. Thrombocytopenia
   8. Infertility, sexual alterations
   9. Neuropathy
C. General interventions
   1. Physiological integrity
      a. Monitor complete blood count (CBC), white blood cell count, platelet count, uric acid level, and electrolytes.
      b. Initiate bleeding precautions if thrombocytopenia occurs.
      c. When the platelet count is less than 50,000 mm³, minor trauma can lead to episodes of prolonged bleeding; when less than 20,000 mm³, spontaneous and uncontrollable bleeding can occur; withhold the medication if the platelet count drops (according to agency policy) and notify the registered nurse (RN) and primary health care provider (PHCP). Bleeding precautions are initiated.
      d. Monitor for petechiae, ecchymosis, bleeding of the gums, and nosebleeds because the decreased platelet count can precipitate bleeding tendencies.
      e. Avoid intramuscular injections, venipunctures, and any invasive procedures as much as possible to prevent bleeding.
      f. Withhold the medication and initiate neutropenic precautions if the segmented neutrophil count decreases below 18%; notify the RN and PHCP.

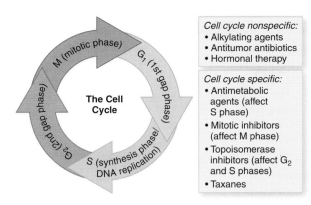

Cell cycle nonspecific:
- Alkylating agents
- Antitumor antibiotics
- Hormonal therapy

Cell cycle specific:
- Antimetabolic agents (affect S phase)
- Mitotic inhibitors (affect M phase)
- Topoisomerase inhibitors (affect G_2 and S phases)
- Taxanes

FIGURE 42.1 The Cell Cycle. *G1*, The cell is preparing for division; *S* (synthesis phase, DNA replication), the cell doubles its DNA content through DNA synthesis; *G2*, the cell produces proteins to be used during cell division and for normal physiological function, after cell division is complete; and *M* (mitotic phase), the single cell splits apart into two cells.

g. Monitor for fever, sore throat, unusual bleeding, and signs/symptoms of infection.

h. Inform the client that loss of appetite also may be the result of taste changes or a bitter taste in the mouth from the medications.

i. Monitor for nausea and vomiting, and provide a high-calorie diet with protein supplements.

j. Administer antiemetics several hours before chemotherapy and for 12 to 48 hours after, as prescribed, because antineoplastic medications stimulate the vomiting center in the brain.

k. Encourage hydration; IV fluids will be administered before and during therapy.

l. Promote a fluid intake of at least 2000 mL/day to maintain adequate renal function.

⚠️ Antineoplastic medication causes the rapid destruction of cells, resulting in the release of uric acid. Allopurinol may be prescribed to lower the serum uric acid level.

2. Safe and effective care environment

a. IV chemotherapy is prepared in an air-vented space (biological safety cabinet); in most health care agencies, it is prepared in the pharmacy.

b. Wear appropriate personal protective equipment (PPE), including gloves, gown, eye protectors, and mask as indicated, to reduce exposure whenever there is a risk of hazardous medications being released into the environment.

c. Nurses who are pregnant need to avoid chemotherapy preparation or the administration of chemotherapy.

d. Discard IV equipment in designated (biohazard) containers.

e. Antineoplastic medication is administered precisely as prescribed to maximize

antineoplastic effects while allowing normal cells to recover.

f. Monitor for phlebitis with IV administration, because these medications may irritate the veins.

g. Vesicants are administered through a central line when possible; if a peripheral line is used, blood return needs to be checked before administration.

h. As prescribed, reduce IV site pain by altering IV rates or warming the injection site to distend the vein and increase blood flow.

i. Monitor for extravasation (leakage of medication into surrounding skin and subcutaneous tissue, which causes tissue necrosis), and notify the RN immediately if this occurs; heat or ice is applied, depending on the medication, and an antidote may be injected into the site.

3. Psychosocial integrity

a. Instruct the client about the possibility of hair loss and that varying degrees of hair loss may occur after the first or second treatment.

b. Discuss the purchase of a wig before treatment starts and consider cutting hair short.

c. Inform the client that new hair growth will occur several months after the final treatment.

d. Instruct the client about the need for contraception because these medications have teratogenic effects.

e. The potential effect of infertility is discussed, which may be irreversible.

f. Encourage pretreatment counseling and encourage sperm banking or preservation of eggs if the client is still of childbearing age.

4. Reinforce health promotion and maintenance teaching

a. Instruct the client, if diarrhea is a problem, to avoid spicy foods and high-fiber foods, and foods that are hot in temperature, which increase peristalsis.

b. Instruct the client to inspect the oral mucosa frequently for erythema and ulcers, rinse the mouth after meals, and carry out good oral hygiene.

c. Instruct the client to use mouth rinses as prescribed for mouth sores if necessary.

d. Instruct the client in the use of antifungal agents for mouth sores, if prescribed, for the development of a fungal infection.

e. Instruct the client to avoid crowds and persons with infections and to report signs of infection such as a low-grade fever, chills, or sore throat.

f. Instruct individuals with colds or infections to avoid visiting the client.

g. Instruct the client to use a soft toothbrush and electric razor to minimize the risk of bleeding.

h. Instruct the client to avoid aspirin-containing products to minimize the risk of bleeding.

i. Instruct to consult the PHCP before receiving vaccinations (live vaccines would not be administered).

D. Anaphylactic reactions

  1. Precautions

    a. Obtain an allergy history.

    b. A test dose is administered when prescribed by the PHCP.

    c. Stay with the client during the administration of medication.

    d. Monitor vital signs.

    e. Have emergency equipment and medications readily available.

    f. Obtain IV access for the administration of emergency medications if needed.

  2. Signs of an anaphylactic reaction

    a. Dyspnea

    b. Chest tightness or pain

    c. Pruritus or urticaria

    d. Tachycardia

    e. Dizziness

    f. Anxiety or agitation

    g. Flushed appearance

    h. Hypotension

    i. Decreased sensorium

    j. Cyanosis

  3. Interventions for an anaphylactic reaction (see **Priority Nursing Actions**)

⚡ PRIORITY NURSING ACTIONS

Anaphylactic Reaction Occurs from Medication

1. Assess respiratory status.
2. Stop the medication.
3. The PHCP is contacted; the Rapid Response Team is also contacted, if necessary.
4. Administer oxygen.
5. Maintain the IV access with normal saline.
6. Administer prescribed emergency medications.
7. Monitor vital signs.
8. Document the event, actions taken, and the client's response.

II. Alkylating Medications (Box 42.1)

A. Description

  1. Break the DNA helix, thereby interfering with DNA replication

  2. Cell cycle phase nonspecific medications

B. Side/adverse effects

  1. Anorexia, nausea, and vomiting may occur.

  2. Stomatitis may occur.

  3. Rash may occur.

  4. Client may feel IV site pain during IV administration.

  5. Busulfan may cause hyperuricemia.

  6. Chlorambucil and mechlorethamine may cause gonadal suppression and hyperuricemia.

BOX 42.1   Alkylating Medications

Nitrogen Mustards
- Bendamustine
- Chlorambucil
- Cyclophosphamide
- Estramustine
- Ifosfamide
- Mechlorethamine
- Melphalan

Nitrosoureas
- Carmustine
- Lomustine
- Streptozocin

Alkylating-Like Medications
- Altretamine
- Busulfan
- Carboplatin
- Cisplatin
- Dacarbazine
- Oxaliplatin
- Temozolomide
- Thiotepa
- Trabectedin

---

7. Cisplatin, a platinum compound, may cause ototoxicity, tinnitus, hypokalemia, hypocalcemia, hypomagnesemia, and nephrotoxicity.

8. Cyclophosphamide may cause alopecia, gonadal suppression, hemorrhagic cystitis, and hematuria.

9. Ifosfamide may cause neurotoxicity.

C. Interventions: Refer to Section I.C. (Antineoplastic Medications—General Interventions).

  1. Monitor results of pulmonary function tests.

  2. Monitor results of chest radiography and renal and liver function studies.

  3. When cisplatin is administered, the client is monitored for dizziness, tinnitus, hearing loss, incoordination, and numbness or tingling of extremities.

  4. Mesna may be administered with ifosfamide to reduce the potential of ifosfamide-induced cystitis.

  5. Reinforce instructions to the client that cyclophosphamide, when prescribed orally, is administered without food.

  6. Reinforce instructions to the client to follow a diet low in purines to alkalinize the urine and lower uric acid blood levels.

  7. Reinforce instructions to the client on how to avoid infection.

  8. Reinforce instructions to the client to report signs of infection or bleeding.

  9. Reinforce instructions to the client about good oral hygiene and use of a soft toothbrush.

BOX 42.2 **Antitumor Antibiotic Medications**

- Bleomycin sulfate
- Dactinomycin
- Daunorubicin
- Doxorubicin
- Epirubicin
- Idarubicin
- Mitomycin
- Mitoxantrone
- Valrubicin

⚠ Cyclophosphamide and ifosfamide are medications that can cause hemorrhagic cystitis. The client is encouraged to drink increased fluids (2 to 3 L/day) during therapy, unless contraindicated.

BOX 42.3 **Antimetabolite Medications**

- Azacitidine
- Capecitabine
- Cladribine
- Clofarabine
- Cytarabine
- Decitabine
- Floxuridine
- Fludarabine
- Fluorouracil
- Gemcitabine
- Hydroxyurea
- Mercaptopurine
- Methotrexate
- Nelarabine
- Pemetrexed
- Pentostatin
- Pralatrexate
- Thioguanine

III. Antitumor Antibiotic Medications (Box 42.2)

A. Description
1. Interfere with DNA and RNA synthesis
2. Cell cycle phase-nonspecific medications

B. Side/adverse effects
1. Nausea and vomiting
2. Fever
3. Bone marrow depression
4. Rash
5. Alopecia
6. Stomatitis
7. Gonadal suppression
8. Hyperuricemia
9. Vesication (blistering of tissue at IV site)
 10. Daunorubicin may cause heart failure and dysrhythmia.
 11. Doxorubicin and idarubicin may cause cardiotoxicity, cardiomyopathy, and electrocardiographic changes. (Dexrazoxane, which is a cardioprotective agent, may be administered with doxorubicin to reduce cardiomyopathy.)
 12. Pulmonary toxicity can occur with bleomycin.

C. Interventions: Refer to Section I.C. (Antineoplastic Medications—General Interventions).
1. Monitor results of pulmonary function tests.
2. Monitor for electrocardiographic changes.
3. Check lung sounds for crackles.
4. Monitor for signs of heart failure, including dyspnea, crackles, peripheral edema, and weight gain.
5. Monitor for results of chest radiography and renal and liver function studies.
6. Monitor for myocardial toxicity, dyspnea, dysrhythmias, hypotension, and weight gain when daunorubicin, doxorubicin, or idarubicin are administered.
 7. Monitor pulmonary status when bleomycin is administered.

IV. Antimetabolite Medications (Box 42.3)

A. Description
1. Antimetabolite medications halt the synthesis of cell protein; their presence impairs cell division.
2. Antimetabolite medications are cell cycle phase-specific and affect the S phase.

B. Side/adverse effects
1. Anorexia, nausea, and vomiting
2. Diarrhea
3. Alopecia
4. Stomatitis
5. Depression of bone marrow
6. Cytarabine may cause alopecia, stomatitis, hyperuricemia, and hepatotoxicity.
 7. Fluorouracil may cause alopecia, stomatitis, diarrhea, phototoxicity reactions, and cerebellar dysfunction.
8. Mercaptopurine may cause hyperuricemia and hepatotoxicity.
 9. Methotrexate may cause alopecia, stomatitis, hyperuricemia, photosensitivity, hepatotoxicity, and hematological, gastrointestinal, and skin toxicity.

C. Interventions: Refer to Section I.C. (Antineoplastic Medications—General Interventions).
1. Monitor renal function studies.
2. Monitor for cerebellar dysfunction.
3. Assess for photosensitivity.
 4. When fluorouracil is administered, monitor for signs of cerebellar dysfunction, such as dizziness, weakness, and ataxia, and monitor for stomatitis and diarrhea, which may necessitate medication discontinuation.
 5. When fluorouracil or methotrexate is administered, instruct the client to use sunscreen and wear protective clothing to prevent photosensitivity reactions.

BOX 42.4 **Mitotic Inhibitors**

Vinca Alkaloids
- Vinblastine sulfate
- Vincristine sulfate
- Vinorelbine

Taxanes
- Cabazitaxel
- Docetaxel
- Paclitaxel

⚠ When methotrexate is administered in large doses, leucovorin may be administered as prescribed to prevent toxicity. This is known as leucovorin rescue.

V. Mitotic Inhibitor Medications (Box 42.4)

A. Description
   1. Mitotic inhibitors prevent mitosis (i.e., cell division) causing cell death.
   2. Mitotic inhibitors are cell cycle phase-specific and act on the M phase.

B. Side/adverse effects
   1. Leukopenia
   2. Neurotoxicity with vincristine manifested as numbness and tingling in the fingers and toes, constipation, and paralytic ileus
   3. Ptosis
   4. Hoarseness
   5. Motor instability
   6. Anorexia, nausea, and vomiting
   7. Peripheral neuropathy
   8. Alopecia
   9. Stomatitis
   10. Hyperuricemia
   11. Phlebitis at IV site

C. Interventions: Refer to Section I.C. (Antineoplastic Medications—General Interventions).
   1. Monitor for hoarseness.
   2. Monitor eyes for ptosis.
   3. Monitor motor stability and initiate safety precautions as necessary.
   4. Monitor for neurotoxicity with vincristine sulfate manifested as numbness and tingling in the fingers and toes.
   5. Monitor for constipation and paralytic ileus.

VI. Topoisomerase Inhibitors (Box 42.5)

A. Description
   1. Block an enzyme needed for DNA synthesis and cell division
   2. Cell cycle phase-specific; act on the G2 and S phases

B. Side/adverse effects
   1. Leukopenia, thrombocytopenia, and anemia
   2. Anorexia, nausea, vomiting
   3. Diarrhea
   4. Alopecia

BOX 42.5 **Topoisomerase Inhibitors**

- Etoposide
- Irinotecan
- Teniposide
- Topotecan

BOX 42.6 **Hormonal Medications and Enzymes**

Estrogens
- Estramustine
- Ethinyl estradiol

Antiestrogens
- Anastrozole
- Exemestane
- Fulvestrant
- Letrozole
- Raloxifene
- Tamoxifen citrate
- Toremifene

Antiandrogens
- Apalutamide
- Bicalutamide
- Darolutamide
- Enzalutamide
- Flutamide
- Goserelin acetate
- Histrelin
- Nilutamide
- Triptorelin

Progestins
Medroxyprogesterone
Megestrol acetate

Other Hormonal Antagonists and Enzymes
- Asparaginase
- Leuprolide acetate
- Mitotane

---

   5. Orthostatic hypotension
   6. Hypersensitivity reaction

C. Interventions: Refer to Section I.C. (Antineoplastic Medications—General Interventions).

VII. Hormonal Medications and Enzymes (Box 42.6)

A. Description
   1. Suppress the immune system and block normal hormones in hormone-sensitive tumors
   2. Change the hormonal balance and slow the growth rate of certain tumors

B. Side/adverse effects
   1. Anorexia, nausea, and vomiting
   2. Leukopenia
   3. Impaired pancreatic function with asparaginase
   4. Sex characteristic alterations
      a. Masculinizing effect in women: Chest and facial hair, menses stops.
      b. Feminine manifestations in men: gynecomastia

BOX 42.7	Immunomodulator Agents

Aldesleukin
Interferon alfa-2a
Interferon alfa-2b
Interferon alfa-n3
Recombinant interferon alfa-2a
Recombinant interferon alfa-2b

Common Monoclonal Antibodies

Bevacizumab
Cetuximab
Ibritumomab
Infliximab
Panitumumab
Pembrolizumab
Rituximab
Trastuzumab

Small Molecule Inhibitors

Bortezomib
Bosutinib
Dasatinib
Erlotinib
Gefitinib
Imatinib
Lapatinib
Nilotinib
Ponatinib
Sorafenib
Sunitinib
Temsirolimus

BOX 42.8	Colony-Stimulating Factors

Granulocyte-Macrophage Colony-Stimulating Factor
- Sargramostim

Granulocyte Colony-Stimulating Factor
- Filgrastim
- Pegfilgrastim

Erythropoietin
- Epoetin alfa
- Darbepoetin alfa

5. Breast swelling
6. Hot flashes
7. Weight gain
8. Hemorrhagic cystitis and hypercholesterolemia, with mitotane
9. Hypertension
10. Thromboembolic disorders
11. Edema
12. Electrolyte imbalances
13. Tamoxifen citrate may cause edema, hypercalcemia, and elevated cholesterol and triglyceride levels.
14. Tamoxifen citrate decreases the effects of estrogen.

C. Interventions: Refer to Section I.C. (Antineoplastic Medications—General Interventions).
   1. Check medications that the client is taking currently.
   2. Monitor serum calcium levels with androgens.
   3. Monitor for signs of alterations in sexual characteristics.
   4. Monitor pancreatic function with asparaginase.
   5. Monitor uric acid and cholesterol levels.
   6. Monitor for signs of hemorrhagic cystitis.

VIII. Immunomodulator Agents: Biological Response Modifiers (Box 42.7)

A. Description
   1. Immunomodulators stimulate the immune system to recognize cancer cells and take action to eliminate or destroy them.
   2. Interleukins help various immune system cells recognize and destroy abnormal body cells.
   3. Interferons slow down tumor cell division, stimulate proliferation, and cause cancer cells to differentiate into nonproliferative forms.

B. Colony-stimulating factors induce more rapid bone marrow recovery after suppression by chemotherapy (Box 42.8).

IX. Targeted Therapy

A. Description
   1. Medications used as targeted therapies are monoclonal antibodies and small-molecule inhibitors that target a cellular element of the cancer cell or antisense medications that work at the gene level.
   2. Examples of monoclonal antibodies are rituximab, trastuzumab, alemtuzumab, bevacizumab, and cetuximab.

B. Adverse effects: Allergic reactions (monoclonal antibodies)

X. Other Antineoplastic Medications

A. Altretamine: Cytotoxic agent used to treat ovarian cancer
B. Denileukin diftitox: Recombinant DNA-derived medication used to treat cutaneous T-cell **lymphoma**
C. Pegaspargase: Used in combination chemotherapies for acute lymphoblastic leukemia in clients unable to take asparaginase
D. Bexarotene: Used to treat advanced-stage cutaneous T-cell **lymphoma**

XI. Medications to Treat Anemia (see Chapter 41 for more information)

A. Iron-deficiency anemia: Iron, oral or intravenous
B. Vitamin B12-deficiency anemia: Vitamin B12, oral or intramuscular
C. Folate-deficiency anemia: Folate, oral
D. Acute blood loss anemia: Blood transfusion, packed red blood cells, platelets, or fresh frozen plasma depending on cause
E. Anemia of chronic disease: Iron, oral or intravenous, erythropoietic growth factors, leukopoietic growth

factors, and thrombopoietic growth factors (see **Chapter 52** for more information).

WHAT WOULD YOU DO?

Answer: For the client receiving an antineoplastic medication with a neutrophil count is less than 18% , the nurse would immediately notify the RN. The RN would withhold the medication. The PHCP is notified for further prescriptions, and neutropenic precautions are initiated to protect the client from infection.

PRACTICE QUESTIONS

1. The nurse is caring for a client who is receiving an intravenous (IV) infusion of an antineoplastic medication. During the infusion, the client complains of pain at the insertion site. During an inspection of the site, the nurse notes redness and swelling. The nurse needs to take which appropriate action?
1. Notify the registered nurse immediately.
2. Administer pain medication to reduce the discomfort.
3. Apply ice and maintain the infusion rate, as prescribed.
4. Elevate the extremity of the IV site, and slow the infusion.

❖ 2. The client with squamous cell carcinoma of the larynx is receiving bleomycin intravenously. The nurse caring for the client anticipates that which diagnostic studies will be prescribed? **Select all that apply.**
❑ 1. Chest x-ray
❑ 2. Echocardiography
❑ 3. Electrocardiography
❑ 4. Cervical radiography
❑ 5. Pulmonary function studies

3. The client with acute myelocytic leukemia is being treated with busulfan. Which laboratory value would the nurse specifically monitor during treatment with this medication?
1. Clotting time
2. Uric acid level
3. Potassium level
4. Blood glucose level

❖ 4. The nurse is assisting with caring for a client with cancer who is receiving cisplatin. Which adverse effects are associated with this medication? **Select all that apply.**
❑ 1. Tinnitus
❑ 2. Ototoxicity
❑ 3. Hyperkalemia

❑ 4. Hypercalcemia
❑ 5. Nephrotoxicity
❑ 6. Hypomagnesemia

❖ 5. The licensed practical nurse (LPN) is assisting the registered nurse (RN) to create a teaching plan for the client receiving an antineoplastic medication. The LPN expects which information to be included? **Select all that apply.**
❑ 1. Rinse mouth after meals and use a soft toothbrush.
❑ 2. Notify the PHCP if the temperature is above 101°F (37.7°C).
❑ 3. Maintain oral hygiene and inspect the mouth for sores daily.
❑ 4. A sore throat is expected so the client would suck on soothing throat lozenges.
❑ 5. Consult with a primary health care provider (PHCP) before receiving immunizations.

6. The client with ovarian cancer is being treated with vincristine. The nurse monitors the client, knowing that which adverse effect is specific to this medication?
1. Diarrhea
2. Hair loss
3. Chest pain
4. Extremity numbness

7. The nurse is reviewing the history and physical examination of a client who will be receiving asparaginase, an antineoplastic agent. The nurse consults with the registered nurse regarding the administration of the medication if which is documented in the client's history?
1. Pancreatitis
2. Diabetes mellitus
3. Myocardial infarction
4. Chronic obstructive pulmonary disease

8. Tamoxifen is prescribed for the client with metastatic breast carcinoma. The nurse understands that which is the **primary** action of this medication?
1. Increase DNA and RNA synthesis
2. Promote the biosynthesis of nucleic acids
3. Increase estrogen concentration and estrogen response
4. Compete with estradiol for binding to estrogen in tissues containing high concentrations of receptors

9. The client with metastatic breast cancer is receiving tamoxifen. The nurse specifically monitors which laboratory value while the client is taking this medication?
1. Glucose level
2. Calcium level
3. Potassium level
4. Prothrombin time

10. The client with small cell lung cancer is being treated with etoposide and the nurse is assisting with caring for the client during administration. The client gets up to use the bathroom and is dizzy and very weak. The nurse understands these symptoms are likely a result of which side/adverse effect that is specifically associated with this medication?

1. Alopecia
2. Chest pain
3. Pulmonary fibrosis
4. Orthostatic hypotension

ANSWERS

1. 1

Rationale: When antineoplastic medications are administered via IV, great care must be taken to prevent extravasation, the condition in which the medication escapes into the tissues surrounding the injection site, because pain, tissue damage, and necrosis can result. The nurse monitors for signs of extravasation, such as redness or swelling at the insertion site. If extravasation occurs, the RN needs to be notified right away and the infusion will be stopped. The nurse will contact the PHCP. Depending on the specific medication, actions are taken to counteract the negative effects. The medication may be aspirated out, ice or warmth applied, and the area infiltrated with a neutralizing agent specific to the medication.
Test-Taking Strategy: Focus on the subject, chemotherapy and extravasation. Note the given information about the insertion site. Think about the definition of extravasation; this will assist to eliminate options 2, 3, and 4 as inappropriate nursing actions.

❖ 2. 1, 5

Rationale: Bleomycin is an antineoplastic medication that can cause interstitial pneumonitis, which can progress to pulmonary fibrosis. During pulmonary fibrosis, the lung tissue becomes very scarred and hard. Pulmonary fibrosis is not reversible and the client is continuously short of breath. Pulmonary function studies and chest x-ray, along with hematological, hepatic, and renal function tests need to be monitored. The nurse needs to monitor lung sounds for dyspnea and adventitious sounds, which could indicate pulmonary toxicity. The medication needs to be discontinued immediately if pulmonary toxicity occurs. Cardiac studies, such as an echocardiogram and electrocardiogram, and a cervical radiograph are unrelated to the specific use of this medication.
Test-Taking Strategy: Focus on the subject and considerations when administering the medication bleomycin. Eliminate options 2 and 3 first because they are cardiac-related and are therefore comparable or alike. From the remaining options, use the ABCs—airway, breathing, and circulation—to direct you to the correct options, the studies related to lung function.

3. 2

Rationale: Busulfan can cause an increase in the uric acid level because of massive cell death of malignant cells. Hyperuricemia can produce uric acid nephropathy, renal stones, and acute kidney injury. Clotting time, potassium, and glucose blood levels are not specifically related to this medication.

Test-Taking Strategy: Focus on the subject, the laboratory value to monitor for busulfan. It is necessary to know the adverse effects associated with this medication. Recalling that busulfan increases the uric acid level will direct you to the correct option.

❖ 4. 1, 2, 5, 6

Rationale: Cisplatin is an alkylating medication. Alkylating medications are cell cycle phase nonspecific and affect the synthesis of DNA by causing its cross-linking to inhibit cell reproduction. Cisplatin may cause ototoxicity, tinnitus, hypokalemia, hypocalcemia, hypomagnesemia, and nephrotoxicity. Amifostine may be administered before cisplatin to reduce the potential for renal toxicity.
Test-Taking Strategy: Note the subject, the adverse effects of cisplatin. Recall that most antineoplastic medications affect the bone marrow and the hematological system. This concept will assist you in determining that *hypo-* rather than *hyper-* conditions would occur. In addition, recall that this medication affects the ears (ototoxicity and tinnitus) and the kidneys (nephrotoxicity).

❖ 5. 1, 3, 5

Rationale: Clients with cancer treated with antineoplastic medications need to be aware of how to care for themselves, and it is important that client teaching is included in the care plan. Because antineoplastic medications affect the bone marrow, clients are often anemic, have lower immunity, and may be at risk for bleeding. Oral hygiene is important, and clients need to inspect their mouths daily, rinse after meals, and use a soft toothbrush. The client would check with the PHCP before receiving any immunizations. The client needs to notify the PHCP if a low-grade temperature such as 99.5°F (39.7°C) or a sore throat occurs. These are often associated with low white blood cell counts.
Test-Taking Strategy: Focus on the subject, a plan of care for the client receiving an antineoplastic medication. Recalling that antineoplastic medications lower the immune response of the body will direct you to the correct options.

6. 4

Rationale: Vincristine is a vinca alkaloid antineoplastic (miotic inhibitor) medication that has an adverse effect, specifically peripheral neuropathy. Peripheral neuropathy can be manifested as numbness and tingling in the fingers and toes. Depression of the Achilles tendon reflex may be the first clinical sign indicating peripheral neuropathy. Constipation, rather than diarrhea, is most likely to occur with this medication, although diarrhea may occur occasionally. Hair loss occurs with nearly all the antineoplastic medications. Chest pain is unrelated to this medication.

Test-Taking Strategy: Focus on the subject, an adverse effect of vincristine. Eliminate options 1 and 2 first because these effects are associated with many of the antineoplastic agents. Note that the question asks for the adverse effect specific to this medication. Correlate peripheral neuropathy with vincristine.

7. 1
Rationale: Asparaginase is an antineoplastic enzyme that is contraindicated if hypersensitivity exists in the case of pancreatitis, or if the client has a history of pancreatitis. The medication impairs pancreatic function, and pancreatic function tests must be performed before therapy begins and when a week or more has elapsed between the administration of doses. The client needs to be monitored for signs of pancreatitis, which include nausea, vomiting, and abdominal pain. The medication may be used for clients with a history of diabetes mellitus, myocardial infarction, or chronic obstructive pulmonary disease.
Test-Taking Strategy: Focus on the subject, a contraindication for asparaginase. It is necessary to know the contraindications associated with this medication. Recall that the exocrine pancreatic cells produce enzymes lipase and amylase; "ase" is the suffix designating an enzyme. Recalling that this medication affects pancreatic function will direct you to the correct option.

8. 4
Rationale: Tamoxifen is an antineoplastic medication that competes with estradiol for binding to estrogen in tissues containing high concentrations of receptors. Tamoxifen reduces DNA synthesis and estrogen response.
Test-Taking Strategy: Note the strategic word, *primary*, and focus on the subject, the action of tamoxifen. Eliminate options 1 and 2 first because they are comparable or alike. Nucleic acids include DNA and RNA. Eliminate option 3 because it is unlikely that the treatment of metastatic breast carcinoma would focus on increasing estrogen concentration and estrogen response.

9. 2
Rationale: Tamoxifen may increase calcium, cholesterol, and triglyceride levels. Before the initiation of therapy, a complete blood count, platelet count, and serum calcium levels would be assessed. These blood levels, along with cholesterol and triglyceride levels, would be monitored periodically during therapy. The nurse would assess for hypercalcemia while the client is taking this medication. Signs of hypercalcemia include increased urine volume, excessive thirst, nausea, vomiting, constipation, hypotonicity of muscles, and deep bone and flank pain. Tamoxifen does not increase glucose or potassium levels, or increase the prothrombin time.
Test-Taking Strategy: Focus on the subject, the laboratory value to monitor for tamoxifen. It is necessary to know the adverse effects associated with this medication. Recalling that this medication causes hypercalcemia will direct you to the correct option.

10. 4
Rationale: A side effect specific to etoposide is orthostatic hypotension. The client's blood pressure is monitored during the infusion. Hair loss occurs with nearly all antineoplastic medications. Chest pain and pulmonary fibrosis are unrelated to this medication.
Test-Taking Strategy: Focus on the subject, a side/adverse effect of etoposide. Note the data in question describes the client as weak and dizzy when getting up. These are symptoms associated with orthostatic hypotension. Eliminate option 1 first because this side effect is associated with many antineoplastic agents. Note that the question asks for the side/adverse effect specific to this medication. Correlate hypotension with etoposide.

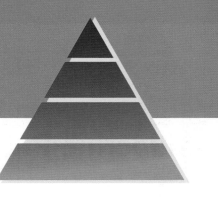

UNIT X

Endocrine Problems of the Adult Client

Pyramid to Success

The endocrine system is made up of organs or glands that secrete hormones and release them directly into the circulation. The endocrine system can be understood easily if you remember that basically one of two situations can occur—hypersecretion or hyposecretion of hormones from the organ or gland. When an excess of the hormone occurs, treatment is aimed at blocking the hormone release through medication or surgery. When a deficit of the hormone exists, treatment is aimed at replacement therapy. Pyramid Points focus on diabetes mellitus, including its prevention, management and self-care, the prevention and treatment of complications, insulin therapy, hypoglycemic and hyperglycemic reactions, and diabetic ketoacidosis; Addison's disease and Addisonian crisis; Cushing's disease or Cushing's syndrome; thyroid disorders and thyroid storm; and care of the client after thyroidectomy or adrenalectomy.

Client Needs: Learning Objectives

Safe and Effective Care Environment
Acting as a client advocate
Collaborating with the interprofessional team and appropriate care providers regarding treatment
Ensuring informed consent for treatments and procedures has been obtained
Establishing priorities of care
Handling hazardous and infectious materials
Maintaining confidentiality related to the health problem
Preventing accidents and client injury
Using medical and surgical asepsis to prevent infection

Client Needs lists modified from: National Council of State Boards of Nursing, Inc. (NCSBN). NCLEX-PN Examination: Test Plan for the National Council Licensure Examination for Practical Nurses, effective April 2020. Chicago: NCSBN.

Health Promotion and Maintenance
Discussing expected body image changes
Identifying lifestyle choices related to treatment
Performing physical assessment/data collection techniques of the endocrine system
Preventing complications
Providing health screening
Teaching about self-care measures

Psychosocial Integrity
Discussing grief and loss issues related to complications of the health problem
Discussing situational role changes related to the health problem
Discussing unexpected body image changes
Identifying coping mechanisms
Monitoring for sensory and perceptual alterations as a result of the health problem
Using support systems

Physiological Integrity
Monitoring for alterations in body systems as a result of the health problem
Monitoring for complications from surgical procedures and health alterations
Monitoring for complications of diagnostic tests, treatments, and procedures
Monitoring for expected outcomes and effects of pharmacological therapy
Monitoring for fluid and electrolyte imbalances that can occur
Monitoring for unexpected response to therapies
Monitoring laboratory values
Preparing the client for diagnostic tests
Providing emergency care to the client
Providing nonpharmacological comfort interventions
Providing nutrition and oral hydration measures

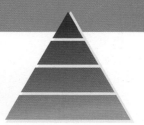
CHAPTER **43**

Endocrine Problems

PRIORITY CONCEPTS Glucose Regulation; Hormonal Regulation

WHAT WOULD YOU DO?

The nurse suspects that a client with pheochromocytoma is developing hypertensive crisis. What would the nurse do? *Answer is located on p. 560.*

I. Anatomy and Physiology of the Endocrine Glands (Box 43.1)

A. Functions
1. Maintenance and regulation of vital functions
2. Response to stress and injury
3. Growth and development
4. Energy metabolism
5. Reproduction
6. Fluid, electrolyte, and acid-base balance

B. Risk factors for endocrine problems (Box 43.2)

C. Hypothalamus (Box 43.3)
1. Portion of the diencephalon of the brain forming the floor and part of the lateral wall of the third ventricle
2. Activates, controls, and integrates the peripheral autonomic nervous system; endocrine processes; and many somatic functions, such as body temperature, sleep, and appetite

D. Pituitary gland (Box 43.4; Fig. 43.1)
1. The master gland; located at the base of the brain
2. Influenced by the hypothalamus; directly affects the function of the other endocrine glands
3. Promotes the growth of body tissue, influences water absorption by the kidney, and controls sexual development and function

E. Adrenal gland
1. One adrenal gland is on top of each kidney.
2. Regulates sodium and electrolyte balance; affects carbohydrate, fat, and protein metabolism; influences the development of sexual characteristics; and sustains the fight-or-flight response
3. Adrenal cortex
    a. The cortex is the outer shell of the adrenal gland.
    b. The cortex synthesizes glucocorticoids and mineralocorticoids and secretes small amounts of sex hormones (androgens, estrogens; Box 43.5).
4. Adrenal medulla
    a. The medulla is the inner core of the adrenal gland.
    b. The medulla works as a part of the sympathetic nervous system and produces epinephrine and norepinephrine.

F. Thyroid gland
1. Located in the anterior part of the neck
2. Controls the rate of body metabolism and growth and produces thyroxine (T_4), triiodothyronine (T_3), and thyrocalcitonin

G. Parathyroid glands
1. Located on the thyroid gland
2. Control calcium and phosphorus metabolism; produce parathyroid hormone (PTH)

H. Pancreas
1. Located posteriorly to the stomach
2. Influences carbohydrate metabolism, indirectly influences fat and protein metabolism, and produces insulin and glucagon

I. Ovaries and testes
1. The ovaries are located in the pelvic cavity and produce estrogen and progesterone.
2. The testes are located in the scrotum, control the development of the secondary sex characteristics, and produce testosterone.

J. Negative feedback loop
1. Regulates hormone secretion by the hypothalamus and pituitary gland
2. Increased amount of target gland hormones in the bloodstream decreases secretion of the same hormone and other hormones that stimulate its release.

II. Diagnostic Tests

A. Stimulation and suppression tests
1. Stimulation tests

a. In the client with suspected underactivity of an endocrine gland, a stimulus may be provided to determine whether the gland is capable of normal hormone production.

b. Measured amounts of selected hormones or substances are administered to stimulate the target gland to produce its hormone.

c. Hormone levels produced by the target gland are measured.

d. Failure of the hormone level to increase with stimulation indicates hypofunction.

2. Suppression tests
   a. Suppression tests are used when hormone levels are high or in the upper range of normal.

BOX 43.1 Endocrine Glands

- Adrenal
- Hypothalamus
- Ovaries
- Pancreas
- Parathyroid
- Pituitary
- Testes
- Thyroid

BOX 43.2 Risk Factors for Endocrine Problems

- Age
- Diet
- Heredity
- Congenital factors
- Trauma
- Environmental factors
- Consequence of surgery or other problems

BOX 43.3 Hypothalamus Hormones

- Corticotropin-releasing hormone
- Gonadotropin-releasing hormone
- Growth hormone-inhibiting hormone
- Growth hormone-releasing hormone
- Melanocyte-inhibiting hormone
- Prolactin-inhibiting hormone
- Thyrotropin-releasing hormone

BOX 43.4 Pituitary Gland Hormones

Anterior Lobe Production
Adrenocorticotropic hormone
Follicle-stimulating hormone
Growth hormone
Luteinizing hormone
Melanocyte-stimulating hormone
Prolactin
Somatotropic growth-stimulating hormone
Thyroid-stimulating hormone

Posterior Lobe
These hormones are produced by the hypothalamus, stored in the posterior lobe, and secreted into the blood when needed.

Oxytocin
Vasopressin, antidiuretic hormone

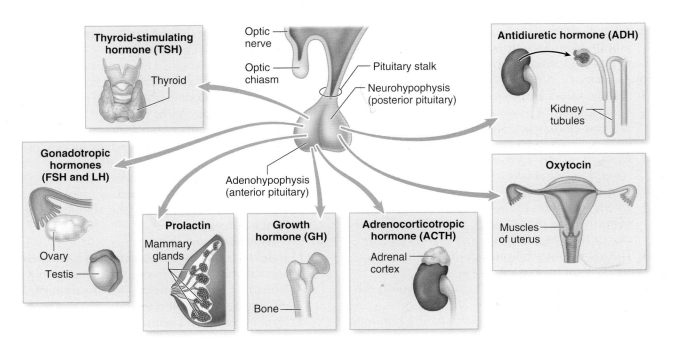

FIGURE 43.1 Pituitary Hormones. *FSH,* Follicle-stimulating hormone; *LH,* luteinizing hormone.

> **BOX 43.5** **Adrenal Cortex**
>
> **Glucocorticoids: Cortisol, Cortisone, Corticosterone**
> Responsible for glucose metabolism, protein metabolism, fluid and electrolyte balance, suppression of the inflammatory response to injury, protective immune response to invasion by infectious agents, and resistance to stress
>
> **Mineralocorticoids: Aldosterone**
> Regulation of electrolyte balance by promoting sodium retention and potassium excretion

  b. Agents that normally induce a suppressed response are administered to determine whether normal negative feedback is intact.
  c. Failure of hormone production to be suppressed during standardized testing indicates hyperfunction.
 3. Overnight dexamethasone suppression test
  a. Used to distinguish between Cushing's syndrome and Cushing's disease
  b. In Cushing's disease, the source of excess cortisol is the pituitary gland rather than the adrenal cortex or exogenous corticosteroid administration.
  c. Dexamethasone, a potent long-acting corticosteroid given at bedtime, would suppress morning cortisol in clients without Cushing's disease by suppressing adrenocorticotropic hormone (ACTH) production; in the client with Cushing's disease, this suppression will not occur.
B. Radioactive iodine uptake
 1. This thyroid function test measures the absorption of an iodine isotope to determine how the thyroid gland is functioning.
 2. A small dose of radioactive iodine is given by mouth or intravenously; the amount of radioactivity is measured in 4 to 6 hours and again at 24 hours.
 3. Normal values are 3% to 10% at 2 to 4 hours and 8% to 25% at 24 hours. Some testing centers only measure at 24 hours. Values may vary depending on the client's iodine intake.
 4. Elevated values indicate hyperthyroidism, decreased iodine intake, or increased iodine excretion.
 5. Decreased values indicate a low T_4 level, the use of antithyroid medications, thyroiditis, myxedema, or hypothyroidism.
 6. The test is contraindicated during pregnancy.
C. T_3 and T_4 resin uptake test
 1. Blood tests are used to diagnose thyroid problems.
 2. T_3 and T_4 regulate thyroid-stimulating hormone (TSH).

 3. Normal values (normal findings vary between laboratory settings)
  a. Triiodothyronine, total T3: 70 ng/dL to 205 ng/dL
  b. Thyroxine, total T4: 5 mcg/dL to 12.0 mcg/dL
  c. Thyroxine, free (FT4): 0.8 ng/dL to 2.8 ng/dL
 4. The T_3 level is elevated in hyperthyroidism, decreases with the aging process, and may be decreased in hypothyroidism.
 5. The T_4 level is elevated in hyperthyroidism and decreased in hypothyroidism.
D. Thyroid-stimulating hormone
 1. Blood test is used to differentiate the diagnosis of primary hypothyroidism.
 2. Normal value is 2 to 10 mcU/L.
 3. Elevated values indicate primary hypothyroidism.
 4. Decreased values indicate hyperthyroidism or secondary hypothyroidism.
E. Thyroid scan
 1. A thyroid scan is performed to identify nodules or growths in the thyroid gland.
 2. A radioisotope of iodine or technetium is administered before scanning the thyroid gland.
 3. Reassure the client that the level of radioactive medication is not dangerous to self or others.
 4. Determine whether the client has received radiographic contrast agents within the past 3 months because these may invalidate the scan.
 5. Check with the primary health care provider (PHCP) regarding discontinuing medications that contain iodine for 14 days before the test and the need to discontinue thyroid medication before the test; check for allergy to iodine.
 6. Reinforce instructions to the client to maintain NPO (nothing by mouth) status after midnight on the day before the test; if iodine is used, the client will fast for an additional 45 minutes after the ingestion of the oral isotope, and the scan will be performed in 24 hours.
 7. If technetium is used, it is administered by the intravenous (IV) route 30 minutes before the scan.
 8. The test is contraindicated during pregnancy and in those with an iodine allergy.
F. Needle aspiration of thyroid tissue
 1. Aspiration of thyroid tissue is done for cytological examination.
 2. No client preparation is necessary; NPO status may or may not be prescribed.
 3. Light pressure is applied to the aspiration site after the procedure.
G. Glycosylated hemoglobin
 1. HgbA1C is blood glucose bound to hemoglobin.
 2. Hemoglobin A1c (glycosylated hemoglobin A; HbA_{1c}) is a reflection of how well blood glucose levels have been controlled for the past 3 to 4 months.
 3. Hyperglycemia in clients with diabetes is usually a cause of an increase in HbA1c.

BOX 43.6 **Pituitary Gland Problems**

Anterior Pituitary
- Hyperpituitarism
- Hypopituitarism

Posterior Pituitary
These problems can be caused by damage to the posterior pituitary or hypothalamus:
- Diabetes insipidus
- Syndrome of inappropriate antidiuretic hormone secretion (SIADH)

---

4. Fasting is not required before the test.

5. Normal reference intervals: 4.0% to 6%, depending on physician preference

6. HgbA1C and estimated average glucose (eAG): Refer to Table 10.3 for these reference intervals.

⚠ Poor glycemic control in a client with diabetes mellitus is usually the cause of an increase in the HbA1c value. An HbA1c level greater than 7.0% is considered poor glycemic control.

H. 24-hour urine collection for vanillylmandelic acid (VMA)

1. Diagnostic tests for pheochromocytoma include a 24-hour urine collection for VMA—a product of catecholamine metabolism, metanephrine, and catecholamines—all of which are elevated in the presence of pheochromocytoma.

2. The normal range of urinary catecholamines:
  a. Epinephrine: <20 mcg/day
  b. Norepinephrine: <100 mcg/day

III. Pituitary Gland Problems (Box 43.6)

A. Hypopituitarism

1. Description: Hyposecretion of one or more of the pituitary hormones caused by tumors, trauma, encephalitis, autoimmunity, or stroke

2. Hormones most often affected are growth hormone (GH) and the gonadotropins (luteinizing hormone, follicle-stimulating hormone), but TSH, ACTH, or antidiuretic hormone (ADH) may be involved.

3. Data collection
  a. Mild to moderate obesity (GH, TSH)
  b. Reduced cardiac output (GH, ADH)
  c. Infertility and sexual dysfunction (gonadotropins, ACTH)
  d. Fatigue, low blood pressure (TSH, ADH, ACTH, GH)
  e. Tumors of the pituitary also may cause headache and visual defects (pituitary is located near the optic nerve).

4. Interventions
  a. Client may need hormone replacement for the specific deficient hormones.

b. Provide emotional support to the client and family.

c. Encourage the client and family to express feelings related to disturbed body image or sexual dysfunction.

d. Reinforce client education regarding the signs/symptoms of both hypofunction and hyperfunction related to insufficient or excess hormone replacement.

B. Hyperpituitarism (Acromegaly)

1. Description: Hypersecretion of GH by the anterior pituitary gland in an adult; caused primarily by pituitary tumors

2. Data collection
  a. Large hands and feet
  b. Thickening and protrusion of the jaw
  c. Arthritic changes and joint pain; impingement syndromes
  d. Visual disturbance
  e. Diaphoresis
  f. Oily, rough skin
  g. Organomegaly
  h. Hypertension atherosclerosis, cardiomegaly, heart failure
  i. Dysphagia
  j. Deepening of the voice
  k. Thickening of the tongue, narrowing of the airway, sleep apnea
  l. Hyperglycemia
  m. Colon polyps, increased colon cancer risk

3. Interventions
  a. Provide pharmacological interventions to suppress GH or block the action of GH.
  b. Prepare the client for radiation of the pituitary gland or for stereotactic radiosurgery, if prescribed.
  c. Prepare the client for hypophysectomy if planned.
  d. Provide pharmacological and nonpharmacological interventions for joint pain.
  e. Provide emotional support to the client and family, and encourage the client and family to express feelings related to disturbed body image.

C. Hypophysectomy (pituitary adenectomy, sublabial transsphenoidal pituitary surgery)

1. Description
  a. The removal of the pituitary tumor via craniotomy or via sublabial transsphenoidal (endoscopic transnasal) approach (the latter approach is preferred because it is associated with fewer complications).
  b. Complications for craniotomy include increased intracranial pressure, bleeding, meningitis, and hypopituitarism.
  c. Complications for the sublabial transsphenoidal surgery include cerebrospinal fluid leak,

infection, diabetes insipidus, and hypopituitarism.

    d. If the sublabial approach is used, an incision is made along the gum line of the inner upper lip.

2. Postoperative interventions

    a. Initiate postoperative care similar to craniotomy care.

    b. Monitor vital signs, neurological status, and level of consciousness.

    c. Elevate the head of the bed.

    d. Monitor for increased intracranial pressure.

    e. Reinforce instructions to the client to avoid sneezing, coughing, and blowing the nose.

    f. Monitor for bleeding.

    g. Monitor for signs of temporary diabetes insipidus; monitor intake and output and report excessive urinary output.

    h. If the entire pituitary is removed, clients will require lifelong replacement of ADH, cortisol, and thyroid hormone.

    i. Monitor for and report signs of infection and meningitis.

    j. Administer antibiotics, analgesics, and antipyretics as prescribed.

    k. Administer oral mouth rinse as prescribed. Clients may be instructed to avoid using a toothbrush or to brush teeth gently with an ultra-soft toothbrush for 10 days to 2 weeks after surgery.

    l. Reinforce instructions to the client regarding the administration of prescribed medications.

⚠ After transsphenoidal hypophysectomy, monitor for and report postnasal drip or clear nasal drainage, which might indicate a cerebrospinal fluid leak. Clear drainage needs to be checked for glucose.

D. Diabetes insipidus

  1. Description

    a. Hyposecretion of ADH caused by stroke, surgery, or trauma, or may be idiopathic

    b. The kidney tubules fail to reabsorb water.

    c. In central diabetes insipidus, there is decreased ADH production.

    d. In nephrogenic diabetes insipidus, ADH production is adequate but the kidneys do not respond appropriately to the ADH.

  2. Data collection

    a. Excretion of large amounts of dilute urine

    b. Polydipsia

    c. Dehydration (decreased skin turgor and dry mucous membranes)

    d. Inability to concentrate urine

    e. A low urinary specific gravity; normal is 1.003 to 1.030

    f. Fatigue

    g. Muscle pain and weakness

    h. Headache

    i. Postural hypotension that may progress to vascular collapse without rehydration

    j. Tachycardia

  3. Interventions

    a. Monitor vital signs and the client's neurological and cardiovascular status.

    b. Provide a safe environment particularly for the client with postural hypotension.

    c. Monitor electrolyte values and for signs of dehydration.

    d. Maintain client intake of adequate fluids; IV hypotonic saline may be prescribed to replace urinary losses.

    e. Monitor intake and output, weight, serum osmolality, and specific gravity of urine for excessive urinary output, weight loss, and low urinary specific gravity.

    f. Reinforce instructions to the client to avoid foods or liquids that produce diuresis.

    g. Vasopressin tannate or desmopressin acetate may be prescribed; these are used when the ADH deficiency is severe or chronic.

    h. Reinforce instructions to the client regarding the administration of medications as prescribed; desmopressin acetate may be administered by subcutaneous injection, intravenously, intranasally, or orally; watch for signs of water intoxication indicating overtreatment.

    i. Reinforce instructions to the client to wear a Medic-Alert bracelet.

E. Syndrome of inappropriate antidiuretic hormone secretion (SIADH)

  1. Description

    a. Condition of hyperfunctioning of the posterior pituitary gland in which excess ADH is released, but not in response to the body's need for it.

    b. Causes include trauma, stroke, malignancy (often in the lungs or pancreas), medication, and stress.

    c. The syndrome results in increased intravascular volume, water intoxication, and dilutional hyponatremia.

    d. May cause cerebral edema and the client is at risk for seizures.

  2. Data collection

    a. Signs of fluid volume overload

    b. Change in the level of consciousness and the client's mental status

    c. Weight gain without edema

    d. Hypertension

    e. Tachycardia

    f. Anorexia, nausea, vomiting

    g. Hyponatremia

    h. Low urinary output and concentrated urine

BOX 43.7 Adrenal Gland Problems

Adrenal Cortex
- Addison's disease
- Primary hyperaldosteronism (Conn's syndrome)
- Cushing's disease
- Cushing's syndrome

Adrenal Medulla
- Pheochromocytoma

TABLE 43.1 Data Collection: Addison's Disease and Cushing's Disease (Cushing's Syndrome)

Addison's Disease	Cushing's Disease and Syndrome
Lethargy, fatigue, and muscle weakness	Generalized muscle wasting and weakness
Gastrointestinal disturbances	Moon face, buffalo hump
Weight loss	Truncal obesity with thin extremities, supraclavicular fat pads; weight gain
Menstrual changes in women; impotence in men	Hirsutism (masculine characteristics in females)
Hypoglycemia, hyponatremia	Hyperglycemia, hypernatremia
Hyperkalemia, hypercalcemia	Hypokalemia, hypocalcemia
Postural hypotension	Hypertension
Hyperpigmentation of the skin (bronzed) with primary disease	Fragile skin that easily bruises; reddish-purple striae on the abdomen and upper thighs

3. Interventions
   a. Monitor vital signs and cardiac and neurological status.
   b. Provide a safe environment, particularly for the client with a change in their level of consciousness or mental status.
   c. Monitor for signs of increased intracranial pressure.
   d. Implement seizure precautions.
   e. Elevate the head of the bed a maximum of 10 degrees to promote venous return and decrease baroreceptor-induced ADH release.
   f. Monitor intake and output and obtain weight daily.
   g. Monitor fluid and electrolyte balance.
   h. Monitor the serum and urine osmolality.
   i. Restrict fluid intake as prescribed.
   j. Assist to administer diuretics and IV fluids (usually normal saline [NS] or hypertonic saline) as prescribed; monitor IV fluids carefully because of the risk for fluid volume overload.
   k. Loop diuretics may be prescribed to promote diuresis, but only if serum sodium is at least 125 mEq/L; potassium replacement may be necessary if loop diuretics are prescribed.
   l. Vasopressin antagonists may be prescribed to decrease the renal response to ADH.

IV. Adrenal Gland Problems (Box 43.7)

A. Adrenal cortex insufficiency (Addison's disease)
   1. Primary adrenal insufficiency
      a. Also known as Addison's disease, refers to hyposecretion of adrenal cortex hormones (glucocorticoids, mineralocorticoids, and androgen); autoimmune destruction is a common cause.
      b. Requires lifelong replacement of glucocorticoids and possibly of mineralocorticoids, if significant hyposecretion occurs; the condition is fatal if left untreated.
   2. Secondary adrenal insufficiency is caused by hyposecretion of ACTH from the anterior pituitary gland; mineralocorticoid release is spared.

3. Loss of glucocorticoids in Addison's disease leads to decreased vascular tone, decreased vascular response to the catecholamines epinephrine and norepinephrine, and decreased gluconeogenesis.
4. In Addison's disease, loss of the mineralocorticoid aldosterone leads to dehydration, hypotension, hyponatremia, and hyperkalemia.
5. Data collection (Table 43.1)
6. Interventions

   a. Monitor vital signs (particularly for hypotension), for weight loss, and intake and output.
   b. Monitor white blood cell (WBC) count; blood glucose; and potassium, sodium, and calcium levels.
   c. Administer glucocorticoid or mineralocorticoid medications as prescribed.
   d. Observe for Addisonian crisis caused by stress, infection, trauma, or surgery.
7. Reinforce client education
   a. Need for lifelong glucocorticoid replacement and possible lifelong mineralocorticoid replacement
   b. Corticosteroid replacement will need to be increased during times of stress.
   c. Avoid individuals with an infection.
   d. Avoid strenuous exercise and stressful situations.
   e. Avoid over-the-counter medications.
   f. Diet needs to be high in protein and carbohydrates; clients taking glucocorticoids would be prescribed calcium and vitamin D supplements to protect against corticosteroid-induced osteoporosis; some clients taking mineralocorticoids may be prescribed a diet high in sodium.

> **BOX 43.8   Addisonian Crisis**
>
> ▪ A life-threatening disorder caused by acute adrenal insufficiency
> ▪ Precipitated by stress, infection, trauma, surgery, or abrupt withdrawal of exogenous corticosteroid use
> ▪ Can cause hyponatremia, hyperkalemia, hypoglycemia, and shock

    g. Wear a MedicAlert bracelet.

    h. Report signs and symptoms of complications such as underreplacement and overreplacement of corticosteroid hormones.

B. Addisonian crisis

  1. Description (Box 43.8)

  2. Data collection

    a. Severe headache

    b. Severe abdominal, leg, and lower back pain

    c. Generalized weakness

    d. Irritability and confusion

    e. Severe hypotension

    f. Shock

  3. Interventions

    a. Prepare to assist the registered nurse (RN) with the administration of IV glucocorticoids, as prescribed.

    b. Prepare to assist the RN with the administration of IV fluids to replace fluids and restore electrolyte balance.

    c. Following resolution of the crisis, administer glucocorticoids and mineralocorticoids orally, as prescribed.

    d. Monitor vital signs, particularly blood pressure.

    e. Monitor neurological status, noting irritability and confusion.

    f. Monitor intake and output.

    g. Monitor laboratory values, particularly sodium, potassium, and blood glucose levels.

    h. Protect the client from infection.

    i. Maintain bed rest and provide a quiet environment.

⚠ Clients taking exogenous corticosteroids need to establish a plan with their PHCP or endocrinologist for increasing their corticosteroids during times of stress.

C. Cushing's syndrome and Cushing's disease (hypercortisolism)

  1. Cushing's syndrome

    a. A metabolic disorder resulting from the chronic and excessive production of cortisol by the adrenal cortex or from the administration of glucocorticoids in large doses for several weeks or longer (exogenous or iatrogenic)

    b. ACTH secreting tumors (most often of the lung, pancreas, or GI tract) can cause Cushing's syndrome.

  2. Cushing's disease is a metabolic disorder characterized by the abnormally increased secretion (endogenous) of cortisol, caused by increased amounts of ACTH secreted by the pituitary gland.

  3. Data collection (see Table 43.1)

  4. Interventions

    a. Monitor vital signs, particularly blood pressure.

    b. Monitor intake and output and weight.

    c. Monitor laboratory values, particularly WBC count, and serum glucose, sodium, potassium, and calcium.

    d. Prepare to assist the RN with the administration of chemotherapeutic agents as prescribed, for inoperable adrenal tumors.

    e. Prepare the client for radiation, as prescribed, if the condition results from a pituitary adenoma.

    f. Prepare the client for the removal of pituitary tumor (hypophysectomy, sublabial transsphenoidal adenectomy), if the condition results from the increased pituitary secretion of ACTH.

    g. Prepare the client for adrenalectomy, if the condition results from an adrenal adenoma; glucocorticoid replacement may be required following adrenalectomy.

    h. Clients requiring lifelong glucocorticoid replacement following adrenalectomy need to obtain instructions from their PHCP about increasing their glucocorticoid prescription during times of stress.

    i. Assess for and protect against postoperative thrombus formation; Cushing's syndrome predisposes to thromboemboli.

    j. Allow the client to discuss feelings related to body appearance.

    k. Instruct the client about the need to wear a MedicAlert bracelet.

⚠ Addison's disease is characterized by the hyposecretion of adrenal cortex hormones (glucocorticoids and mineralocorticoids), whereas Cushing's disease is characterized by a hypersecretion of glucocorticoids.

D. Primary hyperaldosteronism (Conn's syndrome)

  1. Description

    a. Hypersecretion of mineralocorticoids (aldosterone) from the adrenal cortex of the adrenal gland

    b. Most commonly caused by an adenoma

    c. Excess secretion of aldosterone causes sodium and water retention and potassium excretion, leading to hypertension and hypokalemic alkalosis.

2. Data collection
   a. Symptoms related to hypokalemia, hypernatremia, and hypertension
   b. Headache, fatigue, muscle weakness
   c. Cardiac dysrhythmia
   d. Paresthesia, tetany
   e. Change in vision
   f. Glucose intolerance
   g. Elevated serum aldosterone level
3. Interventions
   a. Monitor vital signs, particularly blood pressure.
   b. Monitor for signs of hypokalemia and hypernatremia.
   c. Monitor intake and output and urine for specific gravity.
   d. Monitor for hyperkalemia, particularly for clients with impaired renal function or excessive potassium intake because potassium-retaining diuretics and aldosterone antagonists may be prescribed to promote fluid balance and control hypertension.
   e. Administer potassium supplements, as prescribed, to treat hypokalemia; clients taking potassium-sparing diuretics and potassium supplementation are at risk for hyperkalemia.
   f. Prepare the client for adrenalectomy.
   g. Maintain sodium restriction, if prescribed, preoperatively.
   h. Administer glucocorticoids preoperatively, as prescribed, to prevent adrenal hypofunction and prepare for the stress of surgery.
   i. Monitor the client for adrenal insufficiency postoperatively.
   j. Reinforce instructions to the client regarding the need for glucocorticoid therapy after adrenalectomy.
   k. Reinforce instructions to the client about the need to wear a Medic-Alert bracelet.
E. Pheochromocytoma
1. Description
   a. Catecholamine-producing tumor usually found in the adrenal medulla, but extra-adrenal locations include the chest, bladder, abdomen, and brain; typically a benign tumor, but can be malignant
   b. Excessive amounts of epinephrine and norepinephrine are secreted.
   c. Diagnostic tests include a 24-hour urine collection for VMA.
   d. Surgical removal of the adrenal gland is the primary treatment.
   e. Symptomatic treatment is initiated if surgical removal is not possible.
   f. The complications associated with pheochromocytoma include hypertensive crisis, hypertensive retinopathy and nephropathy, cardiac enlargement and dysrhythmia, heart failure,

myocardial infarction, increased platelet aggregation, and stroke.
   g. Death can occur from shock, stroke, renal failure, dysrhythmia, or dissecting aortic aneurysm.
2. Data collection
   a. Paroxysmal or sustained hypertension
   b. Severe headache
   c. Palpitations
   d. Flushing and profuse diaphoresis
   e. Pain in the chest or abdomen with nausea and vomiting
   f. Heat intolerance
   g. Weight loss
   h. Tremors
   i. Hyperglycemia
3. Interventions
   a. Monitor vital signs, particularly blood pressure and heart rate.
   b. Monitor for hypertensive crisis; monitor for complications that can occur with hypertensive crisis such as stroke, cardiac dysrhythmia, and myocardial infarction.
   c. Reinforce instructions to the client not to smoke, drink caffeine-containing beverages, or change position suddenly.
   d. Prepare to administer a β-adrenergic blocking agent, as prescribed, to control hypertension; α-adrenergic blocking agents are started 7 to 10 days before β-adrenergic blocking agents.
   e. Monitor serum glucose level.
   f. Promote rest and a nonstressful environment.
   g. Provide a diet high in calories, vitamins, and minerals.
   h. Prepare the client for adrenalectomy.

 For the client with pheochromocytoma, avoid stimuli that can precipitate a hypertensive crisis, such as increased abdominal pressure and vigorous abdominal palpation.

F. Adrenalectomy
1. Description (Box 43.9)
2. Preoperative interventions
   a. Monitor electrolyte levels and correct electrolyte imbalances.
   b. Monitor for dysrhythmia.
   c. Monitor for hyperglycemia.
   d. Protect the client from infection.
   e. Administer glucocorticoids, as prescribed.
3. Postoperative interventions
   a. Monitor vital signs.
   b. Monitor intake and output; if the urinary output is less than 30 mL/hr, notify the RN because this may indicate acute kidney injury and impending shock. IV fluids will be prescribed to maintain blood volume.
   c. Monitor weight daily.
   d. Monitor electrolyte and serum glucose levels.

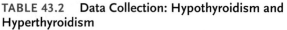

BOX 43.9 **Adrenalectomy**

Surgical removal of an adrenal gland
Lifelong glucocorticoid and mineralocorticoid replacement is necessary with bilateral adrenalectomy.
Temporary glucocorticoid replacement, usually up to 2 years, is necessary after a unilateral adrenalectomy.
Catecholamine levels drop as a result of surgery, which can result in cardiovascular collapse, hypotension, and shock, and the client needs to be monitored closely.
Hemorrhage also can occur because of the high vascularity of the adrenal glands.

TABLE 43.2 **Data Collection: Hypothyroidism and Hyperthyroidism**

Hypothyroidism	Hyperthyroidism
Lethargy and fatigue	Change in personality, such as irritability, agitation, and mood swings
Weakness, muscle aches, paresthesia	Nervousness and fine tremors of the hands
Intolerance to cold	Heat intolerance
Weight gain	Weight loss
Dry skin and hair and loss of body hair	Smooth, soft skin and hair
Bradycardia	Palpitations, cardiac dysrhythmias such as tachycardia or atrial fibrillation
Constipation	Diarrhea
Generalized puffiness and edema around the eyes and face (myxedema)	Protruding eyeballs (exophthalmos) may be present
Forgetfulness and loss of memory	Diaphoresis
Menstrual disturbances	Hypertension
Goiter may or may not be present	Enlarged thyroid gland (goiter)
Cardiac enlargement, tendency to develop heart failure	

   e. Monitor for signs of hemorrhage and shock particularly during the first 24 to 48 hours.
   f. Monitor for manifestations of adrenal insufficiency (see Table 43.1).
   g. Check the dressing for drainage.
   h. Monitor for paralytic ileus.
   i. Administer glucocorticoids and mineralocorticoids, as prescribed.
   j. Administer pain medication as prescribed.
   k. Provide pulmonary interventions to prevent atelectasis (coughing, deep breathing, incentive spirometry, splinting of incision).
   l. Reinforce instructions to the client regarding the importance of hormone replacement therapy following surgery.
  m. Reinforce instructions to the client regarding the signs and symptoms of complications, such as underreplacement and overreplacement of hormones.
   n. Reinforce instructions to the client regarding the need to wear a Medic-Alert bracelet.

V. Thyroid Gland Problems

A. Hypothyroidism
  1. Description
    a. Hypothyroid state resulting from hyposecretion of thyroid hormones and characterized by a decreased rate of body metabolism
    b. The T4 is low and the TSH is elevated.
    c. In primary hypothyroidism, the source of dysfunction is the thyroid gland, and the thyroid cannot produce the necessary amount of hormones. In secondary hypothyroidism, the thyroid is not being stimulated by the pituitary to produce hormones.
  2. Data collection (Table 43.2)
  3. Interventions
    a. Monitor vital signs, including heart rate and rhythm.
    b. Administer thyroid replacement; levothyroxine sodium is most commonly prescribed.

    c. Reinforce instructions to the client about thyroid replacement therapy and about the clinical manifestations of both hypothyroidism and hyperthyroidism related to underreplacement or overreplacement of the hormone.
    d. Reinforce instructions to the client to consume a low-calorie, low-cholesterol, and low-saturated fat diet; discuss a daily exercise program such as walking.
    e. Monitor the client for constipation; provide roughage and fluids to prevent constipation.
    f. Provide a warm environment for the client.
    g. Avoid sedatives and opioid analgesics because of increased sensitivity to these medications; may precipitate myxedema coma.
    h. Monitor for overdose of thyroid medications characterized by tachycardia, chest pain, restlessness, nervousness, and insomnia.
    i. Reinforce instructions to the client to immediately report episodes of chest pain or other signs of overdose.

B. Myxedema coma
  1. Description (Box 43.10)
  2. Data collection
    a. Hypotension
    b. Bradycardia
    c. Hypothermia
    d. Hyponatremia

This rare but serious disorder results from persistently low thyroid production.

Coma can be precipitated by acute illness, rapid withdrawal of thyroid medication, anesthesia and surgery, hypothermia, or the use of sedatives and opioid analgesics.

This acute and life-threatening condition occurs in a client with uncontrollable hyperthyroidism.

It can be caused by manipulation of the thyroid gland during surgery and the release of thyroid hormone into the bloodstream; it also can occur from severe infection and stress.

Antithyroid medications, β-blockers, glucocorticoids, and iodides may be administered to the client before thyroid surgery to prevent its occurrence.

   e. Hypoglycemia
   f. Generalized edema
   g. Respiratory failure
   h. Coma
3. Interventions
   a. Maintain a patent airway.
   b. Institute aspiration precautions.
   c. Monitor IV fluids (normal or hypertonic saline), as prescribed.
   d. Assist RN with the administration of IV levothyroxine sodium, as prescribed.
   e. Assist RN with the administration of IV glucose, as prescribed.
   f. Administer corticosteroids, as prescribed.
   g. Monitor the client's temperature hourly.
   h. Monitor blood pressure frequently.
   i. Keep the client warm.
   j. Monitor for any change in mental status.
   k. Monitor electrolyte and glucose levels.

C. Hyperthyroidism
1. Description
   a. Hyperthyroid state resulting from the hypersecretion of thyroid hormones T_3 and T_4
   b. Characterized by an increased rate of body metabolism
   c. A common cause is Graves' disease, also known as toxic diffuse goiter.
   d. Clinical manifestations are referred to as *thyrotoxicosis.*
   e. T_3 and T_4 are usually elevated and TSH level is low.
2. Data collection (see Table 43.2)
3. Interventions
   a. Provide adequate rest.
   b. Administer sedatives as prescribed.
   c. Provide a cool and quiet environment.
   d. Obtain weight daily.
   e. Provide a high-calorie diet.
   f. Avoid the administration of stimulants.
   g. Administer antithyroid medications, such as methimazole or propylthiouracil, that block thyroid synthesis, as prescribed.
   h. Administer iodine preparations that inhibit the release of thyroid hormone, as prescribed.
   i. Administer propranolol for tachycardia as prescribed.
   j. Prepare the client for radioactive iodine therapy, as prescribed, to destroy thyroid cells.

   k. Prepare the client for subtotal thyroidectomy, if prescribed.
   l. Elevate the head of the bed of a client experiencing exophthalmos; in addition, instruct on a low-salt diet, administer artificial tears, encourage the use of dark glasses, and tape eyelids closed at night if necessary.
   m. Allow the client to express concerns about changes in their body image.
D. Thyroid storm
1. Description (Box 43.11)
2. Data collection
   a. Elevated temperature (fever)
   b. Tachycardia
   c. Systolic hypertension
   d. Nausea, vomiting, diarrhea
   e. Agitation, tremors, anxiety
   f. Irritability, agitation, restlessness, confusion, and seizure as the condition progresses
   g. Delirium and coma
3. Interventions
   a. Maintain a patent airway and adequate ventilation.
   b. Administer antithyroid medications, sodium iodide solution, propranolol, and glucocorticoids as prescribed.
   c. Monitor vital signs.
   d. Monitor continually for cardiac dysrhythmia.
   e. Administer nonsalicylate antipyretics as prescribed (salicylates increase free thyroid hormone levels).
   f. Use a cooling blanket to decrease the client's temperature as prescribed.
E. Thyroidectomy
1. Description
   a. Removal of the thyroid gland
   b. Performed when persistent hyperthyroidism exists
   c. Subtotal thyroidectomy; removal of a portion of the thyroid gland is the preferred surgical intervention.
2. Preoperative interventions
   a. Obtain vital signs and weight.
   b. Monitor electrolyte levels.
   c. Monitor for hyperglycemia.

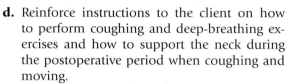

BOX 43.12 **Signs of Tetany**

- Cardiac dysrhythmia
- Carpopedal spasm
- Dysphagia
- Muscle and abdominal cramps
- Numbness and tingling of the face and extremities
- Positive Chvostek's sign
- Positive Trousseau's sign
- Visual disturbance (photophobia)
- Wheezing and dyspnea (bronchospasm, laryngospasm)
- Seizure

d. Reinforce instructions to the client on how to perform coughing and deep-breathing exercises and how to support the neck during the postoperative period when coughing and moving.

e. Assist to administer antithyroid medications, iodides, propranolol, and glucocorticoids as prescribed to prevent the occurrence of thyroid storm.

3. Postoperative interventions

a. Monitor for respiratory distress.

b. Have a tracheotomy set, oxygen, and suction at the bedside.

c. Limit client talking and determine the level of hoarseness.

d. Avoid neck flexion and stress on the suture line.

e. Monitor for laryngeal nerve damage as evidenced by respiratory obstruction, dysphonia, high-pitched voice, stridor, dysphagia, and restlessness.

f. Monitor for signs of hypocalcemia and tetany, which can be the result of trauma to the parathyroid gland (Box 43.12).

g. Assist RN to administer calcium gluconate as prescribed for tetany.

h. Monitor for thyroid storm.

⚠ After thyroidectomy, maintain the client in a semi-Fowler's position. Monitor the surgical site for edema and for signs of bleeding, and check the dressing anteriorly and at the back of the neck. Monitor for inflammation, which could block the airway. An emergency tracheostomy kit must be at the bedside.

VI. Parathyroid Gland Problems

A. Hypoparathyroidism

1. Description

a. Condition caused by hyposecretion of PTH by the parathyroid gland

b. Can occur following thyroidectomy because of the removal of parathyroid tissue

2. Data collection

a. Hypocalcemia and hyperphosphatemia

b. Numbness and tingling in the face

c. Muscle cramps and cramps in the abdomen or in the extremities

d. Positive Trousseau's sign or Chvostek's sign

e. Signs of overt tetany such as bronchospasm, laryngospasm, carpopedal spasm, dysphagia, photophobia, cardiac dysrhythmia, and seizure

f. Hypotension

g. Anxiety, irritability, depression

3. Interventions

a. Monitor vital signs.

b. Monitor for signs of hypocalcemia and tetany.

c. Initiate seizure precautions.

d. Place a tracheotomy set, oxygen, and suction at the bedside.

e. Assist RN with the administration of IV calcium gluconate for hypocalcemia.

f. Provide a high-calcium, low-phosphorus diet.

g. Reinforce instructions to the client regarding the administration of calcium supplements as prescribed.

h. Reinforce instructions to the client regarding the administration of vitamin D supplements as prescribed; vitamin D enhances the absorption of calcium from the GI tract.

i. Reinforce instructions to the client regarding the administration of phosphate binders, as prescribed, to promote the excretion of phosphate through the GI tract.

j. Reinforce instructions to the client in the use of thiazide diuretics, if prescribed, to protect the kidney if vitamin D is also taken.

k. Reinforce instructions to the client to wear a MedicAlert bracelet.

B. Hyperparathyroidism

1. Description: Condition caused by the hypersecretion of PTH by the parathyroid gland

2. Data collection

a. Hypercalcemia and hypophosphatemia

b. Fatigue and muscle weakness

c. Skeletal pain and tenderness

d. Bone deformities that result in pathological fractures

e. Anorexia, nausea, vomiting, epigastric pain

f. Weight loss

g. Constipation

h. Hypertension

i. Cardiac dysrhythmia

j. Renal stones

3. Interventions

a. Monitor vital signs, particularly blood pressure.

b. Monitor for cardiac dysrhythmia.

c. Monitor intake and output and for signs of renal stones.

d. Monitor for skeletal pain; move the client slowly and carefully.

e. Encourage fluid intake.

f. Administer furosemide, as prescribed, to lower calcium levels.

g. Normal saline may be prescribed intravenously to maintain hydration.

h. Assist with the administration of phosphates, which interfere with calcium reabsorption, as prescribed.

i. Assist to administer calcitonin, as prescribed, to decrease skeletal calcium release and increase renal excretion of calcium.

j. Assist with the administration of IV or oral bisphosphonates to inhibit bone resorption.

k. Monitor calcium and phosphorus levels.

l. Prepare the client for parathyroidectomy, as prescribed.

m. Encourage a high-fiber, moderate-calcium diet.

n. Emphasize the importance of an exercise program and avoiding prolonged inactivity.

C. Parathyroidectomy

1. Description: The removal of one or more of the parathyroid glands

    a. Endoscopic radioguided parathyroidectomy with autotransplantation is the most common procedure.

    b. Parathyroid tissue is transplanted in the forearm or near the sternocleidomastoid muscle allowing PTH secretion to continue.

2. Preoperative interventions

    a. Monitor electrolytes, calcium, phosphate, and magnesium levels.

    b. Ensure that calcium levels are decreased to near-normal values.

    c. Inform the client that talking may be painful for the first day or two after surgery.

3. Postoperative interventions

    a. Monitor for respiratory distress.

    b. Place a tracheotomy set, oxygen, and suction at the bedside.

    c. Monitor vital signs.

    d. Position the client in a semi-Fowler's position.

    e. Check the neck dressing for bleeding.

    f. Monitor for hypocalcemic crisis as evidenced by tingling and twitching in the extremities and face.

    g. Monitor for positive Trousseau's sign or Chvostek's sign, which signals the potential for tetany.

    h. Monitor for changes in voice pattern and hoarseness.

    i. Monitor for laryngeal nerve damage.

    j. Reinforce instructions to the client regarding the administration of calcium and vitamin D supplements as prescribed.

VII. Pancreas Problems

A. Diabetes mellitus

1. Description

    a. Chronic disorder of impaired carbohydrate, protein, and lipid metabolism caused by a deficiency of insulin

    b. An absolute or relative deficiency of insulin results in hyperglycemia.

    c. Type 1 diabetes mellitus is a nearly absolute deficiency of insulin (primary beta cell destruction); if insulin is not given, fats are metabolized for energy, which results in ketonemia (acidosis).

    d. Type 2 diabetes mellitus refers to a relative lack of insulin or resistance to the action of insulin; usually insulin is sufficient to stabilize fat and protein metabolism, but not carbohydrate metabolism.

    e. Metabolic syndrome is also known as syndrome X and the individual has coexisting risk factors for developing type 2 diabetes mellitus; these risk factors include abdominal obesity, hyperglycemia, hypertension, high triglyceride level, and a lowered high-density lipoprotein (HDL) cholesterol level.

    f. Diabetes mellitus can lead to chronic health problems and early death as a result of complications that occur in the large and small blood vessels in tissues and organs.

    g. Macrovascular complications include coronary artery disease, cardiomyopathy, hypertension, cerebrovascular disease, and peripheral vascular disease. (Refer to Chapter 49 for information on cardiovascular problems)

    h. Microvascular complications include retinopathy, nephropathy, and neuropathy.

    i. Infection is also a concern because of reduced healing ability.

    j. Male erectile dysfunction can also occur as a result of the disease.

 Obesity is a major risk factor for diabetes mellitus.

2. Data collection

    a. Polyuria, polydipsia, and polyphagia (more common with type 1 diabetes mellitus)

    b. Hyperglycemia

    c. Weight loss (common with type 1 diabetes mellitus, rare with type 2 diabetes mellitus)

    d. Blurred vision

    e. Slow wound healing

    f. Vaginal infections

    g. Weakness and paresthesia

    h. Signs of inadequate circulation to the feet

    i. Signs of accelerated atherosclerosis (renal, cerebral, cardiac, peripheral)

3. Diet
   a. The diabetic client's diet would take into account weight, medication, activity level, and other health problems.
   b. Day-to-day consistency in timing and amount of food intake helps control the blood glucose level.
   c. As prescribed by the PHCP, the client may be advised to follow the recommendations of the American Diabetic Association diet or US dietary guidelines.
   d. Carbohydrate counting may be a simpler approach for some clients; it focuses on the total grams of carbohydrates eaten per meal. The client may be more compliant with carbohydrate counting resulting in better glycemic control; it is usually necessary for clients using intense insulin therapy.
   e. Incorporate the diet into individual client needs, lifestyle, and cultural and socioeconomic patterns.

4. Exercise
   a. Exercise lowers the blood glucose level, encourages weight loss, reduces cardiovascular risks, improves circulation and muscle tone, decreases total cholesterol and triglyceride levels, and decreases insulin resistance and glucose intolerance.
   b. Reinforce instructions to the client regarding dietary adjustments when exercising; dietary adjustments are individualized.
   c. If the client requires extra food during exercise to prevent hypoglycemia, it need not be deducted from the regular meal plan.
   d. If the blood glucose level is greater than 250 mg/dL and urinary ketones (type 1 diabetes mellitus) are present, the client is instructed not to exercise until the blood glucose is closer to normal and urinary ketones are absent.
   e. The client should try to exercise at the same time each day and would exercise when glucose from the meal is peaking, not when insulin or glucose-lowering medications are peaking.
   f. Insulin would not be injected into an area of the body that will be exercised following injection, as exercise speeds absorption.

 Instruct the client with diabetes mellitus to monitor their blood glucose level before, during, and after exercising.

5. Oral hypoglycemic medications: Oral medications are prescribed for clients with type 2 diabetes mellitus when diet and weight control therapy have failed to maintain satisfactory blood glucose levels (see Chapter 44).

6. Insulin (refer to Chapter 44 for additional information on insulin)
   a. Insulin is used to treat type 1 diabetes mellitus and may be used to treat type 2 diabetes mellitus when diet, weight-control therapy, and oral hypoglycemic agents have failed to maintain satisfactory blood glucose levels.
   b. Illness, infection, and stress increase the blood glucose level and the need for insulin; insulin would not be withheld during illness, infection, or stress because hyperglycemia and diabetic ketoacidosis (DKA) can result.
   c. The peak action time of insulin is important to explain to the client because of the possibility of hypoglycemic reactions occurring during that time.

  Regular insulin (U-100 strength) can be administered via IV injection (IV push). Regular insulin (U-100 strength) and the short-duration insulins (lispro, aspart, and glulisine) can be administered via IV infusion.

B. Complications of insulin therapy
   1. Local allergic reactions
      a. Redness, swelling, tenderness, and induration or a wheal at the site of injection may occur 1 to 2 hours after administration.
      b. Reactions usually occur during the early stages of insulin therapy.
      c. Reinforce instructions to the client to cleanse the skin with alcohol before injection.
   2. Insulin lipodystrophy
      a. The development of fibrous fatty masses at the injection site caused by repeated use of an injection site; use of human insulin helps prevent this.
      b. Reinforce instructions to the client to avoid injecting insulin into affected sites.
      c. Reinforce instructions to the client about the importance of rotating insulin injection sites. Systematic rotation within one anatomical area is recommended to prevent lipodystrophy; the client would be instructed not to use the same site more than once in a 2 to 3 week period. Injections need to be 1 ½ inches (3.8 cm) apart within the anatomical area.
   3. Dawn phenomenon
      a. Dawn phenomenon is characterized by hyperglycemia upon morning awakening that results from excessive early morning release of GH and cortisol.
      b. Treatment requires an increase in the client's insulin dose or a change in the time of insulin administration.
   4. Somogyi phenomenon
      a. Normal or elevated blood glucose levels are present at bedtime; hypoglycemia occurs at about 2:00 a.m. to 3:00 a.m., which causes an

increase in the production of counterregulatory hormones.

b. By 7:00 a.m., in response to the counterregulatory hormones, the blood glucose rebounds significantly to the hyperglycemic range.

c. Treatment includes decreasing the evening (predinner or bedtime) dose of intermediate-acting insulin or increasing the bedtime snack, or both.

d. Clients experiencing the Somogyi phenomenon may complain of early morning headaches, night sweats, or nightmares caused by the early morning hypoglycemia.

C. Insulin administration

1. Subcutaneous injections and mixing insulin (see Chapter 44)

2. Insulin pumps

   a. Continuous subcutaneous insulin infusion is administered by an externally worn device that contains a syringe attached to a long, thin, narrow-lumen tube with a needle or Teflon catheter attached to the end.

   b. The client inserts the needle or Teflon catheter into the subcutaneous tissue (usually on the abdomen or upper arm) and secures it with tape or a transparent dressing; the pump is worn on a belt or in a pocket; the needle or Teflon catheter is changed at least every 2 to 3 days.

   c. A continuous basal rate of insulin infuses; in addition, on the basis of the blood glucose level, the anticipated food intake, and the activity level, the client delivers a bolus of insulin before each meal.

   d. Both rapid-acting and regular short-acting insulin (buffered to prevent the precipitation of insulin crystals within the catheter) are appropriate for use in these pumps.

3. Insulin pump and skin sensor

   a. A skin sensor device can be used to monitor the client's blood glucose continuously; the information is transmitted to the pump, determines the need for insulin, and the insulin is then injected.

   b. The pump holds up to a 3-day supply of insulin and can be easily disconnected for activities such as bathing.

4. Pancreas transplants

   a. The goal of pancreatic transplantation is to halt or reverse the complications of diabetes mellitus.

   b. Transplants are performed on a limited number of clients (in general, those clients who are undergoing kidney transplantation simultaneously).

   c. Immunosuppressive therapy is prescribed to prevent and treat rejection.

BOX 43.13 Client Instructions: Self-Monitoring of Blood Glucose Level

Use the proper procedure to obtain the sample for determining the blood glucose level.

Perform the procedure precisely to obtain accurate results.

Follow the manufacturer's instructions for the glucometer.

Wash hands before and after performing the procedure to prevent infection.

Calibrate the monitor as instructed by the manufacturer.

Check the expiration date on the test strips.

If the blood glucose level results do not seem reasonable, reread the instructions, reassess the technique, check the expiration date of the test strips, and perform the procedure again to verify results.

D. Self-monitoring of blood glucose level

1. Self-monitoring provides the client with the current blood glucose level and information to maintain good glycemic control.

2. Some monitoring devices require a finger prick to obtain a drop of blood for testing; devices are also available that do not require a prick to test for glucose.

3. Alternative site testing (obtaining blood from the forearm, upper arm, abdomen, thigh, or calf) is now available using specific measurement devices.

4. Testing via finger or other site pricks needs to be done with caution in clients with diabetic neuropathy.

5. Client instructions (Box 43.13)

E. Urine testing

1. Urine testing for glucose is not a reliable indicator of blood glucose and is not used for monitoring purposes.

2. Reinforce instructions to the client regarding the procedure for testing urine ketones.

3. The presence of ketones may indicate impending ketoacidosis.

4. Urine ketone testing would be performed during illness and whenever the client with type 1 diabetes mellitus has persistently elevated blood glucose levels (higher than 250 mg/dL or as prescribed for 2 consecutive testing periods).

VIII. **Acute Complications of Diabetes Mellitus**

A. Hypoglycemia

1. Description

   a. Hypoglycemia occurs when the blood glucose level falls below 70 mg/dL or when the blood glucose drops rapidly from an elevated level.

   b. Hypoglycemia is caused by too much insulin or oral hypoglycemic agents, too little food, or excessive activity.

   c. The client needs to be instructed to always carry some form of fast-acting simple carbohydrate with him or her (Box 43.14).

BOX 43.14	Simple Carbohydrates to Treat Hypoglycemia

- Commercially prepared glucose tablets
- 6–10 LifeSavers or hard candy
- 4 tsp of sugar
- 4 sugar cubes
- 1 Tbsp of honey or syrup
- ½ cup of fruit juice or regular (nondiet) soft drink
- 8 oz (235 mL) low-fat milk
- 6 saltine crackers
- 3 graham crackers

BOX 43.15	Data Collection: Hypoglycemia

Mild
- Hunger
- Nervousness
- Palpitations
- Sweating
- Tachycardia
- Tremor

Moderate
- Confusion
- Double vision
- Drowsiness
- Emotional changes
- Headache
- Impaired coordination
- Inability to concentrate
- Irrational or irritable behavior
- Light-headedness
- Numbness of the lips and tongue
- Slurred speech

Severe
- Difficulty arousing
- Disoriented behavior
- Loss of consciousness
- Seizure

d. If the client has a hypoglycemic reaction and does not have any of the recommended emergency foods available, any available food should be eaten; high-fat foods slow the absorption of glucose, and the hypoglycemic symptoms may not resolve quickly.

e. Clients who experience frequent episodes of hypoglycemia, older clients, and clients taking β-adrenergic blocking agents may not experience the warning signs of hypoglycemia until the blood glucose level is dangerously low; this phenomenon is termed *hypoglycemia unawareness*.

2. Data collection (Box 43.15)

    a. Mild hypoglycemia: The client remains fully awake but displays adrenergic symptoms; the blood glucose level is usually lower than 70 mg/dL.

    b. Moderate hypoglycemia: The client displays symptoms of worsening hypoglycemia; the blood glucose level is usually less than 54 mg/dL.

    c. Severe hypoglycemia: Client displays severe neuroglycopenic symptoms; the blood glucose level is usually lower than 40 mg/dL.

⚡ PRIORITY NURSING ACTIONS

Suspected Hypoglycemic Reaction (the 15/15 rule)

1. If a blood glucose monitor is readily available, check the client's blood glucose level. If the client is experiencing symptoms suggestive of hypoglycemia such as diaphoresis, hunger, pallor, and shakiness, and a blood glucose monitor is not readily available, assume hypoglycemia and treat accordingly.
2. For the client whose blood glucose is below 70 mg/dL, or for the client with an unknown blood glucose who is exhibiting signs of hypoglycemia, administer 15 g of a carbohydrate such as ½ cup of fruit juice or 15 g of glucose gel.
3. Recheck the blood glucose level in 15 minutes.
4. If the blood glucose remains below 70 mg/dL, administer another 15 g of a simple carbohydrate.
5. Recheck the blood glucose level in 15 minutes; if still below 70 mg/dL, treat with an additional 15 g of a simple carbohydrate.
6. Recheck the blood glucose level in 15 minutes; if still below 70 mg/dL, assist the registered nurse with treating with 25 to 50 mL of 50% IV dextrose or, if no IV equipment is present, treat with 1 mg of glucagon subcutaneously or intramuscularly.
7. After the blood glucose level has recovered, have the client ingest a snack that includes a complex carbohydrate and a protein.
8. Document the client's complaints, actions taken, and outcome.
9. Explore the precipitating cause of the hypoglycemia with the client.

3. Interventions: always follow agency protocols (see **Priority Nursing Actions**)

⚠ Do not attempt to administer oral food or fluids to the client experiencing a severe hypoglycemic reaction who is semiconscious or unconscious and is unable to swallow. This client is at risk for aspiration. For this client, an injection of glucagon is administered subcutaneously or intramuscularly. In the hospital or emergency department, the client may be treated with an IV injection of 25 to 50 mL of 50% dextrose in water.

B. Diabetic ketoacidosis
1. Description (Fig. 43.2)
   a. DKA is a life-threatening complication of type 1 diabetes mellitus that develops when a severe insulin deficiency occurs.

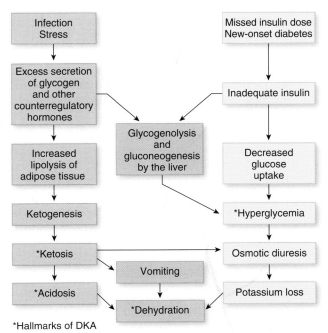

*Hallmarks of DKA

FIGURE 43.2 Pathophysiology of Diabetic Ketoacidosis.

b. The main clinical manifestations include hyperglycemia, dehydration, electrolyte imbalance, ketosis, and acidosis.
2. Data collection (Table 43.3)
3. Interventions
   a. Restore circulating blood volume and protect against cerebral, coronary, and renal hypoperfusion
   b. Dehydration will be treated with rapid IV infusions of 0.9% or 0.45% NS, as prescribed; dextrose is added to IV fluids when the blood glucose level reaches 250 to 300 mg/dL. Too rapid administration of IV fluids, particularly hypotonic solutions, and correcting the blood glucose too rapidly can lead to cerebral edema.
   c. Hyperglycemia will be treated with regular insulin administered intravenously as prescribed.
   d. Correct electrolyte imbalances (potassium level may be elevated as a result of dehydration and acidosis).
   e. Monitor potassium level closely because when the client receives treatment for dehydration and acidosis, the serum potassium will decrease, and potassium replacement may be required.

TABLE 43.3 Differences Between Diabetic Ketoacidosis and Hyperosmolar Hyperglycemic Syndrome

	Diabetic Ketoacidosis (DKA)	Hyperosmolar Hyperglycemic Syndrome
Onset	Sudden	Gradual
Precipitating factors	Infection	Infection
	Other stressors	Other stressors
	Inadequate insulin dose	Poor fluid intake
Manifestations	Ketosis: Kussmaul's respiration, "fruity" breath, nausea, abdominal pain	Altered central nervous system function with neurological symptoms
	Dehydration or electrolyte loss: Polyuria, polydipsia, weight loss, dry skin, sunken eyes, soft eyeballs, lethargy, coma	Dehydration or electrolyte loss: Same as for DKA
Laboratory Findings		
Serum glucose	>300 mg/dL	>600 mg/dL
Osmolarity	Variable	> 350 mOsm/L
Serum ketones	Positive at 1:2 dilution	Negative
Serum pH	<7.35	>7.4
Serum HCO_3	<15 mEq/L	>20 mEq/L
Serum Na	Low, normal, or high	Normal or low
Serum K	Normal; elevated with acidosis, low following dehydration	Normal or low
BUN	>20 mg/dL ; elevated because of dehydration	Elevated
Creatinine	>1.5 mg/dL; elevated because of dehydration	Elevated
Urine ketones	Positive	Negative

BUN, Blood urea nitrogen; *HCO₃,* bicarbonate.
From Ignatavicius D, Workman M: *Medical-surgical nursing: Patient-centered collaborative care,* ed 7, St. Louis, 2013, Saunders.

> **BOX 43.16**   **Client Education: Guidelines During Illness**
>
> Take insulin or oral antidiabetic medications as prescribed.
> Determine the blood glucose level and test the urine for ketones every 3–4 hours.
> If the usual meal plan cannot be followed, substitute soft foods six to eight times a day.
> If vomiting, diarrhea, or fever occurs, consume liquids every 30–60 minutes to prevent dehydration and to provide calories.
> Notify the primary health care provider if vomiting, diarrhea, or fever persists; if blood glucose levels are higher than 250–300 mg/dL; when ketonuria is present for more than 24 hours; when unable to take food or fluids for a period of 4 hours; or when illness persists for more than 2 days.

    f. Cardiac monitoring is necessary for the client with DKA because of the risks associated with abnormal serum potassium levels.

4. Insulin IV administration by the RN

    a. Short-duration insulin only is used.

    b. An IV bolus dose of short-duration regular U-100 insulin (usually 5–10 units) may be prescribed before a continuous infusion is begun.

    c. The prescribed IV dose of insulin for continuous infusion is prepared in 0.9% or 0.45% NS as prescribed.

    d. The insulin infusion is always placed on an IV infusion controller.

    e. Insulin is infused continuously until subcutaneous administration resumes to prevent a rebound of the blood glucose level.

    f. Monitor vital signs.

    g. Monitor urinary output and for signs of fluid overload.

    h. Monitor potassium and glucose levels and for signs of increased intracranial pressure.

    i. The potassium level will fall rapidly within the first hour of treatment as dehydration and acidosis are treated.

    j. Potassium is administered intravenously in a diluted solution as prescribed; ensure adequate renal function before administering potassium.

5. Reinforcement of client education (Box 43.16)

> ⚠ Monitor the client being treated for DKA closely for signs of increased intracranial pressure. If the blood glucose level falls too far or too fast before the brain has time to equilibrate, water is pulled from the blood to the cerebrospinal fluid and the brain, causing cerebral edema and increased intracranial pressure.

C. Hyperosmolar hyperglycemic syndrome (HHS)

  1. Description

    a. Extreme hyperglycemia occurs without ketosis and acidosis.

    b. The syndrome occurs most often among individuals with type 2 diabetes mellitus.

    c. The major difference between HHS and DKA is that ketosis and acidosis do not occur with HHS; enough insulin is present with HHS to prevent the breakdown of fats for energy, thus preventing ketosis.

  2. Data collection (see Table 43.3)

  3. Interventions

    a. Treatment is similar to that for DKA.

    b. Treatment includes fluid replacement, the correction of electrolyte imbalances, and insulin administration.

    c. Fluid replacement in the older client must be done very carefully secondary to the potential for heart failure.

    d. Insulin plays a less critical role in the treatment of HHS than it does for the treatment of DKA because ketosis and acidosis do not occur; rehydration alone may decrease glucose levels.

IX. Chronic Complications of Diabetes Mellitus

A. Diabetic retinopathy

  1. Description

    a. Chronic and progressive impairment of the retinal circulation that eventually causes hemorrhage

    b. Permanent vision changes and blindness can occur.

    c. The client has difficulty with carrying out the daily tasks of blood glucose testing and insulin injections.

  2. Data collection

    a. A change in vision is caused by the rupture of small microaneurysms in retinal blood vessels.

    b. Blurred vision results from macular edema.

    c. Sudden loss of vision results from retinal detachment.

    d. Cataracts result from lens opacity.

  3. Interventions

    a. Maintain safety.

    b. Early prevention via the control of hypertension and blood glucose levels

    c. Photocoagulation (laser therapy) may be done to remove hemorrhagic tissue to decrease scarring and prevent the progression of the disease process.

    d. Vitrectomy may be done to remove vitreous hemorrhages and thus decrease tension on the retina preventing detachment.

    e. Cataract removal with a lens implantation improves vision.

B. Diabetic nephropathy

  1. Description: Progressive decrease in kidney function

  2. Data collection

    a. Microalbuminuria

b. Thirst
c. Fatigue
d. Anemia
e. Weight loss
f. Signs of malnutrition
g. Frequent urinary tract infections
h. Signs of a neurogenic bladder

3. Interventions
   a. Early prevention measures include the control of hypertension and blood glucose levels.
   b. Monitor vital signs.
   c. Monitor intake and output.
   d. Monitor the blood urea nitrogen, creatinine, and urine albumin levels.
   e. Restrict dietary protein, sodium, and potassium intake as prescribed.
   f. Avoid nephrotoxic medications.
   g. Prepare the client for dialysis procedures, if planned.
   h. Prepare the client for kidney transplant, if planned.
   i. Prepare the client for pancreas transplant, if planned.

C. Diabetic neuropathy
   1. Description
      a. A general deterioration of the nervous system throughout the body
      b. Complications include the development of nonhealing ulcers of the feet, gastric paresis, and erectile dysfunction.
   2. Classifications
      a. Focal neuropathy or mononeuropathy: Involves a single nerve or a group of nerves, most frequently cranial nerves III (oculomotor) and VI (abducens), resulting in diplopia
      b. Sensory or peripheral neuropathy: Affects the distal portion of the nerves, most frequently in the lower extremities
      c. Autonomic neuropathy: Symptoms vary according to the organ system involved.
      d. Cardiovascular: Cardiac denervation syndrome (heart rate does not respond to changes in oxygenation needs) and orthostatic hypotension occur.
      e. Pupillary: Pupil does not dilate in response to decreased light.
      f. Gastric: Decreased gastric emptying (gastroparesis)
      g. Urinary: Neurogenic bladder
      h. Skin: Decreased sweating
      i. Adrenal: Hypoglycemic unawareness
      j. Reproductive: Impotence (male) and painful intercourse (female)
   3. Data collection: Findings depend on the classification.
      a. Paresthesia
      b. Decreased or absent reflexes

   c. Decreased sensation to vibration or light touch
   d. Pain, aching, and burning in the lower extremities
   e. Poor peripheral pulses
   f. Skin breakdown and signs of infection
   g. Weakness or loss of sensation in cranial nerves III (oculomotor), IV (trochlear), V (trigeminal), and VI (abducens)
   h. Dizziness and postural hypotension
   i. Nausea and vomiting
   j. Diarrhea or constipation
   k. Incontinence
   l. Dyspareunia
   m. Impotence
   n. Hypoglycemic unawareness

4. Interventions
   a. Early prevention measures include the control of hypertension and blood glucose levels.
   b. Careful foot care is required to prevent trauma (Box 43.17).
   c. Administer medications, as prescribed, for pain relief.
   d. Initiate bladder-training programs.
   e. Reinforce instructions to the client regarding the use of estrogen-containing lubricants for women with dyspareunia.
   f. Prepare the male client with impotence for penile injections or other possible treatment options, as prescribed.
   g. Prepare for surgical decompression of compression lesions related to the cranial nerves as prescribed.

X. Care of the Diabetic Client Undergoing Surgery

A. Preoperative care
   1. Check with the PHCP regarding withholding oral hypoglycemic medications or insulin.
   2. Some long-acting oral antidiabetic medications are discontinued 24 to 48 hours before surgery.
   3. Metformin may need to be discontinued 48 hours before surgery and may not be restarted until renal function is normal postoperatively.
   4. All other oral antidiabetic medications are usually withheld the day of surgery.
   5. Insulin dose may be adjusted or withheld if IV insulin administration during surgery is planned.
   6. Monitor the blood glucose level.
   7. Assist to administer prescribed IV fluids.

B. Postoperative care
   1. Assist the RN with the administration of IV glucose and regular insulin infusions, as prescribed, until the client can tolerate oral feedings.
   2. Administer supplemental short-acting insulin, as prescribed, based on blood glucose results.
   3. Monitor blood glucose levels frequently, especially if the client is receiving parenteral nutrition.

BOX 43.17	Preventive Foot Care Instructions

Provide meticulous skin care and proper foot care.

Inspect feet daily and monitor feet for redness, swelling, or break in skin integrity.

Notify the primary health care provider if redness or a break in the skin occurs.

Avoid thermal injuries from hot water, heating pads, and baths.

Wash feet with warm (not hot) water and dry thoroughly (avoid foot soaks).

Avoid treating corns, blisters, or ingrown toenails.

Do not cross legs or wear tight garments that may constrict blood flow.

Apply moisturizing lotion to the feet, but not between the toes.

Prevent moisture from accumulating between the toes.

Wear loose socks and well-fitting (not tight) shoes; do not go barefoot.

Wear clean cotton socks to keep the feet warm, and change the socks daily.

Avoid wearing the same pair of shoes two days in a row.

Avoid wearing open-toed shoes or shoes with a strap that goes between the toes.

Check shoes for cracks or tears in the lining and for foreign objects before putting them on.

Break in new shoes gradually.

Cut toenails straight across, and smooth nails with an emery board.

Avoid smoking.

---

4. When the client is tolerating food, ensure that the client receives an adequate amount of carbohydrates daily to prevent hypoglycemia.
5. Client is at higher risk for cardiovascular and renal complications postoperatively.
6. Client is also at risk for impaired wound healing.

WHAT WOULD YOU DO?

Answer: Hypertensive crisis can occur as a complication of pheochromocytoma. This can result in stroke, cardiac dysrhythmia, or myocardial infarction. Manifestations include severe headache, extremely high blood pressure (BP), dizziness, blurred vision, shortness of breath, epistaxis (nosebleed), and severe anxiety. If the nurse suspects a hypertensive crisis, the nurse would place the client in a semi-Fowler's position and notify the RN immediately. The PHCP must also be notified immediately, and as prescribed, the nurse needs to prepare to administer oxygen, assist the RN with starting an IV infusion of 0.9% NS solution and infuse it slowly to prevent fluid overload (which would increase blood pressure), assist the RN with the administration of IV medications to lower the BP and monitor it frequently, and also monitor for complications.

PRACTICE QUESTIONS

1. The nurse is caring for a client after a thyroidectomy and notes that calcium gluconate is prescribed. The nurse determines that this medication has been prescribed for which reason?
   1. Treat thyroid storm
   2. Prevent cardiac irritability
   3. Treat hypocalcemic tetany
   4. Stimulate the release of parathyroid hormone

2. The nurse is collecting data regarding a client after a thyroidectomy and notes the development of a hoarse and weak voice. Which nursing action is appropriate?
   1. Check for signs of bleeding.
   2. Administer calcium gluconate.
   3. Notify the registered nurse immediately.
   4. Reassure the client that this is usually a temporary condition.

3. A client is admitted to the emergency department, and a diagnosis of myxedema coma is made. Which action would the nurse prepare to carry out **initially**?
   1. Warm the client.
   2. Maintain a patent airway.
   3. Monitor intravenous fluids.
   4. Administer thyroid hormone.

4. The nurse is assisting with preparing a teaching plan for the client with diabetes mellitus regarding proper foot care. Which instruction would be included in the plan of care?
   1. Soak the feet in hot water.
   2. Avoid using soap to wash the feet.
   3. Apply a moisturizing lotion to dry feet, but not between the toes.
   4. Always have a podiatrist cut your toenails; never cut them yourself.

5. The nurse provides dietary instructions to a client with diabetes mellitus regarding the prescribed diabetic diet. Which statement made by the client indicates the **need for further teaching**?
   1. "I'll eat a balanced meal plan."
   2. "I need to drink diet soft drinks."
   3. "I need to buy special dietetic foods."
   4. "I will snack on fruit instead of cake."

6. A client who has been newly diagnosed with diabetes mellitus has been stabilized with daily insulin injections. Which teaching information would the nurse reinforce upon discharge?
   1. Keep insulin vials refrigerated at all times.
   2. Rotate the insulin injection sites systematically.
   3. Increase the amount of insulin before unusual exercise.
   4. Monitor the urine acetone level to determine the insulin dosage.

7. The nurse reinforces teaching to a client with diabetes mellitus regarding differentiating between hypoglycemia and ketoacidosis. The client demonstrates an understanding of the teaching by stating that glucose will be taken if which symptom develops?
   1. Polyuria
   2. Shakiness
   3. Blurred vision
   4. Fruity breath odor

8. When the nurse is reinforcing instructions to a client who has been newly diagnosed with type 1 diabetes mellitus, which statement by the client would indicate that teaching has been **effective**?
   1. "I will stop taking my insulin if I'm too sick to eat."
   2. "I will decrease my insulin dose during times of illness."
   3. "I will adjust my insulin dose according to the level of glucose in my urine."
   4. "I will notify my primary health care provider if my blood glucose level is consistently greater than 250."

9. The nurse is monitoring a client who has been newly diagnosed with diabetes mellitus for signs of complications. Which statement made by the client would indicate hyperglycemia and thus warrant primary health care provider (PHCP) notification?
   1. "I am urinating a lot."
   2. "My pulse is really slow."
   3. "I am sweating for no reason."
   4. "My blood pressure is really high."

10. The nurse is reinforcing instructions to a client with diabetes mellitus who is recovering from diabetic ketoacidosis (DKA) regarding measures to prevent a recurrence. Which instruction is important for the nurse to emphasize?
    1. Eat six small meals daily.
    2. Test the urine ketone level.
    3. Monitor blood glucose levels frequently.
    4. Receive appropriate follow-up health care.

11. The nurse is reinforcing discharge teaching to a client who has Cushing's syndrome. Which statement by the client indicates that the instructions related to dietary management were understood?
    1. "I can eat foods that contain potassium."
    2. "I will need to limit the amount of protein in my diet."
    3. "I am fortunate that I can eat all the salty foods I enjoy."
    4. "I am fortunate that I do not need to follow any special diet."

❖ 12. The nurse educator is asking the nursing student to recall the signs/symptoms of hypothyroidism. The nurse educator determines that the student understands this disorder if which are included in the student's response? **Select all that apply.**
   ❑ 1. Dry skin
   ❑ 2. Irritability
   ❑ 3. Palpitations
   ❑ 4. Weight loss
   ❑ 5. Constipation
   ❑ 6. Cold intolerance

13. The nurse is caring for a postoperative parathyroidectomy client. Which would require the nurse's **immediate** attention?
    1. Incisional pain
    2. Laryngeal stridor
    3. Difficulty voiding
    4. Abdominal cramps

14. The nurse notes that a client with type 1 diabetes mellitus has lipodystrophy on both upper thighs. Which further information would the nurse obtain from the client during data collection?
    1. Plan for injection rotation
    2. Consistency of aspiration
    3. Preparation of the injection site
    4. Angle at which the medication is administered

15. A client with type 1 diabetes mellitus calls the nurse to report recurrent episodes of hypoglycemia. Which statement by the client indicates a correct understanding of Humulin N insulin and exercise?
    1. "I should not exercise after lunch."
    2. "I should not exercise after breakfast."
    3. "I should not exercise in the late evening."
    4. "I should not exercise in the late afternoon."

ANSWERS

1. 3

Rationale: Hypocalcemia can develop after thyroidectomy if the parathyroid glands are accidentally removed or injured during surgery. Manifestations develop 1 to 7 days after surgery. If the client develops numbness and tingling around the mouth, fingertips, or toes, or muscle spasms or twitching, the primary health care provider is notified immediately. Calcium gluconate must be accessible for the client who underwent thyroidectomy.

Test-Taking Strategy: Focus on the subject, the intended effect of calcium gluconate. Noting the name of the medication (calcium gluconate) would easily direct you to the correct option. Calcium is given if hypocalcemic tetany occurs.

2. 4

Rationale: Weakness and hoarseness of the voice can occur as a result of trauma to the laryngeal nerve. If this develops, the client would be reassured that the problem will subside in a few days. Unnecessary talking would be discouraged. It is not necessary to notify the registered nurse immediately. These signs do not indicate bleeding or the need to administer calcium gluconate.

Test-Taking Strategy: Focus on the subject, postoperative expectations in the client who underwent thyroidectomy. The options of checking for bleeding and administering calcium gluconate can easily be eliminated because they are unrelated to the signs presented in the question. From the remaining options, recall that these signs indicate a temporary condition.

3. 2

Rationale: The initial nursing action would be to maintain a patent airway. Oxygen would be administered, followed by fluid replacement. The nurse would also keep the client warm, monitor intravenous fluids, and administer thyroid hormones.

Test-Taking Strategy: Note the strategic word, *initially*. All of the options are appropriate interventions, but the use of the ABCs—airway, breathing, and circulation—will direct you to the correct option.

4. 3

Rationale: The client would use a moisturizing lotion on his or her feet, but would avoid applying the lotion between the toes. The client would also be instructed not to soak the feet and to avoid hot water to prevent burns. The client may cut the toenails straight across and even with the toe itself, but he or she needs to consult a podiatrist if the toenails are thick or hard to cut or if his or her vision is poor. The client would be instructed to wash the feet daily with a mild soap.

Test-Taking Strategy: Focus on the subject, foot care for the diabetic client. Eliminate the option regarding *hot water* because hot water can cause injury to the client. Eliminate the option stating to *always have a podiatrist cut your toenails* because the word *always* is a closed-ended word. From the remaining options, recalling the concern related to skin infection will assist you with eliminating the option regarding using soap.

5. 3

Rationale: It is important to emphasize to the client and family that they are not eating a diabetic diet, but rather following a balanced meal plan. Adherence to nutrition principles is an important component of diabetic management, and an individualized meal plan would be developed for the client. It is not necessary for the client to purchase special dietetic foods.

Test-Taking Strategy: Note the strategic words, *need for further teaching*. This is a negative event query, which indicates the need to select the incorrect option as the answer. Basic principles related to the diabetic diet will direct you to the correct option.

6. 2

Rationale: Insulin dosages would not be adjusted or increased before unusual exercise. If acetone is found in the urine, it may possibly indicate the need for additional insulin. To minimize the discomfort associated with insulin injections, the insulin needs to be administered at room temperature. Injection sites need to be systematically rotated from one area to another. The client would be instructed to give injections in one area, about 1 inch apart, until the whole area has been used and then to change to another site. This prevents dramatic changes in daily insulin absorption.

Test-Taking Strategy: Focus on the subject, reinforcement of teaching for a client newly diagnosed with diabetes mellitus. Eliminate the option stating to keep insulin vials *refrigerated at all times* first because of the closed-ended word, *all*. Knowledge regarding insulin administration and the significance of acetone in the urine will assist you with eliminating options of increasing insulin and monitoring urine acetone levels.

7. 2

Rationale: Shakiness is a sign of hypoglycemia, and it would indicate the need for food or glucose. Fruity breath odor, blurred vision, and polyuria are signs of hyperglycemia.

Test-Taking Strategy: Knowledge regarding the signs/symptoms of hypoglycemia and hyperglycemia is required to answer this question. Remember that shakiness is a sign of hypoglycemia. The other options are comparable or alike options and are related to hyperglycemia.

8. 4

Rationale: During illness, the client would monitor the blood glucose level, and he or she would notify the primary health care provider (PHCP) if the level is greater than 250 mg/dL. Insulin is not stopped. In fact, insulin may need to be increased during times of illness. Doses would not be adjusted without the PHCP's advice.

Test-Taking Strategy: Note the strategic word, *effective*. Note that options regarding stopping or decreasing insulin doses and adjusting insulin dosage are comparable or alike; therefore, eliminate these options. Recall that serum blood glucose levels would be monitored rather than urine glucose levels because of unreliability issues associated with urine glucose levels.

9. 1

Rationale: The classic symptoms of hyperglycemia include polydipsia, polyuria, and polyphagia. Options 2, 3, and 4 are not signs of hyperglycemia.

Test-Taking Strategy: Focus on the subject, signs of hyperglycemia. Remember the 3 Ps—polyuria, polydipsia, and polyphagia.

10. 3

Rationale: Client education after DKA would emphasize the need for home glucose monitoring four to five times per day. It is also important to instruct the client to notify the PHCP when illness occurs. The presence of urinary ketones indicates that DKA has already occurred. The client needs to eat well-balanced meals with snacks, as prescribed.

Test-Taking Strategy: Focus on the subject, preventing DKA. Recall that the treatment of DKA focuses on the maintenance of an appropriate blood glucose level. Eating six small meals daily is not an accurate component of diabetic care. Receiving follow-up care will not prevent DKA. Testing the urine ketone levels does not prevent DKA, but helps to confirm the diagnosis.

11. 1

Rationale: A diet that is low in calories, carbohydrates, and sodium but ample in protein and potassium content is encouraged for a client with Cushing's syndrome. Such a diet promotes weight loss, the reduction of edema and hypertension, the control of hypokalemia, and the rebuilding of wasted tissue.

Test-Taking Strategy: Focus on the subject, that instructions related to dietary management were understood. Eliminate the option of not needing to follow a special diet because it indicates that no dietary change is necessary. Eliminate the option of limiting protein next because protein is usually only limited in renal problems. Excess sodium is not healthy in general, so eliminate that option.

❖ **12. 1, 5, 6**

Rationale: Signs of hypothyroidism include dry skin, hair, and loss of body hair; constipation; cold intolerance; lethargy and fatigue; weakness; muscle aches; paresthesia; weight gain; bradycardia; generalized puffiness and edema around the eyes and face; forgetfulness; menstrual disturbances; cardiac enlargement; and goiter. Irritability, palpitations, and weight loss are signs of hyperthyroidism.

Test-Taking Strategy: Focus on the subject, hypothyroidism. Note the relationship between *hypo-* in *hypothyroidism* and the correct answers, and recall that everything slows down with hypothyroidism.

13. 2

Rationale: During the postoperative period, the nurse carefully observes the client for signs of hemorrhage, which causes swelling and the compression of adjacent tissue. Laryngeal stridor is a harsh, high-pitched sound heard during inspiration and expiration that is caused by the compression of the trachea and leads to respiratory distress. It is an acute emergency situation that requires immediate attention to avoid the complete obstruction of the airway.

Test-Taking Strategy: Note the strategic word, *immediate*. Focus on the concept of ABCs—airway, breathing, and circulation—and consider the anatomical location of the surgical procedure. The options of incisional pain, difficulty voiding, and abdominal cramps are common postoperative problems that are not life-threatening. Laryngeal stridor addresses the airway and requires immediate attention.

14. 1

Rationale: Lipodystrophy (i.e., the hypertrophy of subcutaneous tissue at the injection site) occurs in some diabetic clients when the same injection sites are used for prolonged periods of time. Thus, clients are instructed to adhere to a rotating injection site plan to avoid tissue changes. Preparation of the site, aspiration, and the angle of insulin administration do not produce tissue damage.

Test-Taking Strategy: Focus on the subject, lipodystrophy. Remember that lipodystrophy is the hypertrophy of subcutaneous tissue at the injection site.

15. 4

Rationale: A hypoglycemic reaction may occur in response to increased exercise. Clients need to avoid exercise during the peak time of insulin. Humulin N insulin peaks between 6 and 14 hours; therefore, late-afternoon exercise would occur during the peak of the medication.

Test-Taking Strategy: Note the subject, the most likely time of a hypoglycemic reaction. Recalling the peak time of Humulin N insulin will direct you to the option of late-afternoon exercise.

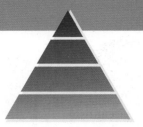

CHAPTER 44

Endocrine Medications

PRIORITY CONCEPTS Glucose Regulation; Hormonal Regulation

WHAT WOULD YOU DO?

The nurse is reviewing the medical record of a client scheduled for a computerized tomography (CT) scan with an intravenous (IV) iodine contrast dye and notes that the client has diabetes mellitus and is taking metformin. What would the nurse do?

Answer is located on p. 573.

I. Pituitary Medications

A. Description
1. The anterior pituitary gland secretes growth hormone (GH), thyroid-stimulating hormone (TSH), adrenocorticotropic hormone (ACTH), prolactin, melanocyte-stimulating hormone (MSH), and gonadotropins (follicle-stimulating hormone [FSH] and luteinizing hormone [LH]).
2. The posterior pituitary gland secretes antidiuretic hormone (vasopressin) and oxytocin.

B. GHs and related medications (Box 44.1)
1. Uses
   a. GHs are used to treat pediatric or adult GH deficiency.
   b. GH receptor antagonists are used to treat acromegaly.
   c. GH releasing factor is used to evaluate anterior pituitary function.
2. Side and adverse effects
   a. May vary depending on the medication
   b. Development of antibodies to GH
   c. Headache, muscle pain, weakness, vertigo
   d. Diarrhea, nausea, abdominal discomfort
   e. Mild hyperglycemia
   f. Hypertension
   g. Weight gain
   h. Allergic reaction (rash, swelling), pain at injection site
   i. Elevated aspartate aminotransferase (AST) and alanine aminotransferase (ALT)

3. Interventions
   a. Check the child's physical growth and compare growth with standards.
   b. Recommend annual bone age determinations for children receiving GHs.
   c. Monitor vital signs, blood glucose levels, AST and ALT levels, and thyroid function tests.
   d. Reinforce teaching to the client and family about the clinical manifestations of hyperglycemia, other side and adverse effects of therapy, and the importance of follow-up regarding periodic blood tests.

II. Antidiuretic Hormones

A. Desmopressin acetate; vasopressin
B. Description
1. Antidiuretic hormones enhance reabsorption of water in the kidneys, promoting an antidiuretic effect and regulating fluid balance.
2. Antidiuretic hormones are used in diabetes insipidus.
3. Vasopressin is used less commonly than desmopressin acetate to treat diabetes insipidus; vasopressin is commonly used to treat septic shock.

C. Side and adverse effects
1. Flushing
2. Headache
3. Nausea and abdominal cramps
4. Water intoxication
5. Hypertension with water intoxication
6. Nasal congestion with nasal administration

D. Interventions
1. Monitor weight.
2. Monitor intake and output and urine osmolality.
3. Monitor electrolyte levels.
4. Monitor for signs of dehydration indicating the need to increase the dosage.
5. Monitor for signs of water intoxication (drowsiness, listlessness, shortness of breath, and headache) indicating need to decrease dosage.
6. Monitor blood pressure.

Growth Hormones
Somatropin
Mecasermin

Growth Hormone Receptor Antagonists
Lanreotide
Octreotide acetate
Pegvisomant
Pasireotide

| BOX 44.2 | Thyroid Hormones |

- Levothyroxine sodium
- Liothyronine sodium
- Thyroid, desiccated

| BOX 44.3 | Antithyroid Medications |

- Methimazole
- Propylthiouracil
- Potassium iodide and strong iodine solution
- Sodium iodide

7. Reinforce instructions to the client in how to use the intranasal medication.
8. Reinforce instructions to the client to weigh himself or herself daily to identify weight gain.
9. Reinforce instructions to the client to report signs of water intoxication or symptoms of headache or shortness of breath.

III. Thyroid Hormones (Box 44.2)

A. Description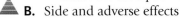
   1. Thyroid hormones control the metabolic rate of tissues and accelerate heat production and oxygen consumption.
   2. Thyroid hormones are used to replace the thyroid hormone deficit in conditions such as hypothyroidism and myxedema coma.
   3. Thyroid hormones enhance the action of oral anticoagulants, sympathomimetics, and antidepressants and decrease the action of insulin, oral hypoglycemics, and digitalis preparations; the action of thyroid hormones is decreased by phenytoin and carbamazepine.
   4. Thyroid hormones need to be given at least 4 hours apart from multivitamins, aluminum hydroxide and magnesium hydroxide, simethicone, calcium carbonate, sevelamer, lanthanum, bile acid sequestrants, iron, and sucralfate, because these medications decrease the absorption of thyroid replacements.

B. Side and adverse effects
   1. Nausea and decreased appetite
   2. Abdominal cramps and diarrhea
   3. Weight loss
   4. Nervousness and tremors
   5. Insomnia
   6. Sweating
   7. Heat intolerance

   8. Tachycardia, dysrhythmia, palpitations, chest pain
   9. Hypertension
   10. Headache
   11. Toxicity: Hyperthyroidism

C. Interventions
   1. The client is assessed for a history of medications currently being taken.
   2. Monitor vital signs.
   3. Monitor weight.
   4. Monitor triiodothyronine, thyroxine, and TSH levels.
   5. Reinforce instructions to the client to take the medication at the same time each day in the morning and without food.
   6. Reinforce instructions to the client in how to monitor the pulse rate.
   7. Inform the client that it is important to discuss which foods to specifically avoid that may inhibit thyroid secretion based on the client's individualized diet plan and medication regimen.
   8. The client is advised to avoid over-the-counter medications.
   9. Reinforce instructions to the client to wear a Medic-Alert bracelet.

⚠ The client taking a thyroid hormone is instructed to report symptoms of hyperthyroidism such as tachycardia, chest pain, palpitations, and excessive sweating. These indicate signs of toxicity.

IV. Antithyroid Medications (Box 44.3)

A. Description
   1. Antithyroid medications inhibit the synthesis of thyroid hormone.
   2. Antithyroid medications are used for hyperthyroidism or Graves' disease.

B. Side and adverse effects
   1. Nausea and vomiting
   2. Diarrhea
   3. Drowsiness, headache, fever
   4. Hypersensitivity with skin rash
   5. Agranulocytosis with leukopenia and thrombocytopenia
   6. Alopecia and hyperpigmentation
   7. Toxicity: Hypothyroidism
   8. Iodism: Characterized by vomiting, abdominal pain, metallic or brassy taste in the mouth, rash; sore gums and salivary glands

BOX 44.4   Medications to Treat Calcium Disorders

Oral Calcium Supplements
- Calcium acetate
- Calcium carbonate
- Calcium citrate
- Calcium glubionate
- Calcium gluconate
- Tribasic calcium phosphate

Vitamin D Supplements
- Cholecalciferol (Vitamin D3)
- Ergocalciferol (Vitamin D2)

Bisphosphonates and Calcium Regulators
- Alendronate sodium
- Calcitonin salmon
- Etidronate disodium
- Ibandronate
- Pamidronate disodium
- Risedronate sodium
- Zoledronic acid

Medications to Treat Hypercalcemia
- Calcitonin
- Cinacalcet hydrochloride
- Doxercalciferol
- Paricalcitol

⚠ Iodism is a concern for clients taking a strong iodine solution also known as Lugol's solution. Because of the risk of iodism, the use of strong iodine solution is limited to about 2 weeks, generally used for clients with hyperthyroidism in preparation for thyroid surgery.

C. Interventions
1. Monitor vital signs.
2. Monitor triiodothyronine, thyroxine, and TSH levels.
3. Monitor weight.
4. Reinforce instructions to the client to take medication with meals to avoid gastrointestinal (GI) upset.
5. Reinforce instructions to the client in how to monitor the pulse rate.
6. Reinforce instructions to the client of side and adverse effects and when to notify the primary health care provider (PHCP).
7. Reinforce instructions to the client regarding the signs of hypothyroidism.
8. Reinforce instructions to the client regarding the importance of medication compliance and that abruptly stopping the medication could cause thyroid storm.
9. Reinforce instructions to the client to monitor for signs and symptoms of thyroid storm (fever, flushed skin, confusion and behavioral changes, tachycardia, dysrhythmias, and signs of heart failure).
10. Reinforce instructions to the client to monitor for signs of iodism.

11. Reinforce instructions to the client to consult the PHCP before eating iodized salt and iodine-rich foods.
12. Reinforce instructions to the client to avoid acetylsalicylic acid (aspirin) and medications containing iodine.

⚠ Methimazole causes agranulocytosis. Therefore, advise the client to contact the PHCP if a fever or sore throat develops.

V. Parathyroid Medications (Box 44.4)

A. Description
1. Parathyroid hormone regulates serum calcium levels.
2. Low serum levels of calcium stimulate parathyroid hormone release.
3. Hyperparathyroidism results in a high serum calcium level and bone demineralization; medication is used to lower the serum calcium level.
4. Hypoparathyroidism results in a low serum calcium level which increases neuromuscular excitability; treatment includes calcium and vitamin D supplements.
5. Calcium salts administered with digoxin increase the risk of digoxin toxicity.
6. Oral calcium salts reduce the absorption of tetracycline hydrochloride.

B. Interventions
1. Monitor electrolyte and calcium levels.
2. Monitor for signs/symptoms of hypocalcemia and hypercalcemia.
3. Monitor for symptoms of tetany in the client with hypocalcemia.
4. Monitor for renal calculi in the client with hypercalcemia.
5. Reinforce instructions to the client regarding the signs and symptoms of hypercalcemia and hypocalcemia.
6. Reinforce instructions to the client to check over-the-counter medication labels for the possibility of calcium content.
7. Reinforce instructions to the client receiving oral calcium supplements to maintain an adequate intake of vitamin D because vitamin D enhances absorption of calcium.
8. Reinforce instructions to the client receiving calcium regulators such as alendronate sodium to swallow the tablet whole with water at least 30 minutes before breakfast and not to lie down for at least 30 minutes.
9. Reinforce instructions to the client using nasal spray of calcitonin to alternate nares.
10. Reinforce instructions to the client using antihypercalcemic agents to avoid foods rich in calcium such as green, leafy vegetables; dairy products; shellfish; and soy.

11. Reinforce instructions to the client not to take other medications within 1 hour of taking a calcium supplement.

12. Reinforce instructions to the client to increase fluid and fiber in the diet to prevent constipation associated with calcium supplements.

VI. Corticosteroids (Mineralocorticoids)

A. Fludrocortisone acetate

B. Description

1. Mineralocorticoids are steroid hormones that enhance the reabsorption of sodium and chloride and promote the excretion of potassium and hydrogen from the renal tubules, thereby helping maintain fluid and electrolyte balance.

2. Mineralocorticoids are used for replacement therapy in primary and secondary adrenal insufficiency in Addison's disease.

C. Side and adverse effects

1. Sodium and water retention, edema, hypertension

2. Hypokalemia

3. Hypocalcemia

4. Osteoporosis, compression fractures

5. Weight gain

6. Heart failure

D. Interventions

1. Monitor vital signs.

2. Monitor intake and output, weight, and for edema.

3. Monitor electrolyte and calcium levels.

4. The client is instructed to take medication with food or milk.

5. The client is instructed to consume a high-potassium diet.

6. The client is instructed to report signs of illness.

7. The client is instructed to notify the PHCP if low blood pressure, weakness, cramping, palpitations, or changes in mental status occur.

8. The client is instructed to wear a MedicAlert bracelet.

 The client taking a corticosteroid is instructed not to stop the medication abruptly because this could result in adrenal insufficiency.

VII. Corticosteroids (Glucocorticoids) (Box 44.5)

A. Description

1. Glucocorticoids affect glucose, protein, and bone metabolism; alter the normal immune response and suppress inflammation; and produce anti-inflammatory, antiallergic, and antistress effects.

2. Glucocorticoids may be used as a replacement in adrenocortical insufficiency.

3. Glucocorticoids are used for their anti-inflammatory and immunosuppressant effects, for both short-term and long-term in the treatment of several nonendocrine disorders.

BOX 44.5 **Corticosteroids: Glucocorticoids**

- Betamethasone
- Cortisone acetate
- Dexamethasone
- Hydrocortisone
- Methylprednisolone
- Prednisolone
- Prednisone
- Triamcinolone

B. Side and adverse effects

1. Hyperglycemia

2. Hypokalemia

3. Hypocalcemia, osteoporosis

4. Sodium and fluid retention

5. Weight gain and edema

6. Mood swings

7. Moon face, buffalo hump, truncal obesity

8. Increased susceptibility to infection and masking of the signs and symptoms of infection

9. Cataracts

10. Hirsutism, acne, fragile skin, bruising

11. Growth retardation in children

12. GI irritation, peptic ulcer, pancreatitis

13. Seizure, psychosis

14. Psychosis (usually occurs with hydrocortisone and dexamethasone in clients receiving very high doses long-term and is most likely due to their effects on blood glucose)

15. Adrenal insufficiency

C. Contraindications and cautions

1. Contraindicated in clients with hypersensitivity, psychosis, and fungal infections

2. Would be used with caution in clients with diabetes mellitus

3. Would be used with extreme caution in clients with infections because they mask the signs/symptoms of an infection

4. They can increase the potency of medications taken concurrently such as aspirin and nonsteroidal anti-inflammatory drugs, thus increasing the risk of GI bleeding and ulceration.

5. Use of potassium-wasting diuretics increases potassium loss resulting in hypokalemia.

6. Dexamethasone decreases the effects of orally administered anticoagulants and antidiabetic agents.

7. Barbiturates, phenytoin, and rifampin decrease the effect of prednisone.

D. Interventions

1. Monitor vital signs.

2. Monitor serum electrolyte and blood glucose level.

3. Monitor for hypokalemia and hyperglycemia.

4. Monitor intake and output, weight, and for edema.

5. Monitor for hypertension.

BOX 44.6 Androgens and Testosterones

Androgen
Methyltestosterone

Testosterone Preparations
Testosterone, pellets
Testosterone, transdermal
Testosterone cypionate
Testosterone enanthate
Testosterone propionate
Testosterone undecanoate
Testosterone, buccal patch
Testosterone, topical gel
Testosterone, nasal gel

---

6. Check medical history for glaucoma, cataracts, peptic ulcer, mental health disorders, or diabetes mellitus.
7. Monitor the older client for signs/symptoms of increased osteoporosis.
8. Check for any change in muscle strength.
9. Prepare a schedule for the client with information on short-term tapered doses.
10. The client is instructed that it is best to take medication in the early morning with food or milk.
11. The client is advised to eat foods high in potassium.
12. The client is instructed to avoid individuals with infections.
13. The client is instructed to inform all PHCPs of the medication regimen.
14. The client is instructed to report signs and symptoms of a medication overdose or **Cushing's syndrome**, including a moon face, puffy eyelids, edema in the feet, increased bruising, dizziness, bleeding, and menstrual irregularities which often result from the large doses of long-term glucocorticoids that may be used to treat nonendocrine conditions.
15. Note that the client may need additional doses during periods of stress such as surgery.
16. The client is instructed not to stop the medication abruptly because abrupt withdrawal can result in severe adrenal insufficiency.
17. The client is advised to consult with the PHCP before receiving vaccinations; live virus vaccines are not to be administered to the client taking glucocorticoids.
18. The client is advised to wear a MedicAlert bracelet.

VIII. Androgens (Box 44.6)

A. Description
1. Used to replace deficient hormones or to treat hormone-sensitive disorders
2. Can cause bleeding if the client is taking oral anticoagulants (increase the effect of anticoagulants)
3. Can cause decreased serum glucose concentration, thereby reducing insulin requirements in the client with diabetes mellitus

4. Hepatotoxic medications are avoided with the use of androgens because of the risk of additive damage to the liver.
5. Androgens usually are avoided in men with known prostate or breast carcinoma because androgens often stimulate growth of these tumors.

B. Side and adverse effects
1. Masculine secondary sexual characteristics (body hair growth, lowered voice, muscle growth)
2. Bladder irritation and urinary tract infections
3. Breast tenderness
4. Gynecomastia
5. Priapism
6. Menstrual irregularities
7. Virilism
8. Sodium and water retention with edema
9. Nausea, vomiting, or diarrhea
10. Acne
11. Changes in libido
12. Hepatotoxicity, jaundice
13. Hypercalcemia

C. Interventions
1. Monitor vital signs.
2. Monitor for edema, weight gain, skin changes.
3. Check mental status and neurological function.
4. Check for signs of liver dysfunction including right upper quadrant abdominal pain, malaise, fever, jaundice, and pruritus.
5. Check for the development of secondary sexual characteristics.
6. The client is instructed to take medication with meals or a snack.
7. The client is instructed to notify the PHCP if priapism develops.
8. The client is instructed to notify the PHCP if fluid retention occurs.
9. Women are instructed to use a nonhormonal contraceptive while on therapy.
10. For women, monitor for menstrual irregularities and decreased breast size.

IX. Estrogens and Progestins

A. Description
1. Estrogens are steroids that stimulate female reproductive tissue.
2. Progestins are steroids that specifically stimulate the uterine lining.
3. Estrogen and progestin preparations may be used to stimulate the endogenous hormones to restore hormonal balance, to treat hormone-sensitive tumors (suppress tumor growth), or for contraception (Boxes 44.7 and 44.8).

B. Contraindications and cautions
1. Estrogens
   a. Estrogens are contraindicated in clients with breast cancer, endometrial hyperplasia, endo-

BOX 44.7 Estrogens

Esterified estrogens
Estradiol
Estrogens, conjugated
Ethinyl estradiol

BOX 44.8 Progestins

- Estradiol/drospirenone
- Estradiol/etonogestrel
- Estradiol/levonorgestrel
- Estradiol/norethindrone
- Estradiol/norgestimate
- Levonorgestrel
- Medroxyprogesterone acetate
- Medroxyprogesterone and conjugated estrogens
- Megestrol acetate
- Norethindrone acetate
- Progesterone

metrial cancer, history of thromboembolism, known or suspected pregnancy, or lactation.

    b. Use estrogens with caution in clients with hypertension, gallbladder disease, or liver or kidney dysfunction.

    c. Estrogens increase the risk of toxicity when used with hepatotoxic medications.

    d. Barbiturates, phenytoin, and rifampin decrease the effectiveness of estrogen.

  2. Progestins are contraindicated in clients with thromboembolic disorders and would be avoided in clients with breast tumors or hepatic disease.

C. Side and adverse effects
  1. Breast tenderness, menstrual changes
  2. Nausea, vomiting, diarrhea
  3. Malaise, depression, excessive irritability
  4. Weight gain
  5. Edema and fluid retention
  6. Atherosclerosis
  7. Hypertension, stroke, myocardial infarction
  8. Thromboembolism (estrogen)
  9. Migraine headaches and vomiting (estrogen)

D. Interventions
  1. Monitor vital signs.
  2. Monitor for hypertension.
  3. Check for edema and weight gain.
  4. The client is advised not to smoke.
  5. The client is advised to undergo routine breast and pelvic examinations.

X. Medications for Diabetes Mellitus

A. Insulin and oral hypoglycemic medications
  1. Description

    a. Insulin increases glucose transport into cells and promotes conversion of glucose to glycogen, decreasing serum glucose levels.

    b. Oral antidiabetic agents act in a number of ways: stimulate the pancreas to produce more insulin, increase the sensitivity of peripheral receptors to insulin, decrease hepatic glucose output, delay intestinal absorption of glucose, enhance the activity of incretins, and promote glucose loss through the kidney.

  2. Contraindications and concerns

 Sulfonylureas can cause a disulfiram-type reaction when alcohol is ingested.

    a. Insulin is contraindicated in clients with hypersensitivity.

    b. Oral antidiabetic agents, except the sodium-glucose cotransporter 2 (SGLT-2) inhibitors, are contraindicated in type 1 diabetes mellitus.

    c. β-Adrenergic blocking agents may mask signs/symptoms of hypoglycemia associated with hypoglycemia-producing medications.

    d. Anticoagulants, chloramphenicol, salicylates, propranolol (Inderal), monoamine oxidase inhibitors, and sulfonamides may cause hypoglycemia.

    e. Corticosteroids, sympathomimetics, thiazide diuretics, phenytoin, thyroid preparations, oral contraceptives, and estrogen compounds may cause hyperglycemia.

    f. Side and adverse effects of the sulfonylureas include GI symptoms and dermatological reactions; hypoglycemia can occur when an excessive dose is administered or when meals are omitted or delayed, food intake is decreased, or activity is increased.

B. Medications for type 2 diabetes mellitus (Table 44.1)
  1. Interventions

 Metformin may need to be withheld temporarily before and for 48 hours after any radiological study that involves the administration of IV contrast dye because of the risk of contrast-induced nephropathy and lactic acidosis. The PHCP needs to be consulted for specific prescriptions.

    a. The client's knowledge of diabetes mellitus and the use of oral antidiabetic agents are assessed.

    b. A medication history regarding the medications that the client is currently taking is obtained.

    c. Monitor vital signs and the blood glucose level.

    d. Reinforce instructions to the client to recognize the signs and symptoms of hypoglycemia and hyperglycemia.

TABLE 44.1 **Medications for Type 2 Diabetes**

Class and Specific Agents	Actions	Major Adverse Effects
Oral Medications		
Biguanide		
Metformin	Decreases glucose production by the liver; increases tissue response to insulin	GI symptoms: decreased appetite, nausea, diarrhea Lactic acidosis (rarely)
Second-Generation Sulfonylureas		
Glimepiride Glipizide Glyburide	Promote insulin secretion by the pancreas; may also increase tissue response to insulin	Hypoglycemia Weight gain
Meglitinides (Glinides)		
Nateglinide Repaglinide	Promote insulin secretion by the pancreas	Hypoglycemia Weight gain
Thiazolidinediones (Glitazones)		
Pioglitazone Rosiglitazone	Decrease insulin resistance, thereby increasing glucose uptake by muscle and adipose tissue and decreasing glucose production by the liver	Hypoglycemia, but only in the presence of excessive insulin Heart failure Bladder cancer Fractures (in women) Ovulation, and thus possible unintended pregnancy
Alpha-Glucosidase Inhibitors		
Acarbose Miglitol	Delay carbohydrate digestion and absorption, thereby decreasing the postprandial rise in blood glucose	GI symptoms: flatulence, cramps, abdominal distention, borborygmus
DPP-4 Inhibitors (Gliptins)		
Alogliptin Linagliptin Saxagliptin Sitagliptin	Enhance the activity of incretins (by inhibiting their breakdown by DPP-4), thereby increasing insulin release, reducing glucagon release, and decreasing hepatic glucose production	Pancreatitis Hypersensitivity reactions
Sodium-Glucose Co-Transporter 2 (SGLT-2) Inhibitors		
Canagliflozin Dapagliflozin Empagliflozin Ertugliflozin (a combination with metformin is available)	Increase glucose excretion via the urine by inhibiting SGLT-2 in the kidney tubules, decreasing glucose levels and inducing weight loss via caloric loss through the urine	Genital mycotic infections Orthostasis
Dopamine Agonist		
Bromocriptine	Activates dopamine receptors in the central nervous system; how it improves glycemic control is unknown	Orthostatic hypotension Exacerbation of psychosis
Non-Insulin Injectable Medications		
Incretin Mimetics		
Exenatide Exenatide extended-release Liraglutide Albiglutide Lixisenatide Dulaglutide	Lower blood glucose by slowing gastric emptying, stimulating glucose-dependent insulin release, suppressing postprandial glucagon release, and reducing appetite	Hypoglycemia GI symptoms: nausea, vomiting, diarrhea Pancreatitis Renal insufficiency
Amylin Mimetics		
Pramlintide	Delays gastric emptying and suppresses glucagon secretion, decreasing the postprandial rise in glucose	Hypoglycemia Nausea Injection-site reactions

GI, Gastrointestinal.
Adapted from Burchum JR, Rosenthal RD: *Lehne's pharmacology for nursing care*, ed 9, St. Louis, 2016, Saunders.

TABLE 44.2   Types of Insulin: Time Course of Activity after Subcutaneous Injection

Generic Name	Time Course		
	Onset (min)	Peak (hr)	Duration (hr)
Short Duration: Rapid Acting			
Insulin lispro	15–30	0.5–2.5	3–6
Insulin aspart	10–20	1–3	3–5
Insulin glulisine	10–15	1–1.5	3–5
Short Duration: Slower Acting			
Regular insulin	30–60	1–5	6–10
Intermediate Duration			
NPH insulin	60–120	6–14	16–24
Long Duration			
Insulin glargine	70	None	18–24
Insulin detemir	60–120	12–24	Varies
Insulin degludec	60-120	None	>40

Adapted from Burchum JR, Rosenthal RD: *Lehne's pharmacology for nursing care*, ed 9, St. Louis, 2016, Saunders.

TABLE 44.3   Premixed Insulin Combinations

Description	Time Course		
	Onset (min)	Peak (hr)	Duration (hr)
70% NPH insulin/30% regular insulin (Humulin)	30–60	1.5–16	10–16
70% NPH insulin/30% regular insulin (Novolin)	30–60	2–12	10–16
50% NPH insulin/50% regular insulin	30–60	2–12	10–16
70% insulin aspart protamine/30% insulin aspart	10–20	1–4	15–18
75% insulin lispro protamine/25% insulin lispro	15–30	1–6.5	10–16
50% insulin lispro protamine/50% insulin lispro	15–30	0.8–4.8	10–16

Use only after the dosages and ratios of the components have been established as correct for the client.
Adapted from Burchum JR, Rosenthal RD: *Lehne's pharmacology for nursing care*, ed 9, St. Louis, 2016, Saunders.

e. Reinforce instructions to the client to avoid over-the-counter medications unless prescribed by the PHCP.

f. Reinforce instructions to the client not to ingest alcohol with sulfonylureas.

g. Reinforce instructions to the client that insulin may be needed during times of increased stress, surgery, or infection.

Avoid exposing insulin to extremes in temperature.
Insulin is not to be frozen, kept in direct sunlight, or in a hot car.
Before injection, insulin needs to be at room temperature.
If a vial of insulin will be used up in 1 month, it may be kept at room temperature; otherwise, the vial would be refrigerated.

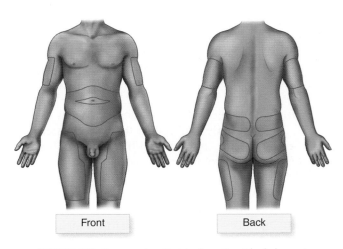

Front   Back

FIGURE 44.1 Common insulin injection sites (shaded areas).

h. Reinforce instructions to the client regarding the necessity of compliance with prescribed medication.

i. Reinforce instructions to the client in how to take each medication, such as with the first bite of a meal for meglitinides and α-glucosidase inhibitors.

j. Reinforce instructions to the client to wear a MedicAlert bracelet.

C. Insulin

1. Insulin primarily acts in the liver, muscle, and adipose tissue by attaching to receptors on cellular membranes and facilitating the passage of glucose, potassium, and magnesium.

2. Insulin is prescribed for clients with type 1 diabetes mellitus, and for clients with type 2 diabetes mellitus whose blood glucose level is not adequately controlled with oral hypoglycemic agents.

3. The onset, peak, and duration of action depend on the insulin type (Tables 44.2 and 44.3).

4. Storing of insulin (Box 44.9)

5. Insulin injection sites

a. The main areas for injections are the abdomen, arms (posterior surface), thighs (anterior surface), and hips (Fig. 44.1).

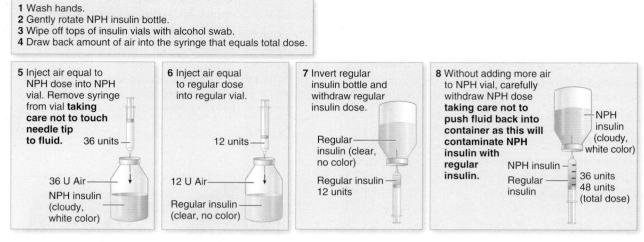

1 Wash hands.
2 Gently rotate NPH insulin bottle.
3 Wipe off tops of insulin vials with alcohol swab.
4 Draw back amount of air into the syringe that equals total dose.

5 Inject air equal to NPH dose into NPH vial. Remove syringe from vial **taking care not to touch needle tip to fluid.** 36 units
36 U Air
NPH insulin (cloudy, white color)

6 Inject air equal to regular dose into regular vial. 12 units
12 U Air
Regular insulin (clear, no color)

7 Invert regular insulin bottle and withdraw regular insulin dose.
Regular insulin (clear, no color)
Regular insulin 12 units

8 Without adding more air to NPH vial, carefully withdraw NPH dose **taking care not to push fluid back into container as this will contaminate NPH insulin with regular insulin.**
NPH insulin (cloudy, white color)
NPH insulin
Regular insulin
36 units
48 units (total dose)

FIGURE 44.2 Steps for mixing insulins.

b. Insulin injected into the abdomen may absorb more evenly and rapidly than at other sites.

c. Systematic rotation within one anatomical area is recommended to prevent lipodystrophy and to promote even absorption; client would be instructed not to use the same site more than once in a 2- to 3-week period.

d. Injections need to be 1 inch to 1.5 inches (2.5–3.8 cm) apart within the anatomical area.

e. Heat, massage, and exercise of the injected area can increase absorption rates and may result in hypoglycemia.

f. Injection into scar tissue may delay absorption of insulin.

6. Administering insulin

 Insulin glargine and insulin detemir cannot be mixed with any other type of insulin.

a. To prevent dosage errors, be certain that there is a match between the insulin concentration noted on the vial and the calibration of units on the insulin syringe. The usual concentration of insulin is U 100 (100 units/mL).

b. The Humulin R brand of regular insulin is the only insulin that is formulated at a U-500 strength. U-500 strength insulin is reserved for clients with severe insulin resistance who require large doses of insulin. A special syringe calibrated for use with U-500 insulin is required.

c. Most insulin syringes have a 27- to 29-gauge needle that is about ½ inch (1.3 cm) long.

d. NPH (neutral protamine Hagedorn) insulin is an insulin suspension; the appearance is cloudy. All other insulin types are solutions; the appearance of all other insulin products is clear.

e. Before use, NPH insulins need to be rotated or rolled between palms to ensure that the insulin suspension is mixed well; otherwise, an inaccurate dose will be drawn; vigorously shaking the bottle will cause bubbles to form. It is not necessary to rotate or roll clear insulins before using.

f. Inject air into the insulin bottle. (A vacuum makes it difficult to draw up the insulin.)

g. When mixing insulins, draw up the shortest-acting insulin first (Fig. 44.2).

h. Short-acting (i.e., regular, lispro, aspart, and glulisine) insulin may be mixed with NPH.

i. A mixed dose of insulin is administered within 5 to 15 minutes of preparation; after this time, the short-acting insulin binds with the NPH insulin and its action is reduced.

j. Aspiration after insertion of the needle is generally not recommended with self-injection of insulin.

k. Insulin is administered at a 45- to 90-degree angle in clients with normal subcutaneous mass and at a 45- to 60-degree angle in thin persons or those with a decreased amount of subcutaneous mass.

 Some rapid- and short-acting insulins can be administered intravenously.

D. Glucagon-like peptide (GLP-1) receptor agonists

1. Noninsulin injectable agents that are analogs of human GLP-1 and have the same effects as the GLP-1 incretin hormone, which are to stimulate glucose level-dependent release of insulin, also then suppress the postprandial release of glucagon to slow gastric emptying and suppress appetite

2. Used for clients with type 2 diabetes mellitus (not recommended for clients taking insulin, nor would clients be taken off of insulin and given a GLP-1 receptor agonist)

3. GLP-1 receptor agonists restore first-phase insulin response (first 10 minutes after food ingestion), lower the production of glucagon after meals, slow gastric emptying (which limits the rise in the blood glucose level after a meal), reduce fasting and postprandial blood glucose levels, and reduce caloric intake resulting in weight loss.

4. Packaged in premeasured doses (pen) that require refrigeration (cannot be frozen)

5. Administered as a subcutaneous injection in the thigh, abdomen, or upper arm. Exenatide is administered twice daily within 60 minutes before morning and evening meals; not taken after meals; if a dose is missed, the treatment regimen is resumed as prescribed with the next scheduled dose. Liraglutide is administered subcutaneously once daily without regard to meals. Albiglutide is injected subcutaneously once weekly.

6. Can cause mild to moderate nausea that abates with use

7. Because delayed gastric emptying slows the absorption of other medications, other prescribed oral medications would be given an hour before injection of these medications.

E. Amylin Mimetic: Pramlintide

1. Synthetic form of amylin, a naturally occurring hormone secreted by the pancreas

2. Used for clients with types 1 and 2 diabetes mellitus who use insulin; administered subcutaneously before meals to lower blood glucose level after meals leading to less fluctuation during the day and better long-term glucose control

3. Associated with an increased risk of insulin-induced severe hypoglycemia, particularly in clients with type 1 diabetes mellitus

4. GI effects, including nausea, can occur.

5. Unopened vials are refrigerated; opened vials can be refrigerated or kept at room temperature for up to 28 days.

6. Reduces postprandial hyperglycemia by delaying gastric emptying and suppressing postprandial glucagon release.

7. Because pramlintide delays gastric emptying, other prescribed oral medications would be given 1 hour before or 2 hours after an injection of pramlintide.

F. Glucagon (also available as GlucaGen)

1. Hormone secreted by the alpha cells of the islets of Langerhans in the pancreas

2. Increases blood glucose level by stimulating glycogenolysis in the liver

3. Can be administered subcutaneously, intramuscularly, or intravenously

4. Used to treat insulin-induced hypoglycemia when the client is semiconscious or unconscious and is unable to ingest liquids

5. The blood glucose level begins to increase within 5 to 20 minutes after administration.

6. The family is instructed in the procedure for administration.

7. See Chapter 43 for additional information regarding interventions for severe hypoglycemia.

WHAT WOULD YOU DO?

Answer: The nurse needs to notify the registered nurse (RN) that the client is taking metformin. The client will need to temporarily discontinue the metformin a day or two before the CT scan and for 48 hours after. IV contrast that contains iodine poses a risk for contrast-induced nephropathy and lactic acidosis. The serum creatinine level is checked before giving IV contrast, and it may also be checked before allowing the client to resume the medication. PHCP prescriptions and agency procedures are followed regarding timelines for discontinuing the medication.

PRACTICE QUESTIONS

1. The nurse is reinforcing teaching for a client regarding how to mix regular insulin and NPH insulin in the same syringe. Which action performed by the client indicates the **need for further teaching**?
   1. Withdraws the NPH insulin first
   2. Withdraws the regular insulin first
   3. Injects air into NPH insulin vial first
   4. Injects an amount of air equal to the desired dose of insulin into the vial

2. The homecare nurse visits a client recently diagnosed with diabetes mellitus who is taking Humulin NPH insulin daily. The client asks the nurse how to store the unopened vials of insulin. The nurse would provide which information?
   1. Freeze the insulin.
   2. Refrigerate the insulin.
   3. Store the insulin in a dark, dry place.
   4. Keep the insulin at room temperature.

❖ 3. The home care nurse is visiting a client who was recently diagnosed with type 2 diabetes mellitus. The client, prescribed repaglinide and metformin, asks the nurse to explain these medications. The nurse would reinforce which instructions to the client? **Select all that apply.**
   ❑ 1. Diarrhea can occur secondary to metformin.
   ❑ 2. The repaglinide is not taken if a meal is skipped.

❑ **3.** The repaglinide is taken 30 minutes before eating.

❑ **4.** Candy or another simple sugar is carried and used to treat mild hypoglycemia episodes.

❑ **5.** Muscle pain is an expected side effect of metformin and may be treated with acetaminophen.

❑ **6.** Metformin increases hepatic glucose production to prevent hypoglycemia associated with repaglinide.

❖ **4.** The nurse is monitoring a client receiving levothyroxine sodium to treat hypothyroidism. Which findings indicate the presence of a side effect associated with this medication? **Select all that apply.**

❑ **1.** Insomnia

❑ **2.** Weight loss

❑ **3.** Bradycardia

❑ **4.** Constipation

❑ **5.** Mild heat intolerance

5. The primary health care provider (PHCP) prescribes exenatide for a client with type 1 diabetes mellitus who takes insulin. The nurse prepares for which **most appropriate** intervention?

1. The medication is administered within 60 minutes before the morning and evening meal.

2. The medication is withheld and the PHCP is called to question the prescription for the client.

3. The client is monitored for gastrointestinal (GI) side effects after administration of the medication.

4. The insulin is withdrawn from the Penlet into an insulin syringe to prepare for administration.

6. A client is taking Humulin NPH insulin daily every morning. The nurse reinforces instructions to the client and would tell the client that which is the **most likely** time for a hypoglycemic reaction to occur?

1. 2 to 4 hours after administration

2. 6 to 14 hours after administration

3. 16 to 18 hours after administration

4. 18 to 24 hours after administration

7. A client with diabetes mellitus visits a healthcare clinic. The client's diabetes mellitus has been previously well controlled with glyburide daily, but recently the fasting blood glucose level has been 180 mg/dL to 200 mg/dL. Which medication, added to the client's regimen, may have contributed to the hyperglycemia?

1. Atenolol

2. Prednisone

3. Phenelzine

4. Allopurinol

8. The home care nurse visits a client at home who has been prescribed prednisone 5 mg orally daily. The nurse reinforces teaching for the client about the medication. Which statement made by the client indicates a **need for further teaching**?

1. "I can take aspirin or my antihistamine if I need it."

2. "I need to take the medication every day at the same time."

3. "I need to avoid coffee, tea, cola, and chocolate in my diet."

4. "If I gain more than 5 pounds a week, I will call my doctor."

9. Desmopressin acetate is prescribed for the treatment of diabetes insipidus. The nurse monitors the client after medication administration for which therapeutic response?

1. Decreased urinary output

2. Decreased blood pressure

3. Decreased peripheral edema

4. Decreased blood glucose level

10. Glimepiride is prescribed for a client with diabetes mellitus. The nurse reinforces instructions for the client and tells the client to avoid which while taking this medication?

1. Alcohol

2. Organ meats

3. Whole-grain cereals

4. Carbonated beverages

ANSWERS

1. 1

Rationale: When preparing a mixture of regular insulin with another insulin preparation, the regular insulin is drawn into the syringe first. This sequence will avoid contaminating the vial of regular insulin with insulin of another type. Options 2, 3, and 4 identify the correct actions for preparing NPH and regular insulin.

Test-Taking Strategy: Note the strategic words, *need for further teaching*. These words indicate a negative event query and ask you to select an option that is an incorrect action. Remember *RN*—draw up the **R**egular insulin before the **N**PH insulin.

2. 2

Rationale: Insulin in unopened vials need to be stored under refrigeration until needed. Vials are not frozen because freezing affects the chemical composition of the insulin. When stored unopened under refrigeration, insulin can be used up to the expiration date on the vial. Freezing insulin, storing insulin in a dark, dry place, and keeping the insulin at room temperature are all incorrect actions.

Test-Taking Strategy: Focus on the subject, how to store unopened vials of insulin. Remembering that insulin is not frozen will assist in eliminating this option. The options for storing insulin at room temperature or in a dark, dry place are comparable or alike and would be eliminated.

❖ **3. 1, 2, 3, 4**
Rationale: Repaglinide is a rapid-acting oral hypoglycemic agent that stimulates pancreatic insulin secretion that is taken 30 minutes before meals and that would be withheld if the client does not eat. Hypoglycemia is a side effect of repaglinide, and the client needs to always be prepared by carrying a simple sugar with her or him at all times. Metformin is an oral hypoglycemic given in combination with repaglinide and works by decreasing hepatic glucose production. A common side effect of metformin is diarrhea. Muscle pain may occur as an adverse effect from metformin, but it also might signify a more serious condition that warrants primary health care provider (PHCP) notification, not the use of acetaminophen.
Test-Taking Strategy: Focus on the subject, client teaching points related to repaglinide and metformin. Also focus on the data in the question and the client's diagnosis to assist in answering the question. Recalling the actions and effects of these medications will assist with answering correctly.

❖ **4. 1, 2, 5**
Rationale: Insomnia, weight loss, and mild heat intolerance are side effects of levothyroxine sodium. Bradycardia and constipation are not side effects associated with this medication, but rather are associated with hypothyroidism, which is the disorder that this medication is prescribed to treat.
Test-Taking Strategy: Focus on the subject, side effects of levothyroxine. Thinking about the pathophysiology of hypothyroidism and the action of the medication will assist you with determining that insomnia, weight loss, and mild heat intolerance are side effects of thyroid hormones.

5. 2
Rationale: Exenatide is an incretin mimetic used for type 2 diabetes mellitus only. It is not recommended for clients taking insulin. Hence, the nurse would hold the medication and question the PHCP regarding this prescription. Although options 1 and 3 are correct statements about the medication, in this situation it would not be administered. The medication is packaged in prefilled pens ready for injection without the need for drawing it up into another syringe.
Test-Taking Strategy: Focus on the subject, type 1 diabetes and exenatide, and note the strategic words, *most appropriate.* Eliminate the option regarding drawing up the medication because the medication is packaged in prefilled pens ready for injection without the need for drawing it up into another syringe. From the remaining options, focus on the data in the question. Although the other options are appropriate when administering this medication, this client would not receive the medication.

6. 2
Rationale: Humulin NPH is an intermediate-acting insulin. The onset of action is 1 to 2 hours, it peaks in 6 to 14 hours, and its duration of action is 16 to 24 hours. Hypoglycemic reactions most likely occur during peak time.
Test-Taking Strategy: Note the strategic words, *most likely,* and focus on the subject, peak time of NPH insulin. Use

knowledge regarding the onset, peak, and duration of action for NPH insulin. Remember that NPH peaks in 6 to 14 hours.

7. 2
Rationale: Prednisone may decrease the effect of oral hypoglycemics, insulin, diuretics, and potassium supplements. Option 1, a β-blocker, and option 3, a monoamine oxidase inhibitor, have their own intrinsic hypoglycemic activity. Option 4 decreases urinary excretion of sulfonylurea agents, causing increased levels of the oral agents, which can lead to hypoglycemia.
Test-Taking Strategy: Focus on the subject, medications that cause an increase in the blood glucose level. Recalling that prednisone decreases the effects of oral hypoglycemics will direct you to the correct option.

8. 1
Rationale: Aspirin and other over-the-counter medications would not be taken unless the client consults with the primary health care provider (PHCP). The client needs to take the medication at the same time every day and needs to be instructed not to stop. A slight weight gain as a result of an improved appetite is expected, but after the dosage is stabilized, a weight gain of 5 lb or more weekly needs to be reported to the PHCP. Caffeine-containing foods and fluids need to be avoided because they may contribute to steroid-ulcer development.
Test-Taking Strategy: Note the strategic words, *need for further teaching.* This indicates a negative event query and a need to select the incorrect statement as the answer. Remember that a client would not take other medications, especially over-the-counter medications, without first consulting with his or her PHCP.

9. 1
Rationale: Desmopressin promotes renal conservation of water. The hormone carries out this action by acting on the collecting ducts of the kidney to increase their permeability to water, which results in increased water reabsorption. The therapeutic effect of this medication would be manifested by a decreased urine output. Options 2, 3, and 4 are unrelated to the effects of this medication.
Test-Taking Strategy: Note the subject, therapeutic response of desmopressin. Focus on the diagnosis in the question to assist in answering the question. Recalling the signs/symptoms related to the loss of large volumes of urine in this disorder will help direct you to the option describing decreased urine output.

10. 1
Rationale: When alcohol is combined with glimepiride, a disulfiram-like reaction may occur. This syndrome includes flushing, palpitations, and nausea. Alcohol can also potentiate the hypoglycemic effects of the medication. Clients need to be instructed to avoid alcohol consumption while taking this medication. The items in options 2, 3, and 4 do not need to be avoided.
Test-Taking Strategy: Focus on the subject, the substance to avoid. Eliminate organ meats, whole-grain cereals, and carbonated beverages because these food items are allowed in a diabetic diet. Remembering that alcohol can affect the action of many medications will assist with directing you to the correct option.

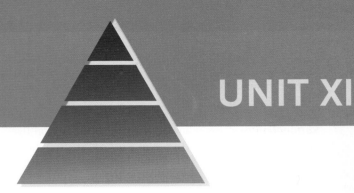

UNIT XI

Gastrointestinal Problems of the Adult Client

Pyramid to Success

Pyramid Points focus on diagnostic tests and nursing care related to the various gastric or intestinal tubes, gastric surgery, cirrhosis, hepatitis, pancreatitis, and colostomy care. Focus on preprocedure and postprocedure care of the client undergoing a gastrointestinal diagnostic test. Remember that an informed consent is required for any invasive procedure. Focus on diet restrictions before and after the diagnostic test and remember that the gag reflex or bowel sounds must return before allowing a client to consume food or fluids. Pyramid Points also include instructions to the client and family regarding the prevention of gastrointestinal problems and the complications associated with the particular problem. Focus on teaching the client and family about diet and nutrition specific to the gastrointestinal problem, tube and wound care, preventing the transmission of infection such as with hepatitis, and care of a colostomy or ileostomy. Remember that body image disturbances can occur in clients with a gastrointestinal alteration. Specific focus relates to the client with a diversion, such as an ileostomy or colostomy; the social isolation issues that can occur; and effective coping strategies.

Client Needs: Learning Objectives

 Safe and Effective Care Environment

Consulting with the interprofessional team regarding the client's care and nutritional status

Ensuring that confidentiality issues related to the gastrointestinal problem are maintained

Ensuring that informed consent for treatments and surgical procedures has been obtained

Establishing priorities of care

Handling infectious drainage and secretions safely

Maintaining standard precautions and other precautions as appropriate

Preventing disease transmission

Suggesting appropriate referrals for homecare and community services

Health Promotion and Maintenance

Performing physical assessment/data collection techniques of the gastrointestinal system

Preventing disease related to the gastrointestinal system

Providing assistance with health screening and health promotion programs related to gastrointestinal disorders

Teaching related to colostomy or ileostomy care

Teaching related to prescribed dietary and other treatment measures

Teaching related to preventing the transmission of disease

Psychosocial Integrity

Assessing coping mechanisms

Considering end-of-life and grief and loss issues

Identifying available support systems

Monitoring for concerns related to body image changes

Physiological Integrity

Administering medications as prescribed specific to the gastrointestinal problem

Assessing for signs and symptoms of infectious diseases of the gastrointestinal tract

Assisting with personal hygiene

Monitoring elimination patterns

Monitoring for complications related to tests, procedures, and surgical interventions

Monitoring for fluid and electrolyte imbalances

Monitoring laboratory values related to gastrointestinal problems

Monitoring parenterally administered fluids, including parenteral nutrition with the registered nurse

Providing adequate nutrition and oral hydration

Providing care for gastrointestinal tubes

Providing nonpharmacological and pharmacological comfort measures

Providing preprocedure and postprocedure care for diagnostic tests related to the gastrointestinal system

Client Needs lists modified from: National Council of State Boards of Nursing, Inc. (NCSBN). *NCLEX-PN Examination: Test Plan for the National Council Licensure Examination for Practical Nurses,* effective April 2020. Chicago: NCSBN.

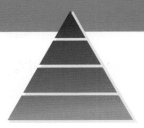

CHAPTER **45**

Gastrointestinal Problems

PRIORITY CONCEPTS **Elimination; Nutrition**

WHAT WOULD YOU DO?

The nurse is preparing a client for a liver biopsy. During review of the client's laboratory results, the nurse notes that the client's prothrombin time is 35 seconds and platelet count is 100,000 mm³. What would the nurse do?
Answer is located on p. 596.

I. Anatomy and Physiology

A. Functions of the gastrointestinal (GI) system
   1. Process food substances
   2. Absorb the products of digestion into the blood
   3. Excrete unabsorbed materials
   4. Provide an environment for microorganisms to synthesize nutrients, such as vitamin K
   5. For risk factors associated with the GI system, see Box 45.1.
B. Mouth
   1. Contains the lips, cheeks, palate, tongue, teeth, salivary glands, muscles, and maxillary bones
   2. Saliva contains the amylase enzyme (ptyalin), which aids in digestion.
C. Esophagus
   1. A collapsible muscular tube about 10 inches (25 cm) long
   2. Carries food from the pharynx to the stomach
D. Stomach
   1. Contains the cardia, fundus, body, and pylorus
   2. Mucous glands are located in the mucosa and prevent autodigestion by providing an alkaline protective covering.
   3. The lower esophageal (cardiac) sphincter prevents reflux of gastric contents into the esophagus.
   4. The pyloric sphincter regulates the rate of stomach emptying into the small intestine.
   5. Hydrochloric acid kills microorganisms, breaks food into small particles, and provides a chemical environment that facilitates gastric enzyme activation.
   6. Pepsin is the chief coenzyme of gastric juice, which converts proteins into proteases and peptones.
   7. Intrinsic factor comes from parietal cells and is necessary for the absorption of vitamin B_{12}.
   8. Gastrin controls gastric acidity.
E. Gallbladder
   1. Stores and concentrates bile and contracts to force bile into the duodenum during the digestion of fats
   2. The cystic duct joins the hepatic duct to form the common bile duct.
   3. The sphincter of Oddi is located at the entrance to the duodenum.
   4. The presence of fatty materials in the duodenum stimulates the liberation of cholecystokinin, which causes contraction of the gallbladder and relaxation of the sphincter of Oddi.
F. Pancreas
   1. Exocrine gland
      a. Secretes sodium bicarbonate to neutralize the acidity of the stomach contents that enter the duodenum
      b. Pancreatic juices contain enzymes for digesting carbohydrates, fats, and proteins.
   2. Endocrine gland
      a. Secretes glucagon to raise the blood glucose level and secretes somatostatin to exert a hypoglycemic effect
      b. The islets of Langerhans secrete insulin.
      c. Insulin is secreted into the bloodstream and is important for carbohydrate metabolism.
G. Pancreatic intestinal juice enzymes
   1. Amylase digests starch to maltose.
   2. Maltase reduces maltose to monosaccharide glucose.
   3. Lactase splits lactose into galactose and glucose.
   4. Sucrase reduces sucrose to fructose and glucose.
   5. Nucleases split nucleic acids to nucleotides.
   6. Enterokinase activates trypsinogen to trypsin.

BOX 45.1	Risk Factors Associated With the Gastrointestinal System

- Allergic reactions to food or medications
- Cardiac, respiratory, and endocrine disorders that may lead to slowed gastrointestinal (GI) movement or constipation
- Chronic alcohol use
- Chronic high stress levels
- Chronic laxative use
- Chronic use of aspirin or nonsteroidal anti-inflammatory drugs (NSAIDs)
- Diabetes mellitus, which may predispose to oral candidal infections or other GI disorders
- Family history of GI disorders
- Long-term GI conditions, such as ulcerative colitis, that may predispose to colorectal cancer
- Neurological disorders that can impair movement, particularly with chewing and swallowing
- Previous abdominal surgery or trauma, which may lead to adhesions
- Tobacco use

BOX 45.2	Common Gastrointestinal System Diagnostic Studies

- Capsule endoscopy
- Endoscopic retrograde cholangiopancreatography (ERCP)
- Endoscopic ultrasound
- Fiberoptic colonoscopy
- Gastric analysis
- Gastrointestinal motility studies
- Hydrogen and urea breath tests
- Laparoscopy: Liver and pancreas laboratory studies
- Liver biopsy
- Paracentesis
- Stool specimens
- Upper gastrointestinal (GI) endoscopy or esophagogastroduodenoscopy
- Upper GI tract study (barium swallow)
- Videofluoroscopic swallowing study

Note: Informed consent is obtained for a diagnostic study that is invasive.

H. Small intestine
  1. The duodenum contains the openings of the bile and pancreatic ducts.
  2. The jejunum is about 8 ft (2.4 m) long.
  3. The ileum is about 12 ft (3.7 m) long.
  4. The small intestine terminates in the cecum.
I. Large intestine
  1. Is about 5 ft (1.5 m) long
  2. Absorbs water and eliminates waste
  3. Intestinal bacteria play a vital role in the synthesis of some B vitamins and vitamin K.
  4. Colon: includes the ascending, transverse, descending, and sigmoid colons and rectum
  5. The ileocecal valve prevents contents of the large intestine from entering the ileum.
  6. The internal and external anal sphincters control the anal canal.
J. Peritoneum: lines the abdominal cavity and forms the mesentery that supports the intestines and blood supply
K. Liver
  1. The largest gland in the body, weighing 3 to 4 lb (1.4–1.8 kg)
  2. Contains Kupffer cells, which remove bacteria in the portal venous blood
  3. Removes excess glucose and amino acids from the portal blood
  4. Synthesizes glucose, amino acids, and fats
  5. Aids in the digestion of fats, carbohydrates, and proteins
  6. Stores and filters blood (200–400 mL of blood stored)
  7. Stores vitamins A, D, and B and iron
  8. The liver secretes bile to emulsify fats (500–1000 mL of bile/day).

  9. Hepatic ducts
    a. Deliver bile to the gallbladder via the cystic duct and to the duodenum via the common bile duct
    b. The common bile duct opens into the duodenum with the pancreatic duct at the ampulla of Vater.
    c. The sphincter prevents the reflux of intestinal contents into the common bile duct and pancreatic duct.

II. Diagnostic Procedures (Box 45.2)
A. Upper GI tract study (barium swallow)
  1. Description: Examination of the upper GI tract under fluoroscopy after the client drinks barium sulfate
  2. Preprocedure: Withhold foods and fluids for 8 hours before the test.
  3. Postprocedure
    a. A laxative may be prescribed.
    b. The client is instructed to increase oral fluid intake to help pass the barium.
    c. Monitor stools for the passage of barium (stools will appear chalky white for 24–72 hours postprocedure) because barium can cause a bowel obstruction.
B. Capsule endoscopy
  1. A procedure that uses a small wireless camera shaped like a medication capsule that the client swallows; the test will detect bleeding or changes in the lining of the small intestine.
  2. The camera travels through the entire digestive tract and sends pictures to a small box that the client wears like a belt; the small box saves the pictures, which are then transferred to a computer for viewing once the test is complete.

3. The client visits the primary health care provider's (PHCP's) office in the morning and swallows the capsule, the recording belt is applied by the office staff, and then the client returns at the end of the day so that pictures can be transferred to the computer.

4. Preprocedure, a bowel preparation will be prescribed; the client will need to maintain a clear liquid diet the evening before the examination; additionally, NPO (nothing by mouth) status is maintained for 3 hours before and after swallowing the capsule (time for NPO status is prescribed by the PHCP, but is usually 2–3 hours).

C. Gastric analysis

1. Description

a. Gastric analysis requires the passage of a nasogastric (NG) tube into the stomach to aspirate gastric contents for the analysis of acidity (pH), appearance, and volume; the entire gastric contents are aspirated, and then specimens are collected every 15 minutes for 1 hour.

b. Medication, such as histamine or pentagastrin, may be administered subcutaneously to stimulate gastric secretions; some medications may produce a flushed feeling.

c. Esophageal reflux of gastric acid may be diagnosed by ambulatory pH monitoring; a probe is placed just above the lower esophageal sphincter (LES) and connected to an external recording device. It provides a computer analysis and graphic display of results.

2. Preprocedure

a. Fasting for at least 12 hours is required before the test.

b. Use of tobacco and chewing gum is avoided for 24 hours before the test.

c. Medications that stimulate gastric secretions are withheld for 24 to 48 hours.

3. Postprocedure

a. Client may resume normal activities.

b. Refrigerate gastric samples if not tested within 4 hours.

D. Upper GI endoscopy

1. Description

a. Also known as esophagogastroduodenoscopy

b. Following sedation, an endoscope is passed down the esophagus to view the gastric wall, sphincters, and duodenum; tissue specimens can be obtained.

2. Preprocedure

a. The client needs to be NPO for 6 to 8 hours before the test.

b. A local anesthetic (spray or gargle) may be administered along with medication that provides moderate sedation just before the scope is inserted.

c. Medication may be administered to reduce secretions, and medication may be administered to relax smooth muscle.

d. The client is positioned on the left side to facilitate saliva drainage and to provide easy access of the endoscope.

e. Airway patency is monitored during the test, and pulse oximetry is used to monitor oxygen saturation; emergency equipment must be readily available.

3. Postprocedure

a. Monitor vital signs.

b. Client needs to be NPO until the gag reflex returns (1–2 hours).

c. Monitor for signs of perforation (pain, bleeding, unusual difficulty with swallowing, elevated temperature).

d. Maintain bed rest for the sedated client until alert.

e. Lozenges, saline gargles, or oral analgesics can relieve a minor sore throat (not given to the client until the gag reflex returns).

E. Fiberoptic colonoscopy

1. Description

a. Colonoscopy is a fiberoptic endoscopy study in which the lining of the large intestine is visually examined; biopsies and polypectomies can be performed.

b. Cardiac and respiratory functions are monitored continuously during the test.

c. Colonoscopy is performed with the client lying on the left side with the knees drawn up to the chest; the position may be changed during the test to facilitate passing of the scope.

2. Preprocedure

a. Adequate cleansing of the colon is necessary, as prescribed by the PHCP.

b. A clear liquid diet is started on the day before the test. Red, orange, and purple (grape) liquids are to be avoided.

c. Consult with the PHCP regarding medications that need to be withheld before the test.

d. The client is NPO for 4 to 6 hours before the test.

e. Moderate sedation is administered intravenously.

f. Medication may be administered to relax smooth muscle.

⚠ The client receiving oral liquid bowel cleansing preparations or enemas is at risk for fluid and electrolyte imbalances.

3. Postprocedure

a. Monitor vital signs.

b. Provide bed rest until alert.

c. Monitor for signs of bowel perforation and peritonitis (Box 45.3).

BOX 45.3 **Signs of Bowel Perforation and Peritonitis**

- Guarding of the abdomen
- Increased fever and chills
- Pallor
- Progressive abdominal distention and abdominal pain
- Restlessness
- Tachycardia and tachypnea

⚠️ Following endoscopic procedures, monitor for the return of a gag reflex before giving the client any oral substance. If the gag reflex has not returned, the client could aspirate.

---

d. Remind the client that passing flatus, abdominal fullness, and mild cramping are expected for several hours.
e. The client is instructed to report any bleeding to the PHCP.

F. Laparoscopy is performed with a fiberoptic laparoscope that allows direct visualization of organs and structures within the abdomen; biopsies may be obtained.

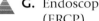 **G.** Endoscopic retrograde cholangiopancreatography (ERCP)
   1. Description
      a. Examination of the hepatobiliary system is performed via a flexible endoscope inserted into the esophagus to the descending duodenum; multiple positions are required during the procedure to pass the endoscope.
      b. If medication is administered before the procedure, the client is monitored closely for signs of respiratory and central nervous system depression, hypotension, oversedation, and vomiting.
   2. Preprocedure
      a. Client is NPO for 6 to 8 hours before the procedure.
      b. Inquire about previous exposure to contrast media and any sensitivities or allergies.
      c. Moderate sedation is administered before the procedure.
   3. Postprocedure
      a. Monitor vital signs.
      b. Monitor for return of gag reflex.
      c. Monitor for signs of perforation or peritonitis (see Box 45.3).

H. Magnetic resonance cholangiopancreatography (MRCP)
   1. Description: Uses magnetic resonance to visualize the biliary and pancreatic ducts in a noninvasive way
   2. Preprocedure and postprocedure: see ERCP

I. Endoscopic ultrasonography
   1. Description: Provides images of the GI wall and digestive organs
   2. Preprocedure and postprocedure: Care is similar to that implemented for endoscopy.

J. Computed tomography (CT) scan
   1. Description
      a. Noninvasive cross-sectional view that can detect tissue densities in the abdomen, including the liver, spleen, pancreas, and biliary tree
      b. Can be performed with or without contrast medium
   2. Preprocedure
      a. Client is NPO for at least 4 hours.
      b. If contrast medium will be used, assess for previous sensitivities and allergies.
   3. Postprocedure: No specific care is required.

K. Paracentesis
   1. Description and preprocedure (see **Priority Nursing Actions**)

⚡ **PRIORITY NURSING ACTIONS**

Paracentesis

1. Ensure that the client understands the procedure and that informed consent has been obtained.
2. Obtain vital signs, including weight, and assist the client to void.
3. Position the client upright.
4. Assist the PHCP, monitor vital signs, and provide comfort and support during the procedure.
5. Apply a dressing to the site of puncture.
6. Monitor vital signs, especially blood pressure and pulse because these parameters provide information on rapid vasodilation postparacentesis; weigh the client postprocedure, and maintain the client on bed rest.
7. Measure the amount of fluid removed.
8. Label and send the fluid for laboratory analysis.
9. Document the event, the client's response, and appearance and amount of fluid removed.

---

2. Postprocedure
   a. Monitor vital signs.
   b. Measure fluid collected, describe, and record.
   c. Label fluid samples and send to the laboratory for analysis.
   d. Apply a dry sterile dressing to the insertion site; monitor the site for bleeding.
   e. Measure abdominal girth and weight.
   f. Monitor for hypovolemia, electrolyte loss, mental status changes, or encephalopathy.

g. Monitor for hematuria caused by bladder trauma.

h. Instruct the client to notify the PHCP if the urine becomes bloody, pink, or red.

⚠️ The rapid removal of fluid from the abdominal cavity during paracentesis leads to decreased abdominal pressure, which can cause vasodilation and resultant shock; therefore, the heart rate and blood pressure need to be monitored closely.

L. Liver biopsy

1. Description: A needle is inserted through the abdominal wall to the liver to obtain a tissue sample for biopsy and microscopic examination.

2. Preprocedure

a. Check results of coagulation tests (prothrombin time, partial thromboplastin time, platelet count).

b. Administer a sedative as prescribed.

c. Note that the client is placed in the supine or left lateral position during the procedure to expose the right side of the upper abdomen.

3. Postprocedure

a. Monitor vital signs.

b. Check biopsy site for bleeding.

c. Monitor for peritonitis (see Box 45.3).

d. Maintain bed rest for several hours as prescribed.

e. Place the client on the right side with a pillow under the costal margin for 2 hours to decrease the risk of bleeding, and instruct the client to avoid coughing and straining.

f. The client is instructed to avoid heavy lifting and strenuous exercise for 1 week.

M. Stool specimens

1. Testing of stool specimens includes inspecting the specimen for consistency and color, and testing for occult blood.

2. Tests for fecal urobilinogen, fat, nitrogen, parasites, pathogens, food substances, and other substances may be performed; these tests require that the specimen be sent to the laboratory.

3. Random specimens are sent promptly to the laboratory.

4. Quantitative 24- to 72-hour collections need to be kept refrigerated until they are taken to the laboratory.

5. Some specimens require that a certain diet be followed or that certain medications be withheld; check agency guidelines regarding specific procedures.

N. Urea breath test

1. The urea breath test detects the presence of *Helicobacter pylori*, the bacteria that cause peptic ulcer disease.

2. The client consumes a capsule of carbon-labeled urea and provides a breath sample 10 to 20 minutes later.

3. Certain medications may need to be avoided before testing and these specific medications to be avoided will be determined by the physician who prescribed the test.

4. *Helicobacter pylori* can also be detected by assessing serum antibody levels.

O. Esophageal pH testing for gastroesophageal reflux disease

1. Used to diagnose or evaluate the treatment for heartburn or reflux disease

2. A probe is inserted into the nostril and is situated in the esophagus.

3. pH is tested over a period of 24-48 hours.

P. Liver and pancreas laboratory studies

1. Liver enzyme levels (alkaline phosphatase [ALP], aspartate aminotransferase [AST], and alanine aminotransferase [ALT]) are elevated with liver damage or biliary obstruction. Normal reference intervals: ALP, 38 to 126 U/L; AST, 0 to 35 U/L; ALT, 4 to 36 U/L.

2. Prothrombin time is prolonged with liver damage. Normal reference interval: 11 to 12.5 seconds.

3. The serum ammonia level assesses the ability of the liver to deaminate protein byproducts. Normal reference interval: 10 to 80 mcg/dL.

4. An increase in cholesterol level indicates pancreatitis or biliary obstruction. Normal reference interval: <200 mg/dL.

5. An increase in bilirubin level indicates liver damage or biliary obstruction. Normal reference intervals: Total, 0.3 to 1.0 mg/dL; indirect, 0.2 to 0.8 mg/dL; direct, 0.1 to 0.3 mg/dL.

6. Increased values for amylase and lipase levels indicate pancreatitis. Normal reference intervals: amylase, 60 to 120 Somogyi units/dL; lipase, 0 to 160 U/L.

III. Data Collection

A. See Chapter 13 for abdominal data collection techniques.

IV. GI Tubes (Refer to Chapter 18)

V. Gastroesophageal Reflux Disease

A. Description

1. The backflow of gastric and duodenal contents into the esophagus

2. The reflux is caused by an incompetent LES, pyloric stenosis, or a motility disorder.

B. Data collection

1. Epigastric pain; heartburn

2. Dyspepsia

3. Nausea; regurgitation

4. Pain and difficulty with swallowing

5. Hypersalivation

C. Interventions

1. The client is instructed to avoid factors that decrease LES pressure or cause esophageal irritation such as peppermint, chocolate, coffee, fried or fatty foods, carbonated beverages, alcoholic beverages, and cigarette smoking.

2. The client is instructed to eat a low-fat, high-fiber diet and to avoid eating and drinking 2 hours before bedtime and wearing tight clothes; also, elevate the head of the bed on 6- to 8-in (15–20 cm) blocks.

3. Avoid the use of anticholinergics, which delay stomach emptying; also, nonsteroidal anti-inflammatory medications (NSAIDs) and other medications that contain acetylsalicylic acid need to be avoided.

4. Reinforce instructions regarding prescribed medications, such as antacids, histamine 2 (H_2)-receptor antagonists, or proton pump inhibitors.

5. Reinforce instructions regarding the administration of prokinetic medications, if prescribed, which accelerate gastric emptying.

6. Surgery may be required in extreme cases when medical management is unsuccessful; this involves fundoplication (wrapping a portion of the gastric fundus around the sphincter area of the esophagus); surgery may be performed by laparoscopy.

VI. Gastritis

A. Description

1. Inflammation of the stomach or gastric mucosa

2. Acute gastritis is caused by the ingestion of food contaminated with disease-causing microorganisms or food that is irritating or too highly seasoned, the overuse of aspirin or other NSAIDs, excessive alcohol intake, bile reflux, or radiation therapy.

3. Chronic gastritis is caused by benign or malignant ulcers or by the bacteria *H. pylori*, and it may be caused by autoimmune diseases, dietary factors, medications, alcohol, smoking, or reflux.

B. Data collection (Box 45.4)

C. Interventions

1. Acute gastritis: Food and fluids may be withheld until symptoms subside; afterward, ice chips can be given, followed by clear liquids, and then solid food.

2. Monitor for signs of hemorrhagic gastritis such as hematemesis, tachycardia, and hypotension, and notify the PHCP if these signs occur.

3. Reinforce instructions to avoid irritating foods, fluids, and other substances such as spicy and highly seasoned foods, caffeine, alcohol, and nicotine.

4. Reinforce instructions on the use of prescribed medications, such as antibiotics and antacids.

BOX 45.4 **Data Collection: Acute and Chronic Gastritis**

Acute
Abdominal discomfort
Anorexia, nausea, vomiting
Headache
Hiccupping
Reflux

Chronic
Anorexia, nausea, vomiting
Belching
Heartburn after eating
Sour taste in the mouth
Vitamin B_{12} deficiency

---

5. Provide the client with information about the importance of vitamin B_{12} injections if a deficiency is present.

VII. Peptic Ulcer Disease

A. Description

1. A peptic ulcer is an ulceration in the mucosal wall of the stomach, pylorus, duodenum, or esophagus in portions accessible to gastric secretions; erosion may extend through the muscle.

2. The ulcer may be referred to as *gastric, duodenal,* or *esophageal,* depending on its location.

3. The most common peptic ulcers are gastric ulcers and duodenal ulcers.

B. Gastric ulcers

1. Description
   a. A gastric ulcer involves ulceration of the mucosal lining that extends to the submucosal layer of the stomach.
   b. Predisposing factors include stress, smoking, the use of corticosteroids, NSAIDs, alcohol, history of gastritis, family history of gastric ulcers, or infection with *H. pylori*.
   c. Complications include hemorrhage, perforation, and pyloric obstruction.

2. Data collection (Box 45.5)

3. Interventions

   a. Monitor vital signs and for signs of bleeding.
   b. Administer small, frequent, bland feedings during the active phase.
   c. Administer H_2-receptor antagonists or proton pump inhibitors, as prescribed, to decrease the secretion of gastric acid.
   d. Administer antacids as prescribed to neutralize gastric secretions.
   e. Administer anticholinergics, as prescribed, to reduce gastric motility.
   f. Administer mucosal barrier protectants as prescribed 1 hour before each meal.

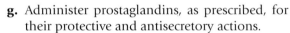

> **BOX 45.5**   **Data Collection: Gastric and Duodenal Ulcers**
>
> **Gastric**
> Gnawing, sharp pain in or to the left of the midepigastric region occurs 30–60 minutes after a meal (food ingestion accentuates the pain).
> Hematemesis is more common than melena.
>
> **Duodenal**
> Burning pain in the midepigastric area 1½–3 hours after a meal and during the night (often awakens the client).
> Melena is more common than hematemesis.
> Pain is often relieved by the ingestion of food.

   g. Administer prostaglandins, as prescribed, for their protective and antisecretory actions.
   4. Client education
     a. Avoid consuming alcohol and substances that contain caffeine or chocolate.
     b. Avoid smoking.
     c. Avoid aspirin or NSAIDs.
     d. Obtain adequate rest and reduce stress.
   5. Interventions during active bleeding
     a. Monitor vital signs closely.
     b. Monitor for signs of dehydration, hypovolemic shock, sepsis, and respiratory insufficiency.
     c. Maintain NPO status and assist with the administration of intravenous (IV) fluid replacement as prescribed; monitor intake and output.
     d. Monitor hemoglobin and hematocrit.
     e. Assist with the administration of blood transfusions, as prescribed.
     f. Prepare to assist with administering medications, as prescribed, to induce vasoconstriction and reduce bleeding.
   6. Surgical interventions
     a. Total **gastrectomy:** Removal of the stomach with attachment of the esophagus to the jejunum or duodenum; also called esophagojejunostomy or esophagoduodenostomy
     b. **Vagotomy:** Surgical division of the vagus nerve to eliminate the vagal impulses that stimulate hydrochloric acid secretion in the stomach
     c. **Gastric resection:** Removal of the lower half of the stomach and usually includes a vagotomy; also called antrectomy
     d. Gastroduodenostomy: Partial gastrectomy, with the remaining segment anastomosed to the duodenum; also called **Billroth I**
     e. Gastrojejunostomy: Partial gastrectomy, with the remaining segment anastomosed to the jejunum; also called **Billroth II**
     f. **Pyloroplasty:** Enlargement of the pylorus to prevent or decrease pyloric obstruction, thereby enhancing gastric emptying

   7. Postoperative interventions
     a. Monitor vital signs.
     b Place in a Fowler's position for comfort and to promote drainage.
     c. Assist to administer fluids and electrolyte replacements intravenously as prescribed; monitor intake and output.
     d. Check bowel sounds.
     e. Monitor NG suction as prescribed.
     f. Maintain NPO status, as prescribed, for 1 to 3 days until **peristalsis** returns.
     g. Progress the diet from NPO, to sips of clear water, to six small bland meals a day, as prescribed, when the bowel sounds return.
     h. Monitor for postoperative complications of hemorrhage, **dumping syndrome**, diarrhea, hypoglycemia, and vitamin B_{12} deficiency.

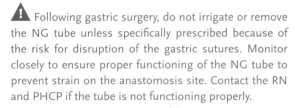

⚠️ Following gastric surgery, do not irrigate or remove the NG tube unless specifically prescribed because of the risk for disruption of the gastric sutures. Monitor closely to ensure proper functioning of the NG tube to prevent strain on the anastomosis site. Contact the RN and PHCP if the tube is not functioning properly.

C. Duodenal ulcers
   1. Description
     a. A duodenal ulcer is a break in the mucosa of the duodenum.
     b. Risk factors and causes include infection with *H. pylori*; alcohol intake; smoking; stress; caffeine; and the use of aspirin, corticosteroids, and NSAIDs.
     c. Complications include bleeding, perforation, gastric outlet obstruction, and intractable disease.
   2. Data collection (see Box 45.5)
   3. Interventions
     a. Monitor vital signs.
     b. Instruct the client about a bland diet, with small frequent meals.
     c. Provide for adequate rest.
     d. Encourage the cessation of smoking.
     e. Reinforce instructions to avoid alcohol intake, caffeine, the use of aspirin, corticosteroids, and NSAIDs.
     f. Administer medications to treat *H. pylori* and antacids to neutralize acid secretions as prescribed.
     g. Administer H_2-receptor antagonists or proton pump inhibitors as prescribed to block the secretion of acid.
   4. Surgical interventions: Surgery is performed only if the ulcer is unresponsive to medications or if hemorrhage, obstruction, or perforation occurs.
D. Dumping syndrome
   1. Description: The rapid emptying of the gastric contents into the small intestine that occurs following gastric resection

BOX 45.6	Client Education: Preventing Dumping Syndrome

- Avoid sugar, salt, and milk.
- Eat a high-protein, high-fat, low-carbohydrate diet.
- Eat small meals, and avoid consuming fluids with meals.
- Lie down after meals.
- Take antispasmodic medications as prescribed to delay gastric emptying.

   2. Data collection
- a. Symptoms occurring 30 minutes after eating
- b. Nausea and vomiting
- c. Feelings of abdominal fullness and abdominal cramping
- d. Diarrhea
- e. Palpitations and tachycardia
- f. Perspiration
- g. Weakness and dizziness
- h. Borborygmi (loud gurgling sounds resulting from bowel hypermotility)

   3. Client education (Box 45.6)

VIII. Vitamin B₁₂ Deficiency

A. Description
1. Vitamin B_{12} deficiency results from an inadequate intake of vitamin B_{12} or a lack of absorption of ingested vitamin B_{12} from the intestinal tract.
2. Pernicious anemia results from a deficiency of intrinsic factor, necessary for intestinal absorption of vitamin B_{12}; gastric disease or surgery can result in a lack of intrinsic factor.

 B. Data collection
1. Severe pallor
2. Fatigue
3. Weight loss
4. Smooth, beefy red tongue
5. Slight jaundice
6. Paresthesia of the hands and feet
7. Gait and balance disturbance

 C. Interventions
1. Increase dietary intake of foods rich in vitamin B_{12} such as meats and liver if the anemia is the result of a dietary deficiency.
2. Administer vitamin B_{12} injections, initially as prescribed weekly and then monthly for maintenance (lifelong) if the anemia is the result of a deficiency of the intrinsic factor, or disease, or surgery of the ileum.

IX. Bariatric Surgery

A. Description
1. Surgical reduction of gastric capacity or absorption ability that may be performed on a client with morbid obesity to produce long-term weight loss

2. Surgery may be performed by laparoscopy; the decision is based on the client's weight, body build, history of abdominal surgery, and current medical disorders.
3. Obese clients are at increased postoperative risk for pulmonary and thromboembolic complications and death.
4. Surgery can prevent complications associated with obesity, such as diabetes mellitus, hypertension, other cardiovascular disorders, and sleep apnea.
5. The client needs to agree to modify his or her lifestyle, lose weight and keep the weight off, and obtain support from available community resources such as the American Society of Bariatric Surgery, or Overeaters Anonymous.

B. Types (Fig. 45.1)

C. Postoperative interventions
1. Care is similar to that for the client undergoing laparoscopic or abdominal surgery.
2. As prescribed, if the client can tolerate water, clear liquids are introduced slowly in 1-ounce (30 mL) cups for each serving once bowel sounds have returned and the client passes flatus.
3. As prescribed, clear fluids are followed by pureed foods, juices, thin soups, and milk 24 to 48 hours after clear fluids are tolerated (the diet is usually limited to liquids or pureed foods for 6 weeks); then the diet is progressed to nutrient-dense regular food.

D. Client teaching points about diet (Box 45.7)

X. Gastric Cancer (see Chapter 41)

XI. Hiatal Hernia

A. Description
1. A hiatal hernia is also known as esophageal or diaphragmatic hernia.
2. A portion of the stomach herniates through the diaphragm and into the thorax.
3. Herniation results from weakening of the muscles of the diaphragm and is aggravated by factors that increase abdominal pressure such as pregnancy, ascites, obesity, tumors, and heavy lifting.
4. Complications include ulceration, hemorrhage, regurgitation, aspiration of stomach contents, strangulation, and incarceration of the stomach in the chest with possible necrosis, peritonitis, and mediastinitis.

B. Data collection
1. Heartburn
2. Regurgitation or vomiting
3. Dysphagia
4. Feeling of fullness

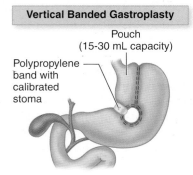

Vertical Banded Gastroplasty

Pouch
(15-30 mL capacity)

Polypropylene
band with
calibrated
stoma

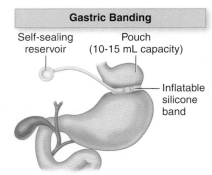

Gastric Banding

Self-sealing
reservoir

Pouch
(10-15 mL capacity)

Inflatable
silicone
band

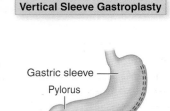

Vertical Sleeve Gastroplasty

Gastric sleeve

Pylorus

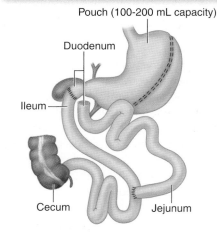

Biliopancreatic Diversion with Duodenal Switch

Pouch (100-200 mL capacity)

Duodenum

Ileum

Cecum   Jejunum

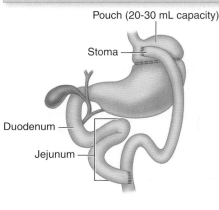

Roux-en-Y Gastric Bypass

Pouch (20-30 mL capacity)

Stoma

Duodenum

Jejunum

FIGURE 45.1 Bariatric surgical procedures.

BOX 45.7   Dietary Measures for the Client Following Bariatric Surgery

Avoid alcohol, high-protein foods, and foods high in sugar and fat.
Eat slowly and chew food well.
Progress food types and amounts as prescribed.
Take nutritional supplements as prescribed, which may include calcium, iron, multivitamins, and vitamin B_{12}.
Monitor and report signs and symptoms of complications, such as dehydration and gastric leak (persistent abdominal pain and nausea and vomiting).

C. Interventions
  1. Medical and surgical management are similar to those for gastroesophageal reflux disease.
  2. Provide small, frequent meals and limit the amount of liquids taken with meals.
  3. The client is advised not to recline for 1 hour after eating.
  4. Avoid anticholinergics, which delay stomach emptying.

XII. Cholecystitis

A. Description
  1. Inflammation of the gallbladder that may occur as an acute or chronic process
  2. Acute inflammation is associated with gallstones (cholelithiasis).

  3. Chronic cholecystitis results when inefficient bile emptying and gallbladder muscle wall disease cause a fibrotic and contracted gallbladder.
  4. Acalculous cholecystitis occurs in the absence of gallstones and is caused by bacterial invasion via the lymphatic or vascular systems.

B. Data collection
  1. Nausea and vomiting
  2. Indigestion
  3. Belching
  4. Flatulence
  5. Epigastric pain that radiates to the right shoulder or scapula
  6. Pain localized in right upper quadrant and triggered by high-fat or high-volume meal
  7. Guarding, rigidity, and rebound tenderness
  8. Mass palpated in the right upper quadrant
  9. Murphy's sign (cannot take a deep breath when the examiner's fingers are passed below the hepatic margin because of pain)
  10. Elevated temperature
  11. Tachycardia
  12. Signs of dehydration

C. Biliary obstruction (choledolithiasis)
  1. Jaundice
  2. Dark orange and foamy urine

3. Steatorrhea and clay-colored feces
4. Pruritus
D. Interventions
1. Maintain NPO status during nausea and vomiting episodes.
2. Maintain NG decompression as prescribed for severe vomiting.
3. Administer antiemetics, as prescribed, for nausea and vomiting.
4. Administer analgesics, as prescribed, to relieve pain and reduce spasm.
5. Administer antispasmodics (anticholinergics), as prescribed, to relax smooth muscle.
6. Reinforce instructions in cases of chronic cholecystitis to eat small, low-fat meals.
7. Reinforce instructions to avoid' gas-forming foods.
8. Prepare the client for nonsurgical and surgical procedures, as prescribed.
E. Surgical interventions
1. **Cholecystectomy** refers to the removal of the gallbladder.
2. **Choledocholithotomy** requires incision into the common bile duct to remove the stone.
3. Surgical procedures may be performed by laparoscopy.
F. Postoperative interventions
1. Monitor for respiratory complications caused by pain at the incisional site.
2. Encourage coughing and deep breathing.
3. Encourage early ambulation.
4. Reinforce instructions about splinting the abdomen to prevent discomfort during coughing.
5. Administer antiemetics as prescribed for nausea and vomiting.
6. Administer analgesics as prescribed for pain relief.
7. Maintain NPO status and NG tube suction as prescribed.
8. Advance diet from clear liquids to solids, when prescribed, and as tolerated by the client.
9. Maintain and monitor drainage from the T-tube, if present (Box 45.8).

XIII. Cirrhosis

A. Description
1. A chronic, progressive disease of the liver characterized by diffuse degeneration and destruction of hepatocytes
2. Repeated destruction of hepatic cells causes the formation of scar tissue.
3. Cirrhosis has many causes and occurs as a result of chronic damage and injury to liver cells; the most common are chronic hepatitis C, alcoholism, nonalcoholic fatty liver disease (NAFLD), and nonalcoholic steatohepatitis (NASH).

BOX 45.8 Care of a T-Tube

Purpose and Description

A T-tube is placed after surgical exploration of the common bile duct. The tube preserves the patency of the duct and ensures drainage of bile until edema resolves and bile is effectively draining into the duodenum. A gravity drainage bag is attached to the T-tube to collect the drainage.

Interventions

Place the client in a semi-Fowler's position to facilitate drainage.

Monitor the amount, color, consistency, and odor of the drainage.

Report sudden increases in bile output to the primary health care provider (PHCP).

Monitor for inflammation and protect the skin from irritation.

Keep the drainage system below the level of the gallbladder.

Monitor for foul odor and purulent drainage, and report its presence to the PHCP.

Avoid irrigation, aspiration, or clamping of the T-tube without a PHCP's prescription.

As prescribed, clamp the tube before a meal and observe for abdominal discomfort and distention, nausea, chills, or fever; unclamp the tube if nausea or vomiting occurs.

B. Complications
1. **Portal hypertension:** A persistent increase in pressure in the portal vein that develops as a result of obstruction to flow
2. **Ascites**
   a. Accumulation of fluid within the peritoneal cavity that results from venous congestion of the hepatic capillaries
   b. Capillary congestion leads to plasma leaking directly from the liver surface and portal vein.
3. Bleeding **esophageal varices:** Fragile, thin-walled, distended esophageal veins that become irritated and rupture
4. Coagulation defects
   a. Decreased synthesis of bile fats in the liver prevents the absorption of fat-soluble vitamins.
   b. Without vitamin K and clotting factors II, VII, IX, and X, the client is prone to bleeding.
5. Jaundice: Occurs because the liver is unable to metabolize bilirubin and because the edema, fibrosis, and scarring of the hepatic bile ducts interfere with normal bile and bilirubin secretion
6. Portal systemic encephalopathy: End-stage hepatic failure characterized by an altered level of consciousness, neurological symptoms, impaired thinking, and neuromuscular disturbances; caused by failure of the diseased liver to detoxify neurotoxic agents such as ammonia
7. Hepatorenal syndrome
   a. Progressive renal failure associated with hepatic failure

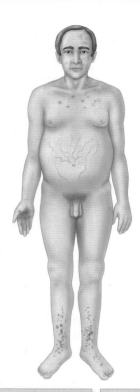

Dermatological Findings

- Axillary and pubic hair changes
- Caput medusae (dilated abdominal veins)*
- Ecchymosis; petechiae*
- Increased skin pigmentation
- Jaundice
- Palmar erythema*
- Pruritus
- Spider angiomas (chest and thorax)*

Endocrine Findings

- Increased aldosterone
- Increased antidiuretic hormone
- Increased circulating estrogens
- Increased glucocorticoids
- Gynecomastia

Immune System Disturbances

- Increased susceptibility to infection
- Leukopenia

Renal Findings

- Hepatorenal syndrome
- Increased urine bilirubin

Fluid and Electrolyte Disturbances

- Ascites
- Decreased effective blood volume
- Hypocalcemia
- Dilutional hyponatremia or hypernatremia
- Hypokalemia
- Peripheral edema
- Water retention

Cardiovascular Findings

- Cardiac dysrhythmias
- Development of collateral circulation
- Fatigue
- Hyperkinetic circulation
- Peripheral edema
- Portal hypertension
- Spider angiomas

Hematological Findings

- Anemia
- Disseminated intravascular coagulation
- Impaired coagulation
- Splenomegaly
- Thrombocytopenia

Neurological Findings

- Asterixis
- Paresthesias of feet
- Peripheral nerve degeneration
- Portal-systemic encephalopathy
- Reversal of sleep-wake pattern
- Sensory disturbances

Pulmonary Findings

- Dyspnea
- Hydrothorax
- Hyperventilation
- Hypoxemia

Gastrointestinal (GI) Findings

- Abdominal pain
- Anorexia
- Ascites
- Clay-colored stools
- Diarrhea
- Esophageal varices
- Fetor hepaticus
- Gallstones
- Gastritis
- Gastrointestinal bleeding
- Hemorrhoidal varices
- Hepatomegaly
- Hiatal hernia
- Hypersplenism
- Malnutrition
- Nausea
- Small nodular liver
- Vomiting

FIGURE 45.2 Clinical picture of a client with liver dysfunction. Manifestations vary according to the progression of the disease. Some dermatological manifestations are noted in color (and marked with asterisks).

   b. Characterized by a sudden decrease in urinary output, elevated blood urea nitrogen and creatinine levels, decreased urine sodium excretion, and increased urine osmolarity

C. Data collection (Fig. 45.2)

D. Interventions

   1. Elevate the head of the bed to minimize shortness of breath.

   2. If ascites and edema are absent and the client does not exhibit signs of impending coma, a high-protein diet supplemented with vitamins is prescribed.

   3. Provide supplemental vitamins (B complex; vitamins A, C, and K, folic acid, and thiamine) as prescribed.

   4. Restrict sodium intake and fluid intake as prescribed.

   5. Initiate enteral feedings or assist with parenteral nutrition as prescribed.

   6. Administer diuretics as prescribed to treat ascites.

   7. Monitor intake and output and electrolyte balance.

   8. Weigh the client and measure abdominal girth daily (Fig. 45.3).

   9. Monitor level of consciousness; monitor for a precoma state (tremors, delirium).

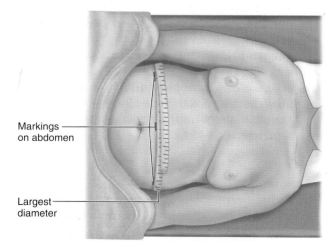

Markings on abdomen

Largest diameter

FIGURE 45.3 How to measure abdominal girth. With the client supine, bring the tape measure around the client and take a measurement at the level of the umbilicus. Before removing the tape, mark the client's abdomen along the sides of tape on the client's flanks (sides) and midline to ensure that later measurements are taken at the same place.

   10. Monitor for asterixis, a coarse tremor characterized by rapid, nonrhythmic extension and flexions in the wrist and fingers (Fig. 45.4).

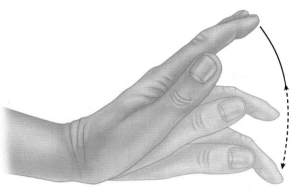

FIGURE 45.4 Eliciting asterixis (flapping tremor). Have the client extend the arm, dorsiflex the wrist, and extend the fingers. Observe for rapid, nonrhythmic extensions and flexions.

11. Monitor for fetor hepaticus—the fruity, musty breath odor of severe chronic liver disease.
12. Assist to maintain gastric intubation to monitor bleeding or esophagogastric balloon tamponade to control bleeding varices if prescribed.
13. Assist with the administration of blood products as prescribed.
14. Monitor coagulation laboratory results; vitamin K may be prescribed.
15. Administer antacids as prescribed.
16. Administer lactulose, as prescribed, which decreases the pH of the bowel, decreases production of ammonia by bacteria in the bowel, and facilitates the excretion of ammonia.
17. Administer antibiotics as prescribed to inhibit protein synthesis in bacteria and decrease the production of ammonia.
18. Avoid medications such as opioids, sedatives, and barbiturates and any hepatotoxic medications or substances.
19. Reinforce instructions about the importance of abstinence of alcohol intake.
20. Prepare the client for paracentesis to remove abdominal fluid.
21. Prepare the client for surgical shunting procedures, if prescribed, to divert fluid from ascites into the venous system.

XIV. Esophageal Varices

A. Description
  1. Dilated and tortuous veins in the submucosa of the esophagus
  2. Caused by portal hypertension, are often associated with liver cirrhosis, and are at high risk for rupture if portal circulation pressure rises
  3. Bleeding varices are an emergency.
  4. The goal of treatment is to control bleeding, prevent complications, and prevent the reoccurrence of bleeding.

B. Data collection
  1. Hematemesis
  2. Melena
  3. Ascites
  4. Jaundice
  5. Hepatomegaly and splenomegaly
  6. Dilated abdominal veins
  7. Signs of shock

⚠ Rupture and resultant hemorrhage of the esophageal varices are a primary concern because they present a life-threatening situation.

C. Interventions
  1. Monitor vital signs.
  2. Elevate the head of the bed.
  3. Monitor for orthostatic hypotension.
  4. Assist with monitoring lung sounds and for the presence of respiratory distress.
  5. Administer oxygen as prescribed to prevent tissue hypoxia.
  6. Monitor level of consciousness.
  7. Maintain NPO status.
  8. IV fluids may be prescribed to restore fluid volume and electrolyte imbalances; monitor intake and output.
  9. Monitor hemoglobin, hematocrit, and coagulation factors.
  10. Assist with the administration of blood transfusions or clotting factors, as prescribed.
  11. Assist in inserting an NG tube or a balloon tamponade as prescribed; balloon tamponade is not used frequently because it is very uncomfortable for the client and its use is associated with complications.
  12. Prepare to assist with administering medications to induce vasoconstriction and reduce bleeding.
  13. Reinforce instructions to avoid activities that will initiate vasovagal responses.
  14. Prepare the client for endoscopic procedures or surgical procedures, as prescribed.

D. Endoscopic injection (sclerotherapy)
  1. The procedure involves the injection of a sclerosing agent into and around bleeding varices.
  2. Complications include chest pain, pleural effusion, aspiration pneumonia, esophageal stricture, and perforation of the esophagus.

E. Endoscopic variceal ligation
  1. The procedure involves ligation of the varices with an elastic rubber band.
  2. Sloughing, followed by superficial ulceration, occurs in the area of ligation within 3 to 7 days.

F. Shunting procedures
  1. Description: Shunt blood away from the esophageal varices
  2. Portacaval shunt involves anastomosis of the portal vein to the inferior vena cava, diverting blood from the portal system to the systemic circulation.
  3. Distal splenorenal shunt
     a. The shunt involves anastomosis of the splenic vein to the left renal vein.
     b. The spleen conducts blood from the high-pressure varices to the low-pressure renal vein.

BOX 45.9 Stages of Viral Hepatitis

Preicteric Stage
The first stage of hepatitis, preceding the appearance of jaundice, includes flu-like symptoms—malaise, fatigue; anorexia, nausea, vomiting, diarrhea; pain—headache, muscle aches, polyarthritis; and elevated serum bilirubin and enzyme levels.

Icteric Stage
The second stage of hepatitis; includes the appearance of jaundice and associated symptoms such as elevated bilirubin levels, dark or tea-colored urine, and clay-colored stools; pruritus; and a decrease in preicteric-phase symptoms.

Posticteric Stage
The convalescent stage of hepatitis, in which the jaundice decreases and the color of the urine and stool returns to normal; energy increases, pain subsides, there is minimal to absent gastrointestinal symptoms, and bilirubin and enzyme levels return to normal.

---

4. Mesocaval shunting involves a side anastomosis of the superior mesenteric vein to the proximal end of the inferior vena cava.
5. Transjugular intrahepatic portosystemic shunt (TIPS)
   a. This nonsurgical procedure uses the normal vascular anatomy of the liver to create a shunt with the use of a metallic stent.
   b. The shunt is between the portal and systemic venous system in the liver and is aimed at relieving portal hypertension.

XV. Hepatitis

A. Description
   1. Inflammation of the liver caused by a virus, bacteria, or exposure to medications or hepatotoxins
   2. The goals of treatment include resting the inflamed liver to reduce metabolic demands and increasing the blood supply, thus promoting cellular regeneration and preventing complications.
B. Types of viral hepatitis include hepatitis A virus (HAV), hepatitis B virus (HBV), hepatitis C virus (HCV), hepatitis D virus (HDV), and hepatitis E virus (HEV).
C. Data collection and stages of viral hepatitis (Box 45.9)

XVI. Hepatitis A

A. Description
   1. Formerly known as infectious hepatitis
   2. Commonly seen during the fall and early winter
B. Individuals at increased risk
   1. Crowded conditions (e.g., daycare and nursing home)
   2. Exposure to poor sanitation
C. Transmission
   1. Fecal-oral route
   2. Person-to-person contact
   3. Parenteral

4. Contaminated fruits, vegetables, or uncooked shellfish
   5. Contaminated water or milk
   6. Poorly washed utensils
D. Incubation and infectious period
   1. Incubation period is 2 to 6 weeks.
   2. Infectious period is 2 to 3 weeks before and 1 week after development of jaundice.
E. Testing
   1. Infection is established by the presence of HAV antibodies (anti-HAV) in the blood.
   2. Immunoglobulins M (IgM) and G (IgG) are normally present in the blood, and increased levels indicate infection and inflammation.
   3. Ongoing inflammation of the liver is evidenced by the presence of elevated IgM antibodies, which persist in the blood for 4 to 6 weeks.
   4. Previous infection is indicated by the presence of elevated IgG antibodies.
F. Complication: Fulminant (severe acute and often fatal) hepatitis
G. Prevention
   1. Strict hand washing
   2. Stool and needle precautions
   3. Treatment of municipal water supplies
   4. Serological screening of food handlers
   5. Hepatitis A vaccine: Two doses are needed at least 6 months apart for lasting protection.
   6. Immune globulin: For individuals exposed to HAV who have never received the hepatitis A vaccine, administer immune globulin during the period of incubation and within 2 weeks of exposure.
   7. Immune globulin and hepatitis A vaccine are recommended for household members and sexual contacts of individuals with hepatitis A.
   8. Preexposure prophylaxis with immune globulin is recommended to individuals traveling to countries with poor or uncertain sanitation conditions.

⚠ Strict and frequent hand washing is key to preventing the spread of all types of hepatitis.

XVII. Hepatitis B

A. Description
   1. Hepatitis B is nonseasonal.
   2. All age groups are affected.
B. Individuals at increased risk
   1. IV drug users
   2. Clients undergoing long-term hemodialysis
   3. Health care personnel
C. Transmission
   1. Blood or body fluid contact
   2. Infected blood products
   3. Infected saliva or semen
   4. Contaminated needles
   5. Sexual contact
   6. Parenteral

7. Perinatal period
8. Blood or body fluid contact at birth
D. Incubation period: 6 to 24 weeks
E. Testing
1. Infection is established by the presence of hepatitis B antigen-antibody systems in the blood.
2. Presence of hepatitis B surface antigen (HBsAg) is the serological marker establishing the diagnosis of hepatitis B.
3. The client is considered infectious if these antigens are present in the blood.
4. If the serological marker (HBsAg) is present after 6 months, it indicates a carrier state or chronic hepatitis.
5. Normally, the serological marker (HBsAg) level declines and disappears after the acute hepatitis B episode.
6. The presence of antibodies to HBsAg (anti-HBs) indicates recovery and immunity to hepatitis B.
7. Hepatitis B early antigen (HBeAg) is detected in the blood about 1 week after the appearance of HBsAg, and its presence determines the infective state of the client.
F. Complications
1. Fulminant hepatitis
2. Chronic liver disease
3. Cirrhosis
4. Primary hepatocellular carcinoma
G. Prevention
1. Strict hand washing
2. Screening blood donors
3. Testing of all pregnant women
4. Needle precautions
5. Avoiding intimate sexual contact if test for HBsAg is positive
6. Hepatitis B vaccine: Adult and pediatric forms; there is also an adult vaccine that protects against hepatitis A and B.
7. Hepatitis B immune globulin is for individuals exposed to HBV through sexual contact or through the percutaneous or transmucosal routes, who have never had hepatitis B and have never received hepatitis B vaccine.

XVIII. Hepatitis C

A. Description
1. HCV infection occurs year-round.
2. Infection can occur in any age group.
3. Infection with HCV is common among drug abusers and is the major cause of posttransfusion hepatitis.
4. Risk factors are similar to those for HBV because hepatitis C is also transmitted parenterally.
B. Individuals at increased risk
1. Parenteral drug users
2. Clients receiving frequent transfusions
3. Health care personnel

C. Transmission: Same as for HBV, primarily through blood
D. Incubation period: 5 to 10 weeks
E. Testing: Anti-HCV is the antibody to HCV and is measured to detect chronic states of hepatitis C.
F. Complications
1. Chronic liver disease
2. Cirrhosis
3. Primary hepatocellular carcinoma
G. Prevention
1. Strict hand washing
2. Needle precautions
3. Screening of blood donors

XIX. Hepatitis D

A. Description
1. HDV is common in the Mediterranean and Middle Eastern areas.
2. HDV occurs with HBV and may cause infection only in the presence of active HBV infection.
3. Coinfection with the delta-agent (HDV) intensifies the acute symptoms of HBV.
4. Transmission and risk of infection are the same as for HBV, via contact with blood and blood products.
5. Prevention of HBV infection with vaccine also prevents HDV infection, because HDV depends on HBV for replication.
B. High-risk individuals
1. Drug users
2. Clients receiving hemodialysis
3. Clients receiving frequent blood transfusions
C. Transmission: Same as for HBV
D. Incubation period: 7 to 8 weeks
E. Testing: Serological HDV determination is made by detection of the HDV antigen (HDAg) early in the course of the infection and by detection of anti-HDV antibody in the later disease stages.
F. Complications
1. Chronic liver disease
2. Fulminant hepatitis
G. Prevention: Because HDV coexists with HBV, the precautions that help prevent HBV are also useful in preventing delta hepatitis.

XX. Hepatitis E

A. Description
1. HEV is a waterborne virus.
2. HEV is prevalent in areas where sewage disposal is inadequate or communal bathing in contaminated rivers is practiced.
3. The risk of infection is the same as for HAV.
4. Infection with HEV presents as a mild disease except in infected women in the third trimester of pregnancy, who have a high mortality rate.

BOX 45.10 **Home Care Instructions for the Client With Hepatitis**

Hand washing must be done frequently.

Do not share bathrooms unless the client strictly adheres to personal hygiene measures.

Individual washcloths, towels, drinking and eating utensils, toothbrushes, and razors need to be labeled and identified.

The client must not prepare food for other family members.

The client needs to avoid alcohol and over-the-counter medications, particularly acetaminophen and sedatives, because these medications are hepatotoxic.

The client would increase activity gradually to prevent fatigue.

The client needs to consume small, frequent, high-carbohydrate, low-fat foods.

The client is not to donate blood.

The client may maintain normal contact with persons as long as proper personal hygiene is maintained.

Close personal contact such as kissing needs to be discouraged until hepatitis B virus (HBV) surface antigen test results are negative.

The client is to avoid sexual activity until HBV surface antigen results are negative.

The client needs to carry a MedicAlert card noting the date of hepatitis onset.

The client needs to inform other health professionals, such as medical or dental personnel, of the onset of hepatitis.

The client needs to keep follow-up appointments with the primary health care provider (PHCP).

B. Individuals with increased risk
  1. Travelers to countries that have a high incidence of HEV such as India, Burma (Myanmar), Afghanistan, Algeria, and Mexico
  2. Eating or drinking of food or water contaminated with the virus
C. Transmission: Same as for HAV
D. Incubation period: 2 to 9 weeks
E. Testing: Specific serological tests for HEV include detection of IgM and IgG antibodies to HEV (anti-HEV).
F. Complications
  1. High mortality rate in pregnant women
  2. Fetal demise
G. Prevention
  1. Strict hand washing
  2. Treatment of water supplies and sanitation measures

XXI. Client and Family Home Care Instructions for Hepatitis
A. See Box 45.10.

XXII. Pancreatitis
A. Description
  1. Acute or chronic inflammation of the pancreas, with associated escape of pancreatic enzymes into surrounding tissue

2. Acute pancreatitis occurs suddenly as one attack or can be recurrent, with resolutions.
3. Chronic pancreatitis is a continual inflammation and destruction of the pancreas, with scar tissue replacing pancreatic tissue.
4. Precipitating factors include trauma, the use of alcohol, biliary tract disease, viral or bacterial disease, hyperlipidemia, hypercalcemia, cholelithiasis, hyperparathyroidism, ischemic vascular disease, and peptic ulcer disease.
B. Acute pancreatitis
  1. Data collection
    a. Abdominal pain, including a sudden onset at the midepigastric or left upper quadrant location with radiation to the back
    b. Pain aggravated by a fatty meal, alcohol, or by lying in a recumbent position
    c. Abdominal tenderness and guarding
    d. Nausea and vomiting
    e. Weight loss
    f. Absent or decreased bowel sounds
    g. Elevated white blood cell count, glucose, bilirubin, alkaline phosphatase, and urinary amylase
    h. Elevated serum lipase and amylase
    i. Cullen's sign
    j. Turner's sign

 Cullen's sign is the discoloration of the abdomen and periumbilical area. Turner's sign is the bluish discoloration of the flanks. Both signs are indicative of pancreatitis.

  2. Interventions
    a Withhold food and fluid during the acute period and maintain hydration with IV fluids as prescribed.
    b. Assist with the administration of parenteral nutrition for severe nutritional depletion.
    c. Administer supplemental preparations and vitamins and minerals to increase caloric intake if prescribed.
    d. An NG tube may be inserted if the client is vomiting or has biliary obstruction or paralytic ileus.
    e. Administer opiates as prescribed for pain.
    f. Administer H_2-receptor antagonists or proton pump inhibitors as prescribed to decrease hydrochloric acid production and prevent activation of pancreatic enzymes.
    g. Reinforce instructions on the importance of avoiding alcohol.
    h. Reinforce instructions on the importance of follow-up visits with the PHCP.
    i. Reinforce instructions to notify the PHCP if acute abdominal pain, jaundice, clay-colored stools, or dark-colored urine develop.

C. Chronic pancreatitis
1. Data collection
   a. Abdominal pain and tenderness
   b. Left upper quadrant mass
   c. Steatorrhea and foul-smelling stools that may increase in volume as pancreatic insufficiency increases
   d. Weight loss
   e. Muscle wasting
   f. Jaundice
   g. Signs/symptoms of diabetes mellitus
2. Interventions
   a. The client is instructed on the prescribed dietary measures (fat and protein intake may be limited).
   b. The client is instructed to avoid heavy meals.
   c. The client is instructed about the importance of avoiding alcohol.
   d. Provide supplemental preparations and vitamins and minerals to increase caloric intake.
   e. Administer pancreatic enzymes, as prescribed, to aid in the digestion and absorption of fat and protein.
   f. Administer insulin or oral hypoglycemic medications, as prescribed, to control diabetes mellitus, if present.
   g. Reinforce instructions on the use of pancreatic enzyme medications.
   h. Reinforce instructions to the client on the treatment plan for glucose management.
   i. Reinforce instructions to notify the PHCP if increased steatorrhea, abdominal distention, cramping, or skin breakdown develops.
   j. Reinforce instructions with regard to the importance of follow-up visits.

XXIII. Pancreatic Tumors, Intestinal Tumors, and Bowel Obstruction
A. See Chapter 41 for more information.

XXIV. Irritable Bowel Syndrome (IBS)
A. Description
1. Functional disorder characterized by chronic or recurrent diarrhea, constipation, and/or abdominal pain and bloating
2. Cause is unclear but may be influenced by environmental, immunological, genetic, hormonal, and stress factors.
B. Interventions
1. Increase dietary fiber.
2. Drink 8 to 10 cups of liquids per day.
3. Medication therapy: Depends on the predominant symptoms of IBS (antidiarrheals *versus* bulk-forming laxatives; lubiprostone or linaclotide for constipation-predominant IBS and alosetron for diarrhea-predominant IBS)

XXV. Ulcerative Colitis
A. Description
1. An ulcerative and inflammatory disease of the bowel that results in poor absorption of nutrients
2. Commonly begins in the rectum and spreads upward toward the cecum
3. The colon becomes edematous and may develop bleeding lesions and ulcers; the ulcers may lead to perforation.
4. Scar tissue develops and causes loss of elasticity and loss of the ability to absorb nutrients.
5. Colitis is characterized by various periods of remission and exacerbation.
6. Acute ulcerative colitis results in vascular congestion, hemorrhage, edema, and ulceration of the bowel mucosa.
7. Chronic ulcerative colitis causes muscular hypertrophy, fat deposits, and fibrous tissue, with bowel thickening, shortening, and narrowing.
B. Data collection
1. Anorexia
2. Weight loss
3. Malaise
4. Abdominal tenderness and cramping
5. Severe diarrhea that may contain blood and mucus
6. Malnutrition, dehydration, and electrolyte imbalances
7. Anemia
8. Vitamin K deficiency
C. Interventions
1. Acute phase: Maintain NPO status and assist to administer fluids and electrolytes intravenously or via parenteral nutrition as prescribed.
2. Restrict the client's activity to reduce intestinal activity.
3. Monitor bowel sounds and for abdominal tenderness and cramping.
4. Monitor stools, noting color, consistency, and the presence or absence of blood.
5. Monitor for bowel perforation, peritonitis (see Box 45.3), and hemorrhage.
6. Following the acute phase, the diet progresses from clear liquids to low-fiber diet as tolerated.
7. Reinforce instructions about diet; usually a low-fiber, high-protein diet with vitamins and iron supplements is prescribed.
8. Reinforce instructions to avoid gas-forming foods, milk products, and foods such as whole-wheat grains, nuts, raw fruits and vegetables, pepper, alcohol, and caffeine-containing products.
9. Reinforce instructions to avoid smoking.
10. Administer medications, as prescribed, which may include a combination of salicylate compounds, corticosteroids, immunosuppressants, and antidiarrheals.

Adult—Gastrointestinal

D. Surgical interventions

1. Performed in extreme cases if medical management is unsuccessful

2. Minimally invasive procedures are considered if the client is a candidate; clients who are obese, have had previous abdominal surgeries, or have adhesions may not be candidates.

3. Minimally invasive procedures can include laparoscopic procedures, robotic-assisted surgery, and natural orifice transluminal endoscopic surgery (NOTES).

4. Restorative proctocolectomy with ileal pouch–anal anastomosis (RPC-IPAA)

   a. Allows for bowel continence

   b. May be performed through laparoscopic procedure

   c. Involves a two-stage procedure that includes removal of the colon and most of the rectum; the anus and anal sphincter remain intact.

   d. An internal pouch known as a reservoir (J-pouch, S-pouch, or pelvic pouch) is created using the small intestine and connected to the anus, followed by creation of a temporary ileostomy through the abdominal skin to allow healing of the internal pouch and all anastomosis sites.

   e. In the second surgical procedure (within 1–2 months), the ileostomy is closed.

5. Total proctocolectomy with permanent ileostomy

   a. Performed if the client is not a candidate for RPC-IPAA or if the client prefers this type of procedure

   b. The procedure involves the removal of the entire colon (colon, rectum, and anus, with anal closure).

   c. The end of the terminal ileum forms the stoma or ostomy, which is located in the right lower quadrant.

6. Preoperative interventions

   a. Consult with an enterostomal therapist to assist with identifying optimal placement of the ostomy.

   b. Reinforce instructions to eat a low-fiber diet for 1 to 2 days before surgery as prescribed.

   c. Parenteral antibiotics are administered 1 hour before the surgical opening.

   d. Address body image concerns and allow the client to express their concerns; a visit from an ostomate may be helpful to the client.

7. Postoperative colostomy interventions

   a. A pouch system with a skin barrier is usually placed on the stoma postoperatively; if a pouch system is not covering the stoma, a petrolatum gauze dressing is placed over it, as prescribed, to keep it moist, followed by a dry sterile dressing.

   b. Monitor the stoma for size, unusual bleeding, or necrotic tissue.

   c. Monitor for color changes in the stoma.

   d. Note that the normal stoma color is pink to bright red and shiny, indicating high vascularity.

   e. Note that a pale pink stoma indicates low hemoglobin and hematocrit levels, and a

---

BOX 45.11   Colostomy Irrigation

Purpose

An enema is given through the stoma to stimulate bowel emptying.

Description

Irrigation is performed by instilling 500–1000 mL of lukewarm tap water through the stoma and allowing the water and stool to drain into a collection bag.

Procedure

- If ambulatory, position the client sitting on the toilet.
- If on bed rest, position the client on his or her side.
- Hang the irrigation bag so that the bottom of the bag is at the level of the client's shoulder or slightly higher.
- Insert the irrigation tube carefully without force.
- Begin the flow of irrigation.
- Clamp the tubing if cramping occurs; release the tubing as cramping subsides.
- Avoid frequent irrigations, which can lead to loss of fluids and electrolytes.
- Perform irrigation at about the same time each day.
- Perform irrigation preferably 1 hour after a meal.
- To enhance effectiveness of the irrigation, massage the abdomen gently.

---

   purple-black stoma indicates compromised circulation, requiring PHCP notification.

   f. Monitor the functioning of the colostomy and check for bowel sounds.

   g. Expect that stool is liquid in the immediate postoperative period but becomes more solid, depending on the area of creation: ascending colon—liquid; transverse colon—loose to semiformed; and descending colon—close to normal.

   h. Monitor the pouch system for proper fit and signs of leakage. Empty the pouch when it is one third full.

   i. Fecal matter should not be allowed to remain on the skin; skin assessment and care are a priority.

   j. Monitor for dehydration and electrolyte imbalance.

   k. Administer analgesics and antibiotics as prescribed.

   l. Reinforce instructions to avoid foods that cause excess gas formation and odor.

   m. Reinforce instructions about stoma care and irrigation, as prescribed (Box 45.11).

   n. Reinforce instructions that normal activities may be resumed when approved by the PHCP.

⚠️ A stoma that is purple-black in color indicates compromised circulation, requiring immediate PHCP notification.

XXVI. Crohn's Disease

A. Description

1. An inflammatory disease that can occur anywhere in the GI tract, but most often affects the terminal ileum and leads to thickening and scarring, a narrowed lumen, fistulas, ulcerations, and abscesses

2. Characterized by remissions and exacerbations

B. Data collection
1. Fever
2. Cramp-like and colicky pain after meals
3. Diarrhea (semisolid), which may contain mucus and pus
4. Abdominal distention
5. Anorexia, nausea, and vomiting
6. Weight loss
7. Anemia
8. Dehydration
9. Electrolyte imbalances
10. Malnutrition (may be worse than that seen in ulcerative colitis)

C. Interventions: Care is similar to the client with ulcerative colitis; however, surgery may be necessary but is avoided for as long as possible because recurrence of the disease process in the same region is likely to occur.

XXVII. Appendicitis

A. Description
1. Inflammation of the appendix
2. When the appendix becomes inflamed or infected, rupture may occur within a matter of hours, leading to peritonitis and sepsis.

B. Data collection
1. Pain in the periumbilical area that descends to the right lower quadrant
2. Abdominal pain that is most intense at McBurney's point
3. Rebound tenderness and abdominal rigidity
4. Low-grade fever
5. Elevated white blood cell count
6. Anorexia, nausea, and vomiting
7. Client in side-lying position, with abdominal guarding and legs flexed
8. Constipation or diarrhea

C. Peritonitis: Inflammation of the peritoneum (see Box 45.3)

D. Appendectomy: Surgical removal of the appendix
1. Preoperative interventions
   a. Maintain NPO status.
   b. Assist with the administration of IV fluids to prevent dehydration.
   c. Monitor for changes in level of pain.
   d. Monitor for signs of ruptured appendix and peritonitis.
   e. Position the client in a right side–lying or low to semi-Fowler's position to promote comfort.
   f. Monitor bowel sounds.
   g. Apply ice packs to the abdomen for 20 to 30 minutes every hour as prescribed.
   h. Assist to administer antibiotics as prescribed.
   i. Avoid laxatives or enemas.

⚠ Avoid the application of heat to the abdomen of a client with appendicitis. Heat can cause rupture of the appendix leading to peritonitis, a life-threatening condition.

2. Postoperative interventions
   a. Monitor temperature for signs of infection.
   b. Monitor incision for signs of infection such as redness, swelling, and pain.
   c. Maintain NPO status until bowel function has returned.
   d. Advance diet gradually as tolerated and as prescribed, when bowel sounds return.
   e. If rupture of the appendix occurred, expect a drain to be inserted, or the incision may be left open to heal from the inside out.
   f. Expect that drainage from the drain may be profuse for the first 12 hours.
   g. Position the client in a right side–lying or low to semi-Fowler's position, with legs flexed, to facilitate drainage.
   h. Change the dressing as prescribed and record the type and amount of drainage.
   i. Perform wound irrigation, if prescribed.
   j. Maintain NG suction and patency of the NG tube if present.
   k. Assist with the administration of antibiotics and analgesics as prescribed.

XXVIII. Diverticulosis and Diverticulitis

A. Diverticulosis
1. Diverticulosis is an outpouching or herniation of the intestinal mucosa.
2. The disorder can occur in any part of the intestine but is most common in the sigmoid colon.

B. Diverticulitis
1. Diverticulitis refers to the inflammation of 1 or more diverticula that occurs from penetration of fecal matter through the thin-walled diverticula and can result in local abscess formation and perforation.
2. A perforated diverticulum can progress to intra-abdominal perforation with generalized peritonitis.

C. Data collection
1. Left lower quadrant abdominal pain that increases with coughing, straining, or lifting
2. Elevated temperature
3. Nausea and vomiting
4. Flatulence
5. Cramp-like pain
6. Abdominal distention and tenderness
7. Palpable, tender rectal mass may be present.
8. Blood in the stools

D. Interventions
1. Provide bed rest during the acute phase.

Adult—Gastrointestinal

2. Maintain NPO status or provide clear liquids during the acute phase as prescribed.
3. Introduce a fiber-containing diet gradually, when the inflammation has resolved.
4. Administer antibiotics, analgesics, and anticholinergics to reduce bowel spasms as prescribed.
5. Reinforce instructions to refrain from lifting, straining, coughing, or bending to avoid increased intra-abdominal pressure.
6. Monitor for perforation, hemorrhage, fistulas, and abscesses.
7. Reinforce instructions to increase fluid intake to 2500 to 3000 mL daily, unless contraindicated.
8. Reinforce instructions to eat soft high-fiber foods, such as whole grains; the client needs to avoid high-fiber foods when inflammation occurs because these foods will irritate the mucosa further.
9. Reinforce instructions to avoid gas-forming foods or foods containing indigestible roughage, seeds, nuts, or popcorn because these food substances become trapped in diverticula and cause inflammation.
10. Reinforce instructions to consume a small amount of bran daily and to take bulk-forming laxatives as prescribed to increase stool mass.

E. Surgical interventions
1. Colon resection with primary anastomosis may be an option.
2. Temporary or permanent colostomy may be required for increased bowel inflammation.

XXIX. Hemorrhoids

A. Description
1. Dilated varicose veins of the anal canal
2. May be internal, external, or prolapsed
3. Internal hemorrhoids lie above the anal sphincter and cannot be seen during inspection of the perianal area.
4. External hemorrhoids lie below the anal sphincter and can be seen during inspection.
5. Prolapsed hemorrhoids can become thrombosed or inflamed.
6. Hemorrhoids are caused by portal hypertension, straining, irritation, or increased venous or abdominal pressure.

B. Data collection
1. Bright red bleeding with defecation
2. Rectal pain
3. Rectal itching

C. Interventions
1. Apply cold packs to the anal/rectal area followed by sitz baths as prescribed.
2. Apply witch hazel soaks and topical anesthetics as prescribed.
3. Encourage a high-fiber diet and fluids to promote bowel movements without straining.
4. Administer stool softeners as prescribed.

D. Surgical interventions: May include ultrasound, sclerotherapy, circular stapling, band ligation, or simple resection of the hemorrhoids (hemorrhoidectomy)

E. Postoperative interventions after hemorrhoidectomy
1. Assist the client into a prone or side-lying position to prevent bleeding.
2. Maintain ice packs over the dressing, as prescribed, until the packing is removed by the PHCP.
3. Monitor for urinary retention.
4. Administer stool softeners as prescribed.
5. Reinforce instructions to increase fluids and high-fiber foods.
6. Reinforce instructions to limit sitting to short periods of time.
7. Reinforce instructions in the use of sitz baths three to four times a day as prescribed.

WHAT WOULD YOU DO?

Answer: Bleeding is a primary concern for a liver biopsy because of the high vascularity of the liver. Therefore, a preprocedure assessment is necessary to check the client's status related to the risk for bleeding. The normal prothrombin time ranges from 11 to 12.5 seconds. Because the client's prothrombin time is prolonged, the client is at risk for bleeding. The normal platelet count is 150,000 to 400,000 mm³. Therefore, the nurse needs to immediately notify the registered nurse (RN) and the primary health care provider (PHCP) of these abnormal laboratory values.

PRACTICE QUESTIONS

1. The nurse is reinforcing teaching to a client about an upcoming colonoscopy procedure. The nurse would include in the instructions that the client will be placed in which position for the procedure?
   1. Left Sims' position
   2. Lithotomy position
   3. Knee-chest position
   4. Right Sims' position

2. The nurse is preparing to perform an abdominal examination. Which step would be taken **first**?
   1. Palpation
   2. Inspection
   3. Percussion
   4. Auscultation

3. The nurse reinforces postoperative liver biopsy instructions to a client. Which would the nurse tell the client?
   1. Avoid alcohol for 8 hours.
   2. Remain NPO for 24 hours.
   3. Lie on the right side for 2 hours.
   4. Save all stools to be checked for blood.

4. The nurse is caring for a client with a diagnosis of chronic gastritis. The nurse anticipates that the client is at risk for which vitamin deficiency?
1. Vitamin A
2. Vitamin C
3. Vitamin E
4. Vitamin B_{12}

5. The nurse is caring for a client after a Billroth II (gastrojejunostomy) procedure. During review of the postoperative prescriptions, which would the nurse clarify?
1. Leg exercises
2. Early ambulation
3. Irrigating the nasogastric (NG) tube
4. Coughing and deep-breathing exercises

6. The nurse is reinforcing discharge instructions to a client after a gastrectomy. Which measure would the nurse include during client teaching to help prevent dumping syndrome?
1. Ambulate after a meal.
2. Eat high-carbohydrate foods.
3. Limit the fluids taken with meals.
4. Sit in a high Fowler's position during meals.

7. The nurse is monitoring a client for the **early** signs/symptoms of dumping syndrome. Which indicates this occurrence?
1. Sweating and pallor
2. Dry skin and stomach pain
3. Bradycardia and indigestion
4. Double vision and chest pain

8. The nurse is reviewing the record of a client with Crohn's disease. Which stool characteristic would the nurse expect to see documented in the record?
1. Diarrhea
2. Constipation
3. Bloody stools
4. Stool constantly oozing from the rectum

9. A client with ascites is scheduled for a paracentesis. The nurse is assisting the primary health care provider (PHCP) with performing the procedure. Which position would the nurse assist the client into for this procedure?
1. Flat
2. Upright
3. Left side–lying
4. Right side–lying

❖ **10.** The nurse is reviewing the prescriptions of a client admitted to the hospital with a diagnosis of acute pancreatitis. Which interventions would the nurse expect to be prescribed? **Select all that apply.**
❑ **1.** Administer antacids, as prescribed.
❑ **2.** Encourage coughing and deep breathing.
❑ **3.** Administer anticholinergics, as prescribed.
❑ **4.** Maintain the client in a supine and flat position.
❑ **5.** Encourage small, frequent, high-calorie feedings.

11. It has been determined that a client with hepatitis has contracted the infection from contaminated food. Which type of hepatitis is this client **most likely** experiencing?
1. Hepatitis A
2. Hepatitis B
3. Hepatitis C
4. Hepatitis D

12. The nurse is reviewing the primary health care provider's (PHCP's) prescriptions written for a client admitted with acute pancreatitis. Which PHCP prescription would the nurse verify if noted in the client's chart?
1. NPO status
2. An anticholinergic medication
3. Position the client supine and flat
4. Prepare to insert a nasogastric (NG) tube

13. A client with hiatal hernia chronically experiences heartburn after meals. Which would the nurse teach the client to avoid?
1. Lying recumbent after meals
2. Eating small, frequent, bland meals
3. Raising the head of the bed on 6-inch blocks
4. Taking histamine receptor antagonist medication, as prescribed

14. The nurse is monitoring for stoma prolapse in a client with a colostomy. Which stoma observation would indicate that a prolapse has occurred?
1. Dark and bluish
2. Sunken and hidden
3. Narrowed and flattened
4. Protruding and swollen

15. An ultrasound of the gallbladder is scheduled for the client with a suspected diagnosis of cholecystitis. Which would the nurse explain to the client about this test?
1. The test is uncomfortable.
2. The test requires that the client be NPO.
3. The test requires the client to lie still for short intervals.
4. The test is preceded by the administration of oral tablets.

ANSWERS

1. 1

Rationale: The client is placed in the left Sims' position for the procedure. This position takes the best advantage of the client's anatomy for ease with introducing the colonoscope. The other options are incorrect.

Test-Taking Strategy: Focus on the subject, position for a colonoscopy. Use concepts related to gastrointestinal (GI) anatomy to answer this question. The position would be the same as that used for giving the client an enema while lying down. When answering factual questions such as these, remember the guiding principles and attempt to visualize the procedure to help you select the correct option.

2. 2

Rationale: The appropriate technique for abdominal examination is inspection, auscultation, percussion, and palpation. Auscultation is performed after inspection and before percussion and palpation to ensure that the motility of the bowel and bowel sounds are not altered. The sequence of maneuvers is inspect, auscultate, percuss, and palpate.

Test-Taking Strategy: Focus on the subject, abdominal examination. Note the strategic word, *first*. Visualize the procedure. Remember that inspection is first, and the sequence for abdominal examination is different from the usual systematic approach.

3. 3

Rationale: To splint the puncture site, the client is kept on the right side for a minimum of 2 hours. It is not necessary to remain NPO for 24 hours. Permission regarding the consumption of alcohol needs to be obtained from the primary health care provider (PHCP). It is not necessary to save all stools.

Test-Taking Strategy: Focus on the subject, a liver biopsy. Recalling the anatomical location of the liver and this procedure will direct you to the correct option.

4. 4

Rationale: Deterioration and atrophy of the lining of the stomach lead to the loss of function of the parietal cells. When the acid secretion decreases, the source of the intrinsic factor is lost, which results in the inability to absorb vitamin B_{12}. This leads to the development of pernicious anemia. Options 1, 2, and 3 are incorrect.

Test-Taking Strategy: Focus on the subject, vitamin deficiency with chronic gastritis. Knowledge regarding the pathophysiology related to the lining of the stomach is required to answer this question. This knowledge will direct you to the correct option.

5. 3

Rationale: In a Billroth II resection, the proximal remnant of the stomach is anastomosed to the proximal jejunum. Patency of the nasogastric (NG) tube is critical for preventing the retention of gastric secretions. However, the nurse would not irrigate or reposition the NG tube after gastric surgery unless specifically prescribed by the primary health care provider (PHCP). In this situation, the nurse would clarify the prescription. Options 1, 2, and 4 are appropriate postoperative interventions.

Test-Taking Strategy: Focus on the subject, care of the client who underwent a Billroth II procedure. Eliminate options 1, 2, and 4 because they are comparable or alike and are general postoperative measures. Also, consider the anatomical location of the surgical procedure to assist with directing you to the correct option.

6. 3

Rationale: The client would be instructed to decrease the amount of fluid taken at meals. The client would also be instructed to avoid high-carbohydrate foods, including fluids such as fruit nectars; assume a low-Fowler's position during meals; lie down for 30 minutes after eating to delay gastric emptying; and take antispasmodics as prescribed.

Test-Taking Strategy: Focus on the subject, dumping syndrome. Eliminate options 1 and 4 first because these measures are comparable or alike and will promote gastric emptying. From the remaining options, select option 3 because this measure will delay gastric emptying.

7. 1

Rationale: Early manifestations occur 5 to 30 minutes after eating. Symptoms include vertigo, tachycardia, syncope, sweating, pallor, palpitations, and the desire to lie down.

Test-Taking Strategy: Focus on the subject, dumping syndrome. Note the strategic word, *early*. Think about the pathophysiology of this disorder to answer correctly. Knowledge regarding the early signs/symptoms associated with dumping syndrome is required to answer this question. Remember, sweating and pallor occur and are early signs of dumping syndrome.

8. 1

Rationale: Crohn's disease is characterized by nonbloody diarrhea of usually not more than four or five stools daily. Over time, the diarrhea episodes increase in frequency, duration, and severity. Options 2, 3, and 4 are not characteristics of Crohn's disease.

Test-Taking Strategy: Focus on the subject, Crohn's disease. Recalling the pathophysiology related to Crohn's disease will direct you to the correct option.

9. 2

Rationale: An upright position allows the intestine to float posteriorly and helps prevent intestinal laceration during catheter insertion. Options 1, 3, and 4 are incorrect positions.

Test-Taking Strategy: Focus on the subject, position for a paracentesis. Visualize this procedure in selecting the correct option. Knowing that fluid will be aspirated from the abdominal cavity will assist with directing you to the correct option.

10. 1, 2, 3 ❖

Rationale: The client with acute pancreatitis is normally placed on an NPO status to rest the pancreas and suppress gastrointestinal (GI) secretions. Because abdominal pain is a prominent symptom of pancreatitis, pain medication will be prescribed. Some clients experience lessened pain by assuming positions that flex the trunk and draw the knees up to the chest. A side-lying position with the head elevated 45 degrees decreases tension on the abdomen and may also help ease the pain. The client is susceptible to respiratory infections because the retroperitoneal fluid raises the diaphragm, which causes the client to take shallow, guarded abdominal breaths. Therefore, measures such as turning, coughing, and deep breathing are instituted. Antacids and anticholinergics may be prescribed to suppress GI secretions.

Test-Taking Strategy: Focus on the subject, interventions associated with acute pancreatitis. Remember the pathophysiology associated with pancreatitis, and note the word *acute* in the question. This will assist in selecting the correct interventions.

11. 1

Rationale: Hepatitis A virus (HAV) is transmitted by the fecal-oral route via contaminated food or infected food handlers. Hepatitis B virus, hepatitis C virus, and hepatitis D virus are most commonly transmitted via infected blood or body fluids.

Test-Taking Strategy: Focus on the subject, transmission of hepatitis, and note the strategic words, *most likely*. Knowledge regarding the modes of transmission of the various types of hepatitis is required to answer this question. Remember, HAV is transmitted by the fecal-oral route via contaminated food or infected food handlers.

12. 3

Rationale: The pain associated with acute pancreatitis is aggravated when the client lies in a supine and flat position. Therefore, the nurse would verify this prescription. Options 1, 2, and 4 are appropriate interventions for the client with acute pancreatitis.

Test-Taking Strategy: Focus on the subject, contraindications in care for the client with acute pancreatitis. Recalling the pathophysiology of this disorder and the measures that relieve pain will direct you to the correct option.

13. 1

Rationale: Hiatal hernia is caused by a protrusion of a portion of the stomach above the diaphragm, where the esophagus

usually is positioned. The client generally experiences pain caused by reflux resulting from ingestion of irritating foods, lying flat following meals or at night, and consuming large or fatty meals. Relief is obtained by eating small, frequent, and bland meals; histamine antagonists and antacids; and elevation of the thorax after meals and during sleep.

Test-Taking Strategy: Focus on the subject, the action to "avoid." This tells you that the correct answer will be the option that represents an aggravating factor for hiatal hernia discomfort. Visualize each option and think about the anatomical location of a hiatal hernia to direct you to the correct option.

14. 4

Rationale: A prolapsed stoma is one in which bowel protrudes through the stoma, with an elongated and swollen appearance. A stoma retraction is characterized by sinking of the stoma. Ischemia of the stoma would be associated with a dusky or bluish color. A stoma with a narrowed opening, either at the level of the skin or fascia, is said to be stenosed.

Test-Taking Strategy: Focusing on the subject, the characteristics of stoma prolapse. Thinking about the definition of *prolapse* will direct you to the correct option.

15. 3

Rationale: Ultrasound of the gallbladder is a noninvasive procedure and is frequently used for emergency diagnosis of acute cholecystitis. The client may need to lie still during the procedure for short intervals of time while visualization of the gallbladder is done. The client may or may not need to be NPO (per PHCP preference), but may be instructed to avoid carbonated beverages for 48 hours before the test to help decrease intestinal gas. It is a painless test and does not require the administration of oral tablets as preparation.

Test-Taking Strategy: Focus on the subject, an ultrasound of the gallbladder. Think about what this diagnostic procedure entails. Visualizing this procedure will direct you to the correct option.

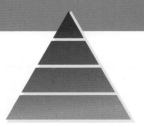

CHAPTER 46

Gastrointestinal Medications

PRIORITY CONCEPTS Inflammation; Tissue Integrity

WHAT WOULD YOU DO?

The nurse checks the ammonia level of a client with hepatic dysfunction who is receiving lactulose and notes that the level is 75 mcg/dL. What would the nurse do?
Answer is located on p. 605.

I. Antacids (Table 46.1 and Fig. 46.1)
A. React with gastric acid to produce neutral salts or salts of low acidity
B. Inactivate pepsin and enhance mucosal protection, but do not coat the ulcer crater
C. These medications are used for peptic ulcer disease and gastroesophageal reflux disease.
D. These medications need to be taken on a regular schedule; some are prescribed to be taken 1 and 3 hours after each meal and at bedtime.
E. To provide maximum benefit, treatment needs to elevate the gastric pH above 5.
F. Antacid tablets need to be chewed thoroughly and followed with a glass of water or milk.
G. Liquid preparations need to be shaken before dispensing.

⚠ To prevent interaction and interference with other medications, allow 1 hour between antacid administration and the administration of other medications.

II. Gastric Protectants
A. Misoprostol
1. An antisecretory medication that enhances mucosal defenses
2. Suppresses secretion of gastric acid and maintains submucosal blood flow by promoting vasodilation
3. Used to prevent gastric ulcers caused by nonsteroidal anti-inflammatory medications and aspirin
4. Administered with meals
5. Causes diarrhea and abdominal pain

6. Contraindicated for use during pregnancy
B. Sucralfate
1. Creates a protective barrier against acid and pepsin
2. Administered orally; needs to be taken on an empty stomach
3. May cause constipation
4. May impede absorption of warfarin sodium, phenytoin, theophylline, digoxin, and some antibiotics; would be administered at least 2 hours apart from these medications

III. Histamine (H₂)-Receptor Antagonists
A. Description
1. Suppress secretion of gastric acid
2. Alleviate symptoms of heartburn and assist with preventing complications associated with peptic ulcer disease
3. Prevent stress ulcers and reduce the recurrence of all ulcers
4. Promote healing in gastroesophageal reflux disease
5. Are contraindicated for use in hypersensitive clients
6. Would be used with caution in clients with impaired renal or hepatic function
B. Cimetidine
1. Can be administered orally, intramuscularly, or intravenously
2. Food reduces the rate of absorption; if taken with meals, absorption will be slowed.
3. Intravenous administration can cause hypotension and dysrhythmia.
4. Antacids can decrease the absorption of oral cimetidine.
5. Cimetidine and antacids need to be administered at least 1 hour apart from each other.
6. Cimetidine passes the blood-brain barrier, and central nervous system side/adverse effects can occur; it may cause mental confusion, agitation, psychosis, depression, anxiety, and disorientation.

600

TABLE 46.1 Classification of Antacids and Considerations

Classification	Considerations
Aluminum compounds	Aluminum hydroxide is used to treat hyperphosphatemia; therefore, it can cause hypophosphatemia. Aluminum hydroxide can reduce the effects of tetracyclines, warfarin sodium, and digoxin and can reduce phosphate absorption and thereby cause hypophosphatemia. Contain significant amounts of sodium; needs to be used with caution in clients with hypertension and heart failure. The most common side effect is constipation.
Magnesium compounds	Magnesium hydroxide is also a saline laxative, and the most prominent side effect is diarrhea; it is usually administered in combination with aluminum hydroxide, an antacid that assists with preventing diarrhea. Magnesium compounds are contraindicated in clients with intestinal obstruction, appendicitis, or undiagnosed abdominal pain. In clients with renal impairment, magnesium can accumulate to high levels, causing signs of toxicity.
Calcium compounds	Calcium carbonate can cause acid rebound. Calcium compounds are rapid-acting and release carbon dioxide in the stomach, causing belching and flatulence. A common side effect is constipation. Milk-alkali syndrome (headache, urinary frequency, anorexia, nausea/vomiting, fatigue) can occur (the client needs to avoid milk products and vitamin D supplements).
Sodium bicarbonate	Has a rapid onset, liberates carbon dioxide, increases intra-abdominal pressure, and promotes flatulence. Would be used with caution in clients with hypertension and heart failure. Can cause systemic alkalosis in clients with renal impairment. Sodium bicarbonate is useful for treating acidosis and elevating urinary pH to promote excretion of acidic medications after overdose.

7. Dosage needs to be reduced in clients with renal impairment.
8. Cimetidine inhibits hepatic drug-metabolizing enzymes and can cause many medication levels to rise; if administered with warfarin sodium, phenytoin, theophylline, or lidocaine, the dosages of these medications would need to be reduced.

C. Famotidine and nizatidine
   1. Famotidine and nizatidine are similar to ranitidine and cimetidine.
   2. These medications do not need to be administered with food.

IV. Proton Pump Inhibitors (Box 46.1)

A. Suppress gastric acid secretion

B. Used to treat active ulcer disease, erosive esophagitis, and pathological hypersecretory conditions

C. Contraindicated in hypersensitivity

D. Common side effects include headache, diarrhea, abdominal pain, and nausea.

V. Medication Regimens to Treat *Helicobacter pylori* Infections (Box 46.2)

A. An antibacterial agent alone is not effective for eradicating *H. pylori* because the bacterium readily becomes resistant to the agent.

B. Triple or quadruple therapy with a variety of medication combinations is used (if triple therapy fails, quadruple therapy is recommended).

VI. Prokinetic Agent

A. Medication: Metoclopramide

B. Stimulates motility of the upper gastrointestinal tract and increases the rate of gastric emptying without stimulating gastric, biliary, or pancreatic secretions

C. Used to treat gastroesophageal reflux and paralytic ileus

D. May cause restlessness, drowsiness, extrapyramidal reactions, dizziness, insomnia, and headache

E. Usually administered 30 minutes before meals and at bedtime

F. Contraindicated in clients with sensitivity and in clients with mechanical obstruction, perforation, or gastrointestinal hemorrhage

G. Can precipitate hypertensive crisis in clients with pheochromocytoma

H. Safety during pregnancy has not been established.

I. Metoclopramide can cause parkinsonian reactions; if this occurs, the medication will be discontinued by the primary health care provider (PHCP).

J. Anticholinergics, such as atropine, and opioid analgesics such as morphine, antagonize the effects of metoclopramide.

K. Alcohol, sedatives, cyclosporine, and tranquilizers produce an additive effect.

VII. Bile Acid Sequestrants (Box 46.3)

A. Act by absorbing and combining with intestinal bile salts, which then are secreted in the feces, preventing intestinal reabsorption

B. Used to treat hypercholesterolemia in adults, biliary obstruction, and pruritus associated with biliary disease

C. With powdered forms, taste and palatability are often reasons for noncompliance and can be improved by the use of flavored products or mixing the medication with various juices.

D. Side and adverse effects include nausea, bloating, constipation, fecal impaction, and intestinal obstruction.

E. Stool softeners and other sources of fiber can be used to abate the gastrointestinal side effects.

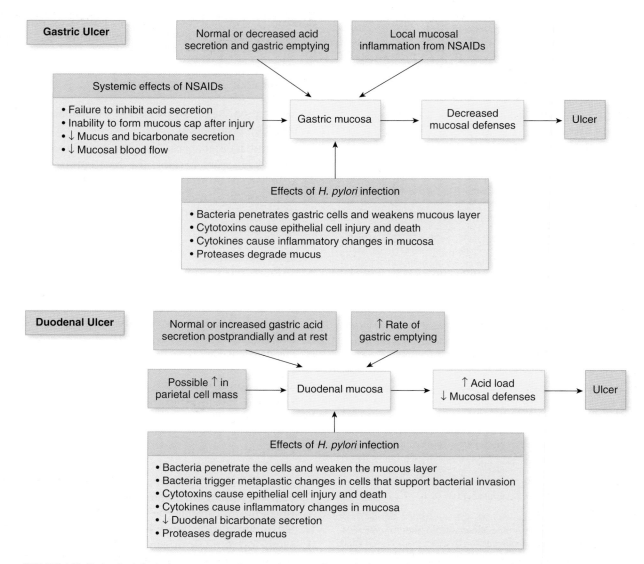

Gastric Ulcer

Systemic effects of NSAIDs
- Failure to inhibit acid secretion
- Inability to form mucous cap after injury
- ↓ Mucus and bicarbonate secretion
- ↓ Mucosal blood flow

Normal or decreased acid secretion and gastric emptying

Local mucosal inflammation from NSAIDs

Gastric mucosa → Decreased mucosal defenses → Ulcer

Effects of *H. pylori* infection
- Bacteria penetrates gastric cells and weakens mucous layer
- Cytotoxins cause epithelial cell injury and death
- Cytokines cause inflammatory changes in mucosa
- Proteases degrade mucus

Duodenal Ulcer

Normal or increased gastric acid secretion postprandially and at rest

↑ Rate of gastric emptying

Possible ↑ in parietal cell mass → Duodenal mucosa → ↑ Acid load ↓ Mucosal defenses → Ulcer

Effects of *H. pylori* infection
- Bacteria penetrate the cells and weaken the mucous layer
- Bacteria trigger metaplastic changes in cells that support bacterial invasion
- Cytotoxins cause epithelial cell injury and death
- Cytokines cause inflammatory changes in mucosa
- ↓ Duodenal bicarbonate secretion
- Proteases degrade mucus

FIGURE 46.1 Pathophysiological components of peptic ulcer. *H. pylori, Helicobacter pylori; NSAIDs,* nonsteroidal anti-inflammatory drugs.

BOX 46.1 Proton Pump Inhibitors

- Esomeprazole
- Dexlansoprazole
- Lansoprazole
- Omeprazole
- Pantoprazole
- Rabeprazole

⚠ Bile acid sequestrants would be used cautiously in clients with suspected bowel obstruction or severe constipation because they can worsen these conditions.

VIII. Treating Hepatic Encephalopathy

A. Medication: Lactulose

B. Used in the prevention and treatment of portal systemic encephalopathy, including hepatic precoma

---

BOX 46.2 Medication Regimens for Treating *Helicobacter pylori* **Infections**

Triple Therapy
Esomeprazole, amoxicillin, clarithromycin
Lansoprazole, amoxicillin, clarithromycin
Esomeprazole, metronidazole, clarithromycin

Quadruple Therapies
Esomeprazole, metronidazole, tetracycline, bismuth subsalicylate

Note: Additional medications may be prescribed for each level of therapy.

BOX 46.3 Bile Acid Sequestrants

- Colesevelam
- Colestipol
- Cholestyramine

and coma; also used in the treatment of chronic constipation

C. Promotes increased **peristalsis** and bowel evacuation, expelling ammonia from the colon and thus lowering the ammonia level (normal ammonia reference interval is 10–80 mcg/dL)

D. Improves protein tolerance in clients with advanced hepatic **cirrhosis**

E. Administered orally in the form of a syrup or rectally

IX. Pancreatic Enzyme Replacements

A. Pancrelipase

B. Used to supplement or replace pancreatic enzymes and thus improve nutritional status and reduce the amount of fatty stools (a deficiency of pancreatic enzymes can compromise digestion, especially the digestion of fats)

C. Would be taken with every meal and snack

D. Side and adverse effects include abdominal cramps or pain, nausea, vomiting, and diarrhea.

E. Products that contain calcium carbonate or magnesium hydroxide interfere with the action of these medications.

X. Treatment for Inflammatory Bowel Disease (Box 46.4)

A. Inflammatory bowel disease has two forms, including **Crohn's disease** and **ulcerative colitis**.

B. Antimicrobials: May be prescribed to prevent or treat secondary infection (see Chapter 60 for information on antimicrobials)

C. 5-Aminosalicylates (5-ASAs): Decrease gastrointestinal inflammation; side and adverse effects include nausea, rash, arthralgia, and hematological disorders.

D. Corticosteroids: Act as anti-inflammatory agents to decrease gastrointestinal inflammation (see Chapter 44 for information on glucocorticoids and corticosteroids)

E. Immunosuppressants: Suppress the immune system; can cause pancreatitis and neutropenia secondary to bone marrow depression, and their use is reserved for those who have not responded to traditional therapies (see Chapter 60 for information on immunosuppressants)

F. Immunomodulators: Monoclonal antibodies that modulate the immune response to induce and maintain remission (see Box 46.4 for specific immunomodulators)

XI. Treatment for Irritable Bowel Syndrome (IBS)

A. IBS is a gastrointestinal disorder that is characterized by crampy abdominal pain accompanied by diarrhea, constipation, or both.

BOX 46.4 **Medications to Treat Inflammatory Bowel Disease**

Antimicrobial
Ciprofloxacin
Clarithromycin
Metronidazole
Rifaximin

5-Aminosalicylates
Balsalazide
Mesalamine
Olsalazine
Sulfasalazine

Corticosteroids
Budesonide
Prednisone
Hydrocortisone

Immunosuppressants
Azathioprine
Cyclosporine
Mercaptopurine
Tacrolimus

Immunomodulators
Adalimumab
Certolizumab
Infliximab
Natalizumab

B. Pharmacological treatment depends on the main symptom: constipation or diarrhea.

C. Constipation-predominant IBS (IBS-C) treatment
1. Bulk-forming laxatives, usually taken at mealtimes with a full glass of water
2. Lubiprostone: Chloride channel activator that increases fluid in the intestines to promote bowel elimination; needs to be taken with food and water
3. Linaclotide: Stimulates receptors in the intestines to promote bowel transit time; taken daily 30 minutes before breakfast
4. See Box 46.6 for a list of additional medications to treat constipation.

D. Diarrhea-predominant IBS (IBS-D) treatment
1. Alosetron
   a. A selective serotonin receptor antagonist
   b. Can cause severe adverse effects such as constipation, impaction, bowel obstruction, perforation of the bowel, and ischemic colitis
   c. A strict risk management procedure needs to be followed, including monitoring for serious adverse effects, reporting them, and immediate discontinuation of the medication if they arise.
2. Antidiarrheal medications: See Box 46.7 for a list of additional medications to treat diarrhea.

BOX 46.5 Commonly Administered Antiemetics

Serotonin Antagonists
Granisetron
Palonosetron
Ondansetron

Glucocorticoids
Dexamethasone
Methylprednisolone

Substance P/Neurokinin-1 Antagonists
Aprepitant
Fosaprepitant
Rolapitant

Benzodiazepine
Lorazepam

Dopamine Antagonists
Phenothiazines
Chlorpromazine
Perphenazine
Prochlorperazine
Promethazine

Butyrophenones
Haloperidol
Droperidol

Others
Amisulpride
Metoclopramide
Trimethobenzamide

Cannabinoids
Dronabinol
Nabilone

Anticholinergics
Scopolamine transdermal

Antihistamines
Dimenhydrinate
Diphenhydramine
Hydroxyzine
Meclizine hydrochloride

Adapted from Lehne R: *Pharmacology for nursing care*, ed 8, Philadelphia, 2013, Saunders.

BOX 46.6 Laxatives

Bulk-Forming
- Methylcellulose
- Polycarbophil
- Psyllium

Stimulants
- Bisacodyl
- Senna

Surfactant
- Docusate sodium

Osmotics
- Magnesium hydroxide
- Magnesium citrate
- Sodium phosphates
- Polyethylene glycol and electrolytes
- Lactulose

BOX 46.7 Medications to Control Diarrhea

Opioids and Related Medications
- Diphenoxylate with atropine sulfate
- Loperamide

Other Antidiarrheals
- Bismuth subsalicylate
- Bulk-forming medications
- Anticholinergic antispasmodics: dicyclomine, glycopyrrolate

---

XII. Antiemetics (Box 46.5)

A. Medications used to control vomiting and motion sickness

B. The choice of the antiemetic is determined by the cause of the nausea and vomiting.

C. Monitor vital signs and intake and output and for signs of dehydration and fluid and electrolyte imbalances.

D. Limit odors in the client's room when the client is nauseated or vomiting.

E. Limit oral intake to clear liquids when the client is nauseated or vomiting.

Antiemetics can cause drowsiness; therefore, a priority intervention is to protect the client from injury.

XIII. Laxatives (Box 46.6)

A. Bulk-forming
  1. Description
    a. Absorb water into the feces and increase bulk to produce large and soft stools
    b. Contraindicated in cases of bowel obstruction
    c. Dependency can occur with long-term use.
  2. Side and adverse effects include gastrointestinal disturbances, dehydration, and electrolyte imbalances.

B. Stimulants: Stimulate motility of large intestine

C. Emollients
  1. Inhibit absorption of water so fecal mass remains large and soft
  2. Used to avoid straining

D. Osmotics: Attract water into the large intestine to produce bulk and stimulate peristalsis

The client receiving a laxative needs to increase fluid intake to prevent dehydration.

XIV. Medications to Control Diarrhea (Box 46.7)

A. Identify and treat the underlying cause and dehydration, replace fluids and electrolytes, relieve abdominal discomfort and cramping, and reduce the passage of stool

B. Opioids

  1. Opioids are effective antidiarrheal medications and decrease intestinal motility and peristalsis.

  2. When poisons, infections, or bacterial toxins are the cause of diarrhea, opioids worsen the condition by delaying the elimination of toxins.

WHAT WOULD YOU DO?

Answer: Lactulose is used in the prevention and treatment of portal systemic encephalopathy, including hepatic precoma and coma. It promotes increased peristalsis and bowel evacuation, expelling ammonia from the colon and thus lowering the ammonia level. The normal ammonia level is 10 to 80 mcg/dL. If the level is 75 mcg /dL, the nurse determines that the medication is effective in lowering the ammonia level. The nurse would report the level to the registered nurse.

PRACTICE QUESTIONS

1. A client with Crohn's disease is scheduled to receive an infusion of infliximab. The nurse assisting with caring for the client would take which action to monitor the **effectiveness** of treatment?

  1. Monitoring the leukocyte count for 2 days after the infusion

  2. Checking the frequency and consistency of bowel movements

  3. Checking serum liver enzyme levels before and after the infusion

  4. Carrying out a Hematest on gastric fluids after the infusion is completed

2. The client has an as needed prescription for loperamide hydrochloride. For which condition would the nurse administer this medication?

  1. Constipation

  2. Acute diarrhea

  3. Abdominal pain

  4. Hematest-positive nasogastric tube drainage

3. The client has an as needed prescription for ondansetron. For which condition would the nurse administer this medication?

  1. Paralytic ileus

  2. Incisional pain

  3. Urinary retention

  4. Nausea and vomiting

4. The client has begun medication therapy with pancrelipase. The nurse evaluates that the medication is having the optimal intended benefit if which effect is observed?

  1. Weight loss

  2. Relief of heartburn

  3. Reduction of steatorrhea

  4. Absence of abdominal pain

5. An older client has recently been taking cimetidine. The nurse needs to monitor the client for which **most** frequent central nervous system side effect of this medication?

  1. Tremors

  2. Dizziness

  3. Confusion

  4. Hallucinations

6. A histamine (H_2)-receptor antagonist will be pre-❖ scribed for a client. The nurse understands that which medications are H_2-receptor antagonists? **Select all that apply.**

  ❏ **1.** Nizatidine

  ❏ **2.** Famotidine

  ❏ **3.** Cimetidine

  ❏ **4.** Esomeprazole

  ❏ **5.** Lansoprazole

7. The client who frequently uses nonsteroidal anti-inflammatory drugs (NSAIDs) has been taking misoprostol. The nurse determines that this medication is having the intended therapeutic effect if which is noted?

  1. Resolved diarrhea

  2. Relief of epigastric pain

  3. Decreased platelet count

  4. Decreased white blood cell count

8. The client has been taking omeprazole for 4 weeks. The nurse evaluates that the client is receiving the optimal intended effect of the medication if the client reports the absence of which symptom?

  1. Diarrhea

  2. Heartburn

  3. Flatulence

  4. Constipation

9. A client with a peptic ulcer is diagnosed with a *H. pylori* infection. The nurse is reinforcing teaching for the client about the medications prescribed, including clarithromycin, esomeprazole, and amoxicillin. Which statement by the client indicates the **best** understanding of the medication regimen?

  1. "My ulcer will heal because these medications will kill the bacteria."

  2. "These medications are only taken when I have pain from my ulcer."

3. "The medications will kill the bacteria and stop the acid production."
4. "These medications will coat the ulcer and decrease the acid production in my stomach."

10. The client with a gastric ulcer has a prescription for sucralfate 1 g by mouth four times daily. The nurse would schedule the medication to be administered at which times?
1. With meals and at bedtime
2. Every 6 hours around the clock
3. One hour after meals and at bedtime
4. One hour before meals and at bedtime

ANSWERS

1. 2
Rationale: The principal manifestations of Crohn's disease are diarrhea and abdominal pain. Infliximab is an immunomodulator that reduces the degree of inflammation in the colon, thereby reducing the diarrhea. Options 1, 3, and 4 are unrelated to this medication.
Test-Taking Strategy: Focus on the subject, Crohn's disease and nursing implications associated with infliximab, and note the strategic word, *effectiveness*. Eliminate option 1 because gastric bleeding is not a characteristic of Crohn's disease. Monitoring the leukocyte count and liver enzyme levels is appropriate when infliximab is given, but not to evaluate the effectiveness of treatment, eliminating options 3 and 4.

2. 2
Rationale: Loperamide is an antidiarrheal agent. It is used to manage acute and also chronic diarrhea in conditions such as inflammatory bowel disease. Loperamide also can be used to reduce the volume of drainage from an ileostomy. It is not used for the conditions in options 1, 3, and 4.
Test-Taking Strategy: Focus on the subject, the intended use of loperamide. Think about the classification of this medication. Recalling that this medication is an antidiarrheal agent will direct you to option 2.

3. 4
Rationale: Ondansetron is an antiemetic used to treat postoperative nausea and vomiting, as well as nausea and vomiting associated with chemotherapy. The other options are incorrect.
Test-Taking Strategy: Focus on the subject, the intended effect of ondansetron. Think about the classification of this medication. Recalling that this medication is an antiemetic will direct you to the correct option.

4. 3
Rationale: Pancrelipase is a pancreatic enzyme used in clients with pancreatitis as a digestive aid. The medication reduces the amount of fatty stools (steatorrhea). Another intended effect could be improved nutritional status. It is not used to treat abdominal pain or heartburn. Its use could result in weight gain but would not result in weight loss if it is aiding in digestion.
Test-Taking Strategy: Focus on the subject, optimal intended effect of the medication as well as the name of the medication. Use knowledge of physiology of the pancreas to assist with directing you to the correct option.

5. 3
Rationale: Cimetidine is a histamine 2 (H_2)-receptor antagonist. Older clients are especially susceptible to the central nervous system side effects of cimetidine. The most frequent of these is confusion. Less common central nervous system side effects include headache, dizziness, drowsiness, and hallucinations.
Test-Taking Strategy: Note the strategic word, *most*. Use knowledge of the older client and medication effects in this population to direct you to the correct option.

❖ **6. 1, 2, 3**
Rationale: H_2-receptor antagonists suppress secretion of gastric acid, alleviate symptoms of heartburn, and assist with preventing complications of peptic ulcer disease. These medications also suppress gastric acid secretions and are used in active ulcer disease, erosive esophagitis, and pathological hypersecretory conditions. The other medications listed are proton pump inhibitors.
Test-Taking Strategy: Focus on the subject, H_2-receptor antagonists. Recalling that these medication names end with *-dine* will assist in answering this question. Also, recall that proton pump inhibitor medication names end with *-zole*.

7. 2
Rationale: The client who frequently uses nonsteroidal anti-inflammatory drugs (NSAIDs) is prone to gastric mucosal injury. Misoprostol is a gastric protectant and is given specifically to prevent this occurrence. Diarrhea can be a side effect of the medication, but it is not an intended effect. Options 3 and 4 are incorrect.
Test-Taking Strategy: Note the subject, intended therapeutic effect of misoprostol. This tells you that the medication is being given to prevent the occurrence of specific symptoms. Recalling that NSAIDs can cause gastric mucosal injury will direct you to the correct option.

8. 2
Rationale: Omeprazole is a proton pump inhibitor classified as an antiulcer agent. The intended effect of the medication is relief of pain from gastric irritation, often called "heartburn" by clients. Omeprazole is not used to treat the conditions identified in options 1, 3, and 4.

Test-Taking Strategy: Focus on the subject, the optimal intended effect of omeprazole. Focus on the name of the medication and note the letters *-zole* in the medication name. Recalling that this medication is a proton pump inhibitor will direct you to the correct option.

9. 3

Rationale: Triple therapy for *H. pylori* infection usually includes two antibacterial drugs and a proton pump inhibitor. Clarithromycin and amoxicillin are antibacterials. Esomeprazole is a proton pump inhibitor. These medications will kill the bacteria and decrease acid production.

Test-Taking Strategy: Note the strategic word, *best*, and focus on the subject, the name of the medications and their actions. Eliminate option 1 because the medications do more than kill the bacteria. These medications are taken not only when there is pain but continually until pain is gone, usually for 1 to 2 weeks. This will eliminate option 2. These medications do not coat the ulcer, eliminating option 4.

10. 4

Rationale: Sucralfate is a gastric protectant. The medication needs to be scheduled for administration 1 hour before meals and at bedtime. The medication is timed to allow it to form a protective coating over the ulcer before food intake stimulates gastric acid production and mechanical irritation. The other options are incorrect.

Test-Taking Strategy: Focus on the subject, scheduling of sucralfate. Focusing on the client's diagnosis, gastric ulcer, and thinking about the pathophysiology associated with a gastric ulcer will assist in directing you to the correct option.

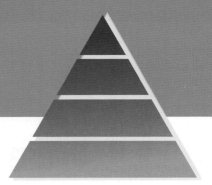

UNIT XII

Respiratory Problems of the Adult Client

 ## Pyramid to Success

The Pyramid to Success focuses on infectious diseases, particularly tuberculosis, and respiratory care in relation to oxygen delivery systems and mechanical ventilation. Pyramid Points also focus on the client with pneumonia, respiratory failure, chronic obstructive pulmonary disease, pneumothorax, influenza, and other respiratory viral infections. The Pyramid to Success includes the care of the client with tuberculosis, especially regarding the importance of the medication regimen, providing adequate nutrition and adequate rest to promote the healing process, and prevention of progression of the health problem. Focus on assisting the client to cope with the social isolation issues that exist during the period of illness and on teaching the client and family the critical measures of screening and preventing respiratory disease. Measures to prevent the transmission of infectious droplet and airborne disease is a priority focus.

 ## Client Needs: Learning Objectives

Safe and Effective Care Environment
Collaborating with the interprofessional team in the management of the respiratory problem
Discussing consultations and referrals related to the respiratory problem
Ensuring that informed consent related to invasive procedures has been obtained
Establishing priorities
Handling infectious materials such as sputum or body fluids safely
Maintaining asepsis when caring for wounds or tracheostomy sites and during mechanical ventilation or suctioning
Maintaining confidentiality related to the respiratory problem

Maintaining droplet and airborne precautions, standard precautions, and other precautions
Health Promotion and Maintenance
Educating the client about adequate fluid and nutritional intake
Educating the client about breathing exercises and respiratory therapy and care
Educating the client about medication administration
Educating the client about the need for follow-up care
Educating the client about the prevention of transmission of infection
Informing the client about health promotion programs
Performing respiratory assessment/data collection techniques
Preventing respiratory problems and infectious diseases
Providing assistance with health screening related to risks for respiratory problems
Psychosocial Integrity
Considering religious, cultural, and spiritual influences when providing care
Discussing body image changes related to respiratory problems
Discussing end-of-life and grief and loss issues
Discussing situational role changes
Identifying coping strategies
Identifying support systems and community resources
Physiological Integrity
Administering medications
Caring for the client that has been placed on mechanical ventilation
Caring for the client receiving respiratory therapy and supplemental oxygen
Managing respiratory illnesses
Monitoring for acid-base imbalances
Monitoring for alterations in body systems
Monitoring for infectious diseases
Providing nutrition and oral hygiene
Providing personal hygiene and promoting rest and sleep
Providing rest and comfort

Client Needs lists modified from: National Council of State Boards of Nursing, Inc. (NCSBN). *NCLEX-PN Examination: Test Plan for the National Council Licensure Examination for Practical Nurses,* effective April 2020. Chicago: NCSBN.

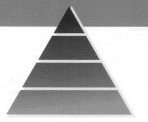

CHAPTER **47**

Respiratory Problems

PRIORITY CONCEPTS **Gas Exchange; Perfusion**

WHAT WOULD YOU DO?

A victim of a gunshot wound to the chest sustained a penetrating injury. The emergency medical response team applied a nonporous dressing over the victim's sucking chest wound at the site of the accident. On arrival at the emergency department, the victim is cyanotic, and the nurse notes subcutaneous emphysema (crepitus) and tracheal deviation away from the affected side. What would the nurse do?

Answer is located on p. 629

I. Anatomy and Physiology

A. Primary functions of the respiratory system
   1. Provides oxygen for metabolism in the tissues
   2. Removes carbon dioxide, the waste product of metabolism
B. Secondary functions of the respiratory system
   1. Facilitates sense of smell
   2. Produces speech
   3. Maintains acid-base balance
   4. Maintains body water levels
   5. Maintains heat balance
C. Upper respiratory tract
   1. Nose: Humidifies, warms, and filters inspired air
   2. Sinuses: Air-filled cavities within the hollow bones that surround the nasal passages and provide resonance during speech
   3. Pharynx
      a. Passageway for the respiratory and digestive tracts located behind the oral and nasal cavities
      b. Divided into the nasopharynx, oropharynx, and laryngopharynx
   4. Larynx
      a. Located just below the pharynx at the root of the tongue; commonly called the *voice box*
      b. Contains two pairs of vocal cords: the false and true cords
      c. The opening between the true vocal cords is the glottis.

d. The glottis plays an important role in coughing, which is the most fundamental defense mechanism of the lungs.
   5. Epiglottis
      a. Leaf-shaped elastic flap structure at the top of the larynx
      b. Prevents food from entering the tracheobronchial tree by closing over the glottis during swallowing
D. Lower respiratory tract
   1. Trachea: Located in front of the esophagus; branches into the right and left mainstem bronchi at the carina
   2. Mainstem bronchi
      a. Begin at the carina
      b. The right bronchus is slightly wider, shorter, and more vertical than the left bronchus.
      c. Divide into secondary or lobar bronchi that enter each of the five lobes of the lung
      d. The bronchi are lined with cilia which propel mucus up and away from the lower airway to the trachea where it can be expectorated or swallowed.
   3. Bronchioles
      a. Branch from the secondary bronchi and subdivide into the small terminal and respiratory bronchioles
      b. The bronchioles contain no cartilage and depend on the elastic recoil of the lung for patency.
      c. The terminal bronchioles contain no cilia and do not participate in gas exchange.
   4. Alveolar ducts and alveoli
      a. *Acinus* (plural, *acini*) is a term used to indicate all structures distal to the terminal bronchiole.
      b. Alveolar ducts branch from the respiratory bronchioles.
      c. Alveolar sacs, which arise from the ducts, contain clusters of alveoli which are the basic units of gas exchange.

d. Type II alveolar cells in the walls of the alveoli secrete surfactant, a phospholipid protein that reduces the surface tension in the alveoli; without surfactant, the alveoli would collapse.

5. Lungs

  a. Located in the pleural cavity in the thorax

  b. Extend from just above the clavicles to the diaphragm, the major muscle of inspiration

  c. The right lung, which is larger than the left, is divided into three lobes: upper, middle, and lower.

  d. The left lung, which is narrower than the right to accommodate the heart, is divided into two lobes.

  e. The respiratory structures are innervated by the phrenic nerve, the vagus nerve, and the thoracic nerves.

  f. The parietal pleura lines the inside of the thoracic cavity, including the upper surface of the diaphragm.

  g. The visceral pleura covers the pulmonary surfaces.

  h. A thin fluid layer, which is produced by the cells lining the pleura, lubricates the visceral pleura and the parietal pleura, allowing them to glide smoothly and painlessly during respiration.

  i. Blood flows throughout the lungs via the pulmonary circulation system.

6. Accessory muscles of respiration include the scalene muscles which elevate the first two ribs; the sternocleidomastoid muscles which raise the sternum; and the trapezius and pectoralis muscles which fix the shoulders.

7. The respiratory process

  a. The diaphragm descends into the abdominal cavity during inspiration causing negative pressure in the lungs.

  b. The negative pressure draws air from the area of greater pressure, the atmosphere, into the area of lesser pressure, the lungs.

  c. In the lungs, air passes through the terminal bronchioles into the alveoli and diffuses into surrounding capillaries, then travels to the rest of the body to oxygenate the body tissues.

  d. At the end of inspiration the diaphragm and intercostal muscles relax and the lungs recoil.

  e. As the lungs recoil, pressure within the lungs becomes greater than the atmospheric pressure causing the air, which now contains the cellular waste products of carbon dioxide and water, to move from the alveoli in the lungs to the atmosphere.

  f. Effective gas exchange depends on distribution of gas (ventilation) and blood (perfusion) in all portions of the lungs.

BOX 47.1   Risk Factors for Respiratory Disorders

- Allergies
- Chest injury
- Crowded living conditions
- Exposure to chemicals and environmental pollutants
- Family history of infectious disease
- Frequent respiratory illness
- Scoliosis and other anatomical/musculoskeletal disorders
- Geographical residence and travel to foreign countries
- Smoking
- Surgery
- Use of chewing tobacco
- Viral syndromes

II. Diagnostic Tests

A. Risk factors for respiratory disorders (Box 47.1)

B. Chest x-ray film (radiograph)

  1. Description: Provides information regarding the anatomical location and appearance of the lungs

  2. Preprocedure

    a. Remove all jewelry and other metal objects from the chest area.

    b. Determine the client's ability to inhale and hold their breath.

  3. Postprocedure: Help the client get dressed.

⚠ Question women regarding pregnancy or the possibility of pregnancy before performing radiography studies.

C. Sputum specimen: Specimen is obtained by expectoration or tracheal suctioning to assist with the identification of organisms or abnormal cells (see **Priority Nursing Actions**).

⚡ PRIORITY NURSING ACTIONS

Respiratory Suctioning Procedure

1. Explain the procedure to the client.
2. Assist the client to an upright position.
3. Perform hand hygiene and don protective garb.
4. Prepare suctioning equipment and turn on the suction.
5. Hyperoxygenate the client.
6. Insert the catheter without suction applied.
7. Once inserted, apply suction intermittently while rotating and withdrawing the catheter.
8. Hyperoxygenate the client.
9. Listen to breath sounds.
10. Document the procedure, client response, and effectiveness.

1. Preprocedure
   a. Determine the specific purpose of specimen collection and check institutional policy for appropriate method for collection.
   b. Obtain an early-morning sterile specimen by suctioning or expectoration after a respiratory treatment, if a treatment is prescribed.
   c. Instruct the client to rinse the mouth with water before collection.
   d. Obtain 15 mL of sputum.
   e. Instruct the client to take several deep breaths and then cough deeply to obtain sputum.
   f. Collect the specimen before the client begins antibiotic therapy. If already started on antibiotic therapy, ensure the laboratory can utilize an antimicrobial removal device when analyzing the specimen.
2. Postprocedure
   a. If a culture of sputum is prescribed, transport the specimen to the laboratory immediately.
   b. Assist the client with mouth care.

⚠ Ensure an informed consent is obtained for any procedure that is invasive. Vital signs are measured before an invasive procedure and monitored postprocedure to detect signs of complications.

D. Laryngoscopy and bronchoscopy
   1. Description: Direct visual examination of the larynx, trachea, and bronchi with a fiberoptic bronchoscope
   2. Preprocedure
      a. Maintain NPO (nothing by mouth) status for the client as prescribed.
      b. Check the results of coagulation studies.
      c. Remove dentures and eyeglasses.
      d. Prepare suction equipment.
      e. Ensure that the client has intravenous (IV) access, and assist to administer medication for sedation as prescribed.
      f. Have emergency resuscitation equipment readily available.
   3. Postprocedure
      a. Maintain the client in the semi-Fowler's position.
      b. Check for the return of the gag reflex.
      c. Maintain NPO status until the gag reflex returns.
      d. Monitor for bloody sputum.
      e. Monitor respiratory status, particularly if sedation has been administered.
      f. Monitor for complications, such as bronchospasm or bronchial perforation, indicated by facial or neck crepitus, dysrhythmia, hemorrhage, hypoxemia, and pneumothorax.
      g. Notify the registered nurse (RN) and primary health care provider (PHCP) if signs of complications occur.

E. Endobronchial ultrasound (EBUS)
   1. Tissue samples are obtained from central lung masses and lymph nodes using a bronchoscope with the help of ultrasound guidance.
   2. Tissue samples are used for diagnosing and staging lung cancer, detecting infections, and identifying inflammatory diseases that affect the lungs, such as sarcoidosis.
   3. Postprocedure, the client is monitored for signs of bleeding and respiratory distress.

F. Pulmonary angiography
   1. Description
      a. A fluoroscopic procedure in which a catheter is inserted through the antecubital or femoral vein into the pulmonary artery, or one of its branches
      b. Involves an injection of iodine, radiopaque, or contrast material
   2. Preprocedure
      a. Check for allergies to iodine, seafood, or other radiopaque dyes.
      b. Maintain NPO status of the client as prescribed.
      c. Check the results of coagulation studies.
      d. Ensure IV access is established.
      e. Assist with the administration of a sedative, as prescribed.
      f. Reinforce instructions about the need to lie still during the procedure.
      g. Tell the client that he or she may feel an urge to cough, flushing, nausea, or a salty taste following injection of the dye.
      h. Have emergency resuscitation equipment available.
   3. Postprocedure
      a. Avoid taking blood pressure measurements for 24 hours in the extremity used for the injection.
      b. Monitor peripheral neurovascular status of the affected extremity.
      c. Check insertion site for bleeding.
      d. Monitor for delayed reaction to the dye.

G. Thoracentesis
   1. Description: Removal of fluid or air from the pleural space via transthoracic aspiration
   2. Preprocedure
      a. Prepare the client for ultrasound or chest radiograph, if prescribed, before the procedure.
      b. Check results of coagulation studies.
      c. Note that the client is positioned sitting upright, with the arms and shoulders supported by a table at the bedside during the procedure.
      d. If the client cannot sit up, place the client ly- ing in bed toward the unaffected side, with the head of the bed elevated.
      e. Instruct the client not to cough, breathe deeply, or move during the procedure.

3. Postprocedure
   a. Monitor respiratory status.
   b. Apply a pressure dressing and check the puncture site for bleeding and crepitus.
   c. Monitor for signs of pneumothorax, air embolism, and pulmonary edema; notify the RN and PHCP if signs of complications occur.

H. Pulmonary function test
   1. Description: Tests used to evaluate lung mechanics, gas exchange, and acid-base disturbance through spirometric measurements, lung volumes, and arterial blood gas levels
   2. Preprocedure
      a. Determine whether an analgesic that may depress the respiratory function is being administered.
      b. Consult with the RN and PHCP regarding withholding bronchodilators before testing, or alternatively, if the testing will be done prior to and after administration of the bronchodilator.
      c. The client is instructed to void before the procedure and to wear loose clothing.
      d. Remove dentures.
      e. Reinforce instructions to the client to refrain from smoking or eating a heavy meal for 4 to 6 hours before the test.
   3. Postprocedure: Client may resume a normal diet and any bronchodilators and respiratory treatments that were withheld before the procedure.

I. Lung biopsy
   1. Description
      a. A transbronchial biopsy and a transbronchial needle aspiration may be performed to obtain tissue for analysis by culture or cytological examination.
      b. An open lung biopsy is performed in the operating room.
   2. Preprocedure
      a. Maintain NPO status before the procedure.
      b. Inform the client that a local anesthetic will be used for a needle biopsy, but a sensation of pressure during needle insertion and aspiration may be felt.
      c. Administer analgesics and sedatives as prescribed.
   3. Postprocedure
      a. Apply a dressing to the biopsy site and monitor for drainage or bleeding.
      b. Monitor for signs of respiratory distress, and notify the RN and PHCP if they occur.
      c. Monitor for signs of pneumothorax and air emboli, and notify the RN and PHCP if they occur.
      d. Prepare the client for chest radiography, if prescribed.

J. Spiral (helical) computed tomography (CT) scan
   1. Frequently used test to diagnose pulmonary embolism

2. IV injection of contrast medium is used; if the client cannot have contrast medium, a ventilation perfusion (V/Q) scan will be done.
   3. The scanner rotates around the body, allowing for a 3-dimensional picture of all regions of the lungs.

K. Ventilation-perfusion (V/Q) lung scan
   1. Description
      a. The perfusion scan evaluates blood flow to the lungs.
      b. The ventilation scan determines the patency of the pulmonary airways and detects abnormalities in ventilation.
      c. A radionuclide may be injected for the procedure.
   2. Preprocedure
      a. Check the client for allergies to dye, iodine, or seafood.
      b. Remove jewelry around the chest area.
      c. Review breathing methods that may be required during testing.
      d. Ensure IV access has been established.
      e. Assist with the administration of a sedative, if prescribed.
      f. Have emergency resuscitation equipment available.
   3. Postprocedure
      a. Monitor the client for reaction to the radionuclide.
      b. Inform the client that the radionuclide clears from the body in about 8 hours.

L. Computed tomography pulmonary angiography
   1. Description
      a. The scan visualizes the pulmonary arteries and blood flow.
      b. Its main use is to diagnose pulmonary embolism and is the preferred method.
      c. A contrast dye is injected.
   2. Preprocedure: Similar to the V/Q lung scan; in addition, renal function should be adequate and dosing of the contrast should be done by a pharmacist.
   3. Postprocedure: Similar to the V/Q lung scan

M. Skin tests: A skin test is an intradermal injection to help diagnose various infectious diseases (Box 47.2).

N. Arterial blood gases (ABGs)
   1. Description: Measurement of the dissolved oxygen and carbon dioxide in the arterial blood helps to indicate the acid-base state and how well the oxygen is being carried to the body.
   2. Preprocedure and postprocedure care and analysis of results: Refer to Chapter 9.

⚠ Avoid suctioning the client before drawing an ABG sample because the suctioning procedure will deplete the client's oxygen resulting in inaccurate ABG results.

BOX 47.2	Skin Test Procedure

1. Determine hypersensitivity or previous reactions to skin tests.
2. Use a skin site that is free of excessive body hair, dermatitis, and blemishes.
3. Apply the injection in the upper one third of the inner surface of the left arm.
4. Circle and mark the injection test site.
5. Document the date, time, and test site.
6. Advise the client not to scratch the test site in order to prevent infection and possible abscess formation.
7. Instruct the client to avoid washing the test site.
8. Interpret the reaction at the injection site between 24 and 72 hours after administration of the test antigen.
9. Check the test site for the amount of induration (hard swelling) in millimeters and for the presence of erythema and vesiculation (small blister-like elevations).

O. Pulse oximetry (see Chapter 10)
P. D-dimer
   1. A blood test that measures clot formation and lysis that results from the degradation of fibrin
   2. Helps to diagnose (a positive test result) the presence of a thrombus in conditions such as deep vein thrombosis, pulmonary embolism, or stroke; it is also used to diagnose disseminated intravascular coagulation (DIC) and to monitor the effectiveness of treatment.
   3. Dependent on laboratory testing, the normal D-dimer level is less than 250 ng/mL.

III. Respiratory Treatments

A. Breathing retraining (Box 47.3)
B. Chest physiotherapy (CPT)
   1. Description: Percussion, vibration, and postural drainage techniques performed over the thorax to loosen secretions in the affected area of the lungs and move them into more central airways
   2. Contraindications
      a. Unstable vital signs
      b. Increased intracranial pressure
      c. Bronchospasm
      d. History of pathological fractures
      e. Rib fractures
      f. Chest incisions
   3. Interventions (Box 47.4)
C. Incentive spirometry (Box 47.5)

IV. Oxygen

▲ **A.** Supplemental oxygen delivery systems (Table 47.1)
   1. Nasal cannula for low flow: Used for the client with chronic airflow limitation and for long-term oxygen use
   2. Nasal high-flow (NHF) respiratory therapy: Used for hypoxemic clients in mild to moderate respiratory depression (Box 47.6)

BOX 47.3	Client Education: Breathing Retraining and Huff Coughing

Breathing Retraining
Includes exercises to decrease the use of the accessory muscles of breathing to decrease fatigue, and to promote CO_2 elimination
The main types of exercises include pursed lip breathing and diaphragmatic breathing.
The client would inhale slowly through the nose.
The client would place the hand over the abdomen while inhaling; the abdomen will expand with inhalation and contract during exhalation.
The client would exhale three times longer than inhalation by blowing through pursed lips.

Huff Coughing
An effective coughing technique that conserves energy, reduces fatigue, and facilitates mobilization of secretions
The client needs to perform three or four deep breaths using pursed lip and diaphragmatic breathing. Leaning slightly forward, the client would cough three or four times during exhalation.
The client may need to splint the thorax or abdomen to achieve a maximum cough.

BOX 47.4	Chest Physiotherapy Procedure

Chest physiotherapy (CPT) is performed in the morning when rising, 1 hour before meals, or 2 to 3 hours after meals.
CPT is stopped if pain occurs.
If the client is receiving a tube feeding, the feeding is stopped and the residual is aspirated before beginning CPT.
A bronchodilator (if prescribed) may be administered 15 minutes before the procedure.
A layer of material (gown or pajamas) is placed between the hands or percussion device and the client's skin.
The client is positioned for postural drainage based on data collection.
The area is percussed for 1–2 minutes.
The same area is vibrated while the client exhales four or five deep breaths.
The client is monitored for respiratory tolerance to the procedure.
The procedure is stopped if cyanosis or exhaustion occurs.
The client's position is maintained for 5–20 minutes after the procedure.
All necessary positions are repeated until the client no longer expectorates mucus.
Sputum is disposed of properly.
Mouth care is provided after the procedure.

   3. Simple face mask: Used for short-term oxygen therapy or to deliver oxygen in an emergency (Fig. 47.1)
   4. Venturi mask: Used for clients at risk for or experiencing acute respiratory failure (Fig. 47.2)

1. Instruct the client to assume a sitting or upright position.
2. Instruct the client to place the mouth tightly around the mouthpiece of the device.
3. Instruct the client on the use of the device; read the manufacturer directions about the device because there are various devices that can achieve lung exercise.
4. Instruct the client to use the device 10 times every hour.

5. **Partial rebreather mask:** Useful when the oxygen concentration needs to be raised; not usually prescribed for a client with chronic obstructive pulmonary disease (COPD)
6. **Nonrebreather mask:** Most frequently used for the client with a deteriorating respiratory status who might require intubation (Fig. 47.3)
7. **Tracheostomy collar and T-bar or T-piece:** Tracheostomy collar is used to deliver high humidity and the desired oxygen to the client with a

TABLE 47.1 Supplemental Oxygen Delivery Systems

Device	Oxygen Delivered	Nursing Considerations
Nasal cannula (nasal prongs)	1–6 L/min for oxygen concentration (FiO_2) of 24% (at 1 L/min) to 44% (at 6 L/min)	Easily tolerated Can dislodge easily Does not get in the way of eating or talking Effective oxygen concentration can be delivered to nose and mouth breathers Ensure that prongs are in the nares with openings facing the client Check the nasal mucosa for irritation from drying effect of higher flow rates Check skin integrity, as tubing can irritate skin Add humidification as prescribed and check water levels
Simple face mask (see Fig. 47.1)	5–8 L/min oxygen flow for FiO_2 of 40%–60% Minimum flow of 5 L/min needed to flush CO_2 from mask	Interferes with eating and talking Can be warm and confining Ensure that mask fits securely over nose and mouth Remove saliva and mucus from the mask Provide skin care to area covered by mask Provide emotional support to decrease anxiety in the client who feels claustrophobic Monitor for risk of aspiration from inability of client to clear mouth—that is, if vomiting occurs
Venturi mask (Ventimask) (Fig. 47.2)	4–10 L/min oxygen flow for FiO_2 of 24%–55% Delivers exact desired selected concentrations of O_2	Keep the air entrapment port for the adapter open and uncovered to ensure adequate oxygen delivery Keep mask snug on the face and ensure tubing is free of kinks because the FiO_2 is altered if kinking occurs or if the mask fits poorly Check the nasal mucosa for irritation; humidity or aerosol can be added to the system as needed
Partial rebreather mask (mask with reservoir bag)	6–15 L/min oxygen flow for FiO_2 of 70%–90%	The client rebreathes one third of the exhaled tidal volume, which is high in oxygen, thus providing a high FiO_2 Adjust flow rate to keep the reservoir bag two thirds full during inspiration Keep mask snug on face Make sure the reservoir bag does not twist or kink Deflation of the bag results in decreased oxygen delivered and rebreathing of exhaled air
Nonrebreather mask (Fig. 47.3)	FiO_2 of 60%–100% at a rate of flow that maintains the bag two thirds full	Adjust flow rate to keep the reservoir bag inflated Keep mask snug on the face Remove mucus and saliva from the mask Provide emotional support to decrease anxiety in the client who feels claustrophobic Ensure that the valves and flaps are intact and functional during each breath (valves would open during expiration and close during inhalation) Make sure the reservoir bag does not twist or kink or that the oxygen source does not disconnect; otherwise, the client will suffocate
Tracheostomy collar and T-bar or T-piece (face tent; face shield) (Fig. 47.4)	The tracheostomy collar can be used to deliver the desired amount of oxygen to a client with a tracheostomy A special adaptor (T-bar or T-piece) can be used to deliver any desired FiO_2 to client with tracheostomy, laryngectomy, or endotracheal tube The face tent provides 8–12 L/min, and the FiO_2 varies because of environmental loss	Ensure that aerosol mist escapes from the vents of the delivery system during inspiration and expiration Empty condensation from the tubing to prevent the client from being lavaged with water and to promote an adequate oxygen flow rate (remove and clean the tubing at least every 4 hours) Keep the exhalation port in the T-piece open and uncovered (if the port is occluded, the client can suffocate) Position the T-piece so that it does not pull on the tracheostomy or endotracheal tube and cause erosion of the skin at the tracheostomy insertion site

FiO_2, Fraction of inspired oxygen.

Comfortably delivers high flows of heated and humidified oxygen through a wide-bore nasal cannula and humidification system

Can deliver nasal flow rates up to 50 to 60 L/min to deliver humidified high-flow oxygen therapy

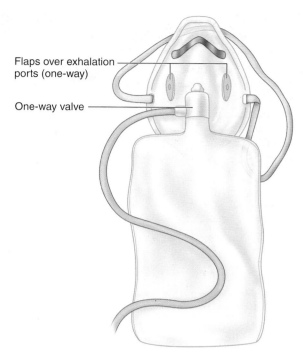

FIG. 47.3 A nonrebreather mask.

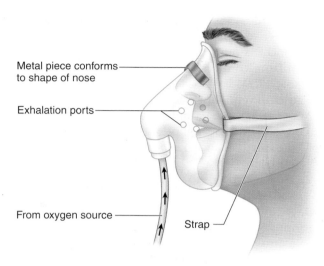

FIG. 47.1 A simple face mask used to deliver oxygen.

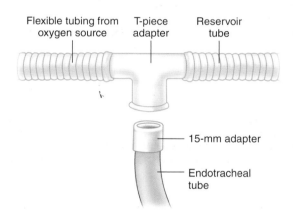

FIG. 47.4 A T-piece apparatus for attachment to an endotracheal tube or tracheostomy tube.

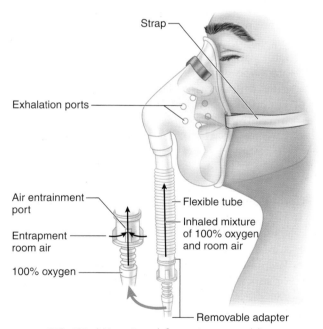

FIG. 47.2 A Venturi mask for precise oxygen delivery.

tracheostomy; the T-bar or T-piece is used to deliver the desired Fio_2 to the client with a tracheostomy, laryngectomy, or endotracheal tube (Fig. 47.4).

8. Face tent: Used instead of a tight-fitting mask for the client who has facial trauma or burns

B. Continuous positive airway pressure (CPAP) and bi-level positive airway pressure (BiPAP)

1. CPAP maintains a set positive airway pressure during inspiration and expiration; beneficial in clients who have obstructive sleep apnea or acute exacerbation COPD.

2. BiPAP provides positive airway pressure during inspiration and ceases airway support during expiration; there is only enough pressure provided during expiration to keep the airways open; usually used if CPAP is ineffective (Fig. 47.5).

3. Both CPAP and BiPAP improve oxygenation through airway support.

C. General interventions

1. Check color, pulse oximetry reading, and vital signs before and during treatment.

2. Place an *Oxygen in Use* sign at the client's bedside.

3. Check for the presence of chronic lung problems before administering oxygen.

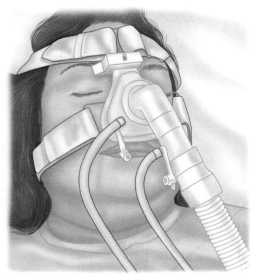

FIG. 47.5 A BiPAP (bilevel positive airway pressure) system using a nasal mask for pressure- and volume-controlled ventilation.

4. Humidify the oxygen if indicated.

5. For specific interventions for each supplemental oxygen delivery system, see Table 47.1.

 A client who is hypoxemic and has chronic hypercapnia may require (per PHCP prescription) low levels of oxygen delivery at 1 to 2 L/min because a low arterial oxygen level is the client's primary drive for breathing.

V. Mechanical Ventilation

A. Description: Used to overcome the client's inability to ventilate or oxygenate adequately. There are a variety of types of mechanical ventilation.

⚠ For a client receiving mechanical ventilation, always check the client first and then check the ventilator. A resuscitation bag must be available at the bedside for all clients receiving mechanical ventilation.

B. Interventions

1. Check vital signs, lung sounds, respiratory status, and breathing patterns (the client will never breathe at a rate lower than the rate set on the ventilator).
2. Monitor skin color particularly in the lips and nail beds.
3. Monitor the chest for bilateral expansion.
4. Obtain pulse oximetry readings.
5. Monitor ABG results.
6. Determine the need for suctioning and observe the type, color, and amount of secretions.
7. Check ventilator settings.
8. Check the level of water in the humidifier and the temperature of the humidification system because extremes in temperature can damage the mucosa in the airway.
9. Ensure that the alarms are set.

10. If a cause for an alarm cannot be determined, ventilate the client manually with a resuscitation bag until the problem is corrected.
11. Empty the ventilator tubing when moisture collects.
12. Turn the client at least every 2 hours or get the client out of bed, as prescribed, to prevent complications of immobility.
13. Have resuscitation equipment available at the bedside.
14. Refer to Chapter 18 for endotracheal tube and tracheostomy tube care.

C. Ventilator controls and settings and descriptions (Table 47.2)

D. Causes of ventilator alarms (Box 47.7)

E. Alarm safety and alarm fatigue

1. It is the responsibility of the nurse to be alert to the sound of an alarm because this signals a client problem.
2. The nurse needs to respond promptly to an alarm and immediately check the client.
3. According to The Joint Commission (TJC), the most common contributing factor related to alarm-related sentinel events is alarm fatigue.
4. Alarm fatigue results when the numerous alarms and the resulting noise tend to desensitize the nursing staff and cause them to ignore alarms or even disable them.
5. Some recommendations of TJC include establishing alarm safety as a facility policy, identifying default alarm settings, identifying the most important alarms to manage, establishing policies and procedures for managing alarms, and staff education.
6. For additional information access: http://www.jointcommission.org/assets/1/18/SEA_50_alarms_4_5_13_FINAL1.PDF.

⚠ Never set ventilator alarm controls to the off position.

F. Complications

1. Hypotension caused by the application of positive pressure, which increases intrathoracic pressure and inhibits blood return to the heart
2. Respiratory complications such as pneumothorax or subcutaneous emphysema as a result of positive pressure
3. Gastrointestinal alterations such as stress ulcers
4. Malnutrition if nutrition is not maintained
5. Infections
6. Muscular deconditioning
7. Ventilator dependence or inability to wean

G. Weaning: Process of going from ventilator dependence to spontaneous breathing

VI. Chest Injuries

A. Rib fracture

1. Description

TABLE 47.2   Ventilator Controls and Settings and Descriptions

Controls and Settings	Descriptions
Tidal volume	The volume of air that the client receives with each breath
Rate	The number of ventilator breaths delivered per minute
Sighs	The volumes of air that are 1.5–2 times the set tidal volume, delivered 6–10 times per hour; may be used to prevent atelectasis
Fraction of inspired oxygen (Fio$_2$)	The oxygen concentration delivered to the client; determined by the client's condition and ABG levels
Peak airway inspiratory pressure	The pressure needed by the ventilator to deliver a set tidal volume at a given compliance Monitoring peak airway inspiratory pressure reflects changes in compliance of the lungs and resistance in the ventilator or client
Continuous positive airway pressure	The application of positive airway pressure throughout the entire respiratory cycle for spontaneously breathing clients Keeps the alveoli open during inspiration and prevents alveolar collapse; used primarily as a weaning modality No ventilator breaths are delivered, but the ventilator delivers oxygen and provides monitoring and an alarm system; the respiratory pattern is determined by the client's efforts
Positive end-expiratory pressure (PEEP)	Positive pressure is exerted during the expiratory phase of ventilation, which improves oxygenation by enhancing gas exchange and preventing atelectasis The need for PEEP indicates a severe gas exchange disturbance Higher levels of PEEP (more than 15 cm H$_2$O) increase the chance of complications, such as barotrauma tension pneumothorax
Pressure support	The application of positive pressure on inspiration that eases the workload of breathing May be used in combination with PEEP as a weaning method As the weaning process continues, the amount of pressure applied to inspiration is gradually decreased

ABG, Arterial blood gas.

BOX 47.7   Causes of Ventilator Alarms

High-Pressure Alarm

Increased secretions are in the airway.

Wheezing or bronchospasm is causing decreased airway size.

The endotracheal tube is displaced.

The endotracheal tube is obstructed as a result of water or a kink in the tubing.

The client coughs, gags, or bites on the oral endotracheal tube.

The client is anxious or fights the ventilator.

Low-Pressure Alarm

Disconnection or leak in the ventilator or in the client's airway cuff occurs.

The client stops spontaneous breathing.

  a. Results from direct blunt chest trauma and causes a potential for intrathoracic injury such as pneumothorax, hemothorax, or pulmonary contusion
  b. Pain with movement, deep breathing, and coughing results in impaired ventilation and inadequate clearance of secretions.
 2. Data collection

  a. Pain and tenderness at the injury site that increases with inspiration
  b. Shallow respirations
  c. Client splints chest
  d. Fractures noted on chest x-ray

3. Interventions
  a. Note that the ribs usually unite spontaneously.
  b. Open reduction and internal fixation of the ribs (rib plating) may be done.
  c. Place the client in the high Fowler's position.
  d. Administer pain medication, as prescribed, to maintain adequate ventilatory status.
  e. Monitor for increased respiratory distress.
  f. Reinforce instructions to the client to self-splint with hands, arms, or a pillow.
  g. Prepare the client for an intercostal nerve block, as prescribed, if the pain is severe.
B. Flail chest
 1. Description
  a. Occurs from blunt chest trauma associated with accidents, which may result in hemothorax and rib fractures
  b. The loose segment of the chest wall becomes paradoxical to the expansion and contraction of the rest of the chest wall.
 2. Data collection
  a. Paradoxical respirations (inward movement of a segment of the thorax during inspiration with outward movement during expiration)
  b. Severe pain in the chest
  c. Dyspnea
  d. Cyanosis
  e. Tachycardia
  f. Hypotension
  g. Tachypnea, shallow respirations
  h. Diminished breath sounds

Adult—Respiratory

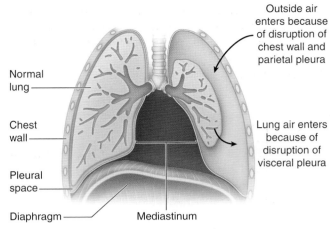

FIG. 47.6 Pneumothorax. Air in the pleural space causes the lungs to collapse around the hilus and may push the mediastinal contents (heart and great vessels) toward the other lung.

BOX 47.8 **Data Collection Findings: Pneumothorax**

- Absent breath sounds on affected side
- Cyanosis
- Decreased chest expansion unilaterally
- Dyspnea
- Hypotension
- Sharp chest pain
- Subcutaneous emphysema as evidenced by crepitus during palpation
- Sucking sound with open chest wound
- Tachycardia
- Tachypnea
- Tracheal deviation to the unaffected side with tension pneumothorax

---

3. Interventions
   a. Maintain the client in a Fowler's position.
   b. Administer humidified oxygen as prescribed.
   c. Monitor for increased respiratory distress.
   d. Encourage coughing and deep breathing.
   e. Administer pain medication as prescribed.
   f. Maintain bed rest and limit activity to reduce oxygen demands.
   g. Prepare for intubation with mechanical ventilation for severe flail chest associated with respiratory failure and shock.
C. Pulmonary contusion
   1. Description
      a. Characterized by interstitial hemorrhage associated with intra-alveolar hemorrhage resulting in decreased pulmonary compliance
      b. The major complication is acute respiratory distress syndrome.
   2. Data collection
      a. Dyspnea
      b. Hypoxemia
      c. Increased bronchial secretions
      d. Hemoptysis
      e. Restlessness
      f. Decreased breath sounds
      g. Crackles and wheezes
   3. Interventions
      a. Maintain a patent airway and adequate ventilation.
      b. Place the client in a Fowler's position.
      c. Administer oxygen as prescribed.
      d. Monitor for increased respiratory distress.
      e. Maintain bed rest and limit activity to reduce oxygen demands.
      f. Prepare for mechanical ventilation if required.
D. Pneumothorax (Fig. 47.6)
   1. Description
      a. Accumulation of atmospheric air in the pleural space, which results in a rise in intrathoracic

pressure and reduced vital capacity, or the greatest amount of air expired from the lungs after taking a deep breath
      b. The loss of negative intrapleural pressure results in collapse of the lung.
      c. A spontaneous pneumothorax occurs with the rupture of a pulmonary bleb, or small air-containing spaces deep in the lung.
      d. An open pneumothorax occurs when an opening through the chest wall allows the entrance of positive atmospheric air pressure into the pleural space.
      e. A tension pneumothorax occurs from a blunt chest injury or from mechanical ventilation when a buildup of positive pressure occurs in the pleural space.
      f. Diagnosis of pneumothorax is made by chest x-ray.
   2. Data collection (Box 47.8)
   3. Interventions
      a. Apply a nonporous dressing over an open chest wound.
      b. Administer oxygen as prescribed.
      c. Place the client in a Fowler's position.
      d. Prepare for chest tube placement, which will remain in place until the lung has expanded fully.
      e. Monitor the chest tube drainage system.
      f. Monitor for subcutaneous emphysema.
      g. Refer to Chapter 18 for information on caring for a client with chest tubes.

⚠ Clients with a respiratory disorder should be positioned with the head of the bed elevated.

VII. Acute Respiratory Failure

A. Description
   1. Occurs when insufficient oxygen is transported to the blood or inadequate carbon dioxide is removed from the lungs and the client's compensatory mechanisms fail

2. Causes include a mechanical abnormality of the lungs or chest wall, a defect in the respiratory control center in the brain, or an impairment in the function of the respiratory muscles.

3. In oxygenation failure, or hypoxemic respiratory failure, oxygen may reach the alveoli but cannot be absorbed or used properly resulting in a PaO_2 less than 60 mm Hg, arterial oxygen saturation (SaO_2) lower than 90%, or partial pressure of arterial carbon dioxide ($PaCO_2$) greater than 50 mm Hg occurring with acidemia.

4. Respiratory failure can be hypoxemic, hypercapnic, or both.

5. Many clients experience both hypoxemic and hypercapnic respiratory failure, and retained carbon dioxide in the alveoli displaces oxygen contributing to the hypoxemia.

6. Manifestations of respiratory failure are related to the extent and rapidity of change in PaO_2 and $PaCO_2$.

B. Data collection
1. Dyspnea
2. Restlessness
3. Confusion
4. Decreased level of consciousness
5. Tachycardia
6. Hypertension
7. Dysrhythmias
8. Alterations in respirations and breath sounds
9. Headache (less common)

C. Interventions
1. Identify and treat the cause of the respiratory failure.
2. Administer oxygen to maintain the PaO_2 level greater than 60 to 70 mm Hg.
3. Place the client in a Fowler's position.
4. Encourage deep breathing.
5. Assist to administer bronchodilators as prescribed.
6. Prepare the client for mechanical ventilation if supplemental oxygen cannot maintain acceptable PaO_2 and $PaCO_2$ levels.

VIII. Acute Respiratory Distress Syndrome

A. Description
1. A form of acute respiratory failure that occurs as a complication of some other condition; it is caused by a diffuse lung injury or critical illness and leads to extravascular lung fluid.
2. The major site of injury is the alveolar capillary membrane.
3. The interstitial edema causes compression and obliteration of the terminal airways and leads to reduced lung volume and compliance.
4. The ABG levels identify respiratory acidosis and hypoxemia that do not respond to an increased percentage of oxygen.
5. The chest x-ray shows bilateral interstitial and alveolar infiltrates; interstitial edema may not be noted until there is a 30% increase in fluid content.

6. Causes include sepsis, fluid overload, shock, trauma, neurological injuries, burns, DIC, drug ingestion, aspiration, and the inhalation of toxic substances.

B. Data collection
1. Tachypnea
2. Dyspnea
3. Decreased breath sounds
4. Deteriorating ABG levels
5. Hypoxemia despite high concentrations of delivered oxygen
6. Decreased pulmonary compliance
7. Pulmonary infiltrates

C. Interventions
1. Identify and treat the cause of the acute respiratory distress syndrome.
2. Administer oxygen as prescribed.
3. Place the client in a Fowler's position.
4. Restrict fluid intake as prescribed.
5. Provide respiratory treatments as prescribed.
6. Administer diuretics, anticoagulants, or corticosteroids as prescribed.
7. Prepare the client for intubation and mechanical ventilation.

IX. Asthma (Fig. 47.7)

A. Description
1. Chronic inflammatory disorder of the airways that causes varying degrees of obstruction in the airways
2. Marked by airway inflammation and hyperresponsiveness to a variety of stimuli or triggers (Box 47.9).
3. Causes recurrent episodes of wheezing, breathlessness, chest tightness, and coughing associated with airflow obstruction that may resolve spontaneously; it is often reversible with treatment.
4. Severity is classified based on the clinical features before treatment.
5. Status asthmaticus is a severe life-threatening asthma episode that is refractory to treatment and may result in pneumothorax, acute cor pulmonale, or respiratory arrest.
6. Refer to Chapter 32 for additional information on asthma.

B. Assessment
1. Restlessness
2. Wheezing or crackles
3. Absent or diminished lung sounds
4. Hyperresonance
5. Use of accessory muscles for breathing
6. Tachypnea with hyperventilation
7. Prolonged exhalation
8. Tachycardia
9. Pulsus paradoxus
10. Diaphoresis
11. Cyanosis

Adult—Respiratory

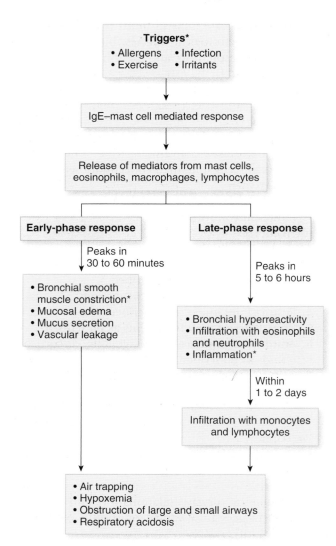

Triggers*
- Allergens
- Infection
- Exercise
- Irritants

↓

IgE–mast cell mediated response

↓

Release of mediators from mast cells, eosinophils, macrophages, lymphocytes

Early-phase response

Peaks in 30 to 60 minutes

- Bronchial smooth muscle constriction*
- Mucosal edema
- Mucus secretion
- Vascular leakage

Late-phase response

Peaks in 5 to 6 hours

- Bronchial hyperreactivity
- Infiltration with eosinophils and neutrophils
- Inflammation*

Within 1 to 2 days

Infiltration with monocytes and lymphocytes

- Air trapping
- Hypoxemia
- Obstruction of large and small airways
- Respiratory acidosis

FIG. 47.7 Pathophysiology in asthma. Stems with asterisks are primary processes. *IgE,* Immunoglobulin E.

12. Decreased oxygen saturation
13. Pulmonary function test results that demonstrate decreased airflow rates

C. Interventions
1. Monitor vital signs.
2. Monitor pulse oximetry.
3. Monitor peak flow.
4. During an acute asthma episode, provide interventions to assist with breathing (Box 47-10).

D. Client education
1. On the intermittent nature of symptoms and need for long-term management
2. To identify possible triggers and measures to prevent episodes
3. About the management of medication and proper administration
4. About the correct use of a peak flowmeter
5. About developing an asthma action plan with the primary PHCP and what to do if an asthma episode occurs

---

BOX 47-9 **Asthma Triggers**

Environmental Factors
- Animal dander
- Cockroaches
- Dust mites
- Exhaust fumes
- Fireplaces
- Molds
- Perfumes or other products with aerosol sprays
- Pollen
- Smoke, including cigarette or cigar smoke
- Sudden weather changes

Physiological Factors
- Cold, dry air
- Gastroesophageal reflux disease (GERD)
- Exercise
- Hormonal changes
- Sinusitis
- Stress
- Viral upper respiratory infection

Medications
- Acetylsalicylic acid (aspirin)
- β-Adrenergic blockers
- Nonsteroidal antiinflammatory drugs

Occupational Exposure Factors
- Agriculture
- Metal salts
- Wood and vegetable dusts
- Industrial chemicals and plastics
- Pharmaceutical drugs

Food Additives
- Sulfites (bisulfites and metabisulfites)
- Beer, wine, dried fruit, shrimp
- Monosodium glutamate
- Tartrazine

From Harding, M. et.al. *Medical-surgical nursing: assessment and management of clinical problems,* ed 11, St. Louis, 2020, Mosby.

BOX 47.10 **Nursing Interventions During an Acute Asthma Episode**

Position the client in a high Fowler's position or sitting to aid in breathing.
Administer oxygen as prescribed.
Stay with the client to decrease anxiety.
Administer bronchodilators as prescribed.
Record the color, amount, and consistency of sputum, if any.
Administer corticosteroids as prescribed.
Auscultate lung sounds before, during, and after treatments.

X. Chronic Obstructive Pulmonary Disease

A. Description
1. Is also known as chronic obstructive lung disease and chronic airflow limitation

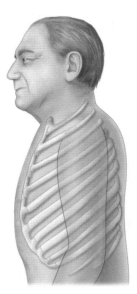

FIG. 47.8 Typical barrel chest in a client with chronic obstructive pulmonary disease.

2. COPD is a disease state characterized by airflow obstruction caused by emphysema or chronic bronchitis.
3. Emphysema is a condition in which the air sacs in the lungs are damaged and enlarged, resulting in hyperinflation and breathlessness.
4. Chronic bronchitis is a condition in which the bronchial tubes become inflamed and excessive mucus production occurs as a result from irritants or injury.
5. Progressive airflow limitation is associated with an abnormal inflammatory response of the lungs and is not completely reversible.
6. COPD leads to pulmonary insufficiency, pulmonary hypertension, and cor pulmonale.

B. Data collection
1. Cough
2. Exertional dyspnea
3. Wheezing and crackles
4. Sputum production
5. Weight loss
6. Barrel chest (emphysema) (Fig. 47.8)
7. Use of accessory muscles for breathing
8. Prolonged expiration
9. Orthopnea
10. Cardiac dysrhythmia
11. Congestion and hyperinflation on chest x-ray film (Fig. 47.9)
12. ABG levels that indicate respiratory acidosis and hypoxemia
13. Pulmonary function tests that demonstrate decreased vital capacity

C. Interventions
1. Monitor vital signs.
2. Administer a concentration of oxygen based on ABG values and oxygen saturation by pulse oximetry as prescribed; usually 1–2 L/min is prescribed

because the stimulus to breathe is a low arterial P_{O_2} instead of an increased P_{CO_2}.
3. Monitor pulse oximetry.
4. Provide respiratory treatments and CPT.
5. Instruct the client in diaphragmatic or abdominal breathing techniques, tripod positioning, and pursed lip breathing techniques, which increase airway pressure and keep air passages open, promoting maximal carbon dioxide expiration.
6. Record the color, amount, and consistency of sputum.
7. Suction fluids from the client's lungs, if necessary, to clear the airway and prevent infection.
8. Monitor weight.
9. Encourage small, frequent meals to maintain nutrition and prevent dyspnea.
10. Provide a high-calorie, high-protein diet with supplements.
11. Encourage fluid intake up to 3000 mL/day to keep secretions thin unless contraindicated.
12. Place the client in a Fowler's position and lean forward to aid in breathing (Fig. 47.10).
13. Allow activity as tolerated.
14. Administer bronchodilators as prescribed, and instruct the client about the use of oral and inhalant medications.
15. Administer corticosteroids, as prescribed, for exacerbation.
16. Administer mucolytics, as prescribed, to thin secretions.
17. Administer antibiotics for infection, if prescribed.

D. Client education (Box 47.11)

BOX 47.11 **Client Education: Chronic Obstructive Pulmonary Disease**

- Adhere to activity limitations, alternating rest periods with activity.
- Avoid gas-producing foods, spicy foods, and extremely hot or cold foods.
- Avoid exposure to individuals with infections, and avoid crowds.
- Avoid extremes in temperature.
- Avoid fireplaces, pets, feather pillows, and other environmental allergens.
- Avoid powerful odors.
- Eliminate smoking and avoid environments with secondary smoke exposure.
- Meet nutritional requirements.
- Receive immunizations as recommended.
- Recognize the signs and symptoms of respiratory infection and hypoxia.
- Use medications and inhalers as prescribed.
- Use oxygen therapy as prescribed.
- Use pursed lip and diaphragmatic or abdominal breathing.
- When dusting, use a wet cloth.

Adult—Respiratory

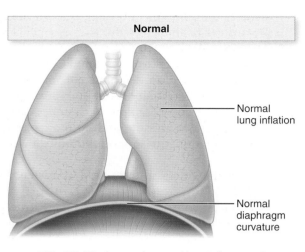

Normal

Normal lung inflation

Normal diaphragm curvature

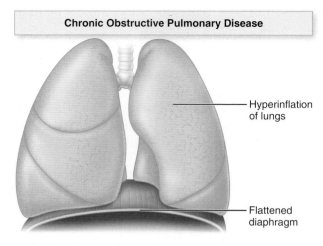

Chronic Obstructive Pulmonary Disease

Hyperinflation of lungs

Flattened diaphragm

FIG. 47.9 Diaphragm shape and lung inflation in the normal client and in the client with chronic obstructive pulmonary disease.

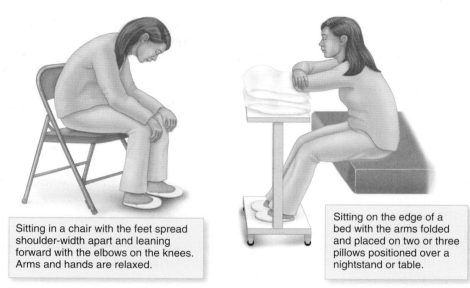

Sitting in a chair with the feet spread shoulder-width apart and leaning forward with the elbows on the knees. Arms and hands are relaxed.

Sitting on the edge of a bed with the arms folded and placed on two or three pillows positioned over a nightstand or table.

FIG. 47.10 Orthopnea positions that clients with chronic obstructive pulmonary disease can assume to ease the work of breathing.

XI. Pneumonia

A. Description
1. An infection of the pulmonary tissue including the interstitial space, the alveoli, and the bronchioles
2. The edema associated with inflammation stiffens the lung, decreases lung compliance and vital capacity, and causes hypoxemia.
3. Pneumonia can be community acquired or hospital acquired.
4. The chest x-ray film shows lobar or segmental consolidation, pulmonary infiltrates, or pleural effusions.
5. A sputum culture identifies the organism.
6. The white blood cell count and erythrocyte sedimentation rate are elevated.

B. Data collection
1. Chills
2. Elevated temperature
3. Pleuritic pain
4. Tachypnea
5. Rhonchi and wheezes
6. Use of accessory muscles for breathing
7. Change in mental status
8. Sputum production

C. Interventions
1. Administer oxygen as prescribed.
2. Monitor respiratory status.
3. Monitor for labored respirations, cyanosis, and cold and clammy skin.
4. Encourage coughing and deep breathing and use of the incentive spirometer.
5. Place the client in the semi-Fowler's position to facilitate breathing and lung expansion.
6. Change the client's position frequently and ambulate as tolerated to mobilize secretions.
7. Provide CPT.
8. Perform nasotracheal suctioning if the client is unable to clear secretions.
9. Monitor pulse oximetry.
10. Monitor and record color, consistency, and amount of sputum.
11. Provide a high-calorie, high-protein diet with small, frequent meals.

12. Encourage fluids up to 3 L/day to thin secretions unless contraindicated.
13. Provide a balance of rest and activity, increasing activity gradually.
14. Administer antibiotics as prescribed.
15. Administer antipyretics, bronchodilators, cough suppressants, mucolytic agents, and expectorants as prescribed.
16. Prevent the spread of infection by hand washing and the proper disposal of secretions.

D. Client education
1. About the importance of rest, proper nutrition, and adequate fluid intake
2. To avoid chilling and exposure to individuals with respiratory infections or viruses
3. Regarding medications and the use of inhalants as prescribed
4. To notify the RN and PHCP if chills, fever, dyspnea, hemoptysis, or increased fatigue occur
5. To receive a pneumococcal vaccine as recommended by the PHCP; refer to the following website for more information: http://www.cdc.gov/vaccines/vpd-vac/pneumo/default.htm.

 Teach clients that using proper hand-washing techniques, disposing of respiratory secretions properly, and receiving vaccines as appropriate will assist with preventing the spread of infection.

XII. Severe Acute Respiratory Syndrome (SARS)

A. Respiratory illness caused by the coronavirus called *SARS-associated coronavirus*
B. The syndrome begins with a fever, an overall feeling of discomfort, body aches, and mild respiratory symptoms.
C. After 2 to 7 days, the client may develop a dry cough and dyspnea.
D. Infection is spread by close person-to-person contact by direct contact with infectious material (respiratory secretions from infected persons or contact with objects contaminated with infectious droplets).
E. Prevention includes avoiding contact with those suspected of having SARS, avoiding travel to countries where an outbreak of SARS exists, avoiding close contact with crowds in areas where SARS exists, and frequent hand washing.

XIII. COVID-19 (Coronavirus)

A. Description
1. The SARS-CoV-2 is the coronavirus that causes COVID-19.
2. Older adults and people who have severe underlying medical conditions like heart or lung disease or diabetes are at higher risk for developing more serious complications from COVID-19 illness.
B. Symptoms
1. People with COVID-19 have had a wide range of symptoms reported, ranging from mild symptoms to severe illness. Symptoms may appear 2-14 days after exposure to the virus. Symptoms can include the following:
   a. Fever or chills
   b. Cough
   c. Shortness of breath or difficulty breathing
   d. Fatigue
   e. Muscle or body aches
   f. Headache
   g. New loss of taste or smell
   h. Sore throat
   i. Congestion or runny nose
   j. Nausea or vomiting
   k. Diarrhea
2. Emergency care should be sought if the person is having difficulty breathing, experiences persistent pain or pressure in the chest, if the person experiences new confusion, is unable to stay awake, or if cyanosis develops.

C. Transmission and prevention
1. COVID-19 may be spread by people who are not showing symptoms.
2. Transmission is from person-to-person and via contact with the virus via respiratory droplets produced when an infected person coughs, sneezes, or talks.
3. These droplets can land in the mouths or noses of people who are nearby or possibly be inhaled into the lungs.
4. Droplet precautions and possibly contact precautions are necessary.
5. Prevention includes avoiding crowds, maintain 6 feet of social distancing especially from sick people, handwashing, use of hand sanitizer, wearing masks, coughing and sneezing into the elbow, keeping the hands away from the face, and keeping surfaces frequently touched cleaned and sanitized daily.
6. Prophylaxis treatment may be recommended for those exposed to coronavirus and may include selected vitamins and minerals and immune system booster supplements; the person should not begin any prophylaxis treatment unless recommended by the primary health care provider.
7. A vaccine for coronavirus is being developed.
D. Treatment
1. Varies depending on the clinical presentation
2. The person needs to report symptoms immediately if coronavirus is suspected and seek treatment from the primary health care provider.
3. The primary health care provider will prescribe treatment based on the most current CDC guidelines for treating coronavirus.
4. For additional information, refer to Centers for Disease Control and Prevention: Coronavirus 2019: https://www.cdc.gov/coronavirus/2019-ncov/hcp/infection-control.html and Centers for Disease

Control and Prevention: Corona virus 2019 (COV-ID-19): https://www.cdc.gov/coronavirus/2019-ncov/faq.html

XIV. Influenza

A. Description
1. Also known as the flu; highly contagious acute viral respiratory infection
2. May be caused by several viruses usually known as types A, B, and C
3. Yearly vaccination is recommended to prevent the disease especially for those who are older than 50 years of age, individuals with chronic illness or who are immunocompromised, those living in institutions, and health care personnel providing direct care to clients (the vaccination is contraindicated in individuals with egg allergies).
4. Additional prevention measures include avoiding those who have developed influenza, frequent and proper hand washing, and cleaning and disinfecting surfaces that have become contaminated with secretions.
5. Avian influenza A (H5N1)
   a. Affects birds; does not usually affect humans; however, human cases have been reported in some countries.
   b. An H5N1 vaccine has been developed for use if a pandemic virus were to emerge.
   c. Reported symptoms are similar to those associated with influenza A, B, and C.
   d. Prevention measures include thoroughly cooking poultry products, avoiding contact with wild animals, frequent and proper hand washing, and cleaning and disinfecting surfaces that have become contaminated with secretions.
6. Swine (H1N1) influenza
   a. A strain of flu that consists of genetic materials from swine, avian, and human influenza viruses
   b. Signs/symptoms are similar to those that present with the seasonal flu; in addition, vomiting and diarrhea commonly occur.
   c. Prevention measures and treatment are the same as for the seasonal flu.

B. Refer to Chapter 37 for information on influenza and Chapter 48 for information on H1N1 vaccines.

C. Data collection
1. Acute onset of fever and muscle aches
2. Headache
3. Fatigue, weakness, anorexia
4. Sore throat, cough, and rhinorrhea

D. Interventions
1. Encourage rest.
2. Encourage fluids to prevent pulmonary complications (unless contraindicated).
3. Monitor lung sounds.
4. Provide supportive therapy such as antipyretics or antitussives as indicated.
5. Administer antiviral medications as prescribed for current strain of influenza (refer to Chapter 48).

XV. Legionnaires Disease

A. Description
1. Acute bacterial infection caused by *Legionella pneumophila*
2. Sources of the organism include contaminated air conditioner cooling tower water and warm stagnant water supplies including water vaporizers, water sonicators, whirlpool spas, and showers.
3. Person-to-person contact does not occur, and the risk for infection is increased by the presence of other conditions.

B. Data collection: Influenza-like symptoms with a high fever, chills, muscle aches, and headache that may progress to dry cough, pleurisy, and sometimes diarrhea

C. Interventions: Treatment is supportive, and antibiotics may be prescribed.

XVI. Pleural Effusion

A. Description
1. Pleural effusion is the collection of fluid in the pleural space.
2. Any condition that interferes with secretion or drainage of fluid in the pleural space will lead to pleural effusion.

B. Data collection
1. Pleuritic pain that is sharp and increases with inspiration
2. Progressive dyspnea with decreased movement of the chest wall on the affected side
3. Dry, nonproductive cough caused by bronchial irritation or mediastinal shift
4. Tachycardia
5. Elevated temperature
6. Decreased breath sounds over affected area
7. Chest x-ray film that shows pleural effusion and a mediastinal shift away from the fluid if the effusion is greater than 250 mL

C. Interventions
1. Identify and treat the underlying cause.
2. Monitor breath sounds.
3. Place the client in a Fowler's position.
4. Encourage coughing and deep breathing.
5. Prepare the client for thoracentesis.
6. If pleural effusion is recurrent, prepare the client for pleurectomy or pleurodesis as prescribed.

D. Pleurectomy
1. Consists of surgically stripping the parietal pleura away from the visceral pleura

2. This produces an intense inflammatory reaction that promotes adhesion formation between the two layers during healing.

E. Pleurodesis

    1. Involves the instillation of a sclerosing substance into the pleural space via a thoracotomy tube

    2. The substance creates an inflammatory response that scleroses tissues together.

XVII. Empyema

A. Description

    1. Collection of pus within the pleural cavity

    2. The fluid is thick, opaque, and foul smelling.

    3. The most common cause is pulmonary infection and lung abscess caused by thoracic surgery or chest trauma in which bacteria are introduced directly into the pleural space.

    4. Treatment focuses on treating the infection, emptying the empyema cavity, reexpanding the lung, and controlling the infection.

B. Data collection

    1. Recent febrile illness or trauma

    2. Chest pain

    3. Cough

    4. Dyspnea

    5. Anorexia and weight loss

    6. Malaise

    7. Elevated temperature and chills

    8. Night sweats

    9. Pleural exudate on chest x-ray

C. Interventions

    1. Monitor breath sounds.

    2. Place the client in a semi-Fowler's or high-Fowler's position.

    3. Encourage coughing and deep breathing.

    4. Administer antibiotics as prescribed.

    5. Instruct the client to splint the chest as necessary.

    6. Assist with thoracentesis or chest tube insertion to promote drainage and lung expansion.

    7. If marked pleural thickening occurs, prepare the client for decortication if prescribed; this surgical procedure involves removal of the restrictive mass of fibrin and inflammatory cells.

XVIII. Pleurisy

A. Description

    1. Inflammation of the visceral and parietal membranes; may be caused by pulmonary infarction or pneumonia

    2. The visceral and parietal membranes rub together during respiration and cause pain.

    3. Pleurisy usually occurs on one side of the chest usually in the lower lateral portions in the chest wall.

B. Data collection

    1. Knife-like pain that is aggravated on deep breathing and coughing

    2. Dyspnea

    3. Pleural friction rub heard on auscultation

C. Interventions

    1. Identify and treat the cause.

    2. Monitor lung sounds.

    3. Administer analgesics as prescribed.

    4. Apply hot or cold applications as prescribed.

    5. Encourage coughing and deep breathing.

    6. Instruct the client to lie on the affected side to splint the chest.

XIX. Pulmonary Embolism

A. Description

    1. Occurs when a thrombus forms (most commonly in a deep vein), detaches, travels to the right side of the heart, and then lodges in a branch of the pulmonary artery

    2. Clients prone to pulmonary embolism are those at risk for deep vein thrombosis including those with prolonged immobilization, surgery, obesity, pregnancy, heart failure, advanced age, or a history of thromboembolism.

    3. Fat emboli can occur as a complication after a fracture of a long bone and can cause pulmonary emboli.

    4. Treatment is aimed at prevention through risk factor recognition and elimination.

 If there is a suspicion for pulmonary embolism, a D-dimer blood test may be prescribed, which measures one of the breakdown products of a blood clot. If normal, then the likelihood of a pulmonary embolism is very low (depending on the laboratory, D-dimer values 250 ng/mL or less are normal). The D-dimer is not diagnostic, but if the D-dimer is not normal, computed tomographic pulmonary angiography is prescribed (unless contraindicated—in which case a ventilation/perfusion scan is performed).

B. Data collection (Box 47.12)

C. Interventions (see Priority Nursing Actions)

BOX 47.12	Data Collection Findings: Pulmonary Embolism

- Apprehension and restlessness
- Blood-tinged sputum
- Chest pain
- Cough
- Crackles and wheezes during auscultation
- Cyanosis
- Distended neck veins
- Dyspnea accompanied by anginal and pleuritic pain, exacerbated by inspiration
- Feeling of impending doom
- Hypotension
- Petechiae over the chest and axilla
- Shallow respirations
- Tachypnea and tachycardia

Adult—Respiratory

⚡ PRIORITY NURSING ACTIONS

Suspected Pulmonary Embolism

1. Notify the Rapid Response Team and PHCP.
2. Reassure the client and elevate the head of the bed.
3. Prepare to administer oxygen.
4. Obtain vital signs and check lung sounds.
5. Prepare to obtain an arterial blood gas.
6. Prepare for the administration of heparin therapy or other therapies.
7. Document the event, interventions taken, and the client's response to treatment.

XX. Lung Cancer and Laryngeal Cancer (see Chapter 41)

XXI. Carbon Monoxide Poisoning (see Chapter 39)

XXII. Histoplasmosis

A. Description
   1. Pulmonary fungal infection caused by spores of *Histoplasma capsulatum*
   2. Transmission occurs by the inhalation of spores, which are commonly found in contaminated soil.
   3. Spores are also usually found in bird droppings.
B. Data collection
   1. Similar to pneumonia
   2. Positive skin test for histoplasmosis
   3. Positive agglutination test
   4. Splenomegaly, hepatomegaly
C. Interventions
   1. Administer oxygen as prescribed.
   2. Monitor breath sounds.
   3. Assist with the administration of antiemetics, antihistamines, antipyretics, and corticosteroids as prescribed.
   4. Assist with the administration of fungicidal medications as prescribed.
   5. Encourage coughing and deep breathing.
   6. Place the client in the semi-Fowler's position.
   7. Monitor vital signs.
   8. Monitor for nephrotoxicity from fungicidal medications.
   9. Instruct the client to wear a mask and spray the floor area with water before sweeping barn and chicken coops.

XXIII. Sarcoidosis

A. Description
   1. Presence of epithelioid cell tubercles in the lung
   2. The cause is unknown, but a high titer of Epstein-Barr virus may be noted.
   3. Viral incidence is highest in African Americans and young adults.

B. Data collection
   1. Night sweats
   2. Fever
   3. Weight loss
   4. Cough and dyspnea
   5. Skin nodules
   6. Polyarthritis
   7. Kveim test: Sarcoid node antigen is injected intradermally and causes a local nodular lesion in about 1 month.
C. Interventions
   1. Administer corticosteroids to control symptoms.
   2. Monitor temperature.
   3. Increase fluid intake.
   4. Provide frequent periods of rest.
   5. Encourage small, nutritious meals.

XXIV. Occupational Lung Disease

A. Description
   1. Caused by exposure to environmental or occupational fumes, dust, vapors, gases, bacterial or fungal antigens, and allergens; can result in acute reversible effects or chronic lung disease
   2. Common disease classifications include occupational asthma, pneumoconiosis (silicosis or coal miner's [black lung] disease), diffuse interstitial fibrosis (asbestosis, talcosis, berylliosis), or extrinsic allergic alveolitis (farmer's lung, bird fancier's lung, or machine operator's lung).
B. Data collection: Signs/symptoms depend on the type of disease and are respiratory symptoms.
C. Interventions
   1. Prevention through the use of respiratory protective devices
   2. Treatment is based on the symptoms experienced by the client.

XXV. Tuberculosis

A. Description
   1. Highly communicable disease caused by *Mycobacterium tuberculosis*
   2. *M. tuberculosis* is a nonmotile, nonsporulating, acid-fast rod that secretes niacin; when the bacillus reaches a susceptible site, it multiplies freely.
   3. Because *M. tuberculosis* is an aerobic bacterium, it primarily affects the pulmonary system especially the upper lobes where the oxygen content is highest, but it also can affect other areas of the body such as the brain, intestines, peritoneum, kidney, joints, and liver.
   4. An exudative response causes a nonspecific pneumonitis and the development of granulomas in the lung tissue.
   5. Tuberculosis has an insidious onset, and many clients are not aware of symptoms until the disease is well advanced.

6. Improper or noncompliant use of treatment programs may cause the development of mutations in the tubercle bacilli resulting in a multidrug-resistant strain of tuberculosis (MDR-TB).

7. The goal of treatment is to prevent transmission, control symptoms, and prevent progression of the disease.

B. Risk factors (Box 47.13)

C. Transmission
1. Via the airborne route by droplet infection
2. When an infected individual coughs, laughs, sneezes, or sings, droplet nuclei containing tuberculosis bacteria enter the air and may be inhaled by others.
3. Identification of those in close contact with the infected individual is important so they can be tested and treated as necessary.
4. When contacts have been identified, these persons are assessed with a tuberculin skin test (TST) and chest x-rays to determine infection with tuberculosis.
5. After the infected individual has received tuberculosis medication for 2 to 3 weeks, the risk of transmission is reduced greatly.

D. Disease progression
1. Droplets enter the lungs, and the bacteria form a tubercle lesion.
2. The defense systems of the body encapsulate the tubercle leaving a scar.
3. If encapsulation does not occur, bacteria may enter the lymph system, travel to the lymph nodes, and cause an inflammatory response called *granulomatous inflammation.*
4. Primary lesions form; the primary lesions may become dormant but can be reactivated and become a secondary infection when reexposed to the bacterium.

BOX 47.13 | **Risk Factors for Tuberculosis**

- Children younger than 5 years of age
- Drinking of unpasteurized milk if the cow is infected with bovine tuberculosis
- Homeless individuals or those from a lower socioeconomic group, minority groups, or immigrant group
- Individuals in constant, frequent contact with an untreated or undiagnosed individual
- Individuals living in crowded areas such as long-term care facilities, prisons, and mental health facilities
- Individuals who are malnourished, have an infection, or an immune dysfunction or human immunodeficiency virus infection; or are immunosuppressed as a result of medication
- Individuals who abuse alcohol or are intravenous (IV) drug users
- Older clients

---

5. In an active phase, tuberculosis can cause necrosis and cavitation in the lesions leading to rupture, the spread of necrotic tissue, and damage to various parts of the body.

E. Client history
1. Past exposure to tuberculosis
2. Client's country of origin and travel to foreign countries in which the incidence of tuberculosis is high
3. Recent history of influenza, pneumonia, febrile illness, cough, or foul-smelling sputum production
4. Previous positive tests for tuberculosis
5. Recent bacille Calmette-Guérin (BCG) vaccine (a vaccine containing attenuated tubercle bacilli that may be given to persons in foreign countries or to persons traveling to foreign countries to produce increased resistance to tuberculosis)

 An individual who has received a BCG vaccine will have a positive TST result and would be evaluated for tuberculosis with a chest x-ray.

F. Clinical manifestations
1. May be asymptomatic during primary infection
2. Fatigue
3. Lethargy
4. Anorexia
5. Weight loss
6. Low-grade fever
7. Chills
8. Night sweats
9. Persistent cough and the production of mucoid and mucopurulent sputum, which is occasionally streaked with blood
10. Chest tightness and a dull, aching chest pain that may accompany the cough

G. Chest data collection
1. A physical examination of the chest does not provide conclusive evidence of tuberculosis.
2. A chest x-ray is not definitive, but the presence of multinodular infiltrates with calcification in the upper lobes suggests tuberculosis.
3. If the disease is active, caseation and inflammation may be seen on the chest x-ray.
4. Advanced disease
   a. Dullness with percussion over the involved parenchymal areas, bronchial breath sounds, rhonchi, and crackles indicate advanced disease.
   b. Partial obstruction of a bronchus caused by endobronchial disease or compression by lymph nodes may produce localized wheezing and dyspnea.

H. QuantiFERON-TB Gold test
1. A blood analysis test by an enzyme-linked immunosorbent assay
2. A sensitive and rapid test (results can be available in 24 hours) that assists in diagnosing the client

TABLE 47.3   Classification of the Tuberculin Skin Test Reaction

Induration = 5 mm or > 5 mm Considered Positive in:	Induration = 10 mm or > 10 mm Considered Positive in:	Induration = 15 mm or > Considered Positive in:
HIV-infected persons Recent contact of a person with TB disease Persons with fibrotic changes on chest x-ray consistent with prior TB Clients with organ transplants Persons immunosuppressed for other reasons	Recent immigrants from high-prevalence countries Injection drug users Residents and employees in high-risk congregate settings Mycobacteriology laboratory personnel Persons with clinical conditions that place them at high risk Children < 4 years of age Infants, children, and adolescents exposed to adults in high-risk categories	Any person, including persons with no known risk factors for TB

HIV, Human immunodeficiency virus; *TB*, tuberculosis.
From Centers for Disease Control and Prevention. *Tuberculosis (TB) Fact Sheets.* Available from: http://www.cdc.gov/tb/publications/factsheets/testing/skintesting.htm.

 I. Sputum cultures

  1. Sputum specimens are obtained for an acid-fast smear.

  2. A sputum culture identifying *M. tuberculosis* confirms the diagnosis.

  3. After medications are started, sputum samples are obtained again to determine the effectiveness of therapy.

  4. Most clients have negative cultures after 3 months of treatment.

 J. Tuberculin skin test (TST) (Table 47.3)

  1. A positive reaction does not mean that active disease is present, but indicates previous exposure to tuberculosis or the presence of inactive (dormant) disease.

  2. Once the test result is positive, it will be positive in future tests.

  3. Skin test interpretation depends on two factors: measurement in millimeters of the induration and the person's risk of being infected with tuberculosis and progression to disease if infected.

  4. Once an individual's skin test is positive, a chest x-ray is necessary to rule out active tuberculosis or to detect old healed lesions.

K. The hospitalized client

  1. The client with active tuberculosis is placed under airborne isolation precautions in a negative pressure room; to maintain negative pressure, the door of the room needs to be tightly closed.

  2. The room would have at least six exchanges of fresh air per hour and would be ventilated to the outside environment if possible.

  3. The nurse wears a particulate filter respirator (a special individually fitted mask) when caring for the client and a gown when a possibility of clothing contamination exists.

  4. Thorough hand washing is required before and after caring for the client.

  5. If the client needs to leave the room for a test or procedure, the client is required to wear a surgical mask.

  6. Respiratory isolation is discontinued when the client is no longer considered infectious.

BOX 47.14   Client Education: Tuberculosis

Provide the client and family with information about tuberculosis and allay concerns about the contagious aspect of the infection.

Instruct the client to follow the medication regimen exactly as prescribed and always to have a supply of the medication on hand.

Advise the client that the medication regimen is continued over 6–12 months, depending on the situation.

Advise the client of the side and adverse effects associated with the medication and ways of minimizing them to ensure compliance.

Reassure the client that after 2–3 weeks of medication therapy, it is unlikely that they will infect anyone.

Inform the client to resume activities gradually.

Instruct the client about the need for adequate nutrition and a well-balanced diet to promote healing and prevent recurrence of the infection.

Instruct the client to increase intake of foods rich in iron, protein, and vitamin C.

Inform the client and family that respiratory isolation is not necessary because family members have already been exposed.

Instruct the client to cover the mouth and nose when coughing or sneezing and confine used tissues to plastic bags.

Instruct the client and family about thorough hand washing.

Inform the client that a sputum culture is needed every 2–4 weeks once medication therapy is initiated.

Inform the client that when the results of three sputum cultures are negative, the client is no longer considered infectious and usually can return to former employment.

Advise the client to avoid excessive exposure to silicone or dust because these substances can cause further lung damage.

Instruct the client regarding the importance of compliance with treatment, follow-up care, and sputum cultures, as prescribed.

  7. After the infected individual has received tuberculosis medication for 2 to 3 weeks, the risk of transmission is reduced greatly.

L. Client education (Box 47.14)

WHAT WOULD YOU DO?

Answer: A tension pneumothorax can occur when there is a buildup of intrathoracic pressure in the pleural space and air cannot escape. One cause is the covering of an open chest wound. Signs include cyanosis, air hunger, restlessness and agitation, tracheal deviation away from the affected side, subcutaneous emphysema, neck vein distension, and hyper-resonance to percussion. The nurse needs to immediately release the chest wound dressing and contact the RN and PHCP. This is a medical emergency requiring possible needle decompression followed by chest tube insertion with a chest drainage system.

PRACTICE QUESTIONS

1. The nurse is reinforcing instructions to a hospitalized client with a diagnosis of emphysema about positions that will enhance the effectiveness of breathing during dyspneic episodes. Which position would the nurse instruct the client to assume?
   1. Side-lying in bed
   2. Sitting in a recliner chair
   3. Sitting up in bed at a 90-degree angle
   4. Sitting on the side of the bed leaning on an over-bed table

2. The nurse is gathering data on a client with a diagnosis of tuberculosis. The nurse would review the results of which diagnostic test to confirm this diagnosis?
   1. Chest x-ray
   2. Bronchoscopy
   3. Sputum culture
   4. Tuberculin skin test

3. The nurse is caring for a client after a bronchoscopy and biopsy. Which finding needs to be reported **immediately** to the primary health care provider (PHCP)?
   1. Dry cough
   2. Hematuria
   3. Bronchospasm
   4. Blood-tinged sputum

❖ 4. The nurse is preparing a list of homecare instructions for the client who has been hospitalized and treated for tuberculosis. Which instructions would the nurse reinforce? **Select all that apply.**
   ❑ 1. Activities need to be resumed gradually.
   ❑ 2. Avoid contact with other individuals except family members for at least 6 months.
   ❑ 3. A sputum culture is needed every 2 to 4 weeks once medication therapy is initiated.
   ❑ 4. Respiratory isolation is not necessary because family members have already been exposed.
   ❑ 5. Cover the mouth and nose when coughing or sneezing and confine used tissues to plastic bags.
   ❑ 6. When one sputum culture is negative, the client is no longer considered infectious and can usually return to his or her former employment.

5. The nurse is instructing a client about pursed lip breathing, and the client asks the nurse about its purpose. The nurse would tell the client that the **primary** purpose of pursed lip breathing is which?
   1. Promote oxygen intake
   2. Strengthen the diaphragm
   3. Strengthen the intercostal muscles
   4. Promote carbon dioxide elimination

6. The low-pressure alarm sounds on the ventilator. The nurse checks the client and then attempts to determine the cause of the alarm but is unsuccessful. Which **initial** action would the nurse take?
   1. Administer oxygen.
   2. Ventilate the client manually.
   3. Check the client's vital signs.
   4. Start cardiopulmonary resuscitation (CPR).

7. The nurse is assigned to care for a client after a left pneumonectomy. Which position is contraindicated for this client?
   1. Lateral position
   2. Low Fowler's position
   3. Semi-Fowler's position
   4. Head of the bed elevation at 40 degrees

8. The nurse is caring for a client after pulmonary angiography via catheter insertion into the left groin. The nurse monitors for an allergic reaction to the contrast medium by observing for the presence of which?
   1. Hypothermia
   2. Respiratory distress
   3. Hematoma in the left groin
   4. Discomfort in the left groin

9. The nurse is reinforcing discharge instructions to the client with pulmonary sarcoidosis. The nurse knows that the client understands the information if the client verbalizes which **early** sign of exacerbation?
   1. Fever
   2. Fatigue
   3. Weight loss
   4. Shortness of breath

10. The nurse is caring for several clients with respiratory disorders. Which client is at least risk for developing a tuberculosis infection?
    1. An uninsured man who is homeless
    2. A woman newly immigrated from another country
    3. A man who is an inspector for the U.S. Postal Service
    4. An older woman admitted from a long-term care facility

❖ 11. The client is diagnosed with pleurisy. The nurse would expect to see which signs/symptoms? **Select all that apply.**
    ❏ 1. Pleural friction rub
    ❏ 2. Sharp, knife-like pain
    ❏ 3. Cyanosis of lips and nailbeds
    ❏ 4. Pain that occurs on both sides of the chest
    ❏ 5. Pain occurs most often during inspiration

12. The nurse notes that a hospitalized client has experienced a positive reaction to the tuberculin skin test. Which action by the nurse is the **priority**?
    1. Report the findings.
    2. Document the finding in the client's record.
    3. Call the employee health service department.
    4. Call the radiology department for a chest x-ray.

13. A client being discharged from the hospital to home with a diagnosis of tuberculosis is worried about the possibility of infecting family members and others. Which information would reassure the client that contaminating family members and others is not likely?

    1. The family does not need therapy, and the client will not be contagious after 1 month of medication therapy.
    2. The family does not need therapy, and the client will not be contagious after 6 consecutive weeks of medication therapy.
    3. The family will receive prophylactic therapy, and the client will not be contagious after 1 continuous week of medication therapy.
    4. The family will receive prophylactic therapy, and the client will not be contagious after 2 to 3 consecutive weeks of medication therapy.

14. The nurse is reinforcing discharge teaching to a client diagnosed with tuberculosis who has been taking medication for 1 1/2 weeks. The nurse knows that the client has understood the information if which statement is made?
    1. "I can't shop at the mall for the next 6 months."
    2. "I need to continue medication therapy for 2 months."
    3. "I can return to work if a sputum culture comes back negative."
    4. "I should not be contagious after 2 to 3 weeks of medication therapy."

15. The nurse is caring for a client with emphysema receiving oxygen. The nurse would consult with the registered nurse if the oxygen flow rate exceeded how many L/min of oxygen?
    1. 1 L/min
    2. 2 L/min
    3. 6 L/min
    4. 10 L/min

ANSWERS

1. 4
Rationale: Positions that will assist the client with breathing include sitting up and leaning on an overbed table, sitting up and resting with the elbows on the knees, or standing or leaning against the wall. The positions in options 1, 2, and 3 will not enhance the effectiveness of breathing.
Test-Taking Strategy: Focus on the subject, positioning for a client with emphysema. Eliminate option 1 because side-lying will not promote appropriate lung expansion. Next, eliminate options 2 and 3 because they are comparable or alike and will restrict lung expansion.

2. 3
Rationale: A definitive diagnosis of tuberculosis is confirmed through culture and isolation of *Mycobacterium tuberculosis*. A presumptive diagnosis is made on the basis of a tuberculin skin test, a sputum smear that is positive for acid-fast bacteria, a chest x-ray, and histological evidence of granulomatous disease on biopsy.

Test-Taking Strategy: Focus on the subject, by noting the word confirm in the question. Confirmation is made by identifying the bacteria, *M. tuberculosis*, which causes the infection. This will direct you to the correct option.

3. 3
Rationale: If a biopsy was performed during a bronchoscopy, blood-streaked sputum is expected for several hours. Frank blood indicates hemorrhage. A dry cough may be expected. The client needs to be assessed for signs of complications, which would include cyanosis, dyspnea, stridor, bronchospasm, hemoptysis, hypotension, tachycardia, and dysrhythmias. Hematuria is unrelated to this procedure.
Test-Taking Strategy: Note the strategic word, *immediately*. Eliminate option 2 first because it is unrelated to the procedure. Next, eliminate option 1 because a dry cough may be expected. Noting that a biopsy has been performed will assist you with eliminating option 4, because blood-streaked sputum would be expected. Note that the correct option relates to the airway.

❖ **4.** 1, 3, 4, 5
Rationale: The nurse would provide the client and family with information about tuberculosis and allay concerns about the contagious aspect of the infection. The client is reassured that after 2 to 3 weeks of medication therapy, it is unlikely that the client will infect anyone. The client is also informed that activities need to be resumed gradually. The client and family are informed that respiratory isolation is not necessary because family members have already been exposed. The client is instructed about thorough hand washing, to cover the mouth and nose when coughing or sneezing, and to confine used tissues to plastic bags. The client is informed that a sputum culture is needed every 2 to 4 weeks once medication is initiated and that when the results of three sputum cultures are negative, the client is no longer considered infectious and can usually return to his or her former employment.
Test-Taking Strategy: Note the subject, homecare instructions for the client with tuberculosis. Knowledge regarding the pathophysiology, transmission, and treatment of tuberculosis is needed to answer this question. Using this knowledge will assist you with directing you to the correct options.

5. 4
Rationale: Pursed lip breathing facilitates maximal expiration for clients with obstructive lung disease and promotes carbon dioxide elimination. This type of breathing allows better expiration by increasing airway pressure, which keeps air passages open during exhalation. Options 1, 2, and 3 are not the purposes of this type of breathing.
Test-Taking Strategy: Focus on the subject, pursed lip breathing, and note the strategic word, *primary*. Visualize the use of this breathing technique to assist with answering correctly. Recalling the respiratory conditions in which this type of breathing is helpful will also assist in directing you to the correct option.

6. 2
Rationale: If an alarm is sounding at any time and the nurse cannot quickly ascertain the problem, the client is disconnected from the ventilator and a manual resuscitation device is used to support respirations until the problem can be corrected. Although oxygen is helpful, it will not provide ventilation to the client. Checking vital signs is not the initial action. There is no reason to begin CPR.
Test-Taking Strategy: Use the concept of ABCs—airway breathing, circulation—and note the strategic word, *initial*. Read the question carefully to note that the subject relates to adequate ventilation of the client. Focusing on this subject will direct you to the correct option.

❖ **7.** 1
Rationale: Complete lateral positioning is contraindicated for a client following pneumonectomy. Because the mediastinum is no longer held in place on both sides by lung tissue, lateral positioning may cause mediastinal shift and compression of the remaining lung. The head of the bed needs to be elevated.
Test-Taking Strategy: Focus on the subject, the position that is contraindicated. Think about what is involved in this surgical procedure. Eliminate options 2, 3, and 4 because they are comparable or alike and all indicate head elevation.

8. 2
Rationale: Signs of allergic reaction to the contrast medium include localized itching and edema, respiratory distress, stridor, and decreased blood pressure. Hypothermia is an unrelated event. Hematoma formation is a complication of the procedure, but does not indicate an allergic reaction. Discomfort is expected.
Test-Taking Strategy: Focus on the subject, an allergic reaction, and use the ABCs—airway, breathing, and circulation. This will direct you to the correct option.

9. 4
Rationale: Shortness of breath is an early sign of exacerbation of pulmonary sarcoidosis. Others include chest pain, hemoptysis, and pneumothorax. Systemic signs/symptoms that occur later include weakness and fatigue, malaise, fever, and weight loss.
Test-Taking Strategy: Note the strategic word, *early*, in the question. Because sarcoidosis is a pulmonary problem, eliminate options 1 and 3 first. Choose option 4 over option 2 because the shortness of breath (and impaired ventilation) appears first and would cause the fatigue as a secondary symptom.

10. 3
Rationale: People at high risk for acquiring tuberculosis include children younger than 5 years of age; homeless individuals or those from a lower socioeconomic group, minority groups, or immigrant group; individuals in constant, frequent contact with an untreated or undiagnosed individual; individuals living in crowded areas such as long-term care facilities, prisons, and mental health facilities; older clients; malnourished individuals, those with an infection, or an immune dysfunction or human immunodeficiency virus infection, or individuals who are immunosuppressed as a result of medication therapy; and individuals who abuse alcohol or are IV drug users.
Test-Taking Strategy: Note the subject, the client at least risk for developing a tuberculosis infection. Begin to answer this question by eliminating options 1 and 2 because immigrants and the medically underserved are more frequently affected by this infection. From the remaining options, note that the postal inspector may or may not come in contact with many people depending on job description. The client from the long-term care facility, however, lives in a group setting, where a large number of people share a common environment 24 hours a day.

11. 1, 2, 5
Rationale: Pleurisy is inflammation of the pleura. The most characteristic symptom of pleurisy is abrupt and severe pain. The pain almost always occurs on one side of the chest. Pleurisy pain is sharp, knife-like, and abrupt in onset and is most evident during inspiration. This causes shallow breathing. A pleural friction rub may be heard.
Test-Taking Strategy: Note the subject, signs/symptoms of pleurisy. Eliminate option 3 first because it is unrelated to pleurisy. Next, eliminate option 4 because the pain almost

always occurs on one side of the chest and clients usually can point to the exact location of the pain.

12. 1

Rationale: The nurse who interprets a tuberculin skin test as positive notifies the PHCP immediately. The PHCP would prescribe a chest x-ray to determine whether the client has clinically active tuberculosis or old healed lesions. A sputum culture would be done to confirm the diagnosis of active tuberculosis. The client is placed on tuberculosis precautions prophylactically until a final diagnosis is made. The findings are documented in the client's record, but this action is not the highest priority. Calling the employee health service would be of no benefit to the client.

Test-Taking Strategy: Note the strategic word, *priority*. Because the nurse may not prescribe diagnostic tests, eliminate option 4 first. Option 3 can be eliminated because calling the employee health service is of no benefit to the client. From the remaining options, notifying the PHCP has a higher priority than the documentation, even though both may be done in the same narrow time period.

13. 4

Rationale: Family members or others who have been in close contact with a client diagnosed with tuberculosis are placed on prophylactic therapy with isoniazid for 6 to 12 months. The client is usually not contagious after taking medication for 2 to 3 consecutive weeks. However, the client needs to take the full course of therapy (for 6 months or longer) to prevent reinfection or drug-resistant tuberculosis.

Test-Taking Strategy: Focus on the subject, treatment of those exposed to tuberculosis and reassuring the client. Recalling that the family requires prophylactic therapy allows you to eliminate options 1 and 2. From the remaining options, it is necessary to know that the client is not contagious after 2 to 3 weeks of therapy.

14. 4

Rationale: The client continues medication therapy for 6 to 12 months depending on the situation. The client is generally considered to not be contagious after 2 to 3 weeks of medication. The client is instructed to wear a mask if there will be exposure to crowds until the medication is effective in preventing transmission. The client is allowed to return to employment when the results of three sputum cultures are negative.

Test-Taking Strategy: Focus on the subject, client understanding of discharge teaching regarding treatment of tuberculosis. Knowing that the medication regimen lasts for at least 6 months helps you eliminate option 2 first. Knowing that three sputum cultures needs to be negative helps you eliminate option 3 next. From the remaining options, recalling that the client is not contagious after 2 to 3 weeks of therapy helps you choose option 4.

15. 2

Rationale: The concentration of oxygen administered is always prescribed by the primary health care provider and is based on ABG values and oxygen saturation by pulse oximetry. Between 1 and 3 L/min of oxygen by nasal cannula may be prescribed and required to raise the PaO_2 level to 60 to 80 mm Hg. However, oxygen is used cautiously in the client with emphysema and would not exceed 2 L/min unless specifically prescribed. Because of the long-standing hypercapnia that occurs in this disorder, the respiratory drive is triggered by low oxygen levels rather than by increased carbon dioxide levels, which is the case in a normal respiratory system.

Test-Taking Strategy: Focus on the subject, oxygen administration with emphysema. Recalling the physiology associated with emphysema is required to answer this question. Remember that oxygen is used cautiously in the client with emphysema and would not exceed 2 L/min unless specifically prescribed.

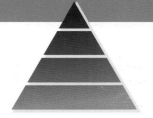

CHAPTER **48**

Respiratory Medications

PRIORITY CONCEPTS Gas Exchange; Infection

WHAT WOULD YOU DO?

A client who has been taking isoniazid for the past 4 months to treat tuberculosis reports to the nurse that they are experiencing a lack of appetite, some nausea, and urine output that is dark in color. What would the nurse do?
Answer is located on p. 645.

I. Medication Inhalation Devices

A. Metered-dose inhaler (MDI): Uses a chemical propellant to push the medication out of the inhaler (Fig. 48.1)

B. Dry powder inhaler (DPI): Delivers medication without using chemical propellants, but it requires strong and fast inhalation

C. Nebulizer: Delivers fine liquid mists of medication through a tube or a mask that fits over the nose and mouth, or with a mouthpiece, using air or oxygen under pressure

D. If two different inhaled medications are prescribed and one of the medications contains a glucocorticoid (corticosteroid), administer the bronchodilator first and the corticosteroid second.

⚠ If two different inhaled medications are prescribed, instruct the client to wait 5 minutes following administration of the first before inhaling the second. If a second dose of the same medication is needed, instruct the client to wait 1 to 2 minutes before taking the second dose.

II. Bronchodilators (Box 48.1)

A. Description

1. Sympathomimetic bronchodilators relax the smooth muscle of the bronchi and dilate the airways of the respiratory tree making air exchange and respiration easier for the client. Examples include β_2-adrenergic agonists such as albuterol.

2. Methylxanthine bronchodilators stimulate the central nervous system (CNS) and respiration, dilate coronary and pulmonary vessels, cause diuresis, and relax smooth muscle.

3. Used to treat acute bronchospasm, acute and chronic asthma, bronchitis, restrictive airway diseases, and reactive airway diseases

4. Contraindicated in individuals with hypersensitivity, peptic ulcer disease, severe cardiac disease and cardiac dysrhythmias, hyperthyroidism, or uncontrolled seizure disorders

5. Used with caution in clients with hypertension, diabetes mellitus, or narrow-angle glaucoma

6. Theophylline increases the risk of digoxin toxicity and decreases the effects of lithium and phenytoin. Theophylline would be the last-line medication.

7. If theophylline and a β_2-adrenergic agonist are administered together, cardiac dysrhythmias may result.

8. Beta blockers, cimetidine, and erythromycin increase the effects of theophylline.

9. Barbiturates and carbamazepine decrease the effects of theophylline.

B. Side and adverse effects

1. Palpitations and tachycardia

2. Dysrhythmia

3. Restlessness, nervousness, tremors

4. Anorexia, nausea, and vomiting

5. Headache and dizziness

6. Hyperglycemia

7. Mouth dryness and throat irritation with inhalers

8. Tolerance and paradoxical bronchoconstriction with inhalers

C. Interventions

1. Monitor vital signs and lung sounds.

2. Monitor for cardiac dysrhythmia.

3. Check for cough, wheezing, decreased breath sounds, and sputum production.

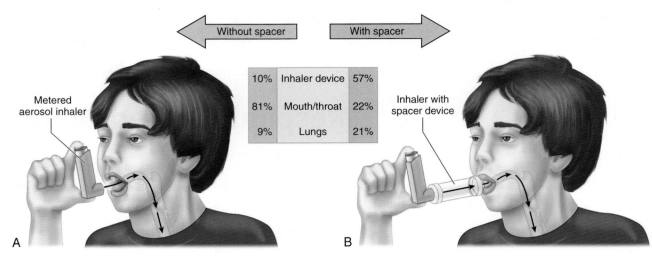

FIGURE 48.1 Distribution of medication with and without a spacer.

4. Monitor for restlessness and confusion.
5. Provide adequate hydration.
6. Administer the medication at regular intervals around the clock to maintain a sustained therapeutic level.
7. Administer oral medications with or after meals to decrease gastrointestinal (GI) irritation.
8. Monitor for therapeutic serum theophylline level of 10 to 20 mcg/mL.
9. Intravenously administered aminophylline or theophylline preparations will be administered slowly and always via an infusion pump.
10. Client education
   a. Not to crush enteric-coated or sustained-release tablets or capsules
   b. To avoid caffeine-containing products such as coffee, tea, cola, and chocolate, as well as over-the-counter medications
   c. About the side and adverse effects of bronchodilators
   d. How to monitor the pulse and to report any abnormalities to the primary health care provider (PHCP)
   e. How to use an inhaler, spacer, or nebulizer (see Fig. 48.1) and how to monitor the amount of medication remaining in an inhaler canister
   f. The importance of smoking cessation and information regarding support resources
   g. To monitor blood glucose level if diabetes mellitus is a coexisting condition
   h. To wear a MedicAlert bracelet, particularly if the client has asthma

 Theophylline toxicity is likely to occur when the serum level is higher than 20 mcg/mL. Early signs of toxicity include restlessness, nervousness, tremors, palpitations, and tachycardia.

III. Anticholinergics (see Box 48.1)
A. Inhaled medications that improve lung function by blocking muscarinic receptors in the bronchi, resulting in bronchodilation
B. Effective for treating chronic obstructive pulmonary disease, allergy-induced asthma, and exercise-induced bronchospasm
C. Side effects include dry mouth and irritation of the pharynx; sucking on sugarless candy will help to relieve symptoms.
D. Systemic anticholinergic effects rarely occur, but can include increased intraocular pressure, blurred vision, tachycardia, cardiovascular events, urinary retention, and constipation.

The client with a peanut allergy would not take ipratropium products because they contain soy lecithin, which is in the same plant family as peanuts.

IV. Glucocorticoids (corticosteroids) (see Box 48.1)
A. Glucocorticoids act as anti-inflammatory agents and reduce edema of the airways; they are used to treat asthma and other inflammatory respiratory conditions.
B. See Chapter 44 for information on glucocorticoids.

V. Leukotriene Modifiers (see Box 48.1)
A. Description
   1. Used in the prophylaxis and treatment of chronic bronchial asthma (not used for acute asthma episodes)
   2. Inhibit bronchoconstriction caused by specific antigens and reduce airway edema and smooth muscle constriction
   3. Contraindicated in clients with hypersensitivity and in breastfeeding mothers
   4. Would be used with caution in clients with impaired hepatic function

BOX 48.1 Medications to Treat Restrictive Airway Disorders

Bronchodilators

β₂-Adrenergic Agonists
Inhaled
Albuterol
Arformoterol
Formoterol
Levalbuterol
Salmeterol

Oral
Albuterol
Terbutaline

Methylxanthines
Aminophylline
Theophylline, oral

Anticholinergics
Ipratropium, inhaled
Tiotropium, inhaled
Aclidinium, inhaled
Revefenacin, inhaled
Umeclidinium, inhaled

Glucocorticoids (Corticosteroids)
Inhaled
Beclomethasone dipropionate
Budesonide
Ciclesonide
Fluticasone propionate
Mometasone furoate

Oral
Prednisone
Prednisolone

Leukotriene Modifiers
Montelukast, oral
Zafirlukast, oral

Inhaled Nonsteroidal Antiallergy Agent
Cromolyn sodium, inhaled

Monoclonal Antibody
Omalizumab

Modified from Burcham JR, Rosenthal LD: *Lehne's Pharmacology for nursing care,* ed 9, St. Louis, 2016, Saunders.

5. Coadministration of inhaled glucocorticoids increases the risk of upper respiratory infection.
B. Side and adverse effects
 1. Headache
 2. Nausea and vomiting
 3. Dyspepsia
 4. Diarrhea
 5. Generalized pain, myalgia
 6. Fever
 7. Dizziness

C. Interventions
 1. Check lung sounds for adventitious breath sounds.
 2. Monitor liver function laboratory values.
 3. Monitor for cyanosis.
D. Client education
 1. To take medication 1 hour before or 2 hours after meals
 2. To increase fluid intake
 3. Not discontinue the medication and to take as prescribed, even during symptom-free periods

VI. Inhaled Nonsteroidal Antiallergy Agent (see Box 48.1)
A. Description
 1. Antiasthmatic, antiallergic, and mast cell stabilizers; inhibit mast cell release after exposure to antigens
 2. Used to treat allergic rhinitis, bronchial asthma, and exercise-induced bronchospasm
 3. Contraindicated in clients with known hypersensitivity
 4. Orally administered cromolyn sodium is used with caution in clients with impaired hepatic or renal function
B. Side and adverse effects
 1. Coughing, sneezing, nasal sting, or bronchospasm after inhalation
 2. Unpleasant taste in the mouth
C. Interventions: Monitor respirations and check lung sounds for rhonchi or wheezing.
D. Client education
 1. To administer oral capsules at least 30 minutes before meals
 2. Not to discontinue the medication abruptly because a rebound asthmatic attack can occur

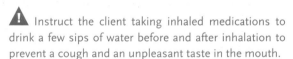 Instruct the client taking inhaled medications to drink a few sips of water before and after inhalation to prevent a cough and an unpleasant taste in the mouth.

VII. Monoclonal Antibody (see Box 48.1)
A. Description
 1. Omalizumab is a recombinant DNA-derived humanized immunoglobulin G (IgG) murine monoclonal antibody that selectively binds to IgE to limit the release of mediators in the allergic response.
 2. Used to treat allergy-related asthma; administered subcutaneously every 2 to 4 weeks
 3. Dose is titrated on the basis of the serum IgE level and body weight.
 4. Contraindicated in those with hypersensitivity to the medication
B. Side and adverse effects
 1. Injection site reactions
 2. Viral infections
 3. Upper respiratory infections

4. Sinusitis
5. Headache
6. Pharyngitis
7. Anaphylaxis
8. Malignancies

C. Interventions
1. Monitor respiratory rate, rhythm, depth, and listen to lung sounds.
2. Check for allergies and/or allergic reaction symptoms such as rash or urticaria.
3. Have medications for the treatment of severe hypersensitivity reactions available during initial administration in case anaphylaxis occurs.

D. Client education
1. That respiratory improvement will not be immediate
2. Not to stop taking or not to decrease the currently prescribed asthma medications unless instructed
3. To avoid live virus vaccines for the duration of treatment

VIII. Antihistamines (Box 48.2)

A. Description
1. Called *histamine antagonists* or H_1 *blockers*; these medications compete with histamine for receptor sites thus preventing a histamine response.
2. When the H_1 receptor is stimulated, the extravascular smooth muscles including those lining the nasal cavity are constricted.
3. Decrease nasopharyngeal, GI, and bronchial secretions by blocking the H_1 receptor
4. Used for the common cold, rhinitis, nausea and vomiting, motion sickness, urticaria, and as a sleep aid
5. Can cause CNS depression if taken with alcohol, opioids, hypnotics, or barbiturates, particularly with first-generation antihistamines
6. Would be used with caution in clients with chronic obstructive pulmonary disease because of their drying effect
7. Diphenhydramine has an anticholinergic effect and needs to be avoided in clients with narrow-angle glaucoma.

B. Side and adverse effects
1. Drowsiness and fatigue
2. Dizziness
3. Urinary retention
4. Blurred vision
5. Wheezing
6. Constipation
7. Dry mouth
8. GI irritation
9. Hypotension
10. Hearing disturbances
11. Photosensitivity
12. Nervousness and irritability
13. Confusion
14. Nightmares

BOX 48.2 Antihistamines

Brompheniramine
Cetirizine
Chlorpheniramine
Clemastine
Cyproheptadine
Desloratadine
Dimenhydrinate
Diphenhydramine
Fexofenadine
Levocetirizine
Loratadine
Olopatadine
Tripolidine

C. Interventions
1. Monitor for signs of urinary dysfunction.
2. Administer with food or milk.
3. Avoid subcutaneous injection; administer by intramuscular injection in a large muscle if the intramuscular route is prescribed.

D. Client education
1. To avoid hazardous activities, alcohol, and other CNS depressants
2. If the medication is being taken for motion sickness, take it 30 minutes before the event and then before meals and at bedtime during the event as prescribed.
3. To suck on hard candy or ice chips for dry mouth

IX. Nasal Decongestants (Box 48.3)

A. Description
1. Include adrenergic, anticholinergic, and corticosteroid medications
2. Shrink nasal mucosal membranes and reduce fluid secretion
3. Used for allergic rhinitis, hay fever, and acute coryza (profuse nasal discharge)
4. Contraindicated or used with extreme caution in clients with hypertension, cardiac disease, hyperthyroidism, or diabetes mellitus

B. Side and adverse effects
1. Nervousness
2. Restlessness, insomnia
3. Hypertension
4. Hyperglycemia

⚠ Nasal decongestants can cause tolerance and rebound nasal congestion (vasodilation) as a result of irritation of the nasal mucosa. Therefore, the client needs to be informed that these medications would not be used for longer than 48 hours.

C. Interventions
1. Monitor for cardiac dysrhythmias.
2. Monitor blood glucose levels.

Adult—Respiratory

BOX 48.3	Nasal Decongestants

Nonglucocorticoids
Oxymetazoline
Phenylephrine hydrochloride
Pseudoephedrine hydrochloride

Glucocorticoids
Beclomethasone
Budesonide
Ciclesonide
Flunisolide
Fluticasone furoate
Fluticasone propionate
Mometasone
Triamcinolone

BOX 48.4	Expectorants and Mucolytic Agents

Expectorant
Guaifenesin

Mucolytic
Acetylcysteine

BOX 48.5	Antitussives

Opioids
Codeine phosphate, codeine sulfate
Hydrocodone

Nonopioids
Benzonatate
Dextromethorphan

D. Client education
   1. To avoid consuming caffeine in large amounts because it can increase restlessness and palpitations
   2. About the importance of limiting the use of nasal sprays and drops to prevent rebound nasal congestion; consider weaning off one nare at a time to prevent this

X. Expectorants and Mucolytic Agents (Box 48.4)
A. Description
   1. Expectorants loosen bronchial secretions so they can be eliminated with coughing; they are used for a dry nonproductive cough and to stimulate bronchial secretions.
   2. Mucolytic agents produce thin mucous secretions to help make the cough more productive.
   3. Mucolytic agents with dextromethorphan would not be used by clients with chronic obstructive pulmonary disease because they suppress the cough.
   4. Acetylcysteine can increase airway resistance and would not be used in clients with asthma. This medication also can be used to prevent liver damage in acetaminophen overdose, as well as protect the kidneys in the event that diagnostic testing requiring contrast dye is done.
B. Side and adverse effects
   1. GI irritation
   2. Rash
   3. Oropharyngeal irritation
C. Interventions
   1. Acetylcysteine is administered by nebulization and would not be mixed with another medication.
   2. If acetylcysteine is administered with a bronchodilator, the bronchodilator needs to be administered 5 minutes before the acetylcysteine.
   3. Monitor for side effects of acetylcysteine such as nausea and vomiting, stomatitis, and runny nose.

D. Client education
   1. To take the medication with a full glass of water to loosen mucus
   2. To maintain adequate fluid intake
   3. To cough and deep breathe

XI. Antitussives (Box 48.5)
A. Description: Act on the cough control center in the medulla to suppress the cough reflex; used for a cough that is nonproductive and irritating
B. Side and adverse effects
   1. Dizziness, drowsiness, sedation
   2. GI irritation, nausea
   3. Dry mouth
   4. Constipation
   5. Respiratory depression
C. Interventions
   1. Encourage the client to take adequate fluids with the medication.
   2. Encourage the client to sleep with the head of the bed elevated.
   3. Note that medication dependency can occur.
   4. Avoid administration to the client with a head injury or a postoperative cranial surgery client.
   5. Avoid administration to the client using opioids, sedative-hypnotics, barbiturates, or antidepressants because CNS depression can occur.
D. Client education
   1. If the cough lasts longer than 1 week and a fever or a rash occurs, notify the PHCP.
   2. Avoid hazardous activities.
   3. Avoid the use of alcohol.

XII. Opioid Antagonists (Box 48.6)
A. Description
   1. Reverses respiratory depression in opioid overdose

BOX 48.6	Opioid Antagonists

Alvimopan
Methylnaltrexone
Naldemedine
Naloxone
Naltrexone

BOX 48.7	First- and Second-Line Medications for Tuberculosis

First-Line Agents
Ethambutol
Isoniazid
Pyrazinamide
Rifampin

Second-Line Agents
Amikacin
Capreomycin sulfate
Cycloserine
Ethionamide
Levofloxacin
Moxifloxacin
p-Aminosalicylic acid
Rifabutin
Rifapentine
Streptomycin

  2. Avoid its use for nonopioid respiratory depression.
  3. Reoccurrence of respiratory depression can occur if duration of opiate exceeds duration of opioid antagonist.
  4. This medication may be prescribed for clients at risk for opioid overdose.
B. Side and adverse effects
  1. Nausea, vomiting
  2. Tremors
  3. Sweating
  4. Increased blood pressure
  5. Tachycardia
C. Interventions
  1. Monitor vital signs, especially respirations.
  2. The registered nurse (RN) is responsible for intravenous administration and for titrating the dose administered every 2 to 5 minutes as prescribed.
  3. Have oxygen and resuscitative equipment available during administration.

XIII. Tuberculosis Medications (Box 48.7)
A. Description
  1. Offers the most effective method for treating the disease and preventing transmission
  2. Treatment of identified lesions depends on whether the individual has active disease or has been exposed to the disease.
  3. Treatment is difficult because the bacterium has a waxy substance on the capsule that makes penetration and destruction difficult.
  4. The use of a multidrug regimen destroys organisms as quickly as possible and minimizes the emergence of drug-resistant organisms.
  5. Active tuberculosis is treated with a combination of medications to which the organism is susceptible.
  6. Individuals with active tuberculosis are treated for 6 to 9 months; however, clients with immunosuppression (e.g., HIV) are treated for a longer period of time.
  7. After the infected individual has received medication for 2 to 3 weeks, the risk of transmission is greatly reduced.
  8. Most clients have negative sputum cultures after 3 months of compliance with medication therapy.
  9. Individuals who have been exposed to active tuberculosis are treated with preventive isoniazid for 9 to 12 months.

B. First- or second-line medications
  1. First-line medications provide the most effective antituberculosis activity.
  2. Second-line medications are used in combination with first-line medications but are more toxic.
  3. Current infecting organisms are proving resistant to standard first-line medications; the resistant organisms develop because individuals with the disease fail to complete the course of treatment so surviving bacteria adapt to the medication and become resistant.
  4. Multidrug therapies are instituted because of the resistant organisms.
C. Multidrug-resistant strain of tuberculosis (MDR-TB)
  1. Resistance occurs when a client receiving two medications (first-line and second-line medications) discontinues one of the medications.
  2. The client briefly experiences some response from the single medication, but then large numbers of resistant organisms begin to grow.
  3. The client, infectious again, transmits the drug-resistant organism to other individuals.
  4. As this event is repeated, an organism develops that is resistant to many of the first-line tuberculosis medications.
D. General client education points on tuberculosis medications
  1. Not to skip doses and to take the medication for the full length of the prescribed therapy
  2. Not to take any other medication without consulting the PHCP
  3. About the importance of follow-up PHCP visits, vision testing, and laboratory tests
  4. To avoid alcohol

5. To take medication on an empty stomach with 8 oz of water 1 hour before or 2 hours after meals and to avoid taking antacids with the medication

6. About the adverse effects that require PHCP notification

7. Inform the client about direct observed therapy (DOT) to ensure adherence to the medication regimen.

XIV. First-Line Medications for Tuberculosis (see Box 48.7)

A. Isoniazid
  1. Description
    a. Bactericidal
    b. Inhibits the synthesis of mycolic acids and acts to kill actively growing organisms in the extracellular environment
    c. Inhibits the growth of dormant organisms in the macrophages and caseating granulomas
    d. Is active only during cell division and is used in combination with other antitubercular medications
  2. Contraindications and cautions
    a. Contraindicated in clients with hypersensitivity or with acute liver disease
    b. Use with caution in clients with chronic liver disease, alcoholism, or renal impairment.
    c. Use with caution in clients taking nicotinic acid.
    d. Use with caution in clients taking hepatotoxic medications because the risk for hepatotoxicity increases.
    e. Alcohol increases the risk of hepatotoxicity.
    f. May increase the risk of toxicity of carbamazepine and phenytoin
    g. Isoniazid may decrease ketoconazole concentrations.
  3. Side and adverse effects
    a. Hypersensitivity reactions
    b. Peripheral neuritis
    c. Neurotoxicity
    d. Hepatotoxicity and hepatitis; increased liver function test levels
    e. Pyridoxine deficiency
    f. Irritation at injection site with intramuscular administration
    g. Nausea and vomiting
    h. Dry mouth
    i. Dizziness
    j. Hyperglycemia
    k. Change in vision
  4. Interventions
    a. Monitor for hypersensitivity.
    b. Monitor for hepatic dysfunction.
    c. Monitor for sensitivity to nicotinic acid.
    d. Monitor liver function test results.
    e. Monitor for signs of hepatitis such as anorexia, nausea, vomiting, weakness, fatigue, dark urine, or jaundice; if these symptoms occur, withhold the medication and notify the RN and PHCP.
    f. Monitor for tingling, numbness, or burning of the extremities.
    g. Monitor mental status.
    h. Monitor for any change in vision and notify the RN of changes.
    i. Monitor for dizziness and initiate safety precautions.
    j. Monitor complete blood count (CBC) and blood glucose level.
    k. Isoniazid is administered 1 hour before or 2 hours after a meal because food may delay absorption.
    i. Isoniazid is administered at least 1 hour before antacids, especially those antacids that contain aluminum.
    m. Pyridoxine is administered as prescribed to reduce the risk of neurotoxicity.

⚠️ Many tuberculosis medications can cause toxic effects such as hepatotoxicity, nephrotoxicity, neurotoxicity, optic neuritis, or ototoxicity. Teach the client about the signs of toxicity and inform the client that the PHCP needs to be notified if any signs arise.

  5. Client education
    a. To avoid tyramine-containing foods because they may cause a reaction such as red and itchy skin, a pounding heartbeat, light-headedness, a hot or clammy feeling, or a headache; if this does occur, the client needs to notify the PHCP
    b. To recognize the signs of neurotoxicity, hepatitis, and hepatotoxicity
    c. To notify the PHCP if signs of neurotoxicity, hepatitis and hepatotoxicity, or a change in vision occurs

B. Rifampin
  1. Description
    a. Inhibits bacterial RNA synthesis
    b. Binds to DNA-dependent RNA polymerase and blocks RNA transcription
    c. Used with at least one other antitubercular medication
  2. Contraindications and cautions
    a. Contraindicated in clients with hypersensitivity
    b. Used with caution in clients with hepatic dysfunction or alcoholism
    c. Use of alcohol or hepatotoxic medications may increase the risk of hepatotoxicity.
    d. Decreases the effects of several medications, including oral anticoagulants, oral hypoglycemics,

chloramphenicol, digoxin, disopyramide phosphate, mexiletine, quinidine polygalacturonate, fluconazole, methadone hydrochloride, phenytoin, and verapamil hydrochloride
3. Side and adverse effects
   a. Hypersensitivity reaction including fever, chills, shivering, headache, muscle and bone pain, and dyspnea
   b. Heartburn, nausea, vomiting, diarrhea
   c. Red-orange–colored body secretions
   d. Change in vision
   e. Hepatotoxicity and hepatitis
   f. Increased uric acid level
   g. Blood dyscrasia
   h. Colitis
4. Interventions
   a. Monitor for hypersensitivity.
   b. Monitor CBC, uric acid, and liver function test results.
   c. Monitor for signs of hepatitis; if they occur, the medication is withheld and the PHCP is notified.
   d. Monitor for signs of colitis.
   e. Monitor for visual changes.
5. Client education
   a. That urine, feces, sweat, and tears will be red-orange and that soft contact lenses can become permanently discolored
   b. To notify the PHCP if jaundice (yellow eyes or skin) develops or if weakness, fatigue, nausea, vomiting, sore throat, fever, or unusual bleeding occurs
C. Ethambutol
   1. Description
      a. Bacteriostatic
      b. Interferes with cell metabolism and multiplication by inhibiting one or more metabolites in susceptible organisms
      c. Inhibits bacterial RNA synthesis and is active only during cell division
      d. Slow-acting so it needs to be administered with other bactericidal agents
   2. Contraindications and cautions
      a. Contraindicated in clients with hypersensitivity or optic neuritis and children younger than 13 years
      b. Used with caution in clients with renal dysfunction, gout, ocular defects, diabetic retinopathy, cataracts, or ocular inflammatory conditions
      c. Used with caution in clients taking neurotoxic medications because the risk for neurotoxicity increases
   3. Side and adverse effects
      a. Hypersensitivity reactions
      b. Anorexia, nausea, vomiting
      c. Dizziness

d. Malaise
e. Mental confusion
f. Joint pain
g. Dermatitis
h. Optic neuritis
i. Peripheral neuritis
j. Thrombocytopenia
k. Increased uric acid level
l. Anaphylactoid reaction
4. Interventions
   a. Monitor the client for hypersensitivity.
   b. Monitor results of CBC, uric acid, and renal and liver function tests.
   c. Monitor for visual changes such as altered color perception and decreased visual acuity; if changes occur, the medication is withheld and the PHCP is notified.
   d. Administer once every 24 hours and administer with food to decrease GI upset.
   e. Monitor uric acid concentration and check for painful or swollen joints or signs of gout.
   f. Monitor intake and output and for adequate renal function.
   g. Monitor mental status.
   h. Monitor for dizziness, and initiate safety precautions.
   i. Monitor for peripheral neuritis (numbness, tingling, or burning of the extremities); if it occurs, the PHCP is notified.
5. Client education
   a. That nausea related to the medication can be prevented by taking the daily dose at bedtime or by taking the prescribed antinausea medications
   b. To notify the PHCP immediately if any visual problems occur, or a rash, swelling and pain in the joints, numbness, tingling, or burning of the hands or feet occurs
D. Pyrazinamide
   1. Description
      a. The exact mechanism of action is unknown.
      b. May be bacteriostatic or bactericidal depending on its concentration at the infection site and susceptibility of infecting organism
      c. Used with at least one other antitubercular medication if ineffectiveness of the primary medication(s) occurs
   2. Contraindications and cautions
      a. Contraindicated in clients with hypersensitivity
      b. Used with caution in clients with diabetes mellitus, renal impairment, or gout, and in children
      c. May decrease the effects of allopurinol, colchicine, and probenecid
      d. Cross-sensitivity is possible with isoniazid, ethionamide, or nicotinic acid.

3. Side and adverse effects
   a. Increases liver function tests and uric acid levels
   b. Arthralgia, myalgia
   c. Photosensitivity
   d. Hepatotoxicity
   e. Thrombocytopenia
4. Interventions
   a. Monitor for hypersensitivity.
   b. Monitor CBC, liver function test results, and uric acid levels.
   c. Observe for hepatotoxic effects; if they occur, the medication is withheld and the PHCP is notified.
   d. Monitor for painful or swollen joints.
   e. Monitor blood glucose level because diabetes mellitus may be difficult to control while client is taking the medication.
5. Client education
   a. To take the medication with food to reduce GI distress
   b. To avoid sunlight or ultraviolet light until photosensitivity is determined

⚠ Some tuberculosis medications can cause red-orange–colored body secretions. The client is informed that this is not a harmful effect but that the secretions can stain and permanently discolor items.

XV. **Second-Line Medications for Tuberculosis (see Box 48.7)**
A. Rifabutin
   1. Description
      a. Inhibits mycobacterial DNA-dependent RNA polymerase and suppresses protein synthesis
      b. Used to prevent disseminated *Mycobacterium avium* complex (MAC) disease in clients with advanced HIV infection
      c. Used to treat active MAC disease and tuberculosis in clients with HIV infection
   2. Cautions
      a. Can affect blood levels of some medications including oral contraceptives and some medications used to treat HIV infection
      b. A nonhormonal method of birth control would be used instead of an oral contraceptive.
   3. Side and adverse effects
      a. Rash
      b. GI disturbances
      c. Neutropenia
      d. Red-orange–colored body secretions
      e. Uveitis
      f. Myositis
      g. Arthralgia
      h. Hepatitis
      i. Chest pain with dyspnea

   j. Flu-like syndrome
   4. Interventions
      a. Observe for hepatotoxic effects; if they occur, the medication is withheld and the PHCP is notified.
      b. Monitor for painful or swollen joints.
      c. Monitor for ocular pain or blurred vision.
   5. Client education: That the medication can be taken without regard to food
B. Rifapentine
   1. Description: Used only for pulmonary tuberculosis
   2. Cautions: Can affect blood levels of some medications including oral contraceptives and warfarin, and some medications used to treat HIV infection
   3. Side and adverse effects
      a. Red-orange–colored body secretions
      b. Hepatotoxicity
   4. Interventions
      a. Monitor baseline liver function studies and monitor throughout therapy.
      b. Observe for hepatotoxic effects; if they occur, the medication is withheld and the PHCP is notified.
   5. Client education
      a. That the medication can be taken without regard to food
      b. To avoid sunlight or ultraviolet light until photosensitivity is determined
      c. That red-orange–colored body secretions may occur
C. Capreomycin sulfate
   1. Description
      a. Mechanism of action is unknown.
      b. Used to treat MDR-TB when significant resistance to other medications is expected
      c. Is administered intramuscularly
   2. Contraindications and cautions
      a. The risk of nephrotoxicity, ototoxicity, and neuromuscular blockade is increased with the use of aminoglycosides or loop diuretics.
      b. Used with caution in clients with renal insufficiency, acoustic nerve impairment, hepatic disorder, myasthenia gravis, or parkinsonism
      c. Not administered to clients receiving streptomycin
   3. Side and adverse effects
      a. Nephrotoxicity
      b. Ototoxicity
      c. Neuromuscular blockade
   4. Interventions
      a. Baseline audiometric testing is performed.
      b. Check renal, hepatic, and electrolyte levels before administration.
      c. Monitor intake and output.

d. Administered intramuscularly deep into a large muscle mass (reconstituted medication may be stored for 48 hours at room temperature).

e. Rotate injection sites.

f. Observe injection site for redness, excessive bleeding, and inflammation.

5. Client education

    a. Not to perform tasks that require mental alertness

    b. To report any hearing loss, balance disturbances, respiratory difficulty, weakness, or signs of hypersensitivity reactions

D. Antibiotics

  1. Description

    a. Aminoglycoside antibiotics or fluoroquinolones are given with at least one other antitubercular medication.

    b. Bactericidal because of receptor-binding action interfering with protein synthesis in susceptible microorganisms

    c. GI disturbances are the most common side effect.

    d. Fluoroquinolones are not recommended for use in children.

  2. Contraindications and cautions

    a. Contraindicated in clients with hypersensitivity, neuromuscular disorders, or eighth cranial nerve damage

    b. Used with caution in the older client, in neonates because of renal insufficiency and immaturity, and in young infants because it may cause CNS depression

    c. The risk of toxicity increases if taken with other aminoglycosides or nephrotoxicity- or ototoxicity-producing medications

  3. Side and adverse effects

    a. Hypersensitivity

    b. Pain and irritation at the injection site

    c. Nephrotoxicity is indicated by increased blood urea nitrogen and serum creatinine levels.

    d. Ototoxicity is indicated by tinnitus, dizziness, ringing or roaring in the ears, and reduced hearing.

    e. Neurotoxicity is indicated by headache, dizziness, lethargy, tremors, and visual disturbances.

    f. Superinfections

  4. Interventions

    a. Monitor for hypersensitivity.

    b. Monitor for ototoxic, neurotoxic, and nephrotoxic reactions.

    c. Monitor liver and renal function test results.

    d. Baseline audiometric test is obtained and repeated every 1 to 2 months because the medication impairs the eighth cranial nerve.

    e. Determine acuteness of hearing.

    f. Monitor for visual changes.

    g. Determine hydration status and maintain adequate hydration during therapy.

    h. Monitor intake and output.

    i. Monitor urinalysis results.

    j. Monitor for superinfection.

  5. Client education: To notify the PHCP if hearing loss, changes in vision, or urinary problems occur

E. Ethionamide

  1. Description

    a. Mechanism of action is unknown.

    b. Used to treat MDR-TB when significant resistance to other medications is expected

  2. Contraindications and cautions

    a. Contraindicated in clients with hypersensitivity

    b. Used with caution in clients with diabetes mellitus or renal dysfunction

  3. Side and adverse effects

    a. Anorexia, nausea, vomiting

    b. Metallic taste in the mouth

    c. Orthostatic hypotension

    d. Jaundice

    e. Change in mental status

    f. Peripheral neuritis

    g. Rash

  4. Interventions

    a. Monitor liver and renal function test results.

    b. Monitor glucose level in the client with diabetes mellitus.

    c. Administered as prescribed to reduce the risk of neurotoxicity

  5. Client education

    a. To take medication with food or meals to minimize GI irritation

    b. To change positions slowly

    c. To report signs of a rash, which can progress to exfoliative dermatitis if the medication is not discontinued

F. Aminosalicylic acid

  1. Description

    a. Inhibits folic acid metabolism in mycobacteria

    b. Used to treat MDR-TB when significant resistance to other medications is expected

  2. Contraindications and cautions

    a. Contraindicated with hypersensitivity to aminosalicylates, salicylates, or compounds containing the para-aminophenol group

    b. Aminobenzoates block the absorption of aminosalicylate sodium.

  3. Side and adverse effects

    a. Hypersensitivity

    b. Bitter taste in the mouth

    c. GI tract irritation

    d. Exfoliative dermatitis

e. Blood dyscrasias

f. Crystalluria

g. Change in thyroid function

4. Interventions

a. Monitor for hypersensitivity.

b. Offer clear water to rinse the mouth and chewing gum or hard candy to alleviate the bitter taste.

c. Encourage fluid intake to prevent crystalluria.

d. Monitor intake and output.

5. Client education

a. To discard the medication and obtain a new supply if a purplish-brown discoloration occurs

b. To take the medication with food

c. That urine may turn red if in contact with hypochlorite bleach, if bleach was used to clean a toilet

d. Not to take aspirin or over-the-counter medications without the PHCP's approval

e. To report signs of a blood dyscrasia such as sore throat or mouth, malaise, fatigue, bruising, or bleeding

G. Cycloserine

1. Description

a. Interferes with cell wall biosynthesis

b. Used to treat MDR-TB when significant resistance to other medications is expected

2. Contraindications and cautions

a. Use of alcohol or ethionamide increases the risk of seizure.

b. Used with caution in clients with seizure disorder, depression, severe anxiety, psychosis, or renal insufficiency, or in clients who use alcohol

3. Side and adverse effects

a. Hypersensitivity

b. CNS reactions

c. Neurotoxicity

d. Seizure

e. Heart failure

f. Headache

g. Vertigo

h. Altered level of consciousness

i. Irritability, nervousness, anxiety

j. Confusion

k. Change in mood, depression, thoughts of suicide

4. Interventions

a. Monitor level of consciousness.

b. Monitor for change in mental status and thought processes.

c. Monitor renal and hepatic function tests.

d. Monitor serum drug level to avoid the risk of neurotoxicity; the peak concentration, measured 2 hours after dosing, should be 25 to 35 mcg/mL.

5. Client education

a. To take the medication after meals to prevent GI upset

b. To report signs of a rash or signs of CNS toxicity

c. To avoid driving or performing tasks that require alertness until the reaction to the medication has been determined

d. About the need for monitoring serum drug levels weekly as prescribed

H. Streptomycin

1. Description

a. An aminoglycoside antibiotic used with at least one other antitubercular medication

b. Bactericidal because of receptor-binding action that interferes with protein synthesis in susceptible organisms

2. Contraindications and cautions

a. Contraindicated in clients with hypersensitivity, myasthenia gravis, parkinsonism, or eighth cranial nerve damage

b. Used with caution in the older client, in neonates because of renal insufficiency and organ immaturity, and in young infants because the medication may cause CNS depression

c. The risk of toxicity increases when streptomycin is taken with other aminoglycosides or nephrotoxicity or ototoxicity-producing medications.

3. Side and adverse effects (Box 48.8)

4. Interventions

a. Monitor for hypersensitivity.

b. Monitor liver and renal function test results.

c. Monitor for ototoxic, neurotoxic, and nephrotoxic reactions.

d. Baseline audiometric testing is performed and repeated every 1 to 2 months because the medication impairs the eighth cranial nerve.

e. Monitor for change in vision.

f. Monitor hydration status and maintain adequate hydration during therapy.

g. Monitor intake and output.

h. Monitor urinalysis results.

i. Monitor for signs of peripheral neuritis.

5. Client education: To notify the PHCP if hearing loss, change in vision, or urinary problems occur

XVI. Influenza Medications

A. Vaccines

1. Description

a. Because the strain of influenza virus is different every year, annual vaccination is recommended (usually sometime during September to April); each time a flu vaccine is administered, the nurse would inform the client of any updated information regarding the vaccine.

BOX 48.8	Side and Adverse Effects of Streptomycin

Nephrotoxicity
Changes in urine output
Decreased appetite
Increased thirst
Nausea, vomiting

Neurotoxicity
Muscle numbness
Seizure
Tingling
Twitching

Vestibular Toxicity
Clumsiness
Dizziness
Unsteadiness

Auditory Toxicity (Ototoxicity)
A full feeling in the ears
Ringing in the ears
Loss of hearing

b. Vaccine is available as inactivated influenza vaccine administered intramuscularly or as a live attenuated influenza vaccine, which is administered nasally.

⚠ The trivalent influenza vaccine includes vaccination against H1N1 and H3N2 strains (influenza A strains) and an influenza B strain. Because the strain of influenza virus is different every year, vaccine components may change. The vaccine is recommended for all individuals unless a contraindication to receiving it exists.

2. Vaccine
   a. The nasal spray (live) vaccine is approved only for healthy people ages 2 through 49.
   b. The nasal spray vaccine is not approved for pregnant women.
   c. The flu shots (inactivated vaccine), depending on the manufacturer, are approved for children as young as 6 months of age and are safe for pregnant women.
   d. The nasal spray contains a live flu virus that has been weakened to the point that it cannot cause the flu; its advantage is that it may elicit a stronger immune response than the flu shot in children who have never had the flu or a flu vaccine before.
   e. The disadvantage of the nasal spray is that it may not be quite as protective as the flu shot for older people who have previously had the flu or a flu vaccine.
   f. All individuals should receive an influenza vaccine. High-priority individuals include pregnant women; household contacts and caregivers of

children younger than 6 months of age; people ages 6 months to 24 years; health care workers and emergency medical personnel; and adults ages 25 to 64 with a chronic medical condition such as asthma, or a weakened immune system that increases the risk of flu complications.

3. Contraindications and cautions
   a. Contraindications of the inactivated vaccine include hypersensitivity, active infection, Guillain-Barré syndrome, active febrile illness, and children younger than 6 months.
   b. Contraindications of the live attenuated vaccine include age younger than 2 years or adults 50 years or older; pregnant women; children or adolescents on long-term aspirin therapy; and those with severe nasal congestion or long-term conditions such as asthma, diabetes mellitus, anemia or blood disorders, or heart, kidney, or lung disease.

4. Side and adverse effects
   a. Inactivated vaccine: Localized pain and swelling at the injection site, general body aches and pains, malaise, fever
   b. Attenuated vaccine: Runny nose or nasal congestion, cough, headache, and sore throat

5. Interventions
   a. The intramuscular route is recommended for the inactivated vaccine; adults and older children need to be vaccinated in the deltoid muscle.
   b. Monitor for side and adverse effects of the vaccine.
   c. Monitor for hypersensitivity reactions in clients receiving vaccination for the first time.

6. Client education
   a. About the importance of an annual vaccination
   b. That the inactivated vaccine contains noninfectious killed viruses and cannot cause influenza
   c. That any respiratory disease unrelated to influenza can occur after the vaccination
   d. That if the attenuated vaccine is received, the virus may be shed in secretions up to 2 days after vaccination
   e. That development of antibodies in adults takes approximately 2 weeks

7. Visit the Centers for Disease Control and Prevention for updates http://www.cdc.gov/flu/protect/vaccine/index.htm

B. Antiviral medications (Table 48.1)
   1. Description
      a. Use during outbreaks of influenza depends on the current strain of influenza.
      b. Diagnosis of influenza needs to include rapid diagnostic tests because symptoms of infection from other pathogens may cause symptoms similar to those of influenza infection.

TABLE 48.1 Side and Adverse Effects of Antiviral Influenza Medications

Antiviral Medications	Side and Adverse Effects
Amantadine	Drowsiness, anxiety, psychosis, depression, hallucinations, tremors, confusion, insomnia, orthostatic hypotension, heart failure, blurred vision, constipation, dry mouth, urinary frequency or retention, leukopenia, photosensitivity, dermatitis
Oseltamivir	Insomnia, diarrhea, abdominal pain, cough
Rimantadine	Depression, hallucinations, tremors, seizures, insomnia, poor concentration, asthenia, gait abnormalities, anxiety, confusion, pallor, palpitations, hypotension, edema, tinnitus, eye pain, constipation, dry mouth, anorexia, abdominal pain, diarrhea, dyspepsia, rash
Zanamivir	Ear, nose, and throat infections; diarrhea; nasal symptoms; cough; sinusitis; bronchitis
Peramivir	Diarrhea, constipation, insomnia, high blood pressure

c. May also be administered as prophylaxis against infection but would not replace vaccination
2. Contraindicated in hypersensitive clients
3. Side and adverse effects (see Table 48.1)
4. Interventions
  a. Administered within 2 days of onset of symptoms and continued for the entire prescription
  b. Monitor for side and adverse effects of specific medications.
5. Client education
  a. That the medication may not prevent the transmission of influenza to others
  b. About the need to adjust activities if dizziness or fatigue occur
  c. About management of side and adverse effects of various medications
  d. To take medication exactly as prescribed and for the duration of prescription

XVII. Pneumococcal Conjugate Vaccine

A. Pneumococcal conjugate vaccine is used for the prevention of invasive pneumococcal disease in infants and children.
B. Pneumococcal polysaccharide vaccine is used for adults and high-risk children older than 2 years.
C. Side and adverse effects include erythema, swelling, pain and tenderness at the injection site, fever, irritability, drowsiness, and reduced appetite.
D. See Chapter 37 for additional information about vaccines for pneumonia.

WHAT WOULD YOU DO?

Answer: An adverse effect of isoniazid is nonviral hepatitis. Manifestations include anorexia, nausea, vomiting, weakness, fatigue, dark urine, or jaundice. If these symptoms occur, the nurse would withhold the medication and notify the RN. The PHCP is also notified. The nurse would also check the client's liver function test results for elevations such as alanine aminotransferase (ALT), the normal level being 4 to 36 units/L; aspartate aminotransferase (AST), the normal level being 0 to 35 units/L; and the total bilirubin level, the normal level being 0.3 to 1.0 mg/dL. If these are elevated, the client could be experiencing nonviral hepatitis.

PRACTICE QUESTIONS

❖ 1. Rifabutin is prescribed for a client with active Mycobacterium avium complex (MAC) disease and tuberculosis. The nurse needs to monitor for which side/adverse effects of the medication? **Select all that apply.**
  ☐ 1. Signs of hepatitis
  ☐ 2. Flu-like syndrome
  ☐ 3. Low neutrophil count
  ☐ 4. Vitamin B$_6$ deficiency
  ☐ 5. Ocular pain or blurred vision
  ☐ 6. Tingling and numbness of the fingers

2. A client has a prescription to take sustained-released guaifenesin every 4 hours, as needed. The nurse determines that the client understands how to **most effectively** use this medication if the client makes which statement?
  1. "I will watch for irritability as a side effect."
  2. "I will take the tablet with a full glass of water."
  3. "I will take an extra dose if the cough is accompanied by fever."
  4. "I will crush the sustained-release tablet if immediate relief is needed."

3. A postoperative client has received a dose of naloxone hydrochloride for respiratory depression shortly after transfer to the nursing unit from the postanesthesia care unit. After administration of the medication, the nurse needs to check the client for which sign/symptom?
  1. Pupillary changes
  2. Scattered lung wheezes
  3. Sudden increase in pain
  4. Sudden episodes of diarrhea

4. A client has been taking isoniazid for 2 months. The client complains to the nurse about numbness, paresthesia, and tingling in the extremities. The nurse interprets that the client is experiencing which problem?
   1. Hypercalcemia
   2. Peripheral neuritis
   3. Small blood vessel spasm
   4. Impaired peripheral circulation

5. A client is to begin a 6-month course of therapy with isoniazid. The nurse would plan to provide which information to the client?
   1. Drink alcohol in small amounts only.
   2. Report yellow eyes or skin immediately.
   3. Increase intake of Swiss or aged cheeses.
   4. Avoid vitamin supplements during therapy.

6. A client has been started on long-term therapy with rifampin. Which information about this medication would the nurse provide to the client?
   1. Always take the medication with food or antacids.
   2. Double-dose the medication if one dose is forgotten.
   3. Red-orange discoloration of sweat, tears, urine, and feces may occur.
   4. May be discontinued independently if symptoms are gone in 3 months

7. The nurse has given a client taking ethambutol information about the medication. The nurse determines that the client understands the instructions if the client states to report which occurrence **immediately**?
   1. Impaired sense of hearing
   2. Problems with visual acuity
   3. Gastrointestinal (GI) side effects
   4. Red-orange discoloration of body secretions

8. Cycloserine is added to the medication regimen for a client with tuberculosis. Which instruction would the nurse reinforce in the client-teaching plan regarding this medication?
   1. To take the medication 1 hour before meals
   2. To return to the clinic weekly for serum drug-level testing
   3. Alcohol intake is acceptable when taking this medication.
   4. Expect to experience skin rashes while taking this medication.

9. A client with tuberculosis is being started on antituberculosis therapy with isoniazid. Before giving the client the first dose, the nurse ensures that which baseline study has been completed?
   1. Electrolyte levels
   2. Coagulation times
   3. Liver enzyme levels
   4. Serum creatinine level

10. A client is receiving acetylcysteine, 20% solution diluted in 0.9% normal saline by nebulizer. The nurse needs to have which item available for a possible adverse event after giving this medication?
    1. Ambu bag
    2. Intubation tray
    3. Nasogastric tube
    4. Suction equipment

ANSWERS

❖ **1. 1, 2, 3, 5**
Rationale: Rifabutin may be prescribed for a client with active MAC disease and tuberculosis. It inhibits mycobacterial DNA–dependent RNA polymerase and suppresses protein synthesis. Side effects include rash, gastrointestinal (GI) disturbances, neutropenia (low neutrophil count), red-orange body secretions, uveitis (blurred vision and eye pain), myositis, arthralgia, hepatitis, chest pain with dyspnea, and flu-like syndrome. Vitamin B_6 deficiency and numbness and tingling in the extremities are associated with the use of isoniazid. Ethambutol also causes peripheral neuritis.
Test-Taking Strategy: Focus on the subject, side and adverse effects of rifabutin. Note the name of the medication to assist in answering the question. Recalling that vitamin B_6 deficiency

and numbness and tingling in the extremities are associated with the use of isoniazid and ethambutol, not rifabutin, will assist in answering.

2. 2
Rationale: Guaifenesin is an expectorant. It needs to be taken with a full glass of water to decrease the viscosity of secretions. Sustained-release preparations are not to be broken open, crushed, or chewed. The medication may occasionally cause dizziness, headache, or drowsiness. The client needs to contact the primary health care provider (PHCP) if the cough lasts longer than 1 week or is accompanied by fever, rash, sore throat, or persistent headache.
Test-Taking Strategy: Note the strategic words, *most effectively*. Begin to answer this question by eliminating option 4 first. Sustained-release preparations are not crushed or

broken. Option 3 is eliminated next because fever indicates infection, and an "extra dose" of an expectorant is not helpful in treating infection. From the remaining options, recalling that increased fluids help liquefy secretions for more effective coughing will direct you to the correct option.

3. 3

Rationale: Naloxone hydrochloride is an antidote to opioids and may also be given to the postoperative client to treat respiratory depression. When given to the postoperative client for respiratory depression, it may also reverse the effects of analgesics. Therefore, the nurse needs to check the client for a sudden increase in the level of pain experienced. Options 1, 2, and 4 are not associated with this medication.

Test-Taking Strategy: Focus on the subject, the purpose and effect of administering naloxone hydrochloride. Recalling that this medication is an antidote to opioid analgesics will assist with directing you to option 3. Remember that this medication will cause sudden pain in the postoperative client or return of pain in the client who received opioid analgesics.

4. 2

Rationale: A common adverse effect of isoniazid is peripheral neuritis. This is manifested by numbness, tingling, and paresthesias in the extremities. This adverse effect can be minimized by pyridoxine (vitamin B_6) intake. Options 1, 3, and 4 are incorrect.

Test-Taking Strategy: Focus on the subject, a problem associated with isoniazid. Options 3 and 4 would not cause the symptoms presented in the question but instead would cause pallor and coolness. From the remaining options, you need to know either that peripheral neuritis is an adverse effect of the medication or that the data in the question do not correlate with hypercalcemia.

5. 2

Rationale: Isoniazid is hepatotoxic, and therefore the client is taught to report signs/symptoms of hepatitis immediately (which include yellow skin and sclera). For the same reason, alcohol needs to be avoided during therapy. The client would avoid intake of Swiss cheese, fish such as tuna, and foods containing tyramine because they may cause a reaction characterized by redness and itching of the skin, flushing, sweating, tachycardia, headache, or light-headedness. The client can avoid developing peripheral neuritis by increasing the intake of pyridoxine (vitamin B_6) during the course of isoniazid therapy.

Test-Taking Strategy: Focus on the subject, signs/symptoms to report associated with use of isoniazid. Alcohol intake is avoided when the client is taking a prescribed medication, so option 1 would be eliminated first. Because the client receiving this medication typically is supplemented with pyridoxine (vitamin B_6), option 4 is incorrect and is eliminated next. From the remaining options, recalling that the medication is hepatotoxic will direct you to the correct option.

6. 3

Rationale: Rifampin needs to be taken exactly as directed. Doses are not to be doubled or skipped. The client would not stop therapy until directed to do so by a PHCP. The medication needs to be administered on an empty stomach unless it causes GI upset, and then it may be taken with food. Antacids,

if prescribed, need to be taken at least 1 hour before the medication. Rifampin causes red-orange discoloration of body secretions and will permanently stain soft contact lenses.

Test-Taking Strategy: Focus on the subject, client teaching associated with rifampin. Use of general medication administration principles will assist with eliminating options 2 and 4. Eliminate option 1 next because of the closed-ended word, *always*.

7. 2

Rationale: Ethambutol causes optic neuritis, which decreases visual acuity and the ability to discriminate between the colors red and green. This poses a potential safety hazard when a client is driving a motor vehicle. The client is taught to report this symptom immediately. The client is also taught to take the medication with food if GI upset occurs. Impaired hearing results from antitubercular therapy with streptomycin. Red-orange discoloration of secretions occurs with rifampin.

Test-Taking Strategy: Focus on the subject, client understanding of instructions given regarding ethambutol. Also note the strategic word, *immediately*. Option 3 is the least likely symptom to report; rather, it would be managed by taking the medication with food. To select from the other options, it is necessary to know that this medication causes optic neuritis, resulting in difficulty with red-green discrimination.

8. 2

Rationale: Cycloserine is an antitubercular medication that requires weekly serum drug level determinations to monitor for the potential of neurotoxicity. Serum drug levels lower than 30 mcg/mL reduce the incidence of neurotoxicity. The medication needs to be taken after meals to prevent GI irritation. The client needs to be instructed to notify the PHCP if a skin rash or signs of central nervous system toxicity are noted. Alcohol must be avoided because it increases the risk of seizure activity.

Test-Taking Strategy: Focus on the subject, client teaching regarding the use of cycloserine. Eliminate options 3 and 4 first, using guidelines related to general medication administration principles. From this point, knowing that the medication level needs to be monitored will assist with selecting the correct option.

9. 3

Rationale: Isoniazid therapy can cause an elevation of hepatic enzyme levels and hepatitis. Therefore, liver enzyme levels are monitored when therapy is initiated and during the first 3 months of therapy. They may be monitored longer in the client who is greater than age 50 or abuses alcohol.

Test-Taking Strategy: Focus on the subject, laboratory monitoring associated with isoniazid. In order to answer this question correctly, it is necessary to know that this medication can be toxic to the liver.

10. 4

Rationale: Acetylcysteine can be given orally or by nasogastric tube to treat acetaminophen overdose, or it may be given by inhalation for use as a mucolytic. The nurse administering this medication as a mucolytic needs to have suction equipment available in case the client cannot manage to clear the increased volume of liquefied secretions.

Test-Taking Strategy: Focus on the subject, equipment necessary in the administration of acetylcysteine. To answer this question, it is necessary to know that acetylcysteine may be given for either acetaminophen overdose or as a mucolytic agent. It is also necessary to know that the inhalation route is only used for mucolytic effects. With this in mind, options 1 and 2 are eliminated because it is unlikely that the client will need resuscitation. Option 3 is eliminated as well because a nasogastric tube may be used in the client with acetaminophen overdose but is not necessary when used as a mucolytic.

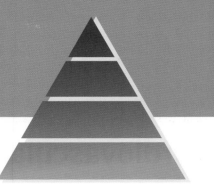

Cardiovascular Problems of the Adult Client

Pyramid to Success

Pyramid Points focus on data related to cardiovascular risks, health screening and promotion and client education, complications of the various cardiovascular health problems, emergency measures, and client education. Focus on the manifestations and treatment in angina, myocardial infarction, heart failure and pulmonary edema, pericarditis, aneurysms, hypertension, and arterial and venous disorders. Focus also on the care of the client following cardiovascular diagnostic treatments and surgical procedures. Note appropriate and therapeutic client positions, particularly with arterial and venous disorders of the extremities. Focus on treatments and medications prescribed for the various cardiovascular health problems and client teaching related to prescribed treatment plans. Be familiar with the components related to cardiac rehabilitation.

Client Needs: Learning Objectives

Safe and Effective Care Environment
  Consulting with the interprofessional health care team
  Establishing priorities
  Maintaining asepsis
  Maintaining standard and other precautions
  Recognizing the need for consultations and referrals
  Upholding client rights
  Verifying that informed consent related to treatments and procedures has been obtained
Health Promotion and Maintenance
  Assisting with providing health screening and health promotion programs

Assisting with mobilizing appropriate community resources
  Client education regarding prevention of cardiovascular health problems
  Discussing alterations in lifestyle
  Identifying risk factors associated with cardiovascular problems
  Implementing cardiovascular data collection techniques
  Preventing cardiovascular health problems
  Promoting cardiac rehabilitation
  Teaching related to diet therapy, exercise, and medications
Psychosocial Integrity
  Assisting the client with accepting lifestyle changes
  Considering religious, spiritual, and cultural influences on health
  Discussing grief and loss and end-of-life issues
  Discussing situational role changes
  Discussing unexpected body image changes
  Identifying coping mechanisms
  Identifying fear, anxiety, and denial
  Identifying support systems
Physiological Integrity
  Administering medications
  Discussing activity limitations and promoting rest and sleep
  Differentiating between the manifestations of angina and myocardial infarction
  Monitoring for complications related to cardiovascular health problems
  Monitoring for therapeutic effects of medications
  Monitoring of cardiac enzyme and troponin levels and other cardiovascular-related laboratory values
  Providing interventions required during emergencies
  Providing nonpharmacological and pharmacological comfort interventions
  Responding to medical emergencies as appropriate

Client Needs lists modified from: National Council of State Boards of Nursing, Inc. (NCSBN). *NCLEX-PN Examination: Test Plan for the National Council Licensure Examination for Practical Nurses,* effective April 2020. Chicago: NCSBN.

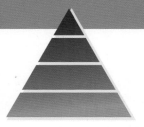

CHAPTER **49**

Cardiovascular Problems

PRIORITY CONCEPTS Health Promotion; Perfusion

WHAT WOULD YOU DO?

A hospitalized client with a diagnosis of abdominal aortic aneurysm suddenly complains of severe back pain and shortness of breath. What would the nurse do?
Answer is located on p. 680

I. Anatomy and Physiology

A. Heart and heart wall layers
  1. The heart is located in the left side of the mediastinum.
  2. The heart consists of three layers.
    a. The epicardium is the outermost layer of the heart.
    b. The myocardium is the middle layer and actual contracting muscle of the heart.
    c. The endocardium is the innermost layer and lines the inner chambers and heart valves.
B. Pericardial sac
  1. Encases and protects the heart from trauma and infection
  2. Has two layers
    a. The parietal pericardium is the tough, fibrous outer membrane that attaches anteriorly to the lower half of the sternum, posteriorly to the thoracic vertebrae, and inferiorly to the diaphragm.
    b. The visceral pericardium is the thin, inner layer that closely adheres to the heart.
  3. The pericardial space is between the parietal and visceral layers. It holds 5 to 20 mL of pericardial fluid, lubricates the pericardial surfaces, and cushions the heart.
C. There are four heart chambers.
  1. The right atrium receives deoxygenated blood from the body via the superior and inferior vena cava.
  2. The right ventricle receives blood from the right atrium and pumps it to the lungs via the pulmonary artery.

3. The left atrium receives oxygenated blood from the lungs via four pulmonary veins.
  4. The left ventricle is the largest and most muscular chamber. It receives oxygenated blood from the lungs via the left atrium and pumps blood into the systemic circulation via the aorta.
D. There are four valves in the heart.
  1. There are two atrioventricular (AV) valves, the tricuspid and the mitral, which lie between the atria and ventricles.
    a. The tricuspid valve is located on the right side of the heart.
    b. The bicuspid (mitral) valve is located on the left side of the heart.
    c. The AV valves close at the beginning of ventricular contraction and prevent blood from flowing back into the atria from the ventricles. These valves open when the ventricle relaxes.
  2. There are two semilunar valves, the pulmonic and the aortic.
    a. The pulmonic semilunar valve lies between the right ventricle and the pulmonary artery.
    b. The aortic semilunar valve lies between the left ventricle and the aorta.
    c. The semilunar valves prevent blood from flowing back into the ventricles during relaxation. They open during ventricular contraction and close when the ventricles begin to relax.
E. Sinoatrial (SA) node
  1. The main pacemaker that initiates each heartbeat
  2. Located at the junction of the superior vena cava and the right atrium
  3. The SA node generates electrical impulses at 60 to 100 beats/min and is controlled by the sympathetic and parasympathetic nervous systems.
F. AV node
  1. Located in the lower aspect of the atrial septum
  2. Receives electrical impulses from the SA node
  3. If the SA node fails, the AV node can initiate and sustain a heart rate of 40 to 60 beats/min.

G. The bundle of His
  1. A continuation of the AV node; located at the interventricular septum
  2. It branches into the right bundle branch, which extends down the right side of the interventricular septum, and the left bundle branch which extends into the left ventricle.
  3. The right and left bundle branches terminate into Purkinje fibers.
H. Purkinje fibers
  1. Purkinje fibers are a diffuse network of conducting strands located beneath the ventricular endocardium.
  2. These fibers spread the wave of depolarization through the ventricles.
  3. Purkinje fibers can act as the pacemaker with a rate between 20 and 40 beats/min when higher pacemakers (such as the SA and AV nodes) fail.
I. Coronary arteries (Fig. 49.1)
  1. The right main coronary artery supplies the right atrium and ventricle, the inferior portion of the left ventricle, the posterior septal wall, and the SA and AV nodes.
  2. The left main coronary artery consists of two major branches, the left anterior descending (LAD) and the circumflex arteries.
  3. The LAD artery supplies blood to the anterior wall of the left ventricle, the anterior ventricular septum, and the apex of the left ventricle.
  4. The circumflex artery supplies blood to the left atrium and the lateral and posterior surfaces of the left ventricle.

⚠ The coronary arteries supply the capillaries of the myocardium with blood. If blockage occurs in these arteries, the client is at risk for myocardial infarction (MI).

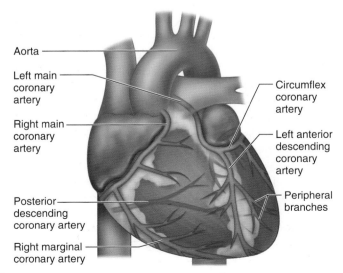

Aorta
Left main coronary artery
Right main coronary artery
Posterior descending coronary artery
Right marginal coronary artery
Circumflex coronary artery
Left anterior descending coronary artery
Peripheral branches

FIGURE 49.1 Coronary arterial system.

J. Heart sounds
  1. The first heart sound (S_1) is heard as the AV valves close and is heard loudest at the apex of the heart.
  2. The second heart sound (S_2) is heard when the semilunar valves close and is heard loudest at the base of the heart.
  3. A third heart sound (S_3) may be heard if ventricular wall compliance is decreased and structures in the ventricular wall vibrate; this can occur in conditions such as heart failure or valvular regurgitation. However, a third heart sound may be normal in individuals younger than 30 years.
  4. A fourth heart sound (S_4) may be heard on atrial systole if resistance to ventricular filling is present; this is an abnormal finding, and the causes include cardiac hypertrophy, disease, or injury to the ventricular wall.
K. Heart rate
  1. The faster the heart rate, the less time the heart has for filling, and the cardiac output decreases.
  2. The normal sinus heart rate is 60 to 100 beats/min.
  3. Sinus tachycardia is a rate greater than 100 beats/min.
  4. Sinus bradycardia is a rate less than 60 beats/min.
L. Autonomic nervous system
  1. Stimulation of sympathetic nerve fibers releases the neurotransmitter norepinephrine, producing an increased heart rate, increased conduction speed through the AV node, increased atrial and ventricular contractility, and peripheral vasoconstriction. Stimulation occurs when a decrease in pressure is detected.
  2. Stimulation of the parasympathetic nerve fibers releases the neurotransmitter acetylcholine, which decreases the heart rate and lessens atrial and ventricular contractility and conductivity. Stimulation occurs when an increase in pressure is detected.
M. Blood pressure (BP) control
  1. Baroreceptors (specialized nerve endings affected by changes in the arterial BP), also called *pressoreceptors*, are located in the walls of the aortic arch and carotid sinuses.
  2. Increases in arterial pressure stimulate baroreceptors, and the heart rate and arterial pressure decrease.
  3. Decreases in arterial pressure reduce stimulation of the baroreceptors, and vasoconstriction and an increase in heart rate occur.
  4. Stretch receptors, located in the vena cava and the right atrium, respond to pressure changes that affect circulatory blood volume.
  5. When the BP decreases as a result of hypovolemia, a sympathetic response occurs causing an increased heart rate and blood vessel

constriction. When the BP increases as a result of hypervolemia, an opposite effect occurs.

6. Antidiuretic hormone (vasopressin) influences BP indirectly by regulating vascular volume.

7. Increases in blood volume result in decreased antidiuretic hormone release, increasing diuresis, and decreasing blood volume and thus decreasing BP.

8. Decreases in blood volume result in increased antidiuretic hormone release. This promotes an increase in blood volume and thus BP.

9. Renin, a potent vasoconstrictor, causes the BP to increase.

10. Renin converts angiotensinogen to angiotensin I; angiotensin I is then converted to angiotensin II in the lungs.

11. Angiotensin II stimulates the release of aldosterone which promotes water and sodium retention by the kidneys; this action increases blood volume and BP.

N. The vascular system

1. Arteries are vessels through which the blood passes away from the heart to various parts of the body. They convey highly oxygenated blood from the left side of the heart to the tissues.

2. Arterioles control the blood flow into the capillaries.

3. Capillaries allow the exchange of fluid and nutrients between the blood and the interstitial spaces.

4. Venules receive blood from the capillary bed and move blood into the veins.

5. Veins transport deoxygenated blood from the tissues back to the right heart and then the lungs for oxygenation.

6. Valves help return blood to the heart against the force of gravity.

7. The lymphatics drain the tissues and return the tissue fluid to the blood.

II. Diagnostic Tests and Procedures (Refer to Chapter 10 for further information on laboratory reference levels)

A. Cardiac markers

1. Troponin
   a. Troponin is composed of three proteins: troponin C, cardiac troponin I, and cardiac troponin T.
   b. A troponin value of 0.05 to 0.49 ng/mL is considered indeterminate; a value greater than 0.50 ng/mL indicates a strong probability of acute myocardial infarction.

2. Creatine kinase, myocardial muscle (CK-MB)
   a. An elevation in value indicates myocardial damage.
   b. An elevation occurs within 4 to 6 hours and peaks 18 to 24 hours following an acute ischemic attack.

c. Normal value (CK-2) in males: 2 to 6 ng/mL; females: 2 to 5 ng/mL.

3. Myoglobin
   a. Myoglobin is an oxygen-binding protein found in cardiac and skeletal muscle.
   b. The level rises within 2 hours after cell death with a rapid decline in the level after 7 hours; however, it is not cardiac specific.

B. Complete blood count

1. The red blood cell count decreases in rheumatic heart disease and infective endocarditis and increases in conditions characterized by inadequate tissue oxygenation.

2. The white blood cell count increases in infectious and inflammatory diseases of the heart and after MI because large numbers of white blood cells are needed to dispose of the necrotic tissue resulting from the infarction.

3. An elevated hematocrit can result from vascular volume depletion.

4. Decreases in hematocrit and hemoglobin can indicate anemia.

C. Blood coagulation factors: An increase in coagulation factors can occur during and after MI which places the client at greater risk of thrombophlebitis and extension of clots in the coronary arteries.

D. Serum lipids (refer to Chapter 10)

1. The lipid profile measures serum cholesterol, triglyceride, and lipoprotein levels.

2. The lipid profile is used to assess the risk of developing coronary artery disease.

3. Lipoprotein-*a* or *Lp(a)*, a modified form of LDL, increases atherosclerotic plaques and increases clots; value should be less than 30 mg/dL.

E. Homocysteine: Elevated levels may increase the risk of cardiovascular disease; normal value is 4.5 to 11.9 mcmol/L (gender and age dependent).

F. Highly sensitive C-reactive protein (hsCRP): Detects an inflammatory process such as that associated with the development of atherothrombosis; a level less than 1 mg/dL is considered low risk, and a level greater than 3 mg/dL places the client at risk for heart disease.

G. Microalbuminuria: A small amount of protein in the urine has been a marker for endothelial dysfunction in cardiovascular disease.

H. Electrolytes (refer to Chapter 8)

1. Potassium
   a. Hypokalemia causes increased cardiac electrical instability, ventricular dysrhythmia, and increased risk of digoxin toxicity.
   b. In hypokalemia, the electrocardiogram (ECG) may show flattening and inversion of the T-wave, the appearance of a U-wave, and ST depression.

    c. Hyperkalemia causes asystole and ventricular dysrhythmia.

    d. In hyperkalemia, the ECG may show tall peaked T-waves, widened QRS complexes, prolonged PR intervals, or flat P-waves.

2. Sodium

    a. Important in controlling contractility of the heart

    b. The serum sodium level decreases with the use of diuretics.

    c. The serum sodium level decreases in heart failure indicating water excess.

3. Calcium

    a. Hypocalcemia can cause ventricular dysrhythmias, prolonged ST and QT interval, and cardiac arrest.

    b. Hypercalcemia can cause a shortened ST segment and widened T-wave, AV block, tachycardia or bradycardia, digitalis hypersensitivity, and cardiac arrest.

4. Phosphorus level: Phosphorus levels need to be interpreted with calcium levels because the kidneys retain or excrete one electrolyte in an inverse relationship to the other.

5. Magnesium

    a. A low magnesium level can cause ventricular tachycardia (VT) and fibrillation.

    b. Electrocardiographic changes that may be observed with hypomagnesemia include tall T-waves and depressed ST segments.

    c. A high magnesium level can cause muscle weakness, hypotension, and bradycardia.

    d. Electrocardiographic changes that may be observed with hypermagnesemia include a prolonged PR interval and widened QRS complex.

⚠ Electrolyte and mineral imbalances can cause cardiac electrical instability that can result in life-threatening dysrhythmia.

I. Blood urea nitrogen: The blood urea nitrogen is elevated in heart disorders that adversely affect renal circulation such as heart failure and cardiogenic shock.

J. Blood glucose: An acute cardiac episode can elevate the blood glucose level.

K. B-type natriuretic peptide (BNP)

    1. BNP is released in response to atrial and ventricular stretch; serves as a marker for heart failure.

    2. BNP levels should be less than 100 ng/mL; the higher the level, the more severe the heart failure.

L. Chest x-ray

    1. Description: Radiography of the chest is done to determine the size, silhouette, and position of the heart.

    2. Interventions

        a. Prepare the client for x-ray film explaining the purpose and procedure.

        b. Remove jewelry.

        c. Ensure that the client is not pregnant.

M. Electrocardiography

    1. Description: This common noninvasive diagnostic test records the electrical activity of the heart and is useful for detecting cardiac dysrhythmia, detecting location and extent of MI, detecting cardiac hypertrophy, and for evaluation of the effectiveness of cardiac medications.

    2. Interventions

        a. Determine the client's ability to lie still. Advise the client to lie still, breathe normally, and refrain from talking during the test.

        b. Reassure the client that an electrical shock will not occur.

        c. Document any cardiac medications the client is taking.

N. Holter monitoring

    1. Description

        a. In this noninvasive test, the client wears a Holter monitor, and an electrocardiographic tracing is recorded continuously over a period of 24 hours or more while the client performs their activities of daily living.

        b. The Holter monitor identifies a dysrhythmia if it occurs and evaluates the effectiveness of antidysrhythmics or pacemaker therapy.

    2. Interventions

        a. Reinforce instructions to the client to resume normal daily activities and to maintain a diary documenting activities and any symptoms that may develop for correlation to the electrocardiographic tracing.

        b. Reinforce instructions to the client to avoid tub baths or showers because they will interfere with the electrocardiographic recorder device.

O. Echocardiography

    1. Description

        a. This noninvasive procedure is based on the principles of ultrasound and evaluates structural and functional changes in the heart.

        b. Heart chamber size is measured, ejection fraction is calculated, and flow gradient across the valves is determined.

        c. A transesophageal echocardiography may be done in which the echocardiogram is done through the esophagus; this is an invasive examination and requires pre- and postprocedure preparation, and care is similar to endoscopy procedures.

    2. Interventions: Determine the client's ability to lie still, and advise the client to lie still, breathe normally, and refrain from talking during the test.

P. Exercise electrocardiography testing (stress test)
  1. Description
      a. This noninvasive test studies the heart during activity and detects and evaluates coronary artery disease.
      b. Treadmill testing is the most commonly used mode of stress testing.
      c. If the client is unable to tolerate exercise, an intravenous (IV) infusion of dipyridamole or dobutamine hydrochloride is given to dilate the coronary arteries and simulate the effect of exercise; the client may need to be NPO (nothing by mouth) for 3 to 6 hours preprocedure.
  2. Preprocedure interventions
      a. Obtain an informed consent if required.
      b. Encourage adequate rest the night before the procedure.
      c. Reinforce instructions to the client about oral intake as prescribed (to maintain an NPO status or eat a light meal 1–2 hours before the procedure).
      d. Reinforce instructions to the client to avoid smoking, alcohol, and caffeine before the procedure.
      e. Reinforce instructions to the client to ask the primary health care provider (PHCP) about taking prescribed medication on the day of the procedure; theophylline products are usually held 12 hours before the test, and calcium channel blockers and beta blockers are usually withheld on the day of the test to allow the heart rate to increase during the stress portion of the test.
      f. Reinforce instructions to the client to wear nonconstrictive, comfortable clothing and supportive rubber-soled shoes for the exercise stress test.
      g. Reinforce instructions to the client to notify the PHCP or cardiologist if any chest pain, dizziness, or shortness of breath occurs during the procedure.
  3. Postprocedure interventions: Instruct the client to avoid taking a hot bath or shower for at least 1 to 2 hours.
Q. Myocardial nuclear perfusion imaging (MNPI)
  1. Description
      a. Nuclear cardiology is the use of radionuclide techniques and scanning in cardiovascular assessment.
      b. The most common tests include technetium pyrophosphate scanning, thallium imaging, and multigated cardiac blood pool imaging; can evaluate cardiac motion and calculate the ejection fraction.
  2. Preprocedure interventions
      a. Obtain informed consent.

      b. Inform the client that a small amount of radioisotope will be injected and that the radiation exposure and risks are minimal.
  3. Postprocedure interventions
      a. Monitor vital signs.
      b. Monitor injection site for bleeding or discomfort.
      c. Inform the client that fatigue is possible.
R. Magnetic resonance imaging (MRI)
  1. Description
      a. This is a noninvasive diagnostic test that produces an image of the heart or great vessels through interaction of magnetic fields, radio waves, and atomic nuclei.
      b. It provides information on chamber size and thickness, valve and ventricular function, and blood flow through the great vessels and coronary arteries.
  2. Preprocedure interventions
      a. Evaluate the client for the presence of a pacemaker or other implanted items that present a contraindication to the test.
      b. Ensure that the client has removed all metallic objects such as watches, jewelry, clothing with metal fasteners, and metal hair fasteners.
      c. Ensure that the client removes all credit cards or the cards will become demagnetized.
      d. Inform the client that he or she may experience claustrophobia while in the scanner.
S. Electrophysiological studies: An invasive procedure in which a programmed electrical stimulation of the heart is induced to cause dysrhythmia and conduction defects; assists in finding an accurate diagnosis and aids in determining treatment
T. Electronic-beam computer tomography scan (EBCT): Determines whether calcifications are present in the arteries; coronary artery calcium (CAC) score is provided (a score higher than 400 requires intensive preventive treatment).
U. Cardiac catheterization

  1. Description
      a. An invasive test involving insertion of a catheter into the heart and surrounding vessels
      b. Obtains information about the structure and performance of the heart chambers and valves and the coronary circulation
  2. Preprocedure interventions
      a. Obtain informed consent.
      b. Monitor for allergies to seafood, iodine, or radiopaque dyes. If allergic, the client may be premedicated with antihistamines and corticosteroids to prevent a reaction.
      c. Withhold solid food for 6 to 8 hours and liquids for 4 hours, as prescribed, to prevent vomiting and aspiration during the procedure.

d. Document the client's height and weight because these data will be needed to determine the amount of dye to be administered.

e. Document baseline vital signs and note the quality and presence of peripheral pulses for postprocedure comparison.

f. Inform the client that a local anesthetic will be administered before catheter insertion.

g. Inform the client that he or she may feel a fluttery feeling as the catheter passes through the heart; a flushed, warm feeling when the dye is injected; a desire to cough; and palpitations caused by heart irritability.

h. Prepare the insertion site by shaving and cleaning with an antiseptic solution, if prescribed.

i. Administer preprocedure medications such as sedatives, if prescribed.

j. Assist to insert an IV line if prescribed.

⚠ If a client taking metformin is scheduled to undergo a procedure requiring the administration of iodine dye, the metformin is withheld 24 to 48 hours (as prescribed) prior because of the risk of lactic acidosis. The medication is not resumed until directed to do so by the PHCP (usually 48 hours after the procedure or after renal function studies are done and the results are evaluated). The client is instructed to check the blood glucose before meals and at bedtime while off the metformin. The PHCP may prescribe sliding scale insulin if blood glucose levels are elevated.

3. Postprocedure interventions

a. Monitor vital signs and cardiac rhythm for dysrhythmia at least every 30 minutes for 2 hours initially.

b. Monitor for chest pain. If dysrhythmia or chest pain occurs, notify the PHCP.

c. Monitor peripheral pulses and the color, warmth, and sensation of the extremity distal to the insertion site at least every 30 minutes for 2 hours initially.

d. Notify the PHCP if the client complains of numbness and tingling; the extremity becomes cool, pale, or cyanotic; or loss of the peripheral pulses occurs. This could indicate clot formation and is an emergency.

e. Monitor the pressure dressing for bleeding or hematoma formation.

f. Apply compression device (if prescribed) to the insertion site to provide additional pressure if required. Utilize air removal device when appropriate and follow specific prescriptions for air removal at specified time intervals.

g. Monitor for bleeding. If bleeding occurs, apply manual pressure immediately and notify the PHCP.

h. Monitor for hematoma. If a hematoma develops, notify the PHCP.

i. Keep extremity extended for 4 to 6 hours, as prescribed, keeping the leg straight to prevent arterial occlusion.

j. Maintain strict bed rest for 6 to 12 hours, as prescribed; however, the client may turn from side to side. Do not elevate the head of the bed more than 15 degrees.

k. If the antecubital vessel was used, immobilize the arm with an armboard.

l. Encourage fluid intake, if not contraindicated, to promote renal excretion of the dye and replace fluid loss caused by the osmotic diuretic effect of the dye.

m. Monitor for nausea, vomiting, rash, or other signs of hypersensitivity to the dye.

V. Intravascular ultrasonography (IVUS): A catheter with a transducer is used as an alternative to injecting a dye into the coronary arteries and detects plaque distribution and composition; it also detects arterial dissection and the degree of stenosis of an occluded artery.

III. Therapeutic Management

A. Percutaneous transluminal coronary angioplasty (PTCA)

1. Description

a. An invasive, nonsurgical technique in which one or more arteries are dilated with a balloon catheter to open the vessel lumen and improve arterial blood flow

b. PTCA may be used for clients with an evolving MI alone or in combination with medications to achieve reperfusion.

c. The client can experience reocclusion after the procedure; thus the procedure may need to be repeated.

d. Complications can include arterial dissection or rupture, embolization of plaque fragments, spasm, and acute MI.

e. A firm commitment is needed on the part of the client to stop smoking, adhere to dietary restrictions, lose weight, alter exercise patterns, and stop any behaviors that could lead to the progression of artery occlusion.

2. Preprocedure interventions

a. Similar to preprocedure interventions for cardiac catheterization

b. The PHCP may prescribe preprocedure medications including acetylsalicylic acid.

c. Reinforce instructions to the client that chest pain may occur during balloon inflation and to report it if it does occur.

3. Postprocedure interventions

a. Similar to postprocedure intervention following cardiac catheterization

b. Administer anticoagulants and antiplatelets, as prescribed, to prevent thrombus formation.

c. IV nitroglycerin may be prescribed to prevent coronary artery vasospasm.

d. Encourage fluids if not contraindicated to enhance renal excretion of dye.

e. Reinforce instructions to the client in the administration of prescribed medications; daily acetylsalicylic acid may be prescribed.

f. Assist the client with planning lifestyle modifications.

B. Laser-assisted angioplasty

  1. Description

    a. A laser probe is advanced through a cannula similar to that used for PTCA.

    b. Used for clients with small occlusions in the distal superficial femoral, proximal popliteal, and common iliac arteries, and in the coronary arteries

    c. Heat from the laser vaporizes the plaque to open the occluded artery.

  2. Preprocedure and postprocedure interventions

    a. Care is similar to that for PTCA.

    b. Monitor for complications of coronary dissection, acute occlusion, perforation, embolism, and MI.

 C. Coronary artery stents

  1. Description

    a. Coronary artery stents are used in conjunction with PTCA to provide a supportive scaffold to eliminate the risk of acute coronary vessel closure and improve long-term patency of the vessel.

    b. A balloon catheter bearing the stent is inserted into the coronary artery and positioned at the site of occlusion. Balloon inflation deploys the stent.

    c. When placed in the coronary artery, the stent reopens the blocked artery.

  2. Preprocedure and postprocedure interventions

    a. Care is similar to that for PTCA.

    b. Acute thrombosis is a major concern following the procedure, and the client is placed on antiplatelet therapy such as clopidogrel and acetylsalicylic acid for several months after the procedure. Length of time of antiplatelet therapy is determined by the type of stent (metal or medication coated) that has been deployed.

    c. Monitor for complications of the procedure such as stent migration or occlusion, coronary artery dissection, and bleeding resulting from anticoagulation.

D. Atherectomy

  1. Description

    a. Atherectomy removes plaque from a coronary artery by the use of a cutting chamber on the inserted catheter or a rotating blade that pulverizes the plaque.

    b. Atherectomy is also used to improve blood flow to ischemic limbs in individuals with peripheral arterial disease.

  2. Preprocedure and postprocedure interventions

    a. Care is similar to that for PTCA.

    b. Monitor for complications of perforation, embolus, and reocclusion.

E. Transmyocardial revascularization

  1. May be used for clients with widespread atherosclerosis involving vessels that are too small and numerous for replacement or balloon catheterization. The procedure is performed through a small chest incision.

  2. Transmyocardial revascularization uses a high-powered laser that creates 20 to 24 channels through the ventricular muscle of the left ventricle, and blood enters these small channels providing the affected region of the heart with oxygenated blood.

  3. The opening on the surface of the heart heals; however, the main channels remain and perfuse the myocardium.

F. Peripheral arterial revascularization

  1. Description

    a. Performed to increase arterial blood flow to the affected limb

    b. Inflow procedures involve bypassing the arterial occlusion above the superficial femoral arteries.

    c. Outflow procedures involve bypassing the arterial occlusions at or below the superficial femoral arteries.

    d. Graft material is sutured above and below the occlusion to facilitate blood flow around the occlusion.

  2. Preoperative interventions

    a. Monitor baseline vital signs and peripheral pulses.

    b. Insert an IV line and urinary catheter as prescribed.

    c. Maintain a central venous catheter and/or arterial line if inserted.

  3. Postoperative interventions

    a. Monitor vital signs and notify the PHCP if changes occur.

    b. Monitor for hypotension, which may indicate hypovolemia or for hypertension which may place stress on the graft and facilitate clot formation.

    c. Maintain bed rest for 24 hours as prescribed.

    d. Instruct the client to keep the affected extremity straight, limit movement, and avoid bending the knee and hip.

    e. Monitor for warmth, redness, and edema, which are often expected outcomes because of increased blood flow.

f. Monitor for graft occlusion, which often occurs within the first 24 hours.

g. Monitor peripheral pulses and for adverse changes in color and temperature of the extremity.

h. Monitor the incision for drainage, warmth, or swelling.

i. Monitor for excessive bleeding. (A small amount of bloody drainage is expected.)

j. Monitor the area over the graft for hardness, tenderness, and warmth which may indicate infection. If this occurs, notify the PHCP immediately.

k. Reinforce instructions to the client about proper foot care and measures to prevent ulcer formation.

l. Assist the client in modifying lifestyle (such as diet) to prevent further plaque formation.

 Following arterial vascularization, monitor for a sharp increase in pain because pain is frequently the first indicator of postoperative graft occlusion. If signs of graft occlusion occur, notify the RN and PHCP immediately.

G. Coronary artery bypass grafting

1. Description

a. The occluded coronary arteries are bypassed with the client's own venous or arterial blood vessels.

b. The saphenous vein, internal mammary artery, or other arteries may be used to bypass lesions in the coronary arteries.

c. Coronary artery bypass grafting is performed when the client does not respond to medical management of coronary artery disease or when vessels are severely occluded.

d. A minimally invasive direct coronary artery bypass (MIDCAB) may be an option for some clients who have a lesion in the LAD artery; a sternal incision is not required (usually a 2-inch [5 cm] left thoracotomy incision is done) and cardiopulmonary bypass is not required in this procedure.

2. Preoperative interventions

a. Familiarize the client and family with the cardiac surgical critical care unit.

b. Inform the client to expect a sternal incision, possible arm or leg incision(s), one or two chest tubes, a Foley catheter, and several IV fluid catheters.

c. Inform the client that an endotracheal tube will be in place and that he or she will be unable to speak.

d. Advise the client that he or she will be placed on mechanical ventilation and to breathe with the ventilator and not fight it.

e. Reinforce instructions to the client to inform the nurse of any postoperative pain because pain medication will be available.

f. Reinforce instructions to the client on how to splint the chest incision, cough and deep breathe, use the incentive spirometer, and perform arm and leg exercises.

g. Encourage the client and family to discuss anxieties and fears related to surgery.

h. Note that prescribed medications may be discontinued preoperatively (usually diuretics 2–3 days before surgery, digoxin 12 hours before surgery, and aspirin and anticoagulants 1 week before surgery).

i. Administer medications as prescribed which may include potassium chloride, antihypertensives, antidysrhythmics, and antibiotics.

3. Transfer of the client from the cardiac surgical unit

a. Monitor vital signs, level of consciousness, and peripheral perfusion. (Alarm safety and alarm fatigue: Refer to Chapter 47.)

b. Monitor for dysrhythmias.

c. Auscultate lungs and monitor respiratory status.

d. Encourage the client to splint the incision, cough and deep breathe, and use the incentive spirometer to raise secretions and prevent atelectasis.

e. Monitor temperature and white blood cell count which indicate infection if elevated after 3 to 4 days.

f. Provide adequate fluids and hydration, as prescribed, to liquefy secretions.

g. Monitor suture line and chest tube insertion sites for redness, purulent discharge, and signs of infection.

h. Monitor sternal suture line for instability, which may indicate an infection.

i. Guide the client to gradually resume activity.

J. Monitor the client for tachycardia, postural (orthostatic) hypotension, and fatigue before, during, and after activity.

k. Discontinue activities if the BP drops more than 10 mm Hg to 20 mm Hg or the pulse increases more than 10 beats/min.

l. Monitor episodes of pain closely.

m. See Box 49.1 for home care instructions.

H. Heart transplantation

1. A donor heart from an individual with a comparable body weight and ABO compatibility is transplanted into a recipient within 6 hours of procurement.

2. The surgeon removes the diseased heart leaving the posterior portion of the atria to serve as an anchor for the new heart.

3. Because a remnant of the client's atria remains, two unrelated P-waves are noted on the ECG.

4. The transplanted heart is denervated and unresponsive to vagal stimulation. Because the heart is denervated, clients do not experience angina.

5. Symptoms of heart rejection include hypotension, dysrhythmia, weakness, fatigue, and dizziness.
6. Endomyocardial biopsies are performed at regular scheduled intervals and whenever rejection is suspected.
7. The client requires lifetime immunosuppressive therapy.
8. Strict aseptic technique and vigilant hand washing must be maintained when caring for the post-transplant client because of increased risk for infection from immunosuppression.
9. The heart rate approximates 100 beats/min and responds slowly to exercise or stress with regard to increases in heart rate, contractility, and cardiac output.

BOX 49.1 Homecare Instructions after Cardiac Surgery

Progressive return to activities at home.

Limiting of pushing or pulling activities for 6 weeks after discharge.

Maintenance of incisional care, and record signs of redness, swelling, or drainage.

Sternotomy incision heals in about 6–8 weeks.

Avoidance of crossing legs. Wear elastic hose if prescribed until edema subsides, and elevating surgical limb (if used to obtain graft) when sitting in a chair.

Use of prescribed medications.

Dietary measures, including the avoidance of saturated fats and cholesterol and the use of salt.

Resumption of sexual intercourse on the advice of the primary health care provider after exercise tolerance is assessed (usually, if the client can walk one block or climb two flights of stairs without symptoms, he or she can resume sexual activity safely)

IV. Cardiac Dysrhythmias

A. Normal sinus rhythm (Fig. 49.2)
  1. Rhythm originates from the SA node.
  2. Atrial and ventricular rhythms are regular at 60 to 100 beats/min.
  3. PR interval and QRS width are within normal limits.

B. Sinus bradycardia
  1. Atrial and ventricular rates are regular and less than 60 beats/min.
  2. PR interval and QRS width are within normal limits.
  3. Note that a low heart rate may be normal for some individuals, such as in athletes.
  4. Treatment may be necessary if the client is symptomatic (signs of decreased cardiac output).
  5. Treatment depends on the cause and may include holding a medication, oxygen, atropine sulfate, or a pacemaker; notify the registered nurse (RN).

C. Sinus tachycardia
  1. Atrial and ventricular rhythms are regular.
  2. Atrial and ventricular rates are 100 to 180 beats/min.
  3. PR interval and QRS width are within normal limits.
  4. Treatment depends on the cause; notify the RN.

D. Atrial fibrillation (Fig. 49.3)
  1. Multiple rapid impulses from many foci depolarize in the atria in a totally disorganized manner at a rate of 350 to 600 times per minute; the atria quiver, which can lead to the formation of thrombi.
  2. Usually no definitive P-wave can be observed—only fibrillatory waves before each QRS.
  3. Treatment includes oxygen, anticoagulants, cardiac medications, and possible cardioversion. Notify the RN.

E. Premature ventricular contractions (PVCs) (Box 49.2 and Fig. 49.4)

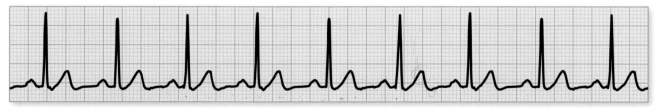

FIGURE 49.2 Normal sinus rhythm.

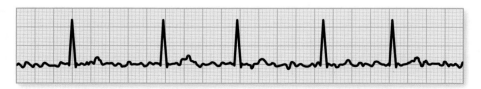

FIGURE 49.3 Atrial dysrhythmias—atrial fibrillation.

1. Early ventricular complexes result from increased irritability of the ventricles.
2. PVCs frequently occur in repetitive patterns such as bigeminy, trigemini, and quadrigeminy.
3. Treatment depends on the cause, and the RN is notified if PVCs occur.

> For the client experiencing PVCs, the PHCP is notified if the client complains of chest pain or if the PVCs increase in frequency, are multifocal, occur on the T-wave (R on T), or occur in runs of VT.

F. Ventricular Tachycardia (VT) (Fig. 49.5)

BOX 49.2   Premature Ventricular Contractions

Bigeminy: Premature ventricular contraction (PVC) every other heartbeat
Trigeminy: PVC every third heartbeat
Quadrigeminy: PVC every fourth heartbeat
Couplet or pair: Two sequential PVCs
Unifocal: Uniform upward or downward deflection arising from the same ectopic focus
Multifocal: Different shapes with the impulse generation from different sites
R-on-T phenomenon: PVC falls on the T wave of the preceding beat and may precipitate ventricular fibrillation

---

1. VT occurs because of a repetitive firing of an irritable ventricular ectopic focus at a rate of 140 to 250 beats/min or more and can lead to cardiac arrest. Notify the RN if VT occurs.
2. A stable client with sustained VT (with pulse and no signs or symptoms of decreased cardiac output) will be treated with oxygen and antidysrhythmics.
3. An unstable client with VT (with pulse and signs/symptoms of decreased cardiac output) will be treated with oxygen and antidysrhythmics and possible synchronized cardioversion. The PHCP may attempt cough cardiopulmonary resuscitation (CPR) by asking the client to cough hard every 1 to 3 seconds.
4. A pulseless client with VT will be treated with defibrillation and CPR.

G. Ventricular fibrillation (VF) (Fig. 49.6)
1. VF is a chaotic rapid rhythm in which the ventricles quiver and there is no cardiac output.
2. Client lacks a pulse, BP, respirations, heart sounds, and is unconscious; VF is fatal if not successfully terminated within 3 to 5 minutes.
3. Treatment includes CPR and immediate defibrillation.

H. Paroxysmal supraventricular tachycardia (PSVT)
1. Sudden, rapid onset of tachycardia originating in the AV node
2. Often begins and ends spontaneously

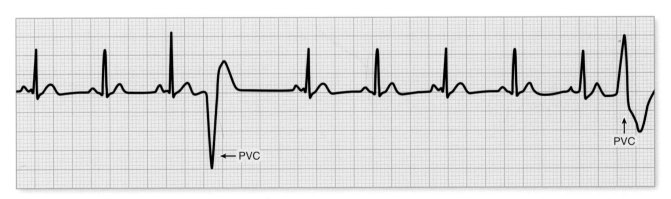

FIGURE 49.4 Normal sinus rhythm with multifocal premature ventricular contractions (one negative and the other positive).

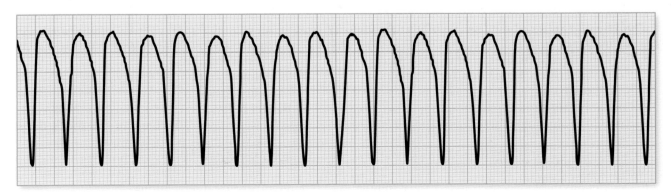

FIGURE 49.5 Ventricular tachycardia.

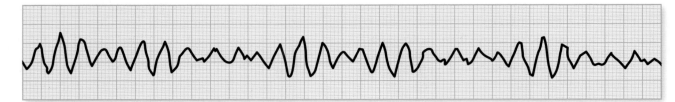

FIGURE 49.6 Ventricular fibrillation.

3. Sometimes excitement, fatigue, caffeine, smoking, or alcohol use precipitates PSVT.

I. Pulseless electrical activity

1. Organized electrical activity noted on the ECG, but there is no mechanical ventricular activity and therefore a pulse does not exist

2. Most common dysrhythmia noted after defibrillation

3. Treated with CPR and antidysrhythmic medications (epinephrine)

J. Guidelines for performing adult CPR

1. Follow CAB (compressions, airway, breathing) guidelines. If a victim is noted not breathing or only gasping, activate the emergency response system and obtain an automated external defibrillator (AED) or monophasic or biphasic defibrillator depending on the setting and equipment available.

2. Check the carotid pulse for a maximum of 10 seconds.

3. If no pulse is felt, begin chest compressions (100–120 per minute) at a depth of 2 inches (5 cm) for 2 minutes or 5 cycles of 30 compressions to 2 ventilations using a barrier device or bag valve mask.

4. To provide ventilations, the head-tilt chin-lift maneuver, or jaw thrust technique is used if neck injury is suspected.

5. Check rhythm and for presence of a pulse every 2 minutes or after 5 cycles (depending on the setting and equipment available, deliver a shock if indicated).

6. Switch compression and ventilation roles if another rescuer is available, to avoid fatigue.

7. Continue this process until the victim gains consciousness, starts breathing, or has a pulse.

8. If the victim has a pulse but is not breathing, continue with rescue breathing until help arrives and advanced cardiovascular life support measures are instituted.

9. For updated information, refer to 2020 American Heart Association Guidelines for Cardiopulmonary Resuscitation and Emergency Cardiovascular Care at https://professional.heart.org/en/science-news/2020-aha-guidelines-for-cpr-and-ecc/.

V. Management of Dysrhythmia

A. Vagal maneuvers

1. Description: Vagal maneuvers induce vagal stimulation of the cardiac conduction system and are used to terminate supraventricular tachydysrhythmia.

2. Carotid sinus massage

a. The PHCP instructs the client to turn the head away from the side to be massaged.

b. The PHCP massages over one carotid artery for a few seconds to determine whether a change in cardiac rhythm occurs.

c. The client needs to be on a cardiac monitor, and an ECG rhythm strip before, during, and after the procedure would be obtained and documented on the chart.

d. Have a defibrillator and resuscitative equipment available.

e. Monitor vital signs, cardiac rhythm, and level of consciousness after the procedure.

3. Valsalva maneuver

a. The PHCP instructs the client to bear down or induces a gag reflex in the client to stimulate a vagal response.

b. Monitor the heart rate, rhythm, and BP.

c. Observe the cardiac monitor for a change in rhythm.

d. Record an electrocardiographic rhythm strip before, during, and after the procedure.

e. Provide an emesis basin if the gag reflex is stimulated, and initiate precautions to prevent aspiration.

f. Have a defibrillator and resuscitative equipment available.

B. Cardioversion

1. Description

a. Cardioversion is synchronized countershock to convert an undesirable rhythm to a stable rhythm.

b. Cardioversion can be an elective procedure performed by the PHCP for stable tachydysrhythmias resistant to medical therapies or an emergent procedure for hemodynamically unstable ventricular or supraventricular tachydysrhythmias.

c. A lower amount of energy is used than with defibrillation.

d. Defibrillator is synchronized to the client's R wave to avoid discharging the shock during the vulnerable period (T wave).

e. If the defibrillator were not synchronized, it could discharge on the T wave and cause VF.

2. Preprocedure interventions

a. Obtain an informed consent if it is an elective procedure.

b. Administer sedation as prescribed.

c. If it is an elective procedure, hold digoxin 48 hours preprocedure as prescribed to prevent postcardioversion ventricular irritability.

d. If it is an elective procedure for atrial fibrillation or atrial flutter, the client would receive anticoagulant therapy for 4 to 6 weeks preprocedure and a transesophageal echocardiogram (TEE) would be performed to rule out clots in the atria before the procedure.

3. During the procedure

a. Ensure that the skin is clean and dry in the area where the electrode paddles/hands off pads will be placed.

b. Stop the oxygen during the procedure to avoid the hazard of fire.

c. Be sure that no one is touching the bed or the client when delivering the countershock (check the entire length of the client three times).

4. Postprocedure interventions

a. Priority data collection includes the ability of the client to maintain airway and breathing.

b. Resume oxygen administration as prescribed.

c. Monitor vital signs.

d. Monitor level of consciousness.

e. Monitor cardiac rhythm.

f. Monitor for indications of successful response such as conversion to sinus rhythm, strong peripheral pulses, an adequate BP, and adequate urine output.

g. Check the skin on the chest for evidence of burns from the edges of the paddles/pads.

C. Defibrillation

1. Defibrillation is an asynchronous countershock used to terminate pulseless VT or VF.

a. The defibrillator is charged to 120 to 200 joules (biphasic) or 360 joules (monophasic) for one countershock from the defibrillator, and then CPR is immediately resumed and continued for 5 cycles or about 2 minutes.

b. The rhythm is rechecked after 2 minutes, and if VF or pulseless VT continues, the defibrillator is charged to give a second shock at the same energy level previously used.

c. Resume CPR after the shock, and continue with the life support protocol.

⚠ Before defibrillating a client, be sure that the oxygen is shut off to avoid the hazard of fire and be sure that no one is touching the bed or the client.

D. Use of pad electrodes

1. One pad is placed at the third intercostal space to the right of the sternum; the other is placed at the fifth intercostal space on the left midaxillary line.

2. Apply firm pressure of at least 25 lb to each of the pads.

3. Be sure that no one is touching the bed or the client when delivering the countershock.

4. Pads for hands-off biphasic defibrillation may be applied in an anterior-posterior position or apex-posterior position, and placement directly over breast tissue needs to be avoided.

E. Automatic external defibrillator (AED)

1. An AED is used by laypersons and emergency medical technicians for prehospital cardiac arrest.

2. Place the client on a firm, dry surface.

3. Turn on the AED and follow the voice prompts.

4. Place the electrode patches in the correct position on the client's chest.

5. Stop CPR.

6. Ensure that no one is touching the client to avoid motion artifact during rhythm analysis.

7. The machine will advise whether a shock is necessary.

8. Shocks are recommended for pulseless VT or VF only (usually 3 shocks are delivered).

9. If unsuccessful, CPR is continued for 1 minute and then another series of shocks is delivered.

F. Automatic implantable cardioverter defibrillator (AICD)

1. Description

a. An AICD monitors cardiac rhythm and detects and terminates episodes of VT and VF.

b. The AICD senses VT or VF and delivers 25 to 30 J up to four times if necessary.

c. An AICD is used in clients with episodes of spontaneous sustained VT or VF unrelated to an MI or in clients whose medication therapy has been unsuccessful in controlling life-threatening dysrhythmia.

d. Transvenous electrode leads are placed in the right atrium and ventricle in contact with the endocardium. Leads are used for sensing, pacing, and delivery of cardioversion or defibrillation.

e. The generator is most commonly implanted in the left pectoral region.

2. Reinforce client education

a. Instruct the client in the basic functions of the AICD.

b. Know the rate cutoff of the AICD and the number of consecutive shocks that it will deliver.

c. Wear loose-fitting clothing over the AICD generator site.

d. Avoid contact sports to prevent trauma to the AICD generator and lead wires.

e. Report any fever, redness, swelling, or drainage from the insertion site.

f. Report symptoms of fainting, nausea, weakness, blackouts, and rapid pulse rates to the PHCP.

g. During shock discharge, the client may feel faint or short of breath.

h. Instruct the client to sit or lie down if he or she feels a shock and to notify the PHCP.

i. Advise the client to maintain a log of the date, time, and activity preceding the shock, the symptoms preceding the shock, and post-shock sensations.

j. Instruct the client and family on how to access the emergency medical system.

k. Encourage the family to learn CPR.

l. Instruct the client to avoid electromagnetic fields directly over the AICD because they can inactivate the device.

m. Instruct the client to move away from a magnetic field immediately if beeping tones are heard, and notify the PHCP.

n. Keep an AICD identification card in the wallet and obtain and wear a MedicAlert bracelet.

o. Inform all PHCPs that an AICD has been inserted. Certain diagnostic tests, such as MRI and procedures using diathermy or electrocautery interfere with AICD function.

VI. Pacemakers

A. Description: a temporary or permanent device that provides electrical stimulation and maintains the heart rate when the client's intrinsic pacemaker fails to provide a perfusing rhythm

B. Settings

1. A synchronous (demand) pacemaker senses the client's rhythm and paces only if the client's intrinsic rate falls below the set pacemaker rate to stimulate depolarization.

2. An asynchronous (fixed rate) pacemaker paces at a preset rate regardless of the client's intrinsic rhythm and is used when the client is asystolic or profoundly bradycardic.

3. Overdrive pacing suppresses the underlying rhythm during tachydysrhythmias so that the sinus node will regain control of the heart.

C. Spikes

1. When a pacing stimulus is delivered to the heart, a spike (straight vertical line) is seen on the monitor or ECG strip.

2. Spikes precede the chamber being paced. A spike preceding a P-wave indicates that the atrium is being paced, and a spike preceding the QRS indicates the ventricle is being paced.

3. An atrial spike followed by a P-wave indicates atrial depolarization, and a ventricular spike followed by a QRS represents ventricular depolarization. This is referred to as "capture."

D. Temporary pacemakers

1. Noninvasive transcutaneous pacing

a. Noninvasive transcutaneous pacing is used as a temporary emergency measure in the profoundly bradycardic or asystolic client until invasive pacing can be initiated.

b. Large electrode pads are placed on the client's chest and back and connected to an external pulse generator.

c. Wash the skin with soap and water before applying electrodes.

d. It is not necessary to shave the hair or apply alcohol or tinctures to the skin.

e. Place the posterior electrode between the spine and left scapula, behind the heart, avoiding placement over bone.

f. Place the anterior electrode between the V_2 and V_5 positions over the heart.

g. Do not place the anterior electrode over female breast tissue; rather, displace breast tissue and place under the breast.

h. Do not take the pulse or BP on the left side. The results will not be accurate because of the muscle twitching and electrical current.

i. Ensure that electrodes are in good contact with the skin.

j. Set pacing rate as prescribed; establish stimulation threshold to ensure capture.

k. If loss of "capture" occurs, check the skin contact of the electrodes and increase the current until "capture" is regained.

l. Evaluate the client for discomfort from cutaneous and muscle stimulation. Administer analgesics as needed.

2. Invasive transvenous pacing

a. Pacing lead wire is placed through the antecubital, femoral, jugular, or subclavian vein into the right atrium or right ventricle so that it is in direct contact with the endocardium.

b. Monitor the pacemaker insertion site.

c. Restrict client movement to prevent lead wire displacement.

3. Invasive epicardial pacing: Applied by using a transthoracic approach. The lead wires are threaded loosely on the epicardial surface of the heart after cardiac surgery.

4. Reducing the risk of microshock

a. Use only inspected and approved equipment.

b. Insulate the exposed portion of wires with plastic or rubber material (fingers of rubber gloves) when wires are not attached to the pulse generator, and cover with nonconductive tape.

c. Ground all electrical equipment using a three-pronged plug.

d. Wear gloves when handling exposed wires.

e. Keep dressings dry.

⚠ Vital signs are monitored and cardiac monitoring is done continuously for the client with a pacemaker.

E. Permanent pacemakers
1. The pulse generator is internal and surgically implanted in a subcutaneous pocket below the clavicle.
2. The leads are passed transvenously via the cephalic or subclavian vein to the endocardium on the right side of the heart. Postoperatively, limitation of arm movement on the operative side is required to prevent lead wire dislodgement.
3. Permanent pacemakers may be single chambered in which the lead wire is placed in the chamber to be paced or dual chambered with lead wires placed in both the right atrium and ventricle.
4. Biventricular pacing of the ventricles allows for synchronized depolarization and is used for moderate to severe heart failure to improve cardiac output.
5. A permanent pacemaker is programmed when inserted and can be reprogrammed if necessary by noninvasive transmission from an external programmer to the implanted generator.
6. Pacemakers are powered by a lithium battery that has an average life span of 10 years, are nuclear powered with a life span of 20 years or longer, or are designed to be recharged externally.
7. Pacemaker function can be checked in the PHCP's office or clinic by a pacemaker interrogator or programmer or from home using telephone transmitter devices.
8. The client may be provided with a device that is placed over the pacemaker battery generator with an attachment to the telephone. The heart rate then can be transmitted to the clinic.

9. Reinforce client teaching as per Box 49.3.

VII. **Coronary Artery Disease**
A. Description
1. Coronary artery disease, also known as coronary heart disease, refers to a narrowing or obstruction of one or more coronary arteries as a result of atherosclerosis, an accumulation of lipid-containing plaque in the arteries (Fig. 49.7).
2. The disease causes decreased perfusion of myocardial tissue and inadequate myocardial oxygen supply leading to hypertension, angina, dysrhythmia, MI, heart failure, and death.
3. Collateral circulation, more than one artery supplying a muscle with blood, is normally present in the coronary arteries, especially in older persons.
4. The development of collateral circulation takes time and develops when chronic ischemia occurs

to meet the metabolic demands. Therefore, an occlusion of a coronary artery in a younger individual is more likely to be lethal than in an older individual.
5. Symptoms occur when the coronary artery is occluded to the point that inadequate blood supply to the muscle occurs causing ischemia.
6. Coronary artery narrowing is significant if the lumen diameter of the left main artery is reduced at least 50% or any major branch is reduced at least 75%.
7. The goal of treatment is to alter the atherosclerotic progression.
B. Data collection
1. Possibly normal findings during asymptomatic periods
2. Chest pain
3. Palpitations
4. Dyspnea
5. Syncope
6. Cough or hemoptysis
7. Excessive fatigue

BOX 49.3 **Pacemakers: Client Education**

Instruct the client about the pacemaker including the programmed rate.
Instruct the client on the signs of battery failure and when to notify the primary health care provider (PHCP).
Instruct the client to report any fever, redness, swelling, or drainage from the insertion site.
Report signs of dizziness, weakness or fatigue, swelling of the ankles or legs, chest pain, or shortness of breath.
Keep a pacemaker identification card in the wallet, and obtain and wear a Medic-Alert bracelet.
Instruct the client on how to take the pulse, to take the pulse daily, and to maintain a diary of pulse rates.
Wear loose-fitting clothing over the pulse generator site.
Avoid contact sports.
Inform all PHCPs that a pacemaker has been inserted.
Instruct the client to inform airport security that he or she has a pacemaker because the pacemaker may set off the security detector.
Instruct the client that most electrical appliances can be used without any interference with the functioning of the pacemaker; however, advise the client not to operate electrical appliances directly over the pacemaker site.
Avoid transmitter towers and antitheft devices in stores.
Instruct the client that if any unusual feelings occur when near any electrical devices to move 5–10 feet away and check the pulse.
Instruct the client about the methods of monitoring the function of the device.
Emphasize the importance of follow-up with the PHCP.
Use cell phones on the side opposite to the pacemaker.

Chronic Causes of Endothelial Injury:
- Hemodynamic factors
- Hyperhomocysteinemia
- Hyperlipidemia
- Hypertension
- Immune reactions
- Smoking
- Toxins
- Viruses

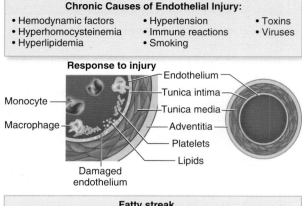

Response to injury

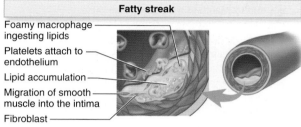

Fatty streak

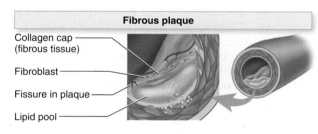

Fibrous plaque

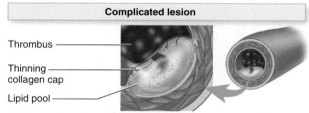

Complicated lesion

FIGURE 49.7 Cross section of an atherosclerotic coronary artery.

C. Diagnostic studies
  1. Electrocardiography
    a. When blood flow is reduced and ischemia occurs, ST segment depression, T-wave inversion, or both are noted. The ST segment returns to normal when the blood flow returns.
    b. With infarction, cell injury results in ST segment elevation followed by T-wave inversion and an abnormal Q-wave.
  2. Cardiac catheterization
    a. Cardiac catheterization provides the most definitive source for diagnosis.
    b. Cardiac catheterization shows the presence of atherosclerotic lesions.
D. Blood lipid levels
  1. Blood lipid levels may be elevated.

2. Cholesterol-lowering medications may be prescribed to reduce the development of atherosclerotic plaques.
E. Interventions
  1. Assist the client with identifying risk factors that can be modified.
  2. Assist the client with identifying barriers to compliance with the therapeutic plan and with identifying methods to overcome such barriers.
  3. Reinforce instructions to the client regarding a low-calorie, low-sodium, low-cholesterol, and low-fat diet with an increase in dietary fiber.
  4. Stress to the client that dietary changes are not temporary and need to be maintained for life.
  5. Teach the client about prescribed medications.
  6. Provide community resources to the client regarding exercise, smoking reduction, and stress reduction as appropriate.
F. Surgical procedures
  1. PTCA to compress the plaque against the walls of the artery and dilate the vessel
  2. Laser angioplasty to vaporize the plaque
  3. Atherectomy to remove the plaque from the artery
  4. Vascular stent to prevent the artery from closing and to prevent restenosis
  5. Coronary artery bypass graft to improve blood flow to the myocardial tissue that is at risk for ischemia or infarction because of the occluded artery
G. Medications
  1. Nitrates to dilate the coronary arteries and decrease **preload** and **afterload**
  2. Calcium channel blockers to dilate coronary arteries and reduce vasospasm
  3. Cholesterol-lowering medications to reduce the development of atherosclerotic plaques
  4. Beta blockers to reduce the BP in individuals who are hypertensive

VIII. Angina

A. Description
  1. Angina is chest pain resulting from myocardial ischemia caused by inadequate myocardial blood and oxygen supply.
  2. Angina is caused by an imbalance between oxygen supply and demand.
  3. Angina causes include obstruction of coronary blood flow because of atherosclerosis, artery spasm, and conditions increasing myocardial oxygen consumption.

⚠️ The goal of treatment for angina is to provide relief of the acute attack, correct the imbalance between myocardial oxygen supply and demand, and prevent the progression of the disease and further attacks to reduce the risk of MI.

B. Patterns of angina
  1. Stable angina
    a. Also called exertional angina
    b. Occurs with activities that involve exertion or emotional stress and is relieved with rest or nitroglycerin
    c. Usually has a stable pattern of onset, duration, severity, and relieving factors
  2. Unstable angina
    a. Also called preinfarction angina
    b. Occurs with an unpredictable degree of exertion or emotion and increases in occurrence, duration, and severity over time
    c. Pain may not be relieved with nitroglycerin.
  3. Variant angina
    a. Also called Prinzmetal's or vasospastic angina
    b. Results from coronary artery spasm
    c. May occur at rest
    d. Attacks may be associated with ST segment elevation noted on the ECG.
  4. Intractable angina is a chronic, incapacitating angina that is unresponsive to interventions.
C. Data collection
  1. Pain (Table 49.1)
  2. Dyspnea
  3. Pallor
  4. Sweating
  5. Palpitations and tachycardia
  6. Dizziness and syncope
  7. Hypertension
  8. Digestive disturbances
D. Diagnostic studies
  1. Electrocardiography: Readings are normal during rest with ST depression and/or T-wave inversion during an episode of pain.
  2. Stress test: Chest pain or changes in the ECG or vital signs during testing may indicate ischemia.
  3. Cardiac enzymes and troponins: Findings are normal in angina.
  4. Cardiac catheterization: Catheterization provides a definitive diagnosis by providing information about the patency of the coronary arteries.

TABLE 49.1   Characteristics of Pain: Angina and Myocardial Infarction

Angina	Myocardial Infarction
Can develop slowly or quickly	Occurs without cause, primarily early in the morning
Usually described as mild or moderate pain	Crushing substernal pain
Substernal, crushing, squeezing pain	May radiate to the jaw, back, and left arm
May radiate to the shoulders, arms, jaw, neck, and back	Lasts 30 minutes or longer
Usually lasts less than 5 minutes; however, can last up to 15–20 minutes	Is unrelieved by rest or nitroglycerin, and relieved only by opioids
Relieved by nitroglycerin or rest	

E. Interventions
  1. Immediate management includes the following:
    a. Monitoring pain; instituting pain relief measures
    b. Administering oxygen by nasal cannula as prescribed
    c. Checking vital signs and providing continuous cardiac monitoring and nitroglycerin as prescribed to dilate the coronary arteries, reduce the oxygen requirements of the myocardium, and relieve the chest pain
    d. Ensuring bed rest is maintained, placing the client in semi-Fowler's position, and staying with the client
    e. Obtaining a 12-lead ECG
    f. Establishing an IV access route
  2. Following the acute episode
    a. See Section VII.E (Coronary Artery Disease, Interventions).
    b. Assist the client to identify angina-precipitating events.
    c. Reinforce instructions to the client to stop activity and rest if chest pain occurs and to take nitroglycerin as prescribed; the client is usually instructed to call emergency medical services if the nitroglycerin does not relieve the pain, and many PHCPs recommend that the client also take an aspirin.
    d. Reinforce instructions to the client regarding prescribed medications.
F. Surgical procedures: See Section VII.F (Coronary Artery Disease, Surgical Procedures).
G. Medications
  1. See Section VII.G (Coronary Artery Disease, Medications).
  2. Antiplatelet therapy may be prescribed that inhibits platelet aggregation and reduces the risk of developing an acute MI.

IX. Myocardial Infarction

A. Description
  1. MI occurs when myocardial tissue is abruptly and severely deprived of oxygen.
  2. Ischemia can lead to necrosis of myocardial tissue if blood flow is not restored.
  3. Infarction does not occur instantly but evolves over several hours.
  4. Obvious physical changes do not occur in the heart until 6 hours after the infarction when the infarcted area appears blue and swollen.
  5. After 48 hours, the infarct turns gray with yellow streaks developing as neutrophils invade the tissue.
  6. By 8 to 10 days after infarction, granulation tissue forms.
  7. Over 2 to 3 months, the necrotic area develops into a scar. Scar tissue permanently changes the size and shape of the entire left ventricle.

8. Not all clients experience the classic symptoms of an MI.
9. Women may experience atypical discomfort, shortness of breath, or fatigue and often present with NSTEMI (non-ST-elevation myocardial infarction) or T-wave inversion.
10. An older client may experience shortness of breath, pulmonary edema, dizziness, altered mental status, or dysrhythmia.

B. Location of MI (see Fig. 49.1)
1. Obstruction of the LAD artery results in anterior or septal MI or both.
2. Obstruction of the circumflex artery results in posterior wall MI or lateral wall MI.
3. Obstruction of the right coronary artery results in inferior wall MI.

C. Risk factors
1. Atherosclerosis
2. Coronary artery disease
3. Elevated cholesterol levels
4. Smoking
5. Hypertension
6. Obesity
7. Physical inactivity
8. Impaired glucose tolerance
9. Stress

D. Diagnostic studies
1. Troponin level
   a. Level rises within 3 hours.
   b. Level remains elevated for up to 7 to 10 days.
2. Total creatine kinase level
   a. Level rises within 6 hours after the onset of chest pain.
   b. Level peaks within 18 hours after damage and death of cardiac tissue.
3. CK-MB isoenzyme
   a. Peak elevation occurs 18 hours after the onset of chest pain.
   b. Level returns to normal 48 to 72 hours later.
4. Myoglobin: Level rises within 2 hours after cell death with a rapid decline in the level after 7 hours.
5. White blood cell count: An elevated white blood cell count appears on the second day after the MI and lasts up to 1 week.
6. ECG
   a. ECG shows either ST elevation MI (STEMI), T-wave inversion, or non-ST elevation MI (NSTEMI); an abnormal Q-wave may also be present.
   b. STEMI is a more serious form of MI than NSTEMI; in STEMI, a coronary artery is completely blocked and a large part of the heart muscle is unable to receive blood. In NSTEMI, the supply of blood to the heart is only partially blocked. Both types are medical emergencies.

   c. Hours to days after the MI, ST and T-wave changes will return to normal, but the Q-wave changes usually remain permanently.
7. Cardiac catheterization may be done emergently to determine the extent and location of obstruction of the coronary arteries; this allows for use of PTCA and restoration of blood flow to the myocardium.
8. Diagnostic tests following the acute stage
   a. Exercise tolerance test or stress test may be prescribed to assess for electrocardiographic changes and ischemia and to evaluate for medical therapy or identify clients who may need invasive therapy.
   b. Thallium scans may be prescribed to assess for ischemia or necrotic muscle tissue.
   c. Multigated cardiac blood pool imaging scans may be used to evaluate left ventricular function.
   d. Cardiac catheterization is performed to determine the extent and location of obstructions of the coronary arteries.

E. Data collection
1. Pain (see Table 49.1)
2. Nausea and vomiting
3. Diaphoresis
4. Dyspnea
5. Dysrhythmia
6. Feelings of fear and anxiety
7. Pallor, cyanosis, and coolness of extremities

F. Complications of MI (Box 49.4)

G. Interventions, acute stage

⚠️ Pain relief increases oxygen supply to the myocardium. Morphine sulfate is administered as a priority for managing pain in the client experiencing an MI.

1. Obtain a description of the chest discomfort.
2. Administer oxygen by nasal cannula, as prescribed, and institute pain relief measures (morphine, nitroglycerin as prescribed).

BOX 49.4	Complications of Myocardial Infarction

Dysrhythmia
Heart failure
Pulmonary edema
Cardiogenic shock
Thrombophlebitis
Pericarditis
Mitral valve insufficiency
Postinfarction angina
Ventricular rupture
Dressler's syndrome (a combination of pericarditis, pericardial effusion, and pleural effusion which can occur several weeks to several months after a myocardial infarction)

3. Monitor vital signs and cardiovascular status and maintain cardiac monitoring.

4. Assess respiratory rate and breath sounds for signs of heart failure, as indicated by the presence of crackles or wheezes or dependent edema.

5. Ensure bed rest and place the client in a semi-Fowler's position to enhance comfort and tissue oxygenation; stay with the client.

6. Assist to establish an IV access route.

7. Obtain a 12-lead ECG.

8. Assist with the administration of thrombolytic therapy, which may be prescribed within the first 6 hours of the coronary event; monitor for signs of bleeding if the client is receiving thrombolytic therapy.

9. Monitor laboratory values as prescribed.

10. Administer β-blockers, as prescribed, to slow the heart rate and increase myocardial perfusion while reducing the force of myocardial contraction.

11. Monitor for cardiac dysrhythmia because tachycardia and PVCs frequently occur in the first few hours after MI. Assist to administer antidysrhythmics as prescribed.

12. Monitor distal peripheral pulses and skin temperature because poor cardiac output may be identified by cool diaphoretic skin and diminished or absent pulses.

13. Monitor BP closely after the administration of medications. If the systolic pressure is lower than 100 mm Hg, or 25 mm Hg lower than the previous reading, lower the head of the bed and notify the PHCP.

14. Provide reassurance to the client and family

H. Interventions following the acute episode
1. Maintain bed rest for the first 24 to 36 hours as prescribed.
2. Allow the client to stand to void or use a bedside commode, if prescribed.
3. Provide range-of-motion exercises to prevent thrombus formation and maintain muscle strength.
4. Progress to dangling legs at the side of the bed or out of bed to the chair for 30 minutes three times a day as prescribed.
5. Progress to ambulation in the client's room, and to the bathroom, and then in the hallway three times a day.
6. Monitor for complications.
7. Administer angiotensin-converting enzyme (ACE) inhibitors, angiotensin-II receptor blockers (ARBs), calcium channel blockers, aspirin, thienopyridines (clopidogrel), and lipid-lowering agents as prescribed.
8. Encourage the client to verbalize feelings regarding the MI.

I. Cardiac rehabilitation: Process of actively assisting the client with cardiac disease to achieve and maintain a vital and productive life within the limitations of their heart disease; also, refer to Section VII.E (Coronary Artery Disease, Interventions)

X. Heart Failure

A. Description
1. Heart failure refers to the inability of the heart to maintain adequate cardiac output to meet the metabolic needs of the body because of impaired pumping ability.
2. Diminished cardiac output results in inadequate peripheral tissue perfusion.
3. Congestion of the lungs and periphery may occur. The client can develop acute pulmonary edema.

B. Classification
1. Acute heart failure occurs suddenly.
2. Chronic heart failure develops over time; however, a client with chronic heart failure can develop an acute episode.

C. Types of heart failure
1. Right ventricular failure/left ventricular failure
   a. Because the two ventricles of the heart represent two separate pumping systems, it is possible for one to fail alone for a short period.
   b. Most heart failure begins with left ventricular failure and progresses to failure of both ventricles.
   c. Acute pulmonary edema—a medical emergency—results from left ventricular failure.
   d. If pulmonary edema is not treated, death will occur from suffocation because the client literally drowns in his or her own fluids.
2. Forward failure/backward failure
   a. In forward failure, an inadequate output of the affected ventricle causes decreased perfusion to vital organs.
   b. In backward failure, blood backs up behind the affected ventricle, causing increased pressure in the atrium behind the affected ventricle.
3. Low output/high output
   a. In low-output failure, not enough cardiac output is available to meet the demands of the body.
   b. High-output failure occurs when a condition causes the heart to work harder to meet the demands of the body.
4. Systolic failure/diastolic failure
   a. Systolic failure leads to problems with contraction and the ejection of blood.
   b. Diastolic failure leads to problems with the heart relaxing and filling with blood.

D. Compensatory mechanisms
1. Compensatory mechanisms act to restore cardiac output to near-normal levels.
2. Initially these mechanisms increase cardiac output; however, they eventually have a damaging effect on pump action.
3. Compensatory mechanisms contribute to an increase in myocardial oxygen consumption; when

TABLE 49.2 **Clinical Manifestations of Right-Sided and Left-Sided Heart Failure**

Right-Sided Heart Failure	Left-Sided Heart Failure
Dependent edema (legs and sacrum)	Signs of pulmonary congestion
Jugular venous distention	Dyspnea
Abdominal distention	Tachypnea
Hepatomegaly	Crackles in the lungs
Splenomegaly	Dry, hacking cough
Anorexia and nausea	Paroxysmal nocturnal dyspnea
Weight gain	Increased BP (from fluid
Nocturnal diuresis	volume excess) or decreased
Swelling of the fingers and hands	BP (from pump failure)
Increased BP (from fluid volume excess) or decreased BP (from pump failure)	

BP, Blood pressure.

this occurs, myocardial reserve is exhausted and clinical manifestations of heart failure develop.

4. Compensatory mechanisms include increased heart rate, improved stroke volume, arterial vasoconstriction, sodium and water retention, and myocardial hypertrophy.

 E. Data collection (Table 49.2)
   1. Right- and left-sided heart failure
   2. Acute pulmonary edema
      a. Severe dyspnea and orthopnea
      b. Tachycardia, tachypnea
      c. Expectoration of large amounts of blood-tinged, frothy sputum
      d. Wheezing and crackles on auscultation, gurgling respirations
      e. Acute anxiety, apprehension, and restlessness
      f. Profuse sweating
      g. Cold, clammy skin
      h. Cyanosis
      i. Nasal flaring, use of accessory breathing muscles

⚠ Signs of left ventricular failure are evident in the pulmonary system. Signs of right ventricular failure are evident in the systemic circulation.

 F. Immediate management of acute episode (see Priority Nursing Actions)

⚡ PRIORITY NURSING ACTIONS

Client Develops Pulmonary Edema

1. Place the client in a high-Fowler's position.
2. Administer oxygen.
3. Check the client quickly, including checking lung sounds.
4. Ensure an intravenous access device is in place.
5. Prepare for the administration of a diuretic and morphine sulfate.
6. Insert a Foley catheter as prescribed.
7. Prepare for intubation and ventilator support, if required.
8. Document the event, actions taken, and the client's response.

BOX 49.5 **Cardiogenic Shock**

Failure of the heart to pump adequately, thereby reducing cardiac output and compromising tissue perfusion.
Necrosis of more than 40% of the left ventricle occurs, usually as a result of the occlusion of major coronary vessels.
The goal of treatment is to maintain tissue oxygenation and perfusion and improve the pumping ability of the heart.

G. Following the acute episode
   1. Encourage the client to verbalize feelings about the lifestyle changes required as a result of their heart failure.
   2. Assist the client with identifying precipitating risk factors of heart failure and methods of eliminating these risk factors.
   3. Reinforce instructions to the client about the prescribed medication regimen, which may include digoxin, a diuretic, an ACE inhibitor, a low-dose β-blocker, and/or a vasodilator.
   4. Advise the client to notify the PHCP if side effects occur from the medications.
   5. Advise the client to avoid over-the-counter medications.
   6. Reinforce instructions to the client to contact the PHCP if he or she is unable to take medications because of illness.
   7. Reinforce instructions to the client to avoid large amounts of caffeine found in coffee, tea, cocoa, chocolate, and some carbonated beverages.
   8. Reinforce instructions to the client about the prescribed low-sodium, low-fat, and low-cholesterol diet.
   9. Provide the client with a list of potassium-rich foods because diuretics can cause hypokalemia (except for potassium-sparing diuretics).
   10. Reinforce instructions to the client regarding fluid restriction, if prescribed, advising the client to spread the fluid out during the day and to suck on hard candy to reduce thirst.
   11. Reinforce instructions to the client to balance periods of activity and rest.
   12. Advise the client to avoid isometric activities which increase pressure in the heart.
   13. Reinforce instructions to the client to monitor daily weight.
   14. Reinforce instructions to the client to report signs of fluid retention such as edema or weight gain.

XI. Cardiogenic Shock (Box 49.5)

XII. Inflammatory Diseases of the Heart

A. Pericarditis
   1. Description
      a. Pericarditis refers to an acute or chronic inflammation of the pericardium.

b. Chronic pericarditis, a chronic inflammatory thickening of the pericardium, constricts the heart causing compression.

c. The pericardial sac becomes inflamed.

d. Pericarditis can result in loss of pericardial elasticity or an accumulation of fluid within the sac.

e. Heart failure or cardiac tamponade may result.

2. Data collection

a. Precordial pain in the anterior chest that radiates to the left side of the neck, shoulder, or back.

b. Pain is grating and is aggravated by breathing (particularly inspiration), coughing, and swallowing.

c. Pain is worse when in the supine position and may be relieved by leaning forward.

d. Pericardial friction rub (scratchy, high-pitched sound) heard during auscultation and produced by the rubbing of the inflamed pericardial layers

e. Fever and chills

f. Fatigue and malaise

g. Elevated white blood cell count

h. ECG changes with acute pericarditis; ST segment elevation with the onset of inflammation; atrial fibrillation is common

i. Signs of right ventricular failure in clients with chronic constrictive pericarditis

3. Interventions

a. Determine the nature of the pain.

b. Position the client in the high-Fowler's position or upright and leaning forward.

c. Deliver oxygen as prescribed.

d. Administer analgesics, nonsteroidal anti-inflammatory drugs, or corticosteroids for pain as prescribed.

e. Auscultate for a pericardial friction rub.

f. Check results of blood culture to identify causative organism.

g. Administer antibiotics for bacterial infection as prescribed.

h. Administer diuretics and digoxin as prescribed to the client with chronic constrictive pericarditis. Surgical incision of the pericardium (pericardiectomy) may be necessary.

I. Monitor for signs of cardiac tamponade, which include pulsus paradoxus, jugular vein distention with clear lung sounds, muffled heart sounds, narrowed **pulse pressure**, tachycardia, and decreased cardiac output.

j. Notify the PHCP if signs of cardiac tamponade occur.

B. Myocarditis

1. Description: An acute or chronic inflammation of the myocardium as a result of pericarditis, systemic infection, or allergic response

2. Data collection

a. Fever

b. Pericardial friction rub

c. A gallop rhythm

d. A murmur that sounds like fluid passing an obstruction

e. Pulsus alternans

f. Signs of heart failure

g. Dyspnea

h. Tachycardia

i. Chest pain

3. Interventions

a. Assist the client to a position of comfort such as sitting up and leaning forward.

b. Administer analgesics, salicylates, and nonsteroidal anti-inflammatory drugs as prescribed to reduce fever and pain.

c. Administer oxygen as prescribed.

d. Provide adequate rest periods.

e. Limit activities to avoid overexertion and to decrease the workload of the heart.

f. Administer digoxin as prescribed, and monitor for signs of digoxin toxicity.

g. Administer antidysrhythmics as prescribed.

h. Administer antibiotics as prescribed to treat the causative organism.

i. Monitor for complications, which can include thrombus, heart failure, or cardiomyopathy.

C. Endocarditis

1. Description

a. Endocarditis refers to an inflammation of the inner lining of the heart and valves.

b. Occurs primarily in clients who are IV drug abusers, have had valve replacements, or have mitral valve prolapse or other structural defects.

c. Ports of entry for the infecting organism include the oral cavity (especially if the client had a dental procedure in the previous 3–6 months), infections (cutaneous, genitourinary, gastrointestinal, and systemic), or surgery or invasive procedures, including IV line placement.

2. Data collection

a. Fever

b. Anorexia, weight loss

c. Fatigue

d. Cardiac murmurs

e. Heart failure

f. Embolic complications from vegetation fragments traveling through the circulation

g. Petechiae

h. Splinter hemorrhages in the nail beds

i. Osler's nodes (reddish tender lesions) on the pads of the fingers, hands, and toes

j. Janeway lesions (nontender hemorrhagic lesions) on the fingers, toes, nose, or ear lobes

k. Splenomegaly

l. Clubbing of the fingers

3. Interventions
  a. Provide adequate rest balanced with activity to prevent thrombus formation.
  b. Maintain antiembolism stockings.
  c. Monitor for signs of heart failure.
  d. Monitor for splenic emboli, as evidenced by sudden abdominal pain radiating to the left shoulder and the presence of rebound abdominal tenderness on palpation.
  e. Monitor for renal emboli, as evidenced by flank pain radiating to the groin, hematuria, and pyuria.
  f. Monitor for confusion, aphasia, or dysphasia which may indicate central nervous system emboli.
  g. Monitor for pulmonary emboli, as evidenced by pleuritic chest pain, dyspnea, and cough.
  h. Monitor skin, mucous membranes, and conjunctiva for petechiae.
  i. Monitor nail beds for splinter hemorrhages.
  j. Monitor for Osler's nodes on the pads of the fingers, hands, and toes.
  k. Monitor for Janeway lesions on the fingers, toes, nose, or earlobes.
  l. Monitor for clubbing of the fingers.
  m. Evaluate blood culture results.
  n. Administer IV antibiotics as prescribed.
  o. Plan and arrange for discharge providing resources required for the continued administration of IV antibiotics.
4. Client education (Box 49.6)

XIII. Cardiac Tamponade (Box 49.7)

XIV. Valvular Heart Disease
A. Description
  1. Valvular heart disease occurs when the heart valves cannot fully open (stenosis) or close completely (insufficiency or regurgitation).
  2. Valvular heart disease prevents efficient blood flow through the heart.
B. Types
  1. Mitral stenosis: Valvular tissue thickens and narrows the valve opening preventing blood flow from the left atrium to left ventricle.
  2. Mitral insufficiency/regurgitation: The valve is incompetent, preventing complete valve closure during systole.
  3. Mitral valve prolapse: Valve leaflets protrude into the left atrium during systole.
  4. Aortic stenosis: Valvular tissue thickens and narrows the valve opening preventing blood flow from the left ventricle into the aorta.
  5. Aortic insufficiency: Valve is incompetent preventing complete valve closure during diastole.
  6. For aortic disorders see Table 49.3.
  7. For tricuspid disorders see Table 49.4.
  8. For pulmonary valve disorders see Table 49.5.
C. Repair procedures
  1. Balloon valvuloplasty
    a. A balloon catheter is passed from the femoral vein through the atrial septum to the mitral valve or through the femoral artery to the aortic valve.

BOX 49.6 Homecare Instructions for the Client with Infective Endocarditis

Teach the client to maintain aseptic technique during setup and administration of IV antibiotics.

Instruct the client to administer IV antibiotics at scheduled times to maintain the blood level.

Instruct the client to monitor IV catheter sites for signs of infection and report immediately to the primary health care provider (PHCP).

Instruct the client to record his or her temperature daily for up to 6 weeks and report fever.

Encourage oral hygiene at least twice a day with a soft toothbrush and rinse well with water after brushing.

Client needs to avoid use of oral irrigation devices and flossing to avoid bacteremia.

Teach the client to thoroughly cleanse any skin lacerations thoroughly and apply an antibiotic ointment as prescribed.

Client needs to inform all PHCPs of a history of endocarditis and request prophylactic antibiotics before every invasive procedure, including dental procedures.

Teach the client to observe for signs/symptoms of embolic phenomena and heart failure.

BOX 49.7 Cardiac Tamponade

A pericardial effusion occurs when the space between the parietal and visceral layers of the pericardium fills with fluid. Pericardial effusion places the client at risk for cardiac tamponade, an accumulation of fluid in the pericardial cavity. Tamponade restricts ventricular filling, and cardiac output drops. Distant, muffled heart sounds are heard.

Acute cardiac tamponade can occur when small volumes (20–50 mL) of fluid accumulate rapidly in the pericardium.

TABLE 49.3 Aortic Valve Disorders

Symptoms	
Aortic Stenosis	**Aortic Insufficiency**
Dyspnea on exertion	Dyspnea
Angina	Angina
Syncope on exertion	Tachycardia
Fatigue	Fatigue
Orthopnea	Orthopnea
Paroxysmal nocturnal dyspnea	Paroxysmal nocturnal dyspnea
Harsh systolic crescendo-decrescendo murmur	Blowing decrescendo diastolic murmur

Interventions
Refer to section on repair procedures
Prepare the client for valve replacement as indicated

TABLE 49.4 Tricuspid Valve Disorders

Symptoms	
Tricuspid Stenosis	**Tricuspid Insufficiency**
Easily fatigued	Asymptomatic in mild situations
Effort intolerance	
Complaints of fluttering sensations in the neck (obstructed venous flow)	Signs of right ventricular failure including ascites, hepatomegaly, peripheral edema
Cyanosis	
Signs of right ventricular failure including ascites, hepatomegaly, peripheral edema, jugular vein distention with clear lung fields	Pleural effusion
	Systolic murmur heard at the left sternal border, fourth intercostal space
Symptoms of decreased cardiac output	
Rumbling diastolic murmur	
Interventions	
Refer to section on repair procedures	
Prepare the client for valve replacement as indicated	

TABLE 49.5 Pulmonary Valve Disorders

Symptoms	
Pulmonary Stenosis	**Pulmonary Insufficiency**
Asymptomatic in a mild condition	Asymptomatic in mild condition
Dyspnea	Dyspnea
Fatigue	Fatigue
Syncope	Syncope
Signs of right ventricular failure including ascites, hepatomegaly, peripheral edema	Signs of right ventricular failure including ascites, hepatomegaly, peripheral edema
Systolic thrill heard at left sternal border	Systolic thrill heard at the left sternal border
Interventions	
Refer to section on repair procedures	Refer to section on repair procedures
Prepare the client for pulmonary valve commissurotomy as indicated	Prepare the client for valve replacement as indicated

b. The balloon is inflated to enlarge the orifice.

c. Institute precautions for arterial puncture if appropriate.

d. Monitor for bleeding from the catheter insertion site.

e. Monitor for signs of systemic emboli.

f. Monitor for signs of a regurgitant valve by monitoring cardiac rhythm, heart sounds, and cardiac output.

2. Mitral annuloplasty: Tightening and suturing the malfunctioning valve annulus to eliminate or greatly reduce regurgitation

3. Commissurotomy/valvotomy

   a. The procedure is accomplished with cardiopulmonary bypass during open heart surgery.

   b. The valve is visualized, thrombi are removed from the atria, fused leaflets are incised, and calcium is débrided from the leaflets, thus widening the orifice.

Adequate rest is important, and fatigue is common.

Anticoagulant therapy is necessary if a mechanical prosthetic valve was inserted.

Instruct the client concerning hazards related to anticoagulant therapy and to notify the primary health care provider (PHCP) if bleeding or excessive bruising occurs.

Instruct the client concerning the importance of good oral hygiene to reduce the risk of infective endocarditis.

Brush teeth twice daily with a soft toothbrush followed by oral rinses.

Avoid irrigation devices, electric toothbrushes, and flossing because these activities can cause the gums to bleed allowing bacteria to enter the mucous membranes and bloodstream.

Monitor incision and report any drainage or redness.

Avoid any dental procedures for 6 months.

Heavy lifting (greater than 10 lb [4.5 kg]) is to be avoided, and be cautious when in an automobile to prevent injury to the sternal incision.

If a prosthetic valve was inserted, a soft audible clicking sound may be heard.

Instruct the client concerning the importance of prophylactic antibiotics before any invasive procedure and the importance of informing all PHCPs of the valvular disease history.

Obtain and wear a MedicAlert bracelet.

D. Valve replacement procedures

   1. Mechanical prosthetic valves: These prosthetic valves are durable.

    Thromboembolism is a problem after valve replacement with a mechanical prosthetic valve, and lifetime anticoagulant therapy is required.

   2. Bioprosthetic valves

      a. Biological grafts are xenografts (valves from other species): porcine valves (pig), bovine valves (cow), or homografts (human cadavers).

      b. The risk of clot formation is small; therefore, long-term anticoagulation is not indicated.

   3. Preoperative interventions: Consult with the PHCP regarding discontinuing anticoagulants 72 hours before surgery.

   4. Postoperative interventions

      a. Monitor closely for signs of bleeding.

      b. Monitor cardiac output and for signs of heart failure.

      c. Administer digoxin as prescribed to maintain cardiac output and prevent atrial fibrillation.

      d. Reinforce client teaching (Box 49.8).

XV. Cardiomyopathy

A. Cardiomyopathy is a subacute or chronic disorder of the heart muscle.

B. Treatment is palliative, not curative, and the client needs to deal with numerous lifestyle changes and a shortened life span.

C. Types, signs/symptoms, and treatment: Refer to Table 49.6.

XVI. Vascular Disorders

A. Venous thrombosis
  1. Description
     a. Thrombus can be associated with an inflammatory process.
     b. When a thrombus develops, inflammation occurs thickening the vein wall and leading to embolization.

  2. Types
     a. Thrombophlebitis: A thrombus associated with inflammation
     b. Phlebothrombosis: A thrombus without inflammation
     c. Phlebitis: Vein inflammation associated with invasive procedures such as IV lines
     d. Deep vein thrombophlebitis: More serious than a superficial thrombophlebitis because of the risk for pulmonary embolism

  3. Risk factors for thrombus formation
     a. Venous stasis from varicose veins, heart failure, and immobility
     b. Hypercoagulability disorders

TABLE 49.6 Pathophysiology, Signs/Symptoms, and Treatment of Cardiomyopathies

| Dilated Cardiomyopathy | Hypertrophic Cardiomyopathy | | Restrictive Cardiomyopathy |
	Nonobstructed	Obstructed	
Pathophysiology			
Fibrosis of myocardium and endocardium Dilated chambers Mural wall thrombi prevalent	Hypertrophy of the walls Hypertrophied septum Relatively small chamber size	Same as for nonobstructed, except for obstruction of left ventricular outflow tract associated with the hypertrophied septum and mitral valve incompetence	Mimics constrictive pericarditis Fibrosed walls cannot expand or contract Chambers narrowed; emboli common
Signs/Symptoms			
Fatigue and weakness Heart failure (left side) Dysrhythmias or heart block Systemic or pulmonary emboli S_3 and S_4 gallops Moderate to severe cardiomegaly	Dyspnea Angina Fatigue, syncope, palpitations Mild cardiomegaly S_4 gallop Ventricular dysrhythmias Sudden death common Heart failure	Same as for nonobstructed except with mitral regurgitation murmur Atrial fibrillation	Dyspnea and fatigue Heart failure (right-sided) Mild to moderate cardiomegaly S_3 and S_4 gallops Heart block Emboli
Treatment			
Symptomatic treatment of heart failure Vasodilators Control of dysrhythmia Surgery: heart transplant	For both: Symptomatic treatment β-Blockers Conversion of atrial fibrillation Surgery: ventriculomyotomy or muscle resection with mitral valve replacement Digoxin, nitrates, and other vasodilators contraindicated with the obstructed form		Supportive treatment of symptoms Treatment of hypertension Conversion from dysrhythmia Exercise restrictions Emergency treatment of acute pulmonary edema

From Ignatavicius D, Workman ML, & Rebar, C: *Medical-surgical nursing: Concepts for interprofessional collaborative care*, ed 9, St. Louis, 2018, Saunders.

   c. Injury to the venous wall from IV injections; administration of vessel irritants (chemotherapy, hypertonic solutions)
   d. Following surgery, particularly orthopedic and abdominal surgery
   e. Pregnancy
   f. Ulcerative colitis
   g. Use of oral contraceptives
   h. Certain malignancies
   i. Fractures or other injuries of the pelvis or lower extremities
B. Phlebitis
   1. Data collection
      a. Red, warm area radiating up the vein of an extremity
      b. Pain and soreness
      c. Swelling
   2. Interventions
      a. Apply warm, moist soaks as prescribed to dilate the vein and promote circulation (check temperature of soak before applying).
      b. Monitor for signs of complications such as tissue necrosis, infection, or pulmonary embolus.
C. Deep vein thrombophlebitis
   1. Data collection
      a. Calf or groin tenderness or pain with or without swelling
      b. Positive Homans' sign may be noted; however, false-positive results are common so this is not a reliable measure.
      c. Warm skin that is tender to touch
   2. Interventions
      a. Provide bed rest as prescribed.
      b. Elevate the affected extremity above the level of the heart as prescribed.
      c. Avoid using the knee gatch or a pillow under the knees.
      d. Do not massage the extremity.
      e. Provide thigh-high or knee-high antiembolism stockings, as prescribed, to reduce venous stasis and to assist in the venous return of blood to the heart; teach how to apply and remove stockings.
      f. Administer an intermittent or continuous warm, moist compress as prescribed.
      g. Palpate the site gently, monitoring for warmth and edema.
      h. Measure and record the circumferences of the thighs and calves.
      i. Monitor for shortness of breath and chest pain, which can indicate pulmonary emboli.
      j. Administer thrombolytic therapy (tissue plasminogen activator) if prescribed, which needs to be initiated within 5 days after the onset of symptoms.
      k. Administer heparin therapy as prescribed to prevent enlargement of the existing clot and prevent the formation of new clots.
      l. Monitor activated partial thromboplastin time during heparin therapy.
      m. Administer warfarin as prescribed following heparin therapy when the symptoms of deep vein thrombophlebitis have resolved.
      n. Monitor prothrombin time and international normalized ratio during warfarin therapy.
      o. Monitor for the hazards and side effects associated with anticoagulant therapy.
      p. Administer analgesics as prescribed to reduce pain.
      q. Reinforce client teaching (Box 49.9).
D. Venous insufficiency
   1. Description
      a. Venous insufficiency results from prolonged venous hypertension which stretches the veins and damages the valves.
      b. The resultant edema and venous stasis cause venous stasis ulcers, swelling, and cellulitis.
      c. Treatment focuses on decreasing edema and promoting venous return from the affected extremity.
      d. Treatment for venous stasis ulcers focuses on healing the ulcer and preventing stasis and ulcer recurrence.

BOX 49.9	Instructions for the Client with Deep Vein Thrombophlebitis

Instruct the client concerning the hazards of anticoagulation therapy.
Recognize the signs/symptoms of bleeding.
Avoid prolonged sitting or standing, constrictive clothing, or crossing of the legs when seated.
Elevate the legs for 10–20 minutes every few hours each day.
Plan a progressive walking program.
Inspect the legs for edema, and measure the circumference of the legs.
Wear antiembolism stockings if they are prescribed.
Avoid smoking.
Avoid any medications unless prescribed by the primary health care provider (PHCP).
Instruct the client concerning the importance of follow-up PHCP visits and laboratory studies.
Obtain and wear a MedicAlert bracelet.

Adult—Cardiovascular

2. Data collection
   a. Stasis dermatitis or brown discoloration along the ankles and extending up to the calf
   b. Edema
   c. Ulcer formation: Edges are uneven, ulcer bed is pink, and granulation is present.
3. Interventions

⚠ For venous insufficiency, leg elevation is usually prescribed to assist with the return of the blood to the heart.

   a. Reinforce instructions to the client to wear elastic or compression stockings during the day and evening if prescribed (instruct the client to put on elastic stockings when awakening, before getting out of bed); it may be necessary to wear the stockings for the remainder of the client's life.
   b. Reinforce instructions to the client to avoid prolonged sitting or standing, constrictive clothing, or crossing legs when seated.
   c. Reinforce instructions to the client to elevate the legs for 10 to 20 minutes every few hours each day.
   d. Reinforce instructions to the client to elevate legs above the level of the heart when in bed.
   e. Reinforce instructions to the client in the use of an intermittent sequential pneumatic compression system, if prescribed. Instruct the ambulatory client to apply the compression system twice daily for 1 hour in the morning and evening.
   f. Advise the client with an open ulcer that the compression system is applied over a dressing.
4. Wound care
   a. Provide care to the wound as prescribed by the PHCP.
   b. Monitor the client's ability to care for the wound and initiate homecare resources as necessary.
   c. If an Unna boot (a dressing constructed of gauze moistened with zinc oxide) is prescribed, the PHCP will change it weekly.
   d. The wound is cleansed with normal saline before application of the Unna boot. Povidone-iodine and hydrogen peroxide are not used because they destroy granulation tissue.
   e. The Unna boot is covered with an elastic wrap that hardens to promote venous return and prevent stasis.
   f. Monitor for signs of arterial occlusion from an Unna boot that may be too tight.
   g. Keep tape off the client's skin.

   h. Occlusive dressings such as polyethylene film or hydrocolloid dressings may be used to cover the ulcer.
5. Medications
   a. Apply topical agents to the wound, as prescribed, to débride the ulcer, eliminate necrotic tissue, and promote healing.
   b. When applying topical agents, apply an oil-based agent such as petroleum jelly on the surrounding skin because débriding agents can injure healthy tissue.
   c. Administer antibiotics as prescribed if infection or cellulitis occurs.

E. Varicose veins
1. Description
   a. Distended, protruding veins that appear darkened and tortuous are evident.
   b. Vein walls weaken and dilate and valves become incompetent.
2. Data collection
   a. Pain in the legs with dull aching after standing
   b. A feeling of fullness in the legs
   c. Ankle edema
3. Trendelenburg test
   a. Place the client in a supine position with the legs elevated.
   b. When the client sits up, if varicosities are present, veins fill from the proximal end. Veins normally fill from the distal end.
4. Interventions
   a. Emphasize the importance of antiembolism stockings as prescribed.
   b. Reinforce instructions to the client to elevate the legs as much as possible.
   c. Reinforce instructions to the client to avoid constrictive clothing and pressure on the legs.
   d. Prepare the client for sclerotherapy or vein stripping as prescribed.
5. Sclerotherapy
   a. A solution is injected into the vein followed by the application of a pressure dressing.
   b. An incision and drainage of the trapped blood in the sclerosed vein are performed 14 to 21 days after the injection, followed by the application of a pressure dressing for 12 to 18 hours.
6. Laser therapy: A laser fiber is used to heat and close the main vessel contributing to the varicosity.
7. Vein stripping: Varicose veins may be removed if they are larger than 4 mm in diameter or if they are in clusters; other treatments are usually tried before vein stripping.

XVII. **Arterial Disorders**

A. Peripheral arterial disease

1. Description
   a. A chronic disorder in which partial or total arterial occlusion deprives the lower extremities of oxygen and nutrients
   b. Tissue damage occurs below the level of the arterial occlusion.
   c. Atherosclerosis is the most common cause of peripheral arterial disease.

2. Data collection
   a. Intermittent claudication (pain in the muscles resulting from an inadequate blood supply)
   b. Rest pain characterized by numbness, burning, or aching in the distal portion of the lower extremities which awakens the client at night and is relieved by placing the extremity in a dependent position
   c. Lower back or buttock discomfort
   d. Loss of hair and dry, scaly skin on the lower extremities
   e. Thickened toenails
   f. Cold and gray-blue skin in the lower extremities
   g. Elevational pallor and dependent rubor in the lower extremities
   h. Decreased or absent peripheral pulses
   i. Signs of arterial ulcer formation occurring on or between the toes or on the upper aspect of the foot that are characterized as painful
   j. BP measurements at the thigh, calf, and ankle are lower than the brachial pressure. (Normally BP readings in the thigh and calf are higher than those in the upper extremities.)

3. Interventions

 Because swelling in the extremities prevents arterial blood flow, the client with peripheral arterial disease is instructed to elevate the feet at rest, but to refrain from elevating them above the level of the heart because extreme elevation slows arterial blood flow to the feet. In severe cases of peripheral arterial disease, clients with edema may sleep with the affected limb hanging from the bed, or they may sit upright (without leg elevation) in a chair for comfort.

   a. Monitor pain.
   b. Monitor the extremities for color, motion and sensation, and pulses.
   c. Obtain BP measurements.
   d. Monitor for signs of ulcer formation or signs of gangrene.
   e. Assist with developing an individualized exercise program, which is initiated gradually and slowly increased. Encourage prescribed exercise, which will improve arterial flow through the development of collateral circulation.
   f. Reinforce instructions to the client to walk to the point of claudication, stop and rest, and then walk a little farther.
   g. Reinforce instructions to the client with peripheral arterial disease to avoid crossing the legs which interferes with blood flow.
   h. Reinforce instructions to the client to avoid exposure of the extremities to cold (causes vasoconstriction) and to wear socks or insulated shoes for warmth at all times.
   i. Reinforce instructions to the client never to apply direct heat to the limb such as with a heating pad or hot water because the decreased sensitivity in the limb will cause burning.
   j. Reinforce instructions to the client to inspect the skin on the extremities daily and to report any signs of skin breakdown.
   k. Reinforce instructions to the client to avoid tobacco and caffeine because of their vasoconstrictive effects.
   l. Reinforce instructions to the client about the use of hemorheologic medications (affect blood flow) and antiplatelet medications as prescribed.

4. Procedures to improve arterial blood flow
   a. Percutaneous transluminal angioplasty with or without intravascular stent
   b. Laser-assisted angioplasty
   c. Atherectomy
   d. Bypass surgery: Inflow procedures bypass the occlusion above the superficial femoral arteries and include aortoiliac, aortofemoral, and axillofemoral bypasses. Outflow procedures bypass the occlusion at or below the superficial femoral arteries and include femoropopliteal and femorotibial bypasses.

B. Raynaud's disease

1. Description
   a. Raynaud's disease refers to the vasospasm of the arterioles and arteries of the upper and lower extremities.
   b. Vasospasm causes constriction of the cutaneous vessels.
   c. Attacks are intermittent and occur with exposure to cold or stress.
   d. Primarily affects fingers, toes, ears, and cheeks

2. Data collection
   a. Blanching of the extremity followed by cyanosis during vasoconstriction
   b. Reddened tissue when the vasospasm is relieved
   c. Numbness, tingling, swelling, and a cold temperature at the affected body part

3. Interventions
   a. Monitor pulses.

b. Administer vasodilators as prescribed.
c. Reinforce instructions to the client regarding medication therapy.
d. Assist the client to identify and avoid precipitating factors such as cold and stress.
e. Reinforce instructions to the client to avoid smoking.
f. Reinforce instructions to the client to wear warm clothing, socks, and gloves in cold weather.
g. Advise the client to avoid injuries to fingers and hands.

C. Buerger's disease (thromboangiitis obliterans)
  1. Description
    a. Buerger's disease is an occlusive disease of the median and small arteries and veins.
    b. The distal upper and lower limbs are affected most commonly.
  2. Data collection
    a. Intermittent claudication
    b. Ischemic pain occurring in the digits while at rest
    c. Aching pain that is more severe at night
    d. Cool, numb, or tingling sensation
    e. Diminished pulses in the distal extremities
    f. Extremities that are cool and red in the dependent position
    g. Development of ulcerations in the extremities
  3. Interventions: See Raynaud's disease.

XVIII. Aortic Aneurysms

A. Description
  1. An aortic aneurysm is an abnormal dilation of the arterial wall caused by localized weakness and stretching in the medial layer or wall of the aorta.
  2. The aneurysm can be located anywhere along the abdominal aorta.
  3. The goal of treatment is to limit the progression of disease by modifying risk factors, controlling the BP to prevent strain on the aneurysm, recognizing symptoms early, and preventing rupture.

B. Types of aortic aneurysm
  1. Fusiform: Diffuse dilation that involves the entire circumference of the arterial segment
  2. Saccular: Distinct localized outpouching of the artery wall
  3. Dissecting: Created when blood separates the layers of the artery wall forming a cavity between them
  4. False (pseudoaneurysm): Occurs when the clot and connective tissue are outside the arterial wall. Pseudoaneurysm occurs as a result of vessel injury or trauma to all three layers of the arterial wall.

C. Data collection
  1. Thoracic aneurysm
    a. Pain extending to neck, shoulders, lower back, or abdomen
    b. Syncope
    c. Dyspnea
    d. Increased pulse

    e. Cyanosis
    f. Weakness
    g. Hoarseness/difficulty swallowing because of pressure from the aneurysm
  2. Abdominal aneurysm
    a. Prominent, pulsating mass in the abdomen, at or above the umbilicus
    b. Systolic bruit over the aorta
    c. Tenderness on deep palpation
    d. Abdominal or lower back pain
  3. Rupturing aneurysm
    a. Severe abdominal or back pain
    b. Lumbar pain radiating to the flank and groin
    c. Hypotension
    d. Increased pulse rate
    e. Signs of shock
    f. Hematoma at flank area
  4. Diagnostic tests
    a. Diagnostic tests are done to confirm the presence, size, and location of the aneurysm.
    b. Tests include abdominal ultrasound, computed tomography scan, and arteriography.
  5. Interventions
    a. Monitor vital signs.
    b. Obtain information regarding back or abdominal pain.
    c. Question the client regarding the sensation of pulsation in the abdomen.
    d. Check peripheral circulation including pulse, temperature, and color.
    e. Observe for signs of rupture.
    f. Note any tenderness over the abdomen.
    g. Monitor for abdominal distention.
    h. Avoid palpating the abdomen if an abdominal aneurysm is suspected.
  6. Nonsurgical interventions
    a. Modify the risk factors.
    b. Reinforce instructions to the client regarding the procedure for monitoring BP.
    c. Reinforce instructions to the client regarding the importance of regular PHCP visits to follow the size of the aneurysm.
    d. Reinforce instructions to the client to notify the PHCP immediately if any of the following occur: severe back or abdominal pain or fullness, soreness over the umbilicus, sudden development of discoloration in the extremities, or a persistent elevation of BP.

 Instruct the client with an aortic aneurysm to immediately report the occurrence of chest or back pain, shortness of breath, difficulty swallowing, or hoarseness.

D. Pharmacological interventions
  1. Administer antihypertensives to maintain the BP within normal limits and prevent strain on the aneurysm.

2. Reinforce instructions to the client regarding the purpose of the medications.
3. Reinforce instructions to the client about the side effects and schedule of the medications.

▲ **E.** Abdominal aortic aneurysm resection
   1. Description: Surgical resection or excision of the aneurysm. The excised section is replaced with a graft that is sewn end to end.
   2. Preoperative interventions
      a. Check all peripheral pulses as a baseline for postoperative comparison.
      b. Instruct the client on coughing and deep-breathing exercises.
   3. Postoperative interventions
      a. Monitor vital signs.
      b. Monitor peripheral pulses distal to the graft site.
      c. Monitor for signs of graft occlusion including changes in pulses, cool to cold extremities below the graft, white or blue extremities or flanks, severe pain, or abdominal distention.
      d. Limit elevation of the head of the bed to 45 degrees to prevent flexion of the graft.
      e. Monitor for hypovolemia and kidney failure resulting from significant blood loss during surgery.
      f. Monitor urine output hourly, and notify the PHCP if it is less than 30 mL/hr to 50 mL/hr.
      g. Monitor serum creatinine and blood urea nitrogen daily.
      h. Monitor respiratory status and auscultate breath sounds to identify respiratory complications.
      i. Encourage turning, coughing, and deep breathing as well as splinting of the incision.
      j. Ambulate as prescribed.
      k. Maintain nasogastric tube to low suction until bowel sounds return.
      l. Monitor bowel sounds and report their return to the PHCP.
      m. Monitor for pain and administer medication as prescribed.
      n. Monitor incision site for bleeding or signs of infection.
      o. Prepare the client for discharge by providing instructions regarding pain management, wound care, and activity restrictions.
      p. Reinforce instructions to the client not to lift objects heavier than 15 lb to 20 lb for 6 to 12 weeks.
      q. Advise the client to avoid activities requiring pushing, pulling, or straining.
      r. Reinforce instructions to the client not to drive a vehicle until approved by the PHCP.

▲ **F.** Thoracic aneurysm repair
   1. Description
      a. A thoracotomy or median sternotomy approach is used to enter the thoracic cavity.
      b. The aneurysm is exposed and excised, and a graft or prosthesis is sewn onto the aorta.
      c. Total cardiopulmonary bypass is necessary for excision of aneurysms in the ascending aorta.
      d. Partial cardiopulmonary bypass is used for clients with an aneurysm in the descending aorta.
   2. Postoperative interventions
      a. Monitor vital signs and neurological and renal status.
      b. Monitor for signs of hemorrhage such as a drop in BP and increased pulse rate and respirations, and report to the PHCP immediately.
      c. Monitor chest tubes for an increase in chest drainage which may indicate bleeding or separation at the graft site.
      d. Monitor sensation and motion of all extremities and notify the PHCP if deficits occur, which can be caused by a lack of blood supply to the spinal cord during surgery.
      e. Monitor respiratory status and auscultate breath sounds to identify respiratory complications.
      f. Encourage turning, coughing, and deep breathing while splinting the incision.
      g. Prepare the client for discharge by providing instructions regarding pain management, wound care, and activity restrictions.
      h. Reinforce instructions to the client not to lift objects heavier than 15 lb to 20 lb for 6 to 12 weeks.
      i. Advise the client to avoid activities requiring pushing, pulling, or straining.
      j. Reinforce instructions to the client not to drive a vehicle until approved by the PHCP.

XIX. Embolectomy ▲

A. Description
   1. Embolectomy is removal of an embolus from an artery using a catheter.
   2. A patch graft may be required to close the artery.

B. Preoperative interventions
   1. Obtain a baseline vascular assessment.
   2. Administer anticoagulants as prescribed.
   3. Administer thrombolytics as prescribed.
   4. Place a bed cradle on the bed.
   5. Avoid bumping or jarring the bed.
   6. Maintain the extremity in slightly dependent position.

C. Postoperative interventions
   1. Monitor cardiac, respiratory, and neurological status.
   2. Monitor the affected extremity for color, temperature, and pulse.
   3. Monitor sensory and motor function of the affected extremity.
   4. Monitor for signs/symptoms of new thrombi or emboli.

5. Administer oxygen as prescribed.
6. Monitor pulse oximetry.
7. Monitor for complications caused by reperfusion of the artery such as spasms and swelling of the skeletal muscles.
8. Monitor for signs of swollen skeletal muscles such as edema, pain during passive movement, poor capillary refill, numbness, and muscle tenseness.
9. Maintain bed rest initially with the client in a semi-Fowler's position.
10. Place a bed cradle on the bed.
11. Check incision site for bleeding or hematoma.
12. Administer anticoagulants as prescribed.
13. Monitor laboratory values related to anticoagulation therapy.
14. Instruct the client to recognize the signs/symptoms of infection and edema.
15. Instruct the client to avoid prolonged sitting or crossing of the legs when sitting.
16. Reinforce instructions to the client to elevate the legs when sitting.
17. Reinforce instructions to the client to ambulate daily.
18. Reinforce instructions to the client about anticoagulant therapy and the hazards associated with anticoagulants.
19. Reinforce instructions to the client to wear antiembolism stockings as prescribed and how to remove and reapply the stockings.

XX. Vena Cava Filter and Ligation of Inferior Vena Cava

A. Vena cava filter: Insertion of an intracaval filter (umbrella) that partially occludes the inferior vena cava and traps emboli to prevent pulmonary emboli
B. Ligation: Suturing or placing clips on the inferior vena cava to prevent pulmonary emboli; performed via abdominal laparotomy
C. Preoperative interventions: If the client has been taking an anticoagulant, consult with the PHCP regarding discontinuation of the medication to prevent hemorrhage.
D. Postoperative interventions: similar to care after embolectomy

XXI. Hypertension

A. Description
1. For an adult (ages 18 years and older), a normal BP is a systolic BP below 120 mm Hg and a diastolic BP below 80 mm Hg.
2. Elevated blood pressure is defined as a systolic BP between 120 and 129 mmHg and a diastolic BP below 80 mmHg.
3. Hypertension (Stage 1) is defined as a systolic BP between 130 mm Hg and 139 mm Hg or a diastolic BP between 80 mm Hg and 89 mm Hg.

4. Hypertension (Stage 2) is defined as a systolic BP of at least 140 mm Hg or a diastolic BP of at least 90 mm Hg.
5. If either the systolic BP or diastolic BP is outside of range, the higher measurement will determine the classification.
6. Hypertension is a major risk factor for coronary, cerebral, renal, and peripheral vascular disease.
7. The disease is initially asymptomatic.
8. The goals of treatment include reduction of the BP and preventing or lessening the extent of organ damage; primary organs affected include the eyes (visual changes), brain (stroke), cardiovascular system (heart failure), and kidneys (hypertensive crisis and renal failure).
9. Nonpharmacological approaches such as lifestyle changes may be prescribed initially; if the BP cannot be decreased after 1–3 months, the client may require pharmacological treatment.

B. Primary or essential hypertension
1. No known cause
2. Risk factors
   a. Aging
   b. Family history
   c. African American race
   d. Obesity
   e. Smoking
   f. Stress
   g. Excessive alcohol
   h. Hyperlipidemia
   i. Increased intake of salt or caffeine

C. Secondary hypertension
1. Treatment depends on the cause and the organs involved.
2. Secondary hypertension occurs as a result of other disorders or conditions.
3. Precipitating disorders or conditions
   a. Cardiovascular disorders
   b. Renal disorders
   c. Endocrine system disorders
   d. Pregnancy
   e. Medications (such as estrogens, glucocorticoids, and mineralocorticoids)

D. Data collection
1. May be asymptomatic
2. Headache
3. Visual disturbances
4. Dizziness
5. Chest pain
6. Tinnitus
7. Flushed face
8. Epistaxis

E. Interventions
1. Goals: One treatment goal is to reduce the BP and another treatment goal is to prevent or lessen the extent of organ damage.

2. Question the client regarding the signs/symptoms indicative of hypertension.
3. Obtain the BP two or more times on both arms with the client supine and standing.
4. Compare the BP with prior documentation.
5. Determine family history of hypertension.
6. Identify current medication therapy.
7. Obtain weight.
8. Evaluate dietary patterns and sodium intake.
9. Monitor for visual changes or retinal damage.
10. Monitor for cardiovascular changes such as distended neck veins, increased heart rate, and dysrhythmia.
11. Evaluate chest x-ray film for heart enlargement.
12. Monitor neurological system.
13. Evaluate renal function.
14. Evaluate results of diagnostic and laboratory studies.

F. Nonpharmacological interventions
   1. Weight reduction, if necessary, or maintenance of ideal weight
   2. Dietary sodium restriction to 2 g daily as prescribed
   3. Moderate intake of alcohol and caffeine-containing products
   4. Initiation of a regular exercise program
   5. Avoidance of smoking
   6. Relaxation techniques and biofeedback therapy
   7. Elimination of unnecessary medications that may contribute to the hypertension

G. Pharmacological interventions
   1. Medication therapy is individualized for each client, and the selection of the medication is based on such factors as the client's age, culture, presence of coexisting conditions, severity of hypertension, and client's preferences.
   2. See Chapter 50 for medications to treat hypertension.

H. See Box 49.10 for client education reinforcement.

▲ XXII. Hypertensive Crisis

A. Description
   1. A hypertensive crisis is an acute and life-threatening condition requiring immediate reduction in BP.
   2. Emergency treatment is required, because target organ damage (brain, heart, kidneys, retina of the eye) can occur quickly.
   3. Death can be caused by stroke, kidney failure, or cardiac disease.

B. Data collection
   1. An extremely high BP and usually the diastolic pressure is greater than 120 mm Hg
   2. Headache
   3. Drowsiness and confusion
   4. Blurred vision
   5. Change in neurological status

BOX 49.10   Client Education for Hypertension

Describe the importance of compliance with the treatment plan.

Describe the disease process, explaining that symptoms usually do not develop until organs have suffered damage.

Initiate and assist the client with planning a regular exercise program, avoiding heavy weight-lifting and isometric exercises.

Emphasize the importance of beginning the exercise program gradually.

Encourage the client to express feelings about daily stress.

Assist the client to identify ways to reduce stress.

Teach relaxation techniques.

Instruct the client on how to incorporate relaxation techniques into the daily living pattern.

Instruct the client and family in the technique for monitoring blood pressure.

Instruct the client to maintain a diary of blood pressure readings.

Emphasize the importance of lifelong medication and the need for follow-up treatment.

Instruct the client and family about the dietary restrictions, which may include sodium, fat, calories, and cholesterol.

Instruct the client on how to shop for and prepare low-sodium meals.

Provide a list of products that contain sodium.

Instruct the client to read labels of products to determine sodium content focusing on substances listed as sodium, NaCl, or MSG (monosodium glutamate).

Instruct the client to bake, roast, or boil foods. Avoid salt in preparation of foods, and avoid using salt at the table.

Instruct the client that fresh foods are best to consume and to avoid canned foods.

Instruct the client about the actions, side effects, and scheduling of medications.

Advise the client that if uncomfortable side effects occur to contact the primary health care provider and not to stop the medication.

Instruct the client to avoid over-the-counter medications.

Stress the importance of follow-up care.

---

6. Tachycardia and tachypnea
7. Dyspnea
8. Cyanosis
9. Seizure

C. Interventions
   1. Maintain a patent airway.
   2. IV antihypertensive medications may be prescribed.
   3. Monitor vital signs, checking the BP every 5 minutes.
   4. Monitor neurological status.
   5. Monitor for hypotension during the administration of antihypertensives. Place the client in a supine position if hypotension occurs.
   6. Have emergency medications and resuscitation equipment readily available.

7. Maintain bed rest with the head of the bed elevated at 45 degrees.
8. Monitor IV therapy, monitoring for fluid overload.
9. Insert a Foley catheter as prescribed.
10. Monitor urinary output, and if oliguria or anuria occurs, notify the PHCP.

WHAT WOULD YOU DO?

Answer: If the client with an abdominal aortic aneurysm suddenly complains of severe back pain and shortness of breath, the nurse would suspect rupture (a surgical emergency) and needs to immediately contact RN and PHCP. The nurse would also obtain information about the back pain, stay with the client while waiting for the arrival of the PHCP, monitor vital signs and neurological status, and provide support to the client. Other signs of rupture include severe abdominal pain or fullness, soreness over the umbilicus, and sudden development of discoloration in the extremities.

PRACTICE QUESTIONS

1. A postcardiac surgery client with a blood urea nitrogen (BUN) level of 45 mg/dL and a serum creatinine level of 2.2 mg/dL has a total 2-hour urine output of 25 mL. The nurse understands that the client is at risk for which condition?
   1. Hypovolemia
   2. Acute kidney injury
   3. Glomerulonephritis
   4. Urinary tract infection

2. The nurse is preparing to ambulate a postoperative client after cardiac surgery. The nurse plans to do which to enable the client to **best** tolerate the ambulation?
   1. Provide the client with a walker.
   2. Remove the telemetry equipment.
   3. Encourage the client to cough and deep breathe.
   4. Premedicate the client with an analgesic before ambulating.

3. A client is wearing a continuous cardiac monitor which begins to alarm at the nurse's station. The nurse sees no electrocardiographic complexes on the screen. The nurse would take which action **first**?
   1. Call a code blue.
   2. Check the client status and lead placement.
   3. Call the primary health care provider (PHCP).
   4. Press the recorder button on the ECG console.

❖ 4. The nurse in a medical unit is caring for a client with heart failure. The client suddenly develops extreme dyspnea, tachycardia, and lung crackles, and the nurse suspects pulmonary edema. The nurse

immediately notifies the registered nurse (RN) and expects which interventions to be prescribed? **Select all that apply.**
   ❑ 1. Administering oxygen
   ❑ 2. Inserting a Foley catheter
   ❑ 3. Administering furosemide
   ❑ 4. Administering morphine sulfate intravenously
   ❑ 5. Transporting the client to the coronary care unit
   ❑ 6. Placing the client in a low-Fowler's side-lying position

5. The nurse is caring for a client on a cardiac monitor who is alone in a room at the end of the hall. The client has a short burst of ventricular tachycardia (VT), followed by ventricular fibrillation (VF). The client suddenly loses consciousness. Which action would the nurse take **first**?
   ❑ 1. Go to the nurse's station quickly and call a code.
   ❑ 2. Run to get a defibrillator from an adjacent nursing unit.
   ❑ 3. Call for help and initiate cardiopulmonary resuscitation (CPR).
   ❑ 4. Start oxygen by cannula at 10 L/min and lower the head of the bed.

6. The nurse is monitoring a client following cardioversion. Which observations would be of **highest priority** to the nurse?
   1. Blood pressure
   2. Status of airway
   3. Oxygen flow rate
   4. Level of consciousness

7. To use an external cardiac defibrillator on a client, which action would be performed to check the cardiac rhythm?
   1. Holding the defibrillator paddles firmly against the chest
   2. Applying the adhesive patch electrodes to the skin and moving away from the client
   3. Applying standard electrocardiographic monitoring leads to the client and observing the rhythm
   4. Connecting standard electrocardiographic electrodes to a transtelephonic monitoring device

8. The nurse is assisting with caring for the client immediately after insertion of a permanent demand pacemaker via the right subclavian vein. The nurse prevents dislodgement of the pacing catheter by implementing which intervention?
   1. Limiting movement and abduction of the left arm
   2. Limiting movement and abduction of the right arm
   3. Assisting the client to get out of bed and ambulate with a walker
   4. Having the physical therapist do active range of motion to the right arm

9. A client diagnosed with thrombophlebitis 1 day ago suddenly complains of chest pain and shortness of breath, and the client is visibly anxious. Which is a life-threatening complication that could be occurring?
   1. Pneumonia
   2. Pulmonary edema
   3. Pulmonary embolism
   4. Myocardial infarction

10. A 24-year-old man seeks medical attention for complaints of claudication in the arch of the foot. The nurse also notes superficial thrombophlebitis of the lower leg. The nurse would check the client's medical history for which finding **next**?
    1. Smoking history
    2. Recent exposure to allergens
    3. History of recent insect bites
    4. Familial tendency toward peripheral vascular disease

11. The nurse has reinforced instructions to the client with Raynaud's disease about self-management of the disease process. The nurse determines that the client **needs further teaching** if the client makes which statement?
    1. "Smoking cessation is very important."
    2. "Moving to a warmer climate would help."
    3. "Sources of caffeine should be eliminated from the diet."
    4. "Taking nifedipine as prescribed will decrease spasms in my blood vessels."

12. A client with myocardial infarction suddenly becomes tachycardic, shows signs of air hunger, and begins coughing frothy, pink-tinged sputum. The nurse listens to breath sounds expecting to hear which breath sounds bilaterally?
    1. Rhonchi
    2. Crackles
    3. Wheezes
    4. Diminished breath sounds

13. The nurse is collecting data on a client with a diagnosis of right-sided heart failure. The nurse would expect to note which specific characteristic of this condition?
    1. Dyspnea
    2. Hacking cough
    3. Dependent edema
    4. Crackles on lung auscultation

14. The nurse is checking the neurovascular status of a client who returned to the surgical nursing unit 4 hours ago after undergoing an aortoiliac bypass graft. The affected leg is warm, and the nurse notes redness and edema. The pedal pulse is palpable and unchanged from admission. Based on this data, the nurse would make which determination about the client's neurovascular status?
    1. Moderately impaired, and the surgeon would be called
    2. Normal, caused by increased blood flow through the leg
    3. Slightly deteriorating, and would be monitored for another hour
    4. Adequate from an arterial approach, but venous complications are arising

❖ 15. The primary health care provider (PHCP) is going to perform carotid massage on a client with rapid rate atrial fibrillation. Which interventions would the nurse anticipate? **Select all that apply.**
    ❑ 1. The client would be placed on a cardiac monitor.
    ❑ 2. The PHCP massages the carotid artery for a full minute.
    ❑ 3. The head would be turned toward the side to be massaged.
    ❑ 4. Rhythm strips would be obtained before, during, and after the procedure.
    ❑ 5. Vital signs, cardiac rhythm, and level of consciousness would be monitored the procedure.

ANSWERS

1. 2
Rationale: The client who undergoes cardiac surgery is at risk for acute kidney injury from poor perfusion, hemolysis, low cardiac output, or vasopressor medication therapy. Kidney injury is signaled by a decreased urine output and increased BUN and creatinine levels. The client may need medications to increase renal perfusion and could need peritoneal dialysis or hemodialysis.
Test-Taking Strategy: Focus on the subject, postoperative laboratory values. The question provides no evidence of any infection, so eliminate options 3 and 4 first. Noting the laboratory values in the question will assist with eliminating option 1.

2. 4
Rationale: The nurse would encourage regular use of pain medication for the first 48 to 72 hours after cardiac surgery because analgesia will promote rest, decrease myocardial oxygen consumption caused by pain, and allow better participation in activities such as coughing, deep breathing, and ambulation.
Test-Taking Strategy: Focus on the subject, ambulating a client after surgery, and note the strategic word, best. The question asks for the *best* action of the nurse to help a client tolerate ambulation. Coughing and deep breathing will not actively help endurance, so eliminate option 3. Eliminate option 2 because removal of telemetry equipment is contraindicated unless prescribed. From the remaining options, noting that the client is postoperative will direct you to option 4.

3. 2

Rationale: Sudden loss of electrocardiographic complexes indicates ventricular asystole or possibly electrode displacement. Checking of the client and equipment is the first action by the nurse.

Test-Taking Strategy: Note the strategic word, *first*. Use the steps of the nursing process, and remember that data collection is the first step. Options 1 and 3 are incorrect because they indicate calling for assistance before collecting data. Option 4 may sound reasonable, but the electrocardiographic monitor automatically starts recording when an alarm sounds. Option 2 is the first action because you would always check the client directly before taking any action.

4. 1, 2, 3, 4

Rationale: Pulmonary edema is a life-threatening event that can result from severe heart failure. During pulmonary edema the left ventricle fails to eject sufficient blood, and pressure increases in the lungs because of the accumulated blood. Oxygen is always prescribed, and the client is placed in a high-Fowler's position to ease the work of breathing. Furosemide, a rapid-acting diuretic, will eliminate accumulated fluid. A Foley catheter is inserted to accurately measure output. Intravenously administered morphine sulfate reduces venous return (preload), decreases anxiety, and reduces the work of breathing. Transporting the client to the coronary care unit is not a priority intervention. In fact, this may not be necessary at all if the client's response to treatment is successful.

Test-Taking Strategy: Focus on the subject, the client's diagnosis. Recalling the pathophysiology associated with pulmonary edema and using the ABCs—airway, breathing, and circulation—will assist you with determining the priority interventions.

5. 3

Rationale: When ventricular fibrillation occurs, the nurse remains with the client and initiates CPR until a defibrillator is available and attached to the client. Options 1, 2, and 4 are incorrect.

Test-Taking Strategy: Note the strategic word, *first*. Eliminate options 1 and 2 first because you would never leave the client alone. From the remaining options, lowering the head of the bed is appropriate (for resuscitation), but the oxygen by cannula at 10 L/min is incorrect. Option 3 is the correct choice.

6. 2

Rationale: Nursing responsibilities after cardioversion include maintenance of a patent airway, oxygen administration, assessment of vital signs and level of consciousness, and dysrhythmia detection. Airway is the priority.

Test-Taking Strategy: Focus on the strategic words, *highest priority*, and use the ABCs—airway, breathing, and circulation—to answer the question. This will direct you to the correct option. Remember, airway comes first.

7. 2

Rationale: The nurse or rescuer puts two large adhesive patch electrodes on the client's chest in the usual defibrillator position. The nurse stops cardiopulmonary resuscitation and orders anyone near the client to move away and not touch the client. The defibrillator then analyzes the rhythm which

may take up to 30 seconds. The machine then indicates if it is necessary to defibrillate. Although automatic external defibrillation can be done transtelephonically, it is done through the use of patch electrodes (not standard electrocardiographic electrodes) that interact via telephone lines to a base station that controls any actual defibrillation. It is not necessary to hold defibrillator paddles against the client's chest with this device.

Test-Taking Strategy: If you are not familiar with this piece of equipment, look first at the word *automatic* in the name. This implies that someone is not as involved in the process as with a conventional defibrillator and thus may help you eliminate option 1. Because standard electrocardiographic monitoring leads are not used (options 3 and 4), you can eliminate these comparable or alike, and incorrect, options. Although automatic external defibrillation can be done transtelephonically, it is done through the use of patch electrodes.

8. 2

Rationale: In the first several hours after insertion of either a permanent or temporary pacemaker, the most common complication is pacing electrode dislodgment. The nurse helps prevent this complication by limiting the client's activities.

Test-Taking Strategy: Focus on the subject, permanent pacemaker insertion. The question tells you that the pacemaker was inserted on the right side. Therefore, to prevent pacing electrode dislodgment, motion needs to be limited on that side. Options 3 and 4 involve movement of the right arm. Limiting the movement of the left arm (option 1) is of no benefit to the client. Thus option 2 is correct.

9. 3

Rationale: Pulmonary embolism is a life-threatening complication of deep vein thrombosis and thrombophlebitis. Chest pain is the most common symptom which is sudden in onset and may be aggravated by breathing. Other signs/symptoms include dyspnea, cough, diaphoresis, and apprehension.

Test-Taking Strategy: Note the data in the question. This question tests your ability to analyze signs/symptoms of pulmonary embolism in a client at risk. Options 2 and 4 would be eliminated because myocardial infarction and pulmonary edema are cardiac-related problems and are therefore comparable or alike. Eliminate option 1 because pneumonia is an infectious process.

10. 1

Rationale: The mixture of arterial and venous manifestations (claudication and phlebitis, respectively) in the young male client suggests thromboangiitis obliterans (Buerger's disease). This is a relatively uncommon disorder characterized by inflammation and thrombosis of smaller arteries and veins. This disorder is typically found in young men who smoke. The cause is unknown but is suspected to have an autoimmune component.

Test-Taking Strategy: Focus on the subject, claudication and phlebitis. You can first eliminate options 2 and 3 because they would most likely cause local skin reactions. Also, note the strategic word, *next*. It is often better to assess a modifiable factor before a nonmodifiable one. This will direct you to the correct option.

11. 2

Rationale: Raynaud's disease responds favorably to the elimination of nicotine and caffeine. Medications such as calcium channel blockers may inhibit vessel spasm and prevent symptoms. Avoiding exposure to cold through a variety of means is very important. However, moving to a warmer climate may not necessarily be beneficial because the symptoms could still occur with the use of air conditioning and during periods of cooler weather. ***Test-Taking Strategy:*** Note the strategic words, *needs further teaching*. These words indicate a negative event query and the need to select the incorrect client statement. All of the options seem reasonable. However, when you analyze each of them, note that relocation is the least favorable of all the options from the viewpoints of practicality and encountering new environmental concerns.

12. 2

Rationale: Pulmonary edema is characterized by extreme breathlessness, dyspnea, air hunger, and production of frothy, pink-tinged sputum. Auscultation of the lungs reveals crackles. Wheezes, rhonchi, and diminished breath sounds are not associated with pulmonary edema. ***Test-Taking Strategy:*** Focus on the data in the question and the subject, breath sounds in a client with pulmonary edema. Recall that fluid produces sounds that are called crackles. This will assist you with eliminating the incorrect options.

13. 3

Rationale: Right-sided heart failure is characterized by signs of systemic congestion that occur as a result of right ventricular failure, fluid retention, and pressure buildup in the venous system. Edema develops in the lower legs and ascends to the thighs and abdominal wall. Other characteristics include jugular (neck vein) congestion, enlarged liver and spleen, anorexia and nausea, distended abdomen, swollen hands and fingers, polyuria at night, and weight gain. Left-sided heart failure produces pulmonary signs. These include dyspnea, crackles on lung auscultation, and a hacking cough. ***Test-Taking Strategy:*** Focus on the subject, right-sided heart failure. Eliminate options 1, 2, and 4 because they are comparable or alike and are pulmonary signs.

14. 2

Rationale: An expected outcome of surgery is warmth, redness, and edema in the surgical extremity caused by increased blood flow. Options 1, 3, and 4 are incorrect. ***Test-Taking Strategy:*** Focus on the subject, aortoiliac bypass graft. Option 1 can be eliminated because the pedal pulse is unchanged. Venous complications from immobilization caused by surgery would not be apparent within 4 hours, so eliminate option 4 next. To choose between options 2 and 3, think about the effects of sudden reperfusion in an ischemic limb. There would be redness from new blood flow and edema from the sudden change in pressure in the blood vessels. Thus option 2 is correct.

15. 1, 4, 5

Rationale: Carotid sinus massage is one maneuver used for vagal stimulation to decrease a rapid heart rate and possibly terminate a tachydysrhythmia. The other maneuvers are the Valsalva maneuver of inducing the gag reflex and asking the client to strain or bear down. Medication therapy is often needed as an adjunct to keep the rate down or maintain the normal rhythm. The client's head needs to be turned away from the side to be massaged in order to provide better access to the carotid artery. The PHCP or cardiologist will massage only one carotid artery for a few seconds to determine whether a change in cardiac rhythm occurs. The client needs to be on a cardiac monitor throughout the procedure and obtain rhythm strips before, during, and after the procedure. ***Test-Taking Strategy:*** Focus on the subject, carotid massage. The client's head needs to be turned away from the side to be massaged in order to provide better access to the carotid artery. This eliminates option 2. The PHCP or cardiologist will massage only one carotid artery for a few seconds to determine whether a change in cardiac rhythm occurs. This eliminates option 3. The client needs to be on a cardiac monitor throughout the procedure and obtain rhythm strips before, during, and after the procedure. Continue to monitor the client's cardiac rhythm as well as vital signs and level of consciousness.

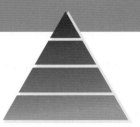
CHAPTER **50**

Cardiovascular Medications

PRIORITY CONCEPTS Clotting; Perfusion

WHAT WOULD YOU DO?

The nurse notes that a client taking warfarin sodium has an international normalized ratio (INR) of 2.8. What would the nurse do?
Answer is located on p. 695.

I. Anticoagulants (Box 50.1)

A. Description
1. Anticoagulants prevent the extension and formation of clots by inhibiting factors in the clotting cascade and decreasing blood coagulability.
2. Anticoagulants are administered when there is evidence or likelihood of clot formation: myocardial infarction, unstable angina, atrial fibrillation, deep vein thrombosis, pulmonary embolism, and the presence of mechanical heart valves.
3. Anticoagulants are contraindicated with active bleeding (except for disseminated intravascular coagulation), bleeding disorders or blood dyscrasias, ulcers, liver and kidney disease, and hemorrhagic brain injuries (Box 50.2).

B. Side and adverse effects
1. Hemorrhage
2. Hematuria
3. Epistaxis
4. Ecchymosis
5. Bleeding gums
6. Thrombocytopenia
7. Hypotension

C. Heparin sodium
1. Description
   a. Heparin prevents thrombin from converting fibrinogen to fibrin.
   b. Heparin prevents thromboembolism.
   c. The therapeutic dose does not dissolve clots but prevents new thrombus formation.
2. Blood levels
   a. The normal activated partial thromboplastin time (aPTT) is 30 to 40 seconds in most

---

BOX 50.1 Anticoagulants

Oral
- Apixaban
- Dabigatran etexilate
- Edoxaban
- Rivaroxaban
- Warfarin sodium

Parenteral
- Argatroban
- Bivalirudin
- Dalteparin
- Desirudin
- Enoxaparin
- Fondaparinux
- Heparin sodium

BOX 50.2 Substances to Avoid with Anticoagulants

- Allopurinol
- Cimetidine
- Corticosteroids
- Fluoroquinolones
- Green, leafy vegetables and other foods high in vitamin K
- Gingko and ginseng (herbs)
- Macrolide antibiotics
- Nonsteroidal anti-inflammatory medications
- Oral hypoglycemic agents
- Phenytoin
- Salicylates
- Sulfonamides

---

laboratories (values depend on reagent and instrumentation used).
   b. To maintain a therapeutic level of anticoagulation when the client is receiving a continuous infusion of heparin, the aPTT would be 1.5 to 2.5 times the normal value. Some agencies use two different protocols, a high-intensity protocol such as for acute coronary syndrome and low-intensity protocol such as for venous

thromboembolism prophylaxis, and the dosages and recommended aPTT ranges are slightly different for the two different protocols.

c. aPTT therapy would be measured every 4 to 6 hours during initial continuous infusion therapy and then daily per agency policy.

d. If the aPTT is too long (level based on agency protocol), the dosage would be lowered.

e. If aPTT is too short (level based on agency protocol), the dosage would be increased.

3. Interventions

a. Monitor aPTT.

b. Monitor platelet count.

c. Observe for bleeding gums, bruises, nosebleeds, hematuria, hematemesis, occult blood in the stool, and petechiae.

d. Instruct client regarding measures to prevent bleeding.

e. The antidote for heparin is protamine sulfate.

f. When heparin is administered subcutaneously, it is injected into the abdomen with a ⅝-inch (16 mm) needle (25–28 gauge) at a 90-degree angle; the injection site must not be aspirated or rubbed.

g. Continuous infusions must be delivered through an infusion pump, and the infusion pump would be preprogrammed to ensure precise rate of delivery.

D. Enoxaparin is a low-molecular-weight heparin

1. Description: Enoxaparin has the same mechanism of action and use as heparin but is not interchangeable. It has a longer half-life than heparin.

2. Interventions

a. Administer enoxaparin only to the recumbent client by subcutaneous injection only in the anterolateral or posterolateral abdominal wall; do not expel the air bubble from the prefilled syringe or aspirate during injection.

b. Monitor the same laboratory values as for heparin and observe for bleeding.

c. The antidote to enoxaparin is protamine sulfate.

E. Warfarin sodium

1. Description

a. Warfarin suppresses coagulation by acting as an antagonist of vitamin K, thereby inhibiting four dependent clotting factors (X, IX, VII, and II).

b. Warfarin prolongs clotting time and is monitored by the prothrombin time (PT) and the international normalized ratio (INR).

c. It is used for long-term anticoagulation, mainly to prevent thromboembolic conditions such as thrombophlebitis, pulmonary embolism, and embolism formation caused by atrial fibrillation, thrombosis, myocardial infarction, or heart valve damage.

2. Blood levels

a. The normal PT is 11 to 12.5 seconds (conventional and SI units).

b. Warfarin sodium prolongs the PT. The therapeutic range is 1.5 to 2 times the control value.

3. INR

a. The normal INR for both conventional and standard units is 0.81 to 1.2 (0.81–1.2).

b. The INR is determined by multiplying the observed PT ratio (the ratio of the client's PT to a control PT) by a correction factor specific to a particular thromboplastin preparation used during testing.

c. The treatment goal is to raise the INR to an appropriate value.

d. An INR of 2 to 3 is appropriate for standard warfarin therapy; an INR of 3 to 4.5 is appropriate for high-dose warfarin therapy.

e. If the PT value is longer than 32 seconds and the INR is greater than 3.0 in a client receiving standard warfarin therapy, initiate bleeding precautions.

f. If the INR is less than the recommended range, warfarin sodium would be increased.

g. Clients may sometimes be prescribed "bridge therapy," whereby heparin sodium is used concurrently with warfarin sodium until the INR reaches the recommended range. Once this occurs, the heparin is discontinued.

4. Interventions

a. Monitor PT and INR.

b. Observe for bleeding gums, bruises, nosebleeds, hematuria, hematemesis, occult blood in the stool, and petechiae.

c. Reinforce instructions to the client regarding measures to prevent bleeding.

d. The antidote for warfarin is phytonadione.

F. Dabigatran etexilate

1. Description

a. Dabigatran etexilate works through direct inhibition of thrombin, preventing the conversion of fibrinogen into fibrin and activation of factor XIII.

b. Current approved use is for clot prevention associated with nonvalvular atrial fibrillation.

c. It is administered in a fixed dose twice daily.

2. Blood levels: No blood testing is required.

3. Interventions: Same as for warfarin except no routine monitoring is required.

II. Thrombolytic Medications (Box 50.3)

A. Description

1. Thrombolytic medications activate plasminogen. Plasminogen generates plasmin (the enzyme that dissolves clots).

Adult—Cardiovascular

BOX 50.3   Thrombolytic Medications

- Alteplase
- Reteplase
- Tenecteplase

---

2. Thrombolytic medications are used early in the course of myocardial infarction (within 4–6 hours of the onset of the infarct) to restore blood flow, limit myocardial damage, preserve left ventricular function, and prevent death.
3. Thrombolytics are also used in arterial thrombosis, deep vein thrombosis, occluded shunts or catheters, and pulmonary emboli.

B. Contraindications
1. Active internal bleeding
2. History of hemorrhagic brain attack (stroke)
3. Intracranial problems including trauma
4. Intracranial or intraspinal surgery within the previous 2 months
5. History of thoracic, pelvic, or abdominal surgery in the previous 10 days
6. History of hepatic or renal disease
7. Uncontrolled hypertension
8. Recent, prolonged cardiopulmonary resuscitation
9. Known allergy to the specific product or any of its preservatives

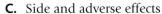 **C.** Side and adverse effects
1. Bleeding
2. Dysrhythmia
3. Allergic reactions

D. Interventions
1. Determine aPTT, PT, fibrinogen level, hematocrit, and platelet count.
2. Monitor the vital signs.
3. Check the pulses.
4. Monitor for bleeding and check all excretions for occult blood.
5. Monitor for neurological changes such as slurred speech, lethargy, confusion, and hemiparesis.
6. Monitor for hypotension and tachycardia.
7. Avoid injections and unnecessary venipunctures if possible.
8. Apply direct pressure over a puncture site for 20 to 30 minutes.
9. The client is handled as little as possible when moving.
10. Reinforce instructions to the client to use an electric razor for shaving and brush teeth gently.
11. The medication is withheld if bleeding develops, and the primary health care provider (PHCP) is notified.
12. Antidote
    a. Aminocaproic acid is the antidote.
    b. Used only in acute, life-threatening conditions

⚠️ Bleeding is the primary concern for a client taking an anticoagulant, thrombolytic, or antiplatelet medication.

BOX 50.4   Antiplatelet Medications

Oral
- Acetylsalicylic acid
- Anagrelide
- Cilostazol
- Clopidogrel
- Dipyridamole
- Ticlopidine
- Ticagrelor
- Pesantine

Parenteral
- Abciximab
- Eptifibatide
- Tirofiban

III. Antiplatelet Medications (Box 50.4)

A. Description
1. Antiplatelet medications inhibit the aggregation of platelets in the clotting process thereby prolonging the bleeding time.
2. Antiplatelet medications may be used with anticoagulants.
3. Used in the prophylaxis of long-term complications after myocardial infarction, coronary revascularization, stents, and stroke.
4. These medications are contraindicated in those with bleeding disorders and known sensitivity.

B. Side and adverse effects
1. Gastrointestinal bleeding
2. Bruising
3. Hematuria
4. Tarry stools

C. Interventions
1. A blood test may be prescribed to determine the client's sensitivity to the medication before beginning administration.
2. Monitor vital signs.
3. The client is instructed to take medication with food if gastrointestinal upset occurs.
4. Monitor the bleeding time.
5. Reinforce instructions to the client to monitor for side and adverse effects related to bleeding and the measures to prevent bleeding.

IV. Cardiac Glycosides

A. Digoxin

B. Description
1. Cardiac glycosides inhibit the sodium-potassium pump, thus increasing intracellular calcium which causes the heart muscle fibers to contract more efficiently.
2. Cardiac glycosides produce a positive inotropic action, which increases the force of myocardial contractions.
3. Cardiac glycosides produce a negative chronotropic action which slows the heart rate.

4. Cardiac glycosides produce a negative dromotropic action that slows conduction velocity through the atrioventricular (AV) node.

5. The increase in myocardial **contractility** increases cardiac, peripheral, and kidney function by increasing **cardiac output**, decreasing **preload**, improving blood flow to the periphery and kidneys, decreasing edema, and increasing fluid excretion. As a result, fluid retention in the lungs and extremities is decreased.

6. Cardiac glycosides are used second line for heart failure (medications affecting the renin angiotensin-aldosterone system are used more often) and cardiogenic shock, atrial tachycardia, atrial fibrillation, and atrial flutter; used less frequently for rate control in atrial dysrhythmia (β-blockers and calcium channel blockers are used more often) (Fig. 50.1).

7. These medications are contraindicated in those with ventricular dysrhythmia and second- or third-degree heart block and need to be used with caution in clients with renal disease, hypothyroidism, and hypokalemia.

C. Side and adverse effects

1. Anorexia, nausea, vomiting, diarrhea
2. Headache
3. Visual disturbances: Diplopia, blurred vision, yellow-green halos, photophobia
4. Drowsiness
5. Bradycardia
6. Fatigue, weakness

⚠ Early signs of digoxin toxicity present as gastrointestinal manifestations (anorexia, nausea, vomiting, diarrhea); then heart rate abnormalities and visual disturbances appear.

D. Interventions

1. Monitor for toxicity as evidenced by anorexia, nausea, vomiting, visual disturbances, confusion, bradycardia, heart block, premature ventricular contractions, and tachydysrhythmia.

2. Monitor serum digoxin level, electrolyte levels, and renal function test results.

3. The therapeutic digoxin range is 0.5 to 2.0 ng/mL. However, a level on the low-end of normal may be preferred to avoid toxicity.

4. An increased risk of toxicity exists in clients with hypercalcemia, hypokalemia, hypomagnesemia, or hypothyroidism.

5. Monitor the potassium level; if hypokalemia occurs (potassium lower than 3.5 mEq/L), notify the PHCP.

6. Reinforce instructions to the client to avoid over-the-counter medications.

7. Monitor the client taking a potassium-wasting diuretic or corticosteroids closely for hypokalemia because the hypokalemia can cause digoxin toxicity.

8. Note that older clients are more sensitive to digoxin toxicity.

9. Advise the client to eat foods high in potassium such as fresh and dried fruits, fruit juices, vegetables, and potatoes.

10. Monitor the apical pulse for 1 full minute; if the apical pulse rate is lower than 60 beats/min, the medication must be withheld and the PHCP notified.

11. Reinforce teaching the client how to measure the pulse and to notify the PHCP if the pulse rate is less than 60 beats/min or more than 100 beats/min.

12. Reinforce teaching the client the signs/symptoms of toxicity.

13. Antidote: Digoxin immune Fab is used in extreme toxicity.

V. Antihypertensive Medications: Diuretics (Box 50.5)

A. Thiazide diuretics (Box 50.6)

1. Description

   a. Thiazide diuretics increase sodium and water excretion by inhibiting sodium reabsorption in the distal tubule of the kidney.

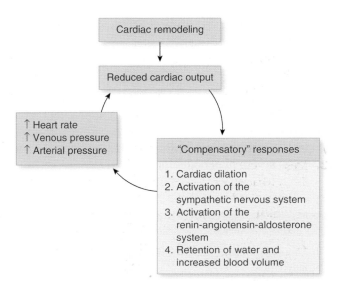

FIGURE 50.1 The vicious cycle of maladaptive compensatory responses to a failing heart.

BOX 50.5 Classifications of Diuretics

- Loop diuretics
- Osmotic diuretics
- Potassium-retaining diuretics
- Thiazide diuretics

BOX 50.6 Thiazide and Thiazide-Like Diuretics

- Chlorothiazide
- Chlorthalidone
- Hydrochlorothiazide
- Indapamide
- Metolazone

    b. Used for hypertension and peripheral edema

    c. Not effective for immediate diuresis

    d. Used in clients with normal renal function (contraindicated in clients with renal failure)

    e. Thiazide diuretics would be used with caution in the client taking lithium because lithium toxicity can occur in the client taking digoxin, corticosteroids, or hypoglycemic medications.

2. Side and adverse effects

    a. Hypercalcemia, hyperglycemia, hyperuricemia

    b. Hypokalemia, hyponatremia

    c. Hypovolemia

    d. Hypotension

    e. Dehydration

    f. Rashes

    g. Photosensitivity

3. Interventions

    a. Monitor vital signs.

    b. Monitor weight.

    c. Monitor urine output.

    d. Monitor electrolyte, glucose, calcium, blood urea nitrogen (BUN), creatinine, and uric acid levels.

    e. Check peripheral extremities for edema.

    f. Reinforce instructions to the client to take the medication in the morning to avoid nocturia and sleep interruption.

    g. Reinforce instructions to the client in how to record the blood pressure (BP).

    h. Reinforce instructions to the client to eat foods high in potassium.

    i. Reinforce instructions to the client in how to take potassium supplements if prescribed.

    j. Reinforce instructions to the client to take medication with food to avoid gastrointestinal upset.

    k. Reinforce instructions to the client to change positions slowly to prevent orthostatic hypotension.

    l. Reinforce instructions to the client to use sunscreen when in direct sunlight because of increased photosensitivity.

    m. Reinforce instructions to the client with diabetes mellitus to have the blood glucose level checked periodically.

B. Loop diuretics (Box 50.7)

1. Description

    a. Loop diuretics inhibit sodium and chloride reabsorption from the loop of Henle and the distal tubule.

    b. Loop diuretics have little effect on the blood glucose level; however, they cause depletion of water and electrolytes, an increase in uric acid levels, and the excretion of calcium.

    c. Loop diuretics are more potent than thiazide diuretics causing rapid diuresis and thus decreasing vascular fluid volume, cardiac output, and BP.

    d. Loop diuretics are used for hypertension, pulmonary edema, edema associated with heart failure, hypercalcemia, and renal disease.

    e. Use loop diuretics with caution in the client taking digoxin or lithium and the client taking aminoglycosides, anticoagulants, corticosteroids, or amphotericin B.

2. Side and adverse effects

    a. Hypokalemia, hyponatremia, hypocalcemia, hypomagnesemia

    b. Thrombocytopenia

    c. Hyperuricemia

    d. Orthostatic hypotension

    e. Rash

    f. Ototoxicity and deafness

    g. Thiamine deficiency

    h. Dehydration

3. Interventions: See Section V.A. (Interventions for thiazide diuretics)

    a. Monitor electrolyte, calcium, magnesium, BUN, creatinine, and uric acid levels.

    b. Monitor for signs of digoxin or lithium toxicity if the client is taking these medications.

    c. Intravenous (IV) furosemide is administered slowly over 1 to 2 minutes, because hearing loss can occur if injected rapidly.

C. Osmotic diuretics (See Chapter 56)

D. Potassium-sparing diuretics (Box 50.8)

1. Description

    a. Potassium-sparing diuretics act on the distal tubule to promote sodium and water excretion and potassium retention.

    b. Used for edema and hypertension, to increase urine output, and to treat fluid retention and overload associated with heart failure, ascites resulting from cirrhosis or nephrotic syndrome, and diuretic-induced hypokalemia.

    c. Potassium-sparing diuretics are contraindicated in severe kidney or hepatic disease and severe hyperkalemia.

BOX 50.7 **Loop Diuretics**

- Bumetanide
- Ethacrynic acid
- Furosemide
- Torsemide

BOX 50.8 **Potassium-Sparing Diuretics**

- Amiloride hydrochloride; hydrochlorothiazide
- Eplerenone
- Spironolactone
- Triamterene

d. Potassium-sparing diuretics would be used with caution in the client with diabetes mellitus, taking antihypertensives or lithium, taking angiotensin-converting enzyme (ACE) inhibitors or potassium supplements because hyperkalemia can result.

⚠ The primary concern with administering potassium-sparing diuretics is hyperkalemia.

2. Side and adverse effects
   a. Hyperkalemia
   b. Nausea, vomiting, diarrhea
   c. Rash
   d. Dizziness, weakness
   e. Headache
   f. Dry mouth
   g. Photosensitivity
   h. Anemia
   i. Thrombocytopenia
3. Interventions
   a. Monitor vital signs.
   b. Monitor urine output.
   c. Monitor for signs/symptoms of hyperkalemia such as nausea, diarrhea, abdominal cramps, tachycardia followed by bradycardia, tall peaked T wave on the electrocardiogram, and oliguria.
   d. Monitor for a potassium level greater than 5.0 mEq/L which indicates hyperkalemia.
   e. Reinforce instructions to the client to avoid foods high in potassium.
   f. Reinforce instructions to the client to avoid exposure to direct sunlight.
   g. Reinforce instructions to the client to monitor for signs of hyperkalemia.
   h. Reinforce instructions to the client to avoid salt substitutes because they contain potassium.
   i. Reinforce instructions to the client to take with or after meals to decrease gastrointestinal irritation.

VI. Peripherally Acting α-Adrenergic Blockers (Box 50.9)

A. Description
   1. These medications decrease sympathetic vasoconstriction by reducing the effects of norepinephrine at peripheral nerve endings resulting in vasodilation and decreased BP.

2. These medications are used to maintain renal blood flow.
3. These medications are used to treat hypertension.

B. Side and adverse effects
   1. Orthostatic hypotension
   2. Reflex tachycardia
   3. Sodium and water retention
   4. Gastrointestinal disturbance
   5. Drowsiness
   6. Nasal congestion
   7. Edema
   8. Weight gain
C. Interventions
   1. Monitor vital signs.
   2. Monitor for fluid retention and edema.
   3. Reinforce instructions to the client to change positions slowly to prevent orthostatic hypotension.
   4. Reinforce instructions to the client in how to monitor the BP.
   5. Reinforce instructions to the client to monitor for edema.
   6. Reinforce instructions to the client to decrease salt intake.
   7. Reinforce instructions to the client to avoid over-the-counter medications.

VII. Centrally Acting Sympatholytics (Adrenergic Blockers) (Box 50.10)

A. Description
   1. Centrally acting sympatholytics stimulate alpha receptors in the central nervous system to inhibit vasoconstriction thus reducing peripheral resistance.
   2. Used to treat hypertension
   3. Contraindicated in impaired liver function
B. Side and adverse effects
   1. Sodium and water retention
   2. Drowsiness, dizziness
   3. Dry mouth
   4. Bradycardia
   5. Edema
   6. Impotence
   7. Hypotension
   8. Depression
C. Interventions
   1. Monitor vital signs.
   2. Reinforce instructions to the client not to discontinue medication because abrupt withdrawal can cause severe rebound hypertension.
   3. Monitor liver function tests.

BOX 50.9	Peripherally Acting α-Adrenergic Blockers

- Doxazosin
- Prazosin
- Terazosin

BOX 50.10	Centrally Acting Sympatholytics

- Clonidine
- Guanfacine
- Methyldopa

Adult—Cardiovascular

VIII. ACE Inhibitors and Angiotensin II Receptor Blockers (ARBs) (Box 50.11)

A. Description
  1. ACE inhibitors prevent peripheral vasoconstriction by blocking conversion of angiotensin I to angiotensin II (AII).
  2. ARBs prevent peripheral vasoconstriction and secretion of aldosterone and block the binding of AII to type 1 AII receptors.
  3. These medications are used to treat hypertension and heart failure. ACE inhibitors are also administered for their cardioprotective effect after myocardial infarction.
  4. Use with potassium supplements and potassium-retaining diuretics is avoided.

B. Side and adverse effects
  1. Nausea, vomiting, diarrhea
  2. Persistent dry cough (ACE inhibitors only)
  3. Hypotension
  4. Hyperkalemia
  5. Tachycardia
  6. Headache
  7. Dizziness, fatigue
  8. Insomnia
  9. Hypoglycemic reaction in the client with diabetes mellitus
  10. Bruising, petechiae, bleeding
  11. Diminished taste (ACE inhibitors)

⚠ A persistent dry cough is a common complaint for those taking an ACE inhibitor, but this often subsides after a few weeks. The client is instructed to contact the PHCP if this occurs and persists.

BOX 50.11   Angiotensin-Converting Enzyme Inhibitors and Angiotensin Receptor Blockers

Angiotensin-Converting Enzyme Inhibitors
- Benazepril
- Captopril
- Enalapril
- Fosinopril
- Lisinopril
- Moexipril
- Perindopril
- Quinapril
- Ramipril
- Trandolapril

Angiotensin II Receptor Blockers
- Azilsartan
- Candesartan
- Eprosartan
- Irbesartan
- Losartan
- Olmesartan
- Telmisartan
- Valsartan

C. Interventions
  1. Monitor vital signs.
  2. Monitor white blood cells, and protein, albumin, BUN, creatinine, and potassium levels.
  3. Monitor for hypoglycemic reactions in the client with diabetes mellitus.
  4. Reinforce instructions to the client to take captopril 20 to 60 minutes before a meal.
  5. Monitor for bruising, petechiae, or bleeding with captopril.
  6. Reinforce instructions to the client not to discontinue medications because rebound hypertension can occur.
  7. Reinforce instructions to the client not to take over-the-counter medications.
  8. Reinforce instructions to the client in how to take the BP.
  9. Reinforce instructions to the client that the taste of food may be diminished during the first month of therapy.
  10. Reinforce instructions to the client to report the side effect of angioedema immediately to the PHCP.

IX. Antianginal Medications (Box 50.12)

A. Nitrates (see **Priority Nursing Actions**)
  1. Description
    a. Nitrates produce vasodilation, decrease preload and **afterload** and reduce myocardial oxygen consumption.
    b. Contraindicated in the client with significant hypotension, increased intracranial pressure, severe anemia, and in those taking medication to treat erectile dysfunction (because of the risk for severe hypotension).
    c. Would be used with caution in cases of severe renal or hepatic disease
    d. Abrupt withdrawal of long-acting preparations is avoided to prevent the rebound effect of severe pain from myocardial ischemia.
  2. Side and adverse effects
    a. Headache
    b. Orthostatic hypotension
    c. Dizziness, weakness
    d. Faintness
    e. Nausea, vomiting
    f. Flushing or pallor

BOX 50.12   Antianginal Medications

- Isosorbide dinitrate
- Isosorbide mononitrate
- Nitroglycerin, sublingual
- Nitroglycerin, translingual
- Nitroglycerin, transdermal patches
- Nitroglycerin ointment
- Intravenous nitroglycerin

g. Dry mouth

h. Reflex tachycardia

3. Sublingual medications

a. Monitor vital signs.

b. Offer sips of water before giving because dryness may inhibit medication absorption.

c. Reinforce instructions to the client to place under the tongue and leave until fully dissolved.

d. Reinforce instructions to the client not to swallow the medication.

e. Reinforce instructions to the client to take 1 tablet for pain and to immediately contact emergency medical services if pain is not relieved; in the hospitalized client, 1 tablet is administered every 5 minutes for a total of three doses and the PHCP is notified immediately if pain is not relieved following the three doses (the BP is checked before each dose administration).

f. The client is informed that a stinging or burning sensation may indicate that the tablet is fresh.

g. Reinforce instructions to the client to store medication in a dark, tightly closed bottle.

h. Reinforce instructions to the client to take acetaminophen for a headache.

4. Translingual medications (spray)

a. Instruct the client to direct the spray against the oral mucosa.

b. Instruct the client to avoid inhaling the spray.

5. Sustained-released medications: The client is instructed to swallow and not chew or crush the medication.

6. Transdermal patch

a. The client is instructed to apply the patch to a hairless area using a new patch and different site each day.

b. As prescribed, the client is instructed to remove the patch after 12 to 14 hours, allowing 10 to 12 "patch-free" hours each day to prevent tolerance.

7. Topical ointments

a. Reinforce instructions to the client to remove the ointment on the skin from the previous dose.

b. Reinforce instructions to the client to squeeze a ribbon of ointment of the prescribed length onto the applicator or dose-measuring paper.

c. Reinforce instructions to the client to spread the ointment over a 2.5 × 3.5-inch (6.5 × 9 cm) area and cover with plastic wrap using either the chest, back, abdomen, upper arm, or anterior thigh (avoid hairy areas).

d. Reinforce instructions to the client to rotate sites and avoid touching the ointment when applying.

8. Patches and ointments

a. Wear gloves when applying.

b. Do not apply on the chest in the area of defibrillator-cardioverter pad placement because skin burns can result if the pads need to be used.

 Instruct the client using nitroglycerin tablets to check the expiration date on the medication bottle because expiration may occur within 6 months of obtaining the medication. The tablets will not relieve the chest pain if they have expired.

X. β-Adrenergic Blockers (Box 50.13)

A. Description

1. β-adrenergic blockers inhibit response to β-adrenergic stimulation thus decreasing cardiac output.

2. β-adrenergic blockers block the release of catecholamines, epinephrine, and norepinephrine,

---

⚡ PRIORITY NURSING ACTIONS

Chest Pain Occurs in a Hospitalized Client with Cardiac Disease: Nitroglycerin

1. The client is quickly assessed, specifically for characteristics of pain, heart rate and rhythm, and BP.
2. A nitroglycerin tablet is administered.
3. The client would not be left alone.
4. The client is reassessed in 5 minutes.
5. Another nitroglycerin tablet is administered if pain is not relieved and the BP is stable.
6. The client is reassessed in 5 minutes.
7. A third nitroglycerin tablet is administered if pain is not relieved and the BP is stable.
8. The client is reassessed in 5 minutes. The PHCP is contacted if the third nitroglycerin tablet does not relieve the pain.
9. The event, actions taken, and the client's response to treatment are documented.

BOX 50.13 β-Adrenergic Blockers

Nonselective (Block β₁ and β₂)
- Carvedilol
- Labetalol
- Nadolol
- Penbutolol
- Pindolol
- Propranolol
- Sotalol

Cardioselective (Block β₁)
- Acebutolol
- Atenolol
- Betaxolol
- Bisoprolol
- Esmolol
- Metoprolol
- Nebivolol

thus decreasing the heart rate and BP; they also decrease the workload of the heart and decrease oxygen demands.

3. Used for angina, dysrhythmia, hypertension, migraine headaches, prevention of myocardial infarction, and glaucoma

4. β-adrenergic blockers are contraindicated in the client with asthma, bradycardia, heart failure (with exceptions), severe renal or hepatic disease, hyperthyroidism, or stroke. Carvedilol, metoprolol, and bisoprolol have been approved for use in heart failure once the client has been stabilized with ACE inhibitor and diuretic therapy.

5. β-adrenergic blockers would be used with caution in the client with diabetes mellitus because the medication may mask the symptoms of hypoglycemia.

6. β-adrenergic blockers need to be used with caution in the client taking antihypertensive medications.

 B. Side and adverse effects
1. Bradycardia
2. Bronchospasm
3. Hypotension
4. Weakness, fatigue
5. Nausea, vomiting
6. Dizziness
7. Hyperglycemia
8. Agranulocytosis
9. Behavioral or psychotic response
10. Depression
11. Nightmares

C. Interventions
1. Monitor vital signs.
2. Withhold the medication if the pulse or BP is not within the prescribed parameters.
3. Monitor for signs of heart failure or worsening heart failure.
4. Check for respiratory distress and for signs of wheezing and dyspnea.
5. Reinforce instructions to the client to report dizziness, light-headedness, or nasal congestion.
6. Reinforce instructions to the client not to stop the medication because rebound hypertension, rebound tachycardia, or an anginal attack can occur.
7. Reinforce instructions to the client taking insulin that the β-adrenergic blocker can mask early signs of hypoglycemia such as tachycardia and nervousness.
8. Reinforce instructions to the client taking insulin to monitor the blood glucose level.
9. Reinforce instructions to the client in how to take pulse and BP.
10. Reinforce instructions to the client to change positions slowly to prevent orthostatic hypotension.
11. Reinforce instructions to the client to avoid over-the-counter medications, especially cold medications and nasal decongestants.

XI. Calcium Channel Blockers (Box 50.14)

A. Description
1. Calcium channel blockers decrease cardiac contractility (negative inotropic effect by relaxing smooth muscle) and the workload of the heart thus decreasing the need for oxygen.
2. Calcium channel blockers promote vasodilation of the coronary and peripheral vessels.
3. Used for angina, dysrhythmia, or hypertension
4. Would be used with caution in the client with heart failure, bradycardia, or AV block

B. Side and adverse effects
1. Bradycardia
2. Hypotension
3. Reflex tachycardia as a result of hypotension
4. Headache
5. Dizziness, light-headedness
6. Fatigue
7. Peripheral edema
8. Constipation
9. Flushing of the skin
10. Changes in liver and kidney function

C. Interventions
1. Monitor vital signs.
2. Monitor for signs of heart failure.
3. Monitor liver enzyme levels.
4. Monitor kidney function tests.
5. Reinforce instructions to the client not to discontinue the medication.
6. Reinforce instructions to the client in how to take a pulse.
7. Reinforce instructions to the client to notify the PHCP if dizziness or fainting occurs.
8. Reinforce instructions to the client to not crush or chew sustained-release tablets.

XII. Peripheral Vasodilators (Box 50.15)

A. Description
1. Peripheral vasodilators decrease peripheral resistance by exerting a direct action on the arteries or the arteries and the veins.
2. Peripheral vasodilators increase blood flow to the extremities and are used in peripheral vascular disorders of venous and arterial vessels.

BOX 50.14 **Calcium Channel Blockers**

- Amlodipine
- Clevidipine
- Diltiazem
- Felodipine
- Isradipine
- Levamlodipine
- Nicardipine
- Nifedipine
- Nimodipine
- Nisoldipine
- Verapamil

BOX 50.15 Vasodilators: Peripheral and Direct-Acting Arteriolar

Peripheral Vasodilators

α-Adrenergic Blockers
- Doxazosin
- Prazosin
- Terazosin

Calcium Channel Blockers
- Diltiazem
- Nifedipine
- Nimodipine
- Verapamil

Hemorheological
- Pentoxifylline (increases microcirculation and tissue perfusion)

Direct-Acting Arteriolar Vasodilators
- Diazoxide
- Fenoldopam
- Hydralazine
- Nitroglycerin
- Sodium nitroprusside

---

3. Peripheral vasodilators are most effective for disorders resulting from vasospasm (Raynaud's disease).
4. These medications may decrease some symptoms of cerebral vascular insufficiency.

B. Side and adverse effects
1. Light-headedness, dizziness
2. Orthostatic hypotension
3. Tachycardia
4. Palpitations
5. Flushing
6. Gastrointestinal distress

C. Interventions
1. Monitor vital signs, especially the BP and heart rate.
2. Monitor for orthostatic hypotension and tachycardia.
3. Monitor for signs of inadequate blood flow to the extremities such as pallor, feeling cold, and pain.
4. Reinforce instructions to the client that it may take up to 3 months for a desired therapeutic response.
5. The client is advised not to smoke because smoking increases vasospasm.
6. Reinforce instructions to the client to avoid aspirin or aspirin-like compounds unless approved by the PHCP.
7. Reinforce instructions to the client to take the medication with meals if gastrointestinal disturbances occur.
8. Reinforce instructions to the client to avoid alcohol because it may cause a hypotensive reaction.
9. The client is encouraged to change positions slowly to avoid orthostatic hypotension.

XIII. Direct-Acting Arteriolar Vasodilators (see Box 50.15)

A. Description
1. Direct-acting vasodilators relax the smooth muscles of the blood vessels, mainly the arteries, causing vasodilation; with vasodilation, the BP drops and sodium and water are retained, resulting in peripheral edema (diuretics may be given to decrease the edema).
2. Direct-acting vasodilators promote an increase in blood flow to the brain and kidneys.
3. These medications are used in the client with moderate to severe hypertension and for acute hypertensive emergencies.

B. Side and adverse effects
1. Hypotension
2. Reflex tachycardia caused by vasodilation and the drop in BP
3. Palpitations
4. Edema
5. Dizziness
6. Headache
7. Nasal congestion
8. Gastrointestinal bleeding
9. Neurological symptoms
10. Confusion
11. With sodium nitroprusside, cyanide toxicity and thiocyanate toxicity can occur.

C. Interventions
1. Monitor vital signs, especially BP.
2. Sodium nitroprusside (administered by the registered nurse [RN])
    a. Monitor cyanide and thiocyanate levels.
    b. Protect from light because the medication decomposes.
    c. When administering, solution must be covered by a dark bag provided by the manufacturer and is stable for 24 hours.
    d. Discard if the medication is red, green, or blue.

⚠ Vasodilators cause orthostatic hypotension. Instruct the client about safety measures when taking these medications, such as the need to rise from a lying to a sitting or standing position slowly.

XIV. Antilipemic Medications (Box 50.16)

A. Description
1. Antilipemic medications reduce serum levels of cholesterol, triglycerides, or low-density lipoprotein.
2. When cholesterol, triglyceride, and low-density lipoprotein levels are elevated, the client is at increased risk for coronary artery disease.
3. In many cases, diet alone will not lower blood lipid levels; therefore, antilipemic medications will be prescribed.

BOX 50.16 Antilipemic Medications

HMG-CoA Reductase Inhibitors
- Atorvastatin
- Fluvastatin
- Lovastatin
- Pitavastatin
- Pravastatin
- Rosuvastatin
- Simvastatin

Other Antilipemic Medications
- Cholestyramine
- Colesevelam
- Colestipol
- Ezetimibe
- Fenofibrate
- Gemfibrozil
- Icosapent
- Lomitapide
- Nicotinic acid
- Omega-3-acid ethyl esters

B. Bile sequestrants (See Chapter 46, Box 46.3)
1. Description
   a. Bind with acids in the intestines, which prevents reabsorption of cholesterol
   b. Would not be used as the only therapy in clients with elevated triglyceride levels because they may raise triglyceride levels
2. Side and adverse effects
   a. Constipation
   b. Gastrointestinal disturbances: Heartburn, nausea, belching, bloating
3. Interventions
   a. Cholestyramine comes in a gritty powder that must be mixed thoroughly in juice or water before administration.
   b. Monitor the client for early signs of peptic ulcer such as nausea and abdominal discomfort followed by abdominal pain and distention.
   c. Reinforce instructions to the client that the medication must be taken with and followed by sufficient fluids.

C. HMG-CoA reductase inhibitors
1. Description
   a. Lovastatin is highly protein bound and must not be administered with anticoagulants.
   b. Lovastatin would not be administered with gemfibrozil.
   c. Lovastatin is administered with caution to the client taking immunosuppressive medications.
2. Side and adverse effects
   a. Nausea
   b. Diarrhea or constipation
   c. Abdominal pain or cramps
   d. Flatulence
   e. Dizziness

f. Headache
g. Blurred vision
h. Rash
i. Pruritus
j. Elevated liver enzyme levels
k. Muscle cramps and fatigue
3. Interventions
   a. Monitor serum liver enzyme levels.
   b. Reinforce instructions to the client to receive an annual eye examination because the medications can cause cataract formation.
   c. If lovastatin is not effective in lowering the lipid level after 3 months, it would be discontinued.

 The client who is taking an antilipemic medication is instructed to report any unexplained muscular pain to the PHCP immediately.

D. Other antilipemic medications (see Box 50.16)
1. Description
   a. Gemfibrozil would not be taken with anticoagulants because they compete for protein sites. If the client is taking an anticoagulant, the anticoagulant dose would be reduced during antilipemic therapy and the INR must be monitored closely.
   b. Do not administer gemfibrozil with HMG-CoA reductase inhibitors because it increases the risk for myositis, myalgias, and rhabdomyolysis.
   c. Fish oil supplements have been associated with a decreased risk for cardiovascular heart disease. Plant stanol and sterol esters and cholestin have been associated with reducing cholesterol levels.
2. Interventions
   a. Monitor vital signs.
   b. Monitor the liver enzyme levels.
   c. Monitor the serum cholesterol and triglyceride levels.
   d. Reinforce instructions to the client to restrict intake of fats, cholesterol, carbohydrates, and alcohol.
   e. Reinforce instructions to the client to follow an exercise program.
   f. Reinforce instructions to the client that it will take several weeks before the lipid level declines.
   g. Reinforce instructions to the client to have an annual eye examination and report any change in vision.
   h. Reinforce instructions to the client with diabetes mellitus who is taking gemfibrozil to monitor their blood glucose level regularly.
   i. Reinforce instructions to the client to increase fluid intake.
   j. Note that nicotinic acid has numerous side effects including gastrointestinal disturbances,

flushing of the skin, elevated liver enzyme levels, hyperglycemia, and hyperuricemia.

k. Reinforce instructions to the client that aspirin or nonsteroidal anti-inflammatory medications taken 30 minutes before may assist with reducing the side effect of cutaneous flushing from nicotinic acid.

l. Reinforce instructions to the client to take nicotinic acid with meals to reduce gastrointestinal discomfort.

WHAT WOULD YOU DO?

Answer: The normal INR is 0.8–1.2. The treatment goal of warfarin sodium is to raise the INR to an appropriate value. An INR of 2–3 is appropriate for most clients, although for some clients the target INR is 3–4.5. If the INR is less than the recommended range, warfarin sodium would be increased. If the INR is greater than the recommended range, warfarin sodium would be reduced. If the INR is 2.8, the nurse would plan to administer the same dosage as prescribed.

PRACTICE QUESTIONS

1. The nurse reinforces discharge instructions to a postoperative client who is taking warfarin sodium. Which statement made by the client reflects the **need for further teaching?**
  1. "I will take my pills every day at the same time."
  2. "I will be certain to avoid alcohol consumption."
  3. "I have already called my family to pick up a MedicAlert bracelet."
  4. "I will take enteric coated aspirin for my headaches because it is coated."

2. A client is receiving digoxin daily. The nurse suspects digoxin toxicity after noting which signs/symptoms? **Select all that apply.**
  ❏ **1.** Visual disturbances
  ❏ **2.** Nausea and vomiting
  ❏ **3.** Apical pulse rate of 63 beats/min
  ❏ **4.** Serum digoxin level of 2.3 ng/mL
  ❏ **5.** Serum potassium level of 3.9 mEq/L

3. Heparin sodium is prescribed for the client. Which laboratory result indicates that the heparin is prescribed at a therapeutic level?
  1. Thrombocyte count of 100,000 mm^3
  2. Prothrombin time (PT) of 21 seconds
  3. International normalized ratio (INR) of 2.3
  4. Activated partial thromboplastin time (aPTT) of 55 seconds

4. The nurse is monitoring a client who is taking propranolol. Which data collection finding would indicate a potential serious complication associated with propranolol?
  1. The development of complaints of insomnia
  2. The development of audible expiratory wheezes
  3. A baseline resting heart rate of 88 beats/min followed by a resting heart rate of 72 beats/min after two doses of the medication
  4. A baseline blood pressure of 150/80 mm Hg followed by a blood pressure of 138/72 mm Hg after two doses of the medication

5. Isosorbide mononitrate is prescribed for a client with angina pectoris. The client tells the nurse that the medication is causing a headache. Which action would the nurse suggest to the client?
  1. Cut the dose in half.
  2. Discontinue the medication.
  3. Take the medication with food.
  4. Contact the primary health care provider (PHCP).

6. A client is diagnosed with an acute myocardial infarction and is receiving tissue plasminogen activator, alteplase. Which action is a **priority** nursing intervention?
  1. Monitor for kidney failure.
  2. Monitor psychosocial status.
  3. Monitor for signs of bleeding.
  4. Have heparin sodium available.

7. A hospitalized client with coronary artery disease complains of substernal chest pain. After checking the client's heart rate and blood pressure, the nurse administers nitroglycerin, 0.4 mg, sublingually. After 5 minutes, the client states, "My chest still hurts." Which appropriate actions would the nurse take? **Select all that apply.**
  ❏ **1.** Call a code blue.
  ❏ **2.** Contact the client's family.
  ❏ **3.** Check the client's pain level.
  ❏ **4.** Check the client's blood pressure.
  ❏ **5.** Administer a second nitroglycerin, 0.4 mg, sublingually.

8. The home health care nurse is visiting a client with elevated triglyceride levels and a serum cholesterol level of 398 mg/dL. The client is taking cholestyramine. Which statement made by the client indicates the **need for further teaching?**
  1. "Constipation and bloating might be a problem."
  2. "I'll continue to watch my diet and reduce my fats."
  3. "Walking a mile each day will help the whole process."
  4. "I'll continue my nicotinic acid from the health food store."

9. A client is taking nicotinic acid for hyperlipidemia, and the nurse reinforces instructions to the client

about the medication. Which statement by the client indicates an understanding of the instructions?
1. "It is not necessary to avoid drinking alcohol."
2. "The medication needs to be taken with meals to decrease flushing."
3. "Clay-colored stools are a common side effect and are not a concern."
4. "Ibuprofen taken 30 minutes before the nicotinic acid will decrease the flushing."

10. The nurse is planning to administer hydrochlorothiazide to a client. Which are concerns related to the administration of this medication?
1. Hypouricemia, hyperkalemia
2. Hypokalemia, hyperglycemia, sulfa allergy
3. Hypokalemia, increased risk of osteoporosis
4. Hyperkalemia, hypoglycemia, penicillin allergy

ANSWERS

1. 4
Rationale: Aspirin-containing products need to be avoided while taking this medication. Alcohol consumption needs to be avoided by a client taking warfarin sodium. Taking prescribed medication at the same time each day increases client compliance. The MedicAlert bracelet provides health care personnel with emergency information.
Test-Taking Strategy: Note the strategic words, *need for further teaching*. These words indicate a negative event query and ask you to select an option that is an incorrect statement. Recalling that warfarin is an anticoagulant and that aspirin is an aspirin-containing product will direct you to the correct option.

❖ 2. 1, 2, 4
Rationale: Signs/symptoms of digoxin toxicity include gastrointestinal signs, bradycardia, visual disturbances, and hypokalemia. A therapeutic serum digoxin level ranges from 0.8 to 2.0 ng/mL. The serum potassium level would be between 3.5 mEq/L and 5.0 mEq/L. The apical pulse must be greater than or equal to 60 beats/min.
Test-Taking Strategy: Focus on the subject, digoxin toxicity. Knowledge of the signs/symptoms of digoxin toxicity is needed to answer correctly.

3. 4
Rationale: The aPTT will assess the therapeutic effect of heparin sodium. The normal aPTT is 30 to 40 seconds. To maintain a therapeutic level, the aPTT would be 1.5 to 2.5 times the normal value. The PT and INR will assess for the therapeutic effect of warfarin sodium. A decreased thrombocyte count can cause bleeding.
Test-Taking Strategy: Note the subject, laboratory values for heparin and warfarin. Eliminate options 2 and 3 because these laboratory values are related to warfarin sodium. Note that option 1 is an unrelated test for monitoring therapeutic values of both heparin sodium and warfarin sodium.

4. 2
Rationale: Audible expiratory wheezes may indicate a serious adverse reaction: bronchospasm. β-blockers may induce this reaction particularly in clients with chronic obstructive pulmonary disease or asthma. Normal decreases in blood pressure and heart rate are expected. Insomnia is a frequent mild side effect and should be monitored.

Test-Taking Strategy: Note the subject, a potential serious complication. Eliminate options 3 and 4 because these are expected effects from the medication. Next, focusing on the subject will direct you to the correct option.

5. 3
Rationale: Isosorbide mononitrate is an antianginal medication. Headache is a frequent side effect of isosorbide mononitrate and usually disappears during continued therapy. If a headache occurs during therapy, the client would be instructed to take the medication with food or meals. It is not necessary to contact the PHCP unless the headaches persist with therapy. It is not appropriate to instruct the client to discontinue therapy or adjust the dosages.
Test-Taking Strategy: Focus on the subject, isosorbide mononitrate and a headache. Eliminate options 1 and 2 first because it is not within the scope of nursing practice to instruct a client to discontinue or adjust dosages. From the remaining options, recalling that the headache can be relieved with the administration of food with the medication will assist in directing you to option 3.

6. 3
Rationale: Tissue plasminogen activator is a thrombolytic. Hemorrhage is a complication of any type of thrombolytic medication. The client is monitored for bleeding. Monitoring for renal failure and monitoring the client's psychosocial status are important but are not the most critical interventions. Heparin is given after thrombolytic therapy, but the question is not asking about follow-up medications.
Test-Taking Strategy: Note the strategic word, *priority*. Think about the action of the medication and remember that bleeding is a priority.

❖ 7. 3, 4, 5
Rationale: The usual guideline for administering nitroglycerin tablets for a hospitalized client with chest pain is to administer one tablet every 5 minutes as needed (PRN) for chest pain for a total dose of three tablets. The registered nurse is notified immediately if a client complains of chest pain. In this situation, because the client is still complaining of chest pain, the nurse would administer a second nitroglycerin tablet. The nurse would check the client's pain level and the client's blood pressure before administering each nitroglycerin dose. There are no data in the question that indicate the need to call a code blue. In addition, it is not necessary to contact the client's family unless the client has requested this.

Test-Taking Strategy: Focus on the data in the question. Use the steps of the nursing process to determine that checking the client's pain level and the client's blood pressure are appropriate actions. Next, recalling the usual guidelines for administering nitroglycerin tablets will assist with determining that an appropriate action is to administer a second nitroglycerin, 0.4 mg, sublingually.

8. 4

Rationale: Nicotinic acid (niacin), even an over-the-counter form, needs to be avoided because it may lead to liver abnormalities. All lipid-lowering medications can also cause liver abnormalities, so a combination of nicotinic acid and cholestyramine resin is to be avoided. Constipation and bloating are the two most common side effects. Walking and the reduction of fats in the diet are therapeutic measures to reduce cholesterol and triglyceride levels.

Test-Taking Strategy: Note the strategic words, *need for further teaching.* These words indicate a negative event query and ask you to select an option that is an incorrect statement. Remembering that over-the-counter medications need to be avoided when a client is taking a prescription medication will direct you to the correct option.

9. 4

Rationale: Flushing is a side effect of this medication. Aspirin or a nonsteroidal anti-inflammatory medication can be taken 30 minutes before taking the medication to decrease flushing. Alcohol consumption needs to be avoided because it will enhance this side effect. The medication needs to be taken with meals; this will decrease gastrointestinal upset. Taking the medication with meals has no effect on the flushing. Clay-colored stools are a sign of hepatic dysfunction and must be immediately reported to the PHCP.

Test-Taking Strategy: Focus on the subject, nicotinic acid (niacin) and flushing. Option 1 can be eliminated because alcohol must be abstained from. Option 2 can be eliminated because taking the medication with meals helps decrease the gastrointestinal symptoms. The clay-colored stools in option 3 are a sign of hepatic dysfunction and must be immediately reported to the PHCP.

10. 2

Rationale: Thiazide diuretics such as hydrochlorothiazide are sulfa-based medications, and a client with a sulfa allergy is at risk for an allergic reaction. Also, clients are at risk for hypokalemia, hyperglycemia, hypercalcemia, hyperlipidemia, and hyperuricemia.

Test-Taking Strategy: Focus on the subject, hydrochlorothiazide. Recalling that thiazide diuretics carry a sulfa ring in their chemical structure will direct you to the correct option.

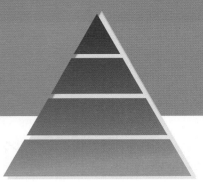

UNIT XIV

Renal and Urinary Problems of the Adult Client

Pyramid to Success

Pyramid Points focus on acute kidney injury and chronic kidney disease, dialysis procedures, and postoperative care following urinary or renal surgery. Be familiar with health problems and diagnostic tests that place the client at risk for acute kidney injury. Focus on the major problems associated with kidney failure and the rationale for the prescribed treatment modalities. Be familiar with the complications associated with hemodialysis and peritoneal dialysis, the specific findings related to complications, and the expected treatment. Focus on the care of a peritoneal catheter and the hemodialysis access device, the complications associated with access devices, and the appropriate nursing interventions if a complication is suspected. Review findings indicating rejection after kidney transplantation. Be familiar with care for the client with urinary or renal calculi and the treatment measures for these health problems.

Client Needs: Learning Objectives

Safe and Effective Care Environment

Consulting with the interprofessional health care team

Establishing priorities

Identifying health problems and diagnostic procedures that increase the risk of developing urinary or renal problems

Identifying the guidelines related to kidney organ donation

Maintaining asepsis related to wound care and dialysis access devices

Maintaining confidentiality related to the renal or urinary problem

Maintaining standard and other precautions related to care for the client

Preventing injury related to complications of the health problem

Upholding client rights

Verifying that informed consent related to diagnostic and surgical procedures has been obtained

Health Promotion and Maintenance

Performing urinary and renal physical data collection techniques

Providing client instructions regarding prescribed treatments related to the urinary or renal health problem

Providing client instructions regarding the prevention of the recurrence of a urinary or renal health problem

Psychosocial Integrity

Assisting the client with using appropriate coping mechanisms

Discussing body image disturbances

Discussing the loss of renal function

Identifying cultural, religious, and spiritual influences on health

Identifying grief and loss and end-of-life issues

Identifying support systems and appropriate community resources

Physiological Integrity

Ensuring elimination measures

Informing the client about diagnostic tests and laboratory results

Monitoring for fluid and electrolyte imbalances and acid-base disorders

Obtaining data indicating rejection of kidney transplant

Preventing complications arising as a result of dialysis

Providing adequate rest and sleep

Providing care related to hemodialysis and peritoneal dialysis and dialysis access devices

Providing care to the client following surgical interventions

Providing comfort interventions

Providing pharmacological therapy

Providing treatment measures for the client with renal or urinary calculi

Teaching the client about the prescribed nutrition and fluid measures

Client Needs lists modified from: National Council of State Boards of Nursing, Inc. (NCSBN). *NCLEX-PN Examination: Test Plan for the National Council Licensure Examination for Practical Nurses*, effective April 2020. Chicago: NCSBN.

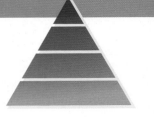

CHAPTER 51

Renal and Urinary Problems

PRIORITY CONCEPTS **Fluids and Electrolytes; Elimination**

WHAT WOULD YOU DO?

The nurse notes that a client with acute kidney injury (AKI) has developed fine crackles in the lung bases bilaterally. What would the nurse do?
Answer is located on p. 724.

I. Anatomy and Physiology

A. Kidney anatomy
1. Each person has two kidneys, which are located behind the peritoneum, attached at the level of the last thoracic and first three lumbar vertebrae on the right and left sides.
2. The kidneys are enclosed in the renal capsule.
3. The renal cortex is the outer layer of the renal capsule and contains blood-filtering structures (glomeruli).
4. The renal medulla is the inner region and contains the renal pyramids and renal tubules.
5. Together, the renal cortex, pyramids, and medulla constitute the parenchyma or functional unit of the kidneys.
6. Nephrons
   a. Located within the parenchyma
   b. Composed of glomeruli and tubules
   c. Selectively secrete and reabsorb ions and filtrates including fluid, waste, electrolytes, acids, and bases

 The nephrons are the functional units of the kidney.

7. Glomerulus
   a. Each nephron contains a tuft of capillaries that filters large plasma proteins and blood cells.
   b. Blood flows into the glomerular capillaries from the afferent arteriole and flows out of the glomerular capillaries into the efferent arteriole.

8. Bowman's capsule
   a. Thin double-walled capsule that surrounds the glomerulus
   b. Fluid and particles from the blood such as electrolytes, glucose, amino acids, and metabolic waste (glomerular filtrate) are filtered through the glomerular membrane into a fluid-filled space in Bowman's capsule (Bowman's space) and then enter the proximal convoluted tubule (PCT).
9. Tubules
   a. The tubules include the PCT, Henle's loop, and the distal convoluted tubule (DCT).
   b. The PCT receives filtrate from the glomerular capsule and reabsorbs water and electrolytes through active and passive transport.
   c. The descending loop of Henle passively reabsorbs water from the filtrate.
   d. The ascending loop of Henle passively reabsorbs sodium and chloride from the filtrate and helps to maintain osmolality.
   e. The DCT actively and passively removes sodium and water.
   f. The filtered fluid is converted to urine in the tubules, and then the urine moves to the pelvis of the kidney.
   g. The urine flows from the pelvis of the kidneys through the ureters and empties into the bladder.

B. Functions of the kidneys
1. Maintain acid-base balance
2. Excrete end products of body metabolism
3. Control fluid and electrolyte balance
4. Excrete bacterial toxins, water-soluble drugs, and drug metabolites
5. Secrete renin to regulate the blood pressure (BP) and erythropoietin to stimulate the bone marrow to produce red blood cells
6. Synthesize vitamin D for calcium absorption and regulation of the parathyroid hormones

699

C. Urine production
  1. As fluid flows through the tubules, water, electrolytes, and solutes are reabsorbed and other solutes such as creatinine, hydrogen ions, and potassium are secreted.
  2. Water and solutes that are not reabsorbed become urine.
  3. The process of selective reabsorption determines the amount of water and solutes to be secreted.
D. Homeostasis of water
  1. The antidiuretic hormone (ADH) is primarily responsible for the reabsorption of water by the kidneys.
  2. ADH is produced by the hypothalamus and secreted from the posterior lobe of the pituitary gland.
  3. Secretion of ADH is stimulated by dehydration or high sodium intake and by a decrease in blood volume.
  4. ADH makes the DCTs and collecting duct permeable to water.
  5. Water is drawn out of the tubules by osmosis and returns to the blood. Concentrated urine remains in the tubule to be excreted.
  6. When ADH is lacking, the client develops diabetes insipidus (DI).
  7. Clients with DI produce large amounts of dilute urine; treatment is necessary because the client cannot drink sufficient water to survive.
E. Homeostasis of sodium
  1. When the amount of sodium increases, extra water is retained to preserve osmotic pressure.
  2. An increase in sodium and water produces an increase in the blood volume and BP.
  3. When BP increases, glomerular filtration increases, and extra water and sodium are lost; blood volume is reduced, returning the BP to normal.
  4. Reabsorption of sodium in the DCT is controlled by the renin-angiotensin system.
  5. Renin, an enzyme, is released from the nephron when the BP or fluid concentration in the DCT is low.
  6. Renin catalyzes the splitting of angiotensin I from angiotensinogen. Angiotensin I converts to angiotensin II as blood flows through the lung.
  7. Angiotensin II, a potent vasoconstrictor, stimulates the secretion of aldosterone.
  8. Aldosterone stimulates the DCTs to reabsorb sodium and secrete potassium.
  9. The additional sodium increases water reabsorption and increases blood volume and BP returning the BP to normal; the stimulus for the secretion of renin is then removed.
F. Homeostasis of potassium
  1. Increase in serum potassium level stimulates the secretion of aldosterone.
  2. Aldosterone stimulates the DCTs to secrete potassium; this action returns the serum potassium concentration to normal.

G. Homeostasis of acidity (pH)
  1. Blood pH is controlled by maintaining the concentration of buffer systems.
  2. Carbonic acid and sodium bicarbonate form the most important buffers for neutralizing acids in the plasma.
  3. The concentration of carbonic acid is controlled by the respiratory system.
  4. The concentration of sodium bicarbonate is controlled by the kidneys.
  5. Normal arterial pH is 7.35 to 7.45, maintained by keeping the ratio of concentrations of sodium bicarbonate to carbon dioxide constant at 20:1.
  6. Strong acids are neutralized by sodium bicarbonate to produce carbonic acid and the sodium salts of the strong acid; this process quickly restores the ratio and thus blood pH.
  7. The carbonic acid dissociates into carbon dioxide and water; because the concentration of carbon dioxide is maintained at a constant level by the respiratory system, the excess carbonic acid is rapidly excreted.
  8. Sodium combined with the strong acid is actively reabsorbed in the DCTs in exchange for hydrogen or potassium ions. The strong acid is neutralized by ammonia and excreted as ammonia or potassium salts.
H. Adrenal glands (refer to Chapter 43 for information about the adrenal glands)
  1. One adrenal gland is on top of each kidney.
  2. The adrenal glands influence BP and sodium and water retention.
I. Bladder
  1. The bladder detrusor muscle is composed of smooth muscle; it distends during bladder filling and contracts during bladder emptying.
  2. The angle of the ureterovesical junction prevents reflux of urine from the bladder to the ureter.
  3. The total safe adult bladder capacity is 400 – 600 mL; normal adult urine output is 1500 mL/day.
J. Prostate gland
  1. The prostate gland surrounds the male urethra.
  2. The prostate gland contains a duct that opens into the prostatic portion of the urethra and secretes the alkaline portion of seminal fluid which protects passing sperm.
K. Risk factors associated with renal problems (Box 51.1)

II. Diagnostic Tests

A. Determination of serum creatinine level
  1. Description: A test that measures the amount of creatinine in the serum; creatinine is an end product of protein and muscle metabolism.
  2. Analysis
    a. Creatinine level reflects glomerular filtration rate (GFR).

<table>
<tr><td colspan="2">BOX 51.1   Risk Factors Associated with Renal Problems</td></tr>
</table>

- Chemical or environmental toxin exposure
- Contact sports
- Diabetes mellitus
- Family history of renal disease
- Frequent urinary tract infections
- Heart failure
- High-sodium diet
- Hypertension
- Medications
- Polycystic kidney disease
- Trauma
- Urolithiasis or nephrolithiasis

TABLE 51.1   **Normal Urinalysis Values**

Color	Amber yellow
Odor	Specific aromatic odor, similar to ammonia
pH	4.6-8.0
Osmolality	300-1300 mOsm/kg
Specific gravity	1.005-1.030
Glucose	Negative
Ketones	Negative
Protein	Negative
Bilirubin	Negative
Casts	Negative
Bacteria	None or < 1000/mL
Hemoglobin	Negative
Myoglobin	Negative
Culture for organisms	Negative

    b. Kidney disease is the only pathological condition that increases the serum creatinine level.
    c. Serum creatinine level increases only when at least 50% of renal function is lost.
    d. Normal reference interval: Male: 0.6 to 1.2 mg/dL; female: 0.5 to 1.1 mg/dL
B. Determination of blood urea nitrogen (BUN) level
  1. Description: A serum test that measures the amount of nitrogenous urea, a by-product of protein metabolism in the liver
  2. Analysis
    a. BUN levels indicate the extent of renal clearance of urea nitrogenous waste products.
    b. An elevation does not always mean kidney disease is present.
    c. Some factors that can elevate the BUN include dehydration, poor renal perfusion, intake of a high-protein diet, infection, stress, corticosteroid use, gastrointestinal (GI) bleeding, and factors that cause muscle breakdown.
    d. Normal reference interval: 10 to 20 mg/dL
C. BUN/creatinine ratio
  1. The BUN is divided by the creatinine level to obtain the ratio; the ratio of BUN to creatinine is usually between 10:1 and 20:1.
  2. When the BUN and serum creatinine levels increase at the same rate, the ratio of the BUN to creatinine remains constant.
  3. Elevated serum creatinine and BUN levels suggest renal dysfunction.
  4. A decreased BUN/creatinine ratio occurs with fluid volume deficit, obstructive uropathy, catabolic state, and a high-protein diet.
  5. An increased BUN/creatinine ratio occurs with fluid volume excess.
D. GFR
  1. A blood test that checks how well the kidneys are working by estimating how much blood passes through the glomeruli every minute

  2. Normal GFR is 125 mL/min in a young adult.
  3. Older people will have lower than normal GFR levels, because GFR decreases with age.
E. Urinalysis: See Table 51.1 for normal urinalysis values.
  1. Description: A urine test for evaluation of the renal system and determination of renal disease
  2. Interventions
    a. Wash perineal area, and use a clean container for collection.
    b. Obtain 10 to 15 mL of the first morning voiding, if possible.
    c. Refrigerated samples may alter the specific gravity.
    d. If the client is menstruating, note this on the laboratory requisition form.
F. A 24-hour urine collection
  1. Check with the laboratory about specific instructions for the client to follow, such as dietary or medication restrictions.
  2. The client is instructed about the urine collection.
  3. At the start time, the client is instructed to void and discard the sample.
  4. Collect all urine at the prescribed time.
  5. Keep the urine specimen on ice or refrigerated and check with the laboratory regarding adding a preservative to the specimen during collection.
  6. At the end of the prescribed time, the client is instructed to empty the bladder and add that urine to the collection container.
G. Specific gravity determination
  1. Description: A urine test that measures the ability of the kidneys to concentrate urine
  2. Interventions
    a. Specific gravity can be measured by a multiple-test dipstick method (most common method),

refractometer (an instrument used in the laboratory setting), or urinometer (least accurate method).

    b. Factors that interfere with an accurate reading include radiopaque contrast agents, glucose, and proteins.

    c. Cold specimens may produce a false high reading.

    d. Normal value is 1.005 to 1.030 (may vary depending on the laboratory).

    e. An increase in specific gravity (more concentrated urine) occurs with insufficient fluid intake, decreased renal perfusion, or increased ADH.

    f. A decrease in specific gravity (less concentrated urine) occurs with increased fluid intake or DI; it may also indicate renal disease or the kidneys' inability to concentrate urine.

 H. Urine culture and sensitivity testing

  1. Description: A urine test that identifies the presence of microorganisms (culture) and determines the specific antibiotics to treat the existing microorganism (sensitivity) appropriately

  2. Interventions

    a. Clean the perineal area and urinary meatus with a bacteriostatic solution.

    b. Collect the midstream sample in a sterile container; if client is unable to obtain a clean catch specimen, a specimen obtained by straight catheterization may be prescribed.

    c. Send the collected specimen to the laboratory immediately.

    d. Identify any sources of potential contaminants during the collection of the specimen such as the hands, skin, clothing, hair, or vaginal or rectal secretions; if contamination occurs, the specimen is discarded and a new specimen needs to be collected.

    e. Urine from the client who drank a very large amount of fluids may be too dilute to provide a positive culture.

 I. Creatinine clearance test

  1. Description

    a. The creatinine clearance test evaluates how well the kidneys remove creatinine from the blood and is an estimate of GFR.

    b. The test includes obtaining a blood sample and timed urine specimens.

    c. Blood is drawn when the urine specimen collection is complete.

    d. The urine specimen for the creatinine clearance is usually collected for 24 hours, but shorter periods (8 or 12 hours) could be prescribed.

⚠ The creatinine clearance test provides the best estimate of the GFR; the normal GFR is 125 mL/min in a young adult. The GFR decreases with age (10% for each decade). By age 65 the GFR is approximately 65 mL/min.

  2. Interventions

    a. Encourage fluids before and during the test.

    b. Reinforce instructions to the client to avoid caffeinated beverages during testing.

    c. Check with the primary health care provider (PHCP) regarding the administration of any prescribed medications during testing.

    d. Reinforce instructions to the client about the urine collection.

    e. At the start time, ask the client to void (or empty the tubing and drainage bag if the client has an indwelling urinary catheter) and discard the first sample.

    f. Collect all urine for the prescribed time.

    g. Keep the urine specimen on ice or refrigerated, and check with the laboratory regarding adding a preservative to the specimen during collection.

    h. At the end of the prescribed time, ask the client to empty the bladder (or empty the tubing and drainage bag if the client has an indwelling urinary catheter) and add that urine to the collection container.

    i. Send the labeled urine specimen to the laboratory.

    j. Document specimen collection, time started and completed, and other pertinent data.

J. KUB (kidneys, ureters, and bladder) radiography

  1. Description: An x-ray film of the urinary system and adjacent structures used to detect urinary calculi or bowel obstruction

  2. Interventions: No specific preparation is necessary.

K. Bladder ultrasonography (bladder scanning)

  1. Bladder ultrasonography is a noninvasive method for measuring the volume of urine in the bladder.

  2. Bladder ultrasonography may be performed to evaluate urinary frequency, inability to urinate, or residual urine (the amount of urine remaining in the bladder after voiding).

L. Intravenous (IV) urography

  1. Description: An x-ray procedure in which an IV injection of a radiopaque dye is used to visualize and identify abnormalities in the renal system

  2. Preprocedure interventions

    a. Verify that an informed consent has been obtained.

    b. Check the client for allergies to iodine, seafood, and radiopaque dyes; contraindications for the test include a positive pregnancy test; cautions include medical history of asthma, significant cardiac disease, renal insufficiency.

    c. Withhold food and fluids for the time prescribed.

    d. Administer laxatives if prescribed.

    e. Inform the client about possible throat irritation, flushing of the face, warmth, or a salty or metallic taste during the test.

3. Postprocedure interventions
   a. Monitor vital signs.
   b. Reinforce instructions to the client to drink at least 1 L of fluid unless contraindicated.
   c. Monitor the venipuncture site for bleeding.
   d. Monitor urinary output.
   e. Monitor for signs of a possible allergic reaction to the dye used during the test, and instruct the client to notify the PHCP if any signs of an allergic reaction occur.
   f. Contrast dye is potentially damaging to kidneys; the risk is greater in older clients and those experiencing dehydration.

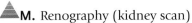 The dye (contrast media) used in IV urography may be nephrotoxic; therefore, encourage increased fluids unless contraindicated, and monitor urinary output. It is essential that preprocedure BUN and creatinine levels are assessed on any client undergoing a procedure in which dye might be injected. The PHCP may institute precautionary measures to prevent AKI or use smaller amounts of the dye.

M. Renography (kidney scan)
   1. Description: An IV injection of a radioisotope for visual imaging of renal blood flow, glomerular filtration, tubular function, and excretion
   2. Preprocedure interventions
      a. Verify that an informed consent has been obtained.
      b. Check for allergies.
      c. Inform the client that the test requires no dietary or activity restrictions.
      d. Reinforce instructions to the client to remain motionless during the test and that imaging may be repeated at various intervals before the test is complete.
   3. Postprocedure interventions
      a. Encourage fluid intake unless contraindicated.
      b. Monitor the client for signs of delayed allergic reaction.
      c. The radioisotope is eliminated in 24 hours; wear gloves for excretion precautions.
      d. Follow standard precautions when caring for incontinent clients, and double-bag client linens per agency policy.
      e. If captopril was administered during the procedure, the client's BP needs to be checked frequently.

N. Cystoscopy and biopsy of the bladder
   1. Description: The bladder mucosa is examined for inflammation, calculi, or tumors by means of a cystoscope; a sample for biopsy may be obtained.
   2. Preprocedure interventions
      a. Verify that an informed consent has been obtained.
      b. If a biopsy is planned, withhold food and fluids for the time prescribed.
      c. If a cystoscopy alone is planned, no special preparation is necessary, and the procedure may be performed in the PHCP's office; postprocedure interventions include increasing fluid intake.
   3. Postprocedure interventions following biopsy
      a. Monitor vital signs.
      b. Increase fluid intake as prescribed.
      c. Monitor intake and output and assess urine characteristics.
      d. Encourage deep-breathing exercises to relieve bladder spasms and administer analgesics as prescribed.
      e. Prepare to administer a sitz bath for back and abdominal pain, if prescribed.
      f. Note that leg cramps are common because of the lithotomy position maintained during the procedure.
      g. Reinforce instructions to the client that burning during urination, pink-tinged or tea-colored urine, and urinary frequency are common after cystoscopy and resolve in a few days.
      h. Monitor for bright red urine or clots, and notify the registered nurse (RN) or PHCP if a fever occurs; an increase in white blood cell (WBC) count suggests infection.

O. Renal biopsy
   1. Description: Insertion of a needle into the kidney to obtain a sample of tissue for examination; usually done percutaneously
   2. Preprocedure interventions
      a. Check vital signs.
      b. Check baseline coagulation studies. The PHCP is notified if abnormal results are noted.
      c. Verify that an informed consent has been obtained.
      d. Withhold food and fluids as prescribed.
   3. Interventions during the procedure: Position the client prone with a pillow under the abdomen and shoulders.
   4. Postprocedure interventions
      a. Monitor vital signs, especially for hypotension and tachycardia, which could indicate bleeding.
      b. Provide pressure to the biopsy site for 30 minutes or as prescribed.
      c. Monitor the hemoglobin and hematocrit levels for any decrease that could indicate bleeding.
      d. Place the client on strict bed rest in the supine position, as prescribed, with a back roll for additional support for 2 to 6 hours after the biopsy.
      e. Check the biopsy site and under the client for bleeding.
      f. Encourage fluid intake of 1500 to 2000 mL as prescribed.

g. Observe the urine for gross and microscopic bleeding.

h. Reinforce instructions to the client to avoid heavy lifting and strenuous activity for 1 to 2 weeks.

i. Reinforce instructions to the client to notify the PHCP if either a temperature greater than 100°F (37.8°C) or hematuria occurs after the first 24 hours post procedure.

III. Acute Kidney Injury

A. Description

1. Acute kidney injury (AKI) is the rapid loss of kidney function from renal cell damage.
2. This occurs abruptly and can be reversible.
3. AKI leads to cell hypoperfusion, cell death, and decompensation of renal function.
4. The prognosis depends on the cause and the condition of the client.
5. Near-normal or normal kidney function may resume gradually.

B. Causes

1. Prenal: Outside the kidney; caused by intravascular volume depletion such as blood loss associated with trauma or surgery, dehydration, decreased cardiac output (as with cardiogenic shock), decreased peripheral vascular resistance, decreased renovascular blood flow, and prerenal infection or obstruction
2. Intrarenal: Within the parenchyma of the kidney; caused by tubular necrosis, prolonged prerenal ischemia, intrarenal infection or obstruction, and nephrotoxicity (Box 51.2)
3. Postrenal: Between the kidney and urethral meatus such as bladder neck obstruction, bladder cancer, calculi, and postrenal infection

C. Phases of AKI and laboratory findings (Box 51.3)

1. Onset: Begins with precipitating event
2. Oliguric phase
   a. For some clients, oliguria does not occur and the urine output is normal; otherwise, the duration of oliguria is 8 to 15 days; the longer the duration, the less chance of recovery.
   b. Sudden decrease in urine output. Urine output is less than 400 mL/day.
   c. Signs of excess fluid volume: hypertension, edema, pleural and pericardial effusions, dysrhythmia, heart failure (HF), and pulmonary edema

---

BOX 51.2 Potentially Nephrotoxic Substances

Medications

Antibiotics: Antimicrobials
- Amphotericin B
- Colistimethate
- Methicillin
- Polymyxin B
- Rifampin
- Sulfonamides
- Tetracycline hydrochloride
- Vancomycin

Aminoglycoside Antibiotics
- Gentamicin
- Kanamycin
- Neomycin
- Netilmicin sulfate
- Tobramycin

Chemotherapy Agents
- Cisplatin
- Cyclophosphamide
- Methotrexate

Nonsteroidal Anti-inflammatory Drugs (NSAIDs)
- Celecoxib
- Flurbiprofen
- Ibuprofen
- Indomethacin
- Ketorolac
- Meclofenamate
- Meloxicam
- Nabumetone

- Naproxen
- Oxaprozin
- Rofecoxib
- Tolmetin

Other Medications
- Acetaminophen
- Captopril
- Cyclosporine
- Fluorinate anesthetics
- Metformin
- D-Penicillamine
- Phenazopyridine hydrochloride
- Quinine

Other Substances
- Organic solvents
- Carbon tetrachloride
- Ethylene glycol

Nonpharmacological Chemical Agents
- Radiographic contrast dye
- Pesticides
- Fungicides
- Myoglobin (from breakdown of skeletal muscle)

Heavy Metals and Ions
- Arsenic
- Bismuth
- Copper sulfate
- Gold salts
- Lead
- Mercuric chloride

Adapted from Ignatavicius D, Workman ML, Rebar CR: *Medical-surgical nursing: Concepts for interprofessional collaborative care*, ed 9, Philadelphia, 2018, Saunders.

BOX 51.3 **Acute Kidney Injury: Phases and Laboratory Findings**

Onset
Begins with precipitating event

Oliguric Phase
Elevated blood urea nitrogen and serum creatinine
Decreased urine specific gravity (prerenal causes) or normal (intrarenal causes)
Decreased glomerular filtration rate (GFR) and creatinine clearance
Hyperkalemia
Normal or decreased serum sodium level
Hypervolemia
Hypocalcemia
Hyperphosphatemia

Diuretic Phase
Gradual decline in blood urea nitrogen and serum creatinine but still elevated
Continued low creatinine clearance with improving GFR
Hypokalemia
Hyponatremia
Hypovolemia

Recovery Phase (Convalescent)
Increased GFR
Stabilization or continual decline in blood urea nitrogen and serum creatinine levels toward normal
Complete recovery may take 1–2 years

---

   d. Signs of uremia: anorexia, nausea, vomiting, and pruritus
   e. Signs of metabolic acidosis: Kussmaul's respirations
   f. Signs of neurological changes: tingling of extremities, drowsiness progressing to disorientation, and then coma

   g. Signs of pericarditis: friction rub, chest pain with inspiration, and low-grade fever
   h. Laboratory analysis (see Box 51.3)
   i. With early recognition or potential for AKI, client may be treated with fluid challenges (IV boluses of 500–1000 mL over 1 hour).
   j. Fluid intake may be restricted. If hypertension is present, daily fluid allowances may be 400 to 1000 mL plus the measured urinary output.
   k. Assist with the administration of medications as prescribed, such as diuretics to increase renal blood flow and diuresis of retained fluid and electrolytes.
  3. Diuretic phase
   a. Urine output rises slowly followed by diuresis (4–5 L/day).
   b. Excessive urine output indicates that damaged nephrons are recovering their ability to excrete wastes.
   c. Dehydration, hypovolemia, hypotension, and tachycardia can occur.

   d. Level of consciousness improves.
   e. Laboratory analysis (see Box 51.3)
   f. IV fluids may be prescribed and may contain electrolytes to replace losses.
  4. Recovery phase (convalescent)
   a. Recovery is a slow process. Complete recovery may take 1 to 2 years.
   b. Urine volume returns to normal.
   c. Memory improves.
   d. Strength increases.
   e. The older adult is less likely than a younger adult to regain full kidney function.
   f. Laboratory analysis (see Box 51.3)
   g. AKI can progress to chronic kidney disease (CKD).

 The signs/symptoms of AKI are primarily caused by the retention of nitrogenous wastes, the retention of fluids, and the inability of the kidneys to regulate electrolytes.

D. Data collection: Obtain objective and subjective data based on characteristics of the phases of AKI (see Box 51.3).
E. Other interventions
  1. Monitor vital signs, especially for signs of hypertension, tachycardia, tachypnea, and an irregular heart rate.
  2. Monitor intake and output (hourly in cases of AKI) and urine color and characteristics.
  3. Monitor daily weight (same scale, same clothes, same time of the day) noting that an increase of 0.5 to 1 lb/day (0.25–0.5 kg/day) indicates fluid retention.
  4. BUN, serum creatinine, and serum electrolyte values are monitored for changes.
  5. Acidosis can occur and may be treated with sodium bicarbonate.
  6. Monitor urinalysis for protein level, hematuria, casts, and specific gravity.
  7. Monitor for altered level of consciousness caused by uremia.
  8. Monitor for signs of infection because the client may not exhibit an elevated temperature or an increased WBC count.
  9. Monitor the lungs for wheezes and rhonchi, and monitor for edema, which can indicate fluid overload.
 10. Administer prescribed diet, which is usually low to moderate protein (to decrease the workload on the kidneys) and high carbohydrate; ill clients may require nutritional support with supplements, enteral feedings, or parenteral nutrition.
 11. Restrict potassium and sodium intake, as prescribed, based on the electrolyte level.
 12. Assist to administer medications as prescribed. Be alert to the metabolic and excretory mechanisms of all prescribed medications.

13. Be alert to nephrotoxic medications that may be prescribed (see Box 51.2).

14. Be alert to the PHCP's adjustment of medication dosages for kidney injury.

15. Assist with the preparation of the client for dialysis, if prescribed. Continuous renal replacement therapy may be used in cases of AKI to treat fluid volume overload or rapidly developing azotemia and metabolic acidosis.

16. Provide emotional support by allowing opportunities for the client to express concerns and fears and encouraging family interactions.

17. Promote consistency in caregivers.

18. Also refer to Section IV.E. in this chapter (Special Problems in Kidney Disease and Interventions).

IV. Chronic Kidney Disease

A. Description

1. CKD is a slow, progressive, and irreversible loss of kidney function with a GFR less than or equal to 60 mL/min for 3 months or longer.

2. Occurs in stages (with loss of 75% of functioning nephrons, the client becomes symptomatic) and eventually results in uremia or end-stage kidney disease (with loss of 90%–95% of functioning nephrons) (Table 51.2)

3. Hypervolemia can occur because of the kidneys' inability to excrete sodium and water, or hypovolemia can occur because of the kidneys' inability to conserve sodium and water.

⚠ CKD affects all major body systems and may require dialysis or kidney transplantation to maintain life.

B. Primary causes

1. May follow AKI

2. Diabetes mellitus or some other metabolic disorder

3. Hypertension

4. Chronic urinary obstruction

5. Recurrent infection

6. Renal artery occlusion

7. An autoimmune disorder

C. Data collection

1. Monitor body systems for the manifestations of CKD.

2. Monitor psychological changes, including emotional lability, withdrawal, depression, anxiety, suicidal behavior, denial, dependence/independence conflict, and any change in body image.

3. Monitor for severe chronic and end-stage kidney disease manifestations (Box 51.4).

D. Interventions

1. Same as the interventions for AKI

2. Administer prescribed diet, usually moderate protein (to decrease the workload on the kidneys), high carbohydrate, low potassium, and low phosphorus.

TABLE 51.2 **Progression of Chronic Kidney Disease**

Signs of CKD	Estimated GFR
Stage 1: At risk; normal kidney function (early kidney disease may or may not be present)	> 90 mL/min
Stage 2: Mild CKD	60–89 mL/min
Stage 3: Moderate CKD	30–59 mL/min
Stage 4: Severe CKD	15–29 mL/min
Stage 5: ESKD	< 15 mL/min

CKD, Chronic kidney disease; *ESKD,* end-stage kidney disease; *GFR,* glomerular filtration rate.
Adapted from Ignatavicius D, Workman ML, Rebar CR: *Medical-surgical nursing: Concepts for interprofessional collaborative care,* ed 9, Philadelphia, 2018, Saunders.

3. Provide oral care to prevent stomatitis and reduce discomfort from mouth sores.

4. Provide skin care to prevent pruritus.

5. Teach the client about fluid, dietary restrictions, and the importance of daily weight measurements.

6. Provide support to promote acceptance of the chronic illness and prepare the client for long-term dialysis and transplantation.

7. Explain to the client about his or her choice to decline dialysis or transplantation; with elderly clients, provide information that says their kidney function is declining and in time may reach end-stage renal disease and require dialysis; encourage healthy lifestyle and discuss choices.

E. Special problems in kidney disease and interventions

1. Activity intolerance and insomnia

a. Fatigue results from anemia and the buildup of wastes from the diseased kidneys.

b. Provide adequate rest periods.

c. Teach the client to plan activities to avoid fatigue.

d. Assist with the administration of mild central nervous system (CNS) depressants, as prescribed, to promote rest.

2. Anemia

a. Anemia results from the decreased secretion of erythropoietin by damaged nephrons, resulting in decreased production of red blood cells.

b. Monitor for decreased hemoglobin and hematocrit levels.

c. Assist with the administration of hematopoietics, such as epoetin alfa or darbepoetin alfa, as prescribed, to promote maturity of the red blood cells.

d. Assist with the administration of folic acid as prescribed.

e. Assist with the administration of oral iron, as prescribed, but not at the same time as phosphate binders.

BOX 51.4 Key Features of Severe Chronic and End-Stage Kidney Disease

Neurological Manifestations
- Lethargy and daytime drowsiness
- Inability to concentrate or decreased attention span
- Seizures
- Coma
- Slurred speech
- Asterixis
- Tremors, twitching, or jerky movements
- Myoclonus
- Ataxia (alteration in gait)
- Paresthesia

Cardiovascular Manifestations
- Cardiomyopathy
- Hypertension
- Peripheral edema
- Heart failure
- Uremic pericarditis
- Pericardial effusion
- Pericardial friction rub
- Cardiac tamponade
- Cardiorenal syndrome

Respiratory Manifestations
- Uremic halitosis
- Tachypnea
- Deep sighing, yawning
- Kussmaul respirations
- Uremic pneumonitis
- Shortness of breath
- Pulmonary edema
- Pleural effusion
- Depressed cough reflex
- Crackles

Hematological Manifestations
- Anemia
- Abnormal bleeding and bruising

Gastrointestinal Manifestations
- Anorexia, nausea, vomiting
- Metallic taste in mouth
- Change in taste acuity and sensation
- Uremic colitis (diarrhea)
- Constipation
- Uremic gastritis (possible gastrointestinal bleeding)

- Uremic fetor
- Stomatitis

Urinary Manifestations
- Polyuria, nocturia (early)
- Oliguria, anuria (later)
- Proteinuria
- Hematuria
- Diluted, straw-like appearance (early)
- Concentrated and cloudy urine appearance (later)

Integumentary Manifestations
- Decreased skin turgor
- Yellow-gray pallor
- Dry skin
- Pruritus
- Ecchymosis
- Purpura
- Soft tissue calcifications
- Uremic frost (late, premorbid)

Musculoskeletal Manifestations
- Muscle weakness and cramping
- Bone pain
- Pathological fractures
- Renal osteodystrophy

Reproductive Manifestations
- Decreased fertility
- Infrequent or absent menses
- Decreased libido
- Impotence
- Sexual dysfunction

Metabolic Manifestations
- Hyperparathyroidism
- Hyperlipidemia
- Alterations in vitamin D, calcium, and phosphorus absorption and metabolism
- Metabolic acidosis
- Hyperkalemia

Psychosocial Manifestations
- Depression
- Fatigue
- Sleep disturbances
- Sexual dysfunction
- Cognitive impairment

Adapted from Ignatavicius D, Workman ML, Rebar CR: *Medical-surgical nursing: Concepts for interprofessional collaborative care*, ed 9, Philadelphia, 2018, Saunders.

    f. Assist with the administration of stool softeners, as prescribed, because of the constipating effects of iron.

    g. Note that oral iron is not well absorbed by the GI tract in CKD and causes nausea and vomiting. Parenteral iron may be used if iron deficiencies persist despite folic acid or oral iron administration.

    h. Assist RN with the administration of a blood transfusion, if prescribed. Blood transfusions are prescribed only when necessary (acute blood loss, symptomatic anemia) because

they decrease the stimulus to produce red blood cells.

    i. Blood transfusions also cause the development of antibodies against human tissues, which can make matching for organ transplantation difficult.

3. GI bleeding

    a. Urea is broken down by the intestinal bacteria to ammonia. Ammonia irritates the GI mucosa causing ulceration and bleeding.

    b. Monitor for decreasing hemoglobin and hematocrit levels.

c. Monitor stools for occult blood.

d. Avoid the administration of acetylsalicylic acid because it is excreted by the kidneys. If administered, aspirin toxicity can occur and prolong the bleeding time.

4. Hyperkalemia

a. Monitor vital signs for hypertension or hypotension and the apical heart rate. An irregular heart rate could indicate dysrhythmia.

b. Monitor the serum potassium level; elevation can cause decreased cardiac output; heart block; fibrillation; or asystole (Fig. 51.1).

c. Provide a low-potassium diet avoiding foods high in potassium. (See Chapter 8 for a listing of foods that are high in potassium.)

d. Assist with the administration of electrolyte-binding and electrolyte-excreting medications such as oral or rectal sodium polystyrene sulfonate, as prescribed, to lower the serum potassium level.

e. Assist with the administration of prescribed medications: 50% dextrose and regular insulin may be prescribed to shift potassium into the cell. IV calcium gluconate may be prescribed to reduce myocardial irritability from hyperkalemia, and IV sodium bicarbonate may be prescribed to correct acidosis.

f. Assist with the administration of prescribed loop diuretics to excrete potassium.

g. Avoid potassium-sparing medications such as spironolactone and triamterene because these medications will increase the potassium level.

h. Assist with the preparation of the client for peritoneal dialysis (PD) or hemodialysis as prescribed.

⚠ Place the client with kidney disease on continuous cardiac monitoring. The client can develop hyperkalemia and is at risk for dysrhythmia.

5. Hypermagnesemia

a. Results from decreased renal excretion of magnesium

b. Monitor cardiac manifestations of bradycardia, peripheral vasodilation, and hypotension.

c. Monitor CNS manifestations of decreased nerve impulse transmission, such as drowsiness or lethargy.

d. Monitor neuromuscular manifestations such as reduced or absent deep tendon reflexes or weak or absent voluntary skeletal muscle contractions.

e. Assist with the administration of loop diuretics as prescribed to excrete magnesium.

f. Assist with the administration of calcium, as prescribed, for resulting cardiac problems.

g. Avoid medications that contain magnesium such as antacids, laxatives, or enemas.

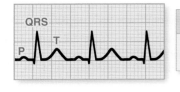

Serum Potassium Level

Normal (3.5-5.0 mEq/L)

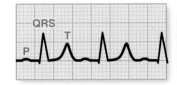

Serum Potassium Level

About 7.0 mEq/L

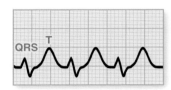

Serum Potassium Level

8.0-9.0 mEq/L

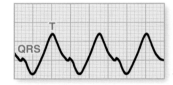

Serum Potassium Level

>10.0 mEq/L

FIGURE 51.1 Cardiac rhythm changes with hyperkalemia.

h. During severe elevations, avoid foods that increase magnesium levels. (See Chapter 8 for a listing of foods that are high in magnesium.)

6. Hyperphosphatemia

a. As the phosphorus level rises, the calcium level drops; this leads to the stimulation of parathyroid hormone causing bone demineralization.

b. Treatment is aimed at lowering the serum phosphorus level.

c. Assist with the administration of phosphate binders with meals, as prescribed, to lower serum phosphate levels.

d. Administer stool softeners and laxatives, as prescribed, because phosphate binders are constipating.

e. Reinforce teaching the client about the need to limit the intake of foods high in phosphorus. (See Chapter 8 for a listing of foods that are high in phosphorus.)

7. Hypertension

a. Caused by failure of the kidneys to maintain BP homeostasis

b. Monitor vital signs for elevated BP.

c. Maintain fluid and sodium restrictions as prescribed.

d. Assist to administer diuretics and antihypertensives as prescribed.

8. Hypervolemia
   a. Monitor vital signs for an elevated BP.
   b. Monitor intake and output and daily weight for indications of fluid retention.
   c. Monitor for periorbital, sacral, and peripheral edema.
   d. Monitor the serum electrolyte levels.
   e. Monitor for hypertension, and notify the PHCP of sustained elevations.
   f. Monitor for signs of HF and pulmonary edema such as restlessness, heightened anxiety, tachycardia, dyspnea, basilar lung crackles, and blood-tinged sputum. Notify the RN or PHCP immediately if signs occur.
   g. Maintain fluid restriction.
   h. Avoid the administration of large amounts of IV fluids.
   i. Assist with the administration of diuretics as prescribed.
   j. Reinforce teaching the client to maintain a low-sodium diet.
   k. Reinforce teaching the client to avoid over-the-counter medications without checking with the PHCP.

9. Hypocalcemia
   a. Occurs as a result of a high phosphorus level and the inability of the diseased kidney to activate vitamin D
   b. The absence of vitamin D causes poor calcium absorption from the intestinal tract.
   c. Monitor serum calcium level.
   d. Administer calcium supplements as prescribed.
   e. Administer activated vitamin D as prescribed.
   f. See Chapter 8 for a listing of foods that are high in calcium.

10. Hypovolemia
    a. Monitor vital signs for hypotension and tachycardia.
    b. Monitor for decreasing intake and output and a reduction in the daily weight.
    c. Monitor for dehydration.
    d. Monitor the electrolyte levels.
    e. Assist with the administration of replacement therapy based on the serum electrolyte level.

11. Infection
    a. The client is at risk for infection caused by a suppressed immune system, dialysis access site, and possible malnutrition.
    b. Monitor for signs of infection.
    c. Avoid urinary catheters when possible; if used, provide catheter care per protocol.
    d. Provide strict asepsis during urinary catheter insertion and other invasive procedures.
    e. Reinforce instructions to the client to avoid fatigue because it decreases body resistance.
    f. Reinforce instructions to the client to avoid persons with infections.
    g. Assist with the administration of antibiotics, as prescribed, monitoring for nephrotoxic effects.

12. Metabolic acidosis
    a. The kidneys are unable to excrete hydrogen ions or manufacture bicarbonate resulting in acidosis.
    b. Assist with the administration of alkalizers, such as sodium bicarbonate, as prescribed.
    c. Note that clients with CKD adjust to low bicarbonate levels and, as a result, do not become acutely ill.

13. Muscle cramps
    a. Occur as a result of electrolyte imbalances and the effects of uremia on peripheral nerves
    b. Monitor serum electrolytes.
    c. Assist with the administration of electrolyte replacements and medications to control muscle cramps as prescribed.
    d. Administer heat and massage as prescribed.

14. Neurological changes
    a. The buildup of active particles and fluids causes changes in the brain cells and leads to confusion and impairment in decision-making ability.
    b. Peripheral neuropathy results from the effects of uremia on the peripheral nerves.
    c. Monitor level of consciousness and for confusion.
    d. Monitor for restless leg syndrome, which is also common during dialysis treatments.
    e. Reinforce teaching the client to examine areas of decreased sensation for signs of injury.

15. Ocular irritation
    a. Calcium deposits in the conjunctiva cause burning and watering of the eyes.
    b. Assist with the administration of medications to control the calcium and phosphate levels as prescribed.
    c. Administer lubricating eye drops.
    d. Protect the client from injury.

16. Potential for injury
    a. The client is at risk for fractures caused by alterations in the absorption of calcium, excretion of phosphate, and altered vitamin D metabolism.
    b. Provide for a safe environment.
    c. Avoid injury; tissue breakdown causes increased serum potassium levels.

17. Pruritus
    a. To rid the body of excess wastes, urate crystals are excreted through the skin causing pruritus.
    b. The deposit of urate crystals (uremic frost) occurs in advanced stages of kidney failure.
    c. Monitor for skin breakdown, rash, and uremic frost.
    d. Provide meticulous skin care and oral hygiene.
    e. Avoid the use of soaps.

f. Assist with the administration of antihistamines and antipruritics, as prescribed, to relieve itching.

g. Reinforce teaching the client to keep the nails trimmed to prevent local infection from scratching.

18. Psychosocial problems

a. Listen to the client's concerns to determine how the client is handling the situation.

b. Allow the client time to mourn the loss of kidney function.

c. With the client's permission, include the family members in discussions of the client's concerns.

d. Reinforce education about treatment options and support the client's decision; elderly clients with CKD may progress slowly toward end-stage kidney disease or require dialysis, and clients may decide on no treatment and opt for end-of-life care.

e. Offer information about support groups.

V. Uremic Syndrome

A. Description: Systemic clinical and laboratory manifestations of severe and/or end-stage kidney disease due to accumulation of nitrogenous waste products in the blood caused by the kidneys' inability to filter out these waste products

B. Data collection

1. Oliguria

2. The presence of protein, red blood cells, and casts in the urine

3. Elevated levels of urea, uric acid, potassium, and magnesium in the urine

4. Hypotension or hypertension

5. Alterations in the level of consciousness

6. Electrolyte imbalances

7. Stomatitis

8. Nausea or vomiting

9. Diarrhea or constipation

C. Interventions

1. Monitor vital signs for hypertension, tachycardia, and an irregular heart rate.

2. Monitor serum electrolyte levels.

3. Monitor intake and output and for oliguria.

4. Provide a limited, but high-quality, protein diet as prescribed.

5. Provide a limited sodium, nitrogen, potassium, and phosphate diet as prescribed.

6. Assist the client with coping mechanisms related to body-image disturbances caused by uremic syndrome.

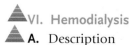
VI. Hemodialysis

A. Description

1. Hemodialysis is an intermittent renal replacement therapy involving the process of cleansing the client's blood.

2. It involves the diffusion of dissolved particles from one fluid compartment into another across a semipermeable membrane. The client's blood flows through one fluid compartment of a dialysis filter, and the dialysate is in another fluid compartment.

B. Functions of hemodialysis

1. Cleanses the blood of accumulated waste products

2. Removes the byproducts of protein metabolism such as urea, creatinine, and uric acid from the blood

3. Removes excess body fluids

4. Maintains or restores the buffer system of the body

5. Corrects electrolyte levels in the body

C. Principles of hemodialysis

1. The semipermeable membrane is made of thin, porous cellophane.

2. The pore size of the membrane allows small particles to pass through, such as urea, creatinine, uric acid, and water molecules.

3. Proteins, bacteria, and some blood cells are too large to pass through the membrane.

4. The client's blood flows into the dialyzer. The movement of substances occurs from the blood to the dialysate by the principles of osmosis, diffusion, and ultrafiltration.

5. Diffusion is the movement of particles from an area of higher concentration to one of lower concentration.

6. Osmosis is the movement of fluids across a semipermeable membrane from an area of lower concentration of particles to an area of higher concentration of particles.

7. Ultrafiltration is the movement of fluid across a semipermeable membrane as a result of an artificially created pressure gradient.

D. Dialysate bath

1. A dialysate bath is composed of water and major electrolytes.

2. Dialysate need not be sterile because bacteria and viruses are too large to pass through the pores of the semipermeable membrane; however, the dialysate must meet specific standards, and water is treated to ensure a safe water supply.

E. Interventions

1. Monitor vital signs before, during, and after dialysis; the client's temperature may elevate because of slight warming of the blood from the dialysis machine. Notify the RN, who will notify the PHCP about excessive temperature elevations because this could indicate sepsis; assist to obtain samples for blood culture as prescribed for excessive temperature elevations.

2. Monitor laboratory values, specifically the BUN, creatinine, and complete blood cell counts before, during, and after dialysis. Alert RN for any abnormal values.

3. Monitor the client for fluid overload before dialysis and fluid volume deficit after dialysis.

4. Weigh the client before and after dialysis to determine fluid loss. Note that the client will not urinate or will urinate small amounts (may be less than 30 mL/hr).

5. Monitor the patency of the blood access device before, during, and after dialysis.

6. Monitor for bleeding. Heparin is added to the dialysis bath to prevent clots from forming within the dialyzer or the blood tubing.

7. Monitor for hypovolemia and shock during dialysis, which can occur from blood loss or excess fluid and electrolyte removal.

8. Provide adequate nutrition. The client may eat before or during dialysis.

9. Identify the client's reactions to the treatment and support coping mechanisms. Encourage independence and involvement in care.

⚠ Withhold antihypertensives and other medications that can affect the BP or result in hypotension until after the hemodialysis treatment. Also withhold medications that could be removed by dialysis such as water-soluble vitamins, certain antibiotics, and digoxin.

VII. Access for Hemodialysis

A. Subclavian and femoral catheter

1. Description

   a. A subclavian (subclavian vein) or femoral (femoral vein) catheter may be inserted for short-term or temporary use in AKI.

   b. The catheter is used until a fistula or graft matures or develops, which is typically 6 weeks or may be required when the client's fistula or graft access has failed because of infection or clotting.

2. Interventions

   a. Monitor the insertion site for hematoma, bleeding, catheter dislodgement, and infection.

   b. These catheters must only be used for dialysis treatments and accessed by dialysis personnel. ⚠

   c. Maintain an occlusive dressing over the catheter insertion site.

3. Subclavian vein catheter

   a. The catheter is usually filled with heparin and capped to maintain patency between dialysis treatments. Heparin is aspirated from the line before dialysis.

   b. The catheter would not be uncapped except for dialysis treatments.

   c. The catheter may be left in place for up to 6 weeks if no complications occur.

4. Femoral vein catheter

   a. Monitor the extremity for circulation, temperature, and pulses. ⚠

   b. Prevent pulling or disconnecting of the catheter when giving care. ⚠

   c. Because the groin is not a clean site, meticulous perineal care is required.

   d. Use an IV infusion pump or controller with microdrip tubing if a heparin infusion through the catheter to maintain patency is prescribed.

⚠ The client with a femoral vein catheter should not sit up more than 45 degrees or lean forward because the catheter may kink and occlude.

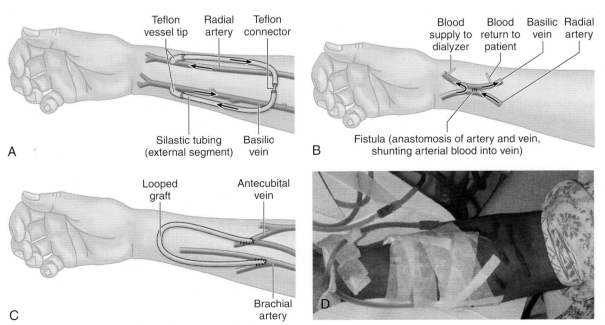

FIGURE 51.2 Vascular access for hemodialysis. (A) External shunt. (B) Internal arteriovenous fistula. (C) Internal arteriovenous graft. (D) A hemodialysis graft while connected to a hemodialysis machine. (D, From Lewis et al., 2011.)

B. External arteriovenous shunt (Fig. 51.2)
 1. Description
   a. Two Silastic cannulas are surgically inserted into an artery and a vein in the forearm or the leg to form an external blood path.
   b. The cannulas are connected to form a U shape. Blood flows from the client's artery through the shunt into the vein.
   c. A tube leading to the membrane compartment of the dialyzer is connected to the arterial cannula.
   d. Blood fills the membrane compartment, passes through the dialyzer, and is returned back to the client through a tube connected to the venous cannula.
   e. When dialysis is complete, the cannulas are clamped and reattached, reforming the U shape.
 2. Advantages
   a. The external arteriovenous shunt can be used immediately after its creation.
   b. No venipuncture is necessary for dialysis.
 3. Disadvantages
   a. Disconnection or dislodgment of the external shunt
   b. Risk of hemorrhage, infection, or clotting
   c. Potential for skin erosion around the catheter site
 4. Interventions
   a. Avoid getting the shunt wet.
   b. A dressing is wrapped completely around the shunt to keep it dry and intact.
   c. Keep cannula clamps at the client's bedside or attached to the arteriovenous dressing for use in the event of accidental disconnection.
   d. Reinforce teaching the client that the shunt extremity must not be used for monitoring BP, drawing blood, placing IV lines, or administering injections.
   e. Fold back the dressing to expose the shunt tubing and check for signs of hemorrhage, infection, or clotting.
   f. Monitor skin integrity around the insertion site.
   g. Auscultate for a bruit and palpate for a thrill, although a bruit may not be heard with the shunt.
   h. Notify the RN immediately who will notify the PHCP if signs of clotting, hemorrhage, or infection occur.
 5. Signs of clotting
   a. Fibrin: white flecks in the tubing
   b. Separation of serum and cells
   c. Absence of a previously heard bruit; thrill absent during palpation
   d. Coolness of the tubing or extremity
   e. Tingling sensation at site or in extremity

C. Internal arteriovenous fistula (see Fig. 51.2)
 1. Description
   a. A permanent access of choice for the client with CKD requiring dialysis

   b. The fistula is created surgically by anastomosis of a large artery and a large vein in the arm.
   c. The flow of arterial blood into the venous system causes the vein to become engorged (matured or developed).
   d. Maturity takes about 4 to 6 weeks depending on the client's ability to do hand-flexing exercises such as "ball squeezing," which will help the fistula to mature.
   e. The fistula is required to be mature before it can be used because the engorged vein is punctured with a large-bore needle for the dialysis procedure.
   f. Subclavian or femoral catheters, peritoneal dialysis, or an external arteriovenous shunt can be used for dialysis while the fistula is maturing or developing.
   g. Avoid taking the BP or performing venipuncture for intravenous access or lab draws to protect the integrity of the fistula.
   h. Fistulas are dressed with pressure dressings after hemodialysis to prevent bleeding. Ensure the removal of the pressure dressing with the prescribed time frame or according to agency policy.
 2. Advantages
   a. Because the fistula is internal, the risks of clotting and bleeding are low.
   b. The fistula can be used indefinitely.
   c. The fistula has a decreased incidence of infection because it is internal and is not exposed.
   d. Once healing has occurred, no external dressing is required.
   e. The fistula allows freedom of movement.
 3. Disadvantages
   a. The fistula cannot be used immediately after insertion so planning ahead for alternate access for dialysis is important.
   b. Needle insertions through the skin and tissues to the fistula are required for dialysis.
   c. Infiltration of the needles during dialysis can occur and cause hematomas.
   d. An aneurysm can form in the fistula.
   e. HF can occur from increased blood flow in the venous system.

⚠ Arterial steal syndrome can develop in a client with an internal arteriovenous fistula. With this complication, too much blood is diverted to the vein and arterial perfusion to the hand is compromised.

D. Internal arteriovenous graft (see Fig. 51.2)
 1. Description
   a. The internal graft may be used for chronic dialysis clients who do not have adequate blood vessels for the creation of a fistula.
   b. An artificial graft made of Gore-Tex or a bovine (cow) carotid artery is used to create an artificial vein for blood flow.

c. The procedure involves the anastomosis of an artery to a vein using an artificial graft.

d. The graft can be used 2 weeks after insertion.

e. Complications of the graft include clotting, aneurysms, and infection.

2. Advantages and disadvantages: Same as for internal arteriovenous fistula

E. Interventions for an arteriovenous fistula and arteriovenous graft

1. Reinforce teaching the client that the extremity must not be used for monitoring BP, drawing blood, placing IV lines, or administering injections; and that the client needs to inform all health care personnel of its presence.

2. Reinforce teaching the client with an arteriovenous fistula to perform hand-flexing exercises, if prescribed, such as "ball squeezing" to promote graft maturity.

3. Palpate pulses below the fistula or graft, and monitor for hand swelling as an indication of ischemia.

4. Note the temperature and capillary refill of the extremity.

5. Monitor for clotting.

a. Complaints of tingling or discomfort in the extremity

b. Inability to palpate a thrill or auscultate a bruit over the fistula or graft

6. Monitor for arterial steal syndrome.

7. Monitor for infection.

8. Monitor lung and heart sounds for signs of HF.

9. Notify the RN immediately who will notify the PHCP if signs of clotting, infection, or arterial steal syndrome occur.

⚠ To ensure patency, palpate for a thrill or auscultate for a bruit over the fistula or graft. Notify the RN and PHCP if a thrill or bruit is absent.

VIII. Complications of Hemodialysis (Box 51.5)

A. If signs of complications occur, the dialysis is slowed or stopped depending on the complication and the PHCP is notified immediately.

B. The nurse stays with the client and monitors the client, including vital signs, and another nurse obtains initial prescriptions from the PHCP.

C. See Priority Nursing Actions for air embolism.

BOX 51.5	Complications of Hemodialysis

- Air embolus
- Disequilibrium syndrome
- Electrolyte alterations
- Encephalopathy
- Hemorrhage
- Hepatitis
- Hypotension
- Sepsis
- Shock

⚡ PRIORITY NURSING ACTIONS

Air Embolism in a Client Receiving Hemodialysis

1. Stop the hemodialysis.
2. Turn the client on the left side with the head down (Trendelenburg).
3. Notify the registered nurse, primary health care provider, and nephrologist.
4. Notify rapid response team for the hospitalized client
5. Administer oxygen.
6. Check vital signs and pulse oximetry.
7. Document the event, actions taken, and the client's response.

IX. Peritoneal Dialysis

A. Description

1. The peritoneum acts as the dialyzing membrane (semipermeable membrane) to achieve dialysis and the membrane is accessed by insertion of a PD catheter through the abdomen.

2. PD works on the principles of osmosis, diffusion, and ultrafiltration; PD occurs via the transfer of fluid and solute from the bloodstream through the peritoneum into the dialysate solution.

3. The peritoneal membrane is large and porous, allowing solutes and fluid to move via osmosis from an area of higher concentration in the body to an area of lower concentration in the dialyzing fluid.

4. The peritoneal cavity is rich in capillaries; therefore, it provides a ready access to the blood supply.

B. Contraindications to PD

1. Peritonitis
2. Recent abdominal surgery
3. Abdominal adhesions
4. Other GI problems such as diverticulosis

C. Access for PD (Fig. 51.3)

1. A siliconized rubber catheter such as a Tenckhoff catheter is surgically inserted into the client's peritoneal cavity to allow infusion of dialysis fluid; the catheter site is covered by a sterile dressing that is changed daily and when soiled or wet.

2. The preferred insertion site is 3 to 5 cm below the umbilicus. This area is relatively avascular and has less fascial resistance.

3. The catheter is tunneled under the skin, through the fat and muscle tissue, and to the peritoneum. It is stabilized with Dacron cuffs in the muscle and under the skin.

4. Over a period of 1 to 2 weeks after insertion, fibroblasts and blood vessels grow around the cuffs, fixing the catheter in place and providing an extra barrier against dialysate leakage and bacterial invasion.

5. If the client is scheduled for transplant surgery, the PD catheter may either be removed or left in place if the need for dialysis is suspected post transplantation.

D. Dialysate solution

1. The dialysate solution is sterile.
2. All dialysis solutions are prescribed by the PHCP; the solution contains electrolytes and minerals and has a specific osmolarity, specific glucose concentration, and other medication additives as prescribed.
3. The higher the glucose concentration, the greater the hypertonicity and the amount of fluid removed during a PD exchange.
4. Increasing the glucose concentration increases the concentration of active particles that cause osmosis, the rate of ultrafiltration, and the amount of fluid removed.
5. If hyperkalemia is not a problem, potassium may be added to each bag of dialysate solution.
6. Heparin is added to the dialysate solution to prevent clotting of the catheter.
7. Prophylactic antibiotics may be added to the dialysate solution to prevent peritonitis.
8. Insulin may be added to the dialysate solution for the client with diabetes mellitus.

E. PD infusion

1. Description
   a. One infusion (fill), dwell, and drain is considered one exchange.
   b. Fill: 1 to 2 L of dialysate, as prescribed, is infused by gravity into the peritoneal space, which usually takes 10 to 20 minutes.
   c. Dwell time: The amount of time that the dialysate solution remains in the peritoneal

cavity is prescribed by the PHCP and can last 20 to 30 minutes to 8 or more hours depending on the type of dialysis used.
   d. Drain (outflow): Fluid drains out of body by gravity into the drainage bag.

2. Interventions before treatment
   a. Monitor vital signs.
   b. Monitor daily weight on the same scale.
   c. Have the client void if possible.
   d. Monitor electrolyte and glucose levels.
   e. Monitor the peritoneal catheter dressing and site.

3. Interventions during treatment
   a. Monitor vital signs.
   b. Monitor for respiratory distress, pain, or discomfort.
   c. Monitor for signs of pulmonary edema.
   d. Monitor for hypotension and hypertension.
   e. Monitor for malaise, nausea, vomiting.
   f. Monitor the catheter site dressing for wetness or bleeding.
   g. Monitor dwell time as prescribed by the PHCP.
   h. Do not allow dwell time to extend beyond the PHCP's prescription because this increases the risk for hyperglycemia.
   i. Initiate outflow; turn the client from side to side if the outflow is slow to start.
   j. Monitor outflow, which would be a continuous stream after the clamp is opened.
   k. Monitor outflow for color and clarity.
   l. Monitor intake and output accurately. If outflow is less than inflow, the difference is equal to the amount absorbed or retained by the client during dialysis and would be counted as intake.

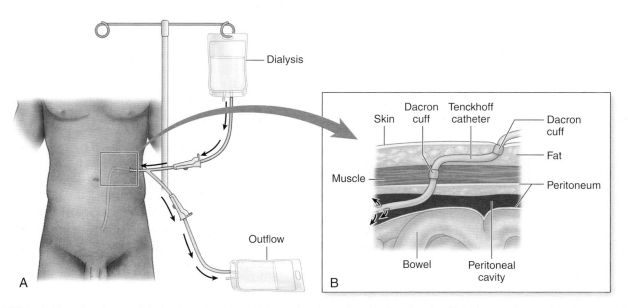

FIGURE 51.3 Manual peritoneal dialysis via an implanted abdominal catheter (Tenckhoff catheter). (A) Dialysate inflow and outflow through implanted abdominal catheter. (B) Implanted abdominal catheter.

m. An outflow greater than inflow needs to be reported to RN and PHCP as well as the appearance of frank blood or cloudiness in outflow.

n. The RN is notified if signs of complications occur.

F. Types of PD

1. Continuous ambulatory peritoneal dialysis (CAPD)

a. Closely resembles renal function because it is a continuous process

b. Does not require a machine for the procedure

c. Promotes client independence

d. The client performs self-dialysis 24 hours a day, 7 days a week.

e. Four dialysis cycles are usually administered in a 24-hour period including an overnight 8-hour dwell time.

f. Dialysate, 1.5 to 2 L, is instilled into the abdomen four times daily and allowed to dwell as prescribed (bags are weighed to determine output); the catheter is clamped, and the bag is rolled up during dwell time.

g. After dwell, the bag is placed lower than the insertion site so that fluid drains by gravity flow.

h. After fluid is drained, the bag is changed, new dialysate is instilled into the abdomen, and the process continues.

i. Between exchanges, the catheter is clamped.

2. Automated PD

a. Automated dialysis requires a peritoneal cycling machine.

b. Automated dialysis can be done as intermittent PD, continuous cycling PD, or nightly PD.

c. The exchanges are automated instead of manual.

X. Complications of Peritoneal Dialysis

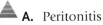 Infection is a concern with PD. Sites of infection are either at the catheter insertion site or in the peritoneum, which can cause peritonitis.

A. Peritonitis

1. Monitor for symptoms of peritonitis: fever, cloudy outflow, rebound abdominal tenderness, abdominal pain, general malaise, nausea, and vomiting.

2. Cloudy or opaque outflow is an early sign of peritonitis.

3. If peritonitis is suspected, obtain a culture of the outflow to determine the infective organism.

4. Assist with the administration of antibiotics as prescribed.

5. Avoid infections by maintaining meticulous sterile technique when connecting and disconnecting PD solution bags and when caring for the catheter insertion site.

6. Prevent the catheter insertion site dressing from becoming wet during care of the client or the dialysis procedure; change the dressing if wet or soiled.

7. Follow institutional procedure for connecting and disconnecting PD solution bags, which may include scrubbing the connection sites with an antiseptic solution.

B. Abdominal pain

1. Peritoneal irritation during inflow commonly causes abdominal cramping and discomfort; the pain usually disappears after 1 to 2 weeks of dialysis.

2. Warm the dialysate before administration using a special dialysate warmer pad, because the cold temperature of the dialysate can cause discomfort.

C. Abnormal outflow characteristics are indicative of complications.

1. Bloody outflow after the first few exchanges indicates vascular complications (the outflow needs to be clear and colorless after the initial exchanges).

2. Brown outflow indicates bowel perforation.

3. Urine-colored outflow indicates bladder perforation.

4. Cloudy outflow indicates peritonitis.

D. Insufficient outflow

1. The main cause of insufficient outflow is a full colon. Encourage a high-fiber diet (because constipation can cause inflow and outflow problems), and administer stool softeners as prescribed.

2. Insufficient outflow may also be caused by catheter migration out of the peritoneal area. If this occurs, an x-ray will be prescribed to evaluate catheter position.

3. Maintain the drainage bag below the client's abdomen.

4. Check for kinks in the tubing.

5. Check for fibrin clots in the tubing, and milk the tubing to dislodge the clot as prescribed.

6. Change the client's outflow position by turning the client to a side-lying position or ambulating the client.

E. Leakage around the catheter site

1. Clear fluid that leaks from the catheter exit site will be noted.

2. It takes 1 to 2 weeks after insertion of the catheter before fibroblasts and blood vessels grow into the catheter cuffs, fixing it in place and providing an extra barrier against dialysate leakage and bacterial invasion.

3. Smaller amounts of dialysate need to be used, and it may take up to 2 weeks for the client to tolerate a full 2-L exchange without leaking around the catheter site.

XI. Continuous Renal Replacement Therapy

A. Continuous renal replacement therapy (CRRT) provides continuous ultrafiltration of extracellular fluid and clearance of urinary toxins over a period of 8 to 24 hours; used primarily for clients in AKI or critically ill clients with CKD who cannot tolerate hemodialysis.

B. Water, electrolytes, and other solutes are removed as the client's blood passes through a hemofilter.

C. Because rapid shifts in fluids and electrolytes typically do not occur, hemofiltration is usually well tolerated by critically ill clients.

D. There are 5 variations of CRRT, some requiring a hemodialysis machine, whereas others rely on the client's BP to power the system.

E. If CRRT does not require a hemodialysis machine, the client's mean arterial BP needs to be maintained above 60 mm Hg and arterial and venous access sites are necessary.

XII. Kidney Transplantation

A. Description
1. A human kidney from a compatible donor is implanted into a recipient.
2. Kidney transplantation is performed for irreversible kidney failure; specific criteria are established for eligibility of a transplant.
3. The recipient needs to take immunosuppressive medications for life.

B. Donors
1. Donors may be living donors (related or unrelated to the client), non–heart-beating donors (NHBDs), or cadaver donors.
2. The most desirable source of kidneys for transplant is living related donors who closely matches the client.
3. NHBDs are those who have been declared dead by cardiopulmonary criteria and have organs harvested immediately after death; these persons have consented previously to organ donation.
4. Cadaver donors are those who have suffered irreversible brain injury; these persons are maintained with mechanical ventilation and must have adequate perfusion to the kidneys.
5. Physical criteria for donors include absence of systemic disease and infection, no history of cancer, no kidney disease or hypertension, and adequate kidney function.
6. Donors are screened for ABO blood group, tissue-specific antigen, human leukocyte antigen suitability, and mixed lymphocyte culture index (histocompatibility); donors are also screened for the presence of any communicable diseases, and they undergo a complete medical evaluation and a nephrology consultation.
7. The donor must be in excellent health with two properly functioning kidneys.
8. The emotional well-being of the donor is determined.

9. Complete understanding of the donation process and outcome by the donor is necessary; usually kidney removal from the donor is done using a laparoscopic procedure.

C. Preoperative interventions
1. Histocompatibility tests will be done by organ bank personnel.
2. Immunosuppressive medications will be administered to the recipient as prescribed.
3. Maintain strict aseptic technique.
4. Assist to verify that hemodialysis of the recipient was completed 24 hours before transplantation.
5. Ensure that the recipient is free of any infections.
6. Monitor renal function studies.
7. Encourage discussion of feelings of the live donor and the recipient.
8. Provide psychological support to the live donor, NHBD, or cadaver donor family and the recipient.

D. Postoperative interventions for the recipient
1. The transplanted kidney is placed in the anterior iliac fossa; usually the recipient's diseased kidneys are left in place, except for those with polycystic kidney disease in which the kidneys are often very enlarged and painful.
2. Urine output usually begins immediately if the donor was a living donor. It is usually delayed for a few days or more with other donor types.
3. Hemodialysis may be performed until adequate kidney function is established.
4. Monitor vital signs for signs of complications such as rejection, thrombosis, renal artery stenosis, or wound problems.
5. Monitor urine output hourly; immediately report an abrupt decrease in urine output.
6. Monitor IV fluids closely; for the first 12 to 24 hours, IV fluid replacement is based on hourly urine output.
7. Assist with the administration of prescribed diuretics and osmotic agents.
8. Monitor daily weight to evaluate fluid status.
9. Monitor daily laboratory results to evaluate renal function, including hematocrit, BUN, and serum creatinine levels; monitor urine for blood and specific gravity.
10. Position the client in the semi-Fowler's position to promote gas exchange, turning from the back to the nonoperative side.
11. Monitor indwelling urinary catheter patency. The indwelling urinary catheter remains in the bladder for 3 to 5 days to allow for anastomosis healing.
12. Note that urine is pink and bloody initially but gradually returns to normal within several days to weeks.
13. Notify the RN, who will notify the PHCP, if gross hematuria and clots are noted in the urine.

14. Monitor the three-way bladder irrigation, if present, for clots; the RN may irrigate the catheter if a PHCP's prescription is present.

 15. Assist with the removal of the indwelling urinary catheter as soon as possible to prevent infection.

16. Maintain aseptic technique and monitor for infection; infection is the primary cause of death in the first year post transplantation.

17. Monitor for bowel sounds and for the passage of flatus; initiate a specific diet and oral fluids, as prescribed, when flatus and bowel sounds return (usually fluids, sodium, and potassium are restricted if the client is oliguric).

18. Maintain good oral hygiene, monitoring for stomatitis and bacterial and fungal infections.

19. Encourage coughing and deep-breathing exercises.

20. Assist with the administration of immunosuppressive medications as prescribed.

21. The client is usually ambulated after 24 hours.

 22. Monitor for signs of organ rejection by monitoring laboratory results.

23. Promote live donor and recipient relationship.

24. Monitor both the donor and recipient for depression.

25. Assist with providing the recipient with instructions following the kidney transplantation (Box 51.6).

 26. Assist the recipient with coping with the body-image disturbances that occur from long-term use of immunosuppressants.

27. Assist with providing information to the recipient of available support groups.

E. Graft rejection: Except in the case of an identical twin donor and recipient, the major postoperative complication of kidney transplantation is graft rejection.

 1. Data collection (Box 51.7)

2. Hyperacute rejection
   a. Hyperacute rejection occurs within 48 hours after the transplant.
   b. Interventions: Removal of rejected kidney

3. Acute rejection
   a. Most common type; occurs most within 1 week postoperatively but can occur any time post transplantation
   b. Interventions: Potentially reversible with increased immunosuppression

4. Chronic rejection
   a. Occurs slowly, months to years after transplant and mimics CKD
   b. Interventions: Immunosuppressive medications and dialysis if necessary

⚠ Except in the case of an identical twin donor and recipient, the major postoperative complication after renal transplant is graft rejection.

XIII. Cystitis (Urinary Tract Infections)

A. Description

1. Cystitis (urinary tract infection [UTI]) refers to an inflammation of the bladder from an infection, obstruction of the urethra, or other irritants.

2. The most common causative organisms are *Escherichia coli*, *Enterobacter*, *Pseudomonas*, and *Serratia* species.

3. Cystitis is more common in women because women have a shorter urethra than men and the urethra in the woman is located close to the rectum.

4. Sexually active and pregnant women are most vulnerable to cystitis.

B. Data collection

1. Frequency and urgency
2. Burning on urination
3. Voiding in small amounts
4. Inability to void
5. Incomplete emptying of the bladder
6. Lower abdominal discomfort or back discomfort; bladder spasms
7. Cloudy, dark, foul-smelling urine
8. Hematuria
9. Malaise, chills, and fever
10. WBC count greater than 10,000 mm³ during urinalysis and culture

---

BOX 51.6 Client Instructions After Kidney Transplantation

Avoid prolonged periods of sitting.
Monitor intake and output.
Recognize the signs/symptoms of infection and rejection.
Use medications as prescribed, and maintain immunosuppressive therapy for life.
Avoid contact sports.
Avoid exposure to persons with infections.
Know the signs/symptoms that require the need to contact the registered nurse (RN), primary health care provider (PHCP), or nephrologist.
Ensure follow-up care.

BOX 51.7 Clinical Signs of Renal Transplant (Graft) Rejection

Fever greater than 100°F (37.8°C)
Pain or tenderness over the grafted kidney
A 2- to 3-lb (0.9–1.4 kg) weight gain in 24 hours
Edema
Hypertension
Malaise
Elevated blood urea nitrogen (BUN) and serum creatinine
Decreased creatinine clearance
Elevated white blood cell count
Rejection indicated by ultrasound or biopsy

Altered mentation is a sign of a UTI in older adults; frequency and urgency may not be specific symptoms of UTI because of urinary elimination changes that occur with aging.

C. Interventions

 1. Before administering prescribed antibiotics, obtain a urine specimen for culture and sensitivity, if prescribed, to identify bacterial growth.

2. Encourage the client to increase fluids up to 3000 mL/day, especially if the client is taking a sulfonamide. Sulfonamides can form crystals in concentrated urine.

3. Assist with the administration of prescribed medications, which may include analgesics, antiseptics, antispasmodics, antibiotics, and antimicrobials.

4. Maintain an acid urine pH (5.5), and instruct the client about foods to consume to maintain acidic urine.

5. Provide heat to the abdomen or sitz baths for complaints of discomfort as prescribed.

6. Note that if the client is prescribed an aminoglycoside, a sulfonamide, or nitrofurantoin, the actions of these medications are decreased by acidic urine.

7. Use sterile technique when inserting a urinary catheter.

8. Provide meticulous perineal care for the client with an indwelling catheter.

9. Discourage caffeine products such as coffee, tea, and cola.

10. Reinforce client education
   a. Avoid alcohol.
   b. Take medications as prescribed.
   c. Take antibiotics on schedule and complete the entire course of medications as prescribed; which medication is prescribed and for how long depends on the client's health condition and the type of bacteria found in the urine.
   d. Repeat the urine culture after treatment.
   e. Prevent recurrence of cystitis (Box 51.8).

XIV. Urosepsis

A. Description
   1. Urosepsis refers to a bacteremia originating in the urinary tract.

BOX 51.8 **Teaching for Prevention of Cystitis**

Use good perineal care, wiping front to back.
Avoid bubble baths, tub baths, and vaginal deodorants or sprays.
Void every 2–3 hours.
Wear cotton pants and avoid wearing tight clothes or pantyhose with slacks.
Avoid sitting in a wet bathing suit for prolonged periods.
If pregnant, void every 2 hours.
If menopausal, use estrogen vaginal creams to restore pH.
Use water-soluble lubricants for intercourse, especially after menopause.
Void and drink a glass of water after intercourse.

---

2. The most common causative organism is *Escherichia coli*.

3. In a client who is immunocompromised, the most common cause is infection from an indwelling urinary catheter or an untreated UTI.

4. The major problem is the ability of this bacterium to develop resistant strains.

5. Urosepsis can lead to septic shock if not treated aggressively.

B. Data collection: Fever is the most common and earliest manifestation.

C. Interventions
   1. Obtain a urine specimen for urine culture and sensitivity before administering antibiotics.
   2. IV antibiotics are administered as prescribed usually until the client has been afebrile for 3 to 5 days.
   3. Assist with the administration of oral antibiotics, as prescribed, after the 3- to 5-day afebrile period.

XV. Urethritis

A. Description
   1. An inflammation of the urethra commonly associated with sexually transmitted infections (STIs); may occur with cystitis
   2. In men, urethritis most often is caused by gonorrhea or chlamydial infection.
   3. In women, urethritis is most often caused by feminine hygiene sprays, perfumed toilet paper or sanitary napkins, spermicidal jelly, UTIs, or changes in the vaginal mucosal lining.

B. Data collection
   1. Pain or burning on urination
   2. Frequency and urgency
   3. Nocturia
   4. Difficulty voiding
   5. Males may have clear to mucopurulent discharge from the penis.
   6. Females may have lower abdominal discomfort.

C. Interventions
   1. Encourage fluid intake.
   2. Assist with preparing the client for testing to determine whether an STI is present.
   3. Assist with the administration of antibiotics as prescribed.
   4. Reinforce instructions to the client in the administration of a sitz bath.
   5. If stricture occurs, prepare the client for dilation of the urethra and instillation of an antiseptic solution.
   6. Reinforce instructions to the female client to avoid the use of perfumed toilet paper or sanitary napkins and feminine hygiene sprays.
   7. Reinforce instructions to the client to avoid intercourse until the symptoms subside or treatment of the STI is complete.

8. Reinforce instructions to the client on STIs if this is the cause.
   a. Prevent STIs by the use of latex condoms or abstinence.
   b. All sexual partners during the 30 days before diagnosis with chlamydial infection need to be notified, examined, and treated if indicated.
   c. Chlamydial infection often coexists with gonorrhea; diagnostic testing is done for both STIs.
   d. Treatment for STIs includes antibiotics as prescribed to treat the causative organism.
   e. The most serious complication of chlamydial infection is sterility.
   f. Follow-up culture may be requested in 4 to 7 days to evaluate the effectiveness of medications.

XVI. Ureteritis

A. Description: An inflammation of the ureter commonly associated with bacterial or viral infections and pyelonephritis

B. Data collection
   1. Dysuria
   2. Frequent urination
   3. Clear to mucopurulent penile discharge in males

C. Interventions
   1. Treatment includes identifying and treating the underlying cause and providing symptomatic relief.
   2. Assist with the administration of metronidazole or clotrimazole, as prescribed, for treating *Trichomonas* infection.
   3. Assist with the administration of nystatin or fluconazole, as prescribed, for treating yeast infections.
   4. Doxycycline or azithromycin may be prescribed for treating chlamydial infections.

XVII. Pyelonephritis

A. Description
   1. An inflammation of the renal pelvis and the parenchyma commonly caused by bacterial invasion
   2. Acute pyelonephritis often occurs after bacterial contamination of the urethra or an invasive procedure of the urinary tract.
   3. Chronic pyelonephritis most commonly occurs after chronic urinary flow obstruction as with reflux or calculi.
   4. *E. coli* is the most common bacterial causative organism.

B. Acute pyelonephritis
   1. Acute pyelonephritis occurs as a new infection or recurs as a relapse of a previous infection.
   2. It can progress to bacteremia or chronic pyelonephritis.

   3. Data collection
      a. Fever and chills
      b. Nausea
      c. Flank pain on the affected side
      d. Costovertebral angle tenderness
      e. Headache
      f. Dysuria
      g. Frequency and urgency
      h. Cloudy, bloody, or foul-smelling urine
      i. Increased WBC in the urine
      j. Tachycardia and tachypnea

C. Chronic pyelonephritis
   1. A slow, progressive disease usually associated with recurrent acute attacks
   2. Causes contraction of the kidney and dysfunctioning of the nephrons, which are replaced by scar tissue
   3. May cause the ureter to become fibrotic and narrowed by strictures
   4. Can lead to AKI or CKD
   5. Data collection
      a. Frequently diagnosed incidentally when a client is being evaluated for hypertension
      b. Inability to conserve sodium
      c. Poor urine-concentrating ability
      d. Pyuria
      e. Azotemia
      f. Proteinuria

D. Interventions
   1. Monitor vital signs especially for elevated temperature.
   2. Encourage fluid intake up to 3000 mL/day to reduce fever and prevent dehydration.
   3. Monitor intake and output (ensure that output is a minimum of 1500 mL every 24 hours).
   4. Monitor weight.
   5. Encourage adequate rest.
   6. Instruct the client in a high-calorie, low-protein diet.
   7. Provide warm, moist compresses to the flank area, and take warm baths to help relieve pain.
   8. Assist to administer analgesics, antipyretics, antibiotics, urinary antiseptics, and antiemetics as prescribed.
   9. Monitor for signs of AKI or CKD.
   10. Encourage follow-up urine culture.

XVIII. Glomerulonephritis (See Chapter 34)

XIX. Nephrotic Syndrome (See Chapter 34)

XX. Polycystic Kidney Disease

A. Description
   1. A cystic formation and hypertrophy of the kidneys that leads to cystic rupture, infection, formation of scar tissue, and damaged nephrons
   2. There is no specific treatment to arrest the progress of the destructive cysts.
   3. The ultimate result of this disease is CKD.

B. Types
   1. Infantile polycystic disease: An inherited autosomal recessive trait that results in the death of the infant within a few months after birth
   2. Adult polycystic disease: An autosomal dominant trait that manifests between 30 and 40 years of age and results in end-stage kidney disease

C. Data collection
   1. Often asymptomatic until the ages of 30 to 40 years
   2. Flank, lumbar, or abdominal pain that worsens with activity and is relieved when lying down
   3. Fever and chills
   4. Recurrent UTI
   5. Hematuria, proteinuria, and pyuria
   6. Calculi
   7. Hypertension
   8. Palpable abdominal masses and enlarged kidneys
   9. Increased abdominal girth

D. Interventions
   1. Monitor for gross hematuria, which indicates cyst rupture.
   2. Increase sodium and water intake because sodium loss rather than retention occurs.
   3. Provide bed rest if ruptured cysts and bleeding occur.
   4. Monitor pain, reinforce instructions on how to use pain medications (avoid nonsteroidal antiinflammatory medications [NSAIDs] and aspirin because of the risk for bleeding), and use dry heat on the abdomen and flank areas for comfort when cysts are infected.
   5. Prevent constipation from pressure of cysts on colon by adequate fiber in diet, stool softeners, adequate fluid intake, and exercise.
   6. Prepare the client for percutaneous cyst puncture for relief of obstruction or drainage of an abscess.
   7. Assist with the administration of antihypertensives as prescribed.
   8. Prevent and/or treat UTIs.
   9. Assist with preparing the client for dialysis or renal transplantation.
   10. Encourage the client to seek genetic counseling.
   11. Provide psychological support to the client and family.
   12. Provide psychosocial support and genetic counseling for family members who may want to donate a kidney.

XXI. Hydronephrosis (Fig. 51.4)

A. Description
   1. The distention of the renal pelvis and calices caused by an obstruction of normal urine flow
   2. The urine becomes trapped proximal to the obstruction.
   3. The causes include calculus, a tumor, scar tissue, ureter obstruction, and hypertrophy of the prostate.

B. Data collection
   1. Hypertension

2. Headache
3. Colicky or dull flank pain that radiates to the groin

C. Interventions
   1. Monitor vital signs frequently.
   2. Monitor for fluid and electrolyte imbalances, including dehydration after the obstruction is relieved.
   3. Monitor for diuresis, which can lead to fluid depletion.
   4. Monitor weight daily.
   5. Monitor urine for specific gravity, albumin, and glucose levels.
   6. Assist with the administration of fluid replacement as prescribed.
   7. Assist with preparing the client for insertion of a nephrostomy tube or a surgical procedure to relieve the obstruction if prescribed.

XXII. Renal Calculi

A. Description
   1. Calculi are stones that can form anywhere in the urinary tract; however, the most frequent site is the kidneys.
   2. Problems resulting from calculi are severe intermittent pain, obstruction, tissue trauma, secondary hemorrhage, and infection.
   3. The stone can be located through radiography of the KUB; IV pyelography; computed tomography (CT) scanning; and renal ultrasonography.
   4. A stone analysis will be done after passage to determine the type of stone and assist with determining treatment.
   5. **Urolithiasis** refers to the formation of urinary calculi.

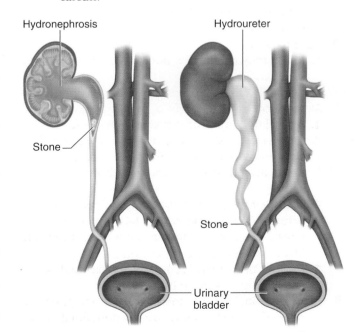

FIGURE 51.4 Hydronephrosis and hydroureter. (From Ignatavicius D, Workman ML, Rebar CR: *Medical-surgical nursing: Concepts for interprofessional collaborative care*, ed 9, Philadelphia, 2018, Saunders.)

6. Nephrolithiasis refers to kidney calculi; these are located in the renal parenchyma.
7. When a calculus occludes the ureter and blocks the flow of urine, the ureter dilates producing hydroureter.
8. If the obstruction is not removed, urinary stasis results in infection, impairment of renal function on the side of the blockage, hydronephrosis, and irreversible kidney damage.

B. Causes
   1. Family history of stone formation
   2. Diet high in calcium, vitamin D, protein, oxalate, purines, or alkali
   3. Obstruction and urinary stasis
   4. Dehydration
   5. Use of diuretics, which can cause volume depletion
   6. UTIs and prolonged urinary catheterization
   7. Immobilization
   8. Hypercalcemia and hyperparathyroidism
   9. Elevated uric acid level such as in gout

C. Data collection
   1. Renal colic, which originates in the lumbar region and radiates around the side and down to the testicle in men and to the bladder in women
   2. Ureteral colic, which radiates toward the genitalia and thigh
   3. Sharp, severe pain of sudden onset
   4. Dull, aching pain in the kidney
   5. Nausea and vomiting, pallor, and diaphoresis during acute pain
   6. Urinary frequency with alternating retention
   7. Signs of a UTI
   8. Low-grade fever
   9. High numbers of red blood cells, WBCs, and bacteria in the urinalysis report
   10. Gross hematuria

D. Interventions
   1. Monitor vital signs, especially the temperature, for signs of infection.
   2. Monitor intake and output.
   3. Monitor for fever, chills, and infection.
   4. Monitor for nausea, vomiting, and diarrhea.
   5. Encourage fluid intake up to 3000 mL/day, unless contraindicated, to facilitate the passage of the stone and prevent infection; monitor for obstruction.
   6. Assist with the administration of IV fluids, as prescribed, if unable to take fluids orally or in adequate amounts to increase the flow of urine and facilitate the passage of the stone.
   7. Provide heat to the flank area as prescribed (massage therapy needs to be avoided).
   8. Assist with the administration of analgesics at regularly scheduled intervals, as prescribed, to relieve pain.
   9. Monitor the client's response to pain medication.
   10. Assist the client with performing relaxation techniques to help with pain relief.
   11. Encourage client ambulation, if stable, to promote the passage of the stone.
   12. Turn and reposition the immobilized client to promote the passage of the stone.
   13. Reinforce instructions to the client about the diet specific to the stone composition if prescribed (Box 51.9).
   14. Prepare the client for surgical procedures if prescribed.

⚠ For the client with renal calculi, strain all urine for the presence of stones and send the stones to the laboratory for analysis.

XXIII. Treatment Options for Renal Calculi (Fig. 51.5)

A. Cystoscopy
   1. Cystoscopy may be done for stones located in the bladder or lower ureter.
   2. No incision is made.
   3. One or two ureteral catheters are inserted past the stone.
   4. The catheters are left in place for 24 hours to drain the urine trapped proximal to the stone and to dilate the ureter.
   5. A continuous chemical irrigation may be prescribed to dissolve the stone.

B. Extracorporeal shock wave lithotripsy (ESWL)
   1. A noninvasive mechanical procedure for breaking up stones located in the kidney or upper ureter so that they can pass spontaneously or be removed by other methods
   2. No incision is made and no drains are placed. A stent may be placed to facilitate passing stone fragments.

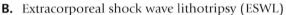

BOX 51.9	**Nutritional Therapy for Calculi**

Purine[a]
High: Sardines, herring, mussels, liver, kidney, goose, venison, meat soups, sweetbreads
Moderate: Chicken, salmon, crab, veal, mutton, bacon, pork, beef, ham

Calcium
High: Milk, cheese, ice cream, yogurt, sauces containing milk; all beans (except green beans), lentils; fish with fine bones (e.g., sardines, kippers, herring, salmon); dried fruits, nuts; cocoa powder, chocolate, cocoa

Oxalate
High: Dark roughage, spinach, rhubarb, asparagus, cabbage, tomatoes, beets, nuts, celery, parsley, runner beans; chocolate, cocoa, instant coffee, cocoa powder, tea; Worcestershire sauce

Note: Depending on the type of calculi, the diet may be modified to decrease foods that are high in the substance that is the cause of the calculi. The client is instructed to follow the primary health care provider's dietary recommendations.
[a] Uric acid is a waste product from purine in food.
Adapted from Lewis SL, Dirksen SR, Heitkemper MM, et al: *Medical surgical nursing: Assessment and management of clinical problems*, ed 8, St. Louis, 2011, Mosby.

3. Fluoroscopy is used to visualize the stone, and ultrasonic waves are delivered to the areas of the stone to disintegrate it.

4. The stones are passed in the urine within a few days.

5. The client is taught to watch for signs of urinary obstruction, bleeding, or hematoma formation.

6. Reinforce instructions to the client to increase fluid intake to flush out the stone fragments.

C. Percutaneous lithotripsy

1. Performed for stones in the bladder, ureter, or kidney

2. An invasive procedure in which a guide is inserted under fluoroscopy near the area of the stone; an ultrasonic wave is aimed at the stone to break it into fragments.

3. Percutaneous lithotripsy may be performed via cystoscopy or nephroscopy.

4. No incision is required for cystoscopy; a small flank incision is needed for nephroscopy.

5. The client may possibly have an indwelling bladder catheter.

6. A nephrostomy tube may be placed to administer chemical irrigations to break up the stone. The nephrostomy tube may remain in place for 1 to 5 days.

7. Encourage the client to drink 3000 to 4000 mL of fluid/day following the procedure as prescribed.

8. Monitor for and instruct the client to observe for complications of infection, hemorrhage, and extravasation of fluid into the retroperitoneal cavity.

D. Ureterolithotomy

1. An open surgical procedure is performed if lithotripsy is not effective for the removal of a stone in the ureter.

2. An incision is made through the lower abdomen or flank and then into the ureter to remove the stone.

3. The client may have a drain, a ureteral stent catheter, and an indwelling bladder catheter.

E. Pyelolithotomy and nephrolithotomy

1. Pyelolithotomy is an incision into the renal pelvis to remove a stone. A large flank incision is required, and the client may have a drain and an indwelling bladder catheter.

2. Nephrolithotomy is an incision into the kidney made to remove a stone. A large flank incision is required, and the client may have a nephrostomy tube and an indwelling bladder catheter.

F. Partial or total nephrectomy

1. Performed for extensive kidney damage, renal infection, severe obstruction from stones or tumors, and the prevention of stone recurrence

2. Monitor the incision particularly if a drain is in place because it will drain large amounts of urine.

3. Protect the skin from urinary drainage, changing dressings frequently if necessary.

4. Monitor the nephrostomy tube, which may be attached to a drainage bag for a continuous flow of urine.

5. The nephrotomy or bladder catheters are not irrigated unless specifically prescribed; if prescribed, this is done by the RN. Monitor the indwelling bladder catheter for drainage.

6. Encourage fluid intake to ensure a urine output of 2500 to 3000 mL/day or more.

XXIV. Kidney Tumors

A. Description

1. Kidney tumors may be benign or malignant, bilateral or unilateral.

2. Common sites of metastasis include bone, lungs, liver, spleen, and the other kidney.

3. The exact cause of renal carcinoma is unknown.

B. Data collection for those with advanced disease

1. Dull flank pain

2. Palpable renal mass

3. Painless gross hematuria

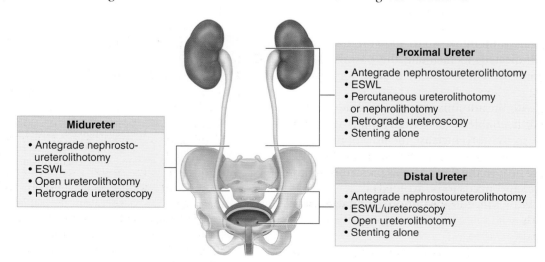

FIGURE 51.5 Treatment options for ureteral stones. *ESWL*, Extracorporeal shock wave lithotripsy.

C. Radical nephrectomy

1. Description

   a. The surgical removal of the entire kidney, adjacent adrenal gland, and renal artery and vein

   b. Radiation therapy and possibly chemotherapy may follow radical nephrectomy.

   c. Before surgery, radiation may be used to embolize (occlude) the arteries supplying the kidney to reduce bleeding during nephrectomy.

2. Postoperative interventions

   a. Monitor vital signs for indicators of bleeding (hypotension and tachycardia).

   b. Monitor for abdominal distention, decreases in urinary output, and alterations in level of consciousness as signs indicative of bleeding. Check the bed linens under the client for bleeding.

   c. Monitor for signs of adrenal insufficiency, which include a large urinary output followed by hypotension and subsequent oliguria.

   d. Assist with the administration of IV fluids and packed red blood cells as prescribed.

   e. Monitor intake and output and daily weight.

   f. Monitor for a urinary output of 30 to 50 mL/hr to ensure adequate renal function.

   g. Maintain the client in a semi-Fowler's position.

   h. If a nephrostomy tube is in place, it is not irrigated (unless specifically prescribed); if prescribed, this is done by the RN.

XXV. Epididymitis

A. Description

1. An acute or chronic inflammation of the epididymis that occurs as a result of a UTI, STI, prostatitis, or from long-term use of an indwelling bladder catheter.

2. The infective organism travels upward through the urethra and ejaculatory duct and along the vas deferens to the epididymis.

B. Data collection

1. Scrotal and groin pain

2. Swelling in the scrotum and groin

3. Pus and bacteria in the urine

4. Fever and chills

5. Abscess development

C. Interventions

1. Encourage fluid intake.

2. Encourage bed rest with the scrotum elevated to prevent traction on the spermatic cord, facilitate drainage, and relieve pain.

3. Reinforce instructions to the client in the intermittent application of cold compresses to the scrotum.

4. Reinforce instructions to the client in the use of sitz baths.

5. Reinforce instructions to the client in the administration of antibiotics for self and sexual partner if the cause is chlamydial or gonorrheal infection.

6. Reinforce instructions to the client to avoid lifting, straining, and sexual contact until the infection subsides.

7. Reinforce instructions to the client to limit the force of the stream because organisms can be forced into the vas deferens and epididymis from strain or pressure during voiding.

8. Reinforce teaching the client that condom use can help to prevent urethritis and epididymitis.

9. Reinforce teaching the client measures to prevent UTI or STI recurrence.

XXVI. Prostatitis

A. Description

1. Inflammation of the prostate gland commonly caused by an infectious agent; may be acute or chronic.

2. The bacterial type occurs as a result of the organism reaching the prostate via the urethra, bladder, bloodstream, or lymphatic channels.

3. The bacterial type usually occurs following a viral illness or a decrease in sexual activity.

B. Data collection

1. Bacterial prostatitis

   a. Client becomes acutely ill.

   b. Fever and chills

   c. Frequency and urgency of urination; dysuria

   d. Perineal and low back pain

   e. Urethral discharge

   f. Prostate is tender, indurated, and warm to touch.

   g. Urethral discharge during palpation of prostate

   h. WBCs found in prostatic secretions

   i. Urine culture is usually positive for gram-negative bacteria, especially after prostate massage.

2. Abacterial prostatitis (most common form of chronic prostatitis)

   a. Backache

   b. Dysuria

   c. Perineal pain

   d. Frequency

   e. Hematuria

   f. Irregularly enlarged, firm, and tender prostate

C. Interventions

1. Encourage adequate fluid intake.

2. Reinforce instructions to the client in the use of sitz baths to promote comfort.

3. Assist with the administration of antibiotics, analgesics, antispasmodics, and stool softeners as prescribed.

4. Inform the client of activities to drain the prostate such as intercourse, masturbation, and prostatic massage.

5. Reinforce instructions to the client to avoid spicy foods, coffee, alcohol, prolonged automobile rides, and sexual intercourse during an acute inflammation.

XXVII. Benign Prostatic Hypertrophy (Hyperplasia)

A. Description

1. Benign prostatic hypertrophy (benign prostatic hyperplasia [BPH]) is a slow enlargement of the prostate gland with hypertrophy and hyperplasia of normal tissue.
2. Enlargement compresses the urethra resulting in partial or complete obstruction.
3. Usually occurs in men older than 50 years

B. Data collection

1. Diminished size and force of urinary stream (early sign of BPH)
2. Urinary urgency and frequency
3. Nocturia
4. Inability to start (hesitancy) or continue a urinary stream
5. Feelings of incomplete bladder emptying
6. Postvoid dribbling from overflow incontinence (later sign)
7. Urinary retention and bladder distention
8. Hematuria
9. Urinary stasis and UTIs
10. Dysuria and bladder pain

C. Interventions

1. Encourage fluid intake of up to 2000 to 3000 mL/day unless contraindicated.
2. Prepare for urinary catheterization to drain the bladder and prevent distention.
3. Avoid administering medications that cause urinary retention, such as anticholinergics, antihistamines, decongestants, and antidepressants.
4. Assist with the administration of medications, as prescribed, to shrink the prostate gland and improve urine flow.
5. Assist with the administration of medications, as prescribed, to relax prostatic smooth muscle and improve urine flow.
6. Reinforce instructions to the client to decrease intake of caffeine and artificial sweeteners and limit spicy or acidic foods.
7. Reinforce instructions to the client to follow a timed voiding schedule.
8. Prepare the client for surgery or invasive procedures as prescribed.

D. Surgical interventions, transurethral resection of the prostate (TURP) and postoperative care (see Chapter 41)

XXVIII. Bladder Cancer (See Chapter 41)

XXIX. Bladder Trauma

A. Description

1. Occurs following a blunt or penetrating injury to the lower abdomen
2. Blunt trauma causes compression of the abdominal wall and bladder.

3. Penetrating wounds occur as a result of a stabbing, gunshot wound, or other objects piercing the abdominal wall.
4. A fractured pelvis that results in bone fragments puncturing the bladder is a common cause of bladder trauma.

B. Data collection

1. Anuria
2. Hematuria
3. Pain below the level of the umbilicus; can radiate to the shoulders
4. Nausea and vomiting

C. Interventions

1. Monitor vital signs.
2. Monitor for hematuria, bleeding, and signs of shock.
3. Promote bed rest.
4. If blood is seen at the meatus, avoid urinary catheterization until a retrograde urethrogram can be performed.
5. Assist with preparing the client for insertion of a suprapubic catheter to aid in urinary drainage if prescribed.
6. Assist with preparing the client for surgical repair of the laceration if indicated.

WHAT WOULD YOU DO?

Answer: AKI is the sudden loss of kidney function caused by renal cell damage from ischemia or toxic substances. It occurs abruptly and can be reversible. AKI leads to hypoperfusion, cell death, and decompensation in renal function. With this disorder, the nurse would monitor for complications such as fluid overload, ascites, pulmonary edema, and heart failure. If fine crackles in the lung bases develop bilaterally, the nurse needs to contact the registered nurse, who will notify the primary health care provider because this could be a sign of one of these complications.

PRACTICE QUESTIONS

❖ **1.** The nurse is caring for the client with epididymitis. Which treatment modalities would be implemented? **Select all that apply.**
 ❑ **1.** Bed rest
 ❑ **2.** Sitz bath
 ❑ **3.** Antibiotics
 ❑ **4.** Heating pad
 ❑ **5.** Scrotal elevation

2. A client has epididymitis as a complication of a urinary tract infection (UTI). The nurse is giving the client instructions to prevent recurrence. The nurse determines that the client **needs further teaching** if the client states the intention to take which action?

1. Drink an increased amount of fluids.
2. Limit the force of the stream during voiding.
3. Continue to take antibiotics until all symptoms are gone.
4. Use condoms to eliminate risk associated with chlamydia and gonorrhea.

3. The nurse is collecting data from a client who has had benign prostatic hyperplasia (BPH) in the past. To determine whether the client is currently experiencing exacerbation of BPH, the nurse would ask the client about the presence of which early symptom?
   1. Nocturia
   2. Urinary retention
   3. Urge incontinence
   4. Decreased force in the stream of urine

4. The nurse is instructing a client with diabetes mellitus about peritoneal dialysis. The nurse tells the client that it is important to maintain the prescribed dwell time for the dialysis because of the risk of which complication?
   1. Peritonitis
   2. Hyperglycemia
   3. Hyperphosphatemia
   4. Disequilibrium syndrome

5. A client with chronic kidney disease has been on dialysis for 3 years. The client is receiving the usual combination of medications for the disease, including aluminum hydroxide as a phosphate-binding agent. The client now has mental cloudiness, dementia, and complaints of bone pain. Which do these data indicate?
   1. Advancing uremia
   2. Phosphate overdose
   3. Folic acid deficiency
   4. Aluminum intoxication

6. A hemodialysis client with a left arm fistula is at risk for arterial steal syndrome. The nurse monitors this client for which signs/symptoms of this disorder?
   1. Edema and purpura of the left arm
   2. Warmth, redness, and pain in the left hand
   3. Aching pain, pallor, and edema of the left arm
   4. Pallor, diminished pulse, and pain in the left hand

7. The nurse is reviewing the medical record of a client with a diagnosis of pyelonephritis. Which health problem noted on the client's record would the nurse identify as a risk factor for this diagnosis?
   1. Hypoglycemia
   2. Diabetes mellitus
   3. Coronary artery disease
   4. Orthostatic hypotension

8. The nurse is reviewing the client's record and notes ❖ that the primary health care provider (PHCP) has documented that the client has a renal disorder. Which laboratory results would indicate a decrease in renal function? **Select all that apply.**
   ❏ 1. Decreased hemoglobin level
   ❏ 2. Elevated serum creatinine level
   ❏ 3. Elevated thrombocyte cell count
   ❏ 4. Decreased red blood cell (RBC) count
   ❏ 5. Elevated blood urea nitrogen (BUN) level

9. A client is scheduled for intravenous pyelography (IVP). Which **priority** nursing action would the nurse take?
   1. Restrict fluids.
   2. Administer a sedative.
   3. Determine if there is a history of allergies.
   4. Administer an oral preparation of radiopaque dye.

10. After a renal biopsy, the client complains of pain at the biopsy site that radiates to the front of the abdomen. Which would this indicate?
    1. Bleeding
    2. Infection
    3. Renal colic
    4. Normal, expected pain

11. The nurse monitoring a client receiving peritoneal ▲ dialysis notes that the client's outflow is less than the inflow. The nurse would take which actions? **Select all that apply.**
    ❏ 1. Contact the nephrologist.
    ❏ 2. Check the level of the drainage bag.
    ❏ 3. Reposition the client to his or her side.
    ❏ 4. Place the client in good body alignment.
    ❏ 5. Check the peritoneal dialysis system for kinks.
    ❏ 6. Increase the flow rate of the peritoneal dialysis solution.

12. A male client has a tentative diagnosis of urethritis. The nurse would assess the client for which manifestations of the disorder?
    1. Hematuria and pyuria
    2. Dysuria and proteinuria
    3. Hematuria and urgency
    4. Dysuria and penile discharge

13. A client with benign prostatic hypertrophy (BPH) undergoes a transurethral resection of the prostate (TURP) and is receiving continuous bladder irrigations postoperatively. Which are the signs/symptoms of transurethral resection (TUR) syndrome?
    1. Tachycardia and diarrhea
    2. Bradycardia and confusion
    3. Increased urinary output and anemia
    4. Decreased urinary output and bladder spasms

14. A client with prostatitis resulting from kidney infection has received instructions on management of the condition at home and prevention of recurrence. Which statement indicates that the client understood the instructions?

1. Stop antibiotic therapy when pain subsides.
2. Exercise as much as possible to stimulate circulation.
3. Use warm sitz baths and analgesics to increase comfort.
4. Keep fluid intake to a minimum to decrease the need to void.

15. The nurse is monitoring an older client suspected of having a urinary tract infection (UTI) for signs of infection. Which sign/symptom is likely to present first?

1. Fever
2. Urgency
3. Confusion
4. Frequency

ANSWERS

❖ **1. 1, 2, 3, 5**

Rationale: Common interventions used in the treatment of epididymitis include bed rest, elevation of the scrotum, ice packs, sitz baths, analgesics, and antibiotics. A heating pad would not be used because direct application of heat could increase blood flow to the area and increase the swelling.

Test-Taking Strategy: Focus on the subject, epididymitis. A sitz bath provides heat that is moist and soothing. However, knowing that direct heat may increase inflammation in tissue that is already at risk will guide you to eliminate option 4 as the item that could increase swelling.

2. 3

Rationale: The client who experiences epididymitis from UTI needs to increase intake of fluids to flush the urinary system. Because organisms can be forced into the vas deferens and epididymis from strain or pressure during voiding, the client needs to limit the force of the stream. Condom use can help to prevent urethritis and epididymitis from STIs. Antibiotics are always taken until the full course of therapy is completed.

Test-Taking Strategy: Note the strategic words, *needs further teaching*. These words indicate a negative event query and the need to select the incorrect client statement. Because option 1 is consistent with good practices in the prevention of UTI, this option can be eliminated first. From the remaining options, it is necessary to know that the force of stream needs to be limited to prevent backflow into the epididymis and that condoms are helpful in preventing this disorder from occurring as a complication of a sexually transmitted infection. Remember that antibiotics are not stopped when symptoms subside and need to be taken until the full course of therapy is completed.

3. 4

Rationale: Decreased force in the stream of urine is an early sign of BPH. The stream later becomes weak and dribbling. The client may then develop hematuria, frequency, urgency, urge incontinence, and nocturia. If untreated, complete obstruction and urinary retention can occur.

Test-Taking Strategy: Note the strategic word, *early*. Option 2 identifies the most extreme symptom and therefore is eliminated first. From the remaining options, focusing on the strategic words and recalling the pathophysiology related to BPH will direct you to the correct option.

4. 2

Rationale: An extended dwell time increases the risk of hyperglycemia in the client with diabetes mellitus as a result of absorption of glucose from the dialysate and electrolyte changes. Diabetic clients may require extra insulin when receiving peritoneal dialysis. Peritonitis is a risk associated with breaks in aseptic technique. Hyperphosphatemia is an electrolyte imbalance that occurs with renal dysfunction. Disequilibrium syndrome is a complication associated with hemodialysis.

Test-Taking Strategy: Focus on the subject, a complication associated with an extended dwell time. Noting the client's diagnosis and recalling that the dialysate solution contains glucose will direct you to the correct option.

5. 4

Rationale: Aluminum intoxication may occur when there is accumulation of aluminum, an ingredient in many phosphate-binding antacids. It results in mental cloudiness, dementia, and bone pain from infiltration of the bone with aluminum. This condition was formerly known as dialysis dementia. It may be treated with aluminum-chelating agents, which make aluminum available to be dialyzed from the body. It can be prevented by avoiding or limiting the use of phosphate-binding agents that contain aluminum.

Test-Taking Strategy: Focus on the subject, aluminum hydroxide. Use knowledge about the manifestations that would occur in each condition presented in the options to answer correctly. Also, note the relation between the medication name in the question and option 4.

6. 4

Rationale: Arterial steal syndrome results from vascular insufficiency after creation of a fistula. The client exhibits pallor and diminished pulse distal to the fistula and complains of pain distal to the fistula, which is caused by tissue ischemia. Warmth, redness, and pain would more likely characterize a problem with infection. Options 2 and 3 are not characteristics of steal syndrome.

Test-Taking Strategy: Focus on the subject, arterial steal syndrome. Think about the name of the condition. Recalling that arterial steal syndrome results from vascular insufficiency will direct you to the correct option.

7. 2

Rationale: Risk factors associated with pyelonephritis include diabetes mellitus, hypertension, chronic renal calculi, chronic cystitis, structural abnormalities of the urinary tract, presence of urinary stones, and indwelling or frequent urinary catheterization.

Test-Taking Strategy: Focus on the subject, pyelonephritis. Eliminate options 1 and 4 first as least likely being associated as risk factors. From the remaining options, remember that diabetes mellitus can cause renal complications. This will direct you to the correct option.

8. 1, 2, 4, 5
Rationale: BUN testing is a frequently used laboratory test to determine renal function. The BUN and serum creatinine levels start to rise when the glomerular filtration rate decreases to less than 40% to 60%. A decreased RBC count as well as a decreased hemoglobin level may be noted if erythropoietic function by the kidney is impaired. Thrombocyte cell counts do not indicate decreased renal function.
Test-Taking Strategy: Focus on the subject, laboratory results indicating a decrease in renal function. Eliminate option 3 because an elevated count is not associated with the renal system. Think about the pathophysiology of renal disease and the organs affected. Also, remember that the BUN and creatinine levels are frequently used laboratory tests to determine renal function.

9. 3
Rationale: An iodine-based dye may be used during the IVP and can cause allergic reactions such as itching, hives, rash, tight feeling in the throat, shortness of breath, and bronchospasm. Checking for allergies is the priority. Options 1, 2, and 4 are unnecessary.
Test-Taking Strategy: Note the strategic word, *priority*, and use the steps of the nursing process as a guide. Options 1, 2, and 4 address implementation. Option 3 is the only option that addresses data collection.

10. 1
Rationale: If pain originates at the biopsy site and begins to radiate to the flank area and around the front of the abdomen, bleeding would be suspected. Hypotension, a decreasing hematocrit, and gross or microscopic hematuria would also indicate bleeding. Signs of infection would not appear immediately after a biopsy. Pain of this nature is not normal. There are no data to support the presence of renal colic.
Test-Taking Strategy: Focusing on the subject, pain at the renal biopsy site, will assist you with eliminating options 3 and 4. Recalling that signs of infection may not appear immediately after biopsy will assist with directing you to option 1 from the remaining choices.

❖11. 2, 3, 4, 5
Rationale: If outflow drainage is inadequate, the nurse attempts to stimulate outflow by changing the client's position. Turning the client to the other side or making sure that the client is in good body alignment may assist with outflow drainage. The drainage bag needs to be lower than the client's abdomen to enhance gravity drainage. The connecting tubing on the peritoneal dialysis system is also checked for kinks or twisting, and the clamps on the system are checked to ensure that they are open. There is no reason to contact the nephrologist. Increasing the flow rate is an inappropriate action and is unassociated with the amount of outflow solution.

Test-Taking Strategy: Focus on the subject, peritoneal dialysis outflow and inflow. Use the principles related to gravity flow and preventing obstruction to flow to answer this question. This will assist you with determining what the correct interventions are.

❖12. 4
Rationale: Urethritis in the male client often results from chlamydial infection and is characterized by dysuria, which is accompanied by a clear to mucopurulent discharge. Because this disorder often coexists with gonorrhea, diagnostic tests are done for both and include culture and rapid assays. Hematuria is not associated with urethritis. Proteinuria is associated with kidney dysfunction.
Test-Taking Strategy: Focus on the subject, manifestations of urethritis. Recalling that urethritis generally is accompanied by dysuria in the male client will assist you in eliminating options 1 and 3. Knowing that the problem originates in the urethra, not the kidneys, will assist you in eliminating option 2, because proteinuria indicates a problem with kidney function.

13. 2
Rationale: TUR syndrome is caused by increased absorption of nonelectrolyte irrigating fluid used during surgery. The client may show signs of cerebral edema and increased intracranial pressure, such as increased blood pressure, bradycardia, confusion, disorientation, muscle twitching, visual disturbances, and nausea and vomiting.
Test-Taking Strategy: Knowledge regarding the subject, TUR syndrome, is required to answer this question. Recalling that increased intracranial pressure is the concern will direct you to option 2.

14. 3
Rationale: Treatment of prostatitis includes medication with antibiotics, analgesics, and stool softeners. The client is also taught to rest, increase fluid intake, and use sitz baths for comfort. Antimicrobial therapy is always continued until the prescription is completely finished.
Test-Taking Strategy: Focus on the subject, prostatitis. Eliminate option 1 first because stopping medication therapy before the end of the course is contraindicated. Option 4 is also eliminated because fluid intake would be increased. From the remaining options, it is necessary to understand that sitz baths provide comfort and that rest is helpful in the healing process. Knowledge of either of these concepts will direct you to option 3.

15. 3
Rationale: In an older client, the only symptom of a UTI may be something as vague as increasing mental confusion or frequent unexplained falls. Frequency and urgency may commonly occur in an older client, and fever can be associated with a variety of conditions.
Test-Taking Strategy: Note the strategic word, *first*. Although all may be signs/symptoms of urinary tract infection, note the client in the question is an older client to determine which one occurs *first*. Eliminate options 2 and 4 because they may commonly occur in an older client. Eliminate option 1 next because fever can be associated with a variety of conditions.

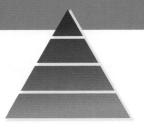

CHAPTER **52**

Renal and Urinary Medications

PRIORITY CONCEPTS Elimination; Safety

WHAT WOULD YOU DO?

A client who is taking ciprofloxacin prescribed for a urinary tract infection complains of dizziness, blurred vision, and sensitivity to light. What would the nurse do?
Answer is located on p. 733.

I. Urinary Tract Antiseptics

A. Description
1. Urinary tract antiseptics inhibit the growth of bacteria in the urine (Box 52.1).
2. Act as disinfectants within the urinary tract
3. Used to treat acute cystitis or urinary tract infections (UTIs)
4. Urinary tract antiseptics do not achieve effective antibacterial concentrations in blood or tissues and therefore cannot be used for infections outside the urinary tract.

B. Side and adverse effects and nursing considerations
1. Fosfomycin
   a. The medication is available as granules that need to be dissolved; instruct the client to mix the contents of one package in about ½ cup (120 mL) of cold water, stir well, and drink all the liquid.
   b. Medications that increase gastrointestinal motility reduce the absorption of Fosfomycin.
2. Methenamine
   a. Used to treat chronic UTIs but not recommended for acute infections
   b. Administer after meals and at bedtime to minimize gastric distress.
   c. Chronic high-dose therapy can cause bladder irritation.
   d. Methenamine can cause crystalluria and should not be used in clients with renal impairment.
   e. Decomposition of the medication generates ammonia; therefore, it would not be used for clients with liver dysfunction.
   f. Methenamine requires acidic urine with a pH of 5.5 or lower.

   g. Increasing fluid intake reduces antibacterial effects by diluting the medication and raising urine pH.
   h. Methenamine would not be combined with sulfonamides because of the risk of crystalluria and urinary tract injury.
   i. Clients taking this medication need to avoid alkalinizing agents including over-the-counter (OTC) antacids containing sodium bicarbonate or sodium carbonate.
3. Nitrofurantoin
   a. Gastrointestinal effects include anorexia, nausea, vomiting, and diarrhea; administration with milk or meals minimizes gastrointestinal distress.
   b. Pulmonary reactions include dyspnea, chest pain, chills, fever, cough, and alveolar infiltrates. These resolve in 2 to 4 days following cessation of treatment.
   c. Hematological effects include agranulocytosis, leukopenia, thrombocytopenia, and megaloblastic anemia.
   d. Peripheral neuropathy effects include muscle weakness, tingling sensations, and numbness.
   e. Neurological effects include headache, vertigo, drowsiness, and nystagmus.
   f. Allergic reactions include anaphylaxis, hives, rash, and tingling sensations around the mouth.
   g. Nitrofurantoin may impart a harmless brown color to the urine.
   h. Nitrofurantoin is contraindicated in clients with renal impairment.
   i. The client is instructed about the expected side effects, signs warranting notification of the primary health care provider (PHCP), and not to take nitrofurantoin with antacids.

II. Fluoroquinolones (Box 52.2)

A. Description: Suppress bacterial growth by inhibiting an enzyme necessary for DNA synthesis; active against a broad spectrum of microbes

---

BOX 52.1   Urinary Tract Antiseptics

- Amoxicillin
- Cefixime
- Fosfomycin
- Methenamine
- Nitrofurantoin

BOX 52.2   Fluoroquinolones

- Ciprofloxacin
- Levofloxacin
- Ofloxacin
- Gatifloxacin

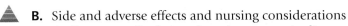 **B.** Side and adverse effects and nursing considerations

1. Can cause dizziness, drowsiness, gastric distress, diarrhea, vaginitis, nausea, and vomiting
2. Adverse effects include psychoses, hallucinations, confusion, tremors, hypersensitivity, and interstitial nephritis.

⚠ With fluoroquinolones, there is an increased risk for tendonitis and tendon rupture. The Achilles tendon is most often involved, but the shoulder and hand tendons can also be affected. Clients at increased risk are those over the age of 60 years, those taking corticosteroids, and clients who have undergone organ transplant.

3. Fluoroquinolones need to be used with caution in clients with hepatic, renal, or central nervous system (CNS) disorders.
4. Monitor client for side effects and adverse effects.
5. Ciprofloxacin, lomefloxacin, and ofloxacin may be taken with or without food.
6. Intravenously administered ciprofloxacin and ofloxacin are infused slowly over 60 minutes to minimize discomfort and vein irritation.
7. The client is advised to report dizziness, light-headedness, visual disturbances, increased light sensitivity, and feelings of depression because these signs could indicate CNS toxicity.
8. The client is informed of signs of hepatic and renal toxicity and the importance of reporting these signs to the PHCP.
9. Avoid ultraviolet light and sun exposure using protective clothing and sunscreen.

⚠ Fluoroquinolones are administered with a full glass of water, and the client is taught that it is necessary to maintain a urine output of at least 1200 to 1500 mL daily to minimize the development of crystalluria.

 III. Sulfonamides (Box 52.3)

A. Description: Suppress bacterial growth by inhibiting the synthesis of folic acid; active against a broad spectrum of microbes; used primarily to treat acute UTIs

---

BOX 52.3   Sulfonamides

- Sulfadiazine
- Sulfasalazine
- Sulfacetamide
- Trimethoprim sulfamethoxazole

B. Side and adverse effects and nursing considerations

1. Hypersensitivity reactions include rash, fever, and photosensitivity.
2. Stevens-Johnson syndrome, the most severe hypersensitivity response, produces symptoms that include widespread lesions of the skin and mucous membranes, fever, malaise, and toxemia.
3. Sulfonamides can cause hemolytic anemia, agranulocytosis, leukopenia, and thrombocytopenia. The client is instructed to notify the PHCP if sore throat or fever occurs.
4. Sulfonamides are administered with caution in clients with renal impairment.
5. Sulfonamides are contraindicated if hypersensitivity exists to sulfonamides, sulfonylureas, or thiazide or loop diuretics.
6. Sulfonamides are contraindicated in infants younger than 2 months and in pregnant women or mothers who are breast-feeding.
7. Sulfonamides can potentiate the effects of warfarin sodium, phenytoin, and orally administered hypoglycemics such as tolbutamide (when combined with sulfonamides, hypoglycemics may require a reduction in dosage).
8. Reinforce instructions to the client to take the medication on an empty stomach with a full glass of water.
9. Reinforce instructions to the client to complete the entire course of prescribed medication.
10. Reinforce instructions to the client to avoid prolonged exposure to sunlight, wear protective clothing, and apply a sunscreen to exposed skin.
11. Adults need to maintain a daily urine output of 1200 mL by consuming 8 to 10 glasses of water each day to minimize the risk of renal damage from the medication.
12. The client is informed that some combination medications of sulfonamides can cause the urine to turn dark brown or red.
13. The sulfonamide combination of trimethoprim-sulfamethoxazole is more effective than either medication alone because it inhibits the sequential steps in bacterial folic acid synthesis.
14. Trimethoprim-sulfamethoxazole is used cautiously with clients experiencing impaired kidney function, folate deficiency, severe allergy, or bronchial asthma.
15. An intravenous (IV) dose of trimethoprimsulfamethoxazole is administered over 60 to 90 minutes and is not mixed with other medications.

Adult—Renal and Urinary

> ### BOX 52.4   Urinary Tract Analgesics
>
> - Pentosan polysulfate sodium
> - Phenazopyridine

> ### BOX 52.5   Anticholinergics-Antispasmodics
>
> - Darifenacin
> - Dicyclomine
> - Oxybutynin chloride
> - Flavoxate
> - Fesoterodine
> - Mirabegron
> - Propantheline
> - Solifenacin
> - Tolterodine
> - Trospium

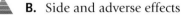 Sulfonamides need to be withheld if a rash is noted. The client is informed to contact the PHCP if a rash appears.

IV. Urinary Tract Analgesics (Box 52.4)

A. Description: A urinary tract analgesic is administered with an antibiotic because the analgesic only treats pain, not the infection.

B. Side and adverse effects
  1. Nausea
  2. Headache
  3. Vertigo

C. Nursing considerations
  1. The client is instructed that the urine will turn red or orange and stain clothing; tears and contact lenses will also become red or orange tinged.
  2. A urinary tract analgesic is contraindicated in clients with renal or hepatic disease.
  3. The medication interferes with accurate urine testing for glucose and ketones.

V. Anticholinergics-Antispasmodics (Box 52.5)

A. Description: Used for overactive bladder (urge incontinence)

B. Side and adverse effects
  1. Anorexia, nausea, vomiting, and dry mouth
  2. Blurred vision
  3. Confusion in older clients
  4. Constipation
  5. Decreased sweating
  6. Dizziness
  7. Drowsiness
  8. Dry eyes
  9. Gastric distress
  10. Headache
  11. Tachycardia
  12. Urinary retention

C. Nursing considerations
  1. Extended-release capsules should not be split, chewed, or crushed.
  2. Tolterodine needs to be used cautiously in clients with narrow-angle glaucoma.
  3. Oxybutynin is not administered to clients with known hypersensitivity, gastrointestinal or genitourinary obstruction, glaucoma, severe colitis, or myasthenia gravis.
  4. Propantheline is not administered to clients with narrow-angle glaucoma, obstructive uropathy, gastrointestinal disease, or ulcerative colitis.
  5. Reinforce instructions to the client to avoid hazardous activities because of the side effects of dizziness and drowsiness.
  6. Monitor intake and output.
  7. Provide gum or hard candy for dry mouth.
  8. Monitor for signs of toxicity (CNS stimulation) such as hypotension, hypertension, confusion, tachycardia, flushed or red face, signs of respiratory depression, nervousness, restlessness, hallucinations, and irritability.

 Antispasmodic medications used to treat overactive bladder (urge incontinence) are not to be used by clients diagnosed with open-angle glaucoma. These medications will block the flow of intraocular fluid and raise the intraocular pressure. This may cause permanent damage to the optic nerve.

VI. Cholinergics

A. Description: Bethanechol chloride is a cholinergic used to increase bladder tone and function and to treat nonobstructive urinary retention and neurogenic bladder.

B. Side and adverse effects
  1. Headache
  2. Hypotension
  3. Flushing and sweating
  4. Increased salivation
  5. Abdominal cramps
  6. Nausea and vomiting
  7. Diarrhea
  8. Urinary urgency
  9. Bronchoconstriction
  10. Transient complete heart block

C. Nursing considerations
  1. Administered on an empty stomach, 1 hour before or 2 hours after meals to lessen nausea and vomiting
  2. Never administered by the intramuscular or IV routes
  3. Monitor intake and output.
  4. Monitor for increased bladder tone and function.
  5. Monitor for cholinergic overdose (excessive salivation, sweating, involuntary urination and defecation, bradycardia, and severe hypotension).

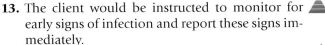

BOX 52.6 Medications for Preventing Organ Rejection

Immunosuppressants
- Cyclosporine
- Everolimus
- Sirolimus
- Tacrolimus

Glucocorticoid
- Prednisone

Cytotoxic Medications
- Azathioprine
- Mercaptopurine
- Mycophenolate mofetil

Antibodies
- Antithymocyte globulin, equine
- Basiliximab

6. Have atropine sulfate (antidote) readily available for IV or subcutaneous administration.

⚠ A cholinergic such as bethanechol chloride is not given to a client who has a urinary stricture or obstruction.

VII. Medications for Preventing Organ Rejection (Box 52.6)

A. Medications include immunosuppressants, corticosteroids, cytotoxic medications, and antibodies.

B. Some medications may be used in combination with one another to produce different actions on the immune system. Combination therapy also allows for the administration of the medications in lower doses, reducing the possibility of side and adverse effects.

C. Cyclosporine

1. Cyclosporine inhibits calcineurin and acts on T lymphocytes to suppress the production of interleukin-2, interferon-γ, and other cytokines.
2. Cyclosporine may be used to prevent rejection of allogeneic kidney, liver, and heart transplants.
3. Prednisone may be administered concurrently.
4. Oral administration of cyclosporine is preferred. IV administration is reserved for clients who cannot take the medication orally.
5. Blood levels of the medication would be measured regularly because of its nephrotoxic effects.
6. The most common adverse effects are nephrotoxicity, infection, hypertension, tremor, and hirsutism.
7. The client is assured that hirsutism is reversible and instructed in the use of a depilatory.
8. Other adverse effects include neurotoxicity, gastrointestinal effects, hyperkalemia, and hyperglycemia.
9. The risk for infection and lymphoma is increased with the use of cyclosporine.
10. Cyclosporine is contraindicated in the presence of hypersensitivity, pregnancy and breast-feeding, recent inoculation with live virus vaccines, and recent contact with an active infection such as chickenpox or herpes zoster.
11. Cyclosporine is embryotoxic; women of childbearing age need to use a mechanical form of contraception and avoid oral contraceptives.
12. The client would be informed about the possibility of renal damage and liver damage and the need for periodic liver function tests and determination of coagulation factors and blood urea nitrogen, serum creatinine, serum potassium, and blood glucose levels.
13. The client would be instructed to monitor for early signs of infection and report these signs immediately.
14. Available in a pill form. If the client is unable to swallow the pill, the client is instructed to dispense the oral liquid medication into a glass container by using a specially calibrated pipette, mix well, and drink immediately; rinse the glass container with diluent and drink it to ensure ingestion of the complete dose; dry the outside of the pipette and return it to its cover for storage.
15. To promote palatability, the client is instructed to mix the liquid medication with milk, chocolate milk, or orange juice just before administration. If client is diabetic, consult with the PCHP.
16. Consuming grapefruit juice is prohibited because it raises cyclosporine levels and increases the risk of toxicity.
17. Ketoconazole, erythromycin, and amphotericin B can elevate cyclosporine levels.
18. Phenytoin, phenobarbital, rifampin, and trimethoprim-sulfamethoxazole can decrease cyclosporine levels.
19. Renal damage can be intensified by the concurrent use of other nephrotoxic medications.

D. Sirolimus

1. Sirolimus is used for the prevention of renal transplant rejection by inhibiting the response of helper T lymphocytes and B lymphocytes to cytokinesis.
2. It may be used with cyclosporine or tacrolimus and corticosteroids.
3. Increases the risk of infection, increases the risk of renal injury, increases the risk of lymphocele (a complication of renal transplant surgery), and raises cholesterol and triglyceride levels
4. Side and adverse effects include rash, acne, anemia, thrombocytopenia, joint pain, diarrhea, and hypokalemia.

E. Tacrolimus

1. Tacrolimus inhibits calcineurin and thereby prevents T cells from producing interleukin-2, interferon-γ, and other cytokines.
2. Tacrolimus is more effective than cyclosporine but is more toxic.

3. Adverse effects are similar to those of cyclosporine and include nephrotoxicity, infection, hypertension, tremor, hirsutism, neurotoxicity, gastrointestinal effects, hyperkalemia, and hyperglycemia.

4. Tacrolimus needs to be used cautiously in immunosuppressed clients and those with renal, hepatic, or pancreatic impairment.

5. Tacrolimus is contraindicated for clients hypersensitive to cyclosporine.

6. Blood glucose levels are monitored and prescribed insulin or oral hypoglycemics are administered.

F. Prednisone

1. Prednisone is a glucocorticoid that inhibits accumulation of inflammatory cells at inflammation sites.

2. Hyperglycemia and hypokalemia can occur with prednisone use. Monitor glucose and serum potassium levels.

3. See Chapter 44 for additional information about prednisone.

G. Azathioprine

1. Azathioprine suppresses cell-mediated and humoral immune responses by inhibiting the proliferation of B- and T-lymphocytes.

2. Can cause neutropenia and thrombocytopenia from bone marrow suppression

3. Contraindicated during pregnancy; associated with an increased incidence of neoplasms

4. Monitor hematocrit, white blood cell count, platelet count, liver enzyme levels, and coagulation factors.

H. Mycophenolate mofetil

1. Mycophenolate mofetil causes selective inhibition of B- and T-lymphocyte proliferation.

2. May be used with cyclosporine or tacrolimus and glucocorticoids for prophylaxis against organ rejection

3. Adverse effects include diarrhea, severe neutropenia, vomiting, and sepsis.

4. Mycophenolate mofetil is associated with an increased risk of infection and malignancies.

5. Absorption is decreased by the use of magnesium and aluminum antacids and cholestyramine.

6. It is contraindicated during pregnancy and breastfeeding.

7. Reinforce instructions to the client to take the medication on an empty stomach and not to open or crush capsules.

8. Reinforce instructions to the client to contact the PHCP for unusual bleeding or bruising, sore throat, mouth sores, abdominal pain, or fever.

 Persons who have undergone organ transplantation, such as a kidney, need to take the prescribed immunosuppressant medications at the same time each day to ensure that the immune system is sufficiently suppressed to prevent organ rejection.

I. Basiliximab

1. Basiliximab binds to interleukin-2 receptors on lymphocytes resulting in diminished cell-mediated immune reactions.

2. Used primarily as an induction agent at the time of transplantation; may be used with other immunosuppressants to prevent acute rejection of transplanted kidneys

3. Administered by the IV route; initial dose is administered within 2 hours before transplantation.

4. Side and adverse effects include headache, insomnia, dizziness, and tremors; chest pain, gastrointestinal distress, edema, shortness of breath, pain in the joints, and slow wound healing can occur.

J. Antithymocyte globulin, equine

1. Antithymocyte globulin, equine, causes a decrease in the number and activity of thymus-derived lymphocytes and is used to suppress organ rejection following renal, liver, bone marrow, and heart transplantation.

2. It is used primarily to treat acute rejection episodes.

3. Before the first infusion, the client needs to undergo intradermal skin testing to determine hypersensitivity.

4. Because this product is made using equine and human blood components, it may carry a risk of transmitting infectious agents such as viruses.

5. Monitor the platelet count and report low counts to the PHCP per agency policy.

6. Arrange for outpatient referral for repeated infusions after discharge.

VIII. Hematopoietic Growth Factors (Box 52.7)

A. Erythropoietic growth factors

1. Stimulate the production of red blood cells

2. Used to treat anemia of **chronic kidney disease**, chemotherapy-induced anemia, anemia caused by zidovudine, and anemia in clients requiring surgery

3. Initial effects can be seen within 1 to 2 weeks and the hematocrit reaches normal levels in 2 to 3 months.

4. The major adverse effect is hypertension.

5. Adverse effects can include heart failure, thrombotic effects such as stroke or myocardial infarction, and cardiac arrest.

B. Leukopoietic growth factors

1. Stimulate the production of white blood cells (leukocytes)

2. Used for clients undergoing myelosuppressive chemotherapy or bone marrow transplantation and those with severe chronic neutropenia

3. Can cause bone pain, leukocytosis, and elevation of plasma uric acid, lactate dehydrogenase, and alkaline phosphatase levels. Long-term therapy has caused splenomegaly.

C. Thrombopoietic growth factor

1. Stimulates the production of platelets

2. Used for clients undergoing myelosuppressive chemotherapy to minimize thrombocytopenia and decrease the need for platelet transfusions

BOX 52.7 Hematopoietic Growth Factors

Erythropoietic Growth Factors
- Epoetin alfa
- Darbepoetin alfa
- Peginesatide

Leukopoietic Growth Factors
- Filgrastim
- Pegfilgrastim
- Sargramostim

BOX 52.8 Medications to Treat Benign Prostatic Hyperplasia

Alpha Blockers
- Alfuzosin
- Doxazosin
- Tamsulosin
- Terazosin
- Silodosin

5a-Alpha Reductase Inhibitors
- Finasteride
- Dutasteride

    3. Adverse effects include fluid retention, cardiac dysrhythmia, conjunctival infection, blurred vision, and papilledema.

IX. Medications for Benign Prostatic Hyperplasia (Box 52.8)

A. Alpha blockers

    1. Relax bladder neck muscles and muscle fibers in the prostate, allowing urine to pass more easily
    2. Adverse effects include dizziness and retrograde ejaculation.

B. 5a-alpha reductase inhibitors
    1. Shrink the prostate by preventing hormone changes that result in growth of the prostate
    2. May take up to 6 months to be effective
    3. Adverse effects include retrograde ejaculation.

WHAT WOULD YOU DO?

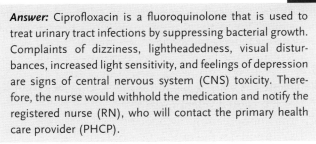

Answer: Ciprofloxacin is a fluoroquinolone that is used to treat urinary tract infections by suppressing bacterial growth. Complaints of dizziness, lightheadedness, visual disturbances, increased light sensitivity, and feelings of depression are signs of central nervous system (CNS) toxicity. Therefore, the nurse would withhold the medication and notify the registered nurse (RN), who will contact the primary health care provider (PHCP).

PRACTICE QUESTIONS

1. The client who has a cold is seen in the emergency department with an inability to void. Because the client has a history of benign prostatic hyperplasia, the nurse determines that the client needs to be questioned about the use of which class of medications?
    1. Diuretics
    2. Antibiotics
    3. Antitussives
    4. Decongestants

2. A sulfonamide is prescribed for a client with a urinary tract infection. During review of the client's record, the nurse notes that the client is taking warfarin sodium daily. Which prescription would the nurse anticipate for this client?
    1. Discontinuation of warfarin sodium
    2. A decrease in the warfarin sodium dosage
    3. An increase in the warfarin sodium dosage
    4. A decrease in the usual dose of the sulfonamide

3. Following kidney transplantation, cyclosporine is prescribed for a client. Which laboratory result would indicate an adverse effect from the use of this medication?
    1. Hemoglobin level of 14.0 g/dL
    2. Creatinine level of 0.6 mg/dL
    3. Blood urea nitrogen level of 25 mg/dL
    4. Fasting blood glucose level of 99 mg/dL

4. Trimethoprim-sulfamethoxazole is prescribed for a client. The nurse would instruct the client to report which symptom if it developed during the course of this medication therapy?
    1. Nausea
    2. Diarrhea
    3. Headache
    4. Sore throat

5. Phenazopyridine hydrochloride is prescribed for a client for symptomatic relief of pain resulting from a lower urinary tract infection. Which instruction would the nurse reinforce to the client?
    1. Take the medication at bedtime.
    2. Take the medication before meals.
    3. Discontinue the medication if a headache occurs.
    4. A reddish-orange discoloration of the urine may occur.

6. Bethanechol chloride is prescribed for a client with urinary retention. Which health problem would be a contraindication to the administration of this medication?
   1. Gastric atony
   2. Urinary strictures
   3. Neurogenic atony
   4. Gastroesophageal reflux

7. The nurse who is administering bethanechol chloride is monitoring for acute toxicity associated with the medication. The nurse would check the client for which sign of toxicity?
   1. Dry skin
   2. Dry mouth
   3. Bradycardia
   4. Signs of dehydration

8. Oxybutynin chloride is prescribed for a client with neurogenic bladder. Which sign would indicate a possible toxic effect related to this medication?
   1. Pallor
   2. Drowsiness

3. Bradycardia
4. Restlessness

9. A client with chronic kidney disease is receiving epoetin alfa. Which laboratory result would indicate a therapeutic effect of the medication?
   1. Hematocrit of 33%
   2. Platelet count of 400,000 mm^3
   3. White blood cell count of 6000 mm^3
   4. Blood urea nitrogen level of 15 mg/dL

10. The nurse is reinforcing discharge instructions to a client receiving sulfadiazine. Which would be included in the list of instructions?
    1. Restrict fluid intake.
    2. Maintain a high fluid intake.
    3. Decrease the dosage when symptoms are improving to prevent an allergic response.
    4. If the urine turns dark brown, call the primary health care provider immediately.

ANSWERS

1. 4
Rationale: Episodes of urinary retention can be triggered by certain medications such as decongestants, anticholinergics, and antidepressants. Diuretics, antibiotics, and antitussives generally do not trigger urinary retention. Retention also can be precipitated by other factors such as alcoholic beverages, infection, bed rest, and becoming chilled.
Test-Taking Strategy: Focus on the subject, medications that cause urinary retention. The question is asking about medications that could exacerbate or contribute to urinary retention. Diuretics would help voiding; therefore, readily eliminate option 1. Antibiotics would have no effect at all, eliminating option 2. From the remaining options, recalling that medications that contain anticholinergics may cause urinary retention will direct you to option 4.

2. 2
Rationale: Sulfonamides can potentiate the effects of warfarin sodium, phenytoin, and orally administered hypoglycemics such as tolbutamide. When an oral anticoagulant is combined with a sulfonamide, a decrease in the anticoagulant dosage may be needed.
Test-Taking Strategy: Focus on the subject, a sulfonamide and interaction with oral anticoagulants. Knowledge about the medication interactions associated with the use of sulfonamides is needed to answer this question. Remember that a sulfonamide can intensify the effects of oral anticoagulants.

3. 3
Rationale: Cyclosporine is an immunosuppressant. Nephrotoxicity can occur from the use of cyclosporine. Nephrotoxicity is evaluated by monitoring for elevated blood

urea nitrogen and serum creatinine levels. The normal blood urea nitrogen level is 10 to 20 mg/dL. The normal creatinine level for a male is 0.6 to 1.2 mg/dL and for a female 0.5 to 1.1 mg/dL. Cyclosporine can lower complete blood cell count levels. A normal hemoglobin is *Male:* 14 to 18 g/dL; *Female:* 12 to 16 g/dL. A normal hemoglobin is not an adverse effect. Cyclosporine does affect the glucose level. The normal fasting glucose is 70 to 99 mg/dL.
Test-Taking Strategy: Focus on the subject, the adverse effects of cyclosporine. Recall that cyclosporine can be nephrotoxic. The correct option is the only one that indicates an increased level of a renal function test. Also, recalling the normal laboratory reference levels will direct you to the correct option, the only abnormal level.

4. 4
Rationale: Clients taking trimethoprim-sulfamethoxazole need to be informed about early signs of blood disorders that can occur from this medication. These include sore throat, fever, and pallor, and the client needs to be instructed to notify the primary health care provider (PHCP) if these symptoms occur. The other options do not require PHCP notification.
Test-Taking Strategy: Focus on the subject, the symptom to be reported. Knowledge that this medication can cause blood dyscrasias will direct you to the correct option.

5. 4
Rationale: The nurse would instruct the client that a reddish-orange discoloration of urine may occur. The nurse also would instruct the client that this discoloration can stain fabric. The medication needs to be taken after meals to reduce the possibility of gastrointestinal upset. A headache is an occasional side effect of the medication and does not warrant discontinuation of the medication.

Test-Taking Strategy: Eliminate options 1 and 2 first because they are comparable or alike in that they address time schedules for the administration of the medication. From the remaining options, eliminate option 3 because the nurse would not advise the client to discontinue this medication.

6. 2
Rationale: Bethanechol chloride can be harmful to clients with urinary tract obstruction or weakness of the bladder wall. The medication has the ability to contract the bladder and thereby increase pressure within the urinary tract. Elevation of pressure within the urinary tract could rupture the bladder in clients with these conditions.
Test-Taking Strategy: Focus on the subject, a contraindication to bethanechol chloride. Noting that the question indicates the medication is used for urinary retention may assist in directing you to the correct option.

7. 3
Rationale: Toxicity (overdose) produces manifestations of excessive muscarinic stimulation such as salivation, sweating, involuntary urination and defecation, bradycardia, and severe hypotension. Treatment includes supportive measures and the administration of atropine sulfate subcutaneously or intravenously.
Test-Taking Strategy: Noting the comparable and alike similarity in options 1, 2, and 4 will assist in eliminating these options. These options all reflect signs of dehydration.

8. 4
Rationale: Toxicity (overdose) of this medication produces central nervous system excitation, such as nervousness, restlessness, hallucinations, and irritability. Other signs of toxicity include hypotension or hypertension, confusion, tachycardia, flushed or red face, and signs of respiratory depression. Drowsiness is a frequent side effect of the medication but does not indicate overdose.

Test-Taking Strategy: Focus on the subject, toxicity associated with oxybutynin chloride. Knowledge regarding the signs/symptoms related to toxicity is required to answer this question. Remember that restlessness is a sign of toxicity.

9. 1
Rationale: Epoetin alfa is synthetic erythropoietin, which the kidneys produce to stimulate red blood cell production in the bone marrow. It is used to treat anemia associated with chronic kidney disease. The normal hematocrit level is *Male:* 42% to 52% ; *Female:* 37% to 47% . Therapeutic effect is seen when the hematocrit reaches between 30% and 33% The normal platelet count is 150,000 to 400,000 mm^3. The normal blood urea nitrogen level is 10 to 20 mg/dL. The normal white blood cell count is 5000 to 10,000 mm^3. Platelet production, white blood cell production, and blood urea nitrogen do not respond to erythropoietin.
Test-Taking Strategy: Focus on the subject, a therapeutic effect. Relate the name of the medication, epoetin alfa, to the potential action or effect of erythropoietin. The only laboratory test that would reflect the effect of this medication is a hematocrit of 33%, found in the correct option.

10. 2
Rationale: Each dose of sulfadiazine needs to be administered with a full glass of water, and the client needs to maintain a high fluid intake. The medication is more soluble in alkaline urine. The client would not be instructed to taper or discontinue the dose. Some forms of sulfadiazine cause urine to turn dark brown or red. This does not indicate the need to notify the PHCP.
Test-Taking Strategy: Focus on the subject, client teaching points related to sulfadiazine. Think about the classification of this medication. Recalling that this medication is used to treat urinary tract infections will direct you to the correct option.

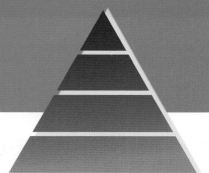

UNIT XV

Eye and Ear Problems of the Adult Client

 ## Pyramid to Success

Pyramid Points focus on safety and nursing interventions for clients with impairment of sight or hearing and on the nursing care related to health problems such as cataracts, glaucoma, and retinal detachment. Communicating with clients who are visually or hearing impaired is also a priority. Emergency interventions for eye and ear problems and injuries are a priority point. Pyramid Points also focus on client instructions related to medication administration, sensory perceptual alterations and safety issues, and available support systems.

Client Needs: Learning Objectives

Safe and Effective Care Environment
Caring for the recipient of a tissue (corneal) donation
Communicating with the interprofessional health care team
Establishing priorities
Maintaining asepsis with procedures and treatments
Maintaining standard and other precautions
Preventing accidents that can occur as a result of sensory impairments
Upholding client rights
Verifying that informed consent for invasive procedures is obtained

Health Promotion and Maintenance
Discussing changes that occur with the aging process
Discussing expected body image changes and self-care deficits

Implementing measures for the prevention and early detection of health problems related to the eye and the ear
Performing physical data collection techniques of the eye and ear
Providing home care instructions following procedures related to the eye and ear
Providing instructions regarding activity limitations or postoperative activities
Providing instructions regarding the administration of eye and ear medications
Teaching regarding the importance of compliance with the prescribed therapy

Psychosocial Integrity
Checking the client's ability to cope with feelings of isolation, fear, or anxiety regarding a possible change in vision and/or hearing status, and loss of independence
Discussing role changes
Identifying family support systems
Informing the client about available community resources
Monitoring for sensory perceptual alterations
Using appropriate communication techniques for impaired vision and hearing

Physiological Integrity
Monitoring for complications related to procedures
Monitoring for expected responses to therapy
Providing care for assistive devices such as eyeglasses, contact lenses, and hearing aids
Taking action in medical emergencies

Client Needs lists modified from: National Council of State Boards of Nursing, Inc. (NCSBN). *NCLEX-PN Examination: Test Plan for the National Council Licensure Examination for Practical Nurses,* effective April 2020. Chicago: NCSBN.

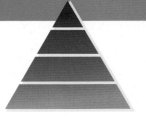

CHAPTER 53

Eye and Ear Problems

PRIORITY CONCEPTS Safety; Sensory Perception

WHAT WOULD YOU DO?

A client enters the emergency department and tells the nurse that they suddenly felt something hit their eye and they now have severe eye pain. The nurse notes an entrance wound in the client's affected eye. What would the nurse do?
Answer is located on p. 751.

I. Anatomy and Physiology of the Eye

A. The eye
  1. The eye is 1 inch (2.5 cm) in diameter and is located in the anterior portion of the orbit.
  2. The orbit is the bony structure of the skull that surrounds the eye and offers protection to the eye.

B. Layers of the eye
  1. External layer
     a. The fibrous coat that supports the eye
     b. Contains the sclera, the fibrous "white of the eye"
     c. Contains the cornea, a dense transparent layer
  2. Middle layer
     a. Called the uveal tract
     b. Consists of the choroid, the ciliary body, and the iris
     c. The choroid is the dark brown membrane located between the sclera and the retina that has dark pigmentation to prevent light from reflecting internally.
     d. The choroid lines most of the sclera and is attached to the retina but can detach easily from the sclera.
     e. The choroid contains many blood vessels and supplies nutrients to the retina.
     f. The ciliary body connects the choroid with the iris and secretes aqueous humor that helps to give the eye its shape. The muscles of the ciliary body control the thickness of the lens.
     g. The iris is the colored portion of the eye, is located in front of the lens, and has a central

circular opening called the pupil. The pupil controls the amount of light (darkness produces dilation and light produces constriction) admitted into the retina.
  3. Internal layer

     a. Consists of the retina, a thin, delicate structure in which the fibers of the optic nerve are distributed
     b. The retina is bordered externally by the choroid and sclera and internally by the vitreous.
     c. The retina is the visual receptive layer of the eye in which light waves are changed into nerve impulses and contains blood vessels and photoreceptors called rods and cones.

C. Vitreous body
  1. Contains a gelatinous substance that occupies the vitreous chamber, which is the space between the lens and the retina
  2. The vitreous body transmits light and gives shape to the posterior eye.

D. Vitreous
  1. Gel-like substance that maintains the shape of the eye
  2. Provides additional physical support to the retina

E. Rods and cones
  1. Rods are responsible for peripheral vision and function at reduced levels of illumination.
  2. Cones function at bright levels of illumination and are responsible for color vision and central vision.

F. Optic disc
  1. The optic disc is a creamy pink to white depressed area in the retina.
  2. The optic nerve enters and exits the eyeball at this area.
  3. This area is called the blind spot because it contains only nerve fibers, lacks photoreceptor cells, and is insensitive to light.

G. Macula lutea
  1. A small, oval, yellowish-pink area located laterally and temporally to the optic disc

2. The central depressed part of the macula is the fovea centralis, the area of sharpest and keenest vision, where most acute vision occurs.

3. Its functions include central vision, night and color vision, and motion detection.

H. Aqueous humor

1. The aqueous humor is a clear, watery fluid that fills the anterior and posterior chambers of the eye.

2. The aqueous humor is produced by the ciliary processes, and the fluid drains into the canal of Schlemm.

3. The anterior chamber lies between the cornea and the iris.

4. The posterior chamber lies between the iris and the lens.

I. Canal of Schlemm: A passageway that extends completely around the eye that permits fluid to drain out of the eye into the systemic circulation so that a constant intraocular pressure (IOP) is maintained.

J. Lens

1. A transparent convex structure behind the iris and in front of the vitreous body

2. The lens bends rays of light so that the light falls on the retina.

3. The curve of the lens changes to focus on near or distant objects.

K. Conjunctiva: The thin, transparent mucous membrane of the eye that lines the posterior surface of each eyelid and is located over the sclera

L. Lacrimal gland

1. The lacrimal gland produces tears.

2. Tears are drained through the punctum into the lacrimal duct and sac.

M. Eye muscles

1. Muscles do not work independently but work with the muscle that produces the opposite movement.

2. Rectus muscles exert their pull when the eye turns temporally.

3. Oblique muscles exert their pull when the eye turns nasally.

N. Nerves

1. Cranial nerve II: Optic nerve (sight)

2. Cranial nerve III: Oculomotor (eye movement)

3. Cranial nerve IV: Trochlear (eye movement)

4. Cranial nerve VI: Abducens (eye movement)

O. Blood vessels

1. The ophthalmic artery is the major artery supplying the structures in the eye.

2. The ophthalmic veins drain the blood from the eye.

II. **Assessment of Vision (See Chapter 13)**

III. **Diagnostic Tests for the Eye**

A. Fluorescein angiography

1. Description

a. A detailed imaging and recording of ocular circulation by a series of photographs taken after the administration of a dye

b. Used to assess problems with retinal circulation, such as those that occur in diabetic retinopathy, retinal bleeding, and macular degeneration

2. Preprocedure interventions

a. Check the client for allergies and previous reactions to dyes.

b. Ensure informed consent has been obtained.

c. A mydriatic medication, which causes pupil dilation, is instilled into the eye 1 hour before the test.

d. The dye is injected into a vein of the client's arm.

e. Inform the client that the dye may cause the skin to appear yellow for several hours after the test and is eliminated gradually through the urine. Urine may be bright green or orange for up to 2 days following the procedure.

f. The client may experience nausea, vomiting, sneezing, paresthesia of the tongue, or pain at the injection site.

g. If hives appear, orally or intramuscularly administered antihistamines such as diphenhydramine are given as prescribed.

3. Postprocedure interventions

a. Encourage rest.

b. Encourage fluid intake to assist in eliminating the dye from the client's system.

c. Remind the client that the yellow skin appearance will disappear.

d. Inform the client that the urine will appear bright green or orange until the dye is excreted.

e. Advise the client to avoid direct sunlight for a few hours after the test and to wear sunglasses if staying indoors is not possible.

f. Inform the client that the photophobia will continue until pupil size returns to normal.

B. Computed tomography (CT)

1. Description

a. The test is performed to examine the eyes, the bony structures around the eye, and the extraocular muscles.

b. Contrast material may be used unless eye trauma is suspected.

2. Interventions

a. No special client preparation or follow-up care is required.

b. Reinforce instructions to the client that he or she will be positioned in a confined space and will need to keep his or her head still during the procedure.

c. Ask about and document allergies and/or previous exposure to contrast.

C. Slit lamp
  1. Description
    a. A slit lamp allows examination of the anterior ocular structures under microscopic magnification.
    b. The client leans on a chin rest to stabilize the head while a narrowed beam of light is aimed so it illuminates only a narrow segment of the eye.
  2. Interventions: Advise the client about the brightness of the light and the need to look forward at a point over the examiner's ear.

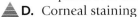 **D.** Corneal staining
  1. Description
    a. A topical dye is instilled into the conjunctival sac to outline irregularities of the corneal surface that are not easily visible.
    b. The eye is viewed through a blue filter, and a bright green color indicates areas of a nonintact corneal epithelium.
  2. Interventions
    a. If the client wears contact lenses, the lenses need to be removed.
    b. Reinforce instructions to the client to blink after the dye has been applied to distribute the dye evenly across the cornea.

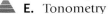 **E.** Tonometry
  1. Description: The test is used primarily to assess for an increase of IOP and potential glaucoma.
  2. Noncontact tonometry
    a. No direct contact with the client's cornea is needed, and no topical eye anesthetic is needed.
    b. A puff of air is directed at the cornea to indent the cornea, which can be unpleasant and may startle the client.
    c. It is a less accurate method of measurement compared with contact tonometry.
  3. Contact tonometry measurement
    a. Requires a topical anesthetic
    b. A flattened cone is brought in contact with the cornea, and the amount of pressure needed to flatten the cornea is measured.
    c. The client needs to be instructed to avoid rubbing the eye after the examination if the eye has been anesthetized because of the potential for scratching the cornea.

  ⚠ Normal IOP is 10 to 21 mm Hg. IOP varies throughout the day and is normally higher in the morning (always document the time of IOP measurement).

F. Ultrasound: Procedure is similar to an ultrasound procedure done in other parts of the body and is done to detect lesions or tumors in the eye.

BOX 53.1	**Risk Factors of Eye Disorders**

Aging process
Congenital
Diabetes mellitus
Hereditary
Medications
Trauma

G. Magnetic resonance imaging (MRI): Similar to an MRI done in other parts of the body; refer to Chapter 55 for additional information on MRI.

IV. Problems of the Eye

A. Risk factors related to eye disorders (Box 53.1)
B. Refractive errors
  1. Description
    a. Refraction is the bending of light rays. Any problem associated with either eye length or refraction can lead to refractive errors.
    b. Myopia (nearsightedness): Refractive ability of the eye is too strong for the eye length; images are bent and fall in front of, not on, the retina.
    c. Hyperopia (farsightedness): Refractive ability of the eye is too weak; images are focused behind the retina.
    d. Presbyopia: Loss of lens elasticity caused by aging; less able to focus the eye for close work, and images fall behind the retina.
    e. Astigmatism: Occurs because of the irregular curvature of the cornea; image focuses at two different points on the retina.
  2. Data collection
    a. Refractive errors are diagnosed through a process called refraction.
    b. The client views an eye chart while various lenses of different strengths are systematically placed in front of the eye and is asked whether each lens sharpens or worsens the vision.
  3. Nonsurgical interventions: Eyeglasses or contact lenses
  4. Surgical interventions
    a. Radial keratotomy: Incisions are made through the peripheral cornea to flatten the cornea, which allows the image to be focused closer to the retina; used to treat myopia.
    b. Photorefractive keratotomy: A laser beam is used to remove small portions of the corneal surface to reshape the cornea to focus an image properly on the retina; used to treat myopia and astigmatism.
    c. Laser in situ keratomileusis (LASIK): The superficial layers of the cornea are lifted as a flap, a laser reshapes the deeper corneal layers, and

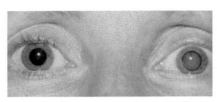

FIGURE 53.1 The cloudy appearance of a lens affected by cataract. (From Patton, Thibodeau, 2018)

then the corneal flap is replaced; used to treat hyperopia, myopia, and astigmatism.

   d. Corneal ring: The shape of the cornea is changed by placing a flexible ring in the outer edges of the cornea; used to treat myopia.

C. Legal blindness

   1. Description: In the client who is **legally blind**, the best visual acuity with corrective lenses in the better eye is 20/200 or less, or the visual field is no greater than 20 degrees in its widest diameter in the better eye.

   2. Interventions

     a. When speaking to the client who has limited sight or is blind, the nurse needs to use a normal tone of voice.

     b. Alert the client when approaching.

     c. Orient the client to the environment.

     d. Use a focal point and provide further orientation to the environment from that focal point; ensure that the client has a clear pathway.

     e. Allow the client to touch objects in the room.

     f. Use the clock placement of foods on the meal tray to orient the client.

     g. Promote independence as much as possible.

     h. Provide radios, televisions, and clocks that give the time orally, or provide a Braille watch.

     i. When ambulating, allow the client to grasp the nurse's arm at the elbow. The nurse keeps his or her arm close to the body so that the client can detect the direction of movement.

     j. Reinforce instructions to the client to remain one step behind the nurse when ambulating.

     k. Reinforce instructions to the client in the use of the cane used for the blind client, which is differentiated from other canes by its straight shape and white color with red tip.

     l. Reinforce instructions to the client that the cane is held in the dominant hand several inches (centimeters) off the floor.

     m. Reinforce instructions to the client that the cane sweeps the ground where the client's foot will be placed next to determine the presence of obstacles.

D. **Cataracts** (Fig. 53.1)

   1. Description

     a. A cataract is opacity of the lens that distorts the image projected onto the retina and that can progress to blindness.

     b. Causes include the aging process (senile cataracts), heredity (congenital cataracts), and injury (traumatic cataracts). Cataracts can also result from another eye disease (secondary cataracts).

     c. Causes of secondary cataracts include diabetes mellitus, maternal rubella, severe myopia, ultraviolet light exposure, and medications such as corticosteroids.

     d. Intervention is indicated when visual acuity has been reduced to a level that the client finds to be unacceptable or adversely affects her or his lifestyle.

   2. Data collection

     a. Blurred vision and decreased color perception are early signs.

     b. Diplopia, reduced visual acuity, absence of the red reflex, and the presence of a white pupil are late signs.

     c. Pain or eye redness is associated with age-related cataract formation.

     d. Loss of vision is gradual.

   3. Interventions

     a. Surgical removal of the lens, one eye at a time, is performed.

     b. With extracapsular extraction, the lens is lifted out without removing the lens capsule. The procedure may be performed by phacoemulsification in which the lens is broken up by ultrasonic vibrations and is extracted.

     c. With intracapsular extraction, the lens and capsule are removed completely.

     d. A partial iridectomy may be performed with the lens extraction to prevent acute secondary glaucoma.

     e. A lens implantation may be performed at the time of the surgical procedure.

   4. Preoperative interventions

     a. Reinforce instructions to the client regarding the postoperative measures, such as the importance of handwashing, and measures to prevent or decrease IOP such as bending over, coughing, straining, or rubbing the eye.

     b. Stress to the client that care after surgery requires instillation of different types of eyedrops several times a day for 2 to 4 weeks.

     c. Administer eye medications preoperatively including **mydriatics** and **cycloplegics** as prescribed.

   5. Postoperative interventions

     a. Elevate the head of the bed 30 to 45 degrees.

     b. Turn the client to the back or nonoperative side.

     c. Provide an eye patch as prescribed. Orient the client to the environment.

     d. Position the client's personal belongings to the nonoperative side.

BOX 53.2	Client Education After Cataract Surgery

Avoid eye straining.

Avoid rubbing or placing pressure on the eyes.

Avoid rapid movements, straining, sneezing, coughing, bending, vomiting, or lifting objects of more than the prescribed weight.

Take measures to prevent constipation.

Follow instructions for dressing changes and prescribed eyedrops and medications.

Wipe excess drainage or tearing with a sterile wet cotton ball from the inner to the outward canthus.

Use an eye shield at bedtime.

If a lens implant is not performed, accommodation is affected and glasses need to be worn at all times.

Cataract glasses act as magnifying glasses and replace central vision only.

Because cataract glasses magnify, objects appear closer; therefore, the client needs to accommodate, judge distance, and climb stairs carefully.

Contact lenses provide sharp visual acuity, but dexterity is needed to insert them.

Eye itching and mild discomfort are normal for a few days after the procedure.

Contact the primary health care provider (PHCP) for any decrease in vision, severe eye pain, or increase in eye discharge.

---

    e. Use side rails for safety (follow agency policies).

    f. Assist with ambulation.

  6. Client education (Box 53.2)

E. Glaucoma

  1. Description

    a. A group of ocular diseases resulting in increased IOP

    b. IOP is the fluid (aqueous humor) pressure within the eye. (Normal IOP is 10–21 mm Hg.)

    c. Increased IOP results from inadequate drainage of aqueous humor from the canal of Schlemm or overproduction of aqueous humor.

    d. The condition damages the optic nerve and can result in blindness.

    e. The gradual loss of visual fields may go unnoticed because central vision is unaffected.

  2. Types

    a. Primary open-angle glaucoma (POAG) results from obstruction to outflow of aqueous humor and is the most common type.

    b. Primary angle-closure glaucoma (PACG) results from blocking the outflow of aqueous humor into the trabecular meshwork; causes include lens or pupil dilation from medications or sympathetic stimulation.

  3. Data collection

    a. Early signs include diminished accommodation and increased IOP.

    b. POAG: painless, and vision changes are slow; results in "tunnel" vision

    c. PACG: blurred vision, halos around lights, and ocular erythema

  4. Acute angle-closure glaucoma

 Acute angle-closure glaucoma is a medical emergency that causes sudden eye pain and possible nausea and vomiting.

    a. Treat acute angle-closure glaucoma as a medical emergency.

    b. Assist to administer medications as prescribed to lower IOP.

    c. Prepare the client for peripheral iridectomy, which allows aqueous humor to flow from the posterior to the anterior chamber.

  5. Interventions for the client with glaucoma

    a. Reinforce instructions to the client on the importance of medications to constrict the pupils (miotics), to decrease the production of aqueous humor (carbonic anhydrase inhibitors), and to decrease the production of aqueous humor and IOP (beta blockers).

    b. Reinforce instructions to the client on the need for lifelong medication use and to wear a MedicAlert bracelet, to avoid anticholinergic medications to prevent increased IOP, and to contact the primary health care provider (PHCP) before taking medications, including over-the-counter medications.

    c. Reinforce instructions to the client to report eye pain, halos around the eyes, and changes in vision to the PHCP.

    d. Reinforce instructions to the client that when maximal medical therapy has failed to halt the progression of visual field loss and optic nerve damage, surgery will be recommended.

    e. Prepare the client for trabeculectomy, as prescribed, which allows drainage of aqueous humor into the conjunctival spaces by the creation of an opening.

F. Retinal detachment

  1. Description

    a. Detachment or separation of the retina from the epithelium

    b. Occurs when the layers of the retina separate because of the accumulation of fluid between them or when both retinal layers elevate away from the choroid as a result of a tumor

    c. Partial detachment becomes complete if untreated.

    d. When detachment becomes complete, blindness occurs.

2. Data collection
   a. Flashes of light
   b. Floaters or black spots (signs of bleeding)
   c. Increase in blurred vision
   d. Sense of a curtain being drawn over the eye
   e. Loss of a portion of the visual field; painless loss of central or peripheral vision

3. Immediate interventions
   a. Provide bed rest.
   b. Cover both eyes with patches, as prescribed, to prevent further detachment.
   c. Speak to the client before approaching.
   d. Position the client's head as prescribed.
   e. Protect the client from injury.
   f. Avoid jerky head movements.
   g. Minimize eye stress.
   h. Assist to prepare the client for a surgical procedure as prescribed.

4. Surgical procedures
   a. Draining fluid from the subretinal space so that the retina can return to the normal position
   b. Sealing retinal breaks by cryosurgery, a cold probe applied to the sclera, to stimulate an inflammatory response leading to adhesions
   c. Diathermy, the use of an electrode needle and heat through the sclera, to stimulate an inflammatory response
   d. Laser therapy to stimulate an inflammatory response and to seal small retinal tears before the detachment occurs
   e. Scleral buckling to hold the choroid and retina together with a splint until scar tissue forms and closes the tear (Fig. 53.2)
   f. Insertion of gas or silicone oil to promote reattachment. These agents float against the retina to hold it in place until healing occurs.

5. Postoperative interventions
   a. Maintain eye patches as prescribed.
   b. Monitor for hemorrhage.
   c. Prevent nausea and vomiting and monitor for restlessness, which can cause hemorrhage.
   d. Monitor for sudden, sharp eye pain (notify the registered nurse [RN] and PHCP).
   e. Encourage deep breathing, but avoid coughing.
   f. Provide bed rest as prescribed.
   g. Position the client as prescribed. (Positioning depends on the location of the detachment.)
   h. Assist with the administration of eye medications as prescribed.
   i. Assist the client with activities of daily living.
   j. Avoid sudden head movements or anything that increases IOP.
   k. Reinforce instructions to the client to limit reading for 3 to 5 weeks.

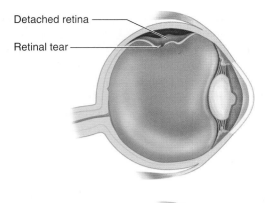
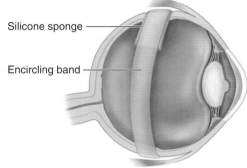

FIGURE 53.2 The scleral buckling procedure for repair of retinal detachment.

   l. Reinforce instructions to the client to avoid squinting, straining and constipation, lifting heavy objects, and bending from the waist.
   m. Reinforce instructions to the client to wear dark glasses during the day and an eye patch at night.
   n. Encourage follow-up care because of the danger of recurrence or occurrence in the other eye.

G. Macular degeneration
   1. A deterioration of the macula, the area of central vision
   2. Can be atrophic (age-related or dry) or exudative (wet)
   3. Age-related: Caused by gradual blocking of retinal capillaries leading to an ischemic and necrotic macula; rods and cones photoreceptors die.
   4. Exudative: Serous detachment of pigment epithelium in the macula occurs, and fluid and blood collect under the macula resulting in scar formation and visual distortion.
   5. Interventions are aimed at maximizing the remaining vision.
   6. Data collection
      a. A decline in central vision
      b. Blurred vision and distortion
   7. Interventions
      a. Initiate strategies to assist with maximizing remaining vision and maintaining independence.

b. Assist with providing referrals to community organizations.

c. Laser therapy or photodynamic therapy may be prescribed to seal the leaking blood vessels in or near the macula.

H. Ocular melanoma

1. Most common malignant eye tumor in adults
2. Tumor usually found in the uveal tract and can spread easily because of rich blood supply
3. Data collection
   a. Tumor can be discovered during routine examination.
   b. If macular area is invaded, blurring of vision occurs.
   c. Increased IOP is present if the canal of Schlemm is invaded.
   d. Change of iris color is noted if the tumor invades the iris.
   e. Ultrasonography may be performed to detect the tumor size and location.
4. Interventions
   a. Enucleation: The entire eyeball is removed surgically and a ball implant is inserted to provide a base for socket prosthesis.
   b. Radiation via a radioactive plaque that is sutured to the sclera. The radioactive plaque remains in place until the prescribed radiation dose is delivered.

I. Enucleation and exenteration

1. Description
   a. Enucleation is the removal of the entire eyeball.
   b. Exenteration is the removal of the eyeball and surrounding tissues and bone.
   c. The procedures are performed for the removal of ocular tumors.
   d. After the eye is removed, a ball implant is inserted to provide a firm base for socket prosthesis and to facilitate the best cosmetic result.
   e. A prosthesis is fitted approximately 1 month after surgery.
2. Preoperative interventions
   a. Provide emotional support to the client.
   b. Encourage the client to verbalize feelings related to loss.
   c. Encourage family support in care.
3. Postoperative interventions
   a. Monitor vital signs.
   b. Monitor a pressure patch or dressing as prescribed.
   c. Report changes in vital signs or the presence of bright red drainage on the pressure patch or dressing.

J. Hyphema

1. Description
   a. The presence of blood in the anterior chamber that occurs as a result of an injury
   b. The condition usually resolves in 5 to 7 days.

2. Interventions
   a. Encourage rest with the client in the semi-Fowler's position.
   b. Avoid sudden eye movements for 3 to 5 days to decrease the likelihood of bleeding.
   c. Assist with the administration of cycloplegic eyedrops, as prescribed, to relax the eye muscles and place the eye at rest.
   d. Reinforce instructions to the client in the use of eye shields or eye patches as prescribed.
   e. Reinforce instructions to the client to restrict reading and limit watching television.

K. Contusions

1. Description
   a. Bleeding into the soft tissue as a result of an injury
   b. A contusion causes a black eye and the discoloration disappears in approximately 10 days.
   c. Pain, photophobia, edema, and diplopia may occur.
2. Interventions
   a. Place ice on the eye immediately.
   b. Reinforce instructions to the client to receive a thorough eye examination.

L. Foreign bodies

1. Description: An object such as dust or dirt that enters the eye and causes irritation
2. Interventions
   a. Have the client look upward, expose the lower lid, wet a cotton-tipped applicator with sterile normal saline, and gently twist the swab over the particle, and remove it.
   b. If the particle cannot be seen, have the client look downward, place a cotton applicator horizontally on the outer surface of the upper eye lid, grasp the lashes, and pull the upper lid outward and over the cotton applicator. If the particle is seen, gently twist a swab over it to remove.

M. Penetrating objects

1. Description: An injury that occurs to the eye in which an object penetrates the eye
2. Interventions
   a. Never remove the object because it may be holding ocular structures in place. The object must be removed by the ophthalmologist.
   b. Cover the object with a cup (paper or plastic), and tape in place.
   c. Do not allow the client to bend over or lie flat, because these positions may move the object.
   d. Do not place pressure on the eye.
   e. The client must be seen by a PHCP and ophthalmologist immediately.
   f. X-rays and CT scans of the orbit are usually performed.

g. MRI is contraindicated because of the possibility of metal-containing projectile movement during the procedure.

N. Chemical burns

1. Description: An eye injury in which a caustic substance enters the eye
2. Interventions (see **Priority Nursing Actions**)

⚡ PRIORITY NURSING ACTIONS

Chemical Eye Injury

1. Irrigate the eye immediately.
2. Check the pH of the eye and continue irrigation until the pH is within normal range (approximately 6.5 to 7.6).
3. Ensure client is examined immediately by an ophthalmologist for assessment of visual acuity.
4. Continue the irrigation as prescribed.
5. Document the event, actions taken, and the client's response.

⚠ If a chemical splash to the eye occurs, treatment must begin immediately; immediately flush the eyes with water for at least 15 to 20 minutes at the scene of the injury, and then the client is brought to the emergency department. If possible, obtain a sample of the chemical involved.

O. Eye (tissue) donation

1. Donor eyes
   a. Donor eyes are obtained from cadavers.
   b. Donor eyes need to be enucleated soon after death and stored in a preserving solution because of rapid endothelial cell death.
   c. Storage, handling, and coordination of donor tissue with surgeons are provided by a network of state eye bank associations.
2. Care to the deceased client as a potential eye donor
   a. The option of eye donation is discussed with the PHCP and family.
   b. Raise the head of the bed 30 degrees.
   c. Instill antibiotic eyedrops as prescribed.
   d. Close the eyes and place a small ice pack as prescribed to the closed eyes.
3. Preoperative care to the recipient of the cornea
   a. Recipient may be told of the tissue (cornea) availability only several hours to 1 day before the surgery.
   b. Assist with alleviating the client's anxiety.
   c. Assess the recipient's eye for signs of infection.
   d. Report the presence of any redness, watery or purulent drainage, or edema around the recipient's eye to the RN and PHCP.
   e. Instill antibiotic drops into the recipient's eye, as prescribed, to reduce the number of microorganisms present.

f. Assist with the administration of fluids and intravenous medications as prescribed.

4. Postoperative care to the recipient
   a. The eye is covered with a pressure patch and protective shield that is left in place for 1 day.
   b. Do not remove or change the dressing without a PHCP's prescription.
   c. Monitor vital signs.
   d. Monitor level of consciousness.
   e. Monitor the eye dressing.
   f. Position the client with the head elevated and on the nonoperative side to reduce IOP.
   g. Orient the client frequently.
   h. Monitor for complications of bleeding, wound leakage, infection, and tissue rejection.
   i. Reinforce instructions to the client on how to apply a patch and eye shield.
   j. Reinforce instructions to the client to wear the eye shield at night for 1 month as prescribed and whenever around small children or pets.
   k. Advise the client not to rub the eye.
   l. Instruct the client to avoid activities that increase IOP.
5. Graft rejection
   a. Rejection can occur at any time.
   b. Inform the client of the signs of rejection.
   c. Signs include redness, swelling, decreased vision, and pain (RSVP).
   d. The eye is treated with topical corticosteroids.

V. Anatomy and Physiology of the Ear

A. Functions
1. Hearing
2. Maintenance of balance

B. External ear (pinna)
1. Embedded in the temporal bone bilaterally at the level of the eyes
2. Extends from the auricle through the external canal to the tympanic membrane (or eardrum), and includes the mastoid process, which is the bony ridge located over the temporal bone

C. Middle ear
1. The middle ear consists of the medial side of the tympanic membrane.
2. The middle ear contains three bony ossicles.
   a. Malleus
   b. Incus
   c. Stapes
3. Functions of the middle ear
   a. Conduct sound vibrations from the outer ear to the central hearing apparatus in the inner ear
   b. Protect the inner ear by reducing the amplitude of loud sounds
   c. The eustachian tube (auditory canal) allows equalization of air pressure on each side of the

tympanic membrane so that the membrane does not rupture.

D. Inner ear

   1. The inner ear contains the semicircular canals, the cochlea, and the distal end of the eighth cranial nerve.

   2. The semicircular canals contain fluid and hair cells connected to sensory nerve fibers of the vestibular portion of the eighth cranial nerve.

   3. The inner ear maintains the sense of balance or equilibrium.

   4. The cochlea is the spiral-shaped organ of hearing.

   5. The organ of Corti (within the cochlea) is the receptor and organ of hearing.

   6. Eighth cranial nerve

     a. The cochlear branch of the nerve transmits neuroimpulses from the cochlea to the brain, where they are interpreted as sound.

     b. The vestibular branch maintains balance and equilibrium.

E. Hearing and equilibrium

   1. The external ear conducts sound waves to the middle ear.

   2. The middle ear, also called the tympanic cavity, conducts sound waves to the inner ear.

   3. The middle ear is filled with air which is kept at atmospheric pressure by the opening of the auditory canal.

   4. The inner ear contains sensory receptors for sound and for equilibrium.

   5. The receptors in the inner ear transmit sound waves and changes in body position as nerve impulses.

VI. **Assessment of the Ear (See Chapter 13)**

VII. **Diagnostic Tests for the Ear**

A. Tomography

   1. Description

     a. Tomography may be performed with or without contrast medium.

     b. Tomography assesses the mastoid, middle ear, and inner ear structures.

     c. Multiple radiographs of the head are obtained.

     d. Tomography is especially helpful in the diagnosis of acoustic tumors.

   2. Interventions

     a. All jewelry is removed.

     b. Lead eye shields are used to cover the cornea to diminish the radiation dose to the eyes.

     c. The client needs to remain still in a supine position.

     d. No follow-up care is required.

     e. If contrast is to be used, assess for allergies or previous response to contrast.

B. Audiometry

   1. Description

     a. Audiometry measures hearing acuity.

     b. Audiometry uses two types: pure tone audiometry and speech audiometry.

     c. Pure tone audiometry is used to identify problems with hearing, speech, music, and other sounds in the environment.

     d. In speech audiometry, the client's ability to hear spoken words is measured.

     e. After testing, audiographic patterns are depicted on a graph to determine the type and level of hearing loss.

   2. Interventions

     a. Inform the client regarding the procedure.

     b. Reinforce instructions to the client to identify the sounds as they are heard.

C. Electronystagmography (ENG)

   1. Description

     a. ENG is a vestibular test that evaluates spontaneous and induced eye movements known as nystagmus.

     b. ENG is used to distinguish between normal nystagmus and medication-induced nystagmus, or nystagmus caused by a lesion in the central or peripheral vestibular pathway.

     c. ENG records changing electrical fields with the movement of the eye, as monitored by electrodes placed on the skin around the eye.

   2. Interventions

     a. The client is instructed to remain NPO (nothing by mouth) for 3 hours before testing and to avoid caffeine-containing beverages for 24 to 48 hours before the test.

     b. Unnecessary medications are omitted for 24 hours before testing.

     c. Instruct the client that this may be a long and tiring procedure.

     d. The client needs to bring prescription eyeglasses to the examination.

     e. The client sits and is instructed to gaze at lights, focus on a moving pattern, focus on a moving point, and then close the eyes.

     f. While sitting in a chair, the client may be rotated to provide information about vestibular function.

     g. In addition, the client's ears are irrigated with cool and warm water, which may cause nausea and vomiting.

     h. After the procedure, the client begins taking clear fluids slowly and cautiously because nausea and vomiting may occur.

     i. Assistance with ambulation may also be necessary after the procedure.

D. MRI: Refer to Chapter 55 for information on MRI.

VIII. Problems of the Ear

A. Risk factors related to ear disorders (Box 53.3)

B. Conductive hearing loss (Fig. 53.3)

  1. Description

    a. Conductive hearing loss occurs when sound waves are blocked to the inner ear fibers because of external ear or middle ear disorders.

    b. Disorders often can be corrected with no damage to hearing or with minimal permanent hearing loss.

  2. Causes

    a. Any inflammatory process or obstruction of the external or middle ear

    b. Tumors

    c. Otosclerosis

    d. A buildup of scar tissue on the ossicles from previous middle ear surgery

C. Sensorineural hearing loss (Fig. 53.3)

  1. Description

    a. Sensorineural hearing loss is a pathological process of the inner ear or of the sensory fibers that lead to the cerebral cortex.

    b. Sensorineural hearing loss is often permanent, and measures need to be taken to reduce further damage.

  2. Causes

    a. Damage to the inner ear structures

    b. Damage to the eighth cranial nerve or the brain itself

    c. Prolonged exposure to loud noise

    d. Medications

    e. Trauma

    f. Inherited disorders

    g. Metabolic and circulatory disorders

    h. Infections

    i. Surgery

    j. Ménière's syndrome

    k. Diabetes mellitus

    l. Myxedema

D. Mixed hearing loss (Fig. 53.3)

  1. Mixed hearing loss is also known as conductive-sensorineural hearing loss.

  2. Client has sensorineural and conductive hearing loss.

E. Central hearing loss: Involves the inability to interpret sound, including speech, as a result of a problem in the brain

F. Signs of hearing loss and facilitating communication (Boxes 53.4 and 53.5) ▲

G. Cochlear implantation ▲

  1. Cochlear implants are used for sensorineural hearing loss.

  2. A small computer converts sound waves into electrical impulses.

BOX 53.3	Risk Factors of Ear Disorders

Aging process
Infection
Medications
Ototoxicity
Trauma
Tumors

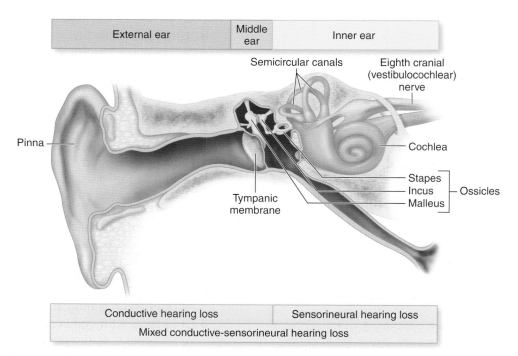

FIGURE 53.3 Anatomy of hearing loss. Hearing loss can be divided into three types: 1. conductive (difficulty in the external or the middle ear); 2. sensorineural (difficulty in the inner ear or acoustic (vestibulocochlear) nerve); and 3. mixed conductive-sensorineural (a combination of the two).

BOX 53.4 Signs of Hearing Loss

Frequently asking others to repeat statements
Straining to hear
Turning head or leaning forward to favor one ear
Shouting during a conversation
Ringing in the ears
Failing to respond when not looking in the direction of the sound
Answering questions incorrectly
Raising the volume of the television or radio
Avoiding large groups
Better understanding of speech when in small groups
Withdrawing from social interactions

BOX 53.5 Facilitation of Communication

Using written words if the client is able to see, read, and write
Providing plenty of light in the room
Getting the attention of the client before beginning to speak
Facing the client when speaking
Talking in a room without distracting noises
Moving close to the client and speaking slowly and clearly
Keeping hands and other objects away from the mouth when talking to the client
Talking in normal volume and lower pitch since shouting is not helpful and higher frequencies are less easily heard
Rephrasing sentences and repeating information
Validating with the client the understanding of statements made by asking the client to repeat what was said
Using lip-reading
Encouraging the client to wear glasses when talking to someone to improve vision for lip reading
Using sign language which combines speech with hand movements that signify letters, words, or phrases
Using telephone amplifiers
Using flashing lights that are activated by ringing of the telephone or doorbell
Using specially trained dogs that help the client to be aware of sound and to alert the client to potential dangers

---

3. Electrodes are placed by the internal ear with a computer device attached to the external ear.
4. Electronic impulses directly stimulate nerve fibers.

H. Hearing aids
   1. Hearing aids are used for the client with conductive hearing loss.
   2. Hearing aids have limited value for the client with sensorineural hearing loss because they only make sounds louder and not clearer.
   3. A difficulty that exists in the use of hearing aids is the amplification of background noise and voices.
   4. Hearing aids are costly and often not covered by insurance. Some clients can obtain hearing aids through a rehabilitation facility or through other resources.
   5. Client education (Box 53.6)

BOX 53.6 Client Education Regarding a Hearing Aid

Begin using the hearing aid slowly to adjust to the device.
Adjust the volume to the minimal hearing level to prevent feedback squeaking.
Concentrate on the sounds that are to be heard and filter out background noise.
Clean the ear mold and cannula per manufacturer's instructions.
Keep the hearing aid dry.
Turn off the hearing aid before removing from the ear to prevent squealing feedback.
Remove the battery when not in use.
Keep extra batteries on hand.
Keep the hearing aid in a safe place.
Prevent hair sprays, oils, or other hair and face products from coming in contact with the receiver of the hearing aid.
Instruct the client to keep the hearing aid in the proper environmental climate, as recommended by the manufacturer, in order to prolong the life of the device.

I. Presbycusis
   1. Description
      a. Presbycusis is a sensorineural hearing loss associated with aging.
      b. Presbycusis leads to degeneration or atrophy of the ganglion cells in the cochlea and a loss of elasticity of the basilar membranes.
      c. Presbycusis leads to compromise of the vascular supply to the inner ear with changes in several areas of the ear structure.
   2. Data collection
      a. Hearing loss is gradual and bilateral.
      b. The client states that he or she has no problem with hearing but cannot understand what the words are.
      c. The client thinks that the speaker is mumbling.

⚠ Teach the client that cotton-tipped applicators must not be inserted into the ear canal, because their use can lead to trauma to the canal and puncture the tympanic membrane.

J. Otitis externa
   1. Description
      a. Otitis externa is an infective inflammatory or allergic response involving the structure of the external auditory canal or the auricles.
      b. An irritating or infective agent comes in contact with the epithelial layer of the external ear.
      c. Contact leads to an allergic response or signs/symptoms of an infection.
      d. The skin becomes red, swollen, and tender to touch during movement.

e. The extensive swelling of the canal can lead to conductive hearing loss because of obstruction.

f. External otitis is more common in children, is termed "swimmer's ear," and occurs more often in hot, humid environments.

g. Prevention includes the elimination of irritating or infecting agents.

2. Data collection
   a. Pain
   b. Itching
   c. Plugged feeling in the ear
   d. Redness and edema
   e. Exudate
   f. Hearing loss

3. Interventions
   a. Apply heat locally for 20 minutes three times a day.
   b. Encourage rest to assist in reducing pain.
   c. Administer antibiotics or corticosteroids as prescribed.
   d. Administer analgesics such as acetaminophen for the pain as prescribed.
   e. Reinforce instructions to the client that the ears would be kept clean and dry.
   f. Reinforce instructions to the client to use earplugs for swimming.
   g. Reinforce instructions to the client that irritating agents such as hair products or headphones need to be discontinued.

K. Otitis media: See Chapter 32
   1. Myringotomy: See Chapter 32
   2. Client education (Box 53.7).

L. Chronic otitis media
   1. Description
      a. Chronic otitis media is a chronic infective, inflammatory, or allergic response involving the structure of the middle ear.
      b. Frequent removal of debris from the canal may be required.
      c. Myringoplasty can reconstruct the tympanic membrane and ossicles and improve conductive hearing loss.
      d. Mastoidectomy may be performed if the infection has spread to involve the mastoid bone.

   ⚠ Monitor the client with otitis media closely for response to treatment. Otic and systemic antibiotics may be used to treat the infection, but often the organism is resistant.

   2. Preoperative interventions
      a. Administer antibiotic drops as prescribed.
      b. Clean the ear of debris as prescribed. Irrigate the ear with a solution as prescribed to restore the normal pH of the ear.
      c. Reinforce instructions to the client to avoid persons with upper respiratory infections,

---

obtain adequate rest, eat a balanced diet, and drink adequate fluids.
   d. Reinforce instructions to the client in deep breathing and coughing. Forceful coughing, which increases pressure in the middle ear, is to be avoided postoperatively.

3. Postoperative interventions
   a. Inform the client that initial hearing after surgery is diminished because of the packing in the ear canal and that hearing improvement will occur after the packing is removed.
   b. Keep the dressing clean and dry.
   c. Keep the client flat with the operative ear up for at least 12 hours as prescribed.
   d. Administer antibiotics as prescribed.

M. Mastoiditis
   1. Description
      a. Mastoiditis may be acute or chronic and results from untreated or inadequately treated chronic or acute otitis media.
      b. The pain is not relieved by myringotomy.

   2. Data collection
      a. Swelling behind the ear and pain with minimal movement of the head
      b. Cellulitis on the skin or external scalp over the mastoid process
      c. A reddened, dull, thick, immobile tympanic membrane with or without perforation
      d. Tender and enlarged postauricular lymph nodes
      e. Low-grade fever

   3. Interventions
      a. Prepare the client for surgical removal of infected material.
      b. Monitor for complications.
      c. Simple or modified radical mastoidectomy with tympanoplasty is the most common treatment.

d. Once infected tissue is removed, the tympanoplasty is performed to reconstruct the ossicles and the tympanic membranes in an attempt to restore normal hearing.

4. Complications

a. Damage to the abducens and facial cranial nerves, exhibited by the inability to look laterally (cranial nerve VI, abducens) and a drooping of the mouth on the affected side (cranial nerve VII, facial)

b. Meningitis

c. Brain abscess

d. Chronic purulent otitis media

e. Wound infections

f. Vertigo, if the infection spreads into the labyrinth

5. Postoperative interventions

a. Monitor for dizziness.

b. Monitor for signs of meningitis as evidenced by a stiff neck and vomiting, and for other complications.

c. Prepare for a wound dressing change 24 hours postoperatively.

d. Monitor the surgical incision for edema, drainage, and redness.

e. Position the client flat with the operative side up.

f. Restrict the client to bed with bedside commode privileges for 24 hours as prescribed.

g. Assist the client with getting out of bed to prevent falling or injuries from dizziness.

h. With reconstruction of the ossicles via a graft, take precautions to prevent dislodging of the graft.

N. Otosclerosis

1. Description

a. A genetic problem of the labyrinthine capsule of the middle ear that results in a bony overgrowth of the tissue surrounding the ossicles

b. Otosclerosis causes the development of irregular areas of new bone formation and causes the fixation of the bones.

c. Stapes fixation leads to a conductive hearing loss.

d. If the disease involves the inner ear, sensorineural hearing loss is present.

e. Bilateral involvement is common, although hearing loss may be worse in one ear.

f. Nonsurgical intervention promotes the improvement of hearing through amplification.

g. Surgical intervention involves removal of the bony growth that is causing the hearing loss.

h. A partial stapedectomy or complete stapedectomy with prosthesis (fenestration) may be performed surgically.

2. Data collection

a. Slowly progressing conductive hearing loss

b. Bilateral hearing loss

c. A ringing or roaring type of constant tinnitus

d. Loud sounds heard in the ear when chewing

e. Pinkish discoloration (Schwartze's sign) of the tympanic membrane, which indicates vascular changes within the ear

O. Fenestration

1. Description

a. Fenestration refers to the removal of the stapes with a small hole drilled in the footplate; a prosthesis is connected between the incus and footplate.

b. Sounds cause the prosthesis to vibrate in the same manner as the stapes.

c. Complications include complete hearing loss, prolonged vertigo, infection, or facial nerve damage.

2. Preoperative interventions

a. Reinforce instructions to the client on measures to prevent middle ear or external ear infections.

b. Reinforce instructions to the client to avoid excessive nose blowing.

3. Postoperative interventions

a. Inform the client that hearing is initially worse after the surgical procedure because of swelling and that no noticeable improvement in hearing may occur for as long as 6 weeks.

b. Inform the client that the Gelfoam ear packing (if used) interferes with hearing but is used to decrease bleeding.

c. Assist with ambulating during the first 1 to 2 days after surgery.

d. Administer antibiotics, antivertiginous, and pain medications as prescribed.

e. Monitor for facial nerve damage, weakness, changes in tactile and taste sensation, vertigo, nausea, and vomiting.

f. Reinforce instructions to the client to move the head slowly when changing positions to prevent vertigo.

g. Reinforce instructions to the client to avoid showering and getting the head and wound wet.

h. Reinforce instructions to the client to avoid using small objects (cotton-tipped applicators) to clean the external ear canal.

i. Reinforce instructions to the client to avoid rapid, extreme changes in pressure caused by quick head movements, sneezing, nose blowing, straining, and changes in altitude.

j. Reinforce instructions to the client to avoid changes in middle ear pressure because they could dislodge the graft or prosthesis.

P. Labyrinthitis

1. Description: Infection of the labyrinth that occurs as a complication of acute or chronic otitis media

Adult—Eye and Ear

2. May result from growth of a cholesteatoma—benign overgrowth of squamous cell epithelium in the middle ear

3. Data collection
   a. Hearing loss that may be permanent on the affected side
   b. Tinnitus
   c. Spontaneous nystagmus to the affected side
   d. Vertigo
   e. Nausea and vomiting

4. Interventions
   a. Monitor for signs of meningitis, the most common complication, as evidenced by headache, stiff neck, and lethargy.
   b. Assist to administer systemic antibiotics as prescribed.
   c. Advise the client to rest in bed in a darkened room.
   d. Assist with the administration of antiemetics and antivertiginous medications as prescribed.
   e. Reinforce instructions to the client that the vertigo subsides as the inflammation resolves.
   f. Reinforce instructions to the client that balance problems that persist may require gait training through physical therapy.

Q. Ménière's syndrome
1. Description
   a. Ménière's syndrome is also called endolymphatic hydrops and refers to dilation of the endolymphatic system by overproduction or decreased reabsorption of endolymphatic fluid.
   b. The syndrome is characterized by tinnitus, unilateral sensorineural hearing loss, and vertigo.
   c. Symptoms occur in attacks and last for several days, and the client becomes totally incapacitated during the attacks.
   d. Initial hearing loss is reversible, but as the frequency of attacks continues, hearing loss becomes permanent.

   ⚠ A priority nursing intervention in the care of a client with Ménière's syndrome is instituting safety measures.

2. Causes
   a. Any factor that increases endolymphatic secretion in the labyrinth
   b. Viral and bacterial infections
   c. Allergic reactions
   d. Biochemical disturbances
   e. Vascular disturbance producing changes in the microcirculation in the labyrinth
   f. Long-term stress may be a possible contributing factor.

3. Data collection
   a. Feelings of fullness in the ear
   b. Tinnitus as a continuous low-pitched roar or humming sound that is present much of the time but worsens just before and during severe attacks
   c. Hearing loss that is worse during an attack
   d. Vertigo as periods of whirling that might cause the client to fall to the ground
   e. Vertigo that is so intense that even while lying down, the client holds the bed or ground in an attempt to prevent the whirling
   f. Nausea and vomiting
   g. Nystagmus
   h. Severe headache

4. Nonsurgical interventions
   a. Prevent injury during vertigo attacks.
   b. Provide bed rest in a quiet environment.
   c. Provide assistance with walking.
   d. Reinforce instructions to the client to move the head slowly to prevent worsening of the vertigo.
   e. Initiate sodium and fluid restrictions as prescribed.
   f. Reinforce instructions to the client to stop smoking.
   g. Reinforce instructions to the client to avoid watching television because the flickering of lights may exacerbate symptoms.
   h. Assist with the administration of nicotinic acid (niacin), as prescribed, for its vasodilatory effect.
   i. Assist with the administration of antihistamines, as prescribed, which will reduce the production of histamine and the inflammation.
   j. Assist to administer antiemetics as prescribed.
   k. Assist to administer tranquilizers and sedatives as prescribed to calm the client and allow him or her to rest and to control vertigo, nausea, and vomiting.
   l. Mild diuretics may be prescribed to decrease endolymph volume.
   m. Inform the client about vestibular rehabilitation as prescribed.

5. Surgical interventions
   a. Surgery is performed when medical therapy is ineffective and the functional level of the client has decreased significantly.
   b. Endolymphatic drainage and insertion of a shunt may be performed early in the course of the disease to assist with the drainage of excess fluids.
   c. A resection of the vestibular nerve or total removal of the labyrinth or a labyrinthectomy may be performed.

6. Postoperative interventions
   a. Monitor packing and dressing on the ear.
   b. Speak to the client on the side of the unaffected ear.
   c. Assist with performing neurological assessments.

d. Maintain side rails as appropriate per agency policy.

e. Assist with ambulating.

f. Encourage the client to use a bedside commode rather than ambulating to the bathroom.

g. Assist with the administration of antivertiginous and antiemetic medications as prescribed.

R. Acoustic neuroma

1. Description

a. Acoustic neuroma is a benign tumor of the vestibular or acoustic nerve.

b. The tumor may cause damage to hearing and to facial movements and sensations.

c. Treatment includes surgical removal of the tumor via craniotomy.

d. Care is taken to preserve the function of the facial nerve.

e. The tumor rarely recurs after surgical removal.

f. Postoperative nursing care is similar to postoperative craniotomy care (see Chapter 55).

 2. Data collection

a. Symptoms usually begin with tinnitus and progress to gradual sensorineural hearing loss.

b. As the tumor enlarges, damage to adjacent cranial nerves occurs.

S. Trauma

1. Description

a. The tympanic membrane has a limited stretching ability and gives way under high pressure.

b. Foreign objects placed in the external canal may exert pressure on the tympanic membrane and cause perforation.

c. If the object continues through the canal, the bony structure of the stapes, incus, and malleus may be damaged.

d. A blunt injury to the basal skull and ear can damage the middle ear structures through fractures extending to the middle ear.

e. Excessive nose blowing and rapid changes of pressure that occur with nonpressurized air flights can increase pressure in the middle ear.

f. Depending on the damage to the ossicles, hearing loss may or may not be reversible.

2. Interventions

a. Tympanic membrane perforations usually heal within 24 hours.

b. Surgical reconstruction of the ossicles and tympanic membrane through tympanoplasty or myringoplasty may be performed to improve hearing.

T. Cerumen and foreign bodies

1. Description

a. Cerumen or wax is the most common cause of impacted canals.

b. Foreign bodies can include vegetables, beads, pencil erasers, insects, or other objects.

2. Data collection

a. Sensation of fullness in the ear with or without hearing loss

b. Pain, itching, or bleeding

3. Cerumen

a. Removal of wax by irrigation may be a slow process.

b. Irrigation is contraindicated in clients with a history of tympanic membrane perforation or otitis media.

c. If prescribed to soften cerumen, glycerin or mineral oil is placed in the ear at bedtime; hydrogen peroxide may also be prescribed.

d. After several days, the ear is irrigated.

e. The maximal amount of solution that would be used for irrigation is 50 to 70 mL.

 Inform the client that ear candles must never be used to remove cerumen. Their use can cause burns and a vacuum effect causing a perforation in the tympanic membrane.

4. Foreign bodies

a. With a foreign object of vegetable matter, irrigation is used with care because this material expands with hydration.

b. Insects are killed before removal unless they can be coaxed out by flashlight or a humming noise; lidocaine may be placed in the ear to relieve pain.

c. Mineral oil or diluted alcohol is instilled to suffocate the insect, which then is removed using ear forceps.

d. A small ear forceps is used to remove the object; care is taken to avoid pushing the object farther into the canal and damaging the tympanic membrane.

WHAT WOULD YOU DO?

Answer: This situation is an emergency. The nurse would immediately accompany the client to a room and notify the registered nurse (RN) and primary health care provider (PHCP) to assess the client. A penetrating eye wound is a serious injury that can cause loss of sight or require loss of the eye (surgical removal). The object is removed only by an ophthalmologist because it may be holding eye structures in place. X-rays and computed tomography (CT) scans of the orbit are usually obtained to ensure that the orbit of the eye is intact and to look for fractures that might entrap orbital muscles. Magnetic resonance imaging (MRI) is contraindicated because of the possibility of metal-containing projectile movement during the procedure. Surgery is usually needed to remove the foreign object.

PRACTICE QUESTIONS

❖ 1. The nurse is preparing to reinforce a teaching plan for a client who is undergoing cataract extraction with intraocular implant. Which home care measures would the nurse include in the plan? **Select all that apply.**

- ❑ 1. To avoid activities that require bending over
- ❑ 2. To contact the surgeon if eye scratchiness occurs
- ❑ 3. To take acetaminophen for minor eye discomfort
- ❑ 4. To place an eye shield on the surgical eye at bedtime
- ❑ 5. That episodes of sudden severe pain in the eye are expected
- ❑ 6. To contact the surgeon if a decrease in visual acuity occurs

2. The nurse is assisting with developing a teaching plan for the client with glaucoma. Which instruction would the nurse suggest to include in the plan of care?
1. Decrease the amount of salt in the diet.
2. Avoid reading the newspaper and watching television.
3. Decrease fluid intake to control the intraocular pressure.
4. Eye medications may need to be administered for the rest of your life.

3. The nurse is assigned to care for a client with a detached retina. Which finding would the nurse expect to be documented in the client's record?
1. Blurred vision
2. Pain in the affected eye
3. A yellow discoloration of the sclera
4. A sense of a curtain falling across the field of vision

❖ 4. The nurse is assigned to care for a client with a diagnosis of detached retina. Which findings would indicate that bleeding has occurred as a result of retinal detachment? **Select all that apply.**

- ❑ 1. Total loss of vision
- ❑ 2. Vision may be cloudy
- ❑ 3. A reddened conjunctiva
- ❑ 4. A sudden sharp pain in the eye
- ❑ 5. Complaints of a burst of black spots or floaters
- ❑ 6. Vision is clear straight ahead but not to the right

5. A client arrives in the emergency department after an automobile crash. The client's forehead hit the steering wheel, and a hyphema has been diagnosed. Which position would the nurse prepare to position the client?
1. Flat on bed rest
2. On bed rest in a semi-Fowler's position
3. In a lateral position on the affected side
4. In a lateral position on the unaffected side

6. A client sustains a contusion of the eyeball after a traumatic injury with a blunt object. The nurse would take which **immediate** action?
1. Apply ice to the affected eye.
2. Irrigate the eye with cool water.
3. Notify the primary health care provider (PHCP).
4. Accompany the client to the emergency department.

7. A client sustains a chemical eye injury from a splash of battery acid. The nurse would prepare the client for which **immediate** measure?
1. Checking visual acuity
2. Covering the eye with a pressure patch
3. Swabbing the eye with antibiotic ointment
4. Irrigating the eye with sterile normal saline

8. The nurse is caring for a client after enucleation and notes the presence of bright red drainage on the dressing. The nurse would take which appropriate action?
1. Document the finding.
2. Continue to monitor vital signs.
3. Report the finding to the registered nurse (RN).
4. Mark the drainage on the dressing and monitor for any increase in bleeding.

9. The nurse is preparing to administer eardrops to an adult client. The nurse administers the eardrops by which technique?
1. Pulling the pinna up and back
2. Pulling the earlobe down and back
3. Tilting the client's head forward and down
4. Instructing the client to stand and lean to one side

10. The nurse is caring for a client who is hearing impaired. The nurse would take which approach to facilitate communication?
1. Speak loudly.
2. Speak frequently.
3. Speak in a normal tone.
4. Speak directly into the impaired ear.

11. A client arrives at the emergency department with a foreign body in the left ear that has been determined to be an insect. Which **initial** intervention would the nurse anticipate to be prescribed?
1. Irrigation of the ear
2. Instillation of antibiotic eardrops
3. Instillation of corticosteroid ointment
4. Instillation of mineral oil or diluted alcohol

12. The nurse notes that the primary health care provider (PHCP) has documented a diagnosis of presbycusis on the client's chart. Which explanation would the nurse give to the client to describe this condition?
1. Tinnitus that occurs with aging

2. Nystagmus that occurs with aging
3. A conductive hearing loss that occurs with aging
4. A sensorineural hearing loss that occurs with aging

13. A client with Ménière's disease is experiencing severe vertigo. The nurse reinforces instructions to the client to do which to assist with controlling the vertigo?
    1. Increase sodium in the diet.
    2. Lie still and watch television.
    3. Avoid sudden head movements.
    4. Increase fluid intake to 3000 mL/day.

14. The nurse is assigned to care for a client hospitalized with Ménière's disease. The nurse expects that

which would **most likely** be prescribed for the client?
1. Low-fat diet
2. Low-sodium diet
3. Low-cholesterol diet
4. Low-carbohydrate diet

15. A client is diagnosed with glaucoma. Which data gathered by the nurse indicate a risk factor associated with glaucoma?
    1. Cardiovascular disease
    2. A history of migraine headaches
    3. Frequent urinary tract infections
    4. Frequent upper respiratory infections

ANSWERS

❖ **1. 1, 3, 4, 6**
Rationale: After eye surgery, some scratchiness and mild eye discomfort may occur in the operative eye and is usually relieved by mild analgesics. If the eye pain becomes severe, the client needs to notify the surgeon because this may indicate hemorrhage, infection, or increased intraocular pressure. The nurse needs to also instruct the client to notify the surgeon of purulent drainage, increased redness, or any decrease in visual acuity. The client is instructed to place an eye shield over the operative eye at bedtime to protect the eye from injury during sleep and to avoid activities that increase intraocular pressure such as bending over.
Test-Taking Strategy: Note the subject of the question, client teaching after cataract extraction with intraocular implant. Recalling that the eye needs to be protected and that a concern is increased intraocular pressure will assist in determining the home care measures to be included in the plan.

2. 4
Rationale: The administration of eyedrops is a critical component of the treatment plan for the client with glaucoma. The client needs to be instructed that medications may need to be taken for the rest of his or her life. Limiting fluids and reducing salt will not decrease intraocular pressure. Option 3 is not necessary.
Test-Taking Strategy: Focus on the subject, glaucoma. Knowing that medications are an integral component of the treatment plan will assist with directing you to the correct option.

3. 4
Rationale: A characteristic clinical manifestation of retinal detachment described by clients is the feeling that a shadow or curtain is falling across the field of vision. There is no pain associated with detachment of the retina. A retinal detachment is an ophthalmic emergency and even more so if visual acuity is still normal. Options 1 and 3 are not specifically associated with a detached retina.
Test-Taking Strategy: Focus on the subject, detached retina. Think about the pathophysiology associated with detached retina. Remember that a characteristic clinical manifestation is the feeling that a shadow or curtain is falling across the field of vision. Retinal detachment can occur suddenly and is an ophthalmic emergency.

❖ **4. 2, 5**
Rationale: Complaints of a sudden burst of black spots or floaters indicate that bleeding has occurred as a result of the detachment. Vision may also be cloudy. Options 1, 3, 4, and 6 are not specifically associated with bleeding as a result of detached retina.
Test-Taking Strategy: Focus on the subject, detached retina and bleeding. Hemorrhage is a serious complication associated with retinal detachment. Remember, complaints of a sudden burst of black spots or floaters and cloudy vision indicate that bleeding has occurred as a result of the detachment.

5. 2
Rationale: A hyphema is the presence of blood in the anterior chamber. It is produced when a force is sufficient to break the integrity of the blood vessels in the eye. It can be caused by direct injury, such as a penetrating injury from a BB pellet, or indirectly, such as from striking the forehead on a steering wheel during an accident. The client is treated by bed rest in a semi-Fowler's position to assist gravity in keeping the hyphema away from the optical center of the cornea.
Test-Taking Strategy: Focus on the subject, hyphema. Think about this type of injury. Eliminate options 1, 3, and 4 because they are comparable or alike. Placing the client flat will produce an increase in pressure at the injured site.

6. 1
Rationale: Treatment for a contusion begins at the time of injury. Ice is applied immediately. The client needs to receive a thorough eye examination to rule out the presence of other eye injuries. Eye irrigation is not indicated in a contusion. Options 3 and 4 will delay immediate treatment. After the application of ice, the PHCP would be notified.
Test-Taking Strategy: Note the strategic word, *immediate*. Noting that the client sustained a contusion to the eye will direct you to the correct option.

7. 4
Rationale: Emergency care after a chemical burn to the eye includes irrigating the eye immediately with sterile normal saline or ocular irrigating solution. The irrigation needs to be maintained for at least 10 minutes. After this emergency treatment, visual acuity is assessed. Options 2 and 3 are not immediate measures.

Test-Taking Strategy: Note the strategic word, *immediate* and focus on the subject, chemical eye injury. Read the question carefully, noting the type of injury to the eye. The question asks about emergency care; therefore, in this type of injury, it is necessary to irrigate the eye first.

8. 3
Rationale: If the nurse notes the presence of bright red drainage on the dressing, it must be reported to the registered nurse because this can indicate hemorrhage. Options 1, 2, and 4 will delay necessary treatment.
Test-Taking Strategy: Note the subject, enucleation. Bright red drainage indicates active bleeding. The registered nurse needs to be notified if this type of drainage occurs.

9. 1
Rationale: For an adult, the nurse tilts the client's head slightly away and pulls the pinna up and back. Asking the client to stand and lean to one side is inappropriate and unsafe.
Test-Taking Strategy: Focus on the subject, administering eardrops. Note that the question addresses an adult client. Use basic knowledge regarding the administration of ear medications in selecting the correct option. In the adult, the pinna is pulled up and back.

10. 3
Rationale: It is important to speak in a normal tone to the client with impaired hearing and avoid shouting. The nurse would talk directly to the client while facing the client and would speak clearly. If the client does not seem to understand what is said, the nurse needs to express it differently. Moving closer to the client and toward the better ear may facilitate communication, but it is important to avoid talking directly into the impaired ear.
Test-Taking Strategy: Focus on the subject, effective communication techniques for the hearing impaired. Knowledge regarding effective communication techniques for the hearing impaired is required to answer this question. Thinking about the effect of each action identified in the options will direct you to the correct option.

11. 4
Rationale: Insects are killed before removal unless they can be coaxed out by a flashlight or a humming noise. Mineral oil or diluted alcohol is instilled into the ear to suffocate the insect, which is then removed by using ear forceps. When the foreign object is vegetable matter, irrigation would not be used because this material expands with hydration and the impaction becomes worse. Options 1, 2, and 3 may be prescribed

after the initial treatment if necessary and if inflammation or infection is a concern.
Test-Taking Strategy: Use knowledge regarding care of the client with a foreign body in the ear to answer this question. Note the strategic word, *initial*. Remember, insects are killed before removal with mineral oil or diluted alcohol.

12. 4
Rationale: Presbycusis is a type of hearing loss that occurs with aging. It is a gradual sensorineural loss caused by nerve degeneration in the inner ear or auditory nerve. Options 1, 2, and 3 are not accurate descriptions.
Test-Taking Strategy: Focus on the subject, presbycusis. Knowledge regarding the description of presbycusis is required to answer this question. Remember, presbycusis is a sensorineural hearing loss that occurs with aging.

13. 3
Rationale: The nurse instructs the client to make slow head movements to prevent worsening of the vertigo. Dietary changes such as salt and fluid restrictions that reduce the amount of endolymphatic fluid are sometimes prescribed. Watching television can increase the vertigo.
Test-Taking Strategy: Identify the subject of the question, *severe vertigo*. Note the relation between severe vertigo and the correct option, avoiding sudden head movements.

14. 2
Rationale: Dietary changes such as salt and fluid restrictions that reduce the amount of endolymphatic fluid are sometimes prescribed. Options 1, 3, and 4 are not specific dietary prescriptions for this condition.
Test-Taking Strategy: Note the strategic words, *most likely* and focus on the subject, Ménière's disease. Recalling the pathophysiology related to Ménière's disease will direct you to the correct option.

15. 1
Rationale: Hypertension, cardiovascular disease, diabetes mellitus, and obesity are associated with the development of glaucoma. Smoking, ingestion of caffeine or large amounts of alcohol, illicit drugs, corticosteroids, altered hormone levels, posture, and eye movements may cause varying transient increases in intraocular pressure.
Test-Taking Strategy: Focus on the subject, glaucoma. Use knowledge regarding the risk factors associated with glaucoma to answer this question. Remember, cardiovascular disease is associated with the development of glaucoma.

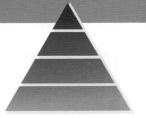

CHAPTER 54

Eye and Ear Medications

PRIORITY CONCEPTS Safety; Sensory Perception

WHAT WOULD YOU DO?

A client who requires the instillation of eyedrops three times daily tells the nurse that he lives alone and is concerned about the ability to administer the drops because his hands are shaky. What would the nurse do?

Answer is located on p. 762.

I. Ophthalmic Medication Administration

A. Guidelines for the use of eye medications
1. Eye medications are usually in the form of drops or ointments.
2. To prevent overflow of medication into the nasal and pharyngeal passages, thus reducing systemic absorption, the client is instructed to apply pressure over the inner canthus next to the nose for 30 to 60 seconds after administration of the medication. The client is instructed to close the eye gently to help distribute the medication (Fig. 54.1).
3. If both an eyedrop and an eye ointment are scheduled to be administered at the same time, the eyedrop is administered first.
4. Hands must be washed and gloves donned before administering eye medications to avoid contaminating the eye or medication dropper or applicator.
5. A separate bottle or tube of medication is used for each client to avoid accidental cross-contamination.
6. The prescribed dose of eye medication is placed in the lower conjunctival sac, never directly onto the cornea.
7. Touching any part of the eye with the dropper or applicator is avoided.
8. Glucocorticoid preparations are administered before other medications.
9. Monitor the pulse of the client receiving an ophthalmic β-blocker. The client is instructed to do the same. The nurse needs to obtain pulse parameters from the primary health care provider (PHCP).
10. Reinforce instructions to the client on how to instill medication correctly, and instillation would be supervised until he or she can do it safely; adaptive devices that position the bottle of eyedrops directly over the eye can also be purchased if instillation is difficult for the client.
11. Reinforce instructions to the client to read the medication labels carefully to ensure administration of the correct medication and correct strength.
12. The client is reminded to keep these medications out of the reach of children.
13. Reinforce instructions to the client to avoid driving or operating hazardous equipment if vision is blurred.
14. The client is informed that he or she may be unable to drive home after an eye examination where a medication to dilate the pupil (mydriatic) or to paralyze the ciliary muscle (cycloplegic) is used.
15. If photophobia occurs, the client is instructed to wear sunglasses and avoid bright lights.
16. Reinforce instructions to the client to administer a missed dose of the eye medication as soon as it is remembered, unless the next dose is scheduled to be administered in 1 to 2 hours.
17. The client with glaucoma is informed that the disorder cannot be cured, only controlled.
18. Reinforce the importance of using medications to treat glaucoma as prescribed and not to discontinue these medications without consulting the PHCP.
19. The client is informed that medications used to treat glaucoma may cause pain and blurred vision, especially when therapy is begun.
20. Reinforce instructions to the client to report the development of any eye irritation.
21. The client using eye gel is instructed to store the gel at room temperature or in the refrigerator but not to freeze it.
22. Reinforce instructions to the client to discard unused eye gel kept at room temperature as recommended by the PHCP and/or the pharmacist.
23. The client is informed that soft contact lenses may absorb certain eye medications and that preserva-

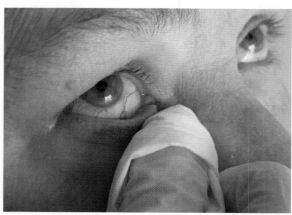

FIGURE 54.1 Applying punctual occlusion to prevent systemic absorption of eyedrops. (From Ignatavicius, Workman, 2018)

tives in eye medications may discolor the contact lenses.

24. The client wearing contact lenses is advised to question the PHCP carefully about special precautions to observe with eye medications.

25. Reinforce instructions to the parents to keep a record of the infant's bowel movements if atropine sulfate eyedrops are being administered as the medication may cause constipation.

26. Bowel sounds of the infant or child receiving atropine sulfate eyedrops are auscultated.

 Because the timing of medication administration is critical, administer eye medications at precise intervals as prescribed; separate the instillation by 3 to 5 minutes if two medications need to be administered at the same time.

B. Instillation of eye medications
  1. Drops
    a. Wash hands.
    b. Put on gloves.
    c. Check the name, strength, and expiration date of the medication.
    d. Instruct the client to tilt the head backward, open the eyes, and look up.
    e. Pull the lower lid down against the cheekbone.
    f. Hold the bottle like a pencil with the tip downward.
    g. Holding the bottle gently rest the wrist of the hand on the client's cheek.
    h. Squeeze the bottle gently to allow the drop to fall into the conjunctival sac.
    i. Reinforce instructions to the client to close the eyes gently and not to squeeze the eyes shut.
    j. Wait 3 to 5 minutes before instilling another drop, if more than one drop is prescribed, to promote maximal absorption of the medication.
    k. Do not allow the medication bottle, dropper, or applicator to come in contact with the eyelid or conjunctival sac.

BOX 54.1   **Mydriatic, Cycloplegic, and Anticholinergic Medications**

- Atropine
- Cyclopentolate
- Homatropine
- Phenylephrine
- Tropicamide

---

    l. To prevent systemic absorption of the medication, apply gentle pressure with a clean tissue to the client's nasolacrimal duct for 30 to 60 seconds (see Fig. 54.1).

  2. Ointments
    a. Reinforce instructions to the client to lie down or tilt head backward and look up.
    b. Hold the ointment tube near but not touching the eye or eyelashes. This action prevents the spread of contaminants from one eye to the other.
    c. Squeeze a thin ribbon of ointment along the lining of the lower conjunctival sac from the inner to the outer canthus.
    d. Reinforce instructions to the client to close the eyes gently, rolling the eyeball in all directions (which increases the contact area of medication to eye).
    e. Reinforce instructions to the client that vision may be blurred by the ointment.
    f. If possible, apply ointment just before bedtime.

II. Mydriatic-Cycloplegic and Anticholinergic Medications (Box 54.1)

A. Description
  1. Mydriatics and cycloplegics dilate the pupils (**mydriasis**) and relax the ciliary muscles (**cycloplegia**).
  2. Anticholinergics block responses of the sphincter muscle in the ciliary body producing mydriasis and cycloplegia.
  3. These medications are used preoperatively or for eye examinations to produce mydriasis.
  4. Mydriatics are contraindicated in glaucoma, cardiac dysrhythmia, and cerebral atherosclerosis and need to be used with caution in the older client and in those with prostatic hypertrophy, diabetes mellitus, or parkinsonism.

B. Side and adverse effects
  1. Tachycardia
  2. Photophobia
  3. Conjunctivitis
  4. Dermatitis
  5. Elevated blood pressure

C. Atropine toxicity
  1. Dry mouth
  2. Blurred vision
  3. Photophobia

4. Tachycardia
5. Fever
6. Urinary retention
7. Constipation
8. Headache, brow pain
9. Confusion
10. Hallucinations, delirium
11. Coma
12. Worsening of glaucoma
D. Systemic reactions to anticholinergics
   1. Dry mouth and skin
   2. Fever
   3. Thirst
   4. Confusion
   5. Hyperactivity
E. Interventions
   1. Monitor for allergic response.
   2. Determine risk for injury.
   3. Check for constipation and urinary retention.
   4. Reinforce instructions to the client that a burning sensation may occur during instillation.
   5. Reinforce instructions to the client not to drive or perform hazardous activities for 24 hours after instillation of the medication unless otherwise directed by the PHCP.
   6. Reinforce instructions to the client to wear sunglasses until the effects of the medication wear off.
   7. Reinforce instructions to the client to notify the PHCP if blurring of vision, loss of sight, difficulty breathing, sweating, or flushing occurs.
   8. Reinforce instructions to the client to report eye pain to the PHCP.

⚠ Mydriatics are contraindicated in clients with glaucoma because of the risk of increased intraocular pressure.

III. Anti-infective Eye Medications (Box 54.2)

A. Description: Anti-infective medications kill or inhibit the growth of bacteria, fungi, and viruses.
B. Side and adverse effects
   1. Superinfection
   2. Global irritation
C. Interventions
   1. Determine risk for injury.
   2. Reinforce instructions to the client on how to apply the eye medication. The client is reminded to clean exudates from the eyes before administering the medication.
   3. The importance of completing the prescribed medication regimen is reinforced.
   4. Reinforce instructions to the client to wash the hands thoroughly and frequently.
   5. The client is advised that if improvement does not occur to notify the PHCP.

IV. Anti-inflammatory Eye Medications (Box 54.3)
A. Description
   1. Anti-inflammatory medications control inflammation, thereby reducing vision loss and scarring.
   2. Anti-inflammatory medications are used for uveitis, allergic conditions, and inflammation of the conjunctiva, cornea, and lids.

BOX 54.2   Anti-Infective Eye Medications

Antibacterials
- Bacitracin
- Chloramphenicol
- Erythromycin
- Moxifloxacin
- Ofloxacin

Aminoglycosides
- Gentamicin sulfate
- Tobramycin

Antifungal
- Natamycin

Antivirals
- Ganciclovir
- Trifluridine

Sulfonamide
- Sulfacetamide

BOX 54.3   Anti-Inflammatory Eye Medications

Corticosteroids
- Dexamethasone
- Difluprednate
- Fluocinolone
- Fluorometholone; sulfacetamide
- Loteprednol etabonate
- Prednisolone, gentamicin
- Triamcinolone

Ophthalmic Immunosuppressant and Anti-inflammatory Agent
- Cyclosporine

Nonsteroidal Anti-inflammatory Agents
- Bromfenac
- Diclofenac
- Flurbiprofen sodium
- Ketorolac tromethamine
- Nepafenac

Mast Cell Stabilizers
- Azelastine hydrochloride
- Cromolyn sodium
- Epinastine
- Ketotifen fumarate
- Nedocromil sodium
- Olopatadine hydrochloride

BOX 54.4   Eye Lubricants

- Carboxymethylcellulose
- Hydroxypropyl methylcellulose
- Petroleum-based ointment
- Polyvinyl alcohol

B. Side and adverse effects
1. Cataracts
2. Increased intraocular pressure
3. Impaired healing
4. Masking signs/symptoms of infection

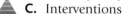 **C. Interventions**
1. Interventions are the same as for anti-infective medications.
2. Note that dexamethasone would not be used for eye abrasions and wounds.

V. Topical Eye Anesthetics

A. Description
1. Topical anesthetics produce corneal anesthesia.
2. Topical anesthetics are used for anesthesia for eye examinations and surgery or to remove foreign bodies from the eye.
3. Do not use discolored solution and store the bottle tightly closed.
4. An example is tetracaine.

B. Side and adverse effects
1. Temporary stinging or burning of the eye
2. Temporary loss of corneal reflex

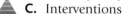 **C. Interventions**
1. Determine risk for injury.
2. Note that these medications would not be given to the client for home use and are not to be self-administered by the client.
3. The client is instructed not to rub or touch the eye while it is anesthetized.
4. Note that the blink reflex is lost temporarily and that the corneal epithelium must be protected.
5. An eye patch is provided to protect the eye from injury until the corneal reflex returns.

VI. Eye Lubricants (Box 54.4)

A. Description
1. Replace tears or add moisture to the eyes.
2. Moisten contact lenses or an artificial eye and protect the eyes during surgery or diagnostic procedures.
3. Used for keratitis, during anesthesia, or for a disorder that results in unconsciousness or decreased blinking

B. Side and adverse effects
1. Burning during instillation
2. Discomfort or pain during instillation
3. Allergic reaction

BOX 54.5   Medications to Treat Glaucoma

Miotics
- Carbachol
- Echothiophate
- Pilocarpine hydrochloride

β-Adrenergic Blocking Eye Medications
- Betaxolol hydrochloride
- Carteolol hydrochloride
- Levobunolol hydrochloride
- Metipranolol
- Timolol maleate

α-Adrenergic Agonists
- Apraclonidine
- Brimonidine

Prostaglandin Analogs
- Latanoprost
- Tafluprost
- Travoprost
- Bimatoprost

Cholinergic Agonists
- Carbachol
- Pilocarpine hydrochloride
- Echothiophate iodide

Carbonic Anhydrase Inhibitors
- Dorzolamide
- Brinzolamide

Rho Kinase Inhibitor
- Netarsudil

C. Interventions
1. The client is informed that burning may occur on instillation.
2. Be alert to allergic responses to the preservatives in the lubricants.

VII. Medications to Treat Glaucoma (Box 54.5)

A. Description
1. These medications reduce intraocular pressure by constricting the pupil and contracting the ciliary muscle, thereby increasing the blood flow to the retina and decreasing retinal damage and loss of vision.
2. These medications open the anterior chamber angle and increase the outflow of aqueous humor.
3. Some may be used to achieve miosis during eye surgery.
4. Contraindicated in clients with retinal detachment, adhesions between the iris and lens, or inflammatory diseases.
5. Used with caution in clients with asthma, hypertension, corneal abrasion, hyperthyroidism, coronary vascular disease, urinary tract obstruction, gastrointestinal obstruction, ulcer disease, parkinsonism, and bradycardia.

B. Side effects
1. Myopia
2. Headache
3. Eye pain
4. Decreased vision in poor light
5. Local irritation
6. Adverse effects
   a. Flushing
   b. Diaphoresis
   c. Gastrointestinal upset and diarrhea
   d. Frequent urination
   e. Increased salivation
   f. Muscle weakness
   g. Respiratory difficulty
7. Toxicity
   a. Vertigo and syncope
   b. Bradycardia and cardiac dysrhythmia
   c. Hypotension
   d. Tremors
   e. Seizure

C. Interventions
1. Monitor vital signs.
2. Determine risk for injury.
3. Monitor the client for degree of diminished vision.
4. Monitor for side and adverse effects and toxic effects.
5. Monitor for postural hypotension, and instruct the client to change positions slowly.
6. Check breath sounds for wheezes and rhonchi because some medications can cause bronchospasms and increased bronchial secretions.
7. Maintain oral hygiene because of the increase in salivation.
8. Have atropine sulfate available as an antidote for pilocarpine.
9. The client or family is instructed regarding the correct administration of eye medications.
10. Reinforce instructions to the client about not stopping the medication suddenly.
11. Reinforce instructions to the client to avoid activities such as driving while vision is impaired.

⚠️ The client with glaucoma is instructed to read labels on over-the-counter medications and avoid atropine-like medications because atropine increases intraocular pressure.

VIII. β-Adrenergic Blocker Eye Medications (see Box 54.5)

A. Description
1. These medications reduce intraocular pressure by decreasing sympathetic impulses and decreasing aqueous humor production without affecting accommodation or pupil size.
2. Are used to treat glaucoma
3. Are contraindicated for a client with asthma or chronic obstructive pulmonary disease because

systemic absorption can cause increased airway resistance
4. Are used with caution in the client receiving oral β-blockers

B. Side and adverse effects
1. Ocular irritation
2. Visual disturbance
3. Bradycardia
4. Hypotension
5. Bronchospasm

C. Interventions
1. Monitor vital signs, especially blood pressure and pulse, before administering medication.
2. Usually, if the pulse is 60 beats/min or less, or if the systolic blood pressure is less than 90 mm Hg, the medication is withheld and the registered nurse (RN) and PHCP are contacted. The nurse needs to obtain pulse parameters from the PHCP for clients receiving ophthalmic β-blockers.
3. The client is instructed to notify the PHCP if shortness of breath occurs.
4. Risk of injury and intake and output is monitored.
5. Reinforce instructions to the client not to discontinue the medication abruptly.
6. Reinforce instructions to the client to change positions slowly because of the potential for orthostatic hypotension.
7. Reinforce instructions to the client to avoid hazardous activities.
8. Reinforce instructions to the client to avoid over-the-counter medications without the PHCP's approval.
9. Clients with diabetes mellitus using β-adrenergic blockers are instructed to monitor their blood glucose levels frequently.

IX. Carbonic Anhydrase Inhibitors (see Box 54.5)

A. Description
1. Carbonic anhydrase inhibitors interfere with the production of carbonic acid, which leads to decreased aqueous humor formation and decreased intraocular pressure.
2. These medications are used for long-term treatment of glaucoma.
3. These medications are contraindicated in the client allergic to sulfonamides.
4. Used with caution for clients with severe renal or liver disease

B. Side and adverse effects
1. Appetite loss
2. Gastrointestinal upset
3. Paresthesia of the fingers, toes, and face
4. Polyuria
5. Hypokalemia
6. Renal calculi
7. Photosensitivity
8. Lethargy and drowsiness
9. Depression

C. Interventions
1. Monitor vital signs.
2. Check visual acuity.
3. Determine risk for injury.
4. Monitor intake and output.
5. Monitor weight.
6. Maintain oral hygiene.
7. Monitor for side effects such as lethargy, anorexia, drowsiness, polyuria, nausea, and vomiting.
8. Monitor electrolyte levels for hypokalemia.
9. Fluid intake is increased unless contraindicated.
10. The client is advised to avoid prolonged exposure to sunlight.
11. The use of artificial tears for dry eyes is encouraged.
12. Reinforce instructions to the client not to discontinue the medication abruptly.
13. Reinforce instructions to the client to avoid hazardous activities while vision is impaired.
14. Reinforce instructions to the client not to wear contact lenses during or within 15 minutes of instilling these medications.

X. Ocusert System

A. Description
1. A thin eye wafer (disk) is impregnated with a time-release dose of pilocarpine.
2. The Ocusert system was devised to overcome the frequent application of pilocarpine.
3. It is placed in the upper or lower cul-de-sac of the eye.
4. The pilocarpine is released over 1 week.
5. The disk is replaced every 7 days.
6. Drawbacks of its use include sudden leakage of pilocarpine, migration of the system over the cornea, and unnoticed loss of the system.

B. Interventions
1. Determine the client's ability to insert the medication disk.
2. Store the medication in the refrigerator.
3. Reinforce instructions to the client to discard damaged or contaminated disks.
4. The client is informed that temporary stinging is expected but to notify the PHCP if blurred vision or brow pain occurs.
5. Reinforce instructions to the client to check for the presence of the disk in the upper and lower cul-de-sac daily, at bedtime, and on arising.
6. Because vision may change in the first few hours after the eye system is inserted, the client is instructed to replace the disk at bedtime.

XI. Osmotic Medications

A. Mannitol
B. Description
1. Lower intraocular pressure
2. Used for the emergency treatment of glaucoma
3. Used preoperatively and postoperatively to decrease vitreous humor volume

C. Side and adverse effects
1. Headache
2. Nausea, vomiting, diarrhea, dehydration
3. Disorientation
4. Electrolyte imbalances
D. Interventions
1. Monitor vital signs.
2. Check visual acuity.
3. Determine risk for injury.
4. Monitor intake and output.
5. Monitor weight.
6. Monitor for electrolyte imbalances.
7. Increase fluid intake unless contraindicated.
8. Monitor for change in level of orientation.

XII. Medications to Treat Macular Degeneration

A. Pegaptanib, ranibizumab, bevacizumab, aflibercept, and verteporfin
B. Description
1. Age-related macular degeneration (ARMD) can be either dry ARMD (atrophic) or wet ARMD (neovascular).
2. Dry ARMD is more common; macular photoreceptors undergo gradual breakdown leading to gradual blurring of central vision.
3. Wet ARMD progresses faster, and macular degeneration is caused by the growth of new subretinal blood vessels, which leads to fluid leakage that lifts the macula and causes permanent injury.
4. Characterized by the presence of drusen (yellow deposits under the retina)
C. Side and adverse effects
1. Endophthalmitis (eye inflammation caused by bacterial, viral, or fungal infection)
2. Blurred vision
3. Cataracts
4. Corneal edema
5. Eye discomfort and discharge
6. Conjunctival hemorrhage
7. Increased intraocular pressure
8. Reduced visual acuity
D. Interventions
1. Reinforce teaching the client about administration of the medications.
2. Reinforce teaching the client about the side effects and the need to notify the PHCP.

XIII. Otic Medication Administration

A. Instillation of ear drops
1. In an adult, pull the pinna up and back to straighten the external canal to instill ear drops.
2. Tilt the client's head in the opposite direction of the affected ear and apply the drops into the ear.
3. With the head tilted, gently move the head back and forth five times.
4. Pull the pinna down and back for infants and children younger than 3 years, up and back for older children.

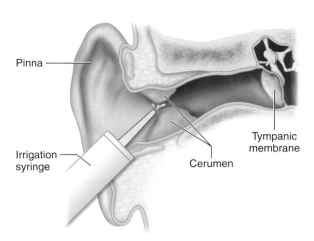

Pinna

Irrigation syringe

Cerumen

Tympanic membrane

FIGURE 54.2 Irrigation of the external canal. Cerumen and debris can be removed from the ear by irrigation with warm water. The stream of water is aimed above or below the impaction to allow back pressure to push it out rather than further down the canal.

 B. Irrigation of the ear (Fig. 54.2)
1. Irrigation of the ear needs to be prescribed by the PHCP.
2. Ensure direct visualization of the tympanic membrane.
3. Warm irrigating solution to 98°F (37.0°C), because solution temperature not close to the client's body temperature will cause ear injury, nausea, vertigo, and nystagmus.
4. Irrigation needs to be done gently to avoid damage to the eardrum.
5. When irrigating, to prevent injury, do not direct irrigation solution directly toward the eardrum but rather toward the wall of the ear canal. In addition, to remove cerumen the solution is directed above or below the impaction toward the wall of the canal to allow back pressure to push the impaction out.
6. During irrigation, the client would be positioned with the ear to be irrigated facing up. Fall precautions must be instituted because the client may get dizzy and an emesis basin needs to be available because vomiting can occur.
C. Systemic medications that affect hearing (Box 54.6)

⚠ If a perforation of the eardrum is suspected, do not perform ear irrigation.

XIV. Anti-infective Ear Medications (Box 54.7)
A. Description
1. Anti-infective medications kill or inhibit the growth of bacteria and are used for otitis media or otitis externa.
2. Anti-infective medications are contraindicated if a prior hypersensitivity exists.
 B. Side and adverse effect: Overgrowth of nonsusceptible organisms

---

BOX 54.6   Medications That Affect Hearing

Antibiotics
- Amikacin
- Chloramphenicol
- Erythromycin
- Gentamicin
- Neomycin
- Streptomycin sulfate
- Tetracycline
- Tobramycin sulfate
- Vancomycin

Diuretics
- Ethacrynic acid
- Furosemide

Others
- Amitriptyline
- Aspirin
- Bleomycin
- Chloroquine
- Cisplatin
- Ibuprofen
- Naproxen
- Nitrogen mustard
- Quinine
- Quinidine
- Sildenafil

BOX 54.7   Anti-Infective Ear Medications

- Acetic acid; aluminum acetate
- Amoxicillin
- Ampicillin
- Cefaclor
- Chloramphenicol
- Ciprofloxacin
- Clarithromycin
- Clindamycin
- Erythromycin
- Gentamicin sulfate otic solution
- Ofloxacin
- Penicillin V potassium
- Trimethoprim; sulfamethoxazole

C. Interventions
1. Monitor vital signs.
2. Check for allergies.
3. Monitor for pain.
4. Monitor for signs of secondary infection.
5. Reinforce instructing the client to report dizziness, fatigue, fever, or sore throat, which may indicate a superimposed infection.
6. Reinforce instructing the client to complete the entire course of the medication.
7. Reinforce instructing the client to keep ear canals dry.

BOX 54.8	Antihistamines and Decongestants

- Brompheniramine
- Cetirizine
- Chlorpheniramine
- Levocetirizine
- Loratadine
- Diphenhydramine
- Fexofenadine
- Phenylephrine
- Pseudoephedrine

XV. Antihistamines and Decongestants (Box 54.8)

A. Description
  1. Produce vasoconstriction.
  2. Stimulate the receptors of the respiratory mucosa.
  3. Reduce respiratory tissue hyperemia and edema to open obstructed eustachian tubes.
  4. These medications may be used for acute otitis media.

B. Side and adverse effects
  1. Drowsiness
  2. Blurred vision
  3. Dry mucous membranes

C. Interventions
  1. The client is informed that drowsiness, blurred vision, and a dry mouth may occur.
  2. Reinforce instructing the client to increase fluid intake unless contraindicated and suck on hard candy to alleviate the dry mouth.
  3. Reinforce instructing the client to avoid hazardous activities if drowsiness occurs.
  4. Reinforce instructions for the client with hypertension to consult the PHCP before the use of these medications.

XVI. Cerumenolytic Medications

A. Carbamide peroxide

B. Description
  1. Emulsify and loosen cerumen deposits
  2. Used to loosen and remove impacted wax from the ear canal

C. Side and adverse effects
  1. Irritation
  2. Redness or swelling of the ear canal

D. Interventions
  1. Reinforce instructing the client not to use drops more often than prescribed.
  2. A cotton plug is moistened with medication before insertion and insert the cotton plug after instilling the ear drops.
  3. Keep the container tightly closed and away from moisture.
  4. Touching the ear with the dropper is avoided.
  5. Thirty minutes after instillation, the ear is gently irrigated as prescribed with warm water, using a soft rubber bulb ear syringe.

  6. Irrigation may be done with hydrogen peroxide solution as prescribed to flush cerumen deposits out of the ear canal.
  7. For a chronic cerumen impaction, one or two drops of mineral oil (if prescribed) will soften the wax.
  8. Reinforce instructing the client to notify the PHCP if redness, pain, or swelling persists.

WHAT WOULD YOU DO?

Answer: If the client lives alone and has a physical condition that may affect instilling the eyedrops, the clinic nurse would assist with the arrangement of a homecare nurse to assess the client and the home situation. If the client is unable to instill eyedrops independently, a friend, neighbor, or family member can be taught the technique if possible. In addition, adaptive equipment that positions the bottle of eyedrops directly over the eye can be purchased and used by the client who has difficulty instilling eyedrops.

PRACTICE QUESTIONS

1. Betaxolol hydrochloride eyedrops have been prescribed for the client with glaucoma. Which nursing action is **most appropriate** related to monitoring for the side/adverse effects of this medication?
  1. Monitoring temperature
  2. Monitoring blood pressure
  3. Checking peripheral pulses
  4. Checking the blood glucose level

2. The nurse assists with preparing the client for ear irrigation as prescribed by the primary health care provider (PHCP). Which action would the nurse plan to take?
  1. Warm the irrigating solution to 98°F (36.6°C).
  2. Position the client with the affected side up after the irrigation.
  3. Direct a slow, steady stream of irrigation solution toward the eardrum.
  4. Assist the client with turning his or her head so that the ear to be irrigated is facing upward.

3. In preparation for cataract surgery, the nurse is to administer cyclopentolate eyedrops. The nurse administers the eyedrops knowing that which is the purpose of this medication?
  1. To produce miosis of the operative eye
  2. To dilate the pupil of the operative eye
  3. To constrict the pupil of the operative eye
  4. To provide lubrication to the operative eye

4. The nurse is providing instructions to a client who will be self-administering eyedrops. To minimize the systemic effects that eyedrops can produce, the client is instructed to perform which action?
   1. Eat before instilling the drops.
   2. Swallow several times after instilling the drops.
   3. Blink vigorously to encourage tearing after instilling the drops.
   4. Occlude the nasolacrimal duct with a finger over the inner canthus for 30 to 60 seconds after instilling the drops.

5. The client is receiving an eyedrop and an eye ointment to the right eye. Which action would the nurse take?
   1. Administer the eyedrop first, followed by the eye ointment.
   2. Administer the eye ointment first, followed by the eyedrop.
   3. Administer the eyedrop, wait 10 minutes, and administer the eye ointment.
   4. Administer the eye ointment, wait 10 minutes, and administer the eyedrop.

6. The nurse is caring for a client with glaucoma. Which medication prescribed for the client would the nurse question?
   1. Betaxolol
   2. Pilocarpine
   3. Atropine sulfate
   4. Pilocarpine hydrochloride

❖ 7. The nurse is preparing to administer eyedrops. Which interventions would the nurse take to administer the drops? **Select all that apply.**
   - ☐ 1. Wash hands.
   - ☐ 2. Put on gloves.
   - ☐ 3. Place the drop in the conjunctival sac.
   - ☐ 4. Pull the lower lid down against the cheekbone.
   - ☐ 5. Instruct the client to squeeze the eyes shut after instilling the eyedrop.
   - ☐ 6. Instruct the client to tilt the head forward, open the eyes, and look down.

8. A client was just admitted to the hospital to rule out a gastrointestinal bleed. The client has brought several bottles of medications prescribed by different specialists. During the admission assessment, the client states, "Lately, I have been hearing some roaring sounds in my ears, especially when I am alone." Which medication would the nurse determine to be the cause of the client's complaint?
   1. Doxycycline
   2. Atropine sulfate
   3. Acetylsalicylic acid
   4. Diltiazem hydrochloride

9. Pilocarpine hydrochloride is prescribed for the client with glaucoma. Which medication would the nurse plan to have available in the event of systemic toxicity?
   1. Metipranolol
   2. Atropine sulfate
   3. Timolol maleate
   4. Carteolol hydrochloride

10. A miotic medication has been prescribed for the client with glaucoma. The client asks the nurse about the purpose of the medication. The nurse would tell the client which purpose?
   1. "The medication will help dilate the eye to prevent an increase in eye pressure."
   2. "The medication will relax the muscles of the eyes and prevent blurred vision."
   3. "The medication causes the pupil to constrict and will lower the pressure in the eye."
   4. "The medication will help block the responses that are sent to the muscles in the eye."

ANSWERS

1. 2
Rationale: Hypotension, dizziness, nausea, diaphoresis, headache, fatigue, constipation, and diarrhea are systemic effects of the medication. Nursing interventions include monitoring the blood pressure for hypotension and assessing the pulse for strength, weakness, irregular rate, and bradycardia. Options 1, 3, and 4 are not specifically associated with this medication.
Test-Taking Strategy: Note the strategic words, *most appropriate*. Use the ABCs—airway, breathing, and circulation—to direct you to the correct option. Although option 3, peripheral pulses, is also related to circulation monitoring, the blood pressure is the umbrella option.

2. 1
Rationale: Irrigation solutions that are not close to the client's body temperature can be uncomfortable and may cause injury, nausea, and vertigo. The client is positioned so that the ear to be irrigated is facing downward because this allows gravity to assist with the removal of the ear wax and solution. After the irrigation, the client is to lie on the affected side to finish draining the irrigating solution. A slow, steady stream of solution needs to be directed toward the upper wall of the ear canal and not toward the eardrum. Too much force could cause the tympanic membrane to rupture.
Test-Taking Strategy: Focus on the subject, ear irrigations. Read each option carefully and remember that the nurse's concern is to prevent damage to the tympanic membrane. In addition,

remember that the client needs to be positioned with the affected side downward to allow drainage of the irrigation solution.

3. 2
Rationale: Cyclopentolate is a rapidly acting mydriatic and cycloplegic medication. Cyclopentolate is effective in 25 to 75 minutes, and accommodation returns in 6 to 24 hours. Cyclopentolate is used for preoperative mydriasis.
Test-Taking Strategy: Options 1 and 4 are comparable or alike and are eliminated first. Miosis refers to a constricted pupil. Note that the question identifies a client being prepared for eye surgery. The pupil would need to be dilated for the surgical procedure.

4. 4
Rationale: Applying pressure on the nasolacrimal duct prevents systemic absorption of the medication. Options 1, 2, and 3 will not prevent systemic absorption.
Test-Taking Strategy: Focus on the subject, administration of eyedrops. Eating and swallowing are comparable or alike and are not related to the systemic absorption of an eye medication. Blinking vigorously to produce tearing may result in the loss of the administered medication.

5. 1
Rationale: When an eyedrop and an eye ointment are scheduled to be administered at the same time, the eyedrop is administered first. Options 2, 3, and 4 are incorrect.
Test-Taking Strategy: Focus on the subject, administration of eyedrops and eye ointments. Recalling the guidelines for administering eye medications will direct you to the correct option.

6. 3
Rationale: Options 1, 2, and 4 are miotic agents used to treat glaucoma. Option 3 is a mydriatic and cycloplegic medication, and its use is contraindicated in clients with glaucoma. Mydriatic medications dilate the pupil and can cause an increase in intraocular pressure in the eye.
Test-Taking Strategy: Focus on the subject, glaucoma. Knowledge regarding the classifications of the medications identified in the options will assist in answering the question. Remember that mydriatics dilate and that these medications are contraindicated in glaucoma.

❖ 7. 1, 2, 3, 4
Rationale: To administer eye medications, the nurse would wash hands and put on gloves. The client is instructed to tilt the head backward, open the eyes, and look up. The nurse pulls the lower lid down against the cheekbone and holds the bottle like a pencil, with the tip downward. Holding the bot-
tle, the nurse gently rests the wrist of the hand on the client's cheek and squeezes the bottle gently to allow the drop to fall into the conjunctival sac. The client is instructed to close the eyes gently and not to squeeze the eyes shut to prevent the loss of medication.
Test-Taking Strategy: Focus on the subject, administering eyedrops. Use guidelines related to standard precautions and visualize this procedure. This will assist in determining the correct interventions.

8. 3
Rationale: Aspirin is contraindicated for gastrointestinal bleeding and is potentially ototoxic. The client would be advised to notify the prescribing primary health care provider so that the medication can be discontinued and/or a substitute that is less toxic to the ear can be taken instead. Options 1, 2, and 4 do not have side effects that are potentially associated with hearing difficulties.
Test-Taking Strategy: Focus on the subject, the client's complaint. Review the classifications and/or therapeutic effects, as well as the side/adverse effects, of each medication in the options. Of the medications identified, only aspirin can cause ototoxicity. In addition, it is contraindicated for a gastrointestinal bleed.

9. 2
Rationale: Systemic absorption of pilocarpine hydrochloride can produce toxicity and includes manifestations of vertigo, bradycardia, tremors, hypotension, and seizure. Atropine sulfate needs to be available in the event of systemic toxicity. Pindolol, timolol maleate, and carteolol hydrochloride are β-blockers.
Test-Taking Strategy: Note that options 1, 3, and 4 are comparable or alike and are β-blockers. Also, remember that atropine sulfate is the antidote for systemic reactions that occur with pilocarpine hydrochloride.

10. 3
Rationale: Miotics cause pupillary constriction and are used to treat glaucoma. They lower the intraocular pressure, thereby increasing blood flow to the retina and decreasing retinal damage and loss of vision. Miotics cause a contraction of the ciliary muscle and a widening of the trabecular meshwork. Options 1, 2, and 4 are incorrect.
Test-Taking Strategy: Focus on the subject, miotic medication. Note that the client has glaucoma. Recall that prevention of increased intraocular pressure is the goal in the client with glaucoma. Options 1, 2, and 4 describe actions related to mydriatic medications, which primarily dilate the pupils and relax the ciliary muscles.

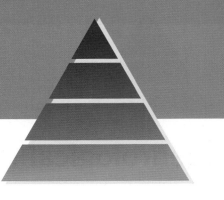

UNIT XVI

Neurological Problems of the Adult Client

 ## Pyramid to Success

Pyramid Points related to neurological health problems focus on nursing care and monitoring for increased intracranial pressure, monitoring level of consciousness, positioning clients, head injuries, spinal cord injuries, spinal shock, autonomic dysreflexia, interventions during a seizure, stroke, Parkinson's disease, and myasthenia gravis. Safety is a priority concern. Pyramid points also focus on immediate interventions for a victim who sustains a neurological injury and immediate interventions if a neurological complication occurs. Focus on the points related to psychosocial effects as a result of neurological problem, such as anxiety, unexpected body image changes, and the appropriate and available support services needed for the client.

 ## Client Needs: Learning Objectives

Safe and Effective Care Environment
Acting as a client advocate
Collaborating with the interprofessional health care team
Discussing necessary referrals to appropriate services
Ensuring that informed consent for invasive procedures has been obtained
Establishing priorities
Maintaining asepsis with procedures and treatments
Maintaining standard, transmission-based, and other precautions
Preventing accidents that can occur as a result of neurological deficits
Upholding client rights

Client Needs lists modified from: National Council of State Boards of Nursing, Inc. (NCSBN). *NCLEX-PN Examination: Test Plan for the National Council Licensure Examination for Practical Nurses,* effective April 2020. Chicago: NCSBN.

Health Promotion and Maintenance
Discussing expected and unexpected body image changes resulting from neurological deficits
Performing neurological data collection using various techniques
Preventing and detecting health problems associated with neurological deficits
Reinforcing homecare instructions regarding care related to the neurological disorder
Teaching about the importance of prescribed therapy

Psychosocial Integrity
Addressing grief and loss issues
Considering the cultural, religious, and spiritual influences of the client when planning care
Determining the client's ability to cope with feelings of isolation and loss of independence
Identifying sensory and perceptual alterations
Identifying support systems and encouraging the use of community resources
Mobilizing coping mechanisms

Physiological Integrity
Administering pharmacological therapy
Maintaining nutrition
Monitoring for alterations in body systems
Monitoring for complications related to treatments and procedures
Monitoring for fluid and electrolyte imbalances
Promoting normal elimination patterns
Promoting self-care measures and maintaining independence as much as is possible
Providing assistive devices for mobility
Providing emergency care
Providing measures to promote comfort

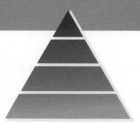

CHAPTER 55

Neurological Problems

PRIORITY CONCEPTS Functional Ability; Intracranial Regulation

WHAT WOULD YOU DO?

The nurse notes that a client who experienced a stroke is sitting in a chair and is leaning to the left with their arm caught in the side of the chair seat. The nurse suspects unilateral body neglect syndrome. What would the nurse do?
Answer is located on p. 788.

I. Anatomy and Physiology of the Brain and Spinal Cord

A. Cerebrum
1. The cerebrum consists of the right and left hemispheres.
2. Each hemisphere receives sensory information from the opposite side of the body and controls the skeletal muscles of the opposite side.
3. The cerebrum governs sensory and motor activity and thought and learning.

B. Cerebral cortex (Box 55.1)
1. The cerebral cortex is the outer gray layer and it is divided into five lobes.
2. It is responsible for the conscious activities of the cerebrum.

C. Basal ganglia: Cell bodies in white matter that help the cerebral cortex in producing smooth voluntary movements

D. Diencephalon
1. Thalamus
   a. Relays sensory impulses to the cortex
   b. Provides a pain gate
   c. Part of the reticular activating system
2. Hypothalamus
3. Regulates autonomic responses of the sympathetic and parasympathetic nervous systems
4. Regulates the stress response, sleep, appetite, body temperature, fluid balance, and emotions
5. Responsible for the production of hormones secreted by the pituitary gland and the hypothalamus

E. Brainstem
1. Midbrain
   a. Responsible for motor coordination
   b. Contains the visual reflex and auditory relay centers
2. Pons: Contains the respiratory centers and regulates breathing
3. Medulla oblongata
   a. Contains all afferent and efferent tracts and contains cardiac, respiratory, vomiting, and vasomotor centers
   b. Controls heart rate, respiration, blood vessel diameter, sneezing, swallowing, vomiting, and coughing

F. Cerebellum: Coordinates smooth muscle movement, posture, equilibrium, and muscle tone

G. Spinal cord
1. Provides neuron and synapse networks to produce involuntary responses to sensory stimulation
2. Controls body movement and regulates visceral function
3. Carries sensory information to and motor information from the brain
4. Extends from the first cervical to the second lumbar vertebra
5. Protected by the meninges, cerebrospinal fluid (CSF), and adipose tissue
6. Horns
   a. Inner column of gray matter contains two anterior and two posterior horns.
   b. Posterior horns connect with afferent (sensory) nerve fibers.
   c. Anterior horns contain efferent (motor) nerve fibers.
7. Nerve tracts
   a. White matter contains the nerve tract.
   b. Ascending tracts (sensory pathway)
   c. Descending tract (motor pathway)

H. Meninges
1. The dura mater is a tough and fibrous membrane.
2. The arachnoid membrane is a delicate membrane and contains CSF.

BOX 55.1 Cerebral Cortex

Frontal Lobe
Broca's area for speech
Motor cortex for voluntary motor function, voluntary eye movement, memory storage, morals, emotions, reasoning and judgment, concentration, and abstraction

Parietal Lobe
Interpretation of taste, pain, touch, temperature, and pressure
Spatial perception

Temporal Lobe
Auditory center
Wernicke's area for sensory and speech

Occipital Lobe
Visual area

Limbic System
Emotional and visceral patterns for survival
Learning and memory

3. The pia mater is a vascular membrane.
4. The subarachnoid space is formed by the arachnoid membrane and the pia mater.

I. Cerebrospinal fluid
  1. Secreted in the ventricles; circulates in the subarachnoid space and through the ventricles to the subarachnoid space of the meninges, where it is reabsorbed
  2. Acts as a protective cushion and aids in the exchange of nutrients and wastes
  3. Normal pressure is 50 to 175 mm H_2O.
  4. Normal volume is 125 to 150 mL.

J. Ventricles
  1. Four ventricles
  2. The ventricles communicate between the subarachnoid spaces and produce and circulate CSF.

K. Blood supply
  1. Right and left internal carotid arteries
  2. Right and left vertebral arteries
  3. These arteries supply the brain via an anastomosis at the base of the brain called the circle of Willis.

L. Neurotransmitters
  1. Acetylcholine
  2. Norepinephrine
  3. Dopamine
  4. Serotonin
  5. Amino acids
  6. Polypeptides

M. Neurons
  1. The neuron consists of cell body, axons, and dendrites.
  2. The cell body contains the nucleus.
  3. Neurons carrying impulses to the central nervous system (CNS) are called *sensory neurons.*

4. Neurons carrying impulses away from the CNS are called *motor neurons.*
5. Synapse is the chemical transmission of impulses from one neuron to another.

N. Axons and dendrites
  1. The axon conducts impulses from the cell body.
  2. The dendrites receive stimuli from the body and transmit them to the axon.
  3. The neurons are protected and insulated by Schwann cells.
  4. The Schwann cell sheath is called the neurolemma.
  5. Neurons do not reproduce after the neonatal period.
  6. If an axon or dendrite is damaged, it will die and be replaced slowly only if the neurolemma is intact and the cell body has not died.

O. Spinal nerves
  1. Human beings have 31 pairs of spinal nerves.
  2. Mixed nerve fibers are formed by the joining of the anterior motor and posterior sensory roots.
  3. Posterior roots contain afferent (sensory) nerve fibers.
  4. Anterior roots contain efferent (motor) nerve fibers.

P. Autonomic nervous system
  1. Sympathetic (adrenergic) fibers dilate pupils, increase heart rate, constrict blood vessels, and relax smooth muscles of the bronchi.
  2. Parasympathetic (cholinergic) fibers produce the opposite effect.

II. Diagnostic Tests

A. Skull and spinal radiography
  1. Description
    a. Radiographs of the skull reveal the size and shape of the skull bones, suture separation in infants, fractures or bony defects, erosion, and calcification.
    b. Spinal radiographs identify fractures, dislocation, compression, curvature, erosion, narrowed spinal cord, and degenerative processes.
  2. Preprocedure interventions
    a. Provide nursing support for the confused, combative, or ventilator-dependent client.
    b. Maintain immobilization of the neck if a spinal fracture is suspected.
    c. Remove metal items from the client.
    d. If the client has thick and heavy hair, this needs to be documented because it could affect interpretation of the x-ray film.
  3. Postprocedure intervention: Maintain immobilization until results are known.

 Always check with the client about the possibility of pregnancy before any radiographic procedures are done.

B. Computed tomography (CT) scan of the brain
1. Description
   a. CT is a type of brain scan that may or may not require injection of a dye.
   b. It is used to detect intracranial bleeding, space-occupying lesions, cerebral edema, infarctions, hydrocephalus, cerebral atrophy, and shifts of brain structures.

> ⚠ Informed consent is needed for any invasive procedure, including procedures that use a contrast medium (dye).

2. Preprocedure interventions
   a. Check for allergies to iodine, contrast dyes, or shellfish if a dye is used.
   b. Assess renal function and verify contrast dose with the pharmacy.
   c. Reinforce instructions to the client on the need to lie still and flat during the test.
   d. Reinforce instructions for the client to hold his or her breath when requested.
   e. Assist with the initiation of an intravenous (IV) line if prescribed.
   f. Remove objects from the head, such as wigs, barrettes, earrings, and hairpins.
   g. Check for claustrophobia.
   h. The client is informed of possible mechanical noises as the scanning occurs.
   i. Inform the client that there may be a hot, flushed sensation and a metallic taste in the mouth when the dye is injected.
   j. Note that some clients may be given the dye even if they report an allergy; they are treated with an antihistamine and corticosteroids before the injection to reduce the severity of a reaction.

> ⚠ Determine the need to withhold metformin if iodinated contrast dye is used for a diagnostic procedure because of the risk for metformin-induced lactic acidosis.

3. Postprocedure interventions
   a. Provide replacement fluids because diuresis from the dye is expected.
   b. Monitor for an allergic reaction to the dye.
   c. Check dye injection site for bleeding or hematoma, and monitor the extremity for color, warmth, and the presence of distal pulses.

C. Magnetic resonance imaging (MRI)
1. Description
   a. MRI is a noninvasive procedure that identifies types of tissues, tumors, and vascular abnormalities.
   b. It is similar to the CT scan but provides more detailed pictures.

2. Preprocedure interventions
   a. Remove all metal objects from the client.
   b. Determine whether the client has a pacemaker, implanted defibrillator, or other metal implant such as a hip prosthesis or vascular clips because these clients cannot have this test performed.
   c. An intermittent infusion device (saline lock) is attached to all IV accesses before the procedure (IV fluid pumps are not allowed in the MRI room).
   d. Provide precautions for the client who is attached to a pulse oximeter because it can cause a burn during testing if coiled around the body or a body part.
   e. Determine whether the client has claustrophobia (unless an open MRI machine is used).
   f. Administer medication as prescribed for the client with claustrophobia.
   g. Determine whether a contrast agent is to be used, and follow the prescription related to the administration of food, fluids, and medications.
   h. Reinforce instructions to the client that he or she will need to remain still during the procedure.

> ⚠ An MRI is contraindicated in a pregnant woman because the increase in amniotic fluid temperature that occurs during the procedure may be harmful to the fetus.

3. Postprocedure interventions
   a. Client may resume normal activities.
   b. Increase fluid and inform client to expect diuresis if a contrast agent was used.

D. Lumbar puncture
1. Description
   a. Insertion of a spinal needle through the L3-L4 interspace into the lumbar subarachnoid space to obtain CSF, measure CSF or pressure, or instill air, dye, or medications.
   b. The test is contraindicated in clients with increased intracranial pressure (ICP) because the procedure will cause a rapid decrease in pressure within the CSF around the spinal cord, leading to brain herniation.
2. Preprocedure interventions: Have the client empty the bladder.
3. Interventions during the procedure
   a. Position the client in a lateral recumbent position and have the client draw their knees up to the abdomen and drop their chin onto their chest. (The prone position may be required for radiologically guided punctures.)
   b. Assist with the collection of specimens (label the specimens in sequence).
   c. Maintain strict asepsis.

4. Postprocedure interventions
  a. Monitor vital signs, lumbar puncture site, neurological signs to check for the presence of leakage of CSF and also monitor for a headache.
  b. Position the client flat as prescribed.
  c. Encourage fluids to replace CSF obtained from the specimen collection or from leakage.
  d. Monitor intake and output (I&O).

E. Cerebral angiography
  1. Description: Injection of a contrast material usually through the femoral artery (or another artery) into the carotid arteries to visualize the cerebral arteries and assess for lesions
  2. Preprocedure interventions
    a. Ensure that informed consent has been obtained.
    b. Check the client for allergies to iodine and shellfish. Check renal function.
    c. Assess for a medication history of anticoagulation therapy; withhold the anticoagulant medication prior to the procedure as prescribed.
    d. Encourage hydration for 2 days before the test.
    e. Maintain the client on NPO (nothing by mouth) status 4 to 6 hours before the test as prescribed.
    f. A neurological assessment is obtained, which will serve as a baseline for postprocedure assessments.
    g. Mark the peripheral pulses.
    h. Remove metal items from the hair.
    i. Assist with the administration of premedication as prescribed.
  3. Postprocedure interventions
    a. Monitor neurological status, vital signs, and neurovascular status of the affected extremity frequently until stable.
    b. Monitor for swelling in the neck and for difficulty swallowing, and notify the primary health care provider (PHCP) if these symptoms occur.
    c. Maintain bed rest for 12 hours as prescribed.
    d. Elevate the head of the bed 15 to 30 degrees only if prescribed.
    e. The head of the bed may be kept flat if the femoral artery is used; always follow the PHCP's prescriptions for positioning.
    f. Check peripheral pulses.
    g. Apply sandbags or another device to immobilize the limb and a pressure dressing to the injection site to decrease bleeding, as prescribed.
    h. Place ice on the puncture site, if prescribed.
    i. Encourage fluid intake.

F. Electroencephalography
  1. Description: A graphic recording of the electrical activity of the superficial layers of the cerebral cortex

  2. Preprocedure interventions
    a. Wash the client's hair.
    b. Inform the client that electrodes are attached to the head and that electricity does not enter the head.
    c. Withhold stimulants, such as coffee, tea, and caffeine beverages; antidepressants; tranquilizers; and possibly antiseizure medications for 24 to 48 hours before the test as prescribed.
    d. Allow the client to have breakfast, if prescribed.
    e. Assist to premedicate for sedation, as prescribed.
  3. Postprocedure interventions
    a. Wash the client's hair.
    b. Maintain side rails (per agency policy) and safety precautions if the client was sedated.

G. Caloric testing (oculovestibular reflex)
  1. Description: Caloric testing provides information about the function of the vestibular portion of the eighth cranial nerve and aids in the diagnosis of cerebellar and brainstem lesions.
  2. Procedure
    a. Patency of the external auditory canal is confirmed.
    b. The client is positioned supine with the head of the bed elevated 30 degrees.
    c. Water that is warmer or cooler than body temperature is infused into the ear.
    d. A normal response is the onset of vertigo and nystagmus (involuntary eye movements) within 20 to 30 seconds.
    e. Absent or disconjugate eye movements indicate brainstem damage.

III. **Neurological Data Collection (refer to Chapter 13 for additional information)**

A. Risk factors
  1. Trauma
  2. Hemorrhage
  3. Tumors
  4. Infection
  5. Toxicity
  6. Metabolic disorder
  7. Hypoxic condition
  8. Hypertension
  9. Stress
  10. Cigarette smoking
  11. Aging process
  12. Chemicals, either ingestion or environmental exposure

 Level of consciousness (LOC) is the most sensitive indicator of neurological status.

B. Vital signs: Monitor for blood pressure or pulse changes, which may indicate increased ICP (rise in blood pressure with widening pulse pressure,

BOX 55.2 Data Collection: Respirations

Cheyne-Stokes
Rhythmic with periods of apnea
Can indicate a metabolic dysfunction or dysfunction in the
cerebral hemisphere or basal ganglia

Neurogenic Hyperventilation
Regular rapid and deep sustained respirations
Indicates a dysfunction in the low midbrain and middle pons

Apneustic
Irregular respirations with pauses at the end of inspiration
and expiration
Indicates a dysfunction in the middle or caudal pons

Ataxic
Totally irregular in rhythm and depth
Indicates a dysfunction in the medulla

Cluster
Clusters of breaths with irregularly spaced pauses
Indicates a dysfunction in the medulla and pons

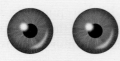

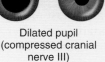

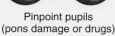

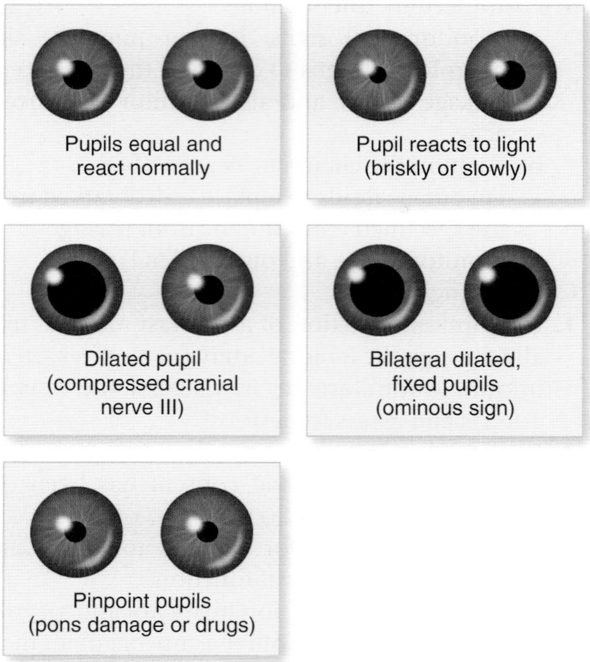

Pupils equal and react normally

Pupil reacts to light (briskly or slowly)

Dilated pupil (compressed cranial nerve III)

Bilateral dilated, fixed pupils (ominous sign)

Pinpoint pupils (pons damage or drugs)

FIGURE 55.1 Pupillary check for size and response.

slowing of the pulse, elevated temperature, abnormal respirations).

C. Respirations (Box 55.2)

D. Temperature
1. An elevated temperature increases the metabolic rate of the brain.
2. An elevation in temperature may indicate a dysfunction of the hypothalamus or brainstem.
3. A slow rise in temperature may indicate infection.

E. Pupils (Fig. 55.1)
1. Unilateral pupil dilation indicates compression of the third cranial nerve.
2. Midposition fixed pupil indicates midbrain injury.
3. Pinpoint fixed pupil indicates pontine damage.
4. See Figure 13.1 for checking extraocular eye movements.

F. Motor function
1. Check muscle tone, including strength and equality.
2. Check for voluntary and involuntary movements and purposeful and nonpurposeful movements.

G. Posturing (see Chapter 35; Fig. 35.3)
1. Posturing indicates a deterioration of the condition.
2. Flexor (decorticate posturing)
   a. The client flexes one or both arms on the chest and may extend the legs stiffly.
   b. Flexor posturing indicates a nonfunctioning cortex.
3. Extensor (decerebrate posturing)
   a. The client stiffly extends one or both arms and possibly the legs.
   b. Extensor posturing indicates a brainstem lesion.

4. Flaccid posturing: The client displays no motor response in any extremity.

H. Reflexes (Box 55.3)

I. Meningeal irritation (Box 55.4)

J. Autonomic system
1. Sympathetic functions/adrenergic responses
   a. Increased pulse and blood pressure
   b. Dilated pupils
   c. Decreased peristalsis
   d. Increased perspiration
   e. Increased respiratory rate
2. Parasympathetic function/cholinergic responses
   a. Decreased pulse and blood pressure
   b. Constricted pupils
   c. Increased salivation
   d. Increased peristalsis
   e. Dilated blood vessels
   f. Bladder contraction

K. Sensory function: touch, pressure, pain

L. Glasgow Coma Scale (Box 55.5)
1. The scale is a method of assessing a client's neurological condition.
2. The scoring system is based on a scale of 3 to 15 points.
3. A score lower than eight indicates that coma is present.

IV. The Unconscious Client

A. Description
1. The unconscious client is in a state of depressed cerebral functioning with unresponsiveness to stimulation of sensory and motor function.

BOX 55.3 Data Collection: Reflexes

Babinski's Reflex
- Dorsiflexion of the big toe and fanning of the other toes; elicited by firmly stroking the lateral aspect of the sole of the foot
- Is a pathological or abnormal reflex in anyone older than 2 years and represents the presence of central nervous system (CNS) disorder

Corneal (Blink) Reflex
- Involuntary closure of the eyelids in response to stimulation of the cornea
- Loss of the blink reflex indicates a dysfunction of cranial nerve V

Gag Reflex
- Contraction of pharyngeal muscle, elicited by touching the back of the throat
- Loss of the gag reflex indicates a dysfunction of cranial nerves IX and X

BOX 55.4 Data Collection: Meningeal Irritation

General Findings
Irritability
Nuchal rigidity
Severe, unrelenting headaches
Generalized muscle aches and pains
Nausea and vomiting
Fever and chills
Tachycardia
Photophobia
Nystagmus
Abnormal pupil reaction and eye movement

Brudzinski's Sign
Involuntary flexion of the hip and knee when the neck is passively flexed; indicates meningeal irritation

Kernig's Sign
Loss of the ability of a supine client to straighten the leg completely when it is fully flexed at the knee and hip; indicates meningeal irritation

Motor Response
Hemiparesis, hemiplegia, and decreased muscle tone
Cranial nerve dysfunction, especially cranial nerves III, IV, VI, VII, and VIII

Memory Changes
Short attention span
Personality and behavioral changes
Bewilderment

BOX 55.5 Glasgow Coma Scale

Score
- The lowest possible score is 3 points (deep coma or death).
- The highest possible score is 15 points (fully awake).

Motor Response Points
Obeys a simple response = 6
Localizes painful stimuli = 5
Normal flexion (withdrawal) = 4
Abnormal flexion (decorticate posturing) = 3
Extensor response (decerebrate posturing) = 2
No motor response to pain = 1

Verbal Response Points
Oriented = 5
Confused conversation = 4
Inappropriate words = 3
Responds with incomprehensible sounds = 2
No verbal response = 1

Eye-Opening Points
Spontaneous = 4
In response to sound = 3
In response to pain = 2
No response even to painful stimuli = 1

Adapted from Ignatavicius D, Workman M: *Medical-surgical nursing: Patient-centered collaborative care*, ed 6, St. Louis, 2010, Saunders.

---

2. Some of the causes include head trauma, cerebral toxins, shock, hemorrhage, tumor, and infection.
B. Data collection
  1. Unarousable
  2. Primitive or no response to painful stimuli
  3. Altered respiration
  4. Decreased cranial nerve and reflex activity
 C. Interventions (Box 55.6)

V. Increased Intracranial Pressure

A. Description
  1. Increased ICP may be caused by trauma, hemorrhage, growths or tumors, hydrocephalus, edema, or inflammation.
  2. Increased ICP can impede circulation to the brain, hinder the absorption of CSF, affect the functioning of nerve cells, and lead to brainstem compression and death.
B. Data collection
  1. Altered LOC, which is the most sensitive and earliest indication of increasing ICP
  2. Headache
  3. Abnormal respirations (see Box 55.2)
  4. Rise in blood pressure with widening pulse pressure
  5. Slowing of pulse
  6. Elevated temperature
  7. Vomiting
  8. Change in pupil size
  9. Late signs of increased ICP, including increased systolic blood pressure, widened pulse pressure, and slowed heart rate
  10. Other late signs include changes in motor function from weakness to hemiplegia, a positive Babinski's reflex, decorticate or decerebrate posturing, and seizures.
C. Interventions
  1. Monitor respiratory status and prevent hypoxia.
  2. The administration of morphine sulfate is avoided to prevent the occurrence of hypoxia.

BOX 55.6 Care of the Unconscious Client

Monitor patency of the airway and keep an airway and emergency equipment at the bedside.

Monitor blood pressure, pulse, and heart sounds.

Monitor respiratory and circulatory status.

Maintain a patent airway and ventilation because a high CO_2 level increases intracranial pressure.

Check lung sounds for the accumulation of secretions; suction fluids from the airway as needed.

Monitor neurological status, including level of consciousness, pupillary reactions, and motor and sensory function, using a coma scale.

Place the client in a semi-Fowler's position (avoid Trendelenburg position).

Change position of the client every 2 hours, avoiding injury when turning.

Use side rails unless contraindicated or according to agency protocol.

Monitor intake and output and daily weight, monitoring for edema and dehydration.

Maintain NPO status until consciousness returns.

Maintain nutrition as prescribed, and monitor fluid and electrolyte balance.

Check the gag and swallow reflex before resuming a diet, and begin the diet with ice chips and fluids when the client becomes alert.

Assist to provide intravenous or enteral feedings as prescribed.

Check bowel sounds.

Monitor elimination patterns.

Monitor for constipation, impaction, and paralytic ileus.

Maintain urinary output to prevent stasis, infection, and calculus formation.

Monitor the status of skin integrity.

Initiate measures to prevent skin breakdown.

Provide frequent mouth care.

Remove dentures and contact lenses.

Check the eyes for the presence of a corneal reflex and irritation, and instill artificial tears or cover the eyes with eye patches.

Monitor drainage from the ears or nose for the presence of cerebrospinal fluid.

Assume that the unconscious client can hear.

Avoid restraints (security devices).

Do not leave the client unattended if unstable.

Initiate seizure precautions if necessary.

Provide range-of-motion exercises to prevent contractures.

Use a footboard or high-top sneakers to prevent foot drop.

Use splints to prevent wrist deformities.

Initiate physical therapy as appropriate.

BOX 55.7 Medications for Intracranial Pressure

Antiseizure

Seizures increase metabolic requirements and cerebral blood flow and volume, thus increasing intracranial pressure.

Antiseizure medications may be given prophylactically to prevent seizures.

Antipyretics and Muscle Relaxants

Temperature reduction decreases metabolism, cerebral blood flow, and thus intracranial pressure.

Antipyretics prevent temperature elevations.

Muscle relaxants prevent shivering.

Blood Pressure Medication

Blood pressure medication may be required to maintain cerebral perfusion at a normal level.

Notify the PHCP if the blood pressure range is less than 100 mm Hg or greater than 150 mm Hg systolic.

Corticosteroids

Corticosteroids stabilize the cell membrane and reduce the leakiness in the blood-brain barrier.

Corticosteroids decrease cerebral edema.

A histamine blocker may be administered to counteract the excess gastric secretion that occurs with the corticosteroid.

Clients need to be withdrawn slowly from corticosteroid therapy to reduce the risk of adrenal crisis.

Intravenous Fluids

Fluids are administered intravenously via an infusion pump to control the amount administered.

Hypertonic intravenous solutions are usually avoided because of the risk of promoting additional cerebral edema.

Hyperosmotic Agent

A hyperosmotic agent increases intravascular pressure by drawing fluid from the interstitial spaces and from the brain cells. Monitor kidney function.

Diuresis is expected.

---

3. Mechanical ventilation is maintained as prescribed; maintaining the $Paco_2$ at 30 to 35 mm Hg will result in vasoconstriction of the cerebral blood vessels, decreased blood flow, and therefore, decreased ICP.

4. Maintain body temperature.

5. Prevent shivering, which can increase ICP.

6. Decrease environmental stimuli.

7. Monitor electrolyte levels and acid–base balance.

8. Monitor I&O.

9. Limit fluid intake to 1200 mL/day as prescribed.

10. Reinforce instructions to the client to avoid straining activities, such as coughing and sneezing.

11. Reinforce instructions to the client to avoid Valsalva maneuver.

⚠ For the client with increased ICP, the head of the bed is elevated 30 to 40 degrees, the Trendelenburg position is avoided, and flexion of the neck and hips is prevented.

D. Medications (Box 55.7)

E. Surgical intervention: See Chapter 35 for additional information on ventriculoperitoneal shunt.

VI. Hyperthermia

A. Description
1. Temperature greater than 105°F (40.6°C), which increases the cerebral metabolism and increases the risk of hypoxia.
2. The causes include infection, heatstroke, exposure to high environmental temperatures, and dysfunction of the thermoregulatory center.

B. Data collection
1. Temperature greater than 105°F (40.6°C)
2. Shivering
3. Nausea and vomiting

C. Interventions
1. Maintain a patent airway.
2. Initiate seizure precautions.
3. Monitor I&O and monitor the skin and mucous membranes for signs of dehydration.
4. Monitor lung sounds.
5. Monitor for dysrhythmia.
6. Check peripheral pulses for systemic blood flow.
7. Induce normothermia with fluids, cool baths, fans, or a hypothermia blanket.

D. Induction of normothermia
1. Prevent shivering, which will increase ICP and oxygen consumption.
2. Assist with the administration of medications, as prescribed, to prevent shivering and to lower body temperature.
3. Monitor neurological status.
4. Monitor for infection and respiratory complications because hypothermia may mask the signs of infection.
5. Monitor for cardiac dysrhythmia.
6. Monitor I&O.
7. Prevent trauma to the skin and tissues.
8. Apply lotion to the skin frequently.
9. Inspect for frostbite if a hypothermia blanket is used.

VII. Traumatic Head Injury

A. Description
1. Head injury is trauma to the skull, resulting in mild to extensive damage to the brain.
2. Immediate complications include cerebral bleeding, hematomas, increased ICP, infections, and seizures.
3. Changes in personality or behavior, cranial nerve deficits, and any other residual deficits depend on the area of the brain damage and the extent of the damage.

B. Types of head injuries (Box 55.8)
1. Open
   a. Scalp lacerations
   b. Fractures in the skull
   c. Interruption of the dura mater
2. Closed
   a. Concussions
   b. Contusions
   c. Fractures

BOX 55.8 **Types of Head Injuries**

Concussion
Concussion is a jarring of the brain within the skull with temporary loss of consciousness.

Contusion
Contusion is a bruising type of injury to the brain tissue.
Contusion may occur along with other neurological injuries, such as with subdural or extradural collections of blood.

Skull Fractures
Linear
Depressed
Compound
Comminuted

Epidural Hematoma
As the most serious type of hematoma, epidural hematoma forms rapidly and results from arterial bleeding.
Epidural hematoma forms between the dura and the skull from a tear in the meningeal artery.
Often associated with temporary loss of consciousness, followed by a lucid period, which rapidly progresses to coma.
Epidural hematoma is a surgical emergency.

Subdural Hematoma
Subdural hematoma forms slowly and results from a venous bleed.
Subdural hematoma occurs under the dura as a result of tears in the veins crossing the subdural space.

Intracerebral Hemorrhage
Intracerebral hemorrhage occurs when a blood vessel within the brain ruptures allowing blood to leak inside the brain.

Subarachnoid Hemorrhage
A subarachnoid hemorrhage refers to bleeding into the subarachnoid space. It may occur as a result of head trauma or spontaneously, such as from a ruptured cerebral aneurysm.

C. Hematoma
1. Description: Hematoma is a collection of blood in the tissues and can occur as a result of a subarachnoid hemorrhage, subdural hemorrhage, or intracerebral hemorrhage.
2. Data collection

   a. Findings depend on the injury.
   b. Clinical manifestations usually result from increased ICP.
   c. Changing neurological signs in the client
   d. Changes in LOC
   e. Airway and breathing pattern changes
   f. Vital sign changes reflecting increasing ICP
   g. Headache, nausea, and vomiting
   h. Visual disturbances, pupillary changes, and papilledema
   i. Nuchal rigidity (not tested until spinal cord injury is ruled out)
   j. CSF drainage from the ears or nose
   k. Weakness and paralysis
   l. Posturing

m. Decreased sensation or absence of feeling
n. Reflex activity changes
o. Seizure activity

> ⚠ CSF can be distinguished from other fluids by the presence of concentric rings (bloody fluid surrounded by a yellow stain, referred to as a "Halo sign" or "double-ring sign") when the fluid is placed on a white sterile background, such as a gauze pad. CSF also tests positive for glucose when tested using a strip test.

3. Interventions
   a. Monitor respiratory status and maintain a patent airway because increased CO_2 levels increase cerebral edema.
   b. Monitor neurological status and vital signs, including temperature.
   c. Monitor for increased ICP.
   d. Maintain head elevation to reduce venous pressure.
   e. Protect the cervical spine, maintain a neutral head position, and prevent neck flexion.
   f. Initiate normothermia measures for increased temperature, and prevent shivering.
   g. Check cranial nerve function, reflexes, and motor and sensory function.
   h. Initiate seizure precautions.
   i. Monitor for pain and restlessness.
   j. Morphine sulfate or other opioid medications may be prescribed to decrease agitation and control restlessness caused by pain for the head-injured client on a ventilator; it is administered with caution because it is a respiratory depressant and may increase ICP.

   k. Monitor for drainage from the nose or ears because this fluid may be CSF; notify the registered nurse immediately if this is noted.

   l. Do not attempt to clean the nose, suction, or allow the client to blow his or her nose if drainage occurs.

   m. Do not clean the ear if drainage is noted, but apply a loose, dry sterile dressing.
   n. Check drainage for presence of CSF.
   o. The PHCP is notified if drainage from the ears or nose occurs and if drainage tests positive for CSF.
   p. Reinforce instructions to the client to avoid coughing because this increases ICP.
   q. Monitor for signs of infection.
   r. Prevent complications of immobility.
   s. The client and family would be informed about possible behavior changes that may occur, including those that are expected and those that need to be reported.
D. Craniotomy
   1. Description
      a. A surgical procedure that involves an incision through the cranium to remove accumulated blood or a tumor

b. Complications of the procedure include increased ICP from cerebral edema, hemorrhage, or obstruction of normal flow of CSF.
c. Additional complications include hematomas, hypovolemic shock, hydrocephalus, respiratory and neurogenic complications, pulmonary edema, and wound infections.
d. Complications related to fluid and electrolyte imbalances include diabetes insipidus and syndrome of inappropriate secretion of antidiuretic hormone (SIADH).
e. Stereotactic radiosurgery (SRS) may be an alternative to traditional surgery and is usually used to treat tumors and arteriovenous malformations.
2. Preoperative interventions
   a. Explain the procedure to the client and family.
   b. Ensure that informed consent has been obtained.
   c. Prepare to shave the client's head as prescribed (usually done in the operating room) and cover the head with appropriate covering.
   d. Stabilize the client before surgery.
3. Postoperative interventions (Box 55.9)
4. Postoperative positioning (Box 55.10)

VIII. Spinal Cord Injury

A. Description
   1. Trauma to the spinal cord causes partial or complete disruption of the nerve tracts and neurons.
   2. The injury can involve contusion, laceration, or compression of the cord.
   3. Spinal cord edema develops; necrosis of the spinal cord can develop as a result of compromised capillary circulation and venous return.
   4. Loss of motor function, sensation, reflex activity, and bowel and bladder control may result.
   5. The most common causes include motor vehicle accidents, falls, sporting and industrial accidents, and gunshot or stab wounds.
   6. Complications related to the injury include respiratory failure, autonomic dysreflexia, spinal shock, further cord damage, and death.
B. Most frequently involved vertebrae
   1. Cervical: C5, C6, and C7
   2. Thoracic: T12
   3. Lumbar: L1
C. Transection of the cord
   1. Complete transection of the cord. The spinal cord is severed completely, with total loss of sensation, movement, and reflex activity below the level of injury.
   2. Partial transection of the cord
      a. The spinal cord is damaged or severed partially.
      b. The symptoms depend on the extent and location of the damage.

BOX 55.9 Nursing Care Following Craniotomy

Monitor vital signs and neurological status every 30–60 minutes.

Monitor for increased intracranial pressure.

Monitor for decreased level of consciousness, motor weakness or paralysis, aphasia, visual changes, and personality changes.

Mechanical ventilation and slight hyperventilation is maintained for the first 24–48 hours as prescribed to prevent increased intracranial pressure.

Check the primary health care provider's (PHCP's) prescriptions regarding client positioning.

Avoid extreme hip or neck flexion, and maintain the head in a midline neutral position.

Provide a quiet environment.

Monitor the head dressing frequently for signs of drainage.

Mark any area of drainage on the dressing at least once each nursing shift for baseline comparison.

Monitor any drains, which may be in place for 24 hours.

Maintain suction on the drain as appropriate; measure drainage every 8 hours, and record the amount and color.

The PHCP is notified if drainage is greater than the normal of 30–50 mL per shift.

The PHCP is notified immediately of excessive amounts of drainage or a saturated head dressing.

Provide basic hygiene.

Record strict measurement of hourly intake and output.

Maintain fluid restriction at 1500 mL/day as prescribed.

Monitor electrolyte values.

Monitor for dysrhythmia, which may occur as a result of fluid and electrolyte imbalance.

Apply ice packs or cool compresses as prescribed. Expect periorbital edema and ecchymosis of one or both eyes, which is not an unusual occurrence.

Provide range-of-motion exercises every 8 hours.

Assist with the administration of antiseizure medications, antacids, corticosteroids, and antibiotics as prescribed.

Assist with the administration of analgesics such as codeine sulfate and acetaminophen (Tylenol) as prescribed for pain.

BOX 55.10 Client Positioning After Craniotomy

Positions prescribed after craniotomy vary with the type of surgery and the specific postoperative surgeon's prescriptions.

Always check the surgeon's prescriptions regarding client positioning.

Incorrect positioning may cause serious and possibly fatal complications.

Removal of a Bone Flap for Decompression

To facilitate brain expansion, the client would be turned from the back to the nonoperative side but not to the side where the operation was performed.

Posterior Fossa Surgery

To protect the operative site from pressure and to minimize tension on the suture line, position the client on the side, with a pillow under the head for support, and not on the back.

Infratentorial Surgery

Infratentorial surgery involves surgery below the tentorium of the brain.

The surgeon may prescribe a flat position without head elevation or may prescribe the head of the bed to be elevated at 30–45 degrees.

Do not elevate the head of the bed in the acute phase of care after surgery without the surgeon's prescription.

Supratentorial Surgery

Supratentorial surgery involves surgery above the tentorium of the brain.

The surgeon may prescribe the head of the bed to be elevated at 30 degrees to promote venous outflow through the jugular veins.

Do not lower the head of the bed in the acute phase of care after surgery without a surgeon's prescription.

---

    c. If the cord has not suffered irreparable damage, early treatment is needed to prevent partial damage from developing into total and permanent damage.

D. Spinal cord syndromes in partial transection or injury (Fig. 55.2)

E. Data collection: Spinal cord injuries (Box 55.11)
  1. Dependent on the level of the cord injury
  2. Level of the spinal cord injury: The lowest spinal cord segment with intact motor and sensory function
  3. Respiratory status changes
  4. Motor and sensory changes below the level of injury

    5. Total sensory loss and motor paralysis below the level of injury
  6. Loss of reflexes below the level of injury
  7. Loss of bladder and bowel control
  8. Urinary retention and bladder distention
  9. Presence of sweat, which does not occur on paralyzed areas

F. Cervical level injuries
  1. Injury at C2 to C3 is usually fatal.
  2. C4 is the major innervation to the diaphragm by the phrenic nerve.
  3. Involvement above C4 causes respiratory difficulty and paralysis of all four extremities.
  4. Client may have movement in the shoulder if the injury is at C5 through C8, and may also have decreased respiratory reserve.

G. Thoracic-level injuries
  1. Loss of movement of the chest, trunk, bowel, bladder, and legs may occur, depending on the level of injury.
  2. Leg paralysis (paraplegia) may occur.

Adult—Neurological

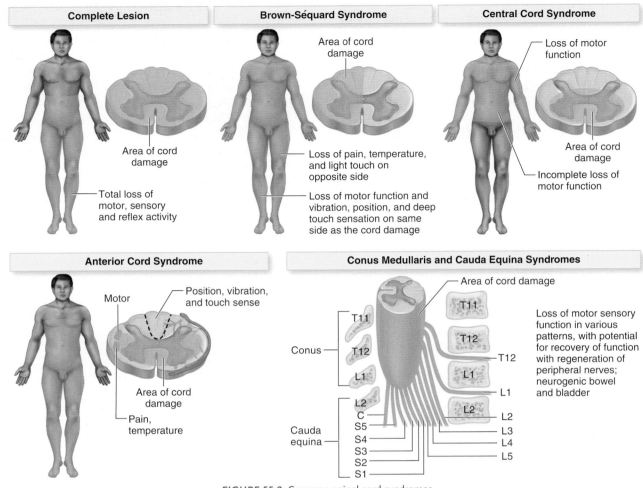

FIGURE 55.2 Common spinal cord syndromes.

BOX 55.11   Effects of Spinal Cord Injury

Tetraplegia (Quadriplegia)
Injury occurring between C1 and C8
Paralysis involving all four extremities

Paraplegia
Injury occurring between T1 and L4
Paralysis involving only the lower extremities

3. Autonomic dysreflexia with lesions or injuries above T6 and in cervical lesions may occur.
4. Visceral distention from a noxious stimulus such as a distended bladder or impacted rectum may cause reactions such as sweating, bradycardia, hypertension, nasal stuffiness, and goose flesh.

H. Lumbar and sacral level injuries
1. Loss of movement and sensation of the lower extremities may occur.
2. S2 and S3 center on micturition; therefore, below this level, the bladder will contract but not empty (neurogenic bladder).

3. Injury above S2 in males allows them to have an erection, but they are unable to ejaculate because of sympathetic nerve damage.
4. Injury between S2 and S4 damages the sympathetic and parasympathetic response, preventing erection or ejaculation.

⚠️ Always suspect spinal cord injury when trauma occurs until this injury is ruled out. Immobilize the client on a spinal backboard with the head in a neutral position to prevent an incomplete injury from becoming complete.

I. Emergency interventions
1. Emergency management is critical because improper movement can cause further damage and loss of neurological function.
2. Monitor the respiratory pattern and maintain a patent airway.
3. Prevent head flexion, rotation, or extension.
4. During immobilization, maintain traction and alignment on the head by placing hands on either side of the head by the ears.
5. Maintain an extended position.

6. Logroll the client.

7. No part of the body should be twisted or turned, and the client is not allowed to assume a sitting position.

8. In the emergency department, a client who has sustained a severe cervical fracture must be placed immediately in skeletal traction via skull tongs or halo traction to immobilize the cervical spine and to reduce the fracture and dislocation.

J. Interventions during hospitalization

1. Respiratory system

   a. Monitor respiratory status because paralysis of the intercostal and abdominal muscles occurs with C4 injuries.

   b. Monitor arterial blood gases and maintain mechanical ventilation if prescribed to prevent respiratory arrest, especially with cervical injuries.

   c. Encourage deep breathing and the use of an incentive spirometer.

   d. Monitor for signs of infection, particularly pneumonia.

2. Cardiovascular system

   a. Monitor for cardiac dysrhythmia.

   b. Monitor for signs of hemorrhage or bleeding around the fracture site.

   c. Monitor for signs of shock, such as hypotension, tachycardia, and a weak and thready pulse.

   d. Monitor the lower extremities for deep vein thrombosis.

   e. Measure circumferences of the calf and thigh to identify increases in size.

   f. Use sequential compression devices (SCDs) as prescribed.

   g. Remove SCDs daily or as prescribed and check the skin integrity.

   h. Monitor for orthostatic hypotension when repositioning the client.

3. Neuromuscular system

   a. Monitor neurological status.

   b. Monitor motor and sensory status to determine the level of injury.

   c. Monitor motor ability by testing the client's ability to squeeze hands, spread the fingers, move the toes, and turn the feet.

   d. Check for the absence of sensation, hyposensation, or hypersensation by pinching the skin or pricking it with a pin, starting at the shoulders and working down the extremities.

   e. Monitor for signs of autonomic dysreflexia and spinal shock.

   f. Immobilize the client to promote healing and prevent further injury.

   g. Monitor pain.

   h. Initiate measures to reduce pain.

   i. Assist with the administration of analgesics as prescribed.

   j. Monitor for complications of immobility.

   k. Prepare the client for decompression laminectomy, spinal fusion, or insertion of instrumentation or rods if prescribed.

   l. Collaborate with the physical therapist and occupational therapist to determine appropriate exercise techniques, check the need for hand and wrist splints, and develop an appropriate plan to prevent foot drop.

4. Gastrointestinal system

   a. Check abdomen for distention and hemorrhage.

   b. Monitor bowel sounds and assess for paralytic ileus.

   c. Prevent constipation.

   d. Initiate a bowel control program as appropriate.

   e. Maintain adequate nutrition and a high-fiber diet.

5. Renal system

   a. Prevent urinary retention.

   b. Initiate a bladder control program as appropriate.

   c. Maintain fluid and electrolyte balance.

   d. Maintain adequate fluid intake of 2000 mL/day.

   e. Monitor for urinary tract infection and calculi.

6. Integumentary system

   a. Check skin integrity.

   b. Turn the client every 2 hours.

7. Psychosocial integrity

   a. Monitor psychosocial status.

   b. Encourage the client to express feelings of anger and depression.

   c. Discuss the client's sexual concerns.

   d. Promote rehabilitation with self-care measures, setting realistic goals based on the client's potential functional level.

   e. Encourage contact with appropriate community resources.

K. Spinal shock and neurogenic shock

1. Description

   a. Spinal shock is a complete but temporary loss of motor, sensory, reflex, and autonomic function that occurs immediately after injury as the cord's response to the injury. It usually lasts less than 48 hours but can continue for several weeks.

   b. Neurogenic shock occurs most commonly in clients with injuries above T6 and usually is experienced soon after the injury. Massive vasodilation occurs leading to pooling of the blood in blood vessels, tissue hypoperfusion, and impaired cellular metabolism.

2. Data collection (Box 55.12)

BOX 55.12 **Manifestations: Neurogenic Shock, Spinal Shock, and Autonomic Dysreflexia**

Neurogenic Shock
Hypotension
Bradycardia

Spinal Shock
Flaccid paralysis
Loss of reflex activity below the level of injury
Bradycardia
Hypotension
Paralytic ileus

Autonomic Dysreflexia
Sudden onset of severe, throbbing headache
Severe hypertension and bradycardia
Flushing above the level of the lesion
Pale extremities below the level of injury
Nasal stuffiness
Nausea
Dilated pupils or blurred vision
Sweating
Piloerection (goose bumps)
Restlessness and a feeling of apprehension

---

 3. Interventions
  a. Monitor for signs of spinal shock following a spinal cord injury.
  b. Monitor for hypotension and bradycardia.
  c. Monitor for reflex activity.
  d. Check bowel sounds.
  e. Monitor for bowel and urinary retention.
  f. Provide supportive measures as prescribed, based on the presence of symptoms.
  g. Monitor for the return of reflexes.
L. Autonomic dysreflexia
  1. Description
    a. Autonomic dysreflexia is also known as autonomic hyperreflexia.
    b. Autonomic dysreflexia generally occurs after the period of spinal shock is resolved and occurs with lesions or injuries above T6 and in cervical lesions.
    c. It is commonly caused by visceral distention from a distended bladder or impacted rectum.
    d. It is a neurological emergency and must be treated immediately to prevent a hypertensive stroke.
  2. Data collection (see Box 55.12)
  3. Interventions (see Priority Nursing Actions)
M. Cervical spine traction for cervical injuries
  1. Description
    a. Skeletal traction is used to stabilize fractures or dislocations of the cervical or upper thoracic spine.

⚡ PRIORITY NURSING ACTIONS

Autonomic Dysreflexia in a Client with a Spinal Cord Injury

1. Raise the head of the bed.
2. Loosen tight clothing on the client.
3. Check for bladder distention or other noxious stimulus and take measures immediately to eliminate the noxious stimulus.
4. Assist with the administration of an antihypertensive medication.
5. Document the occurrence, treatment, and response.

---

  b. Two types of equipment used for cervical traction are skull (cervical) tongs and halo traction (halo fixation device).
2. Skull tongs
  a. Skull tongs are inserted into the outer aspect of the client's skull, and traction is applied.
  b. Weights are attached to the tongs and the client is used as countertraction. The nurse would never add or remove weights.
  c. Monitor the neurological status of the client.
  d. Determine the amount of weight prescribed to be added to the traction.
  e. Ensure that weights hang securely and freely at all times.
  f. Ensure that the ropes for the traction remain within the pulley.
  g. Maintain body alignment and maintain care of the client on a special bed (such as a Roto-Rest bed, or Stryker, or Foster frame), as prescribed.
  h. Turn the client every 2 hours.
  i. Check insertion site of the tongs for infection.
  j. Provide sterile pin site care as prescribed.
3. Halo traction
  a. Halo traction is a static traction device that consists of a headpiece with four pins—two anterior and two posterior—inserted into the client's skull.
  b. The metal halo ring may be attached to a vest (jacket) or cast when the spine is stable, allowing for increased client mobility.
  c. Monitor the client's neurological status for changes in movement or decreased strength.
  d. Never move or turn the client by holding or pulling on the halo traction device.
  e. Check tightness of the jacket by ensuring that one finger can be placed under the jacket.
  f. Check skin integrity to ensure that the jacket or cast is not causing pressure.
  g. Provide sterile pin site care as prescribed.
4. Reinforce client education for the halo traction device (Box 55.13).
5. Initiate interventions in support of the client's self-image.

BOX 55.13 Client Education for a Halo Fixation Device

Notify the primary health care provider (PHCP) if the halo vest (jacket) or ring bolts loosen.

Use fleece or foam inserts to relieve pressure points.

Keep the vest lining dry.

Clean the pin site daily.

Notify the PHCP if redness, swelling, drainage, open areas, pain, tenderness, or a clicking sound occurs from the pin site.

A sponge bath or tub bath is allowed. Showers are prohibited.

Check the skin under the vest daily for breakdown, using a flashlight.

Do not use any products other than shampoo on the hair.

When shampooing the hair, cover the vest with plastic.

When getting out of bed, roll onto the side and push on the mattress with the arms.

Never use the metal frame for turning or lifting.

Use a rolled towel or pillowcase between the back of the neck and the bed or next to the cheek when lying on the side, and raise the head of the bed to increase sleep comfort.

Adapt clothing to fit over the halo device.

Eat foods high in protein and calcium to promote bone healing.

Have the correct-size wrench available at all times for an emergency (tape the wrench to the vest).

If cardiopulmonary resuscitation is required, the anterior portion of the vest will be loosened and the posterior portion will remain in place to provide stability.

---

6. Reinforce teaching the client and family pin site care, care of the vest, and signs/symptoms of infection to report to his or her PHCP.

N. Interventions for thoracic and lumbar and sacral injuries
1. Bed rest
2. Immobilize client with a body cast if prescribed.
3. Monitor for respiratory impairment and paralytic ileus as possible complications of the body cast.
4. Use a brace or corset when the client is out of bed.

O. Surgical interventions for thoracic and lumbar/sacral injuries
1. Decompressive laminectomy
   a. Removal of one or more laminae
   b. Allows for cord expansion from edema; performed if conventional methods fail to prevent neurological deterioration
2. Spinal fusion
   a. Spinal fusion is used for thoracic spinal injuries.
   b. Bone is grafted between the vertebrae for support and to strengthen the back.
3. Postoperative interventions
   a. Monitor for respiratory impairment.
   b. Monitor vital signs, motor function, sensation, and circulatory status in the lower extremities.

c. Encourage breathing exercises.
d. Monitor for signs of fluid and electrolyte imbalance.
e. Observe for complications of immobility.
f. Keep the client in a flat position as prescribed.
g. Provide cast care if the client is in a full body cast.
h. Turn and reposition frequently by logrolling side to back to side, using turning sheets and pillows between the legs to maintain alignment.
i. Assist with the administration of pain medication as prescribed.
j. Maintain an NPO status until the client is passing flatus.
k. Monitor bowel sounds.
l. Provide the use of a fracture bedpan.
m. Monitor I&O.
n. Maintain nutritional status.

P. Medications
1. Dexamethasone
   a. Used for its anti-inflammatory and edema-reducing effects
   b. May interfere with healing
2. Dextran: A plasma expander used to increase capillary blood flow within the spinal cord and to prevent or treat hypotension
3. Baclofen: This medication is used for clients with upper motor neuron injuries to control muscle spasticity.

IX. Cerebral Aneurysm

A. Description: A dilation of the walls of a weakened cerebral artery that can lead to rupture

B. Data collection
1. Headache and pain
2. Irritability
3. Change in vision
4. Tinnitus
5. Hemiparesis
6. Nuchal rigidity
7. Seizure

C. Interventions
1. Maintain a patent airway (suction only with PHCP prescription).
2. Administer oxygen as prescribed.
3. Monitor vital signs and for hypertension or dysrhythmia.
4. Avoid taking the client's temperature via the rectum.
5. Initiate aneurysm precautions (Box 55.14).

X. Seizures

A. Description
1. Seizures are an abnormal, sudden, excessive discharge of electrical activity within the brain.

Adult—Neurological

BOX 55.14   Aneurysm Precautions

Maintain the client on bed rest in a semi-Fowler's or side-lying position.

Maintain a darkened room (subdued lighting and no direct, bright, artificial lights) without stimulation (a private room is optimal).

Provide a quiet environment (avoid activities or startling noises); a telephone in the room is not usually allowed.

Reading, watching television, and listening to music are permitted, provided they do not overstimulate the client.

Limit visitors.

Maintain fluid restrictions.

Provide diet as prescribed; avoid stimulants in the diet.

Prevent any activities that initiate the Valsalva maneuver (straining at stooling, coughing); provide stool softeners to prevent straining.

Administer care gently (e.g., the bath, back rub, range of motion).

Limit invasive procedures.

Maintain normothermia.

Prevent hypertension.

Provide sedation.

Provide pain control.

Assist with the administration of prophylactic antiseizure medications.

Assist with providing deep vein thrombosis prophylaxis as prescribed.

---

2. Epilepsy is a disorder characterized by chronic seizure activity and indicates brain or CNS irritation.

3. Causes include genetic factors, trauma, tumors, circulatory or metabolic disorders, toxicity, and infections.

4. Status epilepticus involves a rapid succession of epileptic spasms without intervals of consciousness; it is a potential complication that can occur with any type of seizure, and brain damage may result.

B. Types of seizures (Box 55.15)

C. Data collection

1. Seizure history
2. Type of seizure
3. Occurrences before, during, and after the seizure
4. Prodromal signs, such as mood changes, irritability, and insomnia

5. Aura: Sensation that warns the client of the impending seizure
6. Loss of motor activity or bowel and bladder function or loss of consciousness during the seizure
7. Occurrences during the postictal state, such as headache, loss of consciousness, sleepiness, and impaired speech or thinking

 D. Interventions

 ⚠️ If the client is having a seizure, maintain a patent airway. Do not force the jaws open or place anything in the client's mouth.

1. Note the time and duration of the seizure.
2. Monitor behavior at the onset of the seizure. Note if the client experienced an aura, a change in facial expression occurred, or a sound or cry occurred from the client.
3. If the client is standing or sitting, place him or her on the floor and protect the head and body.
4. Support airway, breathing, and circulation.
5. Administer oxygen.
6. Prepare to suction secretions.
7. Turn the client to the side to allow secretions to drain while maintaining the airway.
8. Prevent injury during the seizure.
9. Remain with the client.
10. Do not restrain the client.
11. Loosen restrictive clothing.
12. Note the type, character, and progression of the movements during the seizure.
13. Monitor for incontinence.
14. Assist with the administration of IV medications, as prescribed, to stop the seizure.
15. Document the characteristics of the seizure.
16. Provide privacy, if possible.
17. Monitor behavior following the seizure, such as the state of consciousness, motor ability, and speech ability.
18. Reinforce instructions to the client about the importance of lifelong medication and the need for follow-up determination of medication blood levels.
19. Reinforce instructions to the client to avoid alcohol, excessive stress, fatigue, and strobe lights.
20. Encourage the client to contact available community resources, such as the Epilepsy Foundation of America.
21. Encourage the client to wear a MedicAlert bracelet.

XI. Stroke (Brain Attack)

A. Description

1. A stroke or brain attack manifests as a sudden focal neurological deficit and is caused by cerebrovascular disease.
2. Cerebral anoxia lasting longer than 10 minutes causes cerebral infarction with irreversible change.
3. Cerebral edema and congestion cause further dysfunction.
4. Diagnosis is determined by CT scan, electroencephalography, cerebral arteriography, and MRI scan.
5. In most facilities, the type of stroke needs to be determined within a certain time frame after arrival in order for timely treatment to be initiated.
6. Transient ischemic attack (TIA) may be a warning sign of an impending stroke.
7. The permanent disability cannot be determined until the cerebral edema subsides.
8. The order in which function may return is facial, swallowing, lower limb, speech, and arms.
9. Carotid endarterectomy is a surgical intervention used in stroke management and is targeted

BOX 55.15 Types of Seizures

Generalized Seizures

Tonic-Clonic

Tonic-clonic seizures may begin with an aura.

The tonic phase involves the stiffening or rigidity of the muscles of the arms and legs and usually lasts 10–20 seconds, followed by loss of consciousness.

The clonic phase consists of hyperventilation and jerking of the extremities and usually lasts about 30 seconds.

Full recovery from the seizure may take several hours.

Absence

A brief seizure lasts seconds, and the individual may or may not lose consciousness.

No loss or change in muscle tone occurs.

Seizures may occur several times during a day.

The victim appears to be daydreaming.

This type of seizure is more common in children.

Myoclonic

Myoclonic seizures present as a brief generalized jerking or stiffening of extremities.

The victim may fall to the ground from the seizure.

Atonic or Akinetic (Drop Attacks)

An atonic seizure is a sudden momentary loss of muscle tone.

The victim may fall to the ground as a result of the seizure.

Partial Seizures

Simple Partial

The simple partial seizure produces sensory symptoms accompanied by motor symptoms that are localized or confined to a specific area.

The client remains conscious and may report an aura.

Complex Partial

The complex partial seizure is a psychomotor seizure.

The area of the brain most involved is the temporal lobe.

The seizure is characterized by periods of altered behavior of which the client is not aware.

The client loses consciousness for a few seconds.

BOX 55.16 Clinical Manifestations of Stroke Based on Type

Thrombotic Stroke

Typically, there is no decreased level of consciousness within the first 24 hours.

Symptoms get progressively worse as the infarction and edema increase.

Embolic Stroke

Sudden, severe symptoms

Warning signs are less common.

Client remains conscious and may have a headache.

Hemorrhagic Stroke

Sudden onset of symptoms

Symptoms progress over minutes to hours because of the ongoing bleeding.

---

5. Manifestations of different types of stroke are similar and, therefore, it is critical to determine the type of stroke occurring; the type cannot be determined solely based on manifestations and the correct and appropriate treatment for the stroke needs to be initiated.

C. Risk factors
   1. Atherosclerosis
   2. Hypertension
   3. Anticoagulation therapy
   4. Diabetes mellitus
   5. Stress
   6. Obesity
   7. Oral contraceptives

⚠️ A critical factor in the early intervention and treatment of stroke is the accurate identification of stroke manifestations and establishing the onset of the manifestations. Stroke screening scales may be used to quickly identify stroke manifestations. Identification of the type of stroke that is occurring is critical in determining the appropriate treatment, and this is usually done using imaging such as a CT scan.

D. Data collection (Boxes 55.16 and 55.17 and Fig. 55.3)
   1. Findings depend on the area of the brain affected; stroke scales such as the National Institutes of Health Stroke Scale (NIHSS [stroke.nih.gov/resources/scale.htm]) may be used by the health care facility for assessment.
   2. Lesions in the cerebral hemisphere result in manifestations on the contralateral side, which is the side of the body opposite the stroke.
   3. Airway patency is always a priority.
   4. Pulse (may be slow and bounding)
   5. Respirations (Cheyne-Stokes)
   6. Blood pressure (hypertension)
   7. Headache, nausea, and vomiting

at stroke prevention, especially in clients with symptomatic carotid stenosis.

   10. The National Institutes of Health through the National Institute of Neurological Disorders and Stroke (NINDS) developed the "Know Stroke. Know the Signs. Act in Time" campaign devised to help educate the public about the symptoms of stroke and the importance of getting to the hospital quickly (http://www.stroke.nih.gov/).

 B. Causes
   1. Thrombosis
   2. Embolism
   3. Thrombotic and embolic strokes are classified as ischemic strokes.
   4. Hemorrhage from rupture of a vessel; classified as a hemorrhagic stroke

BOX 55.17   Data Collection Findings: Stroke

Agnosia
Inability to recognize and use an object correctly

Apraxia
Called *dyspraxia* if the condition is mild
Characterized by the loss of ability to execute or carry out skilled movements or gestures, despite having the desire and physical ability to perform them

Hemianopsia
Blindness in half of the visual field

Homonymous Hemianopsia
Loss of half of the field of view on the same side in both eyes

Neglect Syndrome (Unilateral Neglect)
Client unaware of the existence of his or her paralyzed side

Proprioception Alterations
Altered position sense that places the client at increased risk of injury
   Note: With visual problems, the client must turn the head to scan the complete range of vision.

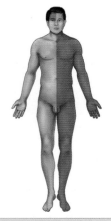 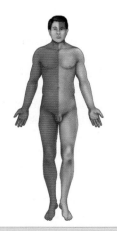

Right-brain damage (stroke on right side of the brain)	**Left-brain damage** (stroke on left side of the brain)
• Impaired judgment • Impaired time concepts • Impulsive, safety problems • Left-sided neglect • Paralyzed left side: hemiplegia • Rapid performance, short attention span • Spatial-perceptual deficits • Tends to deny or minimize problems	• Aware of deficits: depression, anxiety • Impaired comprehension related to language, math • Impaired right/left discrimination • Impaired speech/language aphasias • Paralyzed right side: hemiplegia • Slow performance, cautious

FIGURE 55.3 Manifestations of right brain and left brain stroke.

8. Facial drooping
9. Nuchal rigidity
10. Change in vision
11. Ataxia
12. Dysarthria
13. Dysphagia

14. Change in speech
15. Decreased sensation to pressure, heat, and cold
16. Bowel and bladder dysfunction
17. Paralysis

E. Aphasia
   1. Expressive
      a. Damage occurs in Broca's area of the frontal brain.
      b. The client understands what is said but is unable to communicate verbally.
   2. Receptive
      a. The injury involves Wernicke's area in the temporoparietal area.
      b. The client is unable to understand the spoken and often the written word.
   3. Global or mixed: Language dysfunction occurs during expression and reception.
   4. Interventions for aphasia
      a. Provide repetitive directions.
      b. Break down tasks to one step at a time.
      c. Repeat names of objects frequently used.
      d. Allow time for the client to communicate.
      e. Use a picture board, communication board, or computerized technology.

F. Interventions during the acute phase of stroke
   1. Maintain a patent airway and administer oxygen as prescribed.
   2. Monitor vital signs.
   3. Usually a blood pressure of 150/100 mm Hg, or as prescribed, is maintained to ensure cerebral perfusion.
   4. Suction secretions to prevent aspiration, as prescribed, but never suction nasally or for longer than 10 seconds to prevent increasing ICP.
   5. Monitor for increasing ICP because the client is at most risk during the first 72 hours following the stroke.
   6. Position the client on the side to prevent aspiration, with the head of the bed elevated 15 to 30 degrees as prescribed.
   7. Monitor LOC, pupillary response, motor and sensory response, cranial nerve function, and reflexes.
   8. Maintain a quiet environment.
   9. Insert an indwelling urinary catheter as prescribed.
   10. Assist with the administration of prescribed IV fluids and monitor closely.
   11. Maintain fluid and electrolyte balance.
   12. Assist with the administration of anticoagulants, antiplatelets, diuretics, antihypertensives, and antiseizure medications that may be prescribed.
   13. Establish a form of communication.

G. Interventions in the postacute phase of a stroke
   1. Continue with interventions from the acute phase.
   2. Position the client 2 hours on the unaffected side and 20 minutes on the affected side; the prone position may also be prescribed.
   3. Provide skin, mouth, and eye care.

4. Perform passive range-of-motion exercises to prevent contractures.
5. Place SCDs as prescribed on the client.
6. Monitor the gag reflex and ability to swallow.
7. As prescribed, provide sips of fluids, and slowly advance the diet to foods that are easy to chew and swallow.
8. Provide soft and semisoft foods and flavored, cool or warm, thickened fluids rather than thin liquids because the stroke client is better able to tolerate these types of foods. Speech therapists may do swallow studies to recommend consistency of food and fluids.
9. When the client is eating, position him or her sitting in a chair or sitting up in bed, with the head and neck positioned slightly forward and flexed.
10. Place food in the back of the mouth on the unaffected side to prevent trapping of food in the affected cheek.

H. Interventions in the chronic phase of stroke
   1. Neglect syndrome
      a. The client is unaware of the existence of the paralyzed side (unilateral neglect), which places him or her at risk for injury.
      b. Teach the client to touch and use both sides of the body.
   2. Hemianopsia
      a. The client has blindness in half of the visual field.
      b. Homonymous hemianopsia is blindness in the same visual field of both eyes.
      c. Encourage the client to turn their head to scan the complete range of vision; otherwise, he or she does not see half of the visual field.
   3. Approach the client from the unaffected side.
   4. Place the client's personal objects within the visual field.
   5. Provide eye care for visual deficits.
   6. Place a patch over the affected eye if the client has diplopia.
   7. Increase mobility as tolerated.
   8. Encourage fluid intake and a high-fiber diet.
   9. Administer stool softeners as prescribed.
   10. Encourage the client to express his or her feelings.
   11. Encourage independence in activities of daily living.
   12. Determine the need for assistive devices such as a cane, walker, splints, or braces.
   13. Teach transfer technique from bed to chair and chair to bed.
   14. Provide gait training.
   15. Initiate physical and occupational therapy for assessment and the need for adaptive equipment or other supports for self-care and mobility.
   16. Refer the client to a speech and language pathologist as prescribed.
   17. Encourage the client and family to contact available community resources.

XII. Multiple Sclerosis
A. Description
   1. Multiple sclerosis is a chronic, progressive, noncontagious, degenerative disease of the CNS characterized by demyelinization of the neurons.
   2. It usually occurs between ages 20 and 40 years and consists of periods of remission and exacerbation.
   3. The causes are unknown, but the disease is thought to be a result of an autoimmune response or viral infection.
   4. Precipitating factors include pregnancy, fatigue, stress, infection, and trauma.
   5. Electroencephalogram findings are abnormal.
   6. Results of a lumbar puncture indicates an increased γ-globulin level, but the serum globulin level is normal.

B. Data collection
   1. Fatigue and weakness
   2. Ataxia and vertigo
   3. Tremors and spasticity of the lower extremities
   4. Paresthesia
   5. Blurred vision, diplopia, and transient blindness
   6. Nystagmus
   7. Dysphasia
   8. Decreased perception to pain, touch, and temperature
   9. Bladder and bowel disturbances, including urgency, frequency, retention, and incontinence
   10. Abnormal reflexes, including hyperreflexia, absent reflexes, and a positive Babinski's reflex
   11. Emotional changes such as apathy, euphoria, irritability, and depression
   12. Memory changes and confusion

C. Interventions
   1. Provide energy conservation measures during exacerbation.
   2. Protect the client from injury by providing safety measures.
   3. Place an eye patch on the eye for diplopia.
   4. Monitor for potential complications such as urinary tract infections, calculi, pressure ulcers, respiratory tract infections, and contractures.
   5. Promote regular elimination by bladder and bowel training.
   6. Encourage independence.
   7. Assist the client with establishing a regular exercise and rest program.
   8. Reinforce instructions to the client to balance moderate activity with rest periods.
   9. Assess the need for and provide assistive devices.
   10. Initiate physical and speech therapy.
   11. Reinforce instructions to the client to avoid fatigue, stress, infection, overheating, and chilling.
   12. Reinforce instructions to the client to increase fluid intake and eat a balanced diet, including low-fat, high-fiber foods and foods high in potassium.

13. Reinforce instructions to the client regarding safety measures related to sensory loss, such as regulating the temperature of bathwater and avoiding heating pads.

14. Reinforce instructions to the client regarding safety measures related to motor loss, such as avoiding the use of scatter rugs and using assistive devices.

15. Reinforce instructions to the client in the self-administration of prescribed medications.

16. Provide information about the National Multiple Sclerosis Society: https://www.nationalmssociety.org/.

XIII. Myasthenia Gravis

A. Description

1. Myasthenia gravis is a neuromuscular disease that is characterized by considerable weakness and abnormal fatigue of the voluntary muscles.

2. A defect in the transmission of nerve impulses at the myoneural junction occurs.

3. Causes include insufficient secretion of acetylcholine, excessive secretion of cholinesterase, and unresponsiveness of the muscle fibers to acetylcholine.

B. Data collection

1. Weakness and fatigue

2. Difficulty chewing and swallowing

3. Dysphagia

4. Ptosis

5. Diplopia

6. Weak, hoarse voice

7. Difficulty breathing

8. Diminished breath sounds

9. Respiratory paralysis and failure

C. Interventions

1. Monitor respiratory status and ability to cough and deep breathe adequately.

2. Monitor for respiratory failure.

3. Maintain suctioning and emergency equipment at the bedside.

4. Monitor vital signs.

5. Monitor speech and swallowing abilities to prevent aspiration.

6. Encourage the client to sit up when eating.

7. Assess muscle status.

8. Reinforce instructions to the client to conserve strength.

9. Plan short activities that coincide with times of maximal muscle strength.

10. Monitor for myasthenic and cholinergic crises.

11. Assist with the administration of anticholinesterase medications as prescribed.

12. Reinforce instructions to the client to avoid stress, infection, fatigue, and over-the-counter medications.

13. Reinforce instructions to the client to wear a MedicAlert bracelet.

14. Reinforce instructions to the client about services from the Myasthenia Gravis Foundation.

D. Anticholinesterase medications: Increase levels of acetylcholine at the myoneural junction (see Chapter 56)

E. Myasthenic crisis

1. Description

a. Myasthenic crisis is an acute exacerbation of the disease.

b. The crisis is caused by a rapid, unrecognized progression of the disease; an inadequate amount of medication; infection; fatigue; or stress.

2. Data collection

a. Increased pulse, respirations, and blood pressure

b. Dyspnea, anoxia, and cyanosis

c. Bowel and bladder incontinence

d. Decreased urine output

e. Absent cough and swallow reflex

3. Interventions

a. Monitor for signs of myasthenic crisis.

b. Increase anticholinesterase medication, as prescribed.

F. Cholinergic crisis

1. Description

a. Cholinergic crisis results in depolarization of the motor end plates.

b. The crisis is caused by overmedication with anticholinesterase.

2. Data collection

a. Abdominal cramps

b. Nausea, vomiting, and diarrhea

c. Blurred vision

d. Pallor

e. Facial muscle twitching

f. Hypotension

g. Pupillary miosis

3. Interventions

a. Withhold anticholinesterase medication.

b. Prepare to administer the antidote, atropine sulfate, if prescribed.

G. Acetylcholine receptor antibody (AChR AB, Anti-acetylcholine receptor antibody)

1. This test is performed to diagnose myasthenia gravis (MG) and to monitor response to treatment.

2. The presence of AChR is diagnostic of MG.

a. Normally, no AChR antibody exists in the bloodstream.

b. No fasting is required.

c. False-positive results can occur with other problems such as amyotrophic lateral sclerosis or those exposed to cobra venom.

d. Muscle relaxant and immunosuppressive medications can alter results.

XIV. Parkinson's Disease

A. Description

1. Parkinson's disease is a degenerative disease caused by the depletion of dopamine, which interferes with the inhibition of excitatory impulses, resulting in a dysfunction of the extrapyramidal system.

2. It is a slow, progressive disease that results in a crippling disability.

3. The debilitation can result in falls, self-care deficits, failure of body systems, and depression.

4. Mental deterioration occurs late in the disease.

B. Data collection

1. Bradykinesia, abnormal slowness of movement, and sluggishness of physical and mental responses

2. Akinesia

3. Monotonous speech

4. Handwriting that becomes progressively smaller

5. Tremors in hands and fingers at rest (pill rolling)

6. Tremors increasing when fatigued and decreasing with purposeful activity or sleep

7. Rigidity with jerky movements

8. Restlessness and pacing

9. Blank facial expression; mask-like facies

10. Drooling

11. Difficulty swallowing and speaking

12. Loss of coordination and balance

13. Shuffling steps, stooped position, and propulsive gait

C. Interventions

1. Monitor neurological status.

2. Check ability to swallow and chew.

3. Provide a high-calorie, high-protein, high-fiber soft diet with small, frequent feedings.

4. Increase fluid intake to 2000 mL/day.

5. Monitor for constipation.

6. Promote independence along with safety measures.

7. Avoid rushing the client with activities.

8. Assist with ambulation and provide assistive devices.

9. Reinforce instructions to the client to rock back and forth to initiate movement.

10. Reinforce instructions for the client to wear low-heeled shoes.

11. Encourage the client to lift his or her feet when walking and to avoid prolonged sitting.

12. Provide a firm mattress and position the client prone, without a pillow, to facilitate proper posture.

13. Reinforce instructions for proper posture by teaching the client to hold the hands behind the back to keep the spine and neck erect.

14. Promote physical therapy and rehabilitation.

15. Assist with the administration of antiparkinsonian medications to increase the level of dopamine in the CNS.

16. Reinforce instructions to the client to avoid foods high in vitamin B_6 because they block the effects of antiparkinsonian medications.

17. Reinforce instructions to the client to avoid monoamine oxidase inhibitors because they precipitate hypertensive crisis.

18. See Chapter 56 regarding medication to treat Parkinson's disease.

XV. Trigeminal Neuralgia

A. Description

1. Trigeminal neuralgia is a sensory disorder of the trigeminal (fifth cranial) nerve.

2. It results in severe, recurrent, sharp, facial pain along the trigeminal nerve.

B. Data collection

1. The client has severe pain on the lips, gums, or nose, or across the cheeks.

2. Situations that stimulate symptoms include cold, washing the face, chewing, or food or fluids of extreme temperatures.

C. Interventions

1. Reinforce instructions to the client to avoid hot or cold foods and fluids.

2. Provide small feedings of liquid and soft foods.

3. Reinforce instructions to the client to chew food on the unaffected side.

4. Assist with the administration of medications as prescribed (see Chapter 56).

D. Surgical interventions

1. Microvascular decompression: Surgical relocation of the artery that compresses the trigeminal nerve as it enters the pons; may relieve pain without compromising facial sensation

2. Radiofrequency wave forms: Creates lesions that provide relief from pain without compromising touch or motor function.

3. Rhizotomy: Resection of the root of the nerve to relieve pain

4. Glycerol injection: Destroys the myelinated fibers of the trigeminal nerve (may take up to 3 weeks for pain relief to occur)

XVI. Bell's Palsy (Facial Paralysis)

A. Description

1. Bell's palsy is caused by a lower motor neuron lesion of the seventh cranial nerve that may result from infection, trauma, hemorrhage, meningitis, or a tumor.

2. It results in paralysis of one side of the face.

3. Recovery usually occurs in a few weeks without residual effects.

B. Data collection

1. Flaccid facial muscles

2. Inability to raise the eyebrows, frown, smile, close the eyelids, or puff out the cheeks

3. Upward movement of the eye when attempting to close the eyelid

4. Loss of taste

C. Interventions

1. Encourage the client to do facial exercises to prevent the loss of muscle tone. (A face sling may be prescribed to prevent stretching of weak muscles.)

2. Protect the eyes from dryness and prevent injury.

3. Promote frequent oral care.

4. Reinforce instructions to the client to chew on the unaffected side.

XVII. Guillain-Barré Syndrome

A. Description

1. Guillain-Barré syndrome is an acute infectious neuronitis of the cranial and peripheral nerves.
2. The immune system overreacts to the infection and destroys the myelin sheath.
3. The syndrome is usually preceded by a mild upper respiratory infection or gastroenteritis.
4. Recovery is a slow process and can take years.

⚠️ The major concern associated with Guillain-Barré syndrome is difficulty breathing. Monitor respiratory status closely.

B. Data collection

1. Paresthesia
2. Pain and/or hypersensitivity such as with the weight of bed sheets or other items touching the body
3. Weakness of lower extremities
4. Gradual progressive weakness of the upper extremities and facial muscles
5. Possible progression to respiratory failure
6. Cardiac dysrhythmia
7. CSF that reveals an elevated protein level
8. Abnormal electroencephalogram

C. Interventions

1. Care is directed toward the treatment of symptoms, including pain management.
2. Monitor respiratory status.
3. Provide respiratory treatments.
4. Prepare to initiate respiratory support.
5. Monitor cardiac status.
6. Monitor for complications of immobility.
7. Provide the client and family with support.

XVIII. Amyotrophic Lateral Sclerosis

A. Description

1. Amyotrophic lateral sclerosis is also known as Lou Gehrig's disease.
2. It is a progressive degenerative disease involving the motor system.
3. The sensory and autonomic systems are not involved, and mental status changes do not result from the disease.
4. The cause of the disease may be related to an excess of glutamate, a chemical responsible for relaying messages between the motor neurons.
5. As the disease progresses, muscle weakness and atrophy develop until a flaccid tetraplegia develops.
6. Eventually the respiratory muscles become affected, leading to respiratory compromise, pneumonia, and death.
7. No cure is known, and the treatment is symptomatic.

B. Data collection

1. Respiratory difficulty
2. Fatigue while talking
3. Muscle weakness and atrophy
4. Tongue atrophy
5. Dysphagia
6. Weakness of the hands and arms
7. Fasciculations of the face
8. Nasal quality of speech
9. Dysarthria

C. Interventions

1. Care is directed toward the treatment of symptoms.
2. Monitor the respiratory status and institute measures to prevent aspiration.
3. Provide respiratory treatments.
4. Prepare to initiate respiratory support.
5. Monitor for complications of immobility.
6. Address advance directives as appropriate.
7. Provide the client and family with psychological support.

XIX. Encephalitis

A. Description

1. Encephalitis is an inflammation of the brain parenchyma and often the meninges.
2. It affects the cerebrum, brainstem, and cerebellum.
3. It is most often caused by a viral agent, although bacteria, fungi, or parasites may also be involved.
4. Viral encephalitis is almost always preceded by a viral infection.

B. Transmission

1. Arboviruses can be transmitted to human beings through the bite of an infected mosquito or tick.
2. Echovirus, coxsackievirus, poliovirus, herpes zoster, and viruses that cause mumps and chickenpox are common enteroviruses associated with encephalitis.
3. Herpes simplex virus type 1 can cause viral encephalitis.
4. The organism that causes amebic meningoencephalitis can enter the nasal mucosa of persons swimming in warm fresh water, for example, in a pond or lake.

C. Data collection

1. Presence of cold sores, lesions, or ulcerations of the oral cavity
2. History of insect bites and swimming in freshwater
3. Exposure to infectious diseases
4. Travel to areas where the disease is prevalent
5. Fever
6. Nausea and vomiting
7. Nuchal rigidity
8. Changes in LOC and mental status
9. Signs of increased ICP
10. Motor dysfunction and focal neurological deficits

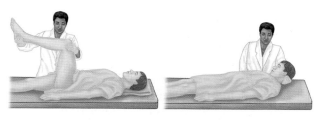

FIGURE 55.4 Kernig's sign and Brudzinski's sign.

D. Interventions
1. Monitor vital and neurological signs.
2. Check LOC using the Glasgow Coma Scale.
3. Monitor for mental status changes and personality and behavior changes.
4. Monitor for signs of increased ICP.
5. Check for the presence of nuchal rigidity and a positive Kernig's sign or Brudzinski's sign, indicating meningeal irritation (Fig. 55.4).
6. Assist the client to turn, cough, and deep breathe frequently.
7. Elevate the head of the bed 30 to 45 degrees.
8. Assess for muscle and neurological deficits.
9. Acyclovir may be prescribed (usually the medication of choice for herpes encephalitis).
10. Assist to initiate rehabilitation as needed for motor dysfunction or neurological deficits.

XX. West Nile Virus
A. Description
1. West Nile virus is a potentially serious illness that affects the CNS.
2. The virus is contracted primarily by the bite of an infected mosquito (mosquitoes become carriers when they feed on infected birds).
3. Symptoms typically develop 3 to 14 days after being bitten by the infected mosquito.
4. Neurological effects can be permanent.
B. Data collection
1. Many individuals will not experience any symptoms.
2. Mild symptoms include fever, headache and body aches, nausea, vomiting, swollen glands, or a rash on the chest, stomach, or back.
3. Severe symptoms include high fever, headache, neck stiffness, stupor, disorientation, tremors, muscle weakness, vision loss, numbness, paralysis, seizure, or coma.
C. Interventions are supportive. There is no specific treatment for the virus.
D. Prevention
1. Use insect repellents containing diethyltoluamide (DEET) when outdoors and wear long sleeves, long pants, and light-colored clothing.
2. Stay indoors at dusk and dawn when mosquitoes are most active.

3. Ensure that mosquito breeding sites are eliminated, such as standing water and water in birdbaths, and keep wading pools empty and on their sides when not in use.

XXI. Meningitis
A. Description
1. Meningitis refers to the inflammation of the arachnoid and pia mater of the brain and spinal cord.
2. It is caused by bacterial and viral organisms, although fungal and protozoan meningitis are also possible.
3. Predisposing factors include skull fractures, brain or spinal surgery, sinus or upper respiratory infections, the use of nasal sprays, and individuals with a compromised immune system.
4. CSF is analyzed to determine the diagnosis and the type of meningitis. In meningitis, CSF is cloudy, with increased protein, increased white blood cells, and decreased glucose counts.
B. Transmission: Occurs in areas of high-population density and crowded living areas such as college dormitories and prisons

⚠️ Transmission of meningitis is by direct contact, including droplet spread.

C. Data collection (see Box 55.4)
1. Mild lethargy; photophobia
2. Deterioration in the LOC
3. Signs of meningeal irritation such as nuchal rigidity and positive Kernig's sign and Brudzinski's sign
4. Red, macular rash with meningococcal meningitis
5. Abdominal and chest pain with viral meningitis
D. Interventions
1. Monitor vital signs and neurological signs.
2. Watch for signs of increasing ICP.
3. Initiate seizure precautions.
4. Monitor for seizure activity.
5. Monitor for signs of meningeal irritation.
6. Assist with performing a cranial nerve assessment.
7. Check peripheral vascular status. (Septic emboli may block circulation.)
8. Maintain isolation precautions as necessary with bacterial meningitis.
9. Maintain urine and stool precautions with viral meningitis.
10. Maintain respiratory isolation for the client with pneumococcal meningitis.
11. Elevate the head of the bed 30 degrees and avoid neck flexion and extreme hip flexion.
12. Prevent stimulation and restrict visitors.
13. Administer analgesics and antibiotics as prescribed.

WHAT WOULD YOU DO?

Answer: Unilateral body neglect syndrome is particularly common with strokes in the right cerebral hemisphere. In this syndrome, the client is unaware of his or her left or paralyzed side and neglects that side. If the nurse makes this observation, the nurse would immediately check the client for signs of injury and provide for a safe environment for the client. The registered nurse (RN) is also notified. The client with this syndrome often indicates that everything is fine and believes that he or she is sitting up straight in the chair. The client would be taught to use both sides of the body and to attend to the affected side first. If the client is experiencing visual problems, the client is taught to turn the head from side to side to expand the visual field.

PRACTICE QUESTIONS

❖ **1.** A client with a seizure disorder is being admitted to the hospital. Which would the nurse plan to implement for this client? **Select all that apply.**
   - ❑ **1.** Pad the bed's side rails
   - ❑ **2.** Place an airway at the bedside
   - ❑ **3.** Place oxygen equipment at the bedside
   - ❑ **4.** Place suction equipment at the bedside
   - ❑ **5.** Tape a padded tongue blade to the wall at the head of the bed

2. The client has just undergone a computed tomography (CT) scan with a contrast medium. Which statement by the client demonstrates an understanding of postprocedure care?
   1. "I need to eat lightly for the remainder of the day."
   2. "I need to rest quietly for the remainder of the day."
   3. "I need to wait to take any medication for at least 4 hours."
   4. "I need to drink extra fluids for the remainder of the day."

3. The nurse is caring for a client with increased intracranial pressure (ICP). Which change in vital signs would occur if ICP is rising?
   1. Increasing temperature, increasing pulse, increasing respirations, decreasing BP
   2. Decreasing temperature, decreasing pulse, increasing respirations, decreasing BP
   3. Decreasing temperature, increasing pulse, decreasing respirations, increasing BP
   4. Increasing temperature, decreasing pulse, decreasing respirations, increasing BP

4. The nurse observes the assistive personnel (AP) positioning the client with increased intracranial pressure (ICP). Which observation would require intervention by the nurse?
   1. The client's head is placed midline
   2. The client's head is turned to the side
   3. The client's neck is in neutral position
   4. The client's head of the bed is elevated 30 to 45 degrees

5. The client recovering from a head injury is arousable and participating in care. The nurse determines that the client understands measures to prevent elevations in intracranial pressure (ICP) if the nurse observes the client doing which activity?
   1. Blowing the nose
   2. Isometric exercises
   3. Coughing vigorously
   4. Exhaling during repositioning

6. The client has clear fluid leaking from the nose after a basilar skull fracture. The nurse determines that this is cerebrospinal fluid (CSF) if the fluid meets which criteria?
   1. It is grossly bloody in appearance and has a pH of 6
   2. It clumps together on the dressing and has a pH of 7
   3. It is clear in appearance and tests negative for glucose
   4. It separates into concentric rings and tests positive for glucose

7. The client is admitted to the hospital for observation with a probable minor head injury after an automobile crash. The nurse expects that the cervical collar will remain in place until which time?
   1. The client is taken for spinal x-rays.
   2. The family comes to visit after surgery.
   3. The nurse needs to provide physical care.
   4. The primary health care provider (PHCP) reviews the x-ray results.

8. The client was seen and treated in the emergency department (ED) for a concussion. Before discharge, the nurse explains the signs/symptoms of a worsening condition. The nurse determines that the family **needs further teaching** if they state they will return to the ED if the client experiences which sign/symptom?
   1. Vomiting
   2. Minor headache
   3. Difficulty speaking
   4. Difficulty awakening

9. The nurse is caring for a client who has undergone craniotomy with a supratentorial incision. The nurse would plan to place the client in which position postoperatively?
   1. Head of bed flat, head and neck midline
   2. Head of bed flat, head turned to the nonoperative side
   3. Head of bed elevated 30 to 45 degrees, head and neck midline
   4. Head of bed elevated 30 to 45 degrees, head turned to the operative side

10. The client with a cervical spine injury has Crutchfield tongs applied in the emergency department. The nurse would perform which **essential** action when caring for this client?
    1. Provide a standard bed frame
    2. Remove the weights to reposition the client
    3. Remove the weights if the client is uncomfortable
    4. Compare the amount of prescribed weights with the amount in use

11. The nurse has provided discharge instructions to a client with an application of a halo device. The nurse determines that the client **needs further teaching** if which statement is made?
    1. "I will use a straw for drinking."
    2. "I will drive only during the daytime."
    3. "I will use caution because the device alters balance."
    4. "I will wash my skin daily under the lamb's wool liner of the vest."

12. The nurse is caring for the client who has suffered spinal cord injury. The nurse further monitors the client for signs of autonomic dysreflexia and suspects this complication if which sign/symptom is noted?

1. Sudden tachycardia
2. Pallor of the face and neck
3. Severe, throbbing headache
4. Severe and sudden hypotension

13. The client with spinal cord injury is prone to experiencing autonomic dysreflexia. The least appropriate measure to minimize the risk of autonomic dysreflexia is which action?
    1. Strictly adhering to a bowel retraining program
    2. Keeping the linen wrinkle-free under the client
    3. Avoiding unnecessary pressure on the lower limbs
    4. Limiting bladder catheterization to once every 12 hours

14. The client with spinal cord injury suddenly experiences an episode of autonomic dysreflexia. After checking vital signs, which **immediate** action would the nurse take?
    1. Raise the head of the bed and remove the noxious stimulus
    2. Lower the head of the bed and remove the noxious stimulus
    3. Lower the head of the bed and administer an antihypertensive agent
    4. Remove the noxious stimulus and administer an antihypertensive agent

15. The client is having a lumbar puncture (LP) performed. The nurse would place the client in which position for the procedure?
    1. Supine, in semi-Fowler's
    2. Prone, in slight Trendelenburg
    3. Prone, with a pillow under the abdomen
    4. Side-lying, with legs pulled up and chin to the chest

ANSWERS

❖ **1. 1, 2, 3, 4**
Rationale: The nurse would plan seizure precautions for a client with a seizure disorder. The precautions include padded side rails and an airway (to maintain airway patency if required), and oxygen and suction equipment at the bedside. Attempts to force a padded tongue blade between clenched teeth may result in injury to the teeth and mouth; therefore, a padded tongue blade is not placed at the bedside.
Test-Taking Strategy: Focus on the subject, preparation for a client being admitted with a seizure disorder. Consider the items that are needed to keep a client safe if a seizure occurs. Eliminate the padded tongue blade as this item could cause injury if placed in the mouth during a seizure.

2. 4
Rationale: After CT scanning, the client may resume all usual activities. The client would be encouraged to take in extra fluids to replace those lost with diuresis from the contrast dye. Options 1, 2, and 3 are unnecessary.

Test-Taking Strategy: Eliminate options 1 and 3 because they are comparable or alike. Next, focus the subject, that a contrast medium was given. This will direct you to the correct option.

3. 4
Rationale: A change in vital signs may be a late sign of increased ICP. Trends include increasing temperature and blood pressure and decreasing pulse and respirations. Respiratory irregularities may also arise.
Test-Taking Strategy: Think about the pathophysiology of increased ICP. If you remember that blood pressure rises, you are able to eliminate options 1 and 2 as comparable or alike. To select from the remaining options, remember that the temperature rises.

4. 2
Rationale: The head of the client with increased ICP would be positioned so that the head is in a neutral, midline position. The nurse would avoid flexing or extending the neck or turning the head side to side. The head of the bed needs to be raised to 30 to 45 degrees. Use of proper

positions promotes venous drainage from the cranium to keep ICP down.

Test-Taking Strategy: Focus on the subject, the need for the nurse to intervene. This indicates a position that interferes with arterial circulation to the brain or with venous drainage from the brain. The only answer that meets one of those criteria is option 2.

5. 4

Rationale: Activities that increase intrathoracic and intra-abdominal pressures cause indirect elevation of the ICP. Some of these activities include isometric exercises, Valsalva maneuver, coughing, sneezing, and blowing the nose. Exhaling during activities such as repositioning or pulling up in bed opens the glottis, which prevents intrathoracic pressure from rising.

Test-Taking Strategy: Focus on the subject, activities that increase intracranial pressure. Evaluate each option in terms of the tension it puts on the body to help you eliminate each of the incorrect options.

6. 4

Rationale: Leakage of CSF from the ears or nose may accompany basilar skull fracture. It can be distinguished from other body fluids because the drainage will separate into bloody and yellow concentric rings on dressing material, which is known as the halo sign. It also tests positive for glucose. Options 1, 2, and 3 are not characteristics of CSF.

Test-Taking Strategy: Focus on the subject, the characteristics of CSF. Recall that CSF contains glucose, whereas other secretions such as mucus do not. Also, remember that CSF separates into rings.

7. 4

Rationale: There is a significant association between cervical spine injury and head injury. For this reason, the nurse leaves any form of spinal immobilization in place until lateral cervical spine x-rays rule out fracture or other damage and the results have been reviewed by the PHCP.

Test-Taking Strategy: Focus on the subject, the client's injury. Remember that the reason for spinal immobilization is to protect the spine from movement, which could cause further damage if the cervical spine were injured. If x-ray results are negative, the PHCP will discontinue the cervical collar.

8. 2

Rationale: A concussion after head injury is a temporary loss of consciousness (from a few seconds to a few minutes) without evidence of structural damage. After concussion, the family is taught to monitor the client and call the primary health care provider or return the client to the emergency department if certain signs/symptoms are noted. These include confusion, difficulty awakening or speaking, one-sided weakness, vomiting, or severe headache. Minor headache is expected.

Test-Taking Strategy: Note the strategic words, *needs further teaching*. These words indicate a negative event query and the need to select the incorrect family statement. Noting the word *minor* in option 2 will direct you to this option.

9. 3

Rationale: Following supratentorial surgery, the head of the bed is kept at a 30- to 45-degree angle. The head and neck would not be angled either anteriorly or laterally, but rather would be kept in a neutral (midline) position. This will promote venous return through the jugular veins, which will help prevent a rise in intracranial pressure.

Test-Taking Strategy: This question tests knowledge of the subject, differences in positioning the craniotomy client with an infratentorial *versus* supratentorial incision. If you remember that with *supra*, one would *keep the head up*, and with *infra*, one would *keep the head down*, options 1 and 2 can be eliminated. Knowing how to position the head for optimal venous drainage helps you select option 3 over option 4.

10. 4

Rationale: Crutchfield tongs are applied after drilling holes in the client's skull under local anesthesia. Weights are attached to the tongs, which exert pulling pressure on the longitudinal axis of the cervical spine. The nurse ensures that weights hang freely and that the amount of weight matches the current prescription. The client with Crutchfield tongs is placed on a Stryker frame or Roto-Rest bed. The nurse does not remove the weights to administer care or change the level of tension or traction based on client comfort level.

Test-Taking Strategy: Note the strategic word, *essential*. Recalling the basic principles of traction care and that weights are not removed will direct you to the correct option.

11. 2

Rationale: Driving is not allowed because the device impairs the range of vision. The halo device alters balance and can cause fatigue because of its weight. The client would cleanse the skin daily under the vest or the device to protect the skin from ulceration and would use powder or lotions sparingly or not at all. The wool liner would be changed if odor becomes a problem. The client needs to have food cut into small pieces to facilitate chewing and use a straw for drinking. Pin care is done as instructed.

Test-Taking Strategy: Note the strategic words, *needs further teaching*. These words indicate a negative event query and the need to select the incorrect client statement. Recall that a halo device is used to allow mobility for the client who needs continuous cervical traction; it maintains the head and spine in a neutral position. With this in mind, select option 2 as the correct option. The inability to turn the head without turning the torso would contraindicate driving.

12. 3

Rationale: The client with spinal cord injury above level T7 is at risk for autonomic dysreflexia. It is characterized by a severe, throbbing headache, flushing of the face and neck, bradycardia, and sudden severe hypertension. Other signs include nasal stuffiness, blurred vision, nausea, and sweating. It is a life-threatening syndrome triggered by a noxious stimulus below the level of the injury.

Test-Taking Strategy: Focus on the subject, autonomic dysreflexia. Remember that autonomic dysreflexia results from the sudden exaggerated response of the sympathetic nervous system to a noxious stimulus. A massive sympathetic nervous system response causes severe hypertension. This would account for the throbbing headache and cause flushing of the face and neck. Baroreceptors sense the sudden hypertension, causing a reflex bradycardia. Also remember that the pulse and blood pressure changes that occur with autonomic dysreflexia are actually the opposite of what would occur with hypovolemic shock.

13. 4

Rationale: The most frequent cause of autonomic dysreflexia is a distended bladder. Straight catheterization would be performed every 4 to 6 hours, and indwelling bladder catheters would be checked frequently for kinks in the tubing. It is not appropriate to catheterize the client every 12 hours. Constipation and fecal impaction are other causes, so maintaining bowel regularity is important. Other causes include stimulation of the skin from tactile, thermal, or painful stimuli. The nurse administers care to minimize risk in these areas.

Test-Taking Strategy: Focus on the subject, the least appropriate action. The least appropriate action is the action that would not be taken. Remember that autonomic dysreflexia is caused by noxious stimuli to the bowel, bladder, or skin. With this in mind, you can eliminate the incorrect options because they are the correct thing to do for the client.

14. 1

Rationale: Key nursing actions are to sit the client up in bed, remove the noxious stimulus, and bring the blood pressure under control with antihypertensive medication per protocol. The nurse can also clearly label the client's chart identifying the risk for autonomic dysreflexia. Client and family would be taught to recognize, and later manage, the signs/symptoms of this syndrome.

Test-Taking Strategy: Note the strategic word, *immediate*. This indicates that this is the first action you would take. If you know to raise the head of the client's bed first (to try to minimize cerebral hypertension), then this eliminates each of the incorrect options.

15. 4

Rationale: The client undergoing a lumbar puncture (LP) is positioned lying on the side, with the knees bent, drawn up to the abdomen, and the chin tucked into the chest. This position helps to open the spaces between the vertebrae.

Test-Taking Strategy: Focus on the subject, positioning for a lumbar puncture (LP). Recall that an LP is the introduction of a needle into the subarachnoid space, so it is reasonable that the position of the client needs to facilitate the procedure. The correct answer is the only position that flexes the vertebrae for easier needle insertion.

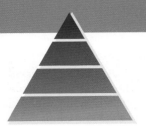

CHAPTER 56

Neurological Medications

PRIORITY CONCEPTS **Intracranial Regulation; Pain**

WHAT WOULD YOU DO?

A client with a traumatic brain injury experiencing restlessness and agitation because of the pain is receiving morphine sulfate. During data collection, the nurse measures the respiratory rate and notes it to be 10 breaths/min. What would the nurse do?
Answer is located on p.800.

I. Antimyasthenic Medications

A. Description
 1. Antimyasthenic medications, also called anticholinesterase medications, relieve muscle weakness associated with myasthenia gravis by blocking acetylcholine breakdown at the neuromuscular junction.
 2. Antimyasthenic medications are used to treat or diagnose myasthenia gravis or distinguish cholinergic crisis from myasthenic crisis.
 3. Neostigmine bromide and pyridostigmine are used to control myasthenic symptoms.
B. Medications (Box 56.1)
C. Side and adverse effects: Cholinergic crisis (Box 56.2)

D. Interventions
 1. Monitor neuromuscular status, including reflexes, muscle strength, and gait.
 2. Monitor the client for signs/symptoms of medication overdose (cholinergic crisis) and underdose (myasthenic crisis).
 3. Reinforce instructions to the client to take medications on time to maintain therapeutic blood level, thus preventing weakness, because weakness can impair the client's ability to breathe and swallow.
 4. Reinforce instructions to the client to take the medication with a small amount of food to prevent gastrointestinal symptoms.

 5. Reinforce instructions to the client to eat 45 to 60 minutes after taking medications to decrease the risk for aspiration.
 6. Reinforce instructions to the client to wear a MedicAlert bracelet.
 7. Note that antimyasthenic therapy is lifelong therapy.
 8. Monitor for medication effectiveness, which is based on the improvement of neuromuscular symptoms or strength without cholinergic signs/symptoms.

II. Multiple Sclerosis Medications

A. Description
 1. Medication therapy is aimed at modifying the disease, treating acute episodes or relapses, and treating associated symptoms.
 2. Disease-modifying medications decrease the frequency and severity of relapses, reduce brain lesions, increase future functional capability, and increase overall quality of life.
 3. The two main groups of disease-modifying medications are immunomodulators and immunosuppressants (Box 56.3).
 4. Treating acute episodes usually consists of giving high-dose glucocorticoid intravenously to suppress inflammation or giving gamma globulin intravenously.
 5. Treating symptoms of multiple sclerosis can be done with a variety of medications and the medication can be changed if unfavorable effects occur.
 6. Box 56.4 identifies medications commonly used to treat symptoms.
B. Side and adverse effects
 1. Immunomodulators: Flu-like reactions, hepatotoxicity, myelosuppression, injection site reactions, depression, and neutralizing antibodies
 2. Immunosuppressants: Myelosuppression, cardiotoxicity, fetal harm, reversible hair loss, injury to the gastrointestinal mucosa, nausea and vomiting, and menstrual irregularities

BOX 56.1 Antimyasthenic Medications

Neostigmine bromide
Pyridostigmine

BOX 56.2 Signs of Cholinergic Crisis

Abdominal cramps
Nausea, vomiting, and diarrhea
Pupillary miosis
Hypotension and dizziness
Increased bronchial secretions
Increased tearing and salivation
Increased perspiration
Increased bronchial secretions
Bronchospasm, wheezing, and bradycardia

BOX 56.3 Medications for Multiple Sclerosis

Immunomodulators
Cladribine
Dimethyl fumarate
Fingolimod
Glatiramer acetate
Interferons (β-1a, 1b, peginterferon β-1a)
Teriflunomide

Immunosuppressant
Mitoxantrone

Monoclonal Antibodies
Alemtuzumab
Natalizumab
Ocrelizumab

Potassium Channel Blockers
Dalfampridine (used to improve walking)

BOX 56.4 Medications to Treat Symptoms of Multiple Sclerosis

Bladder and bowel dysfunction: psyllium, docusate
Fatigue: amantadine, modafinil
Depression: fluoxetine, sertraline
Sexual dysfunction: sildenafil, vardenafil
Neuropathic pain: gabapentin, carbamazepine

Adapted from Burchum JR, Rosenthal LD: *Lehne's pharmacology for nursing care*, ed 10, St. Louis, 2019, Elsevier.

b. Dopaminergic medications are contraindicated in clients with cardiac, renal, or psychiatric disorders.

⚠ Carbidopa-levodopa taken with a monoamine oxidase inhibitor antidepressant can cause a hypertensive crisis.

2. Medications (Box 56.5)
3. Side and adverse effects
   a. Dyskinesia
   b. Involuntary body movements
   c. Chest pain
   d. Nausea and vomiting
   e. Urinary retention
   f. Constipation
   g. Sleep disturbance, insomnia, or periods of sedation
   h. Orthostatic hypotension and dizziness
   i. Confusion
   j. Change in mood, especially depression
   k. Hallucination
   l. Dry mouth
4. Interventions
   a. Monitor vital signs.
   b. Determine risk for injury.
   c. The client is instructed to take the medication with food if nausea or vomiting occurs.
   d. Check for signs/symptoms of parkinsonism, such as rigidity, tremors, akinesia, and bradykinesia, a stooped forward posture, shuffling gait, and masked facies.
   e. Monitor for signs of dyskinesia.
   f. The client is instructed to report side and adverse effects and symptoms of dyskinesia.
   g. Monitor the client for improvement in signs/symptoms of parkinsonism.
   h. The client is instructed to change positions slowly to minimize orthostatic hypotension.
   i. Reinforce instructions to the client to not discontinue the medication abruptly.
   j. Reinforce instructions to the client to avoid alcohol.
   k. The client is informed that urine or perspiration may be discolored and that this is harmless but may stain clothing.

III. Antiparkinsonian Medications

A. Description
1. Antiparkinsonian medications restore the balance of the neurotransmitters acetylcholine and dopamine in the central nervous system (CNS), decreasing and slowing signs/symptoms of Parkinson's disease to maximize the client's functional abilities.
2. These medications include the dopaminergics, which stimulate the dopamine receptors; the anticholinergics, which block the cholinergic receptors; and the catechol-O-methyltransferase inhibitors, which inhibit the metabolism of dopamine in the periphery.

B. Dopaminergic medications
1. Description
   a. Dopaminergic medications stimulate the dopamine receptors and increase the amount of dopamine available in the CNS or enhance neurotransmission of dopamine.

BOX 56.5 **Medications to Treat Parkinson's Disease**

Medications Affecting the Amount of Dopamine

Amantadine
Apomorphine
Bromocriptine
Carbidopa-levodopa
Pramipexole
Rasagiline
Ropinirole
Rotigotine
Safinamide
Selegiline hydrochloride

Anticholinergics

Benztropine mesylate
Trihexyphenidyl hydrochloride

Catechol O-Methyltransferase (COMT) Inhibitors

Carbidopa/levodopa/entacapone
Entacapone
Opicapone
Tolcapone

---

l. The client with diabetes mellitus is advised that glucose testing would not be done by urine testing because the results will not be reliable.

m. Reinforce instructions to the client taking carbidopa-levodopa to divide the total daily prescribed protein intake among all meals of the day. High-protein diets interfere with medication availability to the CNS.

n. When administering carbidopa-levodopa, the client is instructed to avoid excessive vitamin B_6 intake to prevent reaction(s) to the medication.

C. Anticholinergic medications
   1. Description
      a. Anticholinergic medications block the cholinergic receptors in the CNS, thereby suppressing acetylcholine activity.
      b. Anticholinergic medications reduce tremors and drooling but have a minimal effect on bradykinesia, rigidity, and balance abnormalities.

      c. Anticholinergic medications are contraindicated in clients with glaucoma.
      d. The client with chronic obstructive lung disease can develop dry, thick mucus secretions.
   2. Medications (see Box 56.5)

   3. Side and adverse effects
      a. Blurred vision
      b. Dryness of the nose, mouth, throat, and respiratory secretions
      c. Increased pulse rate, palpitations, and dysrhythmia
      d. Constipation
      e. Urinary retention
      f. Restlessness, confusion, depression, and hallucinations

g. Photophobia
4. Interventions
   a. Monitor vital signs.
   b. Determine risk for injury.
   c. Monitor the client for improvement in signs/symptoms.
   d. Check the client's bowel and urinary function, and monitor for urinary retention, constipation, and paralytic ileus.
   e. Monitor for involuntary movements.
   f. The client is encouraged to avoid alcohol, smoking, caffeine, and aspirin to decrease gastric acidity.
   g. Reinforce instructions to the client to consult with the primary health care provider (PHCP) before taking any nonprescription medication(s).
   h. Reinforce instructions to the client to minimize dry mouth by increasing fluid intake and using ice chips, hard candy, or gum.
   i. Reinforce instructions to the client to prevent constipation by increasing fluids and fiber in the diet.
   j. Reinforce instructions to the client to use sunglasses in direct sunlight because of possible photophobia.
   k. Reinforce instructions to the client to have routine eye examinations to assess for intraocular pressure.

 If an anticholinergic medication is discontinued abruptly, the signs/symptoms of parkinsonism, such as rigidity, tremors, akinesia and bradykinesia, a stooped forward posture, shuffling gait, and masked facies may be intensified.

IV. Antiseizure Medications

A. Description
   1. Antiseizure medications are used to depress abnormal neuronal discharge and to suppress the spread of seizure to adjacent neurons.
   2. Antiseizure medications would be used with caution in clients taking anticoagulants, aspirin, sulfonamides, cimetidine, and antipsychotic drugs.
   3. Absorption is decreased with the use of antacids, calcium preparations, and antineoplastic medications.

B. Interventions for clients on antiseizure medications
   1. Initiate seizure precautions.
   2. Monitor urinary output.
   3. Monitor liver and renal function tests and medication blood serum levels.
   4. Monitor for signs of medication toxicity, which would include CNS depression, ataxia, nausea, vomiting, drowsiness, dizziness, restlessness, and visual disturbances.
   5. If a seizure occurs, monitor seizure activity, including location and duration.

BOX 56.6 **Client Education: Antiseizure Medications**

- Take the prescribed medication in the prescribed dose and frequency.
- Take antiseizure medications with food to decrease gastrointestinal irritation, but avoid milk and antacids, which impair absorption.
- If taking liquid medication, shake well before ingesting.
- Do not discontinue the medication(s).
- Avoid alcohol.
- Avoid over-the-counter medications.
- Wear a MedicAlert bracelet.
- Use caution when driving or performing activities that require alertness.
- Maintain good oral hygiene, and use a soft toothbrush.
- Maintain preventive dental checkups.
- Maintain follow-up health care visits with periodic blood studies related to determining toxicity.
- Monitor serum glucose levels (diabetes mellitus).
- Urine may be a harmless pink-red or red-brown in color.
- Report symptoms of sore throat, bruising, and nosebleeds, which may indicate a blood dyscrasia.
- Inform the primary health care provider (PHCP) if side and adverse effects occur, such as gingivitis, nystagmus, slurred speech, rash, or dizziness.

---

6. Protect the client from hazards in the environment during a seizure.

 C. Client education (Box 56.6).

 D. Hydantoins: Fosphenytoin, phenytoin
1. Hydantoins are used to treat partial and generalized tonic-clonic seizures.
2. Phenytoin is also used to treat various types of dysrhythmia.
3. Side and adverse effects
   a. Gingival hyperplasia (reddened gums that bleed easily)
   b. Slurred speech
   c. Confusion
   d. Sedation and drowsiness
   e. Nausea and vomiting
   f. Blurred vision and nystagmus
   g. Headache
   h. Blood dyscrasia: Decreased platelet count and decreased white blood cell count
   i. Elevated blood glucose level
   j. Alopecia or hirsutism
   k. Skin rash or pruritus
4. Interventions
   a. Tube feedings may interfere with the absorption of the enteral form of phenytoin and diminish the effectiveness of the medication; therefore, feedings would be scheduled as far as possible from the time of phenytoin administration.
   b. Monitor therapeutic serum levels to assess for toxicity.

c. Monitor for signs of toxicity.
d. Monitor for ataxia (staggering gait).
e. Reinforce instructions to the client to consult with the PHCP before taking other medications to ensure compatibility with antiseizure medications.

⚠️ Intravenous phenytoin must be given slowly to prevent hypotension and cardiac dysrhythmia. Also, note that oral phenytoin decreases the effectiveness of some birth control pills and can have teratogenic effects if taken during pregnancy.

E. Barbiturates: Amobarbital, phenobarbital
1. Barbiturates are used for tonic-clonic seizures and acute episodes of seizures caused by status epilepticus.
2. Barbiturates may also be used as adjuncts to anesthesia.
3. Side and adverse effects
   a. Sedation, ataxia, and dizziness during initial treatment
   b. Change in mood
   c. Hypotension
   d. Respiratory depression
   e. Tolerance to the medication
F. Benzodiazepines: Clonazepam, clorazepate, diazepam, lorazepam
1. Benzodiazepines are used to treat absence seizures.
2. Diazepam and lorazepam are used to treat status epilepticus, anxiety, and skeletal muscle spasms.
3. Clorazepate is used as adjunctive therapy for partial seizures.
4. Side and adverse effects
   a. Sedation, drowsiness, dizziness, blurred vision
   b. Bradycardia can occur when administered rapidly by the intravenous route.
   c. Medication tolerance and drug dependency
   d. Blood dyscrasia: Decreased platelet count and decreased white blood cell count
   e. Hepatotoxicity

⚠️ Flumazenil reverses the effects of benzodiazepines. It is contraindicated in clients with increased intracranial pressure or status epilepticus who were treated with benzodiazepines, because these problems may recur with reversal.

G. Succinimides: Ethosuximide, methsuximide
1. Succinimides are used to treat absence seizures.
2. Side and adverse effects
   a. Anorexia, nausea, vomiting
   b. Blood dyscrasia
H. Valproates: valproic acid, divalproex sodium
1. Valproates are used to treat tonic-clonic, partial, and myoclonic seizures.

2. Side and adverse effects
   a. Transient nausea, vomiting, and indigestion
   b. Sedation, drowsiness, and dizziness
   c. Pancreatitis
   d. Blood dyscrasias
   e. Hepatotoxicity

 I. Iminostilbenes
   1. Iminostilbenes are used to treat seizure disorders that have not responded to other antiseizure medications.
    2. Iminostilbenes are used to treat trigeminal neuralgia.
   3. Side and adverse effects
      a. Drowsiness
      b. Dizziness
      c. Nausea and vomiting, dry mouth
      d. Constipation or diarrhea
      e. Rash
      f. Visual abnormalities
      g. Blood dyscrasias, agranulocytosis
      h. Headache

J. Other antiseizure medications. (Box 56.7)

V. CNS Stimulants

A. Description
   1. Amphetamines and caffeine stimulate the cerebral cortex of the brain (Box 56.8).
   2. Amphetamines have a high potential for abuse.
   3. Analeptics and caffeine act on the brainstem and medulla to stimulate respiration.
   4. Anorexiants act on the cerebral cortex and hypothalamus to suppress appetite (Box 56.9).
   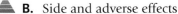 5. CNS stimulants are used to treat narcolepsy and attention-deficit/hyperactivity disorders and are used as adjunctive therapy for exogenous obesity.

B. Side and adverse effects
   1. Irritability
   2. Restlessness
   3. Tremors
   4. Insomnia
   5. Heart palpitations
   6. Tachycardia and dysrhythmia
   7. Hypertension
   8. Dry mouth
   9. Anorexia and weight loss
   10. Abdominal cramping
   11. Diarrhea or constipation
   12. Hepatic failure
   13. Psychoses
   14. Impotence
   15. Dependence and tolerance

C. Interventions
   1. Monitor vital signs.
   2. Monitor mental status.
   3. Document degrees of inattention, impulsivity, hyperactivity, and periods of sleepiness.
   4. Check height, weight, and growth if prescribed for a child.

BOX 56.7   **Other Antiseizure Medications**

Carbamazepine
Gabapentin
Lacosamide
Lamotrigine
Levetiracetam
Oxcarbazepine
Pregabalin
Tiagabine
Topiramate
Zonisamide
Vigabatrin

BOX 56.8   **Amphetamines**

Amphetamine sulfate
Amphetamine/dextroamphetamine
Atomoxetine
Dextroamphetamine sulfate
Dexmethylphenidate
Lisdexamfetamine
Methylphenidate hydrochloride

BOX 56.9   **Anorexiants**

Benzphetamine hydrochloride
Bupropion/naltrexone
Diethylpropion
Lorcaserin
Orlistat
Phendimetrazine
Phentermine hydrochloride
Phentermine/topiramate

---

5. Monitor the complete blood count and white blood cell and platelet counts before and during therapy.
6. Monitor for side and adverse effects.
7. Monitor sleep patterns.
8. Monitor for withdrawal symptoms such as nausea, vomiting, weakness, and headache.
9. Reinforce instructions to the client to take the medication before meals.
10. Reinforce instructions to the client to avoid foods and beverages containing caffeine to prevent additional stimulation.
11. Reinforce instructions to the client to not chew or crush long-acting forms of the medications.
12. Reinforce instructions to the client to read labels on over-the-counter products because many contain caffeine.
13. Reinforce instructions to the client to avoid alcohol.
14. Reinforce instructions to the client not to discontinue the medication abruptly (can produce extreme fatigue and depression).

15. Reinforce instructions to the client to take the last daily dose of the CNS stimulant at least 6 hours before bedtime to prevent insomnia.
16. Monitor for drug dependence and abuse with amphetamines.
17. If a child is taking a CNS stimulant, instruct the parents to notify the school nurse.
18. Monitor for calming effects of CNS stimulants within 3 to 4 weeks for children with attention-deficit/hyperactivity disorder.
19. Monitor growth in the child placed on long-term therapy with methylphenidate hydrochloride or other medication to treat attention-deficit/hyperactivity disorder.

VI. Nonopioid Analgesics

A. Nonsteroidal anti-inflammatory drugs (NSAIDs) (Box 56.10)
   1. Description
      a. NSAIDs are aspirin and aspirin-like medications that inhibit the synthesis of prostaglandins.
      b. The medications act as an analgesic to relieve pain, as an antipyretic to reduce body temperature, and as an anticoagulant to inhibit platelet aggregation.
      c. NSAIDs are used to relieve inflammation and pain and treat rheumatoid arthritis, bursitis, tendinitis, osteoarthritis, and acute gout.
      d. NSAIDs are contraindicated in clients with hypersensitivity or liver or renal disease.
      e. Clients taking anticoagulants should not take aspirin or NSAIDs.
      f. Aspirin and an NSAID should not be taken together because aspirin decreases the blood level and the effectiveness of the NSAID and can increase the risk of bleeding.
      g. NSAIDs can increase the effects of warfarin, sulfonamides, cephalosporins, and phenytoin.
      h. Hypoglycemia can result if ibuprofen is taken with insulin or oral hypoglycemic medication.
      i. A high risk of toxicity exists if ibuprofen is taken concurrently with calcium channel blockers.

 Adolescents and children with flu-like symptoms, viral illnesses, and varicella should not take aspirin because of the risk of Reye's syndrome.

   2. Side and adverse effects (Box 56.11)
   3. Interventions
      a. Check client for allergies.
      b. Obtain a medication history.
      c. Check for history of gastric upset or bleeding, or liver or renal disease.

BOX 56.10 Nonopioid Analgesics

Acetaminophen
Acetaminophen

Aspirin
Aspirin (acetylsalicylic acid; ASA)
Aspirin (acetylsalicylic acid), buffered

Nonsteroidal Anti-Inflammatory Drugs
Ibuprofen
Naproxen

Cyclooxygenase-2 (COX-2) Inhibitor
Celecoxib

Other Nonsteroidal Anti-Inflammatory Drugs
Diclofenac
Diflunisal
Etodolac
Flurbiprofen
Indomethacin
Ketoprofen
Ketorolac
Meclofenamate
Mefenamic acid
Meloxicam
Nabumetone
Oxaprozin
Piroxicam
Sulindac
Tolmetin

BOX 56.11 Side and Adverse Effects of Aspirin and Nonsteroidal Anti-Inflammatory Drugs

Acetylsalicylic Acid
Allergic reactions (anaphylaxis, laryngeal edema)
Bleeding (anemia, hemolysis, increased bleeding time)
Decreased renal function
Dizziness
Drowsiness
Flushing
Gastrointestinal symptoms (distress, heartburn, nausea, vomiting)
Headache
Tinnitus
Visual changes

Nonsteroidal Anti-Inflammatory Drugs
Dysrhythmia
Blood dyscrasias
Cardiovascular thrombotic events
Decreased renal function
Dizziness
Gastric irritation
Hepatotoxicity
Hypotension
Pruritus
Sodium and water retention
Tinnitus

Adult—Neurological

d. Monitor the client for gastrointestinal upset during medication administration.

e. Monitor for edema.

f. Monitor serum salicylate level when the client is taking high doses.

g. Monitor for signs of bleeding such as tarry stools, bleeding gums, petechiae, ecchymosis, and purpura.

h. Reinforce instructions to the client to take the medication with water, milk, or food.

i. An enteric-coated or buffered form of aspirin can be taken to decrease gastric distress.

j. Reinforce instructions to the client that enteric-coated tablets cannot be crushed or broken.

k. Clients taking aspirin would sit upright for 20 to 30 minutes after taking the dose.

l. The client is advised to inform other health care professionals they are taking aspirin.

m. Note that aspirin needs to be discontinued 3 to 7 days before surgery to reduce the risk of bleeding.

n. Reinforce instructions to the client to avoid alcoholic beverages.

B. Acetaminophen

1. Description

a. Acetaminophen inhibits prostaglandin synthesis.

b. Used to decrease pain (mild to moderate) and fever

c. Would not be taken if liver dysfunction exists

2. Side and adverse effects

a. Anorexia, nausea, vomiting

b. Rash

c. Hypoglycemia

d. Oliguria

e. Hepatotoxicity

3. Interventions

a. Monitor vital signs.

b. Check the client for a history of liver and renal dysfunction, alcoholism, and malnutrition.

c. Monitor for hepatic damage, which includes nausea, vomiting, diarrhea, and abdominal pain.

d. Monitor liver enzyme test results.

e. Reinforce instructions to the client that self-medication would not be done longer than 10 days for an adult and 5 days for a child.

f. Note that the antidote for acetaminophen is acetylcysteine.

g. Evaluate for the effectiveness of the medication.

⚠️ Acetaminophen is contraindicated in clients with hepatic or renal disease, alcoholism, and/or hypersensitivity.

VII. Opioid Analgesics

A. Description

1. Opioid analgesics suppress pain impulses but can suppress respiration and coughing by acting on

---

BOX 56.12	Opioid Analgesics

Acetaminophen/hydrocodone
Codeine
Fentanyl
Hydrocodone
Hydromorphone
Meperidine
Methadone
Morphine
Oxycodone
Oxycodone/acetaminophen
Oxymorphone
Tapentadol
Tramadol

---

the respiratory and cough center in the medulla of the brainstem.

2. Can produce euphoria and sedation and cause physical dependence

3. Used for relief of mild, moderate, or severe pain

B. Medications (Box 56.12)

1. Codeine

a. Codeine is also an effective cough suppressant at low doses.

b. Codeine can cause constipation.

2. Hydromorphone

a. Can decrease respiration

b. Can cause constipation

3. Meperidine hydrochloride

a. Can cause hypotension, dizziness, and urinary retention

b. May be used for acute pain and as a preoperative medication

c. May lead to increased intracranial pressure in clients with head injuries

d. Meperidine is contraindicated in clients with head injuries and increased intracranial pressure, respiratory disorders, hypotension, shock, and severe hepatic and renal disease and in clients taking monoamine oxidase inhibitors.

e. Meperidine would not be taken with alcohol or a sedative-hypnotic because it may increase the CNS depression.

f. Meperidine would be used cautiously in children and adults with a seizure disorder or a history of seizures because it decreases the seizure threshold.

4. Morphine

a. Can cause respiratory depression, orthostatic hypotension, and constipation

b. May cause nausea and vomiting because of increased vestibular sensitivity

c. Is used for acute pain caused by myocardial infarction or cancer, for dyspnea caused by pulmonary edema, surgery, and as a preoperative medication

Adult—Neurological

d. Morphine is contraindicated in clients with severe respiratory disorders; head injuries; increased intracranial pressure; severe renal, hepatic, or pulmonary disease; or seizure activity.

e. Morphine is used with caution in clients with shock or blood loss.

⚠ Respiratory depression is the priority concern with opioid analgesics.

5. Nalbuphine is preferable for treating the pain of myocardial infarction because it reduces the oxygen needs of the heart without reducing blood pressure.

6. Methadone

a. Doses of oral concentrate are diluted with at least 90 mL of water.

b. Dispersible tablets are diluted in at least 120 mL of water, orange juice, or acidic fruit beverage.

c. Methadone is used as a replacement medication to treat opiate dependence and to facilitate withdrawal.

7. Hydrocodone/homatropine is frequently used for cough suppression.

⚠ **C.** Interventions for opioid analgesics

1. Monitor vital signs.

2. Check the client thoroughly before administering pain medication.

3. Initiate nursing measures such as massage, distraction, deep breathing and relaxation exercises, the application of heat or cold as prescribed, and providing care and comfort along with administration of the opioid analgesic.

4. Medications are administered 30 to 60 minutes before painful activities.

5. Monitor respiratory rate, and if the rate is less than 12 breaths/min in an adult, withhold the medication, unless ventilatory support is provided or the client has terminal disease (as prescribed).

6. Monitor pulse, and if bradycardia develops, the dose is withheld and the RN and PHCP are notified.

7. Monitor the blood pressure for hypotension.

8. Auscultate breath sounds because opioid analgesics suppress the cough reflex.

9. Activities such as turning, deep breathing, and incentive spirometry to prevent atelectasis and pneumonia are encouraged.

10. Monitor the level of consciousness.

11. Initiate safety precautions such as side rails, a night light, and supervised ambulation.

12. Monitor the intake and output (I&O).

13. Monitor for urinary retention.

14. Reinforce instructions to the client to take oral doses with milk or a snack to reduce gastric irritation.

15. Reinforce instructions to the client to avoid alcohol.

16. Reinforce instructions to the client to avoid activities that require alertness.

BOX 56.13	Opioid Antagonists

Alvimopan
Methylnaltrexone
Naldemedine
Naloxone
Naltrexone
Naloxegol

17. Monitor bowel function for constipation, abdominal distention, and decreased peristalsis.

18. The effectiveness of medication is evaluated.

19. Have the opioid antagonist (e.g. naloxone), oxygen, and resuscitation equipment available (Box 56.13).

D. Morphine

1. Side and adverse effects

a. Respiratory depression

b. Orthostatic hypotension

c. Urinary retention

d. Nausea and vomiting

e. Constipation

f. Sedation, confusion, and hallucinations

g. Cough suppression

h. Constriction of the pupils

i. Miosis

2. Interventions

a. Have naloxone available for overdose.

b. Monitor vital signs and level of consciousness.

c. Compare rate and depth of respirations to the baseline.

d. The medication is withheld if the respiratory rate is less than 12 breaths/min (agency policies are followed). Respirations of less than 10 breaths/min can indicate respiratory distress.

e. Monitor urinary output, which needs to be at least 30 mL/hr.

f. Monitor bowel sounds for decreased peristalsis because constipation can occur.

g. Monitor for pupil changes because pinpoint pupils can indicate morphine overdose.

h. Reinforce instructions to the client to avoid alcohol or CNS depressants because they can cause respiratory depression.

i. Reinforce instructions to the client to report dizziness or difficulty breathing.

j. If taking sustained-release morphine, the client may need short-acting opioid doses for breakthrough pain.

k. The side and adverse effects of the medication are explained to the client and his or her family.

E. Meperidine

1. Side and adverse effects

a Respiratory depression

b. Hypotension and dizziness

c. Tachycardia

d. Drowsiness and confusion

e. Constipation

f Urinary retention
    g. Nausea and vomiting
    h. Seizure
    i. Tremors
  2. Interventions
    a. Monitor vital signs.
    b. Monitor for respiratory depression and hypotension.
    c. Have naloxone available for overdose.
    d. Monitor for urinary retention.
    e. Monitor bowel sounds for decreased peristalsis because constipation can occur.

VIII. Opioid Antagonists
  A. Opioid antagonists (see Box 55.13) are used to treat respiratory depression from opioid overdose.
  B. Interventions
    1. Monitor blood pressure, pulse, and respiratory rate every 5 minutes initially, tapering to every 15 minutes, and then every 30 minutes until the client is stable.
    2. Place the client on a cardiac monitor and monitor cardiac rhythm.
    3. Auscultate breath sounds.
    4. Have resuscitation equipment available.
    5. Do not leave the client unattended.
    6. Monitor the client closely for several hours because when the effects of the antagonist wear off, the client may again display signs of opioid overdose. The onset of naloxone is rapid (less than 1 minute), and it has a short half-life (about 30 minutes).

IX. Osmotic Diuretics
  A. Description
    1. Osmotic diuretics increase the osmotic pressure of the glomerular filtrate, inhibiting reabsorption of water and electrolytes.
    2. Osmotic diuretics are used for oliguria and to prevent renal failure, decrease intracranial pressure, and decrease intraocular pressure in clients with narrow-angle glaucoma.
    3. Mannitol is used with chemotherapy to induce diuresis.
  B. Side and adverse effects
    1. Fluid and electrolyte imbalances
    2. Pulmonary edema from the rapid shifts of fluid
    3. Nausea and vomiting
    4. Headache
    5. Tachycardia from the rapid fluid loss
    6. Hyponatremia and dehydration

  C. Interventions
    1. Monitor vital signs.
    2. Monitor weight.
    3. Monitor urine output.
    4. Monitor electrolyte levels.
    5. Monitor lung and heart sounds for signs of pulmonary edema.
    6. Monitor for signs of dehydration.
    7. Monitor the neurological status.

    8. Monitor for increased intraocular pressure.
    9. Check for signs of decreasing intracranial pressure, if appropriate.
  10. Change the client's position slowly to prevent orthostatic hypotension.
  11. Monitor for crystallization in the vial of mannitol before administering the medication; if crystallization is noted, do not administer the medication from that vial.

WHAT WOULD YOU DO?

Answer: Morphine is an opioid analgesic, of which respiratory depression is an adverse effect. The nurse needs to monitor the respiratory rate closely and if the rate is less than 12 breaths/min in an adult, the nurse needs to withhold the medication and notify the registered nurse.

PRACTICE QUESTIONS

1. The client with myasthenia gravis is suspected of having cholinergic crisis. Which sign/symptom indicates this crisis is taking place?
    1. Ataxia
    2. Mouth sores
    3. Hypothermia
    4. Hypertension

2. The client is receiving meperidine hydrochloride for pain. Which signs/symptoms are side and adverse effects of this medication? **Select all that apply.**
    ❏ **1.** Diarrhea
    ❏ **2.** Tremors
    ❏ **3.** Drowsiness
    ❏ **4.** Hypotension
    ❏ **5.** Urinary frequency
    ❏ **6.** Increased respiratory rate

3. Carbidopa-levodopa is prescribed for a client with Parkinson's disease, and the nurse monitors the client for adverse effects of the medication. Which sign/symptom indicates the client is experiencing an adverse effect?
    1. Pruritus
    2. Tachycardia
    3. Hypertension
    4. Impaired voluntary movements

4. Phenytoin, 100 mg orally three times daily, has been prescribed for a client for seizure control. The nurse reinforces instructions regarding the medication to the client. Which statement by the client indicates an understanding of the instructions?
    1. "I will use a soft toothbrush to brush my teeth."
    2. "It's all right to break the capsules to make it easier for me to swallow them."

3. "If I forget to take my medication, I can wait until the next dose and eliminate that dose."
4. "If my throat becomes sore, it's a normal effect of the medication and it's nothing to be concerned about."

5. The client is taking phenytoin for seizure control, and a blood sample for a serum drug level is drawn. Which laboratory finding indicates a therapeutic serum drug result?
   1. 5 mcg/mL
   2. 15 mcg/mL
   3. 25 mcg/mL
   4. 30 mcg/mL

6. Ibuprofen is prescribed for a client. Which instruction would the nurse give the client about taking this medication?
   1. Take with 8 oz of milk.
   2. Take in the morning after arising.
   3. Take 60 minutes before breakfast.
   4. Take at bedtime on an empty stomach.

7. The nurse is caring for a client who is taking phenytoin for control of seizures. During data collection, the nurse notes that the client is taking birth control pills. Which information would the nurse provide to the client?

1. Pregnancy would be avoided while taking phenytoin.
2. The client may stop taking the phenytoin if it is causing severe gastrointestinal effects.
3. The potential for decreased effectiveness of the birth control pills exists while taking phenytoin.
4. The increased risk of thrombophlebitis exists while taking phenytoin and birth control pills together.

8. The client with trigeminal neuralgia is being treated with carbamazepine. Which laboratory result indicates that the client is experiencing an adverse effect of the medication?
   1. Sodium level, 140 mEq/L
   2. Uric acid level, 5.0 mg/dL
   3. White blood cell count, 3000 mm^3
   4. Blood urea nitrogen (BUN) level, 15 mg/dL

9. The client with myasthenia gravis is receiving pyridostigmine. The nurse monitors for signs/symptoms of cholinergic crisis caused by overdose of the medication. The nurse checks the medication supply to ensure that which medication is available for administration if a cholinergic crisis occurs?
   1. Vitamin K
   2. Acetylcysteine
   3. Atropine sulfate
   4. Protamine sulfate

ANSWERS

1. 4
Rationale: Cholinergic crisis occurs as a result of an overdose of medication. Indications of cholinergic crisis include gastrointestinal disturbances, nausea, vomiting, diarrhea, abdominal cramps, increased salivation and tearing, miosis, hypertension, sweating, and increased bronchial secretions.
Test-Taking Strategy: Note the subject, cholinergic crisis, and recall the signs/symptoms of cholinergic crisis, including hypertension. Note that mouth sores represent a condition that takes time to occur and is not an immediate sign of a crisis.

❖ 2. 2, 3, 4
Rationale: Meperidine hydrochloride is an opioid analgesic. Side and adverse effects include respiratory depression, drowsiness, hypotension, constipation, urinary retention, nausea, vomiting, and tremors.
Test-Taking Strategy: Focus on the subject, side and adverse effects of meperidine hydrochloride. Recalling that this medication is an opioid analgesic and recalling the effects of an opioid analgesic will assist in identifying the side and adverse effects.

3. 4
Rationale: Dyskinesia and impaired voluntary movement may occur with high levodopa dosages. Nausea, anorexia, dizziness, orthostatic hypotension, bradycardia, and akinesia (the temporary muscle weakness that lasts 1 minute to 1 hour, also known as the "on-off phenomenon") are frequent side effects of the medication.
Test-Taking Strategy: Focus on the subject, signs/symptoms of adverse effects associated with carbidopa and levodopa. Options 2 and 3 are cardiac-related options, so these options can be eliminated first as comparable or alike, and not related to the subject. Note that the question asks for an adverse effect; therefore, select option 4 over option 1 as the correct answer.

4. 1
Rationale: Phenytoin is an antiseizure medication. Gingival hyperplasia, bleeding, swelling, and tenderness of the gums can occur with the use of this medication. The client needs to be taught good oral hygiene, gum massage, and the need for regular dentist visits. The client would not skip medication doses because this could precipitate a seizure. Capsules should not be chewed or broken. The client needs to be instructed to report a sore throat, fever, glandular swelling, or any skin reaction because this indicates hematological toxicity.
Test-Taking Strategy: Focus on the subject, an understanding of the instructions. Eliminate option 3 because the client needs to be encouraged to take medications on time. Also, eliminate option 4 because the client needs to report these symptoms to the primary health care provider. From the remaining options, recalling that capsules should not be broken will direct you to option 1.

5. 2

Rationale: The therapeutic serum drug level range for phenytoin is 10 to 20 mcg/mL. Therefore, options 1, 3, and 4 are incorrect.

Test-Taking Strategy: Knowledge regarding the subject, the therapeutic serum range of phenytoin, is required to answer the question. A helpful hint may be to remember that the theophylline therapeutic range and the acetaminophen therapeutic range are similar to the phenytoin therapeutic range. Remembering this may assist you when answering questions related to any of these three medications.

6. 1

Rationale: Ibuprofen is a nonsteroidal anti-inflammatory drug (NSAID). NSAIDs would be given with milk or food to prevent gastrointestinal irritation. Options 2, 3, and 4 are incorrect.

Test-Taking Strategy: Note that options 2, 3, and 4 are comparable or alike. Each of these options indicates administering the medication without food. Remember, NSAIDs can cause gastric irritation.

7. 3

Rationale: Phenytoin enhances the rate of estrogen metabolism, which can decrease the effectiveness of some birth control pills. Options 1, 2, are 4 are not accurate.

Test-Taking Strategy: Recall knowledge of the subject, medication interactions between phenytoin and birth control pills. Option 4 is not an appropriate statement because it would cause anxiety in the client. A client would not be instructed to stop anticonvulsant medication. Pregnancy does not need to be "avoided."

8. 3

Rationale: Adverse effects of carbamazepine appear as blood dyscrasias, including aplastic anemia, agranulocytosis, thrombocytopenia, leukopenia, cardiovascular disturbance, thrombophlebitis, dysrhythmia, and dermatological effects. Options 1, 2, and 4 identify normal laboratory values.

Test-Taking Strategy: Focus on the subject, the medication and normal laboratory values, to answer this question. If you are familiar with normal laboratory values, you will note that the only option that indicates an abnormal value is option 3.

9. 3

Rationale: The antidote for cholinergic crisis is atropine sulfate. Acetylcysteine is the antidote for acetaminophen. Vitamin K is the antidote for warfarin, and protamine sulfate is the antidote for heparin.

Test-Taking Strategy: Knowledge regarding the subject, antidotes for various medications, is needed to answer this question. Remember that atropine sulfate is the antidote for cholinergic crisis.

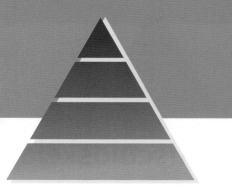

Musculoskeletal Problems of the Adult Client

▲ Pyramid to Success

The Pyramid to Success focuses on the emergency care for a client who sustains a fracture or other musculoskeletal injury, monitoring for complications, and carrying out interventions if complications occur. Nursing care related to casts and traction is emphasized. Skill related to instructing the client in the use of an assistive device such as a cane, walker, or crutches is a Pyramid Point. Pyramid Points also include postoperative care following hip surgery or amputation and care of the client with rheumatoid arthritis or osteoporosis. Focus on the points related to the psychosocial effects as a result of the musculoskeletal problem, such as unexpected body image changes, and the appropriate and available support services needed for the client.

▲ Client Needs: Learning Objectives

Safe and Effective Care Environment
  Communicating with the interprofessional health care team
  Ensuring that informed consent is obtained for treatments and procedures
  Establishing priorities
  Handling hazardous and infectious materials safely
  Maintaining asepsis related to wounds
  Maintaining confidentiality
  Maintaining standard and other precautions
  Preventing accidents and injuries
  Providing physical and occupational therapy referrals
  Upholding client rights
Health Promotion and Maintenance
  Performing data collection techniques related to the musculoskeletal system

  Preventing health problems that occur as a result of the aging process
  Promoting health related to diet and activity
  Providing home care instructions regarding care related to a musculoskeletal problem
  Reinforcing the importance of prescribed therapy
Psychosocial Integrity
  Considering cultural, religious, and spiritual influences
  Discussing situational role changes as a result of the musculoskeletal disorder
  Discussing unexpected body image changes as a result of injury or disease
  Determining the client's ability to cope with mobility limitations and restrictions, feelings of isolation, and loss of independence
  Identifying available support systems and use of community resources
  Identifying sensory and perceptual alterations
  Mobilizing coping mechanisms
Physiological Integrity
  Identifying complications of procedures, injuries, or a fracture
  Providing care related to casts and traction
  Promoting normal elimination patterns
  Promoting self-care measures
  Providing emergency care for a fracture or other injury
  Providing immediate interventions if a complication arises
  Providing measures to promote comfort
  Teaching about the use of assistive devices for mobility such as canes, walkers, and crutches
  Reinforcing measures about pharmacological therapy

Client Needs lists modified from: National Council of State Boards of Nursing, Inc. (NCSBN). *NCLEX-PN Examination: Test Plan for the National Council Licensure Examination for Practical Nurses,* effective April 2020. Chicago: NCSBN.

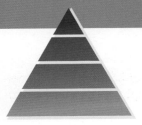
CHAPTER **57**

Musculoskeletal Problems

PRIORITY CONCEPTS Functional Ability; Mobility

WHAT WOULD YOU DO?

The nurse employed in an industrial plant is called to an accident site in the plant in which an employee amputated their index finger on a saw. What would the nurse do?
Answer is located on p. 819.

I. Anatomy and Physiology

A. Skeleton
  1. Axial portion
    a. Cranium
    b. Vertebrae
    c. Ribs
  2. Appendicular portion
    a. Limbs
    b. Shoulders
    c. Hips
B. Types of bones
  1. Types include long, short, flat, and irregular
  2. Spongy bone
    a. Spongy bone is located in the ends of long bones and the center of flat and irregular bones.
    b. Spongy bone can withstand forces applied in many directions.
  3. Dense (compact) bone
    a. Dense bone covers spongy bone
    b. Forms a cylinder around a central marrow cavity
    c. Better able to withstand longitudinal forces than horizontal forces
  4. Characteristics of the bones
    a. Support and protect structures of the body
    b. Provide attachments for muscles, tendons, and ligaments
    c. Contain tissue in the central cavities, which aids in the formation of blood cells
    d. Assist with regulating calcium and phosphate concentrations

5. Bone growth
  a. The length of bone growth results from the ossification of the epiphyseal cartilage at the ends of bones, and bone growth stops between the ages of 18 and 25 years.
  b. The width of bone growth results from the activity of osteoblasts and occurs throughout life but does slow down with aging.

⚠ As aging occurs, bone resorption accelerates, decreasing bone mass and predisposing the client to injury.

C. Types of joints (Table 57.1)
  1. Characteristics of the joints
    a. Allow for the movement between bones
    b. Formed where two bones join
    c. Surfaces are covered with cartilage
    d. Enclosed in a capsule (synovial joints)
    e. Contain a cavity filled with synovial fluid (synovial joints)
    f. Ligaments hold the bone and joint in the correct position.
    g. Articulation is the meeting point of two or more bones.
  2. Synovial fluid
    a. Found in the synovial joint capsule
    b. Formed by the synovial membrane, which lines the joint capsule
    c. Lubricates the cartilage
    d. Provides a cushion against shocks
D. Muscles
  1. Characteristics of muscles
    a. Made up of bundles of muscle fibers
    b. Provide the force to move bones
    c. Assist with maintaining posture
    d. Assist with heat production
  2. The process of contraction and relaxation
    a. Muscle contraction and relaxation require large amounts of adenosine triphosphate.

b. Contraction also requires calcium, which functions as a catalyst.

c. Acetylcholine released by the motor end plate of the motor neuron initiates an action potential.

d. Acetylcholine is then destroyed by acetylcholinesterase.

e. Calcium is required to contract muscle fibers and acts as a catalyst for the enzyme needed for the sliding-together action of actin and myosin.

f. Following contraction, adenosine triphosphate transports calcium out to allow actin and myosin to separate and to allow the muscle to relax.

3. Skeletal muscles

a. Skeletal muscles are attached to two bones by cartilaginous tendons (the connective tissue between tendon or ligament and bone).

b. The point of origin is the point of attachment that does not move.

c. The point of insertion is the point of attachment that moves when the muscle contracts.

d. Skeletal muscles act in groups.

e. Prime movers contract to produce movement.

f. Antagonists relax.

g. Synergists contract to stabilize body movement.

h. Nerves activate and control the muscles.

E. Bone healing

1. Description: Bone union or healing is the process that occurs after the integrity of a bone is interrupted.

2. Stages (Fig. 57.1)

II. Risk Factors Associated with Musculoskeletal Disorders (Box 57.1)

III. Diagnostic Tests

A. Radiographs and magnetic resonance imaging (MRI) (refer to Chapter 55 for information on MRI)

1. Description: Radiography and MRI are commonly used procedures to diagnose disorders of the musculoskeletal system.

2. Interventions

a. Handle injured areas carefully and support extremities above and below the joint.

b. Administer analgesics as prescribed before the procedure, particularly if the client is in pain.

c. Remove any radiopaque and metallic objects, such as jewelry.

d. Ask the client if she is pregnant; MRI may be contraindicated in pregnancy.

e. Shield client's testes, ovaries, or pregnant abdomen.

f. Reinforce instructions to lie still during a radiograph.

g. Inform the client that exposure to radiation is minimal and not dangerous.

h. The nurse needs to wear a lead apron if staying in the room with the client having radiography.

i. Complete screening process per agency policy.

B. Arthrocentesis

1. Description: Arthrocentesis is used to diagnose joint inflammation and infection.

a. Arthrocentesis involves aspirating synovial fluid, blood, or pus via a needle inserted into a joint cavity.

b. Medication, such as corticosteroids, may be instilled into the joint if necessary to alleviate inflammation.

TABLE 57.1	Types of Joints
Type	**Description**
Amphiarthrosis	Cartilaginous joints Slightly movable joints
Diarthrosis	Synovial joints Ball-and-socket joints Permit free movement
Synarthrosis	Fibrous or fixed joints No movement associated with these joints

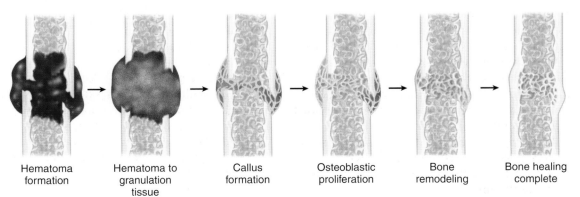

Hematoma formation → Hematoma to granulation tissue → Callus formation → Osteoblastic proliferation → Bone remodeling → Bone healing complete

FIGURE 57.1 The stages of bone healing.

> **BOX 57.1** **Risk Factors Associated with Musculoskeletal Disorders**
>
> Autoimmune disorder
> Calcium deficiency
> Falls
> Hyperuricemia
> Infection
> Medication(s)
> Metabolic disorder
> Neoplastic disorder
> Obesity
> Postmenopausal states
> Trauma and injury

    2. Interventions

      a. Ensure that informed consent has been obtained.

      b. Apply an elastic compression bandage postprocedure as prescribed.

      c. Use ice to decrease pain and swelling.

      d. Pain may worsen after aspirating fluid from the joint; analgesics may be prescribed.

      e. Pain can continue up to 2 days after administration of corticosteroids into a joint.

      f. Reinforce instructions to rest the joint for 8 to 24 hours postprocedure as prescribed.

      g. Reinforce instructions to notify the primary health care provider (PHCP) if a fever, increased redness, or swelling of the joint occurs.

C. Arthroscopy

    1. Description: Arthroscopy is used to diagnose acute and chronic disorders of the joint.

      a. Arthroscopy provides an endoscopic examination of various joints.

      b. Articular cartilage abnormalities can be assessed, loose bodies can be removed, and the cartilage can be trimmed.

      c. A biopsy may be performed during the procedure.

    2. Interventions

      a. Reinforce instructions to fast for 8 to 12 hours before the procedure and ensure that informed consent was obtained.

      b. Administer pain medication as prescribed postprocedure.

      c. Monitor the neurovascular status of the affected extremity.

      d. An elastic compression bandage would be worn for 2 to 4 days as prescribed postprocedure.

      e. Reinforce instructions that walking without weight bearing is usually permitted after sensation returns but to limit activity for 1 to 4 days as prescribed postprocedure.

      f. Reinforce instructions to elevate the extremity as often as possible for 24 hours following the procedure and to place ice on the site to minimize swelling for 12 to 24 hours postprocedure.

      g. Reinforce instructions regarding the use of crutches, which may be used for 5 to 7 days postprocedure for walking.

      h. Advise the client to notify the PHCP if fever or increased knee pain occurs or if edema continues for more than 3 days postprocedure.

D. Bone mineral density measurements

    1. Dual energy x-ray absorptiometry

      a. Measures the bone mass of the spine, wrist and hip bones, and total body

      b. Radiation exposure is minimal

      c. Used to diagnose metabolic bone disease and to monitor changes in bone density with treatment

      d. Inform the client that the procedure is painless.

      e. All metallic objects are removed before the test.

    2. Quantitative ultrasound

      a. Quantitative ultrasound evaluates strength, density, and elasticity of various bones using ultrasound rather than radiation.

      b. Inform the client that the procedure is painless.

E. Bone scan

    1. Description: A bone scan is used to identify, evaluate, and stage bone cancer before and after treatment; it is also used to detect fractures.

      a. Radioisotope is injected intravenously and will collect in areas that indicate abnormal bone metabolism and some fractures, if they exist.

      b. The isotope is excreted in the urine and feces within 48 hours and is not harmful to others.

    2. Interventions

      a. Food and fluid may be withheld before the procedure.

      b. Ensure that informed consent has been obtained.

      c. Remove all jewelry and metal objects.

      d. Following the injection of the radioisotope, the client needs to drink 32 oz of water (if not contraindicated) to promote renal filtering of the excess isotope.

      e. From 1 to 3 hours after the injection, have the client void to clear excess isotope from the bladder before the scanning procedure is completed.

      f. Inform the client of the need to lie supine during the procedure and that the procedure is not painful.

g. Monitor the injection site for redness and swelling.

h. Encourage oral fluid intake after the procedure.

⚠ No special precautions are required after a bone scan because a minimal amount of radioactivity exists in the radioisotope used for the procedure.

F. Bone or muscle biopsy
  1. Description: A biopsy may be performed during surgery or through aspiration or punch or needle biopsy.
  2. Interventions
    a. Ensure that informed consent was obtained.
    b. Monitor for bleeding, swelling, hematoma, or severe pain.
    c. Elevate the site for 24 hours following the procedure to reduce edema.
    d. Apply ice packs as prescribed following the procedure to prevent the development of a hematoma and to decrease site discomfort.
    e. Monitor for signs of infection following the procedure.
    f. Inform the client that mild to moderate discomfort is normal following the procedure.

G. Electromyography (EMG)
  1. Description: An EMG is used to evaluate muscle weakness.
    a. EMG measures electrical potential associated with skeletal muscle contractions.
    b. Needles are inserted into the muscle, and recordings of muscular electrical activity are traced on recording paper through an oscilloscope.

  2. Interventions
    a. Ensure that informed consent was obtained.
    b. Reinforce instructions that the needle insertion is uncomfortable.
    c. Reinforce instructions not to take any stimulants or sedatives for 24 hours before the procedure.
    d. Inform the client that slight bruising may occur at the needle insertion sites.
    e. Mild analgesics can be used for the pain.

IV. Injuries

A. Strains
  1. Strains are an excessive stretching of a muscle or tendon.
  2. Management involves cold and heat applications, exercise with activity limitations, anti-inflammatory medications, and muscle relaxants.
  3. Surgical repair may be required for a severe strain (ruptured muscle or tendon).

B. Sprains
  1. Sprains are an excessive stretching of a ligament, usually caused by a twisting motion, such as in a fall or stepping on an uneven surface.

  2. Sprains are characterized by pain and swelling.
  3. Management involves RICE (rest, ice, a compression bandage, and elevation) to reduce swelling and provide joint support. RICE is considered a first-aid treatment rather than a cure for soft tissue injuries.
  4. Casting may be required for moderate sprains to allow the tear to heal.
  5. Surgery may be necessary for severe ligament damage.

C. Rotator cuff injuries
  1. Musculotendinous or rotator cuff of the shoulder sustains a tear, usually as a result of trauma.
  2. Injury is characterized by shoulder pain and the inability to maintain abduction of the arm at the shoulder (drop arm test).
  3. Management involves nonsteroidal anti-inflammatory drugs (NSAIDs), physical therapy, sling support, and ice/heat applications.

  4. Surgery may be required if medical management is unsuccessful or for those who have a complete tear.

V. Fractures

A. Description: A fracture is a break in the continuity of the bone caused by trauma, twisting as a result of muscle spasm or indirect loss of leverage, or bone decalcification and disease that result in osteopenia.

B. Types of fractures (Box 57.2)

C. Data collection: Fracture of an extremity

  1. Pain or tenderness over the involved area
  2. Decrease or loss of muscular strength or function

BOX 57.2 Types of Fractures

Closed or simple: Skin over the fractured area remains intact.
Comminuted: The bone is splintered or crushed, creating numerous fragments.
Complete: The bone is separated completely by a break into two parts.
Compression: A fractured bone is compressed by other bone.
Depressed: Bone fragments are driven inward.
Greenstick: One side of the bone is broken and the other is bent; these fractures occur most commonly in children.
Impacted: A part of the fractured bone is driven into another bone.
Incomplete: Fracture line does not extend through the full transverse width of the bone.
Oblique: The fracture line runs at an angle across the axis of the bone.
Open or compound: The bone is exposed to air through a break in the skin, and soft tissue injury and infection are common.
Pathological: The fracture results from weakening of the bone structure by pathological processes such as neoplasia; also called spontaneous fracture.
Spiral: The break partially encircles bone.
Transverse: The bone is fractured straight across.

3. Obvious deformity of affected area
4. Creptitation, erythema, edema, or bruising
5. Muscle spasm and neurovascular impairment
D. Initial care of a fracture of an extremity
  1. Immobilize affected extremity with cast or splint.
  2. Check the neurovascular status of the extremity.
  3. Interventions for a fracture include reduction, fixation, traction, and casting.

⚠️ If a compound (open) fracture exists, splint the extremity and cover the wound with a sterile dressing.

E. Reduction restores the bone to proper alignment.
  1. Closed reduction is a nonsurgical intervention that is performed by manual manipulation.
    a. Closed reduction may be performed under local or general anesthesia.
    b. A cast may be applied following reduction.
  2. Open reduction involves a surgical intervention; the fracture may be treated with internal fixation devices.
F. Fixation
  1. Internal fixation follows an open reduction (Fig. 57.2).
    a. Internal fixation involves the application of screws, plates, pins, or intramedullary rods to hold the fragments in alignment.
    b. Internal fixation may involve the removal of damaged bone and replacement with a prosthesis.
    c. Internal fixation provides immediate bone strength.
  2. External fixation is the use of an external frame to stabilize a fracture by attaching skeletal pins through bone fragments to a rigid external support.

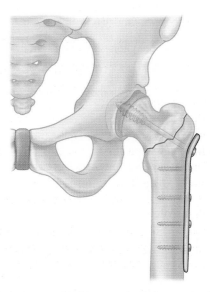

FIGURE 57.2 A compression hip screw used for open reduction with internal fixation.

a. External fixation provides more freedom of movement than with traction.
b. Monitor pin stability and provide pin care to decrease infection risks.
c. Risk of infection exists with both fixation methods.
d. External fixation is commonly used when massive tissue trauma is present.
G. Traction (Fig. 57.3)
  1. Description
    a. Traction is the exertion of a pulling force applied in two directions to reduce and immobilize a fracture.
    b. Traction provides proper bone alignment and reduces muscle spasms.
  2. Interventions
    a. Maintain proper body alignment.
    b. Ensure that the weights hang freely and do not touch the floor.
    c. Do not remove or lift the weights without a PHCP's prescription.
    d. Ensure that pulleys are not obstructed and that ropes in the pulleys move freely.
    e. Place knots in the ropes to prevent slipping.
    f. Check the ropes for fraying.
H. Skeletal traction
  1. Description
    a. Traction is applied mechanically to the bone with pins, wires, or tongs.
    b. Typical weight for skeletal traction is 25 to 40 lb (11–18 kg).
  2. Interventions
    a. Monitor color, motion, and sensation of the affected extremity.
    b. Monitor the insertion sites for redness, swelling, drainage, or increased pain.
    c. Provide insertion site care as prescribed.
  3. Cervical tongs and a halo fixation device (refer to Chapter 55) regarding care of the client with these types of devices)
I. Skin traction
  1. Description: Skin traction is applied by using elastic bandages or an adhesive, foam boot, or sling.
  2. Cervical skin traction relieves muscle spasms and compression in the upper extremities and neck (see Fig. 57.3).
    a. Cervical skin traction uses a head halter and a chin pad to attach the traction.
    b. Use powder to protect the ears from friction rub.
    c. Position the client with the head of the bed elevated 30 to 40 degrees, and attach the weights to a pulley system over the head of the bed.
  3. Buck's (extension) skin traction is used to alleviate muscle spasms and immobilize a lower limb

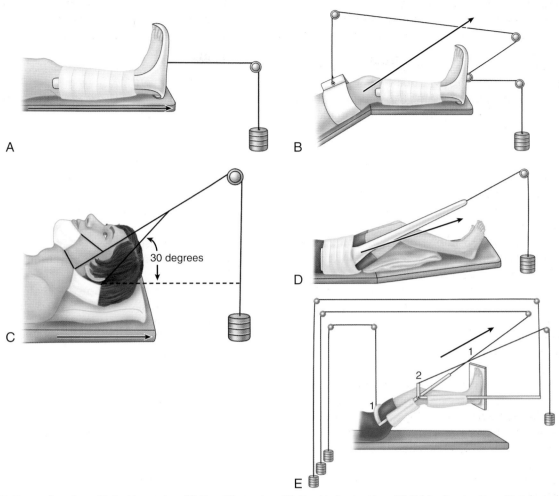

FIGURE 57.3 Types of traction. (A) Buck's traction. (B) Russell's traction. (C) Head halter traction. (D) Pelvic sling traction. (E) Balanced suspension traction.

by maintaining a straight pull on the limb with the use of weights (see Fig. 57.3).

  a. A boot appliance is applied to attach to the traction.

  b. Weight is attached to a pulley; allow the weights to hang freely over the edge of bed.

  c. Not more than 8 to 10 lb (3.5–4.5 kg) of weight would be applied as prescribed.

  d. Elevate the foot of the bed to provide the traction.

4. Russell's skin (sling) traction (see Fig. 57.3 and refer to Chapter 36 regarding information related to this type of traction)

5. Pelvic skin traction is used to relieve low back, hip, or leg pain or to reduce muscle spasm (see Fig. 57.3).

  a. Apply the traction snugly over the pelvis and iliac crest and attach to the weights.

  b. Use measures as prescribed to prevent the client from slipping down in bed.

J. Balanced suspension traction (see Fig. 57.3)

  1. Description

    a. Balanced suspension traction is used with skin or skeletal traction.

    b. It is used to approximate fractures of the femur, tibia, or fibula.

    c. Balanced suspension traction is produced by a counterforce other than the client.

  2. Interventions

    a. Position the client in a low-Fowler's position on either the side or the back.

    b. Maintain a 20-degree angle from the thigh to the bed.

    c. Protect the skin from breakdown.

    d. Provide pin care if pins are used with the skeletal traction.

    e. Clean the pin sites with sterile normal saline and hydrogen peroxide or povidone-iodine as prescribed or per agency policy.

K. Casts

  1. Description: Plaster, fiberglass, or air casts are used to immobilize bones and joints into correct alignment after a fracture or injury.

2. Interventions
   a. Keep the cast and extremity elevated.
   b. Allow a wet plaster cast 24 to 72 hours to dry (synthetic casts dry in 20 minutes).
   c. Handle a wet plaster cast with the palms of the hands (not fingertips) until dry.
   d. Turn the extremity every 1 to 2 hours, unless contraindicated to allow for air circulation and to promote drying of the cast.
   e. Cool setting on a hair dryer can be used to dry a plaster cast (heat cannot be used because the cast heats up and burns the skin).
   f. Monitor closely for circulatory impairment; prepare for bivalving or cutting the cast if circulatory impairment occurs.
   g. Petal the cast or apply moleskin to the edges to protect the client's skin; maintain smooth edges around the cast to prevent crumbling of the cast material.
   h. Monitor for signs of infection such as increased temperature, hot spots on the cast, foul odor, or changes in pain.
   i. If an open draining area exists on the affected extremity, the PHCP will make a cutout portion of the cast known as a *window* for assessment and wound care purposes.
   j. Reinforce instructions not to stick objects inside the cast.
   k. Reinforce teaching the client to keep the cast clean and dry.
   l. Reinforce instructions on isometric exercises to prevent muscle atrophy.

⚠️ Monitor a casted extremity for circulatory impairment such as pain, swelling, discoloration, tingling, numbness, coolness, or diminished pulse. Notify the registered nurse and PHCP immediately if circulatory compromise occurs.

VI. Complications of Fractures (Box 57.3)
A. Fat embolism (see **Priority Nursing Actions**)

⚡ PRIORITY NURSING ACTIONS

Fat Embolism

1. Notify the registered nurse (RN) and primary health care provider (PHCP).
2. Administer oxygen.
3. Monitor vital signs and respiratory status.
4. Assist to monitor prescribed intravenous fluids.
5. Prepare to assist the RN and PHCP with intubation and mechanical ventilation if necessary.
6. Follow up on results of diagnostic tests such as chest x-ray or computed tomography (CT) scan.
7. Document the event, actions taken, and the client's response.

BOX 57.3	Complications of Fractures

- Avascular necrosis
- Compartment syndrome
- Fat embolism
- Infection and osteomyelitis
- Pulmonary embolism

B. Pulmonary embolism
   1. Description: Pulmonary embolism is caused by the movement of foreign particles (blood clot, fat, or air) into the pulmonary circulation.
   2. Data collection
      a. Restlessness and apprehension
      b. Sudden onset of dyspnea and chest pain
      c. Cough, hemoptysis, hypoxemia, or crackles
   3. Interventions
      a. Notify the PHCP immediately if signs of emboli are present.
      b. Administer oxygen and other prescriptions; intravenous (IV) anticoagulant therapy may be prescribed.

C. Compartment syndrome
   1. Description
      a. Tough fascia surrounds muscle groups, forming compartments from which arteries, veins, and nerves enter and exit at opposite ends.
      b. Compartment syndrome occurs when pressure increases within one or more compartments, leading to decreased blood flow, tissue ischemia, and neurovascular impairment.
      c. Within 4 to 6 hours after the onset of compartment syndrome, neurovascular damage may be irreversible if not treated.
   2. Data collection
      a. Unrelieved or increased pain in the limb
      b. Tissue that is distal to the involved area becomes pale, dusky, or edematous
      c. Pain with passive movement and joint dysfunction
      d. Loss of sensation (paresthesia)
      e. Pulselessness (a late sign)
   3. Interventions
      a. Notify the RN and PHCP immediately and prepare to assist the RN.
      b. Continue to elevate the affected extremity.
      c. If severe, assist the PHCP with fasciotomy to relieve pressure and restore tissue perfusion.
      d. Loosen tight dressings or bivalve restrictive cast as prescribed.

D. Infection and osteomyelitis
   1. Description: Infection and osteomyelitis (inflammatory response in bone tissue) can be caused by the introduction of organisms into bones leading to localized bone infection.

2. Data collection
   a. Tachycardia and fever (usually above 101°F [38.3°C])
   b. Erythema and pain in the area surrounding the infection
   c. Leukocytosis and elevated erythrocyte sedimentation rate (ESR)
   d. Confirmed by radiographic assessment, such as plain radiographs, MRI, or bone scan
3. Interventions
   a. Notify the RN and PHCP immediately and prepare to assist the RN.
   b. Initiation of aggressive, long-term IV antibiotic therapy is done. A central venous access line will be likely required.
   c. Hyperbaric oxygen therapy may be prescribed to promote client healing.
   d. Surgery may be performed for resistant osteomyelitis with sequestrectomy and/or bone grafts.

E. Avascular necrosis
1. Description: Occurs when a fracture interrupts the blood supply to a section of bone, leading to bone death
2. Data collection
   a. Pain
   b. Decreased sensation
   c. Confirmed by radiographic assessment, such as radiographs, MRI, or bone scan
3. Interventions
   a. Notify the RN and PHCP if pain or numbness occurs.
   b. Prepare the client for removal of necrotic tissue because it serves as a focus for infection.

VII. Crutch Walking

A. Description
1. An accurate measurement of the client for crutches is important because an incorrect measurement could damage the brachial plexus.

2. The distance between the axillae and the arm pieces on the crutches needs to be two to three finger widths in the axilla space.
3. The elbows would be slightly flexed, 20 to 30 degrees, when the client is walking.
4. When ambulating with the client, stand on the affected side.
5. Reinforce instructions to never rest the axilla on the axillary bars.
6. Reinforce instructions to look up and outward when ambulating and to place the crutches 6 to 10 inches diagonally in front of the foot.
7. Reinforce instructions to stop ambulation if numbness or tingling in the hands or arms occurs.

B. Crutch gaits (Table 57.2)
C. Assisting the client with crutches to sit and stand
1. Place the unaffected leg against the front of the chair.
2. Move the crutches to the affected side, and grasp the arm of the chair with the hand on the unaffected side.
3. Flex the knee of the unaffected leg to lower oneself into the chair while placing the affected leg straight out in front.
4. Reverse the steps to move from a sitting to a standing position.

D. Going up and down stairs
1. Up the stairs
   a. The client moves the unaffected leg up first.
   b. The client moves the affected leg and the crutches up.
2. Down the stairs
   a. The client moves the crutches and the affected leg down.
   b. The client moves the unaffected leg down.

VIII. Canes and Walkers

A. Description: Canes and walkers are made of a lightweight material with a rubber tip at the bottom.

TABLE 57.2 Crutch Gaits

Type of Gait	Use	Procedure
Two-point gait	Used with partial weight-bearing limitations and with bilateral lower extremity prostheses	The crutch on the affected side and the unaffected foot are advanced at the same time.
Three-point gait	Used for partial weight bearing or no weight bearing on the affected leg; requires that the client have strength and balance	Both crutches and the foot of the affected extremity are advanced together, followed by the foot of the unaffected extremity.
Four-point gait	Used if weight bearing is allowed and one foot can be placed in front of the other	The right crutch is advanced, then the left foot, then the left crutch, then the right foot.
Swing-to gait	Used when there is adequate muscle power and balance in the arms and legs	Both crutches are advanced together, then both legs are lifted and placed down on a spot behind the crutches; the feet and crutches form a tripod.
Swing-through gait	Used when there is adequate muscle power and balance in the arms and legs	Both crutches are advanced together, then both legs are lifted through and beyond the crutches and placed down again at a point in front of the crutches.

Adapted from Linton AD: *Introduction to medical-surgical nursing*, ed 6, St. Louis, Saunders, 2016.

B. Interventions
1. Stand at the affected side of the client when ambulating, use of a gait belt may be necessary.
2. The handle would be at the level of the client's greater trochanter.
3. The client's elbow would be flexed at a 15- to 30-degree angle.
4. Reinforce instructions to hold the cane 4 to 6 inches to the side of the foot.
5. Reinforce instructions to hold the cane in the hand on the unaffected side so that the cane and weaker leg can work together with each step.
6. Reinforce instructions to move the cane at the same time as the affected leg.
7. Reinforce instructions to inspect the rubber tips regularly for worn places.

C. Hemicanes or quadripod canes
1. Hemicanes or quadripod canes are used for clients who have the use of only one upper extremity.
2. Hemicanes provide more security than a quadripod cane; however, both types provide more security than a single-tipped cane.
3. Position the cane at the client's unaffected side, with the straight, nonangled side adjacent to the body.
4. Position the cane 6 inches from client's side, with the handgrips level with the greater trochanter.

D. Walker
1. Stand adjacent to the client on the affected side.
2. Reinforce instructions to put all four points of the walker flat on the floor before putting weight on the hand pieces.
3. Reinforce instructions to move the walker forward, followed by the affected or weaker foot and then the unaffected foot.

⚠️ Safety is the priority concern when the client uses an assistive device such as a cane, walker, or crutches. Be sure that the client demonstrates correct use of the device.

IX. Fractured Hip

A. Types
1. Intracapsular (femoral head is broken within the joint capsule)
   a. Femoral head and neck receive decreased blood supply and heal slowly.
   b. Skin traction is applied preoperatively to reduce fracture, immobilize bone, and decrease muscle spasms.
   c. Treatment includes a total hip replacement or open reduction internal fixation (ORIF) with femoral head replacement.

d. To prevent hip displacement postoperatively, avoid extreme hip flexion, and check the surgeon's prescriptions regarding positioning.
2. Extracapsular (fracture is outside the joint capsule)
   a. Fracture can occur at the greater trochanter or can be an intertrochanteric fracture.
   b. Preoperative treatment includes balanced suspension traction or skin traction to relieve muscle spasms and reduce pain.
   c. Surgical treatment includes ORIF with nail plate, screws, pins, or wires.

B. Postoperative interventions
1. Monitor for signs of delirium and institute safety measures.
2. Maintain leg and hip in proper alignment and prevent internal or external rotation; crossing over the midline with the operative leg needs to be avoided to prevent dislocation; avoid extreme hip flexion.
3. Follow the surgeon's prescriptions regarding turning and repositioning; usually, turning to the unaffected side is allowed.
4. Elevate the head of the bed 30 to 45 degrees for meals only.
5. Assist the client with ambulating as prescribed by the surgeon's
6. Weight bearing is usually avoided on the affected leg as prescribed; instruct the client on the use of a walker to avoid weight bearing.
7. Weight bearing is often restricted after an ORIF and may not be restricted after total hip arthroplasty (THA); always refer to the surgeon's prescriptions.
8. Keep the operative leg extended, supported, and elevated when getting the client out of bed.
9. Avoid hip flexion greater than 90 degrees and avoid low chairs when out of bed.
10. Monitor for wound infection or hemorrhage.
11. Perform neurovascular assessment of affected extremity: check color, pulses, capillary refill, movement, and sensation.
12. Maintain the compression of the wound drain to facilitate wound drainage if present.
13. Monitor and record drainage amount, which decreases consistently.
14. Postoperative blood salvage may be done to collect, filter, and reinfuse salvaged blood into the client.
15. Use antiembolism stockings or sequential compression stockings and encourage the client to flex and extend the feet to reduce the risk of deep vein thrombosis (DVT).
16. Reinforce instructions to avoid crossing the legs and activities that require bending over.

17. Physical therapy will be instituted postoperatively with progressive ambulation as prescribed by the surgeon's.

X. Total Knee Replacement

A. Description: Total knee replacement is the implantation of a device to substitute for the femoral condyles and the tibial joint surfaces.

B. Postoperative interventions

1. Monitor surgical incision for drainage and infection.

2. Begin continuous passive motion (CPM) soon after the client is admitted to the postoperative unit.

3. Administer analgesics before CPM to decrease pain.

4. Prepare the client for out-of-bed activities as prescribed; have the client avoid leg dangling.

5. Avoid weight bearing, and instruct the client in the use of the prescribed assistive device, such as a walker or crutches.

6. Postoperative blood salvage to collect, filter, and reinfuse salvaged blood into the client may be prescribed.

7. Administer antibiotics if prescribed within a specified time frame (antibiotics also may be prescribed in the preoperative period).

XI. Joint Dislocation and Subluxation

A. Dislocation: Injury of the ligaments surrounding a joint that leads to displacement or separation of the articular surfaces of the joint

B. Subluxation: Incomplete displacement of joint surfaces when forces disrupt the soft tissue that surrounds the joints

C. Data collection

1. Asymmetry of the contour of affected body parts

2. Pain, tenderness, dysfunction, and swelling

3. Complications include neurovascular compromise, avascular necrosis, and open joint injuries.

4. X-rays are completed to determine joint shifting.

D. Interventions

1. Focus of treatment includes pain relief, joint support, and joint protection.

2. Immediate treatment is done to reduce the dislocation and realign the dislocated joint.

3. Open or closed reduction is done with a postprocedural joint immobilization.

4. IV conscious sedation or local or general anesthesia is used during joint manipulation.

5. Initial activity restriction is followed by gentle range-of-motion activities and a gradual return of activities to normal levels while supporting the affected joint.

6. A weakened joint is prone to recurrent dislocation and may require extended activity restriction.

XII. Herniation: Intervertebral Disk

A. Description: The nucleus of the disk protrudes into the annulus, causing nerve compression.

B. Cervical disk herniation occurs at C5-C6 and C6-C7 interspaces.

1. Cervical disk herniation causes pain radiation to shoulders, arms, hands, scapula, and pectoral muscles.

2. Motor and sensory deficits can include paresthesia, numbness, and weakness of the upper extremities.

3. Interventions

a. Conservative management is used unless the client develops signs of neurological deterioration.

b. Bed rest is prescribed to decrease pressure, inflammation, and pain.

c. Immobilize the cervical area with a cervical collar, traction, or brace, as prescribed.

d. Heat is used to reduce muscle spasms; ice is used to reduce inflammation and swelling.

e. Maintain the head and spine in alignment.

f. Reinforce instructions in the use of analgesics, sedatives, anti-inflammatory agents, and corticosteroids as prescribed.

g. Prepare the client for a corticosteroid injection into the epidural space if prescribed.

h. Assist and instruct client in the use of a cervical collar or cervical traction as prescribed.

4. A cervical collar is used for cervical disk herniation.

a. A cervical collar limits neck movement and holds the head in a neutral or slightly flexed position.

b. The cervical collar may be worn intermittently or 24 hours a day.

c. Inspect skin under the collar for irritation.

d. When prescribed for use and after pain decreases, an exercise plan is designed to strengthen the muscles.

5. Reinforce client education related to cervical disk conditions

a. Avoid flexing, extending, and rotating the neck.

b. Avoid the prone position, and maintain the neck, spine, and hips in neutral position while sleeping.

c. Minimize long periods of sitting.

d. Reinforce instructions regarding medications such as analgesics, sedatives, anti-inflammatory agents, and corticosteroids.

C. Lumbar disk herniation most often occurs at L4-L5 or L5-S1 interspaces.

1. Herniation produces muscle weakness, sensory deficits, and diminished tendon reflexes.

2. The client experiences pain and muscle spasms in the lower back, with radiation of the pain into one hip and down the leg (sciatica).

3. Pain is relieved by bed rest and aggravated by movement, lifting, straining, and coughing.
4. Interventions
   a. Conservative management is indicated unless neurological deterioration or bowel and bladder dysfunction occurs.
   b. Apply moist heat to decrease muscle spasms, and apply ice to decrease inflammation, as prescribed.
   c. Reinforce instructions to sleep on the side, with the knees and hips flexed, and place a pillow between the legs.
   d. Apply pelvic traction as prescribed to relieve muscle spasms and decrease pain.
   e. Begin progressive ambulation as inflammation, edema, and pain subside.
5. Reinforce client education related to lumbar disk conditions
   a. Instruct the client in the use of prescribed medications such as analgesics, muscle relaxants, anti-inflammatory agents, or corticosteroids.
   b. Instruct about application techniques for corsets or braces to maintain immobilization and proper spine alignment.
   c. Instruct on correct posture while sitting, standing, walking, and working.
   d. Instruct on the correct technique to use when lifting objects such as bending knees, maintaining a straight back, and avoiding lifting objects above the elbow level.
   e. Instruct in a weight-control program, as prescribed.
   f. Instruct in an exercise program to strengthen back and abdominal muscles, as prescribed.
D. Disk surgery is used when spinal cord compression is suspected or client symptoms do not respond to conservative treatment.
   1. Postoperative interventions: Cervical disk
      a. Monitor for respiratory difficulty from inflammation or hematoma.
      b. Encourage coughing, deep breathing, and early ambulation, as prescribed.
      c. Monitor for hoarseness and inability to cough effectively, because this may indicate laryngeal nerve damage.
      d. Use throat sprays or lozenges for sore throat, avoiding anesthetic lozenges that may numb the throat and increase choking risks.
      e. Monitor the surgical wound for infection, swelling, redness, drainage, or pain; manage surgical drains accordingly.
      f. Provide a soft diet if the client complains of dysphagia.
      g. Monitor for sudden return of radicular pain, which may indicate cervical spine instability.

2. Postoperative interventions: Lumbar disk
   a. Monitor the surgical dressing for wound drainage and bleeding; maintain surgical drains accordingly.
   b. Monitor lower extremities for sensation, movement, color, temperature, and paresthesia.
   c. Monitor for urinary retention, paralytic ileus, and constipation, which can result from decreased movement, opioid administration, or spinal cord compression.
   d. Prevent constipation by encouraging a high-fiber diet, increased fluid intake, and stool softeners, as prescribed.
   e. Administer opioids and sedatives as prescribed to relieve pain and anxiety.
   f. Assist and instruct the client to apply a prescribed back brace or corset while wearing cotton underwear to prevent skin irritation.
3. Postoperative lumbar disk positioning concerns
   a. In the immediate postoperative period, the client may be expected to lie supine or have other activity restrictions, depending on specific surgical intervention.
   b. Reinforce instructions to avoid spinal flexion or twisting and that the spine needs to be kept aligned.
   c. Reinforce instructions to minimize sitting, which may place a strain on the surgical site.
   d. When the client is lying supine, place a pillow under the neck and slightly flex the knees.
   e. Avoid extreme hip flexion when lying on the side.

⚠ Following disk surgery, instruct the client in correct logrolling techniques for turning and repositioning and for getting out of bed.

XIII. Amputation of a Lower Extremity

A. Description
1. Amputation (Fig. 57.4) is the surgical removal of a limb or part of the limb.
2. Complications include hemorrhage, infection, phantom limb pain, neuroma, and flexion contractures.
B. Postoperative interventions
1. Monitor for signs of complications.
2. Mark bleeding and drainage on the dressing if they occur.
3. Evaluate for phantom limb sensation and pain; explain sensation and pain to the client, and medicate the client as prescribed.
4. To prevent hip flexion contractures, do not elevate the residual limb on a pillow.
5. First 24 hours: Elevate the foot of the bed to reduce edema, and then keep the bed flat to prevent hip flexion contractures, if prescribed by the surgeon.

6. After 24 to 48 hours postoperatively, position the client prone to stretch the muscles and prevent hip flexion contractures, if prescribed.
7. Maintain surgical application of dressing, elastic compression wrap, or elastic stump (residual limb) shrinker, as prescribed, to reduce swelling, minimize pain, and mold the residual limb in preparation for prosthesis (Fig. 57.5).
8. As prescribed, wash the residual limb with mild soap and water and dry completely.
9. Massage the skin toward the suture line to mobilize scar and prevent its adherence to underlying bone.
10. Prepare for the prosthesis and reinforce instructions about progressive resistive techniques by gently pushing the residual limb against pillows and progressing to firmer surfaces.
11. Encourage verbalization regarding loss of the body part, and assist the client with identifying coping mechanisms to deal with the loss.

C. Interventions for below-the-knee amputation
1. Prevent edema.

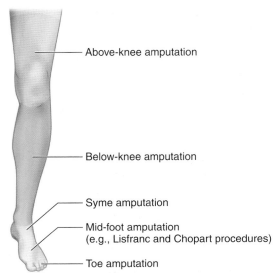

Above-knee amputation

Below-knee amputation

Syme amputation

Mid-foot amputation
(e.g., Lisfranc and Chopart procedures)

Toe amputation

FIGURE 57.4 Common levels of lower-extremity amputation.

2. Do not allow the residual limb to hang over the edge of the bed.
3. Discourage long periods of sitting to lessen complications of knee flexion.
4. Place the client in a prone position throughout the day as prescribed by the surgeon.

D. Interventions for above-the-knee amputation
1. Prevent internal or external rotation of the limb.
2. Place a sandbag, rolled towel, or trochanter roll along the outside of the thigh to prevent external rotation.
3. Place the client in a prone position throughout the day as prescribed by the surgeon.

E. Rehabilitation
1. Instruct the client in the use of a mobility aid such as crutches or a walker.
2. Prepare the residual limb for a prosthesis.
3. Prepare the client for fitting of the residual limb for a prosthesis.
4. Reinforce instructions regarding exercises to maintain range of motion and upper body strengthening.
5. Provide psychosocial support to the client.

F. Traumatic amputation: Emergency care
1. Obtain emergency medical assistance (call 911).
2. Stay with the victim, check the amputation site, and apply direct pressure with gauze or cloth. Do not remove applied pressure dressing to prevent dislodging of a formed clot.
3. Elevate the extremity above heart level.
4. If finger(s) were amputated, place in a watertight sealed plastic bag and place the bag in ice water (not directly on ice) and transport to the emergency department with the victim.

XIV. Rheumatoid Arthritis

A. Description
1. Rheumatoid arthritis is a chronic systemic inflammatory disease (immune complex–disorder); the cause may be related to a combination of environmental and genetic factors.
2. Rheumatoid arthritis leads to destruction of connective tissue and synovial membrane within the joints.

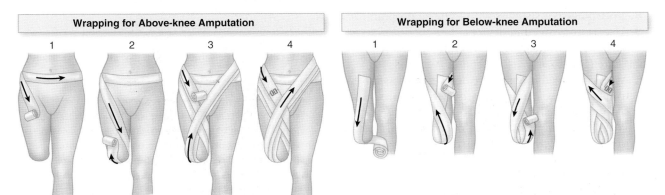

Wrapping for Above-knee Amputation				**Wrapping for Below-knee Amputation**			
1	2	3	4	1	2	3	4

FIGURE 57.5 A common method of wrapping a residual limb. *Left*, Wrapping for above-knee amputation. *Right*, Wrapping for below-knee amputation.

3. Rheumatoid arthritis weakens the joint, leading to dislocation and permanent deformity of the joint.
4. Formation of pannus occurs at the junction of synovial tissue and articular cartilage and projects into the joint cavity, causing necrosis.
5. Exacerbations of disease manifestations occur during periods of physical or emotional stress and fatigue.
6. Vasculitis can impede blood flow, leading to organ or organ system malfunction and failure because of tissue ischemia.

B. Data collection
1. Inflammation, tenderness, and stiffness of the joints
2. Moderate to severe pain with morning stiffness lasting longer than 30 minutes
3. Joint deformities, muscle atrophy, and decreased range of motion in affected joints
4. Spongy, soft feeling in the joints
5. Low-grade temperature, fatigue, and weakness
6. Anorexia, weight loss, and anemia
7. Elevated sedimentation rate and positive rheumatoid factor
8. Radiographic study showing joint deterioration
9. Synovial tissue biopsy reveals inflammation

C. Rheumatoid factor
1. A blood test used to assist with diagnosing rheumatoid arthritis
2. Normal range is 0 to 20 IU/mL

D. Medications: Combination of pharmacological therapies includes NSAIDs, disease-modifying antirheumatic drugs (DMARDs), and glucocorticoids

E. Physical mobility
1. Preserve joint function.
2. Provide range-of-motion exercises to maintain joint motion and muscle strengthening.
3. Balance rest and activity.
4. Splints may be used during acute inflammation to prevent deformity.
5. Prevent flexion contractures.
6. Apply heat or cold therapy to joints as prescribed.
7. Apply paraffin baths and massage as prescribed.
8. Encourage consistency with exercise program.
9. Use joint-protecting devices.
10. Avoid weight bearing on inflamed joints.

F. Self-care (Box 57.4)
1. Assess the need for assistive devices such as raised toilet seats, self-rising chairs, wheelchairs, and scooters to facilitate mobility.
2. Work with the RN and an occupational therapist or PHCP to obtain assistive or adaptive devices.
3. Instruct the client in alternative strategies for providing activities of daily living.

G. Fatigue
1. Identify factors that may contribute to fatigue.
2. Monitor for signs of anemia, and administer iron, folic acid, and vitamins as prescribed.
3. Monitor for medication-related blood loss by testing the stool for occult blood.
4. Reinforce instructions in measures to conserve energy, such as pacing activities and obtaining assistance when possible.

H. Disturbed body image
1. Determine the client's reaction to the body change.
2. Encourage the client to verbalize feelings.
3. Assist the client with self-care activities and grooming.
4. Encourage the client to wear street clothes.

I. Surgical interventions: Minimally invasive procedures may be prescribed.
1. Synovectomy: Surgical removal of the synovia to help maintain joint function
2. Arthrodesis: Bony fusion of a joint to regain some mobility
3. Joint replacement (arthroplasty): Surgical replacement of diseased joints with artificial joints; performed to restore motion to a joint and function to the muscles, ligaments, and other soft tissue structures that control a joint

XV. Osteoarthritis (Degenerative Joint Disease)

A. Description
1. Osteoarthritis is marked by progressive deterioration of the articular cartilage.
2. It causes the formation of bony buildup and the loss of articular cartilage in peripheral and axial joints.
3. Osteoarthritis affects the weight-bearing joints and joints that receive the greatest stress, such as the hips, knees, and lower vertebral column and hands.
4. The cause of primary osteoarthritis is not known. Risk factors include trauma, aging, obesity, genetic changes, and smoking.

BOX 57.4	Client Education for Rheumatoid Arthritis and Degenerative Joint Disease

Assist the client with identifying and correcting safety hazards in their home.
Instruct the client on the correct use of assistive or adaptive devices.
Instruct the client in energy conservation measures.
Review the prescribed exercise program.
Instruct the client to sit in a chair with a high, straight back.
Instruct the client to use only a small pillow when lying down.
Instruct the client on measures to protect the joints.
Instruct the client regarding prescribed medications.
Stress the importance of follow-up visits with the primary health care provider.

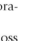

B. Data collection

1. Client experiences joint pain that diminishes after rest and intensifies after activity, noted early in the disease process.
2. As disease progresses, pain occurs with slight motion or even at rest.
3. Symptoms are aggravated by temperature change and climate humidity.
4. Presence of Heberden's nodes or Bouchard's nodes (hands)
5. Joint swelling (may be minimal), crepitus, and limited range of motion
6. Difficulty getting up after prolonged sitting
7. Skeletal muscle disuse atrophy
8. Inability to perform activities of daily living
9. Compression of the spine as manifested by radiating pain, stiffness, and muscle spasms in one or both extremities

C. Pain

1. Administer medications as prescribed such as acetaminophen (Tylenol) or topical applications; if acetaminophen or topical agents do not relieve pain, then NSAIDs may be prescribed. Muscle relaxants may also be prescribed for muscle spasms, especially those occurring in the back.
2. Prepare the client for corticosteroid injections into joints as prescribed.
3. Position the joints in function position and avoid flexion of the knees and hips.
4. Immobilize the affected joint with a splint or brace until inflammation subsides.
5. Avoid large pillows under the head or knees.
6. Provide a bed or foot cradle to keep linen off the feet and legs until inflammation subsides.
7. Reinforce instructions on the importance of moist heat, hot packs or compresses, and paraffin dips as prescribed.
8. Apply cold applications as prescribed when the joint is acutely inflamed.
9. Encourage adequate rest.

D. Nutrition

1. Encourage a well-balanced diet.
2. Maintain weight within normal range to decrease stress on the joints.

E. Physical mobility

1. Reinforce instructions to balance activity with rest while participating in an exercise program that limits stressing affected joints.
2. Reinforce instructions that exercises would be active rather than passive and to stop exercise if pain occurs.
3. Reinforce instructions to limit exercise when joint inflammation is severe.

F. Surgical management: Minimally invasive procedures may be prescribed.

1. Osteotomy: The bone is resected to correct joint deformity, promote realignment, and reduce joint stress.
2. Total joint replacement or arthroplasty
3. Total joint replacement is performed when all measures of pain relief have failed.
4. Hips and knees are replaced most commonly.
5. Total joint replacement is contraindicated in the presence of infection, advanced osteoporosis, or severe joint inflammation.

XVI. Osteoporosis

A. Description

1. Osteoporosis is a metabolic disease characterized by bone demineralization, with loss of calcium and phosphorus salts, leading to fragile bones and the subsequent risk for fractures.
2. Bone resorption accelerates as bone formation slows.
3. Osteoporosis occurs most commonly in the wrist, hip, and vertebral column.
4. Osteoporosis can occur postmenopausally or as a result of a metabolic disorder or calcium deficiency.
5. The client may be asymptomatic until the bones become fragile and a minor injury or movement causes a fracture.
6. Primary osteoporosis
   a. Most often occurs in postmenopausal women; occurs in men with low testosterone levels.
   b. Risk factors include decreased calcium intake, deficient estrogen, and sedentary lifestyle.
7. Secondary osteoporosis
   a. Causes include prolonged therapy with corticosteroids, thyroid-reducing medications, aluminum-containing antacids, or anticonvulsants.
   b. Associated with immobility, alcoholism, malnutrition, or malabsorption
8. Risk factors (Box 57.5)

B. Data collection

1. Possibly asymptomatic
2. Back pain can occur after lifting, bending, or stooping.
3. Back pain that increases with palpation
4. Pelvic or hip pain, especially with weight bearing
5. Problems with balance
6. Decline in height from vertebral compression
7. Kyphosis of the dorsal spine, also known as "Dowager's hump"
8. Degeneration of lower thorax and lumbar vertebrae on radiographic studies

⚠️ The client with osteoporosis is at risk for pathological fractures.

BOX 57.5 **Risk Factors for Osteoporosis**

Cigarette smoking
Early menopause
Excessive use of alcohol
Family history
Female gender
Increasing age
Insufficient intake of calcium
Sedentary lifestyle
Thin, small frame
White (European descent) or Asian race

C. Interventions
1. Determine risk for injury and institute measures to prevent injury in the client's personal environment.
   a. Assist the client with identifying and correcting hazards in his or her environment.
   b. Position household items and furniture to ensure unobstructed walkway.
   c. Use side rails to prevent falls.
   d. Reinforce instructions in the use of assistive devices such as a cane or walker.
   e. Encourage use of a firm mattress.
2. Provide personal care to the client to reduce injuries.
   a. Move the client gently when turning and repositioning.
   b. Assist with ambulation if the client is unsteady.
   c. Provide gentle range-of-motion exercises.
   d. Apply a back brace as prescribed during an acute phase to immobilize the spine and provide spinal column support.
3. Provide client instructions to promote optimal level of health and function.
   a. Reinforce instructions in the use of good body mechanics.
   b. Reinforce instructions regarding exercises to strengthen abdominal and back muscles to improve posture and provide support for the spine.
   c. Reinforce instructions to avoid activities that can cause vertebral compression.
   d. Reinforce instructions to eat a diet high in protein, calcium, vitamins C and D, and iron (see Chapter 11 for foods high in these vitamins and minerals).
   e. Reinforce instructions to avoid alcohol and coffee.
   f. Reinforce instructions to maintain an adequate fluid intake to prevent renal calculi.
4. Administer medication as prescribed to promote bone strength and decrease pain.

XVII. Gout
A. Description
1. Gout is a systemic disease in which urate crystals deposit in joints and other body tissues.
2. Gout results from abnormal amounts of uric acid in the body.
3. Primary gout results from a disorder of purine metabolism.
4. Secondary gout involves excessive uric acid in the blood that is caused by another disease.
B. Phases
1. Asymptomatic: Client has no symptoms, but serum uric acid is elevated.
2. Acute: Client has excruciating pain and inflammation of one or more small joints, especially the great toe.
3. Intermittent: Client has intermittent periods without symptoms between acute attacks.
4. Chronic: Results from repeated episodes of acute gout
   a. Chronic gout results in deposits of urate crystals under the skin.
   b. Chronic gout results in deposits of urate crystals within major organs such as the kidneys, leading to organ dysfunction.
C. Data collection
1. Swelling and inflammation of the joints, leading to excruciating pain
2. Tophi: Hard, irregular-shaped nodules in the skin containing chalky deposits of sodium urate
3. Low-grade fever, malaise, and headache
4. Pruritus from urate crystals in the skin
5. Presence of renal stones from elevated uric acid levels
D. Interventions
1. Provide a low-purine diet as prescribed; foods such as organ meats, wines, and aged cheese would be avoided.
2. Encourage a high fluid intake of 2000 mL/day (unless contraindicated) to prevent stone formation.
3. Encourage a weight-reduction diet if required.
4. Instruct the client to avoid alcohol and starvation diets because they may precipitate a gout attack.
5. Increase urinary pH (above 6) by eating alkaline ash foods.
6. Provide bed rest during acute attacks with affected extremity elevated.
7. Monitor joint range-of-motion ability and appearance of joints.
8. Position the joint in mild flexion during an acute attack.
9. Protect the affected joint from excessive movement or direct contact with sheets or blankets.
10. Provide heat or cold for local treatments to the affected joint as prescribed.

11. Administer medications such as analgesics, anti-inflammatory medications, and uricosuric agents, as prescribed.

WHAT WOULD YOU DO?

Answer: In a traumatic amputation, the nurse would call 911 to transport the victim to the hospital. While awaiting emergency medical assistance, the nurse needs to immediately check the amputation site and apply direct pressure with dry gauze. This pressure dressing is not removed to prevent dislodgment of a formed clot. The extremity is elevated above heart level. The amputated finger is placed in a watertight sealed plastic bag, and the bag is placed in ice water (not directly on ice). The nurse stays with the victim until he or she is transported to the emergency department.

PRACTICE QUESTIONS

1. The nurse is one of several people who witness a vehicle hit a pedestrian at a fairly low speed on a small street. The individual is dazed and tries to get up, and the leg appears fractured. The nurse would plan to perform which action?
1. Try to manually reduce the fracture.
2. Leave the person for a few moments to call an ambulance.
3. Stay with the person and encourage the person to remain still.
4. Assist the person with getting up and walking to the sidewalk.

2. The nurse witnesses a client sustain a fall and suspects that the client's leg may be fractured. Which action is the **priority**?
1. Take a set of vital signs
2. Call the radiology department
3. Immobilize the leg before moving the client
4. Reassure the client that everything will be fine

3. A client with a hip fracture asks the nurse why Buck's extension traction is being applied before surgery. The nurse's response is based on the understanding that Buck's extension traction has which **primary** function?
1. Allows bony healing to begin before surgery
2. Provides rigid immobilization of the fracture site
3. Lengthens the fractured leg to prevent severing of blood vessels
4. Provides comfort by reducing muscle spasms and provides fracture immobilization

4. The nurse is evaluating the pin sites of a client in skeletal traction. The nurse would be least concerned with which finding?

1. Inflammation
2. Serous drainage
3. Pain at a pin site
4. Purulent drainage

5. The nurse is caring for the client who has had skeletal traction applied to the left leg. The client is complaining of severe left leg pain. Which action would the nurse take **first**?
1. Provide pin care
2. Check the client's alignment in bed
3. Medicate the client with an analgesic
4. Call the primary health care provider (PHCP)

6. The nurse has provided instructions regarding specific leg exercises for the client immobilized in right skeletal lower leg traction. The nurse determines that the client **needs further teaching** if the nurse observes the client doing which activity?
1. Pulling up on the trapeze
2. Flexing and extending the feet
3. Doing quadriceps-setting and gluteal-setting exercises
4. Performing active range of motion (ROM) to the right ankle and knee

7. The nurse is checking the casted extremity of a client. The nurse needs to check for which sign indicative of infection?
1. Dependent edema
2. Diminished distal pulse
3. Presence of a "hot spot" on the cast
4. Coolness and pallor of the extremity

8. A client has sustained a closed fracture and has just had a cast applied to the affected arm. The client is complaining of intense pain. The nurse has elevated the limb, applied an ice bag, and administered an analgesic, which was ineffective in relieving the pain. The nurse interprets that this pain may be caused by which condition?
1. Infection under the cast
2. The anxiety of the client
3. Impaired tissue perfusion
4. The newness of the fracture

9. The nurse is assigned to care for a client with multiple traumas who is admitted to the hospital. The client has a leg fracture, and a plaster cast has been applied. In positioning the casted leg, the nurse would perform which intervention?
1. Keep the leg in a level position
2. Elevate the leg for 3 hours, and put it flat for 1 hour
3. Keep the leg level for 3 hours, and elevate it for 1 hour
4. Elevate the leg on pillows continuously for 24 to 48 hours

10. A client is complaining of skin irritation from the edges of a cast applied the previous day. The nurse would plan for which intervention?
1. Massaging the skin at the rim of the cast
2. Petaling the cast edges with adhesive tape
3. Using a rough file to smooth the cast edges
4. Applying lotion to the skin at the rim of the cast

❖ **11.** The nurse is preparing a list of cast care instructions for a client who just had a plaster cast applied to his right forearm. Which instructions would the nurse include on the list? **Select all that apply.**
- ❑ 1. Keep the cast and extremity elevated
- ❑ 2. The cast needs to be kept clean and dry
- ❑ 3. Allow the wet cast 24 to 72 hours to dry
- ❑ 4. Expect tingling and numbness in the extremity
- ❑ 5. Use a hair dryer set on a warm to hot setting to dry the cast
- ❑ 6. Use a soft-padded object that will fit under the cast to scratch the skin under the cast

12. The nurse is planning to reinforce instructions to the client about how to stand on crutches. In the instructions, the nurse would plan to tell the client to place the crutches in which position?
1. 3 inches to the front and side of the client's toes
2. 8 inches to the front and side of the client's toes
3. 15 inches to the front and side of the client's toes
4. 20 inches to the front and side of the client's toes

13. The nurse is evaluating the client's use of a cane for left-sided weakness. The nurse would intervene and correct the client if the nurse observed that the client performed which action?
1. Holds the cane on the right side
2. Moves the cane when the right leg is moved
3. Leans on the cane when the right leg swings through
4. Keeps the cane 6 inches out to the side of the right foot

14. The nurse is caring for a client with a fresh application of a plaster leg cast. The nurse would plan to prevent the development of compartment syndrome by which action?
1. Elevating the limb and covering it with bath blankets
2. Elevating the limb and applying ice to the affected leg
3. Keeping the leg horizontal and applying ice to the affected leg
4. Placing the leg in a slightly dependent position and applying ice

15. A client is being discharged after application of a plaster leg cast. The nurse determines that the client understands proper care of the cast if the client makes which statement?
1. "I need to avoid getting the cast wet."
2. "I will use my fingertips to lift and move the leg."
3. "I need to cover the casted leg with warm blankets."
4. "I can use a padded coat hanger end to scratch under the cast."

ANSWERS

1. 3
Rationale: With a suspected fracture, the client is not moved unless it is dangerous to remain in that spot. The nurse needs to remain with the client and have someone else call for emergency help. A fracture is not reduced at the scene. Before moving the client, the site of the fracture is immobilized to prevent further injury.
Test-Taking Strategy: Focus on the subject, the action to take if a fracture is suspected. Eliminate options 1 and 2 first, because these actions are comparable or alike and could result in further injury to the client. From the remaining options, the most prudent action would be for the nurse to remain with the client and have someone else call for emergency assistance.

2. 3
Rationale: When a fracture is suspected, it is imperative that the area is splinted before the client is moved. Emergency help needs to be called if the client is not hospitalized; a primary health care provider is called for the hospitalized client. The nurse must remain with the client and provide realistic reassurance. The nurse does not prescribe radiology tests.
Test-Taking Strategy: Note the strategic word, *priority*. Eliminate option 2 because the nurse does not prescribe x-rays. Reassuring the client is eliminated next, because the nurse does not tell a client that "everything will be fine." From the remaining options, focus on the data in the question. Immobilizing the limb is imperative for the client's safety, which makes it a better choice than taking vital signs.

3. 4
Rationale: Buck's extension traction is a type of skin traction often applied after hip fracture, before the fracture is reduced in surgery. It reduces muscle spasms and helps immobilize the fracture. It does not lengthen the leg for the purpose of preventing blood vessel severance. It also does not allow for bony healing to begin.
Test-Taking Strategy: Note the strategic word, *primary*, and focus on the subject, the function of Buck's extension traction. Recalling the purpose of traction will assist in eliminating options 1 and 3. From the remaining options, eliminate the option with the words *rigid immobilization*.

4. 2
Rationale: A small amount of serous drainage is expected at pin insertion sites. Signs of infection such as inflammation, purulent drainage, and pain at the pin site are not expected findings and would be reported.
Test-Taking Strategy: Focus on the subject, the finding that the nurse would be least concerned with. Inflammation and

purulent drainage indicate infection and are eliminated first; these options are comparable or alike. To select between the other options, look at them carefully. The complaint of pain is at "a pin site" only. It gives no indication that the pain is related to the fracture or muscle spasm. Because serous drainage is an expected finding, you would select this over the complaint of pain.

5. 2

Rationale: A client who complains of severe pain may need realignment or may have had traction weights prescribed that are too heavy. The nurse realigns the client and, if ineffective, calls the PHCP. Severe leg pain, once traction has been established, indicates a problem. Medicating the client would be done after trying to determine and treat the cause. Providing pin care is unrelated to the problem as described.

Test-Taking Strategy: Note the strategic word, *first*. Use the steps of the nursing process. The option describing checking the client's alignment is the only option that addresses data collection.

6. 4

Rationale: Exercise is indicated within therapeutic limits for the client in skeletal traction to maintain muscle strength and ROM. The client may pull up on the trapeze, perform active ROM with uninvolved joints, and do isometric muscle-setting exercises (e.g., quadriceps- and gluteal-setting exercises). The client may also flex and extend his or her feet. Performing active ROM to the affected leg can be harmful.

Test-Taking Strategy: Note the strategic words, *needs further teaching*. This indicates a negative event query and the need to select the incorrect client action. Options 1 and 3 are most easily identified as correct actions and are therefore eliminated as possible answers. To select between the remaining options, imagine the lines of pull on the fracture site with the movements described. Although flexing and extending the feet do not disrupt the line of pull from the traction, performing active ROM to the affected knee and ankle does.

7. 3

Rationale: Signs/symptoms of infection under a casted area include odor or purulent drainage from the cast or the presence of "hot spots," which are areas of the cast that are warmer than others. The primary health care provider needs to be notified if any of these occur. Signs of impaired circulation in the distal limb include coolness and pallor of the skin, diminished arterial pulse, and edema.

Test-Taking Strategy: Note the subject, a sign of infection. Begin to answer this question by thinking of what you would expect to find with infection: redness, swelling, heat, and purulent drainage. With these in mind, the options of diminished distal pulses and coolness of the extremity can be eliminated. *Dependent edema* is not necessarily indicative of infection; swelling would be continuous. The "hot spot" on the cast could signify infection underneath that area.

8. 3

Rationale: Most pain associated with fractures can be minimized with rest, elevation, application of a cold compress, and administration of analgesics. Pain that is not relieved from these measures needs to be reported to the nurse and primary health care

provider because it may be the result of impaired tissue perfusion, tissue breakdown, or necrosis. Because this is a new closed fracture and cast, infection would not have had time to set in.

Test-Taking Strategy: Focus on the subject, interpretation of the cause of the client's intense pain and the data in the question. The options of anxiety and newness of the fracture can be eliminated first, based on the description in the question. Because the fracture and cast are so new, it is extremely unlikely that infection could have set in. The most likely option is impaired tissue perfusion, because pain from ischemia is not relieved by comfort measures and analgesics.

9. 4

Rationale: A casted extremity is elevated continuously for the first 24 to 48 hours to minimize swelling and to promote venous drainage. Therefore, the other options are incorrect.

Test-Taking Strategy: Focus on the subject, intervention used when positioning a casted leg. Recall that edema sets in after fracture and can be aggravated by casting. For this reason, options 1 and 3 are comparable or alike in keeping the leg level. These are the least helpful and can be eliminated first. There is no useful purpose for the timing in option 2, elevating and then leaving the leg flat.

10. 2

Rationale: The edges of the cast can be petaled with tape to minimize skin irritation. If a client has a cast applied and returns home, the client can be taught to do the same. Massaging and applying lotion will not alleviate the skin irritation from the cast edges. Filing the edges will cause cast material to fall into the cast and could lead to skin irritation under the cast.

Test-Taking Strategy: Focus on the subject, skin irritation. Options 1 and 4 are comparable or alike, and neither helps to get rid of the cause of the irritation, so they are eliminated first. Imagine the use of a "rough file"; it would create plaster chips and dust, which could go underneath the cast.

❖ 11. 1, 2, 3

Rationale: A plaster cast takes 24 to 72 hours to dry (synthetic casts dry in 20 minutes). The cast and extremity may be elevated to reduce edema. A wet cast is handled with the palms of the hands until it is dry, and the extremity is turned (unless contraindicated) so that all sides of the wet cast will dry. A cool setting on the hair dryer can be used to dry a plaster cast (heat cannot be used because the cast heats up and burns the skin). The cast needs to be kept clean and dry, and the client is instructed not to stick anything under the cast because of the risk of breaking skin integrity. The client is instructed to monitor the extremity for circulatory impairment such as pain, swelling, discoloration, tingling, numbness, coolness, or diminished pulse. The primary health care provider is notified immediately if circulatory impairment occurs.

Test-Taking Strategy: Focus on the subject, a plaster cast. Recalling that edema occurs following a fracture and recalling the complications associated with a cast will assist you in answering the question.

12. 2

Rationale: The classic tripod position is taught to the client before giving instructions on gait. The crutches are placed any-

where from 6 to 10 inches in front and to the side of the client, depending on the client's body size. This provides a wide enough base of support to the client and improves balance.
Test-Taking Strategy: Focus on the subject, the safe use of crutches. Three inches and 20 inches seem excessively short and long, respectively; therefore, these options can be eliminated first. Of the remaining options, 8 inches seems more in keeping with the normal length of a stride than 15 inches.

13. 2
Rationale: The cane is held on the stronger side to minimize stress on the affected extremity and provide a wide base of support. The cane is held 6 inches lateral to the fifth great toe. The cane is moved forward with the affected leg. The client leans on the cane for added support, while the stronger side swings through.
Test-Taking Strategy: Note the word, *intervene*. Therefore, the subject of the question is the incorrect client action. Knowing that the cane is held on the stronger side helps you eliminate options 1 and 4 first. To select from the remaining options, recall that the client moves the cane with the weaker leg and leans on it for support when the stronger leg swings through.

14. 2
Rationale: Compartment syndrome is prevented by controlling edema. This is achieved most optimally with elevation and application of ice. Therefore, the other options are incorrect.
Test-Taking Strategy: Focus on the subject, compartment syndrome. Recalling that edema is controlled or prevented with limb elevation helps you eliminate options 3 and 4 first. From the remaining options, think about the effects of ice *versus* bath blankets. Ice will further control edema, but bath blankets will produce heat and prevent air circulation needed for the cast to dry.

15. 1
Rationale: A plaster cast must remain dry to keep its strength. The cast would be handled using the palms of the hands, not the fingertips, until fully dry. Air would circulate freely around the cast to help it dry; the cast also gives off heat as it dries. The client must never scratch under the cast; a cool hair dryer may be used to eliminate itching.
Test-Taking Strategy: Focus on the subject, proper cast care. Knowing that a wet cast can be dented with the fingertips, causing pressure underneath, helps you eliminate option 2 first. Knowing that the cast needs to dry helps you eliminate option 3 next. The option of using a coat hanger is dangerous to skin integrity and is also eliminated. Plaster casts, once they have dried after application, must not become wet.

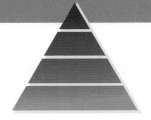

CHAPTER **58**

Musculoskeletal Medications

PRIORITY CONCEPTS Inflammation; Safety

WHAT WOULD YOU DO?

Cyclobenzaprine is prescribed for a client experiencing muscle spasms. The nurse reviews the client's record and notes that the client is currently taking phenelzine. What would the nurse do?
Answer is located on p. 827.

I. Skeletal Muscle Relaxants

A. Description
   1. Skeletal muscle relaxants (Box 58.1) act directly on the neuromuscular junction or act indirectly on the central nervous system (CNS).
   2. Centrally acting muscle relaxants depress neuron activity in the spinal cord or brain.
   3. Peripherally acting muscle relaxants act directly on the skeletal muscles, interfering with calcium release from muscle tubules and thus preventing the fibers from contracting.
   4. Skeletal muscle relaxants are used to prevent or relieve muscle spasms and treat spasticity associated with spinal cord disease or lesions, acute painful musculoskeletal conditions, and chronic debilitating disorders such as multiple sclerosis, brain attacks (stroke), or cerebral palsy.
   5. Skeletal muscle relaxants are contraindicated in clients with severe liver, renal, or heart disease; these medications are often metabolized in the liver or excreted from the kidney.
   6. Skeletal muscle relaxants would not be taken with CNS depressants, such as barbiturates, opioids, alcohol, sedatives, hypnotics, or tricyclic antidepressants, unless specifically prescribed.
B. Side/adverse effects
   1. Dizziness and hypotension
   2. Drowsiness and muscle weakness
   3. Dry mouth
   4. Gastrointestinal upset
   5. Photosensitivity
   6. Liver toxicity

C. Interventions
   1. Obtain a medical history and ask about current medications being taken.
   2. Monitor vital signs.
   3. Monitor for CNS effects.
   4. Determine risk for injury.
   5. Monitor involved joints and muscles for pain and mobility.
   6. Monitor renal function studies.
   7. Reinforce instructions to the client to take the medication with food to decrease gastrointestinal upset.
   8. Reinforce instructions to the client to report side/adverse effects.
   9. Reinforce instructions to the client to avoid alcohol and CNS depressants.
   10. Reinforce instructions to the client to avoid activities requiring alertness such as driving or operating equipment.

 Monitor liver function tests when a client is taking a skeletal muscle relaxant because hepatotoxicity can occur.

D. Nursing considerations
   1. Baclofen
      a. Baclofen causes CNS effects such as drowsiness, dizziness, weakness, fatigue, nausea, constipation, and urinary retention.
      b. Administer with caution in the client with renal or hepatic dysfunction or a seizure disorder.
      c. Baclofen can be administered by the primary health care provider (PHCP) through intrathecal infusion using an implantable pump or by direct intrathecal administration over 1 minute.
      d. The client with an implantable pump is instructed to maintain medication refill appointments to prevent the pump from emptying and experiencing sudden withdrawal symptoms (which could be life threatening).

Adult—Musculoskeletal

| BOX 58.1 | Skeletal Muscle Relaxants |

Baclofen
Carisoprodol
Chlorzoxazone
Cyclobenzaprine
Dantrolene
Diazepam
Metaxalone
Methocarbamol
Orphenadrine
Tizanidine

2. Carisoprodol
   a. The client is advised to take the medication with food to prevent gastrointestinal upset.
   b. Reinforce instructions to the client to report any rash or hypersensitivity to the PHCP.
3. Chlorzoxazone
   a. Monitor the client for hypersensitivity reactions such as urticaria, redness or itching, and possibly angioedema.
   b. Chlorzoxazone may cause malaise and may cause the urine to turn orange or red.
   c. Chlorzoxazone can cause hepatitis and hepatic necrosis.
4. Cyclobenzaprine
   a. Cyclobenzaprine is contraindicated in clients who have received monoamine oxidase inhibitors (MAOIs) within 14 days of initiation of cyclobenzaprine therapy and in clients who have a cardiac disorder.
   b. Cyclobenzaprine has significant anticholinergic (atropine-like) effects and needs to be used with caution in clients with a history of urinary retention, angle-closure glaucoma, or increased intraocular pressure.
   c. Cyclobenzaprine would be used only for short-term therapy (2–3 weeks).
5. Dantrolene
   a. Dantrolene acts directly on skeletal muscles to relieve spasticity.
   b. Liver damage is the most serious adverse effect.
   c. Liver function values would be monitored before the initiation of treatment and during treatment.
   d. Dantrolene can cause gastrointestinal bleeding, urinary frequency, impotence, photosensitivity, rash, and muscle weakness.
   e. Reinforce instructions to the client to wear protective clothing when in the sun.
   f. Reinforce instructions to the client to notify the PHCP if rash, bloody or tarry stools, or yellow discoloration of the skin or eyes occur.

6. Diazepam
   a. Acts in the CNS to suppress spasticity; does not affect skeletal muscle directly
   b. Sedation is a common side effect.
7. Methocarbamol
   a. The parenteral form is contraindicated in clients with renal impairment.
   b. The parenteral form can cause hypotension, bradycardia, anaphylaxis, and seizures, especially when the medication is given too rapidly.
   c. Monitor site for extravasation, which can result in thrombophlebitis and tissue sloughing.
   d. Methocarbamol may cause the urine to turn brown, black, or green.
   e. The client is informed to notify the PHCP if blurred vision, nasal congestion, urticaria, or rash occurs.
8. Tizanidine and metaxalone: Can cause liver damage
9. Orphenadrine has significant anticholinergic (atropine-like) effects and needs to be used with caution in clients with a history of urinary retention, angle-closure glaucoma, or increased intraocular pressure.

 Safety is a primary concern when the client is taking a skeletal muscle relaxant because these medications cause drowsiness.

II. **Antigout Medications**
A. Description
   1. Antigout medications (allopurinol, colchicine, probenecid) reduce uric acid production and increase uric acid excretion (uricosuric) to prevent or relieve gout or to manage hyperuricemia.
   2. Nonsteroidal anti-inflammatory drugs (NSAIDs) are used for their anti-inflammatory effects and to relieve pain during an acute gouty attack (see Chapter 56 for information on NSAIDs).
   3. Glucocorticoids may be prescribed to reduce inflammation during an acute gouty attack (see Chapter 44 for information on glucocorticoids).
   4. Antigout medications need to be used cautiously in clients with gastrointestinal, renal, cardiac, or hepatic disease.
B. Side and adverse effects
   1. Headache
   2. Nausea, vomiting, and diarrhea
   3. Types of blood dyscrasia, such as bone marrow suppression
   4. Flushed skin and rash
   5. Uric acid kidney stones
   6. Sore gums
   7. Metallic taste
C. Interventions
   1. Monitor serum uric acid levels.
   2. Monitor intake and output.

3. Maintain a fluid intake of at least 2000 mL/day to 3000 mL/day to avoid kidney stones.

4. Monitor complete blood cell count and renal and liver function.

5. Reinforce instructions to the client to avoid alcohol and caffeine because these products can increase uric acid levels.

6. The client is encouraged to comply with therapy to prevent elevated uric acid levels, which can trigger a gout attack.

7. Reinforce instructions to the client to avoid foods high in purine as prescribed, such as wine, alcohol, organ meats, sardines, salmon, scallops, and gravy.

8. Reinforce instructions to the client to take the medication with food to decrease gastric irritation.

9. Reinforce instructions to the client to report side/adverse effects to the PHCP.

10. Reinforce instructions to the client not to take aspirin with these medications because the combination could trigger a gout attack.

D. Nursing considerations

1. Allopurinol
   a. Can increase the effect of warfarin and oral hypoglycemic agents
   b. Reinforce instructions to the client not to take large doses of vitamin C while taking allopurinol, because kidney stones may occur.
   c. Hypersensitivity syndrome (rare) can occur and is characterized by rash, fever, eosinophilia, and dysfunction of the liver and kidneys (medication is stopped and the PHCP is notified).
   d. The client is advised to minimize exposure to sunlight and have an annual eye examination because visual changes can occur from prolonged use of allopurinol.

2. Colchicine
   a. Used with caution in older clients, debilitated clients, and clients with cardiac, renal, and/or gastrointestinal disease
   b. If gastrointestinal symptoms occur (nausea, vomiting, diarrhea, and abdominal pain), the medication is stopped and the PHCP is notified.

3. Probenecid
   a. Mild gastrointestinal effects can occur and can be reduced by taking the medication with food.
   b. Aspirin and other salicylates interfere with the uricosuric action of the medication.

⚠️ The concurrent use of antigout medications and aspirin causes elevated uric acid levels; the client would be instructed to take acetaminophen, if prescribed, rather than aspirin.

BOX 58.2 Antiarthritic Medications

Abatacept
Adalimumab
Anakinra
Azathioprine
Cyclosporine
Etanercept
Hydroxychloroquine
Infliximab
Leflunomide
Methotrexate
Penicillamine
Rituximab
Sulfasalazine
Tofacitinib

III. Antiarthritic Medications (Box 58.2)

A. Description (Fig. 58.1)
1. Rheumatoid arthritis occurs as inflammation progresses into the synovia, cartilage, and bone; if this inflammation is not controlled, it will lead to joint destruction, thus affecting client mobility and comfort.
2. The focus of treatment is early diagnosis and aggressive therapy in order to preserve joint function.
3. Medication includes NSAIDs, glucocorticoids, and disease-modifying antirheumatic drugs (DMARDs).
4. Gold salts: Use of gold salts has decreased, but their purpose is to reduce the progression of joint damage caused by arthritic processes. Gold toxicity, characterized by pruritus, rash, metallic taste, stomatitis, and diarrhea, can occur; if toxicity occurs, dimercaprol may be prescribed to enhance gold excretion.

B. DMARDs
1. Description
   a. DMARDs are effective antirheumatic medications that are used to slow the degenerative effects of the disorder.
   b. DMARDs are usually prescribed secondary to NSAIDs but are often the first choice in the treatment of severe arthritis.
   c. Some medications are contraindicated during pregnancy.
2. Common side/adverse effects of DMARDs include injection site inflammation and pain, ecchymosis and edema, pancytopenia and infection, fatigue, headache, nausea, vomiting, flu-like symptoms, and allergic response.
3. Interventions
   a. The client is instructed to monitor for signs of infection and report signs to the PHCP.
   b. Monitor the injection site for signs of irritation, pain, inflammation, and swelling.
   c. Reinforce instructions to the client to consult with the PHCP before receiving live vaccines and to avoid exposure to infections.

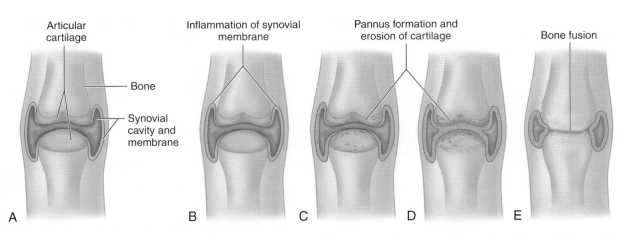

FIGURE 58.1 Progressive joint degeneration in rheumatoid arthritis. (A) Healthy joint. (B) Inflammation of synovial membrane. (C) Onset of pannus formation and cartilage erosion. (D) Pannus formation progresses and cartilage deteriorates further. (E) Complete destruction of joint cavity together with fusion of articulating bones.

  d. The client is informed about the importance of laboratory tests for neutrophil, white blood cell, and platelet counts before the initiation of treatment and during treatment.

4. Anakinra: Injection site reactions are common (pruritus, erythema, rash, pain).

5. Adalimumab
  a. Injection site reactions are common.
  b. Has been associated with neurological injury (numbness, tingling, dizziness, disturbed vision, weakness in the legs)

6. Azathioprine: Immunosuppressive and anti-inflammatory actions; toxic effects include hepatitis and blood dyscrasia.

7. Cyclosporine: Immunosuppressive actions; can cause nephrotoxicity

8. Etanercept
  a. Injection site reactions are common.
  b. Poses a risk for heart failure; has been associated with CNS demyelinating disorders and hematological disorders

9. Hydroxychloroquine sulfate: Associated with retinal damage; the client is informed to contact the PHCP if visual disturbances occur.

10. Leflunomide: Side and adverse effects include diarrhea, respiratory infection, reversible alopecia, rash, and nausea; hepatotoxicity.

11. Methotrexate: Can cause hepatic fibrosis, bone marrow suppression, gastrointestinal ulceration, and pneumonitis

12. Penicillamine: Can cause bone marrow suppression and autoimmune disorders

13. Infliximab: Can cause infusion reactions (fever, chills, pruritus, urticaria, chest pain); hepatotoxicity

14. Rituxan: Can cause increased thirst or urination, swelling of the hands or feet, or tingling of the hands or feet; the PHCP needs to be notified if any of these occur.

15. Sulfasalazine: Can cause gastrointestinal and dermatological reactions, bone marrow suppression, hepatitis
  a. NSAIDs may be prescribed for their anti-inflammatory and analgesic effects. (See Chapter 56 for information on NSAIDs.)
  b. Glucocorticoids may be prescribed for their anti-inflammatory effects. (See Chapter 44 for information on glucocorticoids.)

IV. Medications to Prevent and Treat Osteoporosis

A. Description
1. Osteoporosis is characterized by low bone mass and increased bone fragility.
2. Calcium and vitamin D supplementation can reduce the risk of osteoporosis; calcium maximizes bone growth early in life and maintains bone integrity later in life, and vitamin D ensures calcium absorption. (See Chapter 44 for information on calcium and vitamin D supplements.)
3. Treatment is aimed at reducing the occurrence of fractures by maintaining or increasing bone strength.
4. Medications that decrease bone resorption (antiresorptive) and medications that promote bone formation are used (Box 58.3).
5. Antiresorptive medications include raloxifene, calcitonin, and bisphosphonates.
6. Teriparatide promotes bone growth.

B. Interventions
1. Calcitonin-salmon
  a. Calcitonin is secreted by the thyroid gland and inhibits osteoclastic bone resorption.
  b. Reinforce instructions to the client on how to administer the intranasal or subcutaneous form, depending on the route prescribed.
  c. Intranasal route: Examine the nares for irritation; alternate nostrils for doses.
  d. When calcitonin is taken, it is important to monitor for hypocalcemia.

Abaloparatide
Alendronate
Calcitonin-salmon
Calcium and vitamin D
Denosumab
Ibandronate
Pamidronate
Raloxifene
Risedronate
Romosozumab
Teriparatide
Zoledronic acid

2. Bisphosphonates (see Box 58.3)
   a. Bisphosphonates inhibit osteoclast-mediated bone resorption, thereby increasing total bone mass.
   b. Bisphosphonates include alendronate, risedronate, and ibandronate.
   c. Contraindicated for clients with esophageal disorders that can impede swallowing and for clients who cannot sit or stand for at least 30 minutes (60 minutes with ibandronate)
   d. Adverse effects include esophagitis, muscle pain, and ocular problems; the client is instructed to contact the PHCP if adverse effects occur.

⚠️ Because of the risk of esophagitis, bisphosphonates need to be taken in the morning before eating or drinking with a full glass of water; the client then needs to remain sitting or standing and postpone ingesting anything for at least 30 minutes (60 minutes with ibandronate).

3. Raloxifene
   a. Antiresorptive medication (nonbisphosphonate)
   b. Contraindicated in clients who have a history of venous thrombotic events
   c. Needs to be discontinued 72 hours before prolonged immobilization periods (such as with periods of extended bed rest)
   d. Reinforce instructions to the client to avoid extended periods of restricted activity (such as when traveling).

4. Teriparatide
   a. Teriparatide stimulates new bone formation, thus increasing bone mass.
   b. Teriparatide is a portion of the human parathyroid hormone and works by increasing the action of osteoblasts.
   c. Reserved for use in clients at high risk for fractures

   d. Has been associated with the development of bone cancer

⚠️ NSAIDs such as ibuprofen, indomethacin, and naproxen are commonly used to treat musculoskeletal pain. Acetaminophen may also be used to treat this type of pain and is often considered first-line treatment.

WHAT WOULD YOU DO?

Answer: Cyclobenzaprine is a muscle relaxant and is contraindicated in clients who have received monoamine oxidase inhibitors (MAOIs) within 14 days of initiation of cyclobenzaprine therapy and in clients with cardiac disorders. Phenelzine is a MAOI medication. The nurse would inform the registered nurse and contact the primary health care provider and question the cyclobenzaprine prescription before the initiation of therapy.

PRACTICE QUESTIONS

1. The client has been taking medication for rheumatoid arthritis for 3 weeks. During the administration of etanercept, it is **most important** for the nurse to collect which data?
   1. The white blood cell and platelet counts
   2. A metallic taste in the mouth, with a loss of appetite
   3. Whether the client is experiencing fatigue and joint pain
   4. Whether the client is experiencing itching and edema at the injection site

2. Alendronate is prescribed for a client with osteoporosis and the nurse is providing instructions for the administration of the medication. Which instruction would the nurse reinforce?
   1. Take the medication at bedtime.
   2. Take the medication in the morning with breakfast.
   3. Lie down for 30 minutes after taking the medication.
   4. Take the medication with a full glass of water after rising in the morning.

3. The nurse is monitoring a client receiving baclofen for side effects related to the medication. Which would indicate that the client is experiencing a side effect?
   1. Polyuria
   2. Diarrhea
   3. Drowsiness
   4. Muscular excitability

4. During the monitoring of a client's response to disease-modifying antirheumatic drugs (DMARDs),

which findings would the nurse interpret as acceptable responses? **Select all that apply.**

- ❑ 1. Symptom control during periods of emotional stress
- ❑ 2. Normal white blood cell, platelet, and neutrophil counts
- ❑ 3. Radiological findings that show nonprogression of joint degeneration
- ❑ 4. An increased range of motion in the affected joints 3 months into therapy
- ❑ 5. Inflammation and irritation at the injection site 3 days after injection is given
- ❑ 6. A low-grade temperature when rising in the morning that remains throughout the day

5. A client with acute muscle spasms has been taking baclofen. The client calls the clinic nurse because of continuous feelings of weakness and fatigue and asks the nurse about discontinuing the medication. The nurse would make which appropriate response to the client?
   1. "You should never stop the medication."
   2. "It is best that you taper the dose if you intend to stop the medication."
   3. "It is okay to stop the medication if you think that you can tolerate the muscle spasms."
   4. "Weakness and fatigue commonly occur and will diminish with continued medication use."

6. The nurse is reviewing the laboratory studies on a client receiving dantrolene sodium. Which laboratory test(s) would identify an adverse effect associated with the administration of this medication?
   1. Creatinine
   2. Liver function tests
   3. Blood urea nitrogen
   4. Hematological function tests

7. The nurse is reviewing the record of a client who has been prescribed baclofen. Which disorder would alert the nurse to contact the primary health care provider (PHCP)?
   1. A seizure disorder
   2. Hyperthyroidism
   3. Diabetes mellitus
   4. Coronary artery disease

8. Cyclobenzaprine is prescribed for a client to treat muscle spasms, and the nurse is reviewing the client's record. Which disorder would indicate a need to contact the primary health care provider (PHCP) regarding the administration of this medication?
   1. Glaucoma
   2. Emphysema
   3. Hyperthyroidism
   4. Diabetes mellitus

9. Dantrolene sodium is prescribed for a client experiencing flexor spasms, and the client asks the nurse about the action of the medication. The nurse responds knowing that which is the therapeutic action of this medication?
   1. Depresses spinal reflexes
   2. Acts directly on the skeletal muscle to relieve spasticity
   3. Acts within the spinal cord to suppress hyperactive reflexes
   4. Acts on the central nervous system (CNS) to suppress spasms

10. The nurse is reinforcing discharge instructions to a client receiving baclofen. Which would the nurse include in the instructions?
    1. Restrict fluid intake.
    2. Avoid the use of alcohol.
    3. Stop the medication if diarrhea occurs.
    4. Notify the primary health care provider (PHCP) if fatigue occurs.

ANSWERS

1. 1
Rationale: Infection and suppression can occur as a result of etanercept. Laboratory studies are performed before and during treatment. The appearance of abnormal white blood cell and platelet counts can alert the nurse to a potentially life-threatening infection or potential bleeding. Injection site itching and edema are common occurrences following administration. A metallic taste and loss of appetite are not associated with this medication. Fatigue and joint pain occur with rheumatoid arthritis.
Test-Taking Strategy: Note the strategic words, *most important*. Option 2 can be eliminated because this is not associated with this medication. In early treatment, residual fatigue and joint pain may still be apparent. Option 1 monitors for a hematological disorder, which could indicate a reason for discontinuing this medication and need to be reported.

2. 4
Rationale: Precautions need to be taken with the administration of alendronate to prevent gastrointestinal side/adverse effects (especially esophageal irritation) and to increase absorption of the medication. The medication needs to be taken with a full glass of water after rising in the morning. The client would not eat or drink anything for 30 minutes following administration and would not lie down after taking the medication.
Test-Taking Strategy: Focus on the subject, the administration of alendronate. Recalling that this medication can cause esophageal irritation will direct you to the correct option.

3. 3
Rationale: Baclofen is a CNS depressant and frequently causes drowsiness, dizziness, weakness, and fatigue. It can also cause nausea, constipation, and urinary retention. Clients need to

be warned about the possible reactions. Options 1, 2, and 4 are not side effects.

Test-Taking Strategy: Focus on the subject, side effect of baclofen. Recalling that baclofen is a CNS depressant used to treat muscle spasticity will direct you to the correct option.

❖ **4.** 1, 2, 3, 4

Rationale: Because emotional stress frequently exacerbates the symptoms of rheumatoid arthritis, the absence of symptoms is a positive finding. DMARDs are given to slow progression of joint degeneration. In addition, the improvement in the range of motion after 3 months of therapy with normal blood work is a positive finding. Temperature elevation and inflammation and irritation at the medication injection site could indicate signs of infection.

Test-Taking Strategy: Focus on the subject, acceptable responses to therapy. Recalling that signs of an infection can indicate an unexpected finding will assist you with eliminating options 5 and 6.

5. 4

Rationale: The client would be instructed that symptoms such as drowsiness, weakness, and fatigue are more intense in the early phase of therapy and diminish with continued medication use. The client needs to be instructed never to withdraw or stop the medication abruptly because abrupt withdrawal can cause visual hallucinations, paranoid ideation, and seizures. It is best for the nurse to inform the client that these symptoms will subside and encourage the client to continue the use of the medication.

Test-Taking Strategy: Focus on the subject, the effects of baclofen. Eliminate option 1 first because it is a rather extreme nursing response and uses the closed-ended word, *never.* Next, use general medication guidelines and eliminate options 2 and 3 because these responses do not represent the scope of nursing practice or nursing actions.

6. 2

Rationale: Dose-related liver damage is the most serious adverse effect of dantrolene. To reduce the risk of liver damage, liver function tests would be performed before treatment and periodically throughout the treatment course. It is administered in the lowest effective dosage for the shortest time necessary. Options 1 and 3 are tests that assess kidney function.

Test-Taking Strategy: Focus on the subject, adverse effects of dantrolene. Eliminate options 1 and 3 because they are comparable or alike and assess kidney function. From the remaining options, it is necessary to recall that this medication affects liver function.

7. 1

Rationale: Clients with a seizure disorders may have a lowered seizure threshold when baclofen is administered. Concurrent therapy may require an increase in the anticonvulsive medication. The disorders in options 2, 3, and 4 are not a concern when the client is taking baclofen.

Test-Taking Strategy: Focus on the subject, contraindications of baclofen. Knowledge regarding the contraindications and the cautions associated with the administration of baclofen is required to answer this question. Remember, a lowered seizure threshold can occur when baclofen is administered.

8. 1

Rationale: Because this medication has anticholinergic effects, it needs to be used with caution in clients with a history of urinary retention, angle-closure glaucoma, and increased intraocular pressure. Cyclobenzaprine hydrochloride would be used only for short-term 2- to 3-week therapy. The disorders in options 2, 3, and 4 are not a concern when the client is taking cyclobenzaprine.

Test-Taking Strategy: Focus on the subject, contraindications of cyclobenzaprine. Recalling that this medication has anticholinergic effects will assist with directing you to the correct option.

9. 2

Rationale: Dantrolene acts directly on skeletal muscle to relieve muscle spasticity. The primary action is the suppression of calcium release from the sarcoplasmic reticulum. This in turn decreases the ability of the skeletal muscle to contract. Options 1, 3, and 4 are not actions of the medication.

Test-Taking Strategy: Options 1, 3, and 4 are all comparable or alike in that they address CNS suppression and the depression of reflexes. Therefore, eliminate these options.

10. 2

Rationale: Baclofen is a CNS depressant. The client needs to be cautioned against the use of alcohol and other CNS depressants because baclofen potentiates the depressant activity of these agents. It is not necessary to restrict fluids, but the client would be warned that urinary retention can occur. Constipation rather than diarrhea is an adverse effect of baclofen. Fatigue is related to a CNS effect that is most intense during the early phase of therapy and diminishes with continued medication use. It is not necessary that the client notify the PHCP if fatigue occurs.

Test-Taking Strategy: Focus on the subject, discharge instructions with baclofen. Recalling that baclofen is a CNS depressant will direct you to the correct option. If you were unsure of the correct option, use general principles related to medication administration. Alcohol would be avoided with the use of medications.

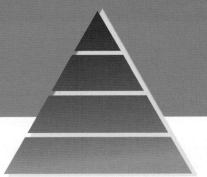

UNIT XVIII

Immune Problems of the Adult Client

Pyramid to Success

Pyramid Points focus on hypersensitivity and anaphylaxis and the effects of and complications associated with an immune deficiency. Specific focus relates to the nursing care related to the health problem, the effect of the treatment on the client, and client adaptation. Human immunodeficiency virus (HIV) and acquired immunodeficiency syndrome (AIDS) is a Pyramid focus, along with protecting the client from infection and preventing the transmission of infection to other individuals. Psychosocial issues relate to social isolation and the body image disturbances that can occur as a result of the immune disorder.

Client Needs: Learning Objectives

Safe and Effective Care Environment

Acting as an advocate related to the client's decisions

Addressing advance directives

Consulting with the interprofessional health care team

Ensuring that informed consent for treatments and procedures has been obtained

Establishing priorities

Handling hazardous and infectious materials safely

Implementing standard and other precautions

Maintaining asepsis

Maintaining confidentiality regarding diagnosis

Preventing infection

Upholding client rights

Client Needs lists modified from: National Council of State Boards of Nursing, Inc. (NCSBN). *NCLEX-PN Examination: Test Plan for the National Council Licensure Examination for Practical Nurses,* effective April 2020. Chicago: NCSBN.

Health Promotion and Maintenance

Assisting with providing health promotion programs

Ensuring that the client receives recommended immunizations

Implementing health screening measures

Monitoring for expected body image changes

Performing physical data collection techniques related to the immune system

Preventing disease related to infection

Respecting client lifestyle choices

Psychosocial Integrity

Assisting in mobilizing appropriate support and resource systems

Assisting the client and family to cope

Assisting the client to cope, adapt, and solve problems during illness or stressful events

Considering religious, spiritual, and cultural preferences

Discussing grief and loss related to death and the dying process

Promoting a positive environment to maintain optimal quality of life

Physiological Integrity

Managing medical emergencies

Managing pain

Monitoring for the expected and unexpected responses to treatments

Promoting nutrition

Protecting the client from infection

Providing basic care and comfort

Reviewing diagnostic test and laboratory test results

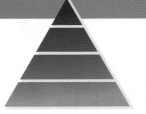

CHAPTER **59**

Immune Problems

PRIORITY CONCEPTS Immunity; Infection

WHAT WOULD YOU DO?

The nurse notes that a client with scleroderma (systemic sclerosis) is having difficulty swallowing. What would the nurse do?
Answer is located on p. 839.

I. Functions of the Immune System (Fig. 59.1)

A. Provides protection against invasion from microorganisms from outside the body

B. Protects the body from internal threats and maintains the internal environment by removing dead or damaged cells

II. Immune Response

A. T lymphocytes and B lymphocytes

  1. Lymphocytes are produced in the bone marrow and migrate to lymphoid tissue, where they remain dormant until they need to form sensitized lymphocytes for cellular immunity or antibodies for humoral immunity.

  2. Some B lymphocytes lie dormant until a specific antigen enters the body, at which time they greatly increase in number and are available for defense.

  3. Types of T lymphocytes include helper/inducer, suppressor, and cytotoxic/cytolytic.

  4. T- and B- lymphocytes are necessary for a normal immune response.

B. Humoral response

  1. Humoral response is immediate.

  2. This type of response provides protection against acute, rapidly developing bacterial and viral infections.

C. Cellular response

  1. Cellular response is delayed and is called *delayed hypersensitivity.*

  2. This type of response is active against slowly developing bacterial infections and is involved in the autoimmune response, some allergic reactions, and the rejection of foreign cells.

III. Immunity

A. Innate immunity

  1. Innate immunity is also called *native* or *natural immunity.*

  2. Is present at birth and includes biochemical, physical, and mechanical barriers of defense, in addition to the inflammatory response

B. Acquired immunity

  1. Acquired or adaptive immunity is received passively from the mother's antibodies, animal serum, or antibodies produced in response to an infection.

  2. Immunization produces active acquired immunity.

IV. Immunizations: Refer to Chapter 37 for information about immunizations.

V. Laboratory Studies

A. Antinuclear antibody (ANA) determination

  1. The ANA determination refers to a blood test used in the differential diagnosis of rheumatic diseases and for the detection of antinucleoprotein factors and patterns associated with certain autoimmune diseases.

  2. The test is negative at 1:40 dilution, depending on the laboratory.

  3. A positive result does not necessarily confirm a disease.

  4. The ANA titer is positive in most individuals diagnosed with systemic lupus erythematosus (SLE); it may also be positive in individuals with systemic sclerosis (scleroderma) or rheumatoid arthritis.

B. Anti-dsDNA antibody test

  1. The anti-dsDNA (double-stranded DNA) antibody test is a blood test done specifically to identify or differentiate DNA antibodies found in SLE.

831

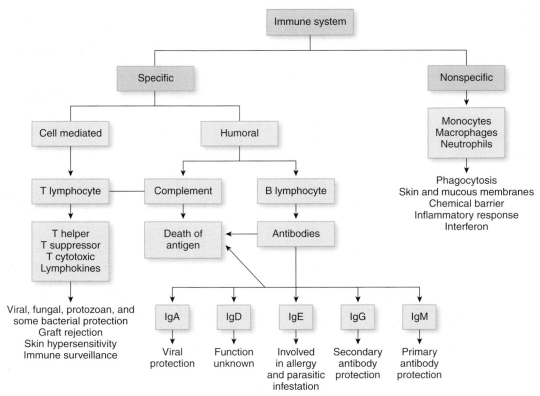

FIGURE 59.1 Components of the immune system. *Ig*, Immunoglobulin.

2. The test supports a diagnosis, monitors disease activity and response to therapy, and establishes a prognosis for SLE.

3. Values: negative, lower than 70 IU/mL by enzyme-linked immunosorbent assay (ELISA)

C. Human immunodeficiency virus (HIV) testing
1. CD4+ T-cell count
   a. Monitors the progression of HIV
   b. As the disease progresses, usually the number of CD4+ T cells decreases, with a resultant decrease in immunity.
   c. The normal CD4+ T-cell count is between 500 cells/L and 1600 cells/L.
   d. In general, the immune system remains healthy with CD4+ T-cell counts higher than 500 cells/L.
   e. Immune system problems occur when the CD4+ T-cell count is between 200 cells/L and 499 cells/L.
   f. Severe immune system problems occur when the CD4+ T-cell count is lower than 200 cells/L.
2. CD4-to-CD8 ratio
   a. Monitors progression of HIV
   b. Normal ratio is approximately 2:1.
3. Viral culture involves placing the infected client's blood cells in a culture medium and measuring the amount of reverse transcriptase activity over a specified period of time.

4. Viral load testing measures the presence of HIV viral genetic material (RNA) or another viral protein in the client's blood.

5. The p24 antigen assay quantifies the amount of HIV viral core protein in the client's serum.

6. Oral testing for HIV
   a. Uses a device that is placed against the gum and cheek for 2 minutes
   b. Fluid (not saliva) is drawn into an absorbable pad, which, in an HIV-positive individual, contains antibodies.
   c. The pad is placed in a solution and a specified observable change is noted if the test result is positive.
   d. If the result is positive, a blood test is needed to confirm the results.

7. Home test kits for HIV: These kits are available and the individual needs to follow the specific instructions (a drop of blood is placed on a test card with a special code number). Results are received by calling a telephone number and entering a special code number.

8. Nursing considerations
   a. Maintain issues of confidentiality surrounding HIV and acquired immunodeficiency syndrome (AIDS) testing.
   b. Follow prescribed state regulations and protocols related to reporting positive test results.

D. Skin testing

1. Description
   a. The administration of an allergen to the surface of the skin or into the dermis
   b. Administered by patch, scratch, or intradermal techniques
2. Preprocedure interventions
    a. Discontinue systemic corticosteroids or antihistamine therapy 5 days before the test, as prescribed.
   b. Ensure informed consent has been obtained.
3. Postprocedure interventions
   a. Record the site, date, and time of the test.
   b. Record the date and the time for follow-up site reading.
   c. Have client remain in waiting room or office for at least 30 minutes after the injection to monitor for adverse effects.
   d. Inspect the site for erythema, papules, vesicles, edema, and wheal.
   e. Measure flare along with the wheal, and document size and other findings; a wheal of 0.5 cm in diameter or greater is considered positive.
   f. Provide the client with a list of potential allergens, if identified.

 Have resuscitation equipment available if skin testing is performed because the allergen may induce an anaphylactic reaction.

 VI. Hypersensitivity and Allergy

A. Description
1. An allergy is an abnormal, individual response to certain substances that normally do not trigger such an exaggerated reaction.
2. With some types of allergies, a reaction occurs on a second and subsequent contact with the allergen.
3. Skin testing may be done to determine the allergen.

B. Data collection
1. History of exposure to allergen(s)
2. Itching, tearing, and burning of the eyes and skin
3. Rash(es)
4. Nose twitching and nasal stuffiness

C. Interventions
1. Identification of the specific allergen
2. Management of the symptoms with antihistamines, anti-inflammatory agents, or corticosteroids
3. Ointments, creams, wet compresses, and soothing baths for local reactions
4. Desensitization programs may be recommended.

 VII. Anaphylaxis

A. Description
1. Anaphylaxis is a serious and immediate hypersensitivity reaction with the release of histamine from the damaged cells.

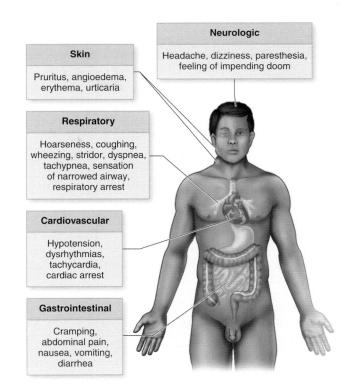

FIGURE 59.2 Clinical manifestations of a systemic anaphylactic reaction.

2. Anaphylaxis can be systemic or cutaneous (localized).

B. Data collection (Fig. 59.2)

⚡ PRIORITY NURSING ACTIONS

Anaphylaxis Reaction

1. Quickly check respiratory status and maintain a patent airway.
2. Call the registered nurse (RN), who will contact the primary health care provider (PHCP) or rapid response team.
3. Administer oxygen.
4. Assist the RN with preparing to start an intravenous (IV) line and infuse normal saline.
5. Prepare the administration of diphenhydramine and epinephrine.
6. Document the event, actions taken, and the client's response.

C. Interventions (see **Priority Nursing Actions**)

VIII. Latex Allergy

A. Description
1. Latex allergy is a hypersensitivity to latex.
2. The source of the allergic reaction is thought to be the proteins in the natural rubber latex or the various chemicals used in the manufacturing process of latex gloves.

BOX 59.1 Products That May Contain Natural Rubber Latex

Ace bandages (brown)
Adhesive or elastic bandages
Ambu bag
Balloons
Blood pressure cuff (tubing and bladder)
Catheter leg bag straps
Catheters
Condoms
Diaphragms
Elastic pressure stockings
Electrocardiogram pads
Feminine hygiene pads
Gloves
Intravenous catheters, tubing, and rubber injection ports
Nasogastric tubes
Pads for crutches
Prepackaged enema kits
Rubber stoppers on medication vials
Stethoscopes
Syringes

Note: Health care agencies use as many nonlatex products as possible and have nonlatex supplies available for clients with a latex allergy.

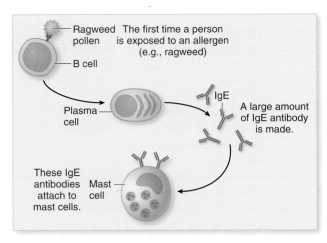

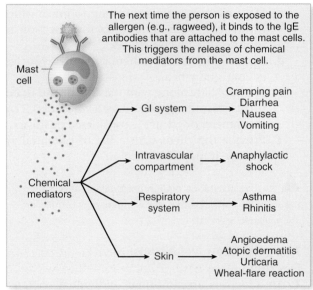

FIGURE 59.3 Steps in a type I allergic reaction.

3. Symptoms of the allergy can range from mild contact dermatitis to moderately severe symptoms of rhinitis, conjunctivitis, urticaria, and bronchospasm to severe life-threatening anaphylaxis.

B. Common routes of exposure (Box 59.1)
  1. Cutaneous: Natural latex gloves and latex balloons
  2. Percutaneous and parenteral: IV lines and catheters; hemodialysis equipment
  3. Mucosal: Use of latex condoms, catheters, airways, and nipples
  4. Aerosol: Aerosolization of powder from latex gloves can occur when gloves are dispensed from the box or when gloves are removed from the hands.

C. At-risk individuals
  1. Health care workers
  2. Individuals who work in the rubber industry
  3. Individuals having multiple surgeries
  4. Individuals with spina bifida
  5. Individuals who wear gloves frequently such as food handlers, hairdressers, and auto mechanics
  6. Individuals allergic to kiwis, bananas, pineapples, tropical fruits, grapes, avocados, potatoes, hazelnuts, and water chestnuts

D. Data collection
  1. Anaphylaxis or type I hypersensitivity is a response to natural rubber latex (Fig. 59.3).
  2. A delayed type IV hypersensitivity reaction can occur within 6 to 48 hours following exposure;

symptoms of contact dermatitis include pruritus, edema, erythema, vesicles, papules, and crusting and thickening of the skin.

E. Interventions (Box 59.2)

IX. Immunodeficiency

A. Description
  1. Immunodeficiency is the absence or inadequate production of immune bodies.
  2. The disorder can be congenital (primary) or acquired (secondary).
  3. Treatment depends on the inadequacy of immune bodies and its primary cause.

B. Data collection
  1. Factors that decrease immune function
  2. Frequent infection
  3. Nutritional status
  4. Medication history, such as use of corticosteroids for long periods
  5. History of alcohol or drug abuse

C. Interventions

1. Protect the client from infection.
2. Promote a balanced diet with adequate nutrition.
3. Use strict aseptic technique for all procedures.
4. Provide psychosocial care regarding lifestyle changes and role changes.
5. Reinforce instructions to the client regarding measures to prevent infection and to wear a MedicAlert bracelet.

 The priority concern for a client with immunodeficiency is infection.

 X. Autoimmune Disease

A. Description: The body is unable to recognize its own cells as a part of itself. Autoimmune disease can affect collagenous tissue.

B. Systemic lupus erythematosus (SLE)

1. Description
   a. A chronic progressive systemic inflammatory disease that can cause major organs and systems to fail
   b. Connective tissue and fibrin deposits collect in the blood vessels on collagen fibers and organs.
   c. The deposits lead to necrosis and inflammation of the blood vessels, lymph nodes, the gastrointestinal tract, and pleura.
   d. No cure for the disease is known, but remission is frequently experienced by clients who manage their care well.

2. Causes
   a. The cause of SLE is unknown, but it is thought to result from a defect in the immunological mechanisms and to have a genetic origin.
   b. Precipitating factors include medications, stress, genetic factors, sunlight or ultraviolet light, and pregnancy.
   c. Discoid lupus erythematosus is possible with some medications but totally disappears after the medication is stopped; the only manifestation is the skin rash that occurs in lupus.

3. Data collection
   a. Identify precipitating factors.
   b. Erythema of the face (malar rash; also called a butterfly rash)
   c. Dry, scaly, raised rash on the face or upper body
   d. Fever
   e. Weakness, malaise, and fatigue
   f. Anorexia
   g. Weight loss
   h. Photosensitivity
   i. Joint pain
   j. Erythema of the palms
   k. Anemia
   l. Positive antinuclear antibody (ANA) test and lupus erythematosus (LE) preparation
   m. Elevated sedimentation rate (ESR) and C-reactive protein

4. Interventions
   a. Monitor skin integrity and provide frequent oral care.
   b. Instruct the client to clean the skin with a mild soap, avoiding harsh and perfumed substances.
   c. Assist with the use of ointments and creams for the rash as prescribed.
   d. Identify factors contributing to fatigue.
   e. Administer iron, folic acid, or vitamin supplements as prescribed, if anemia occurs.
   f. Provide a high-vitamin and high-iron diet.
   g. Provide a high-protein diet if there is no evidence of kidney disease.
   h. Reinforce instructions regarding measures to conserve energy, such as pacing activities and balancing rest with exercise.
   i. Administer topical or systemic corticosteroids, salicylates, and nonsteroidal anti-inflammatory drugs, as prescribed, for pain and inflammation.
   j. Monitor intake and output, and the client's daily weight for signs of fluid overload if corticosteroids are used.
   k. Reinforce instructions to the client to avoid exposure to sunlight and ultraviolet light.
   l. Monitor for proteinuria and red blood cell casts in the urine.
   m. Monitor for bruising, bleeding, and injury.
   n. Assist with plasmapheresis, as prescribed, to remove autoantibodies and immune complexes from the blood before organ damage occurs.
   o. Monitor for signs of organ involvement such as pleuritis, nephritis, pericarditis, coronary artery disease, hypertension, neuritis, anemia, and peritonitis.
   p. Note that lupus nephritis occurs early in the disease process.
   q. Provide supportive therapy as major organs become affected.

   r. Provide emotional support and encourage the client to verbalize feelings.

   s. Provide information regarding support groups and encourage the use of community resources.

 For the client with SLE, monitor the blood urea nitrogen and creatinine level frequently for signs of renal impairment.

C. Scleroderma (systemic sclerosis)

  1. Description

    a. Scleroderma is a chronic connective tissue disease similar to SLE that is characterized by inflammation, fibrosis, and sclerosis.

    b. This disorder affects the connective tissue throughout the body.

    c. It causes fibrotic changes involving the skin, synovial membranes, esophagus, heart, lungs, kidneys, and gastrointestinal tract.

    d. Treatment is directed toward forcing the disease into remission and slowing its progress.

  2. Data collection

    a. Pain

    b. Stiffness and muscle weakness

    c. Pitting edema of the hands and fingers that progresses to the rest of the body

    d. Skin tissue is tight, shiny, hard, and thick, and it loses its elasticity and adheres to underlying structures.

    e. Dysphagia

    f. Decreased range of motion

    g. Joint contractures

    h. Inability to perform activities of daily living

  3. Interventions

    a. Encourage activity as tolerated.

    b. Maintain a constant room temperature.

    c. Provide small, frequent meals, while eliminating foods that stimulate gastric secretions, such as spicy foods, caffeine, and alcohol.

    d. Monitor for esophageal involvement; if present, advise the client to sit up for 1 to 2 hours after meals.

    e. Provide supportive therapy as the major organs become affected.

    f. Administer corticosteroids as prescribed for inflammation.

    g. Provide emotional support and encourage the use of resources as necessary.

D. Polyarteritis nodosa

  1. Description

    a. Polyarteritis nodosa is a collagen disease and a form of systemic vasculitis that causes inflammation of the arteries in visceral organs, brain, and skin.

    b. Treatment is similar to the treatment for SLE.

    c. Polyarteritis nodosa affects middle-aged men.

    d. The cause is unknown and prognosis is poor.

    e. Renal disorders and cardiac involvement are the most frequent causes of death.

  2. Data collection

    a. Malaise, weakness, low-grade fever

    b. Severe abdominal pain

    c. Bloody diarrhea

    d. Weight loss

    e. Elevated sedimentation rate

  3. Interventions: Refer to interventions for SLE.

E. Pemphigus

  1. Description

    a. Pemphigus is a rare autoimmune disease that occurs predominantly between middle and old age.

    b. The cause is unknown and the disorder is potentially fatal.

    c. Treatment is aimed at suppressing the immune response that causes blister formation.

  2. Data collection

    a. Fragile, partial-thickness lesions bleed, weep, and form crusts when bullae are disrupted.

    b. Debilitation, malaise, pain, and dysphagia

    c. Nikolsky's sign: Separation of the epidermis caused by rubbing the skin

    d. Leukocytosis, eosinophilia, foul-smelling discharge from skin

  3. Interventions

    a. Provide supportive care.

    b. Provide oral hygiene and increase fluid intake, unless contraindicated.

    c. Soothe oral lesions as prescribed, and assist with soothing baths as prescribed for relief of symptoms.

    d. Topical or systemic antibiotics may be prescribed for secondary infections.

    e. Corticosteroids and cytotoxic agents may be prescribed to bring about remission.

XI. Goodpasture's Syndrome

A. Description

  1. Goodpasture's syndrome is an autoimmune disorder; autoantibodies are made against the glomerular basement membrane and alveolar basement membrane.

  2. Most common in males and young adults who smoke, and the exact cause is unknown

  3. The lungs and the kidneys are affected primarily, and the disorder is usually not diagnosed until significant pulmonary or renal involvement occurs.

B. Data collection

  1. Clinical manifestations indicating pulmonary and renal involvement

  2. Shortness of breath

  3. Hemoptysis

  4. Decreased urine output

  5. Edema and weight gain

  6. Hypertension and tachycardia

C. Interventions
1. Focus on suppressing the autoimmune response with medications such as corticosteroids and on plasmapheresis (filtration of the plasma to remove some proteins) to remove the autoantibodies.
2. Provide supportive therapy for pulmonary and renal involvement.

 XII. Lyme Disease
A. Description
1. Lyme disease is an infection caused by the spirochete *Borrelia burgdorferi*, acquired from a tick bite (ticks live in wooded areas and survive by attaching to a host).
2. Infection with the spirochete stimulates inflammatory cytokines and autoimmune mechanisms.
 B. Data collection (Box 59.3)
1. The typical ring-shaped rash of Lyme disease does not occur in all clients. Many clients never develop a rash.
2. If a rash does occur, it can occur anywhere on the body, not only at the site of the bite.
 C. Interventions
1. Gently remove the tick with tweezers, wash skin with antiseptic, and dispose of the tick by flushing it down the toilet; the tick may also be disposed of by placing it in a sealed jar so that the PHCP can inspect it and determine its type.
2. Obtain a blood test 4 to 6 weeks after a bite to detect the presence of the disease (testing before this time is not reliable).
3. Reinforce instructions to the client regarding the administration of antibiotics; these are initiated immediately (even before the blood testing results are known).

BOX 59.3 Data Collection and Stages of Lyme Disease

First Stage
Symptoms can occur several days to months following the bite.
A small red pimple develops that spreads into a ring-shaped rash.
Rash may be large or small or may not occur at all.
Flu-like symptoms occur, such as headache, stiff neck, muscle aches, and fatigue.

Second Stage
This stage occurs several weeks following the bite.
Joint pain occurs.
Neurological complications occur.
Cardiac complications occur.

Third Stage
Large joints become involved.
Arthritis progresses.

---

4. Instruct the client to avoid areas that contain ticks, such as wooded grassy areas, especially in the summer months.
5. Instruct the client to wear long-sleeved tops, long pants, closed shoes, and hats while outside.
6. Instruct the client to spray the body with tick repellent containing DEET before going outside.
7. Instruct the client to examine the body when returning inside for the presence of ticks.

XIII. Immunodeficiency Syndrome
A. Acquired immunodeficiency syndrome (AIDS)
1. AIDS is a viral disease caused by HIV that destroys T-cells, thereby increasing susceptibility to infection and malignancy (Fig. 59.4).

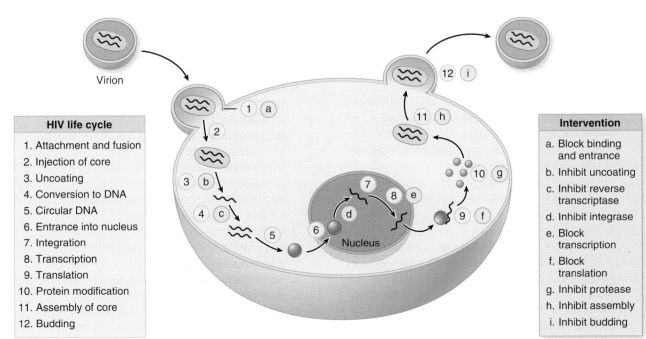

HIV life cycle	Intervention
1. Attachment and fusion	a. Block binding and entrance
2. Injection of core	b. Inhibit uncoating
3. Uncoating	c. Inhibit reverse transcriptase
4. Conversion to DNA	d. Inhibit integrase
5. Circular DNA	e. Block transcription
6. Entrance into nucleus	f. Block translation
7. Integration	g. Inhibit protease
8. Transcription	h. Inhibit assembly
9. Translation	i. Inhibit budding
10. Protein modification	
11. Assembly of core	
12. Budding	

FIGURE 59.4 The life cycle of human immunodeficiency virus (HIV).

2. The syndrome is manifested clinically by opportunistic infection and unusual neoplasms.
3. AIDS is considered a chronic illness.
4. The disease has a long incubation period, sometimes up to 10 years or longer.
5. Manifestations may not appear until late in the infection.

B. Diagnosis and monitoring the client with AIDS: Refer to Box 59.4 for tests used to evaluate the progression of HIV infection.

C. High-risk groups
1. Heterosexual or homosexual contact with high-risk individuals
2. IV drug abusers, especially in those who share needles
3. Persons receiving blood products
4. Health care workers
5. Babies born to infected mothers

D. Data collection
1. Malaise, fever, anorexia, weight loss, influenza-like symptoms
2. Lymphadenopathy of at least 3 months
3. Leukopenia
4. Diarrhea
5. Fatigue
6. Night sweats
7. Presence of opportunistic infections
8. Protozoal infections (*Pneumocystis jiroveci* pneumonia, a major source of mortality)
9. Neoplasms (Kaposi's sarcoma, purplish/red lesions of internal organs and skin), B-cell non-Hodgkin's lymphoma, cervical cancer)
10. Fungal infections (candidiasis, histoplasmosis)
11. Viral infections (cytomegalovirus, herpes simplex)
12. Bacterial infections

E. Interventions
1. Provide respiratory support.
2. Administer oxygen and respiratory treatments as prescribed.
3. Provide psychosocial support as needed.
4. Maintain fluid and electrolyte balance.
5. Monitor for signs of infection and implement protective isolation precautions as needed.
6. Prevent the spread of infection.
7. Initiate standard and other precautions as necessary.
8. Provide comfort as necessary.
9. Provide meticulous skin care.
10. Provide adequate nutritional support as prescribed.

XIV. Kaposi's sarcoma

A. Description: Skin lesions that occur primarily in individuals with a compromised immune system
B. Data collection
1. Kaposi's sarcoma is a slow-growing tumor that appears as a raised, oblong, purplish/reddish-brown lesion; may be tender or nontender.

BOX 59.4 Tests Used to Evaluate Progression of Human Immunodeficiency Virus Infection

Complete Blood Cell Count
White blood cell (WBC) count normal to decreased
Lymphopenia (<30% of the normal number of WBCs)
Thrombocytopenia (decreased platelet count)

Lymphocyte Screen
Reduced CD4+/CD8+ T-cell ratio
CD4+ (helper) lymphocytes decreased
CD8+ lymphocytes increased

Quantitative Immunoglobulin
Immunoglobulin G (IgG) increased
IgA frequently increased

Chemistry Panel
Lactate dehydrogenase increased (all fractions)
Serum albumin decreased
Total protein increased
Cholesterol decreased
AST and ALT elevated

Anergy Panel
Nonreactive (anergic) or poorly reactive to infectious agents or environmental materials (e.g., pokeweed, phytohemagglutinin mitogens and antigens, mumps, *Candida*)

Hepatitis B Surface Antigen
To detect the presence of hepatitis B

Blood Cultures
To detect septicemia

Chest Radiograph
To detect *Pneumocystis jiroveci* infection or tuberculosis

From Copstead L, Banasik J: *Pathophysiology*, ed 5, St. Louis, 2014, Saunders. *ALT*, Alanine aminotransferase; *AST*, aspartate aminotransferase; *WBC*, white blood cell.

---

2. Organ involvement includes the lymph nodes, airways, lungs, or any part of the gastrointestinal tract from the mouth to anus.
3. Interventions
   a. Maintain standard and other precautions as necessary.
   b. Provide protective isolation if the immune system is depressed.
   c. Prepare the client for radiation therapy or chemotherapy, as prescribed.
   d. Immunotherapy may be prescribed to stabilize the immune system.

XV. Posttransplantation Immunodeficiency

A. Description
1. Secondary immunodeficiency is immunosuppression caused by therapeutic agents.
2. The client needs to take immunosuppression agents for the rest of his or her life posttransplantation

to decrease rejection of the transplanted organ or tissue.

B. Diagnosis and monitoring of posttransplantation clients
  1. Check renal and hepatic function.
  2. Monitor the complete cell count with differential to monitor for signs of infection.
  3. Check all body secretions periodically for blood.

C. High-risk clients
  1. Clients with a history of malignancy or premalignancy have an increased susceptibility to malignancy if immunosuppressed.
  2. Clients with recent infection or exposure to tuberculosis, herpes zoster, or chickenpox have a high risk for severe generalized disease when taking immunosuppressive agents.

D. Data collection
  1. Monitor for signs of opportunistic infections.
  2. Monitor nutritional status.
  3. Monitor for signs of rejection (signs will depend on the organ or tissue transplant).

E. Interventions
  1. Strict aseptic technique is necessary.
  2. Reinforce teaching regarding asepsis and the signs of infection and rejection.
  3. Institute protective isolation precautions necessary.
  4. Provide psychosocial support as needed.
  5. Reinforce client teaching about immunosuppressants.

WHAT WOULD YOU DO?

Answer: Major organ damage can occur with diffuse scleroderma, with esophageal involvement being one complication. The nurse would continuously monitor the client's ability to swallow. If esophageal involvement is suspected, the nurse would collaborate with the RN and PHCP about scheduling a swallowing study. The nurse would also assist with collaboration with the nutritionist about dietary changes, such as the need for small, frequent meals and minimizing the intake of foods and liquids that stimulate gastric secretion (spicy foods, caffeine, alcohol). The client needs to also sit up for 1 to 2 hours after meals.

PRACTICE QUESTIONS

1. Which individual is least at risk for the development of Kaposi's sarcoma?
  1. A kidney transplant client
  2. A male with a history of same-sex partners
  3. A client receiving antineoplastic medications

  4. An individual working in an environment where exposure to asbestos exists

2. The nurse prepares to give a bath and change the bed linens for a client with cutaneous Kaposi's sarcoma lesions. The lesions are open and draining a scant amount of serous fluid. Which would the nurse incorporate in the plan during the bathing of this client?
  1. Wearing gloves
  2. Wearing a gown and gloves
  3. Wearing a gown, gloves, and a mask
  4. Wearing a gown and gloves to change the bed linens and gloves only for the bath

3. The client is suspected of having systemic lupus erythematous (SLE). The nurse monitors the client, knowing that which is one of the **initial** characteristic signs of SLE?
  1. Weight gain
  2. Subnormal temperature
  3. Elevated red blood cell count
  4. Rash on the face across the nose and on the cheeks

4. The client diagnosed with pemphigus is being seen in the clinic regularly. The nurse would plan care based on which description of this condition?
  1. The presence of tiny red vesicles
  2. An autoimmune disease that causes blistering in the epidermis
  3. The presence of skin vesicles found along the nerve caused by a virus
  4. The presence of red, raised papules and large plaques covered by silvery scales

❖ **5.** Which interventions would be implemented in the care of a client at high risk for an allergic response to a latex allergy? **Select all that apply.**
  ❑ **1.** Use nonlatex gloves.
  ❑ **2.** Use medications from glass ampules.
  ❑ **3.** Place the client in a private room only.
  ❑ **4.** Do not puncture rubber stoppers with needles.
  ❑ **5.** Keep a latex-safe supply cart available in the client's area.
  ❑ **6.** Use a blood pressure cuff from an electronic device only to measure the blood pressure.

6. The nurse is assisting with planning the care of a client with a diagnosis of immunodeficiency. The nurse would incorporate which intervention as a **priority** in the plan of care?
  1. Protecting the client from infection
  2. Providing emotional support to decrease fear
  3. Encouraging discussion about lifestyle changes
  4. Identifying factors that decreased the immune function

7. The client calls the office of the primary health care provider (PHCP) and states to the nurse that he was just stung by a bumblebee while gardening. The client is afraid of a severe reaction because their neighbor experienced such a reaction just one week ago. Which would be the appropriate nursing action?
   1. Advise the client to soak the site in hydrogen peroxide.
   2. Ask the client if they ever sustained a bee sting in the past.
   3. Tell the client to call an ambulance for transport to the emergency room.
   4. Tell the client not to worry about the sting unless difficulty with breathing occurs.

8. The nurse is assisting with the administration of immunizations at a health care clinic. The nurse would understand that immunization provides which protection?
   1. Protection from all diseases
   2. Innate immunity from disease
   3. Natural immunity from disease
   4. Acquired immunity from disease

9. The nurse is assigned to care for a client diagnosed with systemic lupus erythematosus (SLE). The nurse would plan care considering which factor regarding this diagnosis?
   1. A local rash occurs as a result of allergy.
   2. It is a disease caused by overexposure to sunlight.
   3. A continuous release of histamine in the body causes the disease.
   4. It is an inflammatory disease of collagen contained in connective tissue.

10. The camp nurse prepares to instruct a group of children about Lyme disease. Which information would the nurse include in the instructions?
    1. Lyme disease is caused by a tick carried by deer.
    2. Lyme disease is caused by contamination from cat feces.
    3. Lyme disease can be contagious by skin contact with an infected individual.
    4. Lyme disease can be caused by the inhalation of spores from bird droppings.

11. The client is diagnosed with stage I of Lyme disease. The nurse would check the client for which characteristic of this stage?
    1. Arthralgia
    2. Flu-like symptoms
    3. Enlarged and inflamed joints
    4. Signs of a neurological disorder

12. The client arrives at the health care clinic and states to the nurse that they were just bitten by a tick and would like to be tested for Lyme disease. The client tells the nurse that they removed the tick and flushed it down the toilet. Which nursing action is appropriate?
    1. Refer the client for a blood test immediately.
    2. Inform the client that there is not a test available for Lyme disease.
    3. Tell the client that testing is not necessary unless arthralgia develops.
    4. Instruct the client to return in 4 to 6 weeks to be tested, because testing before this time is not reliable.

13. The nurse, a Cub Scout leader, is preparing a group of Cub Scouts for an overnight camping trip and instructs them about the methods to prevent Lyme disease. Which statement by one of the Cub Scouts indicates a **need for further teaching**?
    1. "I need to bring a hat to wear during the trip."
    2. "I will wear long-sleeved tops and long pants."
    3. "I will not use insect repellent because it will attract the ticks."
    4. "I need to wear closed shoes and socks that can be pulled up over my pants."

14. The client with acquired immunodeficiency syndrome (AIDS) is diagnosed with cutaneous Kaposi's sarcoma. Based on this diagnosis, the nurse would determine that this has been confirmed by which finding?
    1. Swelling in the genital area
    2. Swelling in the lower extremities
    3. Punch biopsy of the cutaneous lesions
    4. Appearance of reddish-blue lesions on the skin

15. The client brought to the emergency department is experiencing an anaphylactic reaction from eating shellfish. The nurse needs to implement which **immediate** action?
    1. Administering epinephrine
    2. Maintaining a patent airway
    3. Administering a corticosteroid
    4. Instructing the client on the importance of obtaining a MedicAlert bracelet

ANSWERS

1. 4

Rationale: Kaposi's sarcoma is a vascular malignancy that presents as a skin disorder and is a common acquired immunodeficiency syndrome indicator. It is seen frequently in men with a history of same-sex partners. Although the cause of Kaposi's sarcoma is not known, it is considered to be the result of an alteration or failure in the immune system. The renal transplant client and the client receiving antineoplastic medications are at risk for immunosuppression. Exposure to asbestos is not related to the development of Kaposi's sarcoma.

Test-Taking Strategy: Note the subject, the client least at risk for Kaposi's sarcoma. Option 2 can be eliminated easily. Note that options 1 and 3 are comparable or alike; these clients are at risk for immunosuppression.

2. 2

Rationale: Gowns and gloves are required if the nurse anticipates contact with soiled items, such as wound drainage, or while caring for a client who is incontinent with diarrhea or a client who has an ileostomy or colostomy. Masks are not required unless droplet or airborne precautions are necessary. Regardless of the amount of wound drainage, a gown and gloves needs to be worn.

Test-Taking Strategy: Focus on the subject, preventing disease transmission. Think about the method of transmission of infection when answering a question of this type. Read the question, noting that the tasks presented in this case are bathing and changing bed linens. Eliminate option 3 because the method of transmission is not respiratory. Eliminate options 1 and 4 because neither provides adequate protection based on the method of transmission.

3. 4

Rationale: Skin lesions or a rash on the face across the bridge of the nose and on the cheeks is an initial characteristic sign of systemic lupus erythematous (SLE). Fever and weight loss may also occur. Anemia is most likely to occur later in SLE.

Test-Taking Strategy: Focus on the subject, the characteristics of SLE and note the strategic word, *initial*. Recalling the characteristic butterfly rash associated with SLE will direct you to the correct option.

4. 2

Rationale: Pemphigus is an autoimmune disease that causes blistering in the epidermis. The client has large flaccid blisters (bullae). Because the blisters are in the epidermis, they have a thin covering of skin and break easily, leaving large denuded areas of skin. During the initial examination, clients may have crusting areas instead of intact blisters. Option 1 describes eczema, option 3 describes herpes zoster, and option 4 describes psoriasis.

Test-Taking Strategy: Focus on the subject, signs/symptoms of pemphigus. Recalling that pemphigus vulgaris is an autoimmune disorder will direct you to the correct option.

❖ **5. 1, 2, 4, 5**

Rationale: If a client is allergic to latex and is at high risk for an allergic response, the nurse would use nonlatex gloves and latex-safe supplies and would keep a latex-safe supply cart available in the client's area. Any supplies or materials that contain latex would be avoided. These include blood pressure cuffs and medication bottles with rubber stoppers that require puncture with a needle. It is not necessary to place the client in a private room.

Test-Taking Strategy: Focus on the subject, the client at high risk for an allergic response to a latex allergy. Recalling that items that contain rubber are likely to contain latex will direct you to the correct interventions. Also noting the closed-ended word, *only*, in options 3 and 6 will assist in eliminating these options.

6. 1

Rationale: The client with immunodeficiency has inadequate or absent immune bodies and is at risk for infection. The priority nursing intervention would be to protect the client from infection. Options 2, 3, and 4 may be components of care but are not the priority.

Test-Taking Strategy: Use Maslow's hierarchy of needs theory and focus on the strategic word, *priority*. Remember that physiological needs are the priority. This will direct you to the correct option.

7. 2

Rationale: In some types of allergies, a reaction occurs only on second and subsequent contacts with the allergen. Therefore, the appropriate action would be to ask the client if he ever received a bee sting in the past. Option 1 is not appropriate advice. Option 3 is unnecessary. The client would not be told "not to worry."

Test-Taking Strategy: Use the steps of the nursing process. Option 2 is the only option that addresses data collection.

8. 4

Rationale: Acquired immunity can occur by receiving an immunization that causes antibodies to a specific pathogen to form. Natural (innate) immunity is present at birth. No immunization protects the client from all diseases.

Test-Taking Strategy: Eliminate option 1 first because of the closed-ended word, *all*. Next eliminate options 2 and 3 because they are comparable or alike and the same type of immunity.

9. 4

Rationale: SLE is an inflammatory disease of collagen contained in connective tissue. Options 1, 2, and 3 are not associated with this disease.

Test-Taking Strategy: Focus on the subject, the characteristics of SLE. Eliminate option 1 because SLE is a systemic disorder, not a local one. Next, eliminate option 3 because of its similarity to option 1. From the remaining options, select option 4 because of its systemic characteristic.

10. 1

Rationale: Lyme disease is a multisystem infection that results from a bite by a tick carried by several species of deer. Persons bitten by *Ixodes* ticks can be infected with the spirochete *Borrelia burgdorferi*. Lyme disease cannot be transmitted from one person to another. Toxoplasmosis is caused from the ingestion of cysts from contaminated cat feces. Histoplasmosis is caused by the inhalation of spores from bat or bird droppings.

Test-Taking Strategy: Focus on the subject, the characteristics and transmission of Lyme disease. Recalling that this disease is caused by a bite will assist in eliminating the incorrect options.

11. 2

Rationale: The hallmark of stage I is the development of a skin rash within 2 to 30 days of infection, generally at the site of the tick bite. The rash develops into a concentric ring, giving it a bull's-eye appearance. The lesion enlarges up to 50 cm to 60 cm, and smaller lesions develop farther away from the original tick bite. In stage I, most infected persons develop flu-like symptoms that last 7 to 10 days; these symptoms may reoccur later. Arthralgia and joint enlargements are most likely to occur in stage III. Neurological deficits occur in stage II.

Test-Taking Strategy: Eliminate options 1 and 3 first because they are comparable or alike. Next, note that the question asks for the characteristics of stage I. From the remaining two options, select the least serious one because the subject of the question relates to stage I. Expect neurological disorders to occur with progression of the disease.

12. 4

Rationale: A blood test is available to detect Lyme disease; however, the test is not reliable if performed before 4 to 6 weeks following the tick bite. Antibody formation takes place in the following manner: immunoglobulin M is detected 3 to 4 weeks after Lyme disease onset, peaks at 6 to 8 weeks, and then gradually disappears; immunoglobulin G is detected 2 to 3 months after infection and may remain elevated for years. Options 1, 2, and 3 are incorrect.

Test-Taking Strategy: Focus on the subject, the instruction for the client who was bitten by a tick. Eliminate option 1 first. The word *immediately* would indicate that this is potentially an incorrect option. A blood test is available; therefore, eliminate option 2. Eliminate option 3 because treatment would begin before the arthralgia develops.

13. 3

Rationale: In the prevention of Lyme disease, individuals need to be instructed to use an insect repellent on the skin and clothes when in an area where ticks are likely to be found. Long-sleeved tops and long pants, closed shoes, and a hat or cap need to be worn. If possible, one needs to avoid heavily wooded areas or areas with thick underbrush. Socks can be pulled up and over the pant legs to prevent ticks from entering under clothing.

Test-Taking Strategy: The strategic words, *need for further teaching*, indicate a negative event query and ask you to select an option that is an incorrect statement. Note that option 3 uses the words *will not*. Reading carefully will assist with directing you to this option.

14. 3

Rationale: Kaposi's sarcoma lesions begin as red, dark blue, or purple macules on the lower legs that change into plaques. These large plaques ulcerate or open and drain. The lesions spread by metastasis through the upper body and then to the face and oral mucosa. They can move to the lymphatic system, lungs, and gastrointestinal tract. Late disease results in swelling and pain in the lower extremities, penis, scrotum, or face. Diagnosis is made by punch biopsy of cutaneous lesions and biopsy of pulmonary and gastrointestinal lesions.

Test-Taking Strategy: Focus on the subject, diagnosing Kaposi's sarcoma. Eliminate options 1 and 2 first because these symptoms occur late in the development of Kaposi's sarcoma. From the remaining options, note the word *confirmed*. This word will assist with directing you to the option that will confirm the diagnosis: the biopsy of the lesions.

15. 2

Rationale: If the client experiences an anaphylactic reaction, the immediate action would be to maintain a patent airway. The client then would receive epinephrine. Corticosteroids may also be prescribed. The client will need to be instructed about obtaining and wearing a MedicAlert bracelet, but this is not the immediate action.

Test-Taking Strategy: Note the strategic word, *immediate*. Use the ABCs—airway, breathing, and circulation—to answer the question. Airway is always the priority.

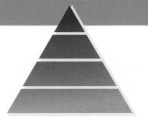

CHAPTER **60**

Immunological Medications

PRIORITY CONCEPTS **Immunity; Safety**

WHAT WOULD YOU DO?

A hospitalized client who is receiving ceftriaxone to treat an infection develops severe diarrhea. What would the nurse do?

Answer is located on p. 846.

I. **Human Immunodeficiency Virus (HIV) and Acquired Immunodeficiency Syndrome (AIDS)**

A. Medications include nucleoside-nucleotide reverse transcriptase inhibitors (NRTIs), nonnucleoside reverse transcriptase inhibitors (NNRTIs), protease inhibitors (PIs), and fusion inhibitors (Box 60.1).

B. NRTIs and NNRTIs work by inhibiting the activity of reverse transcriptase.

C. PIs work by interfering with the activity of the enzyme protease.

D. Fusion inhibitors work by inhibiting the binding of HIV to cells.

E. Standard treatment consists of using three or four medications in regimens known as highly active antiretroviral therapy (HAART); this therapy is not curative but can delay or reverse loss of immune function, preserve health, and prolong life.

F. Other medications include those that are used to treat complications or opportunistic infections that may develop (see Box 60.1).

G. NRTIs

1. Abacavir: Can cause nausea; monitor for hypersensitivity reaction, including fever, nausea, vomiting, diarrhea, lethargy, malaise, sore throat, shortness of breath, cough, and rash.

2. Abacavir/lamivudine: In addition to the effects that can occur from abacavir and lamivudine, hypersensitivity reactions, lactic acidosis, and severe hepatomegaly can occur.

3. Didanosine: Can cause nausea, diarrhea, peripheral neuropathy, hepatotoxicity, and pancreatitis

4. Emtricitabine: Can cause headache, diarrhea, nausea, rash, hyperpigmentation of the palms and soles, lactic acidosis, and severe hepatomegaly

5. Emtricitabine/tenofovir: In addition to the effects that can occur from emtricitabine and tenofovir, lactic acidosis and severe hepatomegaly can occur.

6. Lamivudine: Causes nausea and nasal congestion

7. Lamivudine/zidovudine: Can cause anemia and neutropenia and lactic acidosis with hepatomegaly

8. Lamivudine/zidovudine/abacavir: In addition to the effects that can occur from lamivudine, zidovudine, and abacavir, hypersensitivity reactions, anemia, neutropenia, lactic acidosis, and severe hepatomegaly can occur.

9. Stavudine: Can cause peripheral neuropathy and pancreatitis

10. Tenofovir: Can cause nausea and vomiting

11. Zidovudine: Can cause nausea, vomiting, anemia, leukopenia, myopathy, fatigue, and headache

H. NNRTIs

1. Delavirdine: Can cause rash, liver function changes, and pruritus

2. Efavirenz: Can cause rash, dizziness, confusion, difficulty concentrating, strange dreams, and encephalopathy

3. Etravirine: Can cause rash, gastrointestinal disturbance, headache, hypertension, and peripheral neuropathy

4. Nevirapine: Can cause rash, Stevens-Johnson syndrome, hepatitis, and increased transaminase levels

5. Rilpivirine: Can cause headache, nausea, stomach pain, dizziness, and feeling sleepy during the daytime

I. Protease inhibitors (PIs)

1. Atazanavir: Can cause nausea, headache, infection, vomiting, diarrhea, drowsiness, insomnia, fever, hyperglycemia, hyperlipidemia, and increased bleeding in clients with hemophilia

2. Darunavir: Can cause diarrhea, nausea, vomiting, heartburn, stomach pain, headache, rash, and changes in the shape and location of body fat

---

BOX 60.1 **Medications for Human Immunodeficiency Virus and Acquired Immunodeficiency Syndrome**

Nucleoside-Nucleotide Reverse Transcriptase Inhibitors (NRTIs)
Abacavir
Abacavir/lamivudine
Didanosine
Emtricitabine
Emtricitabine/tenofovir
Lamivudine
Lamivudine/zidovudine
Lamivudine/zidovudine/abacavir
Stavudine
Tenofovir
Zidovudine

Nonnucleoside Reverse Transcriptase Inhibitors (NNRTIs)
Delavirdine
Doravine
Efavirenz
Etravirine
Nevirapine
Rilpivirine

Protease Inhibitors (PIs)
Atazanavir
Darunavir
Fosamprenavir
Indinavir
Lopinavir/ritonavir
Nelfinavir
Ritonavir
Saquinavir
Tipranavir

Integrase Inhibitor
Raltegravir
Dolutegravir
Elvitegravir

Fusion Inhibitor
Enfuvirtide

Chemokine Receptor 5 (CCR5) Antagonist
Maraviroc

Anti-inflammatory Medication
Sulfasalazine

Anti-infective Medications
Atovaquone
Metronidazole
Pentamidine isethionate
Sulfamethoxazole/trimethoprim

Antifungal Medications
Amphotericin B
Fluconazole
Ketoconazole
Itraconazole
Voriconazole

Antiviral Medications
Acyclovir
Foscarnet
Ganciclovir
Valacyclovir

---

3. Fosamprenavir: Can cause nausea, vomiting, headache, altered taste sensations, perioral paresthesia, rashes, and altered liver function
4. Indinavir: Can cause nausea, diarrhea, hyperbilirubinemia, nephritis, and kidney stones
5. Lopinavir/ritonavir combination: Can cause nausea, diarrhea, altered taste sensations, circumoral paresthesia, and hepatitis
6. Nelfinavir: Can cause nausea, flatulence, and diarrhea
7. Ritonavir: Can cause nausea, vomiting, diarrhea, altered taste sensations, circumoral paresthesia, hepatitis, and increased triglyceride levels
8. Saquinavir: Can cause nausea, diarrhea, photosensitivity, and headache
9. Tipranavir: Hepatotoxicity (liver damage); can also cause nausea, vomiting, diarrhea, headache, and fatigue

J. Integrase inhibitors
   1. Stop HIV replication and is used in combination with other antiretroviral medications
   2. Common side/adverse effects include nausea, diarrhea, fatigue, headache, and itching.

K. Fusion inhibitor: Enfuviritide can cause skin irritation at injection site, fatigue, nausea, insomnia, and peripheral neuropathy.
L. Chemokine receptor 5 (CCR5) antagonist: Maraviroc
   1. Binds with CCR5 and blocks viral entry
   2. Most common side/adverse effects are cough, dizziness, pyrexia, rash, abdominal pain, musculoskeletal symptoms, and upper respiratory tract infections; liver injury and cardiovascular events have occurred in some clients.
M. Anti-infective and anti-inflammatory medications: Used to treat opportunistic infections such as *Pneumocystis jiroveci* pneumonia; *Toxoplasma* encephalitis is treated with sulfamethoxazole-trimethoprim (see Box 60.1).
N. Antifungal medications: Used to treat candidiasis, cryptococcal meningitis (see Box 60.1)
O. Antiviral medications: Used to treat cytomegalovirus retinitis, herpes simplex, varicella-zoster virus (see Box 60.1)

⚠ The client with HIV or AIDS is at high risk for the development of opportunistic infections.

BOX 60.2 Immunosuppressants

Calcineurin Inhibitors
Cyclosporine
Tacrolimus

Cytotoxic Medications
Azathioprine
Cyclophosphamide
Methotrexate
Mycophenolate mofetil
Mycophenolic acid

Antibodies
Basiliximab
Lymphocyte immune globulin, antithymocyte globulin
Muromonab-CD3
Rh₀(D) immune globulin

Other
Sirolimus
Everolimus

Glucocorticoids
See Chapter 44.

 II. Immunosuppressants (Box 60.2)

A. Description: Immunosuppressants are used for transplant recipients to prevent organ or tissue rejection and to treat autoimmune disorders such as systemic lupus erythematosus.

B. Cyclosporine
  1. Used for the prevention of rejection following allogeneic organ transplantation
  2. Usually administered with a glucocorticoid and another immunosuppressant
  3. Most common adverse effects are nephrotoxicity, infection, hypertension, and hirsutism.

C. Tacrolimus
  1. Used for prevention of rejection following liver or kidney transplantation
  2. Adverse effects include nephrotoxicity, neurotoxicity, gastrointestinal effects, hypertension, hyperkalemia, hyperglycemia, hirsutism, and gum hyperplasia.

D. Azathioprine
  1. Generally used with renal transplant recipients
  2. Can cause neutropenia and thrombocytopenia

E. Cyclophosphamide
  1. Used for its immunosuppressant action to treat autoimmune disorders
  2. Can cause neutropenia and hemorrhagic cystitis

F. Methotrexate
  1. Used for its immunosuppressant action to treat autoimmune disorders
  2. Can cause hepatic fibrosis and cirrhosis, bone marrow suppression, ulcerative stomatitis, and renal damage

G. Mycophenolate mofetil and mycophenolic acid
  1. Used to prevent rejection following kidney, heart, and liver transplantation
  2. Can cause diarrhea, vomiting, neutropenia, sepsis; increases risk of infection and malignancies, especially lymphomas

H. Basiliximab
  1. Used to prevent rejection following kidney transplantation
  2. Can cause severe acute hypersensitivity reactions including anaphylaxis

I. Lymphocyte immune globulin, antithymocyte globulin
  1. Used to prevent rejection following kidney, heart, liver, and bone marrow transplantation
  2. Side/adverse effects include fever, chills, leukopenia, and skin reactions.
  3. Can cause anaphylactoid reactions

J. Sirolimus
  1. Used to prevent renal transplant rejection
  2. Increases the risk of infection; raises cholesterol and triglyceride levels; can cause renal injury
  3. Can cause anaphylactoid reactions
  4. Other side/adverse effects include rash, acne, anemia, thrombocytopenia, joint pain, diarrhea, and hypokalemia.

 Monitor the client taking an immunosuppressant closely for signs of infection.

III. Immunizations (see Chapter 37)

IV. Antimicrobials (Box 60.3)

A. Inhibit the growth of bacteria

B. Include medication classifications of aminoglycosides, cephalosporins, fluoroquinolones, macrolides, lincosamides, monobactams, penicillins and penicillinase-resistant penicillins, sulfonamides, streptogramins, tetracyclines, antimycobacterials, antifungals (see Box 60.3)

C. Adverse effects (Table 60.1)

D. Nursing considerations
  1. Check for allergies.
  2. Monitor appropriate laboratory values before therapy, as appropriate, and during therapy to assess for adverse effects.
  3. Monitor for adverse effects and report to the primary health care provider (PHCP) if any occur.
  4. The appropriate method of administration is determined and instructions are provided to the client.
  5. Monitor intake and output.
  6. Encourage fluid intake (unless contraindicated).
  7. Initiate safety precautions because of possible central nervous system effects.
  8. Reinforce teaching the client about the medication and how to take it; the importance of completing the full prescribed course is emphasized.

BOX 60.3   Antimicrobials

Aminoglycosides
Amikacin
Gentamicin
Neomycin
Streptomycin
Tobramycin

Antimycobacterials
Antituberculosis agents
(see Chapter 48)
Leprostatics: Clofazimine,
Thalidomide

Antifungal Medications
Amphotericin B
Fluconazole
Ketoconazole
Itraconazole
Posaconazole
Voriconazole

Antiviral Medications
Acyclovir
Famciclovir
Foscarnet
Ganciclovir
Valacyclovir

Cephalosporins
Cefaclor
Cefadroxil
Cefazolin
Cefdinir
Cefditoren
Cefepime
Cefexime
Cefotaxime
Cefotetan
Cefoxitin
Cefpodoxime
Cefprozil
Ceftazidime
Ceftibuten
Ceftriaxone
Cefuroxime
Cephalexin

Fluoroquinolones
Ciprofloxacin
Gemifloxacin

Levofloxacin
Moxifloxacin
Ofloxacin

Lincosamides
Clindamycin
Lincomycin

Macrolides
Azithromycin
Clarithromycin
Erythromycin
Fidaxomicin

Monobactam
Aztreonam

Penicillins
Amoxicillin
Ampicillin
Penicillin G
Penicillin V
Piperacillin

Penicillinase-Resistant Penicillins
Dicloxacillin
Nafcillin
Oxacillin

Sulfonamides
Sulfadiazine
Sulfamethoxazole
Sulfasalazine
Sulfisoxazole
Trimethoprim/sulfamethoxazole

Stretogramins
Pristinamycin
Virginiamycin
Quinupristin/dalfopristin

Tetracyclines
Demeclocycline
Doxycycline
Minocycline
Tetracycline

TABLE 60.1   Antibiotics and their Adverse Effects

Classification	Adverse Effects
Aminoglycosides	Ototoxicity Confusion, disorientation Renal toxicity Gastrointestinal irritation Palpitations, blood pressure changes Hypersensitivity reactions
Cephalosporins	Gastrointestinal disturbances Pseudomembranous colitis Headache, dizziness, lethargy, paresthesia Nephrotoxicity Superinfections
Fluoroquinolones	Headache, dizziness, insomnia, depression Gastrointestinal effects Bone marrow depression Fever, rash, photosensitivity
Macrolides	Gastrointestinal effects Pseudomembranous colitis Confusion Superinfections Hypersensitivity reactions
Lincosamides	Gastrointestinal effects Pseudomembranous colitis Bone marrow depression
Monobactams	Gastrointestinal effects Hepatotoxicity Allergic reactions
Penicillins and penicillinase-resistant penicillins	Gastrointestinal effects, including sore mouth and furry tongue Superinfections Hypersensitivity reactions, including anaphylaxis
Sulfonamides	Gastrointestinal effects Hepatotoxicity Nephrotoxicity Bone marrow depression Dermatological effects, including hypersensitivity and photosensitivity Headache, dizziness, vertigo, ataxia, depression, seizures
Tetracyclines	Gastrointestinal effects Hepatotoxicity Teeth (staining) and bone damage Superinfections Dermatological reactions, including rash and photosensitivity Hypersensitivity reactions
Antimycobacterials, leprostatics	Gastrointestinal effects Neuritis, dizziness, headache, malaise, drowsiness, hallucinations
Antifungals	Gastrointestinal effects Headache, rash, anemia, hepatotoxicity, hearing loss, peripheral neuritis

WHAT WOULD YOU DO?

Answer: Ceftriaxone is a cephalosporin. Some adverse effects include gastrointestinal disturbances, pseudomembranous colitis, and superinfections. If the client develops severe diarrhea, the nurse needs to notify the registered nurse immediately and contact the PHCP immediately because of the potential development of an adverse effect. In some situations, antibiotic-associated gastrointestinal disturbances such as diarrhea may require contact precautions.

PRACTICE QUESTIONS

❖ **1.** The client diagnosed with acquired immunodeficiency syndrome (AIDS) is taking nevirapine. The nurse would monitor for which side/adverse effects of the medication? **Select all that apply.**
   - ❑ **1.** Rash
   - ❑ **2.** Hepatotoxicity
   - ❑ **3.** Hyperglycemia
   - ❑ **4.** Peripheral neuropathy
   - ❑ **5.** Reduced bone mineral density

2. The client diagnosed with acquired immunodeficiency syndrome (AIDS) has begun therapy with zidovudine. The nurse would monitor which laboratory result during treatment with this medication?
   - **1.** Blood culture
   - **2.** Blood glucose level
   - **3.** Blood urea nitrogen
   - **4.** Complete blood count

3. The nurse is reviewing the results of serum laboratory studies drawn on a client diagnosed with acquired immunodeficiency syndrome (AIDS) who is receiving didanosine. The nurse determines that the client may have the medication discontinued by the primary health care provider (PHCP) if which significantly elevated result is noted?
   - **1.** Serum protein
   - **2.** Blood glucose
   - **3.** Serum amylase
   - **4.** Serum creatinine

4. The nurse is caring for a postrenal transplantation client with a prescription for cyclosporine. If the nurse notes an increase in one of the client's vital signs and the client is complaining of a headache, which vital sign is **most likely** increased?
   - **1.** Pulse
   - **2.** Respirations
   - **3.** Blood pressure
   - **4.** Pulse oximetry

5. Amikacin is prescribed for a client with a diagnosed bacterial infection. The nurse instructs the client to contact the primary health care provider (PHCP) **immediately** if which occurs?
   - **1.** Nausea
   - **2.** Lethargy
   - **3.** Hearing loss
   - **4.** Muscle aches

6. The nurse is assigned to care for the client diagnosed with cytomegalovirus retinitis and acquired immunodeficiency syndrome (AIDS) who is receiving foscarnet. The nurse would monitor the results of which laboratory study while the client is taking this medication?
   - **1.** CD4+ cell count
   - **2.** Lymphocyte count
   - **3.** Serum albumin level
   - **4.** Serum creatinine level

7. The client with diagnosed acquired immunodeficiency syndrome (AIDS) and *Pneumocystis jiroveci* infection has been receiving pentamidine. The client develops a temperature of 101°F (38.3°C). The nurse continues to monitor the client, knowing that this sign would **most likely** indicate which condition?
   - **1.** The dose of the medication is too low.
   - **2.** The client is experiencing toxic effects of the medication.
   - **3.** The client has developed inadequacy of thermoregulation.
   - **4.** A result of another infection caused by the leukopenic effects of the medication.

8. Saquinavir is prescribed for the client who is diagnosed with human immunodeficiency virus (HIV) seropositive. The nurse would reinforce medication instructions about which health care measure to the client?
   - **1.** Avoid sun exposure.
   - **2.** Eat low-calorie foods.
   - **3.** Eat foods that are low in fat.
   - **4.** Take the medication on an empty stomach.

❖ **9.** Ketoconazole is prescribed for a client with a diagnosis of candidiasis. Which interventions would the nurse include when administering this medication? **Select all that apply.**
   - ❑ **1.** Restrict fluid intake.
   - ❑ **2.** Monitor liver function studies.
   - ❑ **3.** Instruct the client to avoid alcohol.
   - ❑ **4.** Administer the medication with an antacid.
   - ❑ **5.** Instruct the client to avoid exposure to the sun.
   - ❑ **6.** Administer the medication on an empty stomach.

10. The client who is diagnosed with human immunodeficiency virus (HIV) seropositive has been taking stavudine. The nurse would monitor which parameter closely while the client is taking this medication?
   - **1.** Gait
   - **2.** Appetite
   - **3.** Level of consciousness
   - **4.** Hemoglobin and hematocrit blood levels

ANSWERS

❖ **1. 1, 2**

Rationale: Nevirapine is an nonnucleoside reverse transcriptase inhibitors (NNRTIs), that is used to treat HIV infection. It is used in combination with other antiretroviral medications to treat HIV. Adverse effects include rash, Stevens-Johnson syndrome, hepatitis, and increased transaminase levels. Hyperglycemia, peripheral neuropathy, and reduced bone density are not side/adverse effects of this medication.

Test-Taking Strategy: Focus on the subject, side/adverse effects of nevirapine. Hyperglycemia, peripheral neuropathy, and reduced bone mineral density are not common side/adverse effects of commonly prescribed medications. Remember that rash, Stevens-Johnson syndrome, hepatitis, and increased transaminase levels are side/adverse effects of nevirapine.

2. 4

Rationale: A common side/adverse effect of therapy with zidovudine is leukopenia and anemia. The nurse monitors the complete blood count results for these changes. Options 1, 2, and 3 are unrelated to the use of this medication.

Test-Taking Strategy: Focus on the subject, zidovudine. Recalling that zidovudine causes leukopenia and anemia will direct you to the correct option.

3. 3

Rationale: Didanosine can cause pancreatitis. A serum amylase level that is increased 1.5 to 2 times the normal may signify pancreatitis in the client with AIDS and is potentially fatal. The medication may have to be discontinued. The medication is also hepatotoxic and can result in liver failure.

Test-Taking Strategy: Focus on the subject, adverse effects of didanosine. Recalling that this medication can cause damage to the pancreas and is hepatotoxic will direct you to the correct option.

4. 3

Rationale: Hypertension can occur in a client taking cyclosporine, and because this client is also complaining of a headache, the blood pressure is the vital sign to be monitored most closely. Other adverse effects include infection, nephrotoxicity, and hirsutism. Options 1, 2, and 4 are unrelated to the use of this medication.

Test-Taking Strategy: Note the strategic words, *most likely*. Focus on the subject, cyclosporine, and note the data in the question. Recall that this medication can cause hypertension, which can be manifested by a headache.

5. 3

Rationale: Amikacin is an aminoglycoside. Adverse effects of aminoglycosides include ototoxicity (hearing problems), confusion, disorientation, gastrointestinal irritation, palpitations, blood pressure changes, nephrotoxicity, and hypersensitivity. The nurse instructs the client to report hearing loss to the PHCP immediately. Lethargy and muscle aches are not associated with the use of this medication. It is not necessary to contact the PHCP immediately if nausea occurs. If nausea persists or results in vomiting, the PHCP needs to be notified.

Test-Taking Strategy: Note the strategic word, *immediately*, and focus on the subject, contacting the PHCP for an adverse effect of amikacin. Nausea, lethargy, and muscle aches do not usually require immediate contact of the PHCP. Recalling that this medication is an aminoglycoside (most aminoglycoside medication names end in the letters -*cin*) and that aminoglycosides are ototoxic will direct you to the correct option.

6. 4

Rationale: Foscarnet is toxic to the kidneys. Serum creatinine is monitored before therapy, two to three times per week during induction therapy, and at least weekly during maintenance therapy. Foscarnet may also cause decreased levels of calcium, magnesium, phosphorus, and potassium. Thus these levels are also measured with the same frequency.

Test-Taking Strategy: Focus on the subject, monitoring laboratory results for a client taking foscarnet. CD4+ counts, serum albumin, and lymphocyte counts are not monitored frequently during use of most medications. Recalling that this medication is nephrotoxic will direct you to the correct option.

7. 4

Rationale: Frequent side/adverse effects of this medication include leukopenia, thrombocytopenia, and anemia. The client needs to be monitored routinely for signs/symptoms of infection. Options 1, 2, and 3 are inaccurate interpretations.

Test-Taking Strategy: Note the strategic words, *most likely*. Focus on the subject, the client develops a temperature of 101°F (38.3°C) while taking pentamidine. Note the relationship between these words and the correct option. Also note that low medication dose, toxic effects, and inadequacy of thermoregulation are not common side/adverse effects of commonly used medications.

8. 1

Rationale: Saquinavir is an antiretroviral protease inhibitor (PI) used with other antiretroviral medications to manage HIV infection. Saquinavir is administered with meals and is best absorbed if the client consumes high-calorie, high-fat meals. Saquinavir can cause photosensitivity, and the nurse would instruct the client to avoid sun exposure.

Test-Taking Strategy: Focus on the subject, instructions to the client taking saquinavir. Options 2 and 3 can be eliminated first, knowing that these dietary measures would not likely be prescribed for this client. From the remaining options, you need to know that this medication can cause photosensitivity.

9. 2, 3, 5 ❖

Rationale: Ketoconazole is an antifungal medication. It is administered with food (not on an empty stomach), and antacids are avoided for 2 hours after taking the medication to ensure absorption. The medication is hepatotoxic, and the nurse monitors liver function studies. The client is instructed to avoid exposure to the sun because the medication increases photosensitivity. The client is also instructed to avoid alcohol. There is no reason for the client to restrict fluid intake. In fact, this could be harmful to the client.

Test-Taking Strategy: Focus on the subject, interventions when administering ketoconazole. Use general medication guidelines to assist in selecting the correct interventions. Also remember that this medication is administered with food and that it is hepatotoxic.

10. 1
Rationale: Stavudine is an antiretroviral used to manage HIV infection in clients who do not respond to or who cannot tolerate conventional therapy. The medication can cause peripheral neuropathy, and the nurse would monitor the client's gait closely and ask the client about paresthesia. Options 2, 3, and 4 are unrelated to the use of this medication.

Test-Taking Strategy: Focus on the subject, side/adverse effects of stavudine. Recalling that this medication causes peripheral neuropathy will direct you to the correct option.

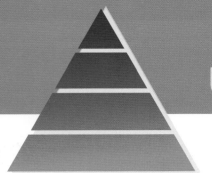

Mental Health Problems of the Adult Client

Pyramid to Success

The Pyramid to Success focuses on the therapeutic nurse–client relationship, client rights, hospital admission procedures, the ethical and legal issues related to the care of a client with a mental health problem, and grief and loss. Pyramid Points also focus on crisis intervention and coping. Care for a client with an addiction, such as an eating disorder, substance abuse disorder, or gambling disorder, is another focus area. Additional areas of focus include anxiety, depression, suicide, abuse and neglect, bullying, violence, rape crisis interventions, posttraumatic stress disorder, moral injury, obsessive-compulsive disorders, schizophrenia, and bipolar disorders. Pyramid Points also address the use of medications prescribed for a client with a mental health problem.

Client Needs: Learning Objectives

Safe and Effective Care Environment
Ensuring client advocacy
Ensuring that informed consent related to treatments, such as restraints (security devices) or seclusion has been obtained
Implementing legal responsibilities related to reporting incidences of abuse, neglect, or violence
Maintaining confidentiality
Providing safety to the client and others
Upholding client rights
Using restraints (security devices) and seclusion appropriately and safely

Health Promotion and Maintenance
Assisting with providing health promotion programs related to addictions
Identifying community resources for the client

Identifying individual lifestyle choices
Performing psychosocial data collection techniques

Psychosocial Integrity
Addressing grief and loss issues
Assisting with crisis intervention
Caring for the client who has been sexually abused or raped
Considering religious, cultural, and spiritual influences on health
Developing a therapeutic nurse-client relationship
Identifying abuse and neglect situations
Monitoring for addictions
Identifying coping mechanisms
Identifying domestic violence situations
Identifying support system
Implementing behavioral interventions as prescribed
Providing a therapeutic milieu
Teaching stress-management techniques

Physiological Integrity
Monitoring for abusive and self-destructive behavior
Monitoring elimination patterns
Monitoring for alterations in body systems related to substance abuse
Monitoring for expected and untoward effects of medications
Monitoring for potential complications related to medications and treatments, such as electroconvulsive therapy
Monitoring laboratory values related to medication therapy
Monitoring rest and sleep patterns
Providing adequate nutrition
Providing personal hygiene measures
Treating physical injuries from abuse or self-destructive behavior

Client Needs lists modified from: National Council of State Boards of Nursing, Inc. (NCSBN). NCLEX-PN Examination: Test Plan for the National Council Licensure Examination for Practical Nurses, effective April 2020. Chicago: NCSBN.

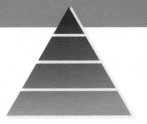

CHAPTER 61

Foundations of Mental Health Nursing

PRIORITY CONCEPTS Caregiving; Coping

WHAT WOULD YOU DO?

A client needs assistance with their use of coping mechanisms to decrease anxiety. What would the nurse do?
Answer is located on p. 858.

 I. The Nurse–Client Relationship

A. Principles
1. Genuineness, respect, and empathic understanding are characteristics important to the development of a therapeutic nurse–client relationship.
2. The client would be cared for in a holistic manner.
3. The nurse considers the client's cultural and spiritual beliefs and values when assessing the client's response to the nurse-client relationship and his or her adaptation to stressors.
4. Appropriate limits and boundaries define and facilitate a therapeutic nurse–client relationship.
5. Honest and open communication is an important cornerstone for the development of trust—an underpinning of the therapeutic nurse–client relationship.
6. The nurse uses therapeutic communication techniques to encourage the client to express thoughts and feelings as they address identified problem areas.
7. The nurse respects the client's confidentiality and limits discussion of the client to members of the treatment team.
8. The goal of the nurse–client relationship is to assist the client with developing problem-solving and coping mechanisms.

⚠ The nurse needs to consider the cultural, religious, and spiritual practices of the client and whether these practices may give the client hope, comfort, and support while healing.

B. Phases of a therapeutic nurse–client relationship
1. Preinteraction phase
   a. The preinteraction phase begins before the nurse's first contact with the client.
   b. Develops appropriate physical and interpersonal environment (seating, lighting) to promote comfort and facilitate collaboration
   c. Anticipates potential client issues
   d. Prepares for client interaction
   e. Determines how to initially approach client
   f. The nurse needs to consider her or his own preconceived ideas, stereotypes, biases, and values that may impinge on the nurse–client relationship.
2. Orientation or introductory phase
   a. Acceptance, trust, and boundaries are established.
   b. Introduces herself or himself to the client by using first and last name and designation
   c. Expectations and the time frame of the relationship are identified (establishing a contract).
   d. Identifies client's strengths and needs
   e. Collects data to identify the client's problem and plan client-centered goals
   f. Termination and separation of the relationship are discussed in anticipation of the time-limited nature of the relationship.
3. Working phase
   a. Exploring, focusing on, and evaluating the client's concerns and problems occur; an attitude of acceptance and active listening assists the client with expressing their thoughts and feelings.
   b. Actively problem solves with the client
   c. Uses interpersonal strategies to help the client identify effective coping strategies
   d. Encourages self-direction and self-management whenever possible to promote health and wellness
4. Termination or separation phase
   a. Prepare the client for termination and separation during initial contact.
   b. Evaluates progress and achievement of goals

c. Identifies responses related to termination and separation, such as anger, distancing from the relationship, a return of symptoms, and dependency

d. Encourage the client to express feelings about termination.

e. Identify the client's strengths and anticipated needs for follow-up care.

f. Refers the client to community resources and/or other support systems

C. Family as an extension of the client

1. Family members would be viewed as collaborators in the management of a client's mental health needs (maintain confidentiality as necessary).

2. Competence and caring focused toward family members can enhance the nurse's ability to identify client and family needs and to select and implement effective interventions directed toward promoting adaptive functioning.

3. Nurses have a professional obligation to be aware of and sensitive to the cultural, ethnic, religious, and spiritual factors that affect the structure and resulting needs of the client and his or her family.

4. Educating family members regarding the client's mental health problems, identification of symptoms, and effective management of maladaptive behaviors plays a vital role in the client's quality of life.

D. Impact of culture, ethnicity, and spirituality on client care

1. Cultural competency allows the nurse to recognize the uniqueness of each client and the impact that culture, values, religious and spiritual beliefs have on an individual's mental health, as well as the treatment required for an existing mental health problem.

2. A client's culture, ethnicity, values, religious and spiritual belief systems can affect all aspects of mental health care, including medication therapies, and can act as either protective or risk factors when dealing with the development and/or treatment of mental health problems.

3. Nurses must be aware of the impact that their own culture, religious and spiritual beliefs, and values have on the care they provide and avoid biases.

4. The treatment plan must be agreed upon by both client and nurse and must take into consideration the needs of the client whenever possible.

II. Therapeutic Communication Process

A. Principles

1. Communication includes verbal and nonverbal expression.

2. Successful communication includes appropriateness, efficiency, flexibility, and feedback.

3. Anxiety in the nurse or client impedes communication.

4. Communication needs to be goal-directed and within a professional framework.

B. Therapeutic and nontherapeutic communication techniques (Table 61.1)

III. Mental Health

A. Mental health is a lifelong process of successful adaptation to a changing internal and external environment.

B. The mentally healthy individual is *in contact with reality*, is able to relate to people and situations in their environment, and can resolve conflicts within a problem-solving framework.

C. The mentally healthy individual has psychobiological resilience.

IV. Mental Health Problem

A. Description

1. A mental health problem can cause the loss of ability to respond to the internal and external environment in ways that are in harmony with oneself or the expectations of society.

2. It is characterized by thought, or behavior patterns that impair functioning and cause distress.

B. Personality characteristics

1. Self-concept is distorted.

2. Perception of strengths and weaknesses is unrealistic.

3. Thoughts and perceptions may not be reality-based.

4. The ability to find meaning and purpose in life may be impaired.

5. Life direction and productivity may be disturbed.

6. Meeting one's own needs may be problematic.

7. Excessive reliance or preoccupation on the thoughts, opinions, and actions of self or others may be present.

C. Adaptations to stress

1. The individual's sense of self-control may be affected.

2. Perception of the environment may be distorted.

3. Coping mechanisms may not exist or may be ineffective.

D. Interpersonal relationships

1. Interpersonal relationships may be minimally existent or may be negatively affected.

2. The ability to enjoy sustained intimacy in relationships is impaired.

V. Coping and Defense Mechanisms

A. Coping mechanisms

1. Coping involves any effort to decrease anxiety.

2. Coping mechanisms can be constructive or destructive, task or problem oriented in relation to direct problem solving, cognitively oriented in an attempt to neutralize the meaning of the

TABLE 61.1   Therapeutic (Effective) and Nontherapeutic (Ineffective) Communication Techniques

Therapeutic Techniques

Technique	Description
Active listening	Carefully noting what the client is saying and observing the client's nonverbal behavior
Broad openings	Encouraging the client to select topics for discussion
Clarifying	Providing a means for making the message clearer, correcting any misunderstandings, and promoting mutual understanding
Focusing	Directing the conversation on the topic being discussed
Informing	Giving information to the client
Offering self to help	Includes staying with the client, talking to the client, and offering to help the client
Open-ended questions	Encouraging conversation because these questions require more than one-word answers
Paraphrasing	Restating in different words what the client said
Reflecting	Directing the client's question or statement back to the client for consideration
Restating	Repeating what the client has said and directing the statement back to the client to provide the client the opportunity to agree or disagree or to clarify the message further
Silence	Allowing time for formulating thoughts
Summarizing	Stating briefly what was discussed during the conversation
Validating	Verifying that both the nurse and the client are interpreting the topic or message in the same way

Nontherapeutic Techniques

Technique	Description
Approval	Implying that the client is thinking or doing the right thing and is not thinking or doing what is wrong; this may direct the client to focus on thinking or behavior that pleases the nurse
Asking excessive questions	Demanding information from the client without respect for the client's willingness or readiness to respond
Changing the subject	Avoiding addressing the client's thoughts, feelings, or concerns; implying that the client's statement is not important
Closed-ended questions	Questions that ask for specific information such as a "yes" or "no" answer and therefore inhibit communication
Disagreeing	Opposing the client's thinking or opinions, implying that the client is wrong
Disapproving	Indicating a negative value judgment about the client's behavior or thoughts
False reassurance	Making a statement that implies that the client has no reason to be worried or concerned, belittling a client's concerns
Giving advice	Assuming that the client cannot think for herself or himself, which inhibits problem solving and fosters dependence
Minimizing the client's feelings	Making a statement that implies that the client's feelings are not important
Parroting	Repeating the client's words before determining what the client has said
Placing the client's feelings on hold	Avoiding addressing the client's thoughts, feelings, or concerns; making a statement that places the responsibility of addressing the client's thoughts, feelings, or concerns elsewhere or on another person
Value judgments	Making a comment that addresses the client's morals; this can make the client feel angry or guilty or as though she or he is not being supported.
"Why?" questions	Cause the client to feel defensive, because many times she or he does not know the reason "why"; these types of questions also often imply criticism.

From Stuart, G: *Principles and practice of psychiatric* nursing, ed 10, St. Louis, 2013, Mosby, p. 226.

TABLE 61.2   Defense Mechanisms

Defense Mechanism	Example
Compensation: Putting forth extra effort to counterbalance perceived deficiencies by emphasizing strengths	A businessman perceives his small physical stature negatively. He tries to overcome this by being aggressive, forceful, and controlling in business dealings.
Conversion: The expression of emotional conflicts through physical symptoms that have no organic cause	A young man develops chronic abdominal pain after an emotionally traumatic event. There was no identifiable cause found for his symptoms.
Denial: Ignoring the existence of unpleasant or intolerable thoughts, feelings, needs, or impulse	A 42-year old female has just been told that her breast biopsy indicates a malignancy. When her husband visits her that evening, she tells him that no one has discussed the laboratory results with her.
Displacement: Feelings about a person, object, or situation are directed to another less threatening person, object, or situation	A 4-year old boy is angry because he has just been punished by his mother for drawing on his bedroom walls. He begins to play war with his soldier toys and has them fight each other.
Dissociation: The blocking of an anxiety-provoking event or period of time from the consciousness, memory, or perception to compartmentalize uncomfortable or unpleasant aspects of oneself	A man is brought to the emergency room by the police and is unable to explain who he is and where he lives or works.
Identification: The conscious or unconscious attempt to change oneself to resemble an admired person	A 15-year old female has her hair styled like that of her young English teacher, whom she admires.
Intellectualization: Excessive reasoning of an event based solely on facts without involving feelings or emotion; the thinking is disconnected from feelings, and situations are dealt with at a cognitive level.	A woman avoids dealing with her anxiety in shopping malls by explaining that shopping is a frivolous waste of time and money.
Introjection: A type of identification in which the individual incorporates the traits or values of another into herself or himself	An 8-year old boy tells his 3-year old sister, "Don't scribble in your book of nursery rhymes. Just look at the pretty pictures," thus expressing his parents' values.
Isolation: Response in which a person blocks feelings associated with an unpleasant experience	A medical student dissects a cadaver for her anatomy course without being disturbed by thoughts of death.
Projection: Transferring one's internal feelings, thoughts, and unacceptable ideas and traits to someone else	A young woman who denies she has sexual feelings about a co-worker accuses him without basis of trying to seduce her.
Rationalization: An attempt to make unacceptable feelings and behaviors acceptable by justifying the behavior	A student fails an examination and complains that the lectures were not well organized or clearly presented.
Reaction formation: Developing conscious attitudes and behaviors and acting out behaviors opposite to what one really feels	A married woman who feels attracted to one of her husband's friends treats him rudely.
Regression: Returning to an earlier developmental stage and pattern of behavior to express an impulse to deal with anxiety	A four-year old girl who has been toilet trained for more than 1 year begins to wet her pants again when her new baby brother is brought home from the hospital.
Repression: An unconscious process in which the client blocks undesirable and unacceptable thoughts or ideas from conscious expression	A man does not recall hitting his wife when she was pregnant.

From Stuart, G: *Principles and practice of psychiatric* nursing, ed 10, St. Louis, 2013, Mosby, p. 226.

problem, or defense or emotion oriented, thus regulating the response to protect oneself.

B. Defense mechanisms
1. As anxiety increases, the individual copes by using defense mechanisms.
2. A defense mechanism is a coping mechanism used in an effort to protect the individual from feelings of anxiety; as anxiety increases and becomes overwhelming, the individual copes by using defense mechanisms to protect the ego and decrease anxiety (Table 61.2).

⚠️ Coping and defense mechanisms are used by the client as protection from unmanageable stress and to decrease anxiety.

C. Interventions
1. Assist the client with identifying the source of anxiety and explore methods to reduce anxiety.
2. Assess the client's use of defense mechanisms.
3. Facilitate the appropriate use of defense mechanisms.
4. Determine whether the defense mechanisms used by the client are effective for him or her or create additional distress.
5. Avoid arguing or criticizing the client's behavior and use of defense mechanisms.
6. Do not take defense coping mechanisms away until client has established more appropriate coping strategies to effectively deal with stressors.

VI. Diagnostic and Statistical Manual of Mental Health Disorders

A. The *Diagnostic and Statistical Manual of Mental Health Disorders*, published by the American Psychiatric Association, provides guidelines for health care personnel for identifying and categorizing mental health problems.

B. The manual is a system used in clinical, research, and education settings, in which diagnostic criteria are included for each mental health problem.

C. Dual diagnosis: Refers to the client who has both a mental health problem and a substance-related problem; also known as comorbidity or co-occurring problems

D. See American Psychiatric Association for updates: http://www.dsm5.org/Pages/Default.aspx

 ## VII. Types of Mental Health Admissions and Discharges

A. Voluntary admission
   1. The client (or the client's guardian) seeks admission for care.
   2. The voluntary client is free to sign out of the hospital with psychiatrist (primary health care provider [PHCP]) notification and prescription.
   3. Detaining a voluntary client against his or her will is termed false imprisonment.
   4. Civil rights are retained fully by the client. For a list of rights see http://www.cchr.org/about-us/mental-health-declaration-of-human-rights.html.

 B. Right to confidentiality
   1. A client has a right to confidentiality regarding his or her medical information. The Health Insurance Portability and Accountability Act (HIPAA) of 1996 ensures client confidentiality with regard to release and electronic transmission of data.
   2. Information sometimes must be released in life-threatening situations without the client's consent.
   3. In the event of a specific threat against an identified individual, the health care professional has a legal obligation to warn intended victim(s) of a client's threats of harm.

⚠ Except in an emergency situation, client information can be released only with the client's informed consent, which specifies the information that can be released and the time frame for which the release is valid.

C. Involuntary admission
   1. Involuntary admission may be necessary when a person is mentally ill, is a danger to self or others, or is in need of mental health treatment or physical care.
   2. Involuntary admission occurs when a person is admitted or detained involuntarily for mental health treatment because of actual or imminent danger to self or others; the person's condition is deteriorating and they require hospitalization.
   3. The client who is admitted involuntarily retains his or her right to informed consent.
   4. The client retains the right to refuse treatment, including medications, unless a separate and specific treatment order is obtained from the court.
   5. The client loses the right to refuse treatment when the client poses an immediate danger to self or others, requiring immediate action by the interprofessional health care team.
   6. Depending on the jurisdiction, an order from an external board such as a court or from the psychiatrist or PHCP is required for an involuntary admission, except in the case of an emergency, which does not allow time to obtain the necessary order from the board; in the case of all involuntary admissions, legal counsel must be provided for the client. In this situation, the client may be held for a 72-hour period until further evaluation is completed.
   7. A hearing is held by an external board within a specified time for clients admitted involuntarily; the specific time period varies by state. The psychiatrist or PHCP may also be the person making decisions surrounding client discourse, depending on state guidelines.
   8. In most states, a client can institute a hearing to seek an expedient judicial discharge (a writ of habeas corpus).
   9. At the hearing, a determination is made as to whether the client may be released from the hospital or detained for further treatment and evaluation, or committed to a mental health facility for an undetermined time period.
   10. A client has the right to treatment in the least restrictive treatment environment; if treatment objectives can be achieved by court-ordered treatment to an outpatient facility as opposed to an inpatient facility, the client has the right to be treated in the outpatient setting.
   11. A client is considered legally competent unless he or she has been declared incompetent through a legal hearing separate from the involuntary commitment hearing.
   12. In the course of providing nursing care and carrying out medical prescriptions, if the nurse believes that a client lacks competency to make informed decisions, action would be initiated to determine whether a legal guardian or substitute decision-maker needs to be appointed by the court.

D. Release from the hospital
   1. Description
      a. In some, but not all jurisdictions, a client may be released voluntarily, against medical advice, or with conditions (conditional release).

It is important to be familiar with the laws in the area in which you work regarding conditional release.

b. A client who sought voluntary admission has the right to receive release upon request.

2. Voluntary release

a. In the absence of an act of self-harm or danger to others, a voluntary client should never be detained.

b. If a voluntary client wishes to be discharged from treatment, but is considered potentially dangerous to self or others, the PHCP can prescribe for the client to be detained while legal proceedings for involuntary status are sought. In other states, the PHCP places them on a 72-hour hold while further evaluation occurs.

c. Some states provide for conditional release of involuntarily hospitalized clients; this enables the treating PHCP to prescribe continued treatment on an outpatient basis as opposed to discharging the client to follow-up on his or her own initiative. Community treatment prescription may also be instituted depending on the facility and state.

d. Conditional release usually involves outpatient treatment for a specified period to determine the client's compliance with medication protocol, ability to meet basic needs, and ability to reintegrate into the community.

e. An involuntary client who is released conditionally may be reinstitutionalized while the commitment is still in effect without recommencement of formal admission procedures.

3. Discharge planning and follow-up care

a. Discharge is the termination of the client-institution relationship.

b. The release may be prescribed by the psychiatrist, external board, or administration for involuntarily admitted clients and may be requested by voluntary clients at any time.

c. In most states, the client can institute an external board hearing to seek an expedient judicial discharge (writ of habeas corpus).

d. Discharge planning and follow-up care are important for the continued well-being of the client with a mental health problem.

e. After-care case managers are used to facilitate the client's adaptation back into the community and provide early referral if the treatment plan is unsuccessful.

VIII. Types of Therapy for Care

A. Milieu therapy

1. The milieu refers to the safe physical and social environment in which an individual is receiving treatment.

2. Safety is the most important priority in managing the milieu, and all encounters with the client have the goal of being "therapeutic."

3. All members of the interprofessional health care team contribute to the planning and functioning of the milieu and are significant and valuable to the client's successful treatment outcomes; the team generally includes a registered nurse (RN), social worker, exercise therapist, recreational therapist, psychologist, psychiatrist, occupational therapist, and clinical nurse specialist or nurse practitioner.

4. Community meetings, activity groups, social skills groups, and physical exercise programs are included to accomplish treatment goals.

5. One-to-one relationships are used to examine client behaviors, feelings, and interactions within the context of the therapeutic group activities.

⚠ The focus of milieu therapy is to empower the client through involvement in setting his or her own goals and to develop purposeful relationships with the staff to assist with meeting those goals.

B. Interpersonal psychotherapy

1. A treatment modality that uses a therapeutic relationship to modify the client's feelings, attitudes, and behaviors and work within an agreed upon time frame to help meet the client's goals

2. Therapeutic communication forms the foundation of the therapist-client relationship, and this relationship is used as a way for the client to examine other relationships in his or her life.

3. Supportive level of psychotherapy

a. Brief therapy or may extend over a period of years, allowing the client to express feelings, explore alternatives, and make decisions in a safe, caring environment.

b. No plan exists to introduce new methods of coping; instead, the therapist reinforces the client's existing coping mechanisms.

4. Re-educative level of psychotherapy

a. The client explores alternatives in a planned, systematic way; this requires a longer period of therapy than supportive therapy.

b. The client agrees upon and specifies desired changes of behavior and learning new ways of perceiving and behaving.

c. Techniques may include short-term psychotherapy, reality therapy, cognitive restructuring, behavior modification, and development of coping skills.

5. Reconstructive level of psychotherapy

a. Emotional and cognitive restructuring of self takes place.

b. Positive outcomes include a greater understanding of self and others, more emotional freedom, and the development of potential abilities.

C. Behavior therapy
   1. A treatment approach that uses the principles of Skinnerian (operant conditioning) or Pavlovian (classical conditioning) behavior therapy to bring about behavioral change; the belief is that most behaviors are learned.
   2. Operant conditioning refers to the manipulation of selected reinforcers to elicit and strengthen desired behavioral responses; the reinforcer refers to the consequence of the behavior, which is defined as anything that increases the occurrence of a behavior.
   3. In classical conditioning (respondent conditioning), the individual responds to a stimulus but is basically a passive agent.
   4. Desensitization is a form of behavior therapy whereby exposure to increasing increments of a feared stimulus is paired with increasing levels of relaxation, which helps to reduce the intensity of fear to a more tolerable level.
   5. Aversion therapy is a form of behavior therapy; its goal is to have the client give up an undesirable habit or behavior by causing them to associate it with an unpleasant effect.
   6. Modeling is a behavior therapy whereby the therapist acts as a role model for specific identified behaviors so that the client learns through imitation.

D. Cognitive therapy
   1. An active, directive, time-limited, structured approach used to treat various mental health problems including anxiety and depressive problems
   2. It is based on the principle that how individuals feel and behave is determined by how they think about the world and their place in it; their cognitions are based on the attitudes or assumptions developed from previous experience.
   3. Therapeutic techniques are designed to identify, reality-test, and correct distorted conceptualizations and the dysfunctional beliefs underlying these cognitions.
   4. The therapist helps the individual to change the way he or she thinks thereby reducing symptoms.

E. Group development and group therapy
   1. Involves a leader such as a therapist, nurse, or other designated health care team member and, ideally, five to eight members working on their individual goals within the context of a group, which presumably increases the opportunity for feedback and support.
   2. Initial development of the group
      a. Characterized by superficial rather than open and trusting communication
      b. Members become acquainted with each other and search for similarities among themselves.

c. Members may be unclear about the purpose or goals of the group.
      d. Group norms, roles, and responsibilities are established.
      e. The work of termination begins and is expanded upon throughout the duration of the group.
   3. Working in the group
      a. The real work of the group is accomplished.
      b. Members are familiar with one another, the group leader, and the group roles and they feel free to address and attempt to solve their problems.
      c. Both conflict and cooperation surface during the group's work as the members learn to work with one another.
   4. Termination of the group
      a. Begins with the initial meeting
      b. Members' feelings are explored regarding their accomplishments and the impending termination of the group.
      c. The termination stage provides an opportunity for members to learn to deal more realistically and comfortably with this normal part of human experience.
   5. Self-help or support groups (Box 61.1)

⚠️ Support groups are based on the premise that individuals who have experienced and are insightful concerning a problem are able to help others who have a similar problem.

F. Family therapy
   1. Family therapy is a specific intervention mode based on the premise that the member with the presenting symptoms signals the presence of problems in the entire family; this premise also

BOX 61.1	**Examples of Self-Help or Support Groups**

Adult Children of Alcoholics
Al-Anon
Alcoholics Anonymous
Bereavement groups
Cancer support groups
Codependents Anonymous
Gamblers Anonymous
Groups to help deal with unexpected body image changes, such as mastectomy or colostomy
Groups to help deal with caring for family members
Mental illness support groups
Narcotics Anonymous
Overeaters Anonymous
Parents without Partners
Recovery groups, such as for those who have experienced trauma
Smoking cessation groups

assumes that a change in one member will bring about changes in other members.

2. The therapist works to assist family members to identify and express their thoughts and feelings; define family roles and rules; try new, more productive styles of relating; and restore strength to the family.

WHAT WOULD YOU DO?

Answer: A coping mechanism involves any effort to decrease anxiety and can be constructive or destructive, task oriented, or defense oriented. The nurse would first help the client with identifying the source of anxiety. Next, the nurse would explore with the client various methods to reduce anxiety, such as relaxation methods. A defense mechanism is a coping mechanism used in an effort to protect the individual from feelings of anxiety; as anxiety increases and becomes overwhelming, the individual copes by using defense mechanisms to protect the ego and decrease anxiety. If this occurs, the nurse would facilitate appropriate and constructive use of the defense mechanism and determine whether the defense mechanism used by the client is effective for him or her, or if it creates additional distress. The nurse must never criticize the client's behavior or the use of defense mechanisms.

PRACTICE QUESTIONS

1. The nurse is assigned to care for a client experiencing disturbed thought processes. The nurse is told that the client believes that their food is being poisoned. Which communication technique would the nurse plan to use to encourage the client to eat?
   1. Open-ended questions and silence
   2. Focusing on self-disclosure regarding food preferences
   3. Stating the reasons that the client may not want to eat
   4. Offering opinions about the necessity of adequate nutrition

2. The nurse is assigned to care for a client admitted to the hospital after sustaining an injury from a house fire. The client attempted to save a neighbor involved in the fire, but despite the client's efforts, the neighbor died. Which action would the nurse take to enable the client to work through the meaning of the crisis?
   1. Identifying the client's ability to function
   2. Identifying the client's potential for self-harm
   3. Inquiring about the client's feelings that may affect coping
   4. Inquiring about the client's perception of the cause of the neighbor's death

3. The nurse is assisting with the data collection on a client admitted to the psychiatric unit. After review of the obtained data, the nurse would identify which as a **priority** concern?
   1. The client's report of not eating or sleeping
   2. The presence of bruises on the client's body
   3. The client's report of self-destructive thoughts
   4. The family member is disapproving of the treatment.

4. Laboratory work is prescribed for a client who has been experiencing delusions. When the laboratory technician approaches the client to obtain a specimen of the client's blood, the client begins to shout, "You're all vampires. Let me out of here!" The nurse present at the time would respond with which question or statement?
   1. "The technician is not going to hurt you but is going to help."
   2. "Are you fearful and think that others may want to hurt you?"
   3. "What makes you think that the technician wants to hurt you?"
   4. "The technician will leave and come back later for your blood."

5. An intoxicated client is brought to the emergency department by local police. The client is told that the primary health care provider (PHCP) will be in to see the client in about 30 minutes. The client becomes very loud and offensive and wants to be seen by the PHCP immediately. The nurse assisting to care for the client would take which appropriate nursing intervention?
   1. Watch the behavior escalate before intervening.
   2. Attempt to talk with the client to de-escalate the behavior.
   3. Offer to take the client to an examination room until he or she can be treated.
   4. Inform the client that he or she will be asked to leave if the behavior continues.

6. A client is admitted to a psychiatric unit for treatment of a psychotic disorder. The client is at the locked exit door and is shouting, "Let me out! There's nothing wrong with me! I don't belong here!" The nurse identifies this behavior as which defense mechanism?
   1. Denial
   2. Projection
   3. Regression
   4. Rationalization

7. A client says to the nurse, "I'm going to die, and I wish my family would stop hoping for a 'cure'! I get so angry when they carry on like this! After all, I'm

the one who's dying." Which therapeutic response would the nurse make to the client?
1. "Have you shared your feelings with your family?"
2. "I think we should talk more about your anger with your family."
3. "You're feeling angry that your family continues to hope for you to be 'cured'?"
4. "Well, it sounds like you're being pretty pessimistic. After all, years ago people died of pneumonia."

8. The nurse in a psychiatric unit is assigned to care for a client admitted to the unit 2 days ago. During review of the client's record, the nurse notes that the admission was a voluntary one. Based on this type of admission, which would the nurse expect to note?
1. The client will be angry and will refuse care.
2. The client will participate in the treatment plan.
3. The client will be very resistant to treatment measures.
4. The client's family will be very resistant to treatment measures.

9. The nurse enters a client's room, and the client immediately demands to be released from the hospital. During review of the client's record, the nurse notes that the client was admitted 2 days ago for the treatment of an anxiety disorder and that the admission was a voluntary one. The nurse reports the findings to the RN and expects that the RN will take which action?
1. Call the client's family.
2. Persuade the client to stay a few more days.
3. Contact the primary health care provider (PHCP).
4. Tell the client that discharge is not possible at this time.

10. A client is admitted to the psychiatric nursing unit. When collecting data from the client, the nurse notes that the client was admitted on an involuntary status. Based on this type of admission, which would the nurse expect to note?
1. The client presents a harm to self.
2. The client requested the admission.
3. The client consented to the admission.
4. The client provided written application to the facility for admission.

11. Following a group therapy session, a client approaches the nurse and verbalizes a need for seclusion because of uncontrollable feelings. The nurse reports the findings to the RN and expects that the RN will take which action?
1. Call the client's family.
2. Place the client in seclusion immediately.

3. Inform the client that seclusion has not been prescribed.
4. Get a written prescription from the primary health care provider (PHCP) and obtain an informed consent.

12. The nurse is providing care for a client admitted to the hospital with a diagnosis of anxiety disorder. The nurse is talking with the client, and the client says, "I have a secret that I want to tell you. You won't tell anyone about it, will you?" Which is the appropriate nursing response?
1. "No, I won't tell anyone."
2. "I cannot promise to keep a secret."
3. "If you tell me the secret, I will tell it to your doctor."
4. "If you tell me the secret, I will need to document it in your record."

13. The nurse in the mental health unit reviews the therapeutic and nontherapeutic communication techniques with a nursing student. Which are therapeutic communication techniques? **Select all that apply.**
☐ 1. Restating
☐ 2. Listening
☐ 3. Asking the client, "Why?"
☐ 4. Maintaining neutral responses
☐ 5. Giving advice, approval, or disapproval
☐ 6. Providing acknowledgment and feedback

14. The nurse is preparing a client for the termination phase of the nurse–client relationship. Which task would the nurse appropriately plan for during this phase?
1. Plan short-term goals.
2. Identify expected outcomes.
3. Assist with making appropriate referrals.
4. Assist with developing realistic solutions.

15. The psychiatric nurse is greeted by a neighbor in a local grocery store. The neighbor says to the nurse, "How is Carol doing? She is my best friend and is seen at your clinic every week." Which is the appropriate nursing response?
1. "I cannot discuss any client situation with you."
2. "I'm not supposed to discuss this, but because you are my neighbor, I can tell you that she is doing great!"
3. "You may want to know about Carol, so you need to ask her yourself so you can get the story firsthand."
4. "I'm not supposed to discuss this, but because you are my neighbor, I can tell you that she really has some problems!"

ANSWERS

1. 1

Rationale: Open-ended questions and silence are strategies used to encourage clients to discuss their problem. Options 3 and 4 do not encourage the client to express feelings. The nurse would not offer opinions and would not state the reasons, but would encourage the client to identify the reasons for their behavior. Option 2 is not a client-centered intervention.

Test-Taking Strategy: Focus on the subject, communication techniques. Eliminate options 3 and 4 first because they do not support client expression of feelings. Eliminate option 2 next because it is not a client-centered intervention. Focusing on the client's feelings will direct you to option 1.

2. 3

Rationale: The client must first deal with feelings and negative responses before the client is able to work through the meaning of the crisis. Option 3 pertains directly to the client's feelings. Options 1, 2, and 4 do not directly address the client's feelings.

Test-Taking Strategy: Focus on the subject, adjustment to a crisis. Focusing on the feelings of the client will direct you to the correct option.

3. 3

Rationale: The client's thoughts are extremely important when verbalized. Self-destructive thoughts are the highest priority. Options 1, 2, and 4 will all affect the treatment of the client but are not of greatest importance at this time.

Test-Taking Strategy: The client is the focus of the question; therefore, eliminate option 4. Focus on the strategic word, *priority*, and use prioritizing skills. Remember, if the client verbalizes self-destructive thoughts, it is a priority concern.

4. 2

Rationale: Option 2 is the only option that recognizes the client's need. This response helps the client focus on the emotion underlying the delusion but does not argue with it. If the nurse attempts to change the client's mind, the delusion may, in fact, be even more strongly held. Options 1, 3, and 4 do not focus on the client's feelings.

Test-Taking Strategy: Use therapeutic communication techniques. This will direct you to option 2. In addition, option 2 focuses on the client's feelings.

5. 3

Rationale: Safety of the client, other clients, and staff is of prime concern. Option 3 is in effect an isolation technique that allows for separation from others and provides for a less stimulating environment where the client can maintain dignity. When dealing with an impaired individual, trying to talk may be out of the question. Waiting to intervene could cause the client to become even more agitated and a threat to others. Option 4 would only further aggravate an already agitated individual.

Test-Taking Strategy: Focus on the subject of the question, dealing with a loud and offensive client. Noting that the client is intoxicated will assist with directing you to option 3. Option 3 most directly addresses the situation and the behavior and feelings of the client.

6. 1

Rationale: Denial is the refusal to admit to a painful reality and is treated as if it does not exist. In projection, a person unconsciously rejects emotionally unacceptable features and attributes them to other people, objects, or situations. In regression, the client returns to an earlier, more comforting, although less mature, way of behaving. Rationalization is justifying the unacceptable attributes about oneself.

Test-Taking Strategy: Focus on the subject, the use of a defense mechanism. Note the words, *"There's nothing wrong with me!"* Select the option that recognizes the client's attempt to avoid looking at the reality of the situation.

7. 3

Rationale: Reflection is the therapeutic communication technique that redirects the client's feelings back to validate what the client is saying. In option 2, the nurse attempts to use focusing, but the attempt to discuss central issues is premature. In option 4, the nurse makes a judgment and is nontherapeutic in the one-on-one relationship. In option 1, the nurse is attempting to assess the client's ability to openly discuss feelings with family members. Although this may be appropriate, the timing is somewhat premature and closes off facilitation of the client's feelings.

Test-Taking Strategy: Use therapeutic communication techniques. Note that option 3 uses the therapeutic technique of reflection and focuses on the client's feelings. Options 1, 2, and 4 are nontherapeutic at this time.

8. 2

Rationale: Generally, voluntary admission is sought by the client or client's guardian. If the client seeks voluntary admission, the most likely expectation is that the client will participate in the treatment program. Options 1 and 3 are not likely for a client seeking voluntary admission. Option 4 is not centered on the individual client.

Test-Taking Strategy: Note the subject, voluntary admission. This will direct you to option 2. In addition, note that options 1, 3, and 4 are comparable or alike.

9. 3

Rationale: Generally, voluntary admission is sought by the client or client's guardian. Voluntary clients have the right to demand and obtain release. The best nursing action is to contact the PHCP. Option 1 violates client confidentiality. Option 2 is not therapeutic or appropriate. Option 4 does not apply to a voluntary admission status.

Test-Taking Strategy: Focus on the subject, voluntary admission. Noting the type of hospital admission will assist you with eliminating option 4. It is inappropriate to "persuade" a client to stay in the hospital. Option 1 would be eliminated simply based on the issues of client rights and confidentiality.

10. 1

Rationale: Involuntary admission is made without the client's consent. Involuntary admission is necessary when a person is a danger to self or others or is in need of psychiatric treatment or physical care. Options 2, 3, and 4 describe the process of voluntary admission.

Test-Taking Strategy: Note the subject, involuntary status. This would direct you to the correct option. Also, note that options 2, 3, and 4 are comparable or alike.

11. 4

Rationale: A client may request to be secluded or restrained. Federal laws require the consent of the client unless an emergency situation exists in which an immediate risk to the client or others can be documented. The use of seclusion and restraint is permitted only with the written prescription of the PHCP, which must be reviewed and renewed every 24 hours, depending on state law requirements. It must also specify the type of restraint to be used.

Test-Taking Strategy: Focus on the subject, procedures for seclusion. There is no reason to call the family at this time; therefore, eliminate option 1. Knowing that a PHCP's written prescription is necessary in this situation will assist you with eliminating option 2. Option 3 is not the best choice because this information, if given to a client experiencing uncontrollable feelings, may cause escalation of the feelings.

12. 2

Rationale: The nurse would never promise to keep a secret. Secrets are appropriate in a social relationship but not in a therapeutic one. The nurse needs to be honest with the client and tell the client that a promise cannot be made to keep the secret.

Test-Taking Strategy: Use therapeutic communication techniques and think about safety. Option 1 can be eliminated because it is inappropriate. Also, options 3 and 4 are not only inappropriate but are threatening to an extent and may even block further communication.

❖ **13. 1, 2, 4, 6**

Rationale: Some therapeutic communication techniques include listening, maintaining silence, maintaining neutral responses, using broad openings and open-ended questions, focusing and refocusing, restating, clarifying and validating, sharing perceptions, reflecting, providing acknowledgment and feedback, giving information and presenting reality, encouraging formulation of a plan of action, providing nonverbal encouragement, and summarizing. Asking why, giving advice, and approving or disapproving are nontherapeutic.

Test-Taking Strategy: Think about the use of therapeutic communication techniques. This will assist you with selecting the correct answers.

14. 3

Rationale: Tasks of the termination phase include evaluating client performance, evaluating achievement of expected outcomes, evaluating future needs, making appropriate referrals, and dealing with the common behaviors associated with termination. Options 1, 2, and 4 identify the tasks of the working phase of the relationship.

Test-Taking Strategy: Focus on the subject, the tasks of the termination phase. Thinking about the definition of *termination* would direct you to the correct option.

15. 1

Rationale: The nurse is required to maintain confidentiality regarding clients and their care. Confidentiality is basic to the therapeutic relationship and is a client's right. Option 3 is correct in a sense, but it is a rather blunt statement. Both options 2 and 4 identify statements that do not maintain client confidentiality.

Test-Taking Strategy: Focus on the subject, maintaining confidentiality. This would assist you with eliminating options 2 and 4. From the remaining options, select option 1 over option 3 because it is most direct and correct. Option 3 is a rather blunt and somewhat rude statement.

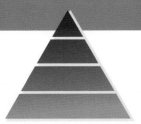

CHAPTER **62**

Mental Health Problems

PRIORITY CONCEPTS Mobd and Affect; Safety

WHAT WOULD YOU DO?

A client is experiencing visual hallucinations. What would the nurse do?
Answer is located on p. 877.

I. Anxiety

A. Description
  1. Anxiety is a normal response to stress.
  2. A subjective experience that includes feelings of apprehension, uneasiness, uncertainty, or dread
  3. Occurs as a result of a threat that may be misperceived or misinterpreted, or a threat to identity or self-esteem
  4. May result when values are threatened, or preceding new experiences

B. Types of anxiety
  1. Normal: A healthy type of anxiety
  2. Acute: Precipitated by imminent loss or change that threatens one's sense of security
  3. Chronic: Anxiety that persists as a characteristic response to daily activities

C. Levels of anxiety
  1. Mild
    a. Associated with the tension of everyday life
    b. Increased ability to grasp information
    c. Sense of sight and sound are increased.
    d. The perceptual field is increased.
    e. Can be motivating, produce growth, enhance creativity, and increase learning
    f. Physical symptoms may include restlessness, irritability, or mild tension.
  2. Moderate
    a. The focus is on immediate concerns.
    b. Moderate anxiety narrows the perceptual field.
    c. Sense of sight and sound diminish as selective inattentiveness occurs.
    d. Learning and problem solving still occur.
    e. Physical symptoms include increased heart rate, perspiration, gastric discomfort, headache, urinary urgency, and/or mild tremors.

  3. Severe
    a. Severe anxiety is a feeling that something bad is about to happen.
    b. A significant narrowing in the perceptual field occurs.
    c. Focus is on minute or scattered details.
    d. All behavior is aimed at relieving the anxiety.
    e. Learning and problem solving are not possible.
    f. Actions are aimed at reducing or alleviating anxiety.
    g. Physical symptoms are caused by stimulation of the sympathetic nervous system (e.g., headache, nausea, dizziness, sleep disturbances), increased tremors, pounding heart rate and hyperventilation.
    h. The individual needs direction to focus.
  4. Panic
    a. Panic is associated with dread and terror and a sense of impending doom.
    b. Disorganization, difficulty perceiving reality, and inability to concentrate
    c. The individual is unable to communicate or function effectively.
    d. Loss of rational thoughts with distorted perception occurs.
    e. Increased motor activity (pacing, shouting, screaming) or withdrawal
    f. If prolonged, panic can lead to exhaustion and death.
    g. Impulsive and erratic behavior

D. Interventions: General nursing measures (see Priority Nursing Actions)
  1. Recognize the anxiety.
  2. Establish trust.
  3. Protect the client.
  4. Do not criticize **coping mechanisms**.
  5. Do not force the client into situations that provoke anxiety.
  6. Modify the environment by setting limits or limiting interaction with others.
  7. Provide creative outlets.

8. Monitor for signs of impending destructive behavior.
9. Promote relaxation techniques such as breathing exercises or guided imagery.
10. Monitor vital signs and administer antianxiety medications as prescribed.

⚡ PRIORITY NURSING ACTIONS

Anxiety in a Client

1. Provide a calm environment, decrease environmental stimuli, and stay with the client.
2. Ask the client to identify what and how he or she feels.
3. Encourage the client to describe and discuss his or her feelings.
4. Help the client identify the cause(s) of the feelings if he or she is having difficulty doing so.
5. Listen to the client for expressions of helplessness and hopelessness.
6. Document the event, significant information, actions taken and follow-up actions, and the client's response.

⚠ The immediate nursing action for a client with anxiety is to decrease stimuli in the environment and provide a calm and quiet environment.

E. Interventions: Mild to moderate levels
  1. Help the client to identify the source of their anxiety.
  2. Encourage the client to talk about feelings and concerns.
  3. Help the client to identify thoughts and feelings that occurred before the onset of anxiety.
  4. Encourage problem solving.
  5. Encourage gross motor exercise.
F. Interventions: Severe to panic levels
  1. Ensure safety.
  2. Reduce the anxiety quickly.
  3. Use a calm manner.
  4. Always remain with the client.
  5. Minimize environmental stimuli.
  6. Provide clear, simple statements.
  7. Use a low-pitched voice.
  8. Attend to the physical needs of the client.
  9. Provide gross motor activity.
  10. Administer antianxiety medications as prescribed.

II. Generalized Anxiety Disorder

A. Description
  1. An unrealistic anxiety about everyday worries that persists more days than not, over the last 6 months, and that is not associated with another mental health or medical problem
  2. Physical symptoms occur.

B. Data collection
  1. Restlessness and inability to relax
  2. Episodes of trembling and shakiness
  3. Chronic muscular tension
  4. Dizziness
  5. Inability to concentrate
  6. Chronic fatigue and sleep problems
  7. Inability to recognize the connection between the anxiety and physical symptoms
  8. Client is focused on the physical discomfort.
C. Unexpected and expected panic attacks
  1. Description
    a. Most extreme level of anxiety resulting in disturbed behavior
    b. Produces a sudden onset of feelings of intense apprehension and dread
    c. The cause usually cannot be identified.
    d. Severe, recurrent, intermittent anxiety attacks lasting 5 to 30 minutes occur.
  2. Data collection
    a. Choking sensation
    b. Labored breathing
    c. Pounding heart
    d. Chest pain
    e. Dizziness
    f. Nausea
    g. Blurred vision
    h. Diaphoresis
    i. Numbness or tingling of the extremities
    j. A sense of unreality and helplessness
    k. A fear of being trapped
    l. A fear of dying
  3. Interventions (Refer to Section I.D.)

III. Posttraumatic Stress Disorder

A. Description: After experiencing a psychologically traumatic event, the individual is prone to reexperience the event and have recurrent and intrusive dreams or flashbacks.
B. Diagnosis: Symptoms last at least 1 month and can occur months or years after the traumatizing events.
C. Stressors
  1. Natural disaster
  2. Terrorist attack
  3. Combat experiences
  4. Accidents
  5. Rape
  6. Crime or violence
  7. Sexual, physical, and emotional **abuse**
  8. Reexperiencing the event as flashbacks
D. Data collection
  1. Avoidance or numbness
  2. Irritability or outbursts of anger
  3. Detachment
  4. Depression that may involve suicidal thoughts
  5. Anxiety

6. Sleep disturbances and nightmares
7. Flashbacks of the event
8. Hypervigilance and exaggerated startle response
9. Guilt about surviving the event
10. Poor concentration and avoidance of activities that trigger the memory of the event

E. Interventions (Box 62.1)

⚠ Clients dealing with cancer may develop post-traumatic stress disorder (PTSD). It can be triggered by the diagnosis, pain, tests and test results, treatment, length of treatment, recurring cancer, or fear of its return. The symptoms of PTSD are similar to those of PTSD disorder but are generally not as severe.

IV. Moral Injury

A. Description
1. Occurs as a result of acting, witnessing behaviors, or failing to prevent behaviors that are in conflict with one's own deeply held values and moral beliefs
2. Moral injury is not currently considered a mental problem; it has similarities and differences when compared to PTSD.
3. Moral injury is similar to PTSD in that both begin with an event that is harmful to self or others and is often life-threatening. Other similarities include guilt, shame, betrayal, and loss of trust that occurs.
4. Hyperarousal and a fear-based reaction that occurs in PTSD is not characteristic of moral injury; in addition, it is possible to have moral injury and not meet the criteria for PTSD.

BOX 62.1   Interventions for Posttraumatic Stress Disorder

Be nonjudgmental and supportive.
Assure the client that his or her feelings and behaviors are normal reactions.
Assist the client with recognizing the association between his or her feelings and behaviors and the trauma experience.
Encourage the client to express his or her feelings. Provide individual therapy that addresses loss of control or anger issues.
Monitor for suicidal risk.
Assist the client with developing adaptive coping mechanisms and using relaxation techniques.
Encourage the use of support groups.
Facilitate a progressive review of the trauma experience (called flooding).
Encourage the client to establish and reestablish relationships.
Inform the client that hypnotherapy or systematic desensitization may be used as a form of treatment.

---

5. Most research on moral injury has been with Service members and Veterans because of their exposure to war and combat situations.
6. Other research on moral injury has been among health care workers, including the effects of a health care crisis, such as COVID-19. For additional information refer to Watson, P., Norman, S. & Maguen, S. Hamblen, J. (2020). Moral injury in health care workers, US Department of Veterans Affairs at https://www.ptsd.va.gov/professional/treat/cooccurring/moral_injury_hcw.asp.

B. Data collection
1. Assess for depression and self-injurious behaviors as a priority.
2. Guilt: the person feels as though they did something bad.
3. Shame: the person believes they are bad because of what they did.
4. Disgust: when the person recalls memories of the act
5. Anger: as a response to a loss or betrayal
6. Inability to self-forgive for the act, witnessing the act, or failing to prevent the act

C. Interventions
1. An accepting, nonjudgmental approach is important because the person may be concerned about a nurse's or therapist's reaction and sometimes the person may feel as though they don't deserve to feel better; assess the client for these self-beliefs.
2. Goals include to build resilience, manage stress, improve well-being.
3. Assess for depression and self-injurious behaviors.
4. Self-report questionnaires to assess moral injury in war-related experiences may be useful for certain clients.
5. It may be difficult for an individual to share morally injurious acts because of their guilt, shame, and disgust; one on one therapy may be a safe environment initially, but the treatment plan should be decided by the client.
6. Group therapy may be helpful because individuals who have experienced similar injuries can share and communicate their emotions and pain.
7. Cognitive processing therapy may assist with addressing beliefs about self and working through beliefs that may underlie the guilt, shame, or betrayal, such as doing something differently during the trauma.
8. Other therapies being researched include Acceptance and Commitment Therapy, Adaptive Disclosure, Impact of Killing Intervention, Trauma Informed Guilt Reduction Therapy, and Building Spiritual Strength.
9. For additional information about moral injury and therapies refer to: Norman, S. & Maguen, S.

(2020). Moral injury, US Department of Veterans Affairs at https://www.ptsd.va.gov/professional/treat/cooccurring/moral_injury.asp.

V. Specific Phobias

A. Description
1. Irrational fear of an object, activity or situation that persists and that leads to avoidance
2. Associated with panic-level anxiety if the object, situation, or activity cannot be avoided
3. Defense mechanisms commonly used include repression and displacement.

B. Types (Box 62.2)

C. Interventions
1. Identify the basis of the anxiety.
2. Allow the client to verbalize feelings about the anxiety-producing object or situation. Frequently talking about the feared object is the first step in the desensitization process.
3. Teach relaxation techniques, such as breathing exercises, muscle relaxation exercises, and visualization of pleasant situations.
4. Promote desensitization by gradually introducing the individual to the feared object or situation in small doses.

⚠ Always stay with the client experiencing anxiety to promote safety and security. Never force the client to have contact with the phobic object or situation.

VI. Obsessive-Compulsive and Related Disorders

A. Obsessions: Preoccupation with persistently intrusive thoughts, impulses, and images and ideas

B. Compulsions: The performance of rituals or repetitive behaviors an individual is driven to perform to prevent some event, divert unacceptable thoughts and decrease anxiety. Obsessions and compulsions often occur together and can disrupt normal daily activities.

C. Anxiety occurs when one resists obsessions or compulsions, and from being powerless to resist the thoughts or rituals.

D. Obsessive thoughts can involve issues of violence, aggression, sexual behavior, orderliness, or religion and can uncontrollably interrupt conscious thoughts and the ability to function.

E. Compulsive behavior patterns (behaviors or rituals)
1. Compulsive behavior patterns decrease the anxiety.
2. The patterns are associated with the obsessive thoughts.
3. The patterns neutralize the thought.
4. During stressful times the ritualistic behavior increases.
5. Defense mechanisms include repression, displacement, and undoing.

F. Related disorders
1. Hoarding disorder
2. Excoriation (skin-picking) disorder
3. Substance or medication-induced obsessive-compulsive and related disorder
4. Obsessive-compulsive and related disorder due to another medical condition
5. Trichotillomania (hair-pulling disorder)

G. Interventions (Box 62.3)

VII. Somatic Symptom Disorders and Related Disorders

A. Description
1. Somatic symptom disorders are characterized by a combination of persistent worry or complaints and an associative maladaptive response regarding physical illness without supporting physical findings and medical diagnosis.

BOX 62.2 Types of Phobias

Acrophobia: Fear of heights
Agoraphobia: Fear of open spaces
Astraphobia: Fear of electrical storms
Claustrophobia: Fear of closed spaces
Hematophobia: Fear of blood
Hydrophobia: Fear of water
Monophobia: Fear of being alone
Mysophobia: Fear of dirt or germs
Nyctophobia: Fear of darkness
Pyrophobia: Fear of fires
Social phobia: Fear of situations in which one might be embarrassed or criticized and the fear of making a fool of oneself
Xenophobia: Fear of strangers
Zoophobia: Fear of animals

BOX 62.3 Interventions for Obsessive-Compulsive Disorder

Ensure that basic needs (food, rest, grooming) are met.
Identify the situations that precipitate the compulsive behavior; encourage the client to verbalize concerns and feelings.
Be empathetic toward the client, and be aware of his or her need to perform the compulsive behavior.
Do not interrupt the compulsive behaviors unless they jeopardize the safety of the client or others (provide for client safety related to the behavior).
Allow time for the client to perform the compulsive behavior, but set limits on behaviors that may interfere with the client's physical well-being to protect the client from physical harm.
Implement a schedule for the client that distracts from the behaviors (structure simple activities, games, or tasks for the client).
Recognize and reinforce positive nonritualistic behaviors.

2. The client focuses on the physical signs/symptoms and is unable to control the signs/symptoms.
3. The physical signs/symptoms increase with psychosocial stressors and result in a high level of functional impairment.
4. The anxiety is redirected into a somatic concern.
5. The client may unconsciously use somatization for secondary gains such as increased attention and decreased responsibilities.

B. Conversion disorder (functional neurological symptom disorder)

1. Description
   a. The sudden onset of a neurological symptom or a deficit in the absence of a neurological cause or diagnosis
   b. Conversion disorder is an expression of a psychological conflict or need.
   c. The most common conversion symptoms are blindness, deafness, numbness, paralysis, gait disturbance, and the inability to talk.
   d. Conversion disorder has no organic cause.
   e. Symptoms are beyond the conscious control of the client and are directly related to conflict.
   f. The development of physical symptoms reduces anxiety.

2. Data collection
   a. A physiological cause for symptoms is ruled out.
   b. Unconcerned with symptoms
   c. Physical limitations or disability
   d. Feelings of guilty, anxiety, or frustration
   e. Low self-esteem and feelings of inadequacy
   f. Unexpressed anger or conflict
   g. Secondary gain
   h. History of physical or sexual abuse

C. Interventions

1. Obtain a nursing history and check for physical problems.
2. Explore with the client the needs being met by the physical symptoms.
3. Assist the client with identifying alternative ways of meeting needs.
4. Assist the client with relating their feelings and conflicts to the physical symptoms.
5. Convey understanding that the physical symptoms are real to the client.
6. Assure the client that physical illness has been ruled out.
7. Explore the source of anxiety and stimulate verbalization of anxiety.
8. Encourage the use of relaxation techniques as the anxiety increases.
9. Use a pain assessment scale if the client complains of pain, and implement pain-reduction measures as required.

10. Report and assess any new physical complaint.
11. Encourage diversionary activities.
12. Provide positive feedback.
13. Assist the client with recognizing his or her own feelings and emotions.
14. Assist to administer antianxiety medications if prescribed.

⚠ For a client with a somatic symptom disorder, allow a specific time period for the client to discuss physical complaints because the client will feel less threatened if this behavior is limited rather than stopped completely. However, avoid responding with positive reinforcement about the physical complaints.

VIII. Dissociative Disorder

A. Description

1. Dissociative disorder is a disruption in integrative functions of memory, consciousness, or identity.
2. Dissociative disorder is associated with exposure to an extremely traumatic event.

B. Dissociative identity disorder (DID), formerly called *multiple personality disorder*

1. Description
   a. Two or more fully developed distinct and unique personalities exist within the client and recurrently control behavior.
   b. The host is the primary personality, and the other personalities are referred to as *alters.*
   c. Alter personalities may take full control of the client, one at a time, and may or may not be aware of one another.
   d. The alters may be aware of the host, but the host is not usually aware of the alter(s).

2. Data collection
   a. The client may have an inability to recall important information (unrelated to ordinary forgetfulness).
   b. Transition from one personality to another is related to stress or a traumatic event and is sudden.
   c. Dissociation is used as a method of distancing and defending oneself from anxiety and traumatizing experiences.

C. Dissociative amnesia

1. Description
   a. The inability to recall important personal information because it provokes anxiety; often due to trauma
   b. Memory impairment may range from partial to almost complete.
   c. The client may assume a new identity in a new environment, may drift from place to place, develop few relationships, and then return home unable to remember the amnesia.

2. Data collection
   a. Localized: The client blocks out all memories about a specified period.
   b. Selective: The client recalls some but not all memories about a specified period.
   c. Generalized: The client has a loss of all memory about past life.

D. Depersonalization/derealization disorder:
   1. Description: An altered self-perception in which one's own reality is temporarily lost or changed
   2. Data collection
      a. Feelings of detachment
      b. Intact reality testing

E. Interventions
   1. Develop a trusting relationship with the client.
   2. Encourage verbal expression of painful experiences, anxieties, and concerns.
   3. Explore methods of coping.
   4. Identify sources of conflict.
   5. Focus on the client's strengths and skills.
   6. Orient the client.
   7. Implement stress-reduction techniques.
   8. Plan for individual, group, and/or family psychotherapy to integrate dissociated aspects of personality or memory and expand self-awareness.
   9. Provide nondemanding, simple routines.
   10. Allow the client to progress at his or her own pace.

IX. Mood Disorders

A. Bipolar and related disorders
   1. Description: (Box 62.4)
      a. Bipolar disorder is characterized by extreme changes in mood, energy, and the ability to function.
      b. The classifications of bipolar include Bipolar I disorder, Bipolar II disorder, cyclothymic disorder, and mixed features.
      c. Bipolar I disorder: Most severe form characterized by severe mood episodes from mania to depression
      d. Bipolar II disorder: A milder form of mood elevation; there are milder episodes of hypomania that alternate with periods of severe depression.
      e. Cyclothymic disorder: Brief periods of hypomanic symptoms occur alternating with brief periods of depressive symptoms that are not as extensive or as long-lasting as seen in full hypomanic episodes or full depressive episodes.
      f. Mixed features: The occurrence of simultaneous symptoms of opposite mood polarities during manic, hypomanic, or depressive episodes. Its features are high energy, sleeplessness, and racing thoughts. At the same time, the individual may feel hopeless, despairing, irritable, and suicidal.

BOX 62.4 Data Collection: Bipolar Disorder

Mania
Becomes angry quickly
Delusional self-confidence
Constantly pushing limits, manipulating, and finding fault
Euphoric with intense feelings of well-being
Demonstrates little or no inhibition
Distracted by environmental stimuli
Extroverted personality
Flight of ideas
Grandiose and persecutory delusions
High and unstable affect
Significant decrease in appetite
Inability to eat or sleep because of involvement in more important things
Inappropriate affect
Dress that is inappropriately bizarre, loud, and/or colorful
Makeup is colorful or overdone
Initiation of activity
Pressured and/or clanging speech
Restlessness
Sexually promiscuous
Unlimited energy
Urgent motor activity

Depression
Increased or decreased appetite
Decrease in activities of daily living
Decreased emotion and physical activity
Easily fatigued
Inability to make decisions
Poor concentration
Internalizing hostility
Introverted personality
Social isolation and withdrawn from groups
Lack of energy
Lack of initiative
Lack of self-confidence and low self-esteem
Lack of sexual interest
Psychomotor retardation
Suicidal thinking

---

   g. The medication of choice has traditionally been lithium carbonate, which can be toxic and requires regular monitoring of serum lithium levels to help keep the medication's therapeutic index level appropriate; a stable intake of adequate dietary sodium and fluid (2 to 3L daily) must be maintained to avoid toxicity.
   h. Other medications may be prescribed both to reduce the symptoms of acute bipolar manic episodes and for maintenance therapy.
   i. Antianxiety agents may be prescribed to assist in managing the psychomotor agitation characteristic of mania; these medications would be avoided in clients with a history of substance abuse.

j. Atypical antipsychotic medications may be prescribed for both their sedative and mood stabilizing effects.

2. Data collection
   a. Assist to monitor whether client is a danger to self or others.
   b. Check for alcohol or substance use/misuse.
   c. Mood
   d. Behavior
   e. Speech (flight of ideas, tangential)
   f. Cognitive functioning
   e. Inflated self-regard (delusions of grandeur)
   h. Sleeping pattern
   i. Impulse control

3. Interventions for mania (Box 62.5)
   a. Remove hazardous objects from the environment (this would be done for all clients).
   b. Monitor the client closely for fatigue.
   c. Provide frequent rest periods and monitor the client's sleep patterns; use comfort measures to promote sleep.
   d. Provide a private room if possible.
   e. Encourage the client to ventilate feelings.
   f. Use calm, slow interactions.
   g. Help the client focus on one topic during the conversation.
   h. Ignore or distract the client from grandiose thinking; present reality to the client.
   i. Do not argue with the client.
   j. Limit group activities and assess the client's tolerance level; solitary activities may be necessary.
   k. Provide high-calorie finger foods and fluids.
   l. Reduce environmental stimuli.
   m. Set limits on inappropriate behaviors.
   n. Provide physical activities and outlets for tension.
   o. Avoid competitive games.
   p. Provide gross motor activities such as walking.
   q. Provide structured activities or one-to-one activities with the nurse.
   r. Provide simple and direct explanations for routine procedures.
   s. Supervise the administration of medication; monitor for noncompliance.

▲ X. Depressive Disorders

A. Description
   1. Depression affects feelings, thoughts, and behaviors.
   2. It can occur after a loss, including loss of self-esteem, the end of a significant relationship, the death of a loved one, or a traumatic event.
   3. The loss is followed by grief and mourning; if this process does not resolve, depression results.

| BOX 62.5 | Dealing with Inappropriate Behaviors Associated with Bipolar Disorder |

Aggressive Behavior

Assist the client with identifying feelings of frustration and aggression.

Encourage the client to talk out instead of acting out feelings of frustration.

Assist the client with identifying precipitating events or situations that lead to aggressive behavior.

Describe the consequences of the behavior for self and others.

Assist with identifying previous coping mechanisms.

Assist the client with problem-solving techniques to cope with frustration or aggression.

De-escalation Techniques

Maintain safety for the client, other clients, and self.

Respect personal space and use a nonaggressive posture.

Use a calm approach and communicate with a calm, clear tone of voice (be assertive, not aggressive).

Determine what the client considers to be his or her need.

Avoid verbal struggles; agree or agree to disagree.

Be concise.

Listen closely to what client is saying.

Provide the client with clear options that deal with the client's behavior.

Offer choices and optimism.

Assist the client with problem solving and decision making regarding the options.

Debrief the client and staff.

Manipulative Behavior

Set clear, consistent, realistic, and enforceable limits, and communicate expected behaviors.

Be clear about the consequences associated with exceeding set limits, and follow through with the consequences in a nonpunitive manner if necessary.

Discuss the client's behavior in a nonjudgmental and non-threatening manner.

Avoid power struggles with the client (avoid arguing with the client).

Assist the client in developing means of setting limits on personal behavior.

---

4. Depression may be mild, moderate, or severe.
5. Treatment includes counseling, antidepressant medication, and electroconvulsive therapy (ECT).
6. See Box 62.4 for general data collection findings.

B. Mild depression
   1. Mild depression is triggered by an external event and follows the normal grief reaction.
   2. Mild depression lasts less than 2 weeks.
   3. Feeling sad
   4. Feeling let down or disappointed
   5. Mild alternations in sleep patterns
   6. Feeling less alert
   7. Irritability
   8. Disinterested in spending time with others
   9. Increased or decreased appetite

10. Increased used of substances such as alcohol or drugs

C. Moderate depression

    1. Moderate depression persists over time.

    2. The person experiences a sense of change and often seeks help.

    3. Despondent and gloomy

    4. Dejected

    5. Low self-esteem

    6. Helplessness and powerlessness

    7. May experience intense anxiety and anger

    8. Diurnal variation: The person may feel better at a certain time of day.

    9. Slow thought processes and difficulty in concentrating

    10. Rumination: Persistent thinking about and discussion of a particular subject

    11. Negative thinking and suicidal thoughts (see Chapter 64)

    12. Sleep disturbances, early-morning awakening, or oversleeping

    13. Social withdrawal

    14. Anorexia, weight loss or gain, and fatigue

    15. Somatic complaints

    16. Moving or talking more slowly

    17. Increased use of substances such as alcohol or drugs

D. Major depressive disorder

    1. Depressed mood or loss of pleasure in activities for at least 2 weeks

    2. Impaired social, occupational, and/or educational functioning

    3. Mood changes from person's baseline

    4. Daily, experiences at least five of the following symptoms:

        a. Irritability or depressed mood most of the day, nearly every day (subjective report or observation of others)

        b. Decreased interest or pleasure in most activities

        c. Significant weight change (5%) or change in appetite

        d. Change in activity level

        e. Fatigue or loss of energy

        f. Guilt/worthlessness

        g. Diminished ability to think or concentrate, or more indecisive

        h. Thoughts of suicide

E Interventions (Box 62.6)

⚠ For a client at risk for self-harm, ask the client directly, "Have you thought of hurting yourself?"

XI. Electroconvulsive Therapy (ECT)

A. Description

    1. ECT is an effective treatment for depression (not a cure); a small amount of electrical current is delivered through electrodes attached to the temples that causes a brief seizure within the brain; outward movement is usually a slight movement of hands, feet, or a toe because premedication is given to relax the muscles. In addition, a short-acting anesthetic is given.

BOX 62.6 Interventions for Depressed Clients

Risk for Harm

Assess for homicidal and suicidal ideation.

Provide safety from suicidal actions (be certain that there are no harmful objects in the environment).

Do not leave the client alone for extended periods.

If the client has a suicidal plan, place on one-to-one supervision.

Activities

Use gentle encouragement to participate in activities of daily living and unit therapies.

Do not push decision making or making complex choices; make decisions that the client is not ready to make.

Provide achievable activities in which the client can achieve success (focus on strengths).

Begin the client with one-to-one activities.

Provide activities for easy mastery to increase self-esteem and help in alleviating guilt feelings and activities that do not require a great deal of concentration (simple card games, drawing).

Engage the client in gross motor activities (walking).

Eventually bring the client into small group activities and then into large groups.

Nutrition

Monitor nutritional intake and weight. Offer small, high-calorie, high-protein snacks and fluids throughout the day.

Stay with the client during meals to accurately assess intake and to assist in ensuring adequate nutritional intake.

Hygiene Care

Monitor for general hygiene and self-care deficits; deficits may indicate worsening depression.

Provide prompts to encourage activities of daily living.

Sleep Patterns

Monitor sleep patterns.

Decrease environmental stimuli at bedtime.

Encourage relaxation techniques.

Spend time with the client before bedtime to increase comfort and minimize feelings of loneliness and isolation.

Altered Thought Processes

Remind the client of times when he or she felt better and was successful.

Spend time with the client to convey the client's worth and value.

Encourage the client to discuss losses or changes in the life situation.

Encourage the client to express sadness or anger and allow adequate time for verbal responses.

Respond to anger therapeutically.

BOX 62.7 Electroconvulsive Therapy: Indications for Use

When antidepressant medications have no effect.
When there is a need for a rapid, definitive response, such as when a client is suicidal or homicidal.
When the client is in extreme agitation or stupor.
When the risks of other treatments outweigh the risk of electroconvulsive therapy (ECT).
When the client has a history of poor medication response, a history of good ECT response, or both.
When the client prefers ECT as a treatment.

---

2. The usual course is 6 to 12 treatments given every 2 to 5 days; maintenance ECT once a month may help to decrease the relapse rate for a client with recurrent depression.
3. ECT is not always effective in clients with dysthymic depression, depression and personality disorders, drug dependence, or depression secondary to situational or social difficulties.
4. At-risk clients include clients with recent myocardial infarction, brain attack (stroke), or intracranial mass lesions.

B. Uses (Box 62.7)
　1. Clients with severe depressive and bipolar depressive disorders, especially while psychotic symptoms are present, such as delusions of guilt, somatic delusions, and delusions of infidelity
　2. Clients who have depression with marked psychomotor retardation and stupor
　3. Manic clients whose conditions are resistant to lithium and antipsychotic medications and clients who are rapid cyclers (a client with a bipolar disorder who has many episodes of mood swings close together)
　4. Clients with schizophrenia (especially catatonia), clients with schizoaffective syndromes and psychotic clients

C. Preprocedure: Follow facility protocols
　1. Explain the procedure to the client.
　2. Encourage the client to discuss feelings, including myths regarding ECT.
　3. Teach the client and family what to expect.
　4. Informed consent must be obtained when voluntary clients are being treated.
　5. For involuntary clients, when informed consent cannot be obtained, permission may be obtained from the next of kin, although in some states the permission for ECT must be obtained from the court.
　6. Maintain NPO status after midnight or at least 4 hours before treatment, as prescribed.
　7. Baseline vital signs are taken.
　8. The client is requested to void.
　9. Hairpins, contact lenses, and dentures are removed.
　10. Administer preprocedure medication as pre-scribed.

D. During the procedure: Follow facility protocols
　1. As the intravenous line is inserted, electroencephalographic and electrocardiographic electrodes are attached.
　2. The blood pressure, pulse, and oxygen saturation are monitored throughout the treatment.
　3. A blood pressure cuff is placed around one ankle and inflated to block the medication from entering the foot. When the procedure begins, seizure activity can be monitored by watching for movement in that foot.
　4. Medications administered may include a short-acting anesthetic and a muscle relaxant.
　5. Oxygen is administered by face mask.
　6. An airway or mouth guard is placed to prevent biting the tongue.
　7. An electrical stimulus is administered; a brief seizure occurs.

E. Postprocedure: Follow facility protocols
　1. The client is transported to a recovery room with the blood pressure cuff and oximeter in place, where oxygen, suction, and other emergency equipment are available.
　2. Client wakes up about 15 minutes after procedure.
　3. When the client is awake, talk to the client and take vital signs.
　4. The client may be confused and disoriented for several hours; provide frequent orientation (brief, distinct, and simple) and reassurance.
　5. The client returns to the nursing unit when at least a 90% oxygen saturation level is maintained, vital signs are stable, and mental status is satisfactory.
　6. Check for a gag reflex before giving the client fluids, food, or medication.

F. Potential side effects
　1. Include confusion, disorientation, and short-term memory loss.
　2. The client may be confused and disoriented when awakening.
　3. Other side effects include headache, hypotension, muscle soreness, nausea, and tachycardia.
　4. Memory deficits may occur, but memory usually recovers completely, although some clients have memory loss lasting 6 months.

⚠ Monitor both a depressed client and a client who has recently been prescribed an antidepressant medication closely for signs of suicidal ideation. If the client presents with increased energy, monitor closely because it could mean that the client now has the energy to perform the suicide act.

XII. Schizophrenia

A. Description
　1. Schizophrenia is a group of mental health problems characterized by psychotic features

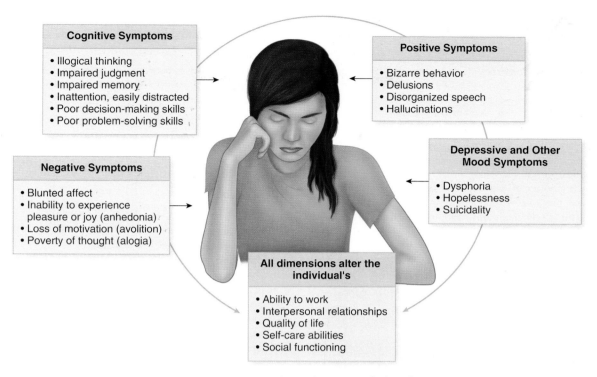

Cognitive Symptoms

- Illogical thinking
- Impaired judgment
- Impaired memory
- Inattention, easily distracted
- Poor decision-making skills
- Poor problem-solving skills

Positive Symptoms

- Bizarre behavior
- Delusions
- Disorganized speech
- Hallucinations

Negative Symptoms

- Blunted affect
- Inability to experience pleasure or joy (anhedonia)
- Loss of motivation (avolition)
- Poverty of thought (alogia)

Depressive and Other Mood Symptoms

- Dysphoria
- Hopelessness
- Suicidality

All dimensions alter the individual's

- Ability to work
- Interpersonal relationships
- Quality of life
- Self-care abilities
- Social functioning

FIGURE 62.1 Treatment-relevant dimensions of schizophrenia.

(hallucinations and delusions), disordered thought processes, and disrupted interpersonal relationships.

2. Disturbances in affect, mood, behavior, and thought processes occur.

3. Treatment with medication controls abnormal motor activity and other symptoms associated with the mental health problem.

B. Data collection (Fig. 62.1)

1. Physical characteristics

a. Unkempt appearance; may neglect hygiene, eating, sleeping, and elimination

b. Body image distortions

c. May be preoccupied with somatic complaints

2. Motor activity

a. Catatonic posturing: Holding bizarre postures for long periods

b. Catatonic excitement: Moving excitedly with no environmental stimuli present

c. Waxy flexibility: Having one's arms or legs placed in a certain position and holding that same position for hours

d. Possible total immobilization

e. Inability to respond to commands or responding only to commands

f. Echolalia: Repeating the speech of another person

g. Repetitive or stereotyped movements

h. Echopraxia: Repeating the movements of another person

i. Motor activity that may be increased as evidenced by agitation, pacing, inability to sleep, loss of appetite and weight, and impulsiveness

j. Possible inability to initiate activity (anergia)

3. Emotional characteristics

a. Mistrust may be present.

b. View of the world as threatening and unsafe

c. Affect may be blunted, flat, or inappropriate.

d. May display feelings of ambivalence, helplessness, anxiety, anger, guilt, or depression in response to hallucinations, delusions, or as a result of the grief related to losses imposed by this illness

4. Compulsive rituals: Performed as an attempt to solve conflicting feelings by constant, repetitive activity

5. Overcompliance: Attempt to deny responsibility for any action by doing only what another instructs exactly

6. Affective disturbances

a. Flat or incongruent affect or inappropriate affect

b. Altered thought processes

7. Abnormal thought processes (Box 62.8)

a. Impaired reality testing

b. Fragmentation of thoughts

c. Thought blocking

d. Loose associations

e. Echolalia: pathological repeating of another's words

f. Distorted perception of the environment

g. Neologisms: Made-up words that have meaning only to the client

h. Magical thinking

i. Inability to conceptualize meaning in words or thoughts

BOX 62.8   Abnormal Thought Processes

Description

Abnormal thought processes displayed by a client with a mental health problem

Types

Circumstantiality

Before getting to the point or answering a question, the individual gets caught up in countless details and explanations.

Confabulation

Filling a memory gap with detailed fantasy believed by the teller. The purpose of confabulation is to maintain self-esteem. This is seen in organic conditions such as Korsakoff's psychosis.

Flight of Ideas

A constant flow of speech in which the individual jumps from one topic to another in rapid succession. A connection between topics exists, although it is sometimes difficult to identify. This is seen in manic states.

Looseness of Association

Haphazard, illogical, and confused thinking and interrupted connections in thought. This is seen mostly in schizophrenic disorders.

Neologisms

Words that an individual makes up that only have meaning for the individual. This is often part of a delusional system.

Thought Blocking

A sudden cessation of a thought in the middle of a sentence; the client is unable to continue the train of thought. Often sudden new thoughts come up unrelated to the topic.

Word Salad

A mixture of words and phrases that have no meaning

BOX 62.9   Delusions

Description

A false belief held to be true even when there is evidence to the contrary.

Types

Grandeur

The false belief that one is a powerful and important person.

Jealousy

The false belief that one's partner or mate is being unfaithful.

Persecution

The thought that one is being singled out for harm by others.

Interventions

Ask the client to describe the delusion.

Be open and honest during interactions to reduce suspiciousness.

Focus the conversation on reality-based topics rather than the delusion.

Encourage the client to express feelings and focus on the feelings that the delusions generate.

If the client obsesses on the delusion, set firm limits on the amount of time for talking about the delusion.

Do not argue with the client or try to convince him or her that the delusions are false.

Validate if part of the delusion is real.

---

    j. Inability to organize facts logically

    k. Delusions associated with thought processes or content

  8. Types of delusions (Box 62.9)

    a. Loss of reference, in which the client believes that certain events, situations, or interactions, are related directly to self

    b. Delusions of persecution, in which the client believes that she or he is being harassed, threatened, or persecuted by some powerful force

    c. Delusions of grandeur, in which the client attaches special significance to self in relation to others or the universe, and has an exaggerated sense of self that has no basis in reality

    d. Somatic delusions, in which the client believes that her or his body is changing or responding in an unusual way, which has no basis in reality

  9. Perceptual distortions

    a. Illusions that may be brief experiences with a misinterpretation or misperception of reality

    b. Hallucinations (five senses) such as perceiving objects, sensations, or images with no basis in reality (Box 62.10)

  10. Language and communication disturbances (Box 62.11)

    a. Related to disorders in thought process

    b. Inability to organize language

    c. Inappropriate response to a situation

    d. A single word or phrase that may represent the whole meaning of the conversation such that the client may feel that he or she has communicated adequately

    e. Development of a private language

    f. Difficulty in communicating clearly

C. Interventions: Schizophrenia (Box 62.12)

D. Interventions: Active hallucinations

  1. Monitor for hallucination cues and assess content of hallucinations.

  2. Intervene with one-on-one contact.

  3. Decrease stimuli or move the client to another area.

  4. Avoid conveying to the client that others are also experiencing the hallucination.

  5. Respond verbally to anything real that the client talks about.

  6. Avoid touching the client.

  7. Encourage the client to express feelings.

  8. During a hallucination, attempt to engage the client's attention through a concrete activity.

BOX 62.10   Hallucinations

Description

A sense (occurs with one of the five senses) perception for which no external stimuli exist. This can have an organic or functional cause.

Types

Auditory

Hearing voices when none are present.

Gustatory

Experiencing taste in the absence of stimuli.

Olfactory

Smelling smells that do not exist.

Tactile

Feeling touch sensations in the absence of stimuli.

Visual

Seeing things that are not there.

Interventions

Ask the client directly about the hallucination.

Avoid reacting to the hallucination as if it were real.

Decrease stimuli or move the client to another area.

Do not negate the client's experience.

Focus on reality-based topics.

Attempt to engage the client's attention through a concrete activity.

Respond verbally to anything real that the client talks about.

Avoid touching the client.

Monitor for signs of increasing anxiety or agitation, which may indicate that the hallucinations are increasing.

BOX 62.11   Language and Communication Disturbances

Alogia (poverty of speech): Reduced volume or lack of spontaneous comments and overly brief responses

Associative looseness: Confused thinking that is manifested as illogical speech and reasoning that is not bound to reality.

Clang association: Repetition of words or phrases that are similar in sound but in no other way

Echolalia: Repetition of words or phrases heard from another person

Mutism: Absence of verbal speech

Neologism: A new word devised that has special meaning only to the client

Pressured speech: Speaking as if the words are being forced out quickly

Religiosity: Excessive preoccupation with religious ideas

Tangentiality: Digression from one topic to another without ever completing the thought or reaching a conclusion

Verbigeration: Purposeless repetition of words or phrases

Word salad (Schizophasia): Form of speech in which words or phrases are connected meaninglessly

BOX 62.12   Interventions for Schizophrenia

Assess the client's physical needs.

Set limits on the client's behaviors when it interferes with others and becomes disruptive.

Maintain a safe environment.

Initiate one-on-one interaction and progress to small groups as tolerated.

Spend time with the client even if he or she is unable to respond.

Monitor for altered thought processes.

Maintain ego boundaries and avoid touching the client.

Avoid an overly warm approach. A neutral approach is less threatening.

Do not make promises to the client that cannot be kept.

Establish daily routines.

Assist the client to improve grooming and accept responsibility for personal care.

Sit with the client in silence if necessary.

Provide brief and frequent contact with the client.

Tell the client when you are leaving.

Tell the client when you do not understand.

Do not "go along" with the client's delusions or hallucinations.

Provide simple, concrete activities, such as puzzles or word games.

Reorient the client as necessary.

Help the client establish what is real and unreal.

Stay with the client if he or she is frightened.

Speak to the client in a simple, direct, and concise manner.

Reassure the client that the environment is safe.

Remove the client from group situations if the client's behavior is too bizarre, disturbing, or dangerous to others.

Set realistic goals.

Initially, do not offer choices to the client, and gradually assist him or her in making decisions.

Use canned or packaged food, especially with the paranoid schizophrenic client.

Provide a music device at night for insomnia.

Decrease excessive stimuli in the environment.

Monitor for suicide risk.

Assist the client to use alternative means to express feelings through music or art therapy or writing.

9. Accept and do not joke about or judge the client's behavior.
10. Provide easy activities and a structured environment with routine activities of daily living.
11. Monitor for signs of increasing fear, anxiety, or agitation.
12. Decrease stimuli as needed.
13. Administer medications as prescribed.

⚠ For a client with hallucinations, safety is the first priority. Ensure that the client does not have an auditory command telling him or her to harm self or others.

E Interventions: Delusions
1. Interact based on reality.
2. Encourage the client to express feelings.
3. Do not dispute the client or try to convince the client that delusions are false.
4. Initially, begin activities on a one-on-one basis.
5. Alter hospital routines as necessary, such as using canned or packaged food or food from home.
6. Recognize accomplishments and provide positive feedback for success.

XIII. Personality Disorders

A. Description
1. Personality disorders involve the consistent expression of various inflexible maladaptive behavior patterns or traits that may impair functioning and relationships.
2. The client usually remains in touch with reality and typically has a lack of insight in self-identity and interpersonal behavior (empathy or intimacy).
3. Stress exacerbates manifestations of the personality disorder.
4. Not directly associated with the effects of substance misuse or a general medical condition, such as severe head injury

B. Characteristics
1. Poor impulse control:
   a. Acting out to manage internal pain
   b. Forms of acting out include physical and verbal attacks, such as yelling and swearing, and self-injurious behaviors, such as cutting own skin, banging the head, punching self, manipulation, substance abuse, promiscuous sexual behaviors, and **suicide attempts**.
   c. The client may be preoccupied with such things as self, religion, or sex.
2. Mood characteristics
   a. May experience abandonment and depression
   b. Moods may include rage, guilt, fear, and emptiness.
3. Impaired judgment
   a. Difficulty with problem solving
   b. Inability to perceive the consequences of behavior
4. Impaired reality testing: Distortion of reality and often projection of own feelings onto others
5. Impaired object relations: Rigid and inflexible, with difficulty in intimate relationships
6. Impaired self-perception: Distorted self-perception and experience of self-hate or self-idealization
7. Impaired thought processes
   a. Difficulty concentrating
   b. Impaired memory
   c. Concrete or diffuse thinking

8. Impaired stimulus barrier
   a. Inability to regulate incoming sensory stimuli
   b. Increased excitability
   c. Poor attention span
   d. Excessive response to noise and light
   e. Agitation
   f. Insomnia

C. Cluster A personality disorders types include the odd types: schizoid, schizotypal, and paranoid.
1. Schizoid personality disorder is characterized by an inability to form warm, close social relationships.
   a. Social detachment and lack of close relationships
   b. Interest in solitary activities
   c. Aloofness and indifference
   d. Restricted expression of emotions
   e. Lack of interest in others
2. Schizotypal personality disorder is characterized by the display of abnormal or highly unusual thoughts, perceptions, speech, and behavior patterns.
   a. Suspiciousness and paranoia
   b. Unable to understand how behaviors impact others
   c. Eccentricity
   d. Magical thinking
   e. Odd thinking and speech
   f. Relationship deficits
   g. Blunted affect
   h. Reclusiveness
3. Paranoid personality disorder is characterized by suspiciousness and mistrust of others (Box 62.13).
   a. May be suspicious and distrusting
   b. May be argumentative
   c. May be hostile or aloof
   d. May be rigid, critical, and controlling of others
   e. May have thoughts of grandiosity

⚠ Do not whisper or laugh in front of a client with a paranoid disorder because the client will think that you are talking about or laughing at him or her; this increases the paranoia.

D. Cluster B personality disorders include the dramatic, emotional, erratic types: histrionic, narcissistic, borderline, and antisocial.
1. Histrionic personality disorder is characterized by overly dramatic and intensely expressive behavior.
   a. Lively and dramatic and enjoys being the center of attention
   b. Has poor and shallow interpersonal relationships
   c. May be sexually seductive or provocative
   d. Dramatizes her or his life and may appear theatrical
   e. Overly concerned with appearance
   f. Easily bored

BOX 62.13 Interventions for Paranoia

Assess for suicide risk.
Diminish suspicious behavior.
Avoid direct eye contact.
Establish a trusting relationship.
Turn off television, radios, and computer screens.
Promote increased self-esteem.
Remain calm, nonthreatening, and nonjudgmental.
Provide continuity of care.
Respond honestly to the client.
Follow through on commitments made to the client.
Acknowledge the client's feelings, but tell him or her that you do not share his or her interpretation of an event.
Provide a daily schedule of activities.
Assist the client to identify diversionary activities.
Gradually introduce the client to groups.
Refocus conversation to reality-based topics.
Use role playing to help the client identify thoughts and feelings.
Provide positive reinforcement for successes.
Do not argue with delusions.
Use concrete, specific words.
Do not be secretive with the client.
Do not whisper in the client's presence.
Assure the client that he or she will be safe.
Involve the client in noncompetitive tasks.
Provide the client opportunity to complete small tasks.
Monitor eating, drinking, sleeping, and elimination patterns.
Limit physical contact.
Monitor for agitation and decrease stimuli as needed.

2. Narcissistic personality disorder is characterized by an increased sense of self-importance, preoccupation with fantasies and a sense of unlimited success.
   a. Need for admiration and inflation of accomplishments
   b. Overestimation of abilities and underestimations of contributions of others
   c. Lack of empathy and sensitivity to others
3. Borderline personality disorder is characterized by instability in interpersonal relationships, unstable mood and self-image, and impulsive and unpredictable behavior.
   a. Poor self-regard or unstable self-image
   b. Lack of self-direction
   c. Unstable or intense personal relationships
   d. Lack of empathy toward the needs and feelings of others
   e. Extreme shifts in mood
   f. Impulsive
   g. Engages in risk-taking behaviors
   h. Argumentative and hostile in response to perceived slights or insults
   i. Depression
   j. Manipulation

   k. Intense feelings of anxiety in response to stress
   l. Chronic feelings of emptiness and intense fear of being rejected
   m. Splitting: sees others as all good or all bad; creates conflict between individuals by playing one person against another
4. Antisocial personality disorder is comprised of a pattern of irresponsible and antisocial behavior, selfishness, an inability to maintain lasting relationships, poor sexual adjustment, a failure to accept social norms, and a tendency toward irritability and aggressiveness.
   a. Perceives the world as hostile
   b. Lack of empathy and feelings of remorse
   c. Egocentrism; focused on personal gratification
   d. Deceitful and manipulative
   e. Irresponsible
   f. Impulsive and engages in risk-taking behaviors
   g. Persistent or frequent feelings of anger
   h. Refusal to conform to social rules and normative behavior

E. Cluster C personality disorders include the anxious, fearful types of personality disorders: obsessive-compulsive personality, avoidant, and dependent.
   1. Obsessive-compulsive personality disorder is characterized by difficulty expressing warm and tender emotions, perfectionism, stubbornness, the need to control others, and a devotion to work.
      a. Perfectionist with unreasonably high expectations of self
      b. Inflexible and preoccupied with details and rules
      c. Sense of self derived primarily from work
      d. Social and personal relationships viewed as secondary to work and productivity
      e. Difficulty understanding the ideas, feelings, and behaviors of others
      f. Engages in rituals
   2. Avoidant personality disorder is characterized by social withdrawal and extreme sensitivity to potential rejection.
      a. Feelings of inadequacy
      b. Hypersensitive to reactions of others and poor reactions to criticism
      c. Social isolation
      d. Lack of support system
   3. Dependent personality disorder is characterized by intense lack of self-confidence and low self-esteem, and lack of ability to function independently, such that the individual passively allows others to make decisions and assume responsibility for major areas in the person's life. The dependent client has great difficulty making decisions.

F. General interventions for the client with a personality disorder
1. Maintain safety against self-destructive behaviors.
2. Allow the client to make choices and be as independent as possible.
3. Encourage the client to discuss feelings rather than act them out.
4. Ensure health care team is consistent with information and with responses to the client's acting-out behaviors.
5. Discuss expectations and responsibilities with the client.
6. Discuss the consequences that follow certain behaviors.
7. Inform the client that harm to self, others, and property is unacceptable.
8. Identify splitting behavior.
9. Assist the client with dealing directly with anger.
10. Encourage the client to keep a journal recording daily feelings.
11. Encourage the client to participate in group activities, and praise nonmanipulative behavior.
12. Set and maintain limits to decrease manipulative behavior.
13. Remove the client from group situations in which attention-seeking behaviors occur.
14. Provide realistic praise for positive behaviors in social situations.

XIV. Neurodevelopmental Disorders

A. Autism: Refer to Chapter 35.
B. Attention-deficit/hyperactivity disorder Refer to Chapter 35.

XV. Neurocognitive disorders

A. Dementia and Alzheimer's disease
1. Dementia
   a. Dementia is a syndrome with progressive deterioration in intellectual functioning; secondary to structural or functional changes.
   b. Long- and short-term memory losses occur with impairment in judgment, abstract thinking, problem-solving ability, and behavior.
   c. Dementia results in a self-care deficit.
   d. Dementia-like symptoms can be a result of physiological conditions, and such conditions must be ruled out initially.
   e. The most common type of dementia is Alzheimer's disease.
2. Alzheimer's disease (Box 62.14)
   a. Alzheimer's disease is an irreversible form of senile dementia from nerve cell deterioration.

BOX 62.14	Alzheimer's Disease

Agnosia: Failure to recognize or identify objects despite intact sensory function
Amnesia: Loss of memory caused by brain degeneration
Aphasia: Language disturbance in understanding and expressing the spoken word
Apraxia: Inability to perform motor activities despite intact motor function

---

   b. Individuals with Alzheimer's disease experience cognitive deterioration and progressive loss of ability to carry out activities of daily living.
   c. The client experiences a steady decline in physical and mental functioning and usually requires long-term care facility placement in the final stages of the illness.
   d. Stages and major characteristics of Alzheimer's disease: stage 1 (mild): forgetfulness; stage 2 (moderate): confusion; stage 3 (moderate to severe): ambulatory dementia; and stage 4 (late): end stage.
3. Interventions
   a. Identify and reinforce retained skills.
   b. Provide continuity of care.
   c. Orient the client to the environment.
   d. Furnish the environment with familiar possessions.
   e. Acknowledge the client's feelings.
   f. Help the client and family members manage memory deficits and behavior changes.
   g. Encourage the family members to express feelings about caregiving.
   h. Provide the caregiver support and identify the resources and support groups available.
   i. Monitor activities of daily living.
   j. Remind the client how to perform self-care activities.
   k. Help the client maintain independence.
   l. Provide the client with consistent routines.
   m. Provide exercise such as walking with an escort.
   n. Avoid activities that tax the memory.
   o. Allow the client plenty of time to complete a task.
   p. Use constant encouragement in a simple step-by-step approach.
   q. Provide activities that distract and occupy time, such as listening to music, coloring, and watching television.
   r. Provide the client with mental stimulation with simple games or activities.
4. Wandering
   a. Provide a safe environment free of clutter and hazardous items.

b. Provide safe ambulation, including comfortable and well-fitting shoes, mobility aids.
c. Provide close and frequent supervision.
d. Close and secure doors.
e. Use identification bracelets and electronic surveillance.
f. Encourage rest periods in the afternoon, because wandering worsens at night.
g. Provide regular supervised exercise or walking programs.
h. Sundown syndrome (sundowning) is characterized by a pronounced increase in symptoms and problem behaviors in the evening.

⚠ Providing a safe environment is a priority in the care of a client with Alzheimer's disease.

5. Communication disorders
   a. Disorders include language disorder (expressive–receptive disorder), speech sound disorder (phonological disorder), childhood-onset fluency disorder (stuttering disorder), and social communication disorder (impaired social communication).
   b. Adapt to the communication level of the client.
   c. Pay attention to nonverbal cues.
   d. Use a firm volume and a low-pitched voice to communicate.
   e. Stand directly in front of the client and maintain eye contact.
   f. Give ample time for the client to respond.
   g. Use a calm and reassuring voice; do not speak loudly unless the client is hearing impaired.
   h. Use pantomime gestures if the client is unable to understand spoken words.
   i. Speak slowly and clearly, using short words and simple sentences.
   j. Ask only one question at a time and give one direction at a time.
   k. Repeat questions if necessary but do not rephrase.
   l. Provide alternative means of communication.
   m. Minimize external noise or distractions when communicating.
6. Impaired judgment
   a. Remove throw rugs, toxic substances, and dangerous electrical appliances from the environment.
   b. Reduce hot water heater temperature.
7. Altered thought processes
   a. Call the client by name.
   b. Orient the client frequently.
   c. Use familiar objects in the room.
   d. Place a calendar and clock in a visible place.
   e. Maintain familiar routines.
   f. Allow the client to reminisce.
   g. Make tasks simple.

h. Allow time for the client to complete a task.
i. Provide positive reinforcement for positive behaviors.
8. Altered sleep patterns
   a. Allow the client to wander in a safe place until he or she becomes tired.
   b. Prevent shadows in the room by using indirect light.
   c. Avoid the use of hypnotics because they cause confusion and aggravate the sundown effect.
9. Agitation
   a. Assess the precipitant of the agitation.
   b. Reassure the client.
   c. Remove items that can be hazardous during the time of agitation.
   d. Approach the client slowly and calmly from the front, and then speak, gesture, and move slowly.
   e. Remove client to a less stressful environment; decrease excess stimuli.
   f. Use touch gently.
   g. Do not argue with the client or force client to do something.

WHAT WOULD YOU DO?

Answer: If a client is actively hallucinating, the nurse would intervene with one-on-one contact. The nurse would ask the client directly about the hallucination and avoid reacting to the hallucination as if it were real. The nurse would decrease stimuli or move the client to another area and avoid indicating to the client that others also are experiencing the hallucination. The nurse would encourage the client to express feelings, focus on reality-based topics, and respond verbally to anything real that the client talks about. The nurse also avoids touching the client. During a hallucination, the nurse also would attempt to engage the client's attention through a concrete activity and monitor for signs of increasing anxiety or agitation, which may indicate that the hallucinations are increasing.

PRACTICE QUESTIONS

1. A client with delirium becomes agitated and confused at night. The **best initial** intervention by the nurse is which action?
   1. Move the client next to the nurse's station.
   2. Use a night light and turn off the television.
   3. Keep the television and a soft light on during the night.
   4. Play soft music during the night and maintain a well-lit room.

2. The nurse is collecting data on a client who is actively hallucinating. Which nursing statement would be therapeutic at this time?

1. "I know you feel 'they are out to get you,' but it's not true."
2. "I can hear the voice, and she wants you to come to dinner."
3. "Sometimes people hear things or voices others can't hear."
4. "I talked to the voices you're hearing and they won't hurt you now."

3. The nurse is caring for a client with a diagnosis of depression. The nurse monitors for signs of constipation and urinary retention, knowing that these problems are likely caused by which situation?
   1. Poor dietary choices
   2. Lack of exercise and poor diet
   3. Inadequate dietary intake and dehydration
   4. Psychomotor retardation and side effects of medication

4. A client is admitted to the inpatient unit and is being considered for electroconvulsive therapy (ECT). The client appears calm, but the family is hypervigilant and anxious. The client's mother begins to cry and states, "My child's brain will be destroyed. How can the doctor do this?" The nurse would make which therapeutic response?
   1. "It sounds as though you need to speak to the psychiatrist."
   2. "Perhaps you'd like to see the ECT room and speak to the staff."
   3. "Your child has decided to have this treatment. You should be supportive of the decision."
   4. "It sounds as though you have some concerns about the ECT procedure. Why don't we sit down together and discuss any concerns you may have?"

❖ 5. Which nursing interventions are appropriate for a hospitalized client with mania who is exhibiting manipulative behavior? **Select all that apply.**
   ❏ 1. Communicate expected behaviors to the client.
   ❏ 2. Follow through about the consequences of behavior in a nonpunitive manner.
   ❏ 3. Ensure that the client knows that he or she is not in charge of the nursing unit.
   ❏ 4. Assist the client with developing a means of setting limits on personal behavior.
   ❏ 5. Enforce rules and inform the client that he or she will not be allowed to attend therapy groups.
   ❏ 6. Be clear with the client regarding the consequences of exceeding limits set regarding behavior.

6. The nurse is preparing for the hospital discharge of a client with a history of command hallucinations to harm self or others. The nurse instructs the client about interventions for hallucinations and anxiety and determines that the client understands the interventions when the client makes which statement?
   1. "My medications won't make me anxious."
   2. "I'll go to a support group and talk so that I won't hurt anyone."
   3. "I won't get anxious or hear things if I get enough sleep and eat well."
   4. "I can call my therapist when I'm hallucinating so I can talk about my feelings and plans and not hurt anyone."

7. The nurse observes that a client is psychotic, pacing, and agitated and is making aggressive gestures. The client's speech pattern is rapid, and the client's effect is belligerent. Based on these observations, which is the nurse's **immediate priority** of care?
   1. Provide safety for the client and other clients on the unit.
   2. Provide the clients on the unit with a sense of comfort and safety.
   3. Assist the staff with caring for the client in a controlled environment.
   4. Offer the client a less-stimulating area to calm down and gain control.

8. The nurse is caring for a client diagnosed with catatonic stupor. The client is lying on the bed, with the body pulled into a fetal position. Which is the appropriate nursing intervention?
   1. Ask direct questions to encourage talking.
   2. Leave the client alone and intermittently check on them.
   3. Sit beside the client in silence and verbalize occasional open-ended questions.
   4. Take the client into the dayroom with other clients so they can help watch him.

9. A mother of a teenage client with an anxiety disorder is concerned about her daughter's progress during discharge. She states that her daughter "stashes food, eats all the wrong things that make her hyperactive," and "hangs out with the wrong crowd." While helping the mother prepare for her daughter's discharge, the nurse would make which suggestion?
   1. The mother should restrict the daughter's socializing time with her friends.
   2. The mother should restrict the amount of chocolate and caffeine products in the home.
   3. The mother should keep her daughter out of school until she can adjust to the school environment.
   4. The mother should consider taking time off of work to help her daughter readjust to the home environment.

10. A client is unwilling to leave the house for fear of "doing something crazy in public." Because of this fear, the client remains homebound except when accompanied outside by the spouse. The spouse asks the nurse, "What is the name of my wife's disorder?" Which answer would the nurse give to the spouse?
1. Agoraphobia
2. Hematophobia
3. Claustrophobia
4. Hypochondriasis

11. A client has reported that crying spells have been a major problem over the past several weeks and that the doctor said depression is probably the reason. The nurse observes that the client is sitting slumped in the chair, and the clothes that the client is wearing do not fit well. The nurse interprets that further data collection would focus on which assessment?
1. Weight loss
2. Sleep pattern
3. Medication compliance
4. Onset of the crying spells

12. A client was admitted to a medical unit with acute blindness. Many tests are performed, and there seems to be no organic reason why this client cannot see. The nurse later learns that the client became blind after witnessing a hit-and-run car crash in which a family of three was killed. The nurse suspects that the client may be experiencing which diagnosis?
1. Psychosis
2. Repression
3. Conversion disorder
4. Dissociative disorder

13. A manic client announces to everyone in the dayroom that a stripper is coming to perform that evening. When the psychiatric nurse's aide firmly states that the client's behavior is not appropriate, the manic client becomes verbally abusive and threatens physical violence to the nurse's aide. Based on the analysis of this situation, the nurse determines that the appropriate action would be which intervention?
1. Escort the manic client to his or her room.
2. Orient the client to time, person, and place.
3. Tell the client that the behavior is not appropriate.
4. Tell the client that smoking privileges are revoked for 24 hours.

14. The nurse notes documentation in a client's record that the client is experiencing delusions of persecution. The nurse recognizes that these types of delusions are characteristic of which thoughts?
1. The false belief that one is a very powerful person
2. The false belief that one is a very important person
3. The false belief that one's partner is being unfaithful
4. The false belief that one is being singled out for harm by others

15. A client who is diagnosed with pedophilia and recently has been paroled as a sex offender says, "I'm in treatment and I have served my time. Now this group has posters all over the neighborhood with my photograph and details of my crime." Which is an appropriate response by the nurse?
1. "When children are hurt the way you hurt them, people want you isolated."
2. "You're lucky it doesn't escalate into something pretty scary after your crime."
3. "You understand that people fear for their children, but you're feeling unfairly treated?"
4. "You seem angry, but you have committed serious crimes against several children, so your neighbors are frightened."

ANSWERS

1. 2

Rationale: It is important to provide a consistent daily routine and a low-stimulation environment when the client is agitated and confused. Noise levels, including a radio and television, may add to the confusion and disorientation. Moving the client next to the nurses' station is not the initial intervention.

Test-Taking Strategy: Note the strategic words, *best* and *initial*, in the question. Eliminate options 3 and 4 first because they are comparable or alike. From the remaining options, recalling that a low-stimulation environment is best will direct you to option 2.

2. 3

Rationale: It is important for the nurse to reinforce reality with the client. Options 1, 2, and 4 do not reinforce reality but reinforce the hallucination that the voices are real.

Test-Taking Strategy: Focus on the subject, hallucinations, and note that options 1, 2, and 4 all indicate reinforcement to the client that the voices are real. Option 3 is the only statement that indicates reality.

3. 4

Rationale: In this situation, urinary retention is most likely caused by medications. Option 4 is the only option that addresses both constipation and urinary retention. Constipation can be related to inadequate food intake, lack of exercise, and poor diet.

Test-Taking Strategy: Note that the question addresses both constipation and urinary retention. Options 1, 2, and 3 are all comparable or alike and address diet. Option 4 addresses both concerns of constipation and urinary retention.

4. 4

Rationale: The nurse needs to encourage the family and client to verbalize their fears and concerns. Option 4 is the only option that encourages verbalization. Options 1, 2, and 3 avoid dealing with the client or family concerns.

Test-Taking Strategy: Focus on the subject, a therapeutic response. Use therapeutic communication techniques and focus on the client's and family's feelings and concerns. This will direct you to the correct option.

❖ **5. 1, 2, 4, 6**

Rationale: Interventions for dealing with the client exhibiting manipulative behavior include setting clear, consistent, and enforceable limits on manipulative behaviors; being clear with the client regarding the consequences of exceeding limits set; following through with the consequences in a nonpunitive manner; and assisting the client with developing a means for setting limits on personal behaviors. Enforcing rules and informing the client that he or she will not be allowed to attend therapy groups are violations of a client's rights. Ensuring that the client knows that he or she is not in charge of the nursing unit is inappropriate; power struggles need to be avoided.

Test-Taking Strategy: Focus on the subject, manipulative behavior. Recalling clients' rights and that power struggles need to be avoided will assist with selecting the correct interventions.

6. 4

Rationale: There may be an increased risk for impulsive and/or aggressive behavior if a client is receiving command hallucinations to harm self or others. Talking about the auditory hallucinations can interfere with the subvocal muscular activity associated with a hallucination. Option 4 is a specific agreement to seek help and evidences self-responsible commitment and control over his or her own behavior.

Test-Taking Strategy: Focus on the subject, hallucinations to harm self or others. Note the relationship between the word, *hallucinations,* in the question and the information in the correct option.

7. 1

Rationale: Safety of the client and other clients is the priority. Option 1 is the only option that addresses the client and other clients' safety needs. Option 2 addresses other clients' needs. Option 3 is not client centered. Option 4 addresses the client's needs.

Test-Taking Strategy: Note the strategic words, *immediate priority,* and focus on the subject, safety. Option 1 is the umbrella option and addresses the safety of all.

8. 3

Rationale: Clients with catatonic stupor may be immobile and mute and may require consistent, repeated approaches. The nurse facilitates communication with the client by sitting in silence, asking open-ended questions, and pausing to pro-

vide opportunities for the client to respond. The nurse would not leave the client alone. Fortunately, with pharmacotherapy and improved individual management, severe catatonic symptoms rarely occur. Option 4 relies on other clients to care for this one, which is an inappropriate expectation. Asking direct questions of this client is not therapeutic. Option 3 is the best action because it provides for client supervision and communication as appropriate.

Test-Taking Strategy: Focus on the subject, catatonic stupor. Eliminate option 1 because asking direct questions of this client is not therapeutic. Eliminate option 2 because the nurse would not leave the client alone. Eliminate option 4 next because this action relies on other clients to care for this one.

9. 2

Rationale: Clients with anxiety disorder need to abstain from or limit their intake of caffeine, chocolate, and alcohol. These products have the potential of increasing anxiety. Options 1 and 3 are unreasonable and are an unhealthy approach. It may not be realistic for a family member to take time away from work.

Test-Taking Strategy: Options 1, 3, and 4 are comparable or alike and are concerned with monitoring or curtailing the client's physical activities. Option 2 addresses preparation of the client's environment and focuses on the concern or subject expressed in the question.

10. 1

Rationale: Agoraphobia is a fear of being alone in open or public places where escape might be difficult. Agoraphobia includes experiencing fear or a sense of helplessness or embarrassment if a phobic attack occurs. Avoidance of such situations usually results in the reduction of social and professional interactions. Hematophobia is the fear of blood. Claustrophobia is a fear of closed-in places. Clients with somatic symptom disorder focus their anxiety on physical complaints and are preoccupied with their health.

Test-Taking Strategy: Focus on the data in the question, client is unwilling to go out of the house. Recalling the specific types of phobias and associated client behaviors will direct you to the correct option.

11. 1

Rationale: All the options are possible issues to address; however, the weight loss is the first item that needs further data collection because ill-fitting clothing could indicate a problem with nutrition. The client has already told the nurse that the crying spells have been a problem. Medication or sleep patterns are not mentioned or addressed in the question.

Test-Taking Strategy: Use Maslow's Hierarchy of Needs Theory to answer the question. Focusing on the data in the question will assist in eliminating the incorrect options.

12. 3

Rationale: A conversion disorder is the alteration or loss of a physical function that cannot be explained by any known pathophysiological mechanism. It is thought to be an expression of a psychological need or conflict. In this situation, the client witnessed an accident that was so psychologically painful that the client became blind. A dissociative disorder is a disturbance or alteration in the normally integrative functions of identity, memory, or consciousness. Psychosis is a state in which a person's mental capacity to recognize reality, communicate, and relate to others is impaired, thus interfering with the person's capacity to deal with life's demands. Repression is a coping mechanism in which unacceptable feelings are kept out of awareness.

Test-Taking Strategy: Focus on the subject, blindness with no organic reason. Noting that the client evidences no organic reason to account for the blindness will direct you to the correct option.

13. 1

Rationale: The client is at risk for injury to self and others and therefore would be escorted out of the dayroom. Option 4 may increase the agitation that already exists in this client. Orientation will not halt the behavior. Telling the client that the behavior is not appropriate has already been attempted by the psychiatric nurse's aide.

Test-Taking Strategy: Focus on the data in the question and the subject, therapeutic interventions for the manic client. Options 2, 3, and 4 will not deescalate the client's agitation.

14. 4

Rationale: A delusion is a false belief held to be true even when there is evidence to the contrary. A delusion of persecution is the thought that one is being singled out for harm by others. A delusion of grandeur is the false belief that he or she is a very powerful and important person. A delusion of jealousy is the false belief that one's partner is being unfaithful.

Test-Taking Strategy: Eliminate options 1 and 2 first because they are comparable or alike. From the remaining options, note the relationship between the word, *persecution*, in the question and the description in option 4.

15. 3

Rationale: Focusing and verbalizing the implied concern is the therapeutic response because it assists the client to clarify thinking and to reexamine what the client is really saying. Option 3 is the only option that reflects the use of this therapeutic communication technique. Option 1 is insensitive and anxiety-provoking. Option 2 gives advice and does not facilitate the client's expression of feelings. Option 4 does not facilitate the client's expression of feelings.

Test-Taking Strategy: Use therapeutic communication techniques to answer the question. Remembering to focus on the client's feelings and concerns will direct you to the correct option.

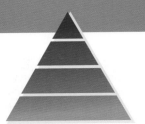

CHAPTER **63**

Mental Health

Addictions

PRIORITY CONCEPTS **Addiction; Coping**

The nurse notes that a client is experiencing signs of alcohol withdrawal delirium. What would the nurse do?
Answer is located on p. 888.

I. **Eating Disorders**

A. Description: Characterized by uncertain selfidentification and grossly disturbed eating habits

B. Compulsive overeating
1. Compulsive overeating is binge-like overeating without purging.
2. Food consumption is out of the individual's control and occurs in a stereotyped fashion.
3. Repulsed by eating, that is, the eating relieves tension but does not produce pleasure
4. Aware that eating patterns are abnormal and feels depressed after eating
5. Eats secretly during a binge and consumes high-calorie and easily digestible food
6. Repeatedly tries to diet but without success
7. Feels helpless and hopeless about weight
8. Responds to feelings of guilt, anger, depression, boredom, loneliness, inadequacy, or ambivalence by eating

C. Anorexia nervosa
1. Description
   a. Onset often is associated with a stressful life event.
   b. Intensely fears obesity
   c. Body image is distorted, and a disturbed self-concept is common.
   d. Preoccupied with foods that prevent weight gain and has a phobia against foods that produce weight gain
   e. The eating disorder can be life-threatening.
   f. Death can occur from starvation, suicide, cardiomyopathies, or electrolyte imbalance.
2. Data collection
   a. Appetite loss and refusal to eat
   b. Appetite denial

c. Feelings of lack of control
d. Compulsive exercising
e. Overachiever and perfectionist
f. Physical alterations: Many occur and can include decreased temperature, pulse, and blood pressure; weight loss; gastrointestinal disturbances such as constipation; teeth and gum deterioration; esophageal varices from induced vomiting; electrolyte imbalances; dry, scaly skin; presence of lanugo on extremities; sleep disturbances; hormone deficiencies; amenorrhea for at least three consecutive menstrual periods; cyanosis and numbness of extremities; and bone degeneration.

D. Bulimia nervosa
1. Description
   a. Repeated episodes of excessive and uncontrollable consumption of large amounts of food (binges) followed by inappropriate compensatory actions such as self-induced vomiting, misuse of cathartics (e.g., laxatives), diuretics, and/or self-starvation
   b. Most clients remain within a normal weight range, but feel that their lives are dominated by the eating-related conflict.
2. Data collection
   a. Preoccupied with body shape and weight
   b. Preoccupation with thoughts of food
   c. Extreme fear of gaining weight
   d. Consumption of high-calorie foods in secret; guilt about secretive eating
   e. Binge-purge syndrome
   f. Attempts to lose weight through diets, vomiting, enemas, cathartics, and amphetamines or diuretics
   g. Monitor nutritional status and the severity of any medical problems
   h. Has need for control yet experiences feelings of powerlessness or loss of control
   i. Low self-esteem
   j. Poor interpersonal relationships
   k. Decreased or absent interest in sex

l. Mood swings
m. Electrolyte imbalances
n. Physical alterations: Similar to those that occur with anorexia nervosa
o. Important to ask questions about their perception of the problem and eating habits

E. Interventions: Clients with an eating disorder
1. Assess nutritional status and the severity of any medical problems.
2. Establish a one-to-one therapeutic relationship with the client; the nurse needs to establish trust and recognize any client reluctance to establish a relationship.
3. Establish a plan concerning the nutritional plan for the day.
4. Assist with identifying precipitants to the eating disorder.
5. Encourage the client to express feelings about the eating behavior and about how the client feels about his/her body.
6. Be accepting and nonjudgmental.
7. Work on exploring self-concept and establishing identity.
8. Implement behavior modification techniques.
9. Individual, group, and family therapy
10. If in a health care facility, supervise during mealtimes and for a specified period after meals and monitor intake and output; set a time limit for each meal and provide a pleasant, relaxed environment for eating.
11. Monitor for signs of physical complications related to the eating disorder.
12. When a client's weight is below ideal body weight, medical intervention is necessary.
13. Weigh daily at the same time, using the same scale, after the client voids (weighing each day may decrease anxiety for some clients); when weighing the client, ensure that the client is wearing the same clothing as when the previous weight was taken.
14. Monitor and restore fluid and electrolyte balance.
15. Monitor elimination patterns.
16. Monitor and limit the client's activity level (anorexia nervosa and bulimia nervosa).
17. Encourage the client to participate in diversional activities.
18. Assess suicidal potential.
19. Administer antidepressant medication if prescribed.
20. Encourage psychotherapy.
21. Refer the client to support groups.

II. Substance Use Disorders

A. Description: Substance use disorders (**addiction**) cause cognitive, behavioral, and physiological changes (Box 63.1).

BOX 63.1 CAGE Screening Test

C Have you ever felt the need to *cut down* on your drinking/drug use?
A Have you ever been *annoyed* by criticism of your drinking/drug use?
G Have you ever felt *guilty* about something you have done when you were drinking or taking drugs?
E Have you ever had an *eye opener*: drinking or taking drugs first thing in the morning to get going or to avoid withdrawal symptoms?

B. Substance dependence
1. Substance dependence is a pattern of repeated use of a substance, which usually results in tolerance, withdrawal symptoms, and compulsive drug-taking behavior.
2. Substances are taken in larger amounts and over longer periods than was intended.
3. There is a desire to cut down, but efforts to decrease or discontinue use are unsuccessful.
4. Daily activities revolve around the use of a substance.

⚠ Screening tools are available to assess a substance abuse disorder, such as the Michigan Alcohol Screening Test (MAST), Drug Abuse Screening Test (DAST), and CAGE screening questionnaire.

C. Substance tolerance refers to the need for increased amounts of the substance to achieve the desired effect.
D. Substance misuse
1. Uses substances recurrently
2. Recurrent, significant harmful consequences related to the use of substances are experienced.
3. Involvement with the legal system is common; the client may have legal issues to deal with and resolve.
E. Substance withdrawal
1. Physiological and substance-specific cognitive symptoms occur.
2. Substance withdrawal occurs when an individual experiences a decrease in blood levels of a substance on which the individual is physiologically dependent.
F. Other factors to consider in the client with a substance-related disorder
1. Rebellion and peer group pressure in adolescence may contribute to the onset of substance use.
2. Substance use may become a **coping mechanism** for decreasing physical and emotional pain.
3. Depression may precede or occur as a result of or in association with substance use.
4. Grief and loss may be associated with substance use.

G. Dysfunctional behaviors related to substance misuse
1. Preoccupation with obtaining and using substance
2. Manipulation to avoid consequences of behavior
3. Impulsiveness
4. Anger, including physical and verbal abuse
5. Avoidance of relationships outside the family unit
6. Relationships within the family become dysfunctional as the children take on atypical roles to protect family unit
7. Sense of self-importance and requiring special treatment
8. Denial; blaming everything but the substance use for his or her problems
9. Uses rationalization and projection to justify unacceptable behaviors
10. Low self-esteem
11. Depression
12. Codependency issues
    a. Codependency refers to the presence of coexisting behaviors present in a significant other, which serves to enable the addict or alcoholic to continue the irresponsible patterns of use without experiencing consequences.
    b. Examples of codependency: Paying bills for which the addict or alcoholic is responsible, bailing the addict or alcoholic out of jail, and helping the addict or alcoholic call in sick to their employment agency
    c. It is important to address codependency issues with the family to maximize the chance for recovery of the client with the addiction and the person with the codependent behaviors.

III. Alcohol Misuse

A. Description
1. Alcohol is a central nervous system (CNS) depressant affecting all body tissues.
2. Physical dependence is a biological need for alcohol to avoid physical withdrawal symptoms, whereas psychological dependence refers to craving for the subjective effect of alcohol.

B. Risk factors
1. Biological predisposition. Cultural, genetic and familial predisposition may be a risk factor.
2. Depressed and highly anxious characteristics
3. Low self-esteem
4. Poor self-control
5. History of rebelliousness, poor school performance, or delinquency
6. Poor parental relationships

C. Data collection
1. Slurred speech
2. Uncoordinated movements
3. Unsteady gait
4. Restlessness

5. Confusion
6. Sneaking drinks, drinking in the morning, and experiencing blackouts
7. Binge drinking
8. Arguments about drinking
9. Missing work
10. Increased tolerance to alcohol
11. Intoxication, with blood alcohol content (BAC) of 0.1% (100 mg alcohol/dL blood) or greater (legal BAC may vary state to state)

⚠ Part of data collection needs to include the type of alcohol, how much, for how long, and date and when last consumed.

D. Psychological symptoms
1. Depression
2. Irritable, belligerent, and hostile
3. Suspiciousness
4. Rationalization
5. Isolation
6. Decrease in inhibitions
7. Decrease in self-esteem
8. Denial that a problem exists

E. Complications associated with chronic alcohol use
1. Vitamin deficiencies
    a. Vitamin B deficiency causing peripheral neuropathies
    b. Thiamine deficiency causing Korsakoff's syndrome (a form of amnesia)
2. Alcohol-induced persistent amnesic disorder causing severe memory problems
3. Wernicke's encephalopathy (degenerative condition of the brain) causing confusion, ataxia, and abnormal eye movements
4. Hepatitis; cirrhosis of the liver
5. Esophagitis and gastritis
6. Pancreatitis
7. Anemia
8. Immune system dysfunction
9. Brain damage
10. Peripheral neuropathy
11. Cardiac problems

IV. Alcohol Withdrawal

A. Description
1. Early signs develop within a few hours after cessation of alcohol intake.
2. These signs peak after 24 to 48 hours and then rapidly disappear, unless the withdrawal progresses to alcohol withdrawal delirium.
3. At the onset of withdrawal (Box 63.2), follow agency protocol using specified withdrawal assessment scales as indicated by unit or agency policy.
4. Chlordiazepoxide may be prescribed for acute alcohol withdrawal and is usually given orally, unless a more immediate onset is required.

BOX 63.2	Early Signs of Alcohol Withdrawal

Anorexia (nausea and vomiting may occur)
Anxiety
Easily startled
Hyperalertness
Hypertension
Insomnia
Irritability
Jerky movements
Possibly experiences hallucinations, illusions, or vivid nightmares
Possibly reports a feeling of "shaking inside"
Seizures (usually appear 7–48 hours after cessation of alcohol)
Tachycardia
Tremors

BOX 63.3	Manifestations of Alcohol Withdrawal Delirium

Agitation
Anorexia
Anxiety
Delirium
Diaphoresis
Disorientation with fluctuating levels of consciousness
Fever (temperature of 100°F [37.8°C]–103°F [39.4°C])
Hallucinations and delusions
Insomnia
Tachycardia and hypertension

   5. Benzodiazepines would decrease the withdrawal symptoms because of cross tolerance (see Chapter 65 for a list of benzodiazepines).
   6. An intramuscular injection of vitamin B_1 (thiamine) followed by several days of oral administration is usually prescribed to prevent Wernicke's encephalopathy.
B. Withdrawal delirium (Box 63.3)

⚠ Withdrawal delirium is a medical emergency. Death can occur from myocardial infarction, fat emboli, peripheral vascular collapse, electrolyte imbalance, aspiration pneumonia, or suicide.

C. Interventions
   1. Provide care in a nonjudgmental manner.
   2. Check the client frequently.
   3. Monitor vital signs and neurological signs (every 15 minutes) and provide one-to-one supervision.
   4. Serum electrolytes, including glucose and magnesium, will be monitored.
   5. Provide a quiet, nonstimulating environment. Encourage family members (one at a time) to stay with the client to minimize anxiety.
   6. Orient frequently.
   7. Explain all treatments and procedures in a quiet and simple manner.
   8. Initiate seizure precautions.
   9. Assist with the administration of sedating or anticonvulsant medication as prescribed.
   10. Provide small, frequent, high-carbohydrate foods (administer antiemetic before meals as needed).
   11. Monitor intake and output.
   12. Assist with the administration of vitamins (multivitamin, vitamin B complex including thiamine, and vitamin C).
   13. Assist the client with activities of daily living and assist with ambulation if stable.
   14. Allow to express fears.

D. Medication therapy for alcohol abuse and alcohol dependence
   1. Description: Medication is prescribed only for those individuals who have stopped drinking.
   2. Naltrexone: Works by blocking the "high" feeling in the brain that people experience when they drink alcohol
   3. Acamprosate: Works by reducing the physical distress and emotional discomfort people usually experience when they quit drinking
   4. Disulfiram: Works by causing a severe adverse reaction when someone taking the medication consumes alcohol
E. Disulfiram therapy
   1. Description
      a. The client must abstain from alcohol for at least 12 hours before the initial dose is administered.
      b. Adverse effects usually begin within several minutes to 30 minutes after consuming alcohol and may last from 30 minutes up to 2 hours.
      c. Alcohol consumption is avoided for up to 14 days after disulfiram therapy has been discontinued because it places the client at risk for a disulfiram-alcohol reaction.
   2. Adverse reactions
      a. Facial flushing
      b. Sweating
      c. Throbbing headache
      d. Neck pain
      e. Nausea and vomiting
      f. Hypotension
      g. Tachycardia
      h. Respiratory distress
      i. Fatigue
   3. Client education
      a. Inform the client about the effects of the medication.
      b. Ensure that the client agrees to abstain from alcohol and any substances that contain alcohol.
      c. Inform the client that the effects of the medication may occur for several days after discontinuance.

BOX 63.4   **Managing the Client Who Abuses Alcohol**

Direct the client's focus to the substance abuse problem.

Identify with the client those situations that precipitate angry feelings.

Set limits on manipulative behavior and verbal and physical abuse.

Hold the client firmly to reasonable limits, consistently reinforcing rules, with equitable consequences for breaking rules.

Hold the client accountable for all behaviors

Assist with motivational interviewing to assist client to explore strengths and weaknesses.

Encourage focusing on strengths if the client is losing control.

Encourage the client to participate in group therapy and support groups.

BOX 63.5   **Therapies for Substance Abuse Clients and Their Families**

Behavior therapy (including cognitive behavior therapy [CBT]), aversion conditioning with medication

Hospitalization

Psychotherapy (individual, group, family)

12-Step support groups such as Alcoholics Anonymous; Narcotics Anonymous; Pills Anonymous; Al-Anon, Al-a-Teen, or Narc-Anon (for family members and friends of alcoholics or addicts); and Adult Children of Alcoholics

Transitional living programs (halfway houses)

F. Managing the client who abuses alcohol (Boxes 63.4 and 63.5)

⚠ Inform the client who is taking disulfiram to avoid the use of substances that contain alcohol, such as cough medicines, rubbing compounds, vinegar, mouthwashes, and aftershave lotions. The client needs to read the labels of all products.

V. Drug Dependency

A. CNS depressants

1. CNS depressants can include alcohol, benzodiazepines, and barbiturates, and other substances that act as a depressant, sedative, or hypnotic.
2. Intoxication can produce drowsiness, hypotension, incoordination and unsteady gait, slurred speech, impairment of memory, and irritability.
3. Overdose can produce cardiovascular or respiratory depression, coma, shock, seizures, and death.
4. Overdose: If the client is awake, vomiting is induced and activated charcoal is administered. If the client is comatose, airway establishment and maintenance and gastric lavage with activated charcoal are the priorities. Seizure precautions are indicated.

BOX 63.6   **Intoxication: Central Nervous System Stimulants**

Dilated pupils

Euphoria

Hypertension

Impaired judgment and social or occupational functioning

Insomnia

Nausea and vomiting

Paranoia, delusions, or hallucinations

Potential for violence

Tachycardia

---

5. Intravenous flumazenil may be used during a benzodiazepine overdose to reverse the effects.
6. Withdrawal effects include nausea, vomiting, tachycardia, diaphoresis, irritability, tremors, insomnia, and seizures. Withdrawal needs to be treated with a carefully titrated similar drug (abrupt withdrawal can lead to death).
7. Withdrawal from CNS depressants such as barbiturates is generally treated with a barbiturate such as phenobarbital or a long-acting benzodiazepine.

B. CNS stimulants

1. CNS stimulants can include amphetamines, cocaine, and crack, and other stimulants.
2. Intoxication (Box 63.6)
3. Overdose can produce respiratory distress, ataxia, hyperpyrexia, seizure, coma, brain attack (stroke), myocardial infarction, and death.
4. Overdose is treated with antipsychotics and management of associated effects.
5. Withdrawal effects include fatigue, depression, agitation, apathy, anxiety, insomnia, disorientation, lethargy, and craving.
6. Withdrawal is treated with antidepressants, a dopamine agonist, or bromocriptine; severe depression and suicidal ideation can accompany stimulant withdrawal.

C. Opioids

1. Opioids can include opium, heroin, meperidine, morphine sulfate, codeine sulfate, methadone, hydromorphone, and fentanyl.
2. Intoxication (Box 63.7)
3. Overdose can produce respiratory depression, coma, shock, seizure, and death.
4. Overdose is treated with an opioid antagonist such as naloxone.
5. Withdrawal effects include yawning, insomnia, irritability, rhinorrhea, diaphoresis, cramps, nausea and vomiting, muscle aches, chills, fever, lacrimation, and diarrhea.
6. Withdrawal may be treated by methadone detoxification or tapering dosage with other opioids.

7. Clonidine, an a-adrenergic blocker, assists in reducing the severity of sympathetic nervous system–generated withdrawal discomfort.

8. Specific measures for symptom management may also be used, such as antidiarrheal agents and acetaminophen for muscle aches.

D. Hallucinogens

1. Hallucinogens include substances such as lysergic acid diethylamide (LSD), mescaline (peyote), psilocybin (mushrooms), and phencyclidine (PCP).

2. Intoxication (Box 63.8)

3. Overdose of LSD, peyote, and psilocybin include psychosis, brain damage, and death; effects of PCP include psychosis, hypertensive crisis, hyperthermia, seizures, and respiratory arrest.

4. Treatment (LSD, peyote, psilocybin) involves low environmental stimuli (speak slowly, clearly, and in a low voice) and medications to treat anxiety.

5. Treatment (PCP) involve possible gastric lavage (if alert); treatment to acidify urine to assist in excreting the drug; and interventions to treat behavioral disturbances, hyperthermia, hypertension, and respiratory distress.

6. Management of withdrawal is primarily supportive and may include medications to target particular problem behaviors, such as agitation.

⚠ Flashbacks, which are unexpected reexperiences of the effects of taking a hallucinogenic drug, can occur for extended periods of time after its original use. Safety during flashbacks is a priority.

E. Inhalants

1. Inhalants can include gases or liquids such as butane, paint thinner, paint and wax removers, airplane glue, nail polish remover, and nitrous oxide.

2. Intoxication (Box 63.9)

3. Overdose can cause damage to the nervous system and death.

4. Withdrawal management is mainly supportive, including treating affected body systems.

F. Marijuana (Cannabis sativa)

1. Generally is smoked but can be ingested; may be legally prescribed in certain states and in some states and provinces is legal without prescription

2. Causes euphoria, detachment, relaxation, talkativeness, slowed perception of time, anxiety, and paranoia

3. Long-term dependence can result in lethargy, amotivation syndrome, difficulty concentrating, memory loss, and possibly chronic respiratory problems.

4. Withdrawal management is mainly supportive.

G. Other recreational and club drugs

⚠ There are many types of illegal street drugs that are harmful. The nurse needs to be knowledgeable about the physiological effects of these various drugs, be able to recognize the signs associated with their use, and be prepared to provide immediate treatment.

1. Can include methylenedioxymethamphetamine (MDMA, ecstasy), γ-hydroxybutyrate (GHB) methamphetamine (crank, meth, crystal meth), and ketamine (special K)

2. Effects include euphoria, increased energy, increased self-confidence, and increased sociability.

3. Adverse effects include hyperthermia, rhabdomyolysis, renal failure, hepatotoxicity, depression, panic attacks, psychosis, cardiovascular collapse, and death.

BOX 63.7 Intoxication: Opioids

Constricted pupils
Decreased respirations
Drowsiness
Euphoria
Hypotension
Impaired memory, attention, and judgment
Psychomotor retardation
Slurred speech

BOX 63.8 Intoxication: Hallucinogens

Agitation and belligerence
Anxiety and depression
Bizarre, regressive, or violent behavior
Blank stare
Diaphoresis
Dilated pupils
Elevated vital signs including blood pressure
Hallucinations
Impaired judgment and social and occupational functioning
Incoordination
Muscular rigidity and chronic jerking
Paranoia
Seizures
Tachycardia
Tremors

BOX 63.9 Intoxication: Inhalants

Enhancement of sexual pleasure
Euphoria
Excitation followed by drowsiness, light-headedness, disinhibition, and agitation
Giggling and laughter

4. Programs for addiction also address nicotine withdrawal and the pharmacological and psychotherapeutic interventions for this problem, such as nicotine patches, nicotine inhalers, and bupropion for the reduction of withdrawal and cravings.

5. The use of anabolic steroids has been noted in the media to be the cause of adverse events, including death.

H. Interventions: Withdrawal (Box 63.10)
1. Initiate seizure precautions.
2. Hydrate the client.
3. Monitor vital signs every hour; include cardiac monitoring and diagnostic tests such as electrocardiogram and cardiac markers because of the risk of cardiac damage with certain drugs.
4. Monitor intake and output.
5. Orient the client frequently.
6. Maintain minimal stimuli.
7. Approach the client in an accepting and nonjudgmental manner.
8. Direct the client's focus to the substance abuse problem.
9. Assist the client with identifying situations that precipitate angry feelings.
10. Assist the client with dealing with their emotions.
11. Limit blame-placing or rationalizing to explain the substance abuse problem.
12. Assist the client to use assertive techniques rather than manipulation to meet needs.
13. Set limits on manipulative behavior and verbal and physical abuse.
14. Maintain firm and reasonable limits, consistently reinforcing rules, with reasonable consequences for breaking rules.
15. Hold the client accountable for all behaviors.
16. Assist the client with exploring strengths and weaknesses.
17. Encourage focusing on strengths if the client is losing control.
18. Encourage the client to participate in unit activities.
19. Encourage the client to participate in group therapy and support groups.

I. Dual diagnosis
1. Sometimes the use of alcohol and drugs masks underlying psychiatric pathology
2. Psychiatric pathology may also be precipitated by substance use and misuse.
3. When psychiatric disorders and substance misuse are present together, it is often referred to as *dual diagnosis*.

J. Addiction and abuse in health care professionals: Suspicious signs
1. Frequently reporting that drugs have been wasted without being witnessed by another nurse
2. Administering maximum dosages of controlled substances when other nurses do not administer the maximum dose
3. A variance in usual pain relief in the absence of a change in dosage or frequency in their clients
4. Work patterns include the following: always volunteering to carry opioid (narcotic) drug cabinet or drawer keys; choosing shifts in which less supervision is present; or choosing work areas in which the use of controlled substances is high, such as critical care units, operating rooms, anesthesia units, and trauma units.
5. Nurses have a professional and ethical obligation to report impaired co-workers.
6. Most impaired nurses are able to return to work through the State Board of Nursing assistance and monitoring programs. Such programs usually require strict adherence to clearly stated rules and regular reports and drug screens.

BOX 63.10   Withdrawal: Nursing Care

Obtain information regarding the drug type and amount consumed.
Check vital signs.
Remove unnecessary objects from the environment.
Provide one-to-one supervision if necessary.
Provide a quiet, calm environment with minimal stimuli.
Maintain client orientation.
Ensure the client's safety by implementing seizure precautions.
Use security devices if necessary and prescribed, to prevent the client from harming self and others.
Provide for physical needs.
Provide food and fluids as tolerated.
Assist with the administration of medications as prescribed to decrease withdrawal symptoms.
Collect blood and urine samples for drug screening.

WHAT WOULD YOU DO?

Answer: The nurse would immediately contact the PHCP if signs of alcohol withdrawal delirium occur, and the nurse would follow agency protocol using specified assessment scales. One-to-one supervision needs to be provided to ensure safety. The nurse would provide care in a nonjudgmental manner and monitor vital signs and neurological signs (every 15 minutes). The environment needs to be quiet and nonstimulating, and a family member would be encouraged to stay with the client to minimize anxiety. The nurse would orient the client frequently, explain all treatments and procedures in a quiet and simple manner, initiate seizure precautions, and administer sedating or anticonvulsant medication as prescribed. In addition, the nurse would provide small, frequent, high-carbohydrate foods (administer antiemetic before meals as needed).

PRACTICE QUESTIONS

1. The nurse is caring for a female client who was recently admitted to the hospital for anorexia nervosa. The nurse enters the client's room and notes that the client is doing vigorous push-ups. Which nursing action is appropriate?
   1. Interrupt the client and weigh her immediately.
   2. Interrupt the client and offer to take her for a walk.
   3. Allow the client to complete her exercise program.
   4. Tell the client that she is not allowed to exercise vigorously.

❖ 2. Which are appropriate interventions for caring for the client undergoing alcohol withdrawal? **Select all that apply.**
   - ❏ 1. Monitor vital signs.
   - ❏ 2. Maintain an NPO status.
   - ❏ 3. Provide a safe environment.
   - ❏ 4. Address hallucinations therapeutically.
   - ❏ 5. Provide stimulation in the environment.
   - ❏ 6 Provide reality orientation as appropriate.

3. The nursing student is creating a plan of care for the hospitalized client with bulimia nervosa. The nursing instructor intervenes if the student documents which intervention in the plan that is not specific to this disorder?
   1. Monitor intake and output.
   2. Monitor electrolyte levels.
   3. Observe for excessive exercise.
   4. Monitor for the use of laxatives and diuretics.

4. The nurse is monitoring a client who abuses alcohol for signs of alcohol withdrawal delirium. The nurse would monitor for which symptoms?
   1. Hypotension, ataxia, vomiting
   2. Stupor, agitation, muscular rigidity
   3. Hypotension, bradycardia, agitation
   4. Hypertension, disorientation, hallucinations

5. The spouse of a client admitted to the hospital for alcohol withdrawal says to the nurse, "I need to get out of this bad situation." The **most** helpful response by the nurse would be which statement?
   1. "Why don't you tell your husband about this?"
   2. "This is not the best time to make that decision."
   3. "What do you find difficult about this situation?"
   4. "I agree with you. You need to get out of this situation."

6. The nurse is caring for a client who is suspected of being dependent on drugs. Which question would be appropriate for the nurse to ask when collecting data from the client regarding drug abuse?

1. "Why did you get started on these drugs?"
2. "How much do you use and what effect does it have on you?"
3. "How long did you think you could take these drugs without someone finding out?"
4. The nurse does not ask any questions because of fear that the client is in denial and will throw the nurse out of the room.

7. A client who has been drinking alcohol on a regular basis admits to having "a problem" and is asking for assistance with the problem. The nurse would encourage the client to attend which community group?
   1. Al-Anon
   2. Fresh Start
   3. Families Anonymous
   4. Alcoholics Anonymous

8. A client with a diagnosis of anorexia nervosa, who is in a state of starvation, is in a two-bed hospital room. A newly admitted client will be assigned to this client's room. Which client would be an appropriate choice as this client's roommate?
   1. A client with pneumonia
   2. A client receiving diagnostic tests
   3. A client who thrives on managing others
   4. A client who could benefit from the client's assistance at mealtimes

9. The nurse is assigned to care for a client at risk for alcohol withdrawal. The client's spouse asks the nurse, "When will the first signs of withdrawal appear?" The nurse would give which reply?
   1. "In 7 days"
   2. "In 14 days"
   3. "In 21 days"
   4. "Within a few hours"

10. The nurse determines that the wife of an alcoholic client is benefiting from attending an Al-Anon group when the nurse hears the wife make which statement?
   1. "I no longer feel that I deserve the beatings my husband inflicts on me."
   2. "My attendance at the meetings has helped me to see that I provoke my husband's violence."
   3. "I enjoy attending the meetings because they get me out of the house and away from my husband."
   4. "I can tolerate my husband's destructive behaviors now that I know they are common for alcoholics."

11. A female client with anorexia nervosa is a member of a support group. The client has verbalized that she would like to buy some new clothes, but her finances are limited. Group members have brought some used clothes for the client to replace her old

clothes. The client believes that the new clothes were much too tight, so she has reduced her calorie intake to 800 calories daily. The nurse identifies this behavior as which finding?
1. Normal
2. Regressive
3. Indicative of the client's ambivalence
4. Evidence of the client's altered and distorted body image

12. A hospitalized client with a history of alcohol abuse tells the nurse, "I am leaving now. I have to go. I don't want any more treatment. I have things that I have to do right away." The client has not been discharged. In fact, the client is scheduled for an important diagnostic test to be performed in 1 hour. After the nurse discusses the client's concerns with the client, the client dresses and begins to walk out of the hospital room. Which is the appropriate nursing action?
1. Call the nursing supervisor.
2. Call security to block all exit areas.
3. Tell the client that she cannot return to this hospital again if she leaves now.
4. Restrain the client until the primary health care provider (PHCP) can be reached.

13. The nursing student is asked to identify the characteristics of bulimia nervosa. Which characteristic if identified by the student indicates a **need to further research** the disorder?

1. Dental erosion
2. Electrolyte imbalances
3. Enlarged parotid glands
4. Body weight well below ideal range

14. The nurse is caring for a client who has a history of opioid abuse and is monitoring the client for signs of withdrawal. Which manifestations are specifically associated with withdrawal from opioids?
1. Dilated pupils, tachycardia, and diaphoresis
2. Yawning, irritability, diaphoresis, cramps, and diarrhea
3. Tachycardia, hypertension, sweating, and marked tremors
4. Depressed feelings, high drug craving, fatigue, and agitation

15. The nurse is monitoring the behavior of the client and understands that the client with anorexia nervosa manages anxiety by which action?
1. Engaging in immoral acts
2. Always reinforcing self-approval
3. Observing rigid rules and regulations
4. Having the need to always make the right decision

ANSWERS

1. 2
Rationale: Clients with anorexia nervosa are frequently preoccupied with vigorous exercise and push themselves beyond normal limits to work off caloric intake. The nurse needs to provide for appropriate exercise as well as place limits on vigorous activities. Options 1, 3, and 4 are inappropriate nursing actions.
Test-Taking Strategy: Focus on the subject, anorexia nervosa. Recalling that the nurse needs to set firm limits with clients who have this disorder will direct you to option 2.

2. 1, 3, 4, 6
Rationale: When the client is experiencing withdrawal from alcohol, the priority for care is to prevent the client from harming himself or herself or others. The nurse would provide a low-stimulation environment to maintain the client in as calm a state as possible. The nurse would monitor the vital signs closely and report abnormal findings. The nurse would frequently reorient the client to reality and would address hallucinations therapeutically. Adequate nutritional and fluid intake must be maintained.
Test-Taking Strategy: Use therapeutic communication techniques to assist with selecting the correct interventions. Also, recalling the characteristics associated with alcohol withdrawal will assist you with answering correctly.

3. 3
Rationale: Excessive exercise is a characteristic of anorexia nervosa, not bulimia nervosa. Frequent vomiting, in addition to laxative and diuretic abuse, may lead to dehydration and electrolyte imbalance. Monitoring for both dehydration and electrolyte imbalance is an important nursing action. Option 3 is the only option that is not associated with care of the client with bulimia.
Test-Taking Strategy: Note the words, *not specific to this disorder*, in the question. This word indicates the need to select the incorrect intervention. Options 1, 2, and 4 are comparable or alike and directly or indirectly infer concern about fluid and electrolyte balance. Option 3 is different from the other options.

4. 4
Rationale: The symptoms associated with alcohol withdrawal delirium typically are anxiety, insomnia, anorexia, hypertension, disorientation, visual or tactile hallucinations, agitation, fever, and delusions.
Test-Taking Strategy: Focus on the subject, signs of alcohol withdrawal. Review each option carefully to ensure that all the symptoms are contained in the correct option. Eliminate options 1 and 3 first, knowing that hypertension rather than hypotension occurs. From the remaining options, recalling that the client who is stuporous is not likely to exhibit agitation will direct you to option 4.

5. 3

Rationale: The most helpful response is the one that encourages the client to problem solve. Giving advice implies that the nurse knows what is best and can also foster dependency. The nurse would not agree with the client, nor would the nurse request that the client provide explanations.

Test-Taking Strategy: Note the strategic word, *most*. Use therapeutic communication techniques. Eliminate option 1 because of the word *why*, which would be avoided in communication. Eliminate option 2 because this option places the client's feelings on hold. Eliminate option 4 because the nurse is agreeing with the client. Option 3 is the only option that addresses the client's feelings.

6. 2

Rationale: Whenever the nurse collects data from a client who is dependent on drugs, it is best for the nurse to attempt to elicit information by being nonjudgmental and direct. Option 1 is incorrect because it is judgmental, off focus, and reflects the nurse's bias. Option 3 is incorrect because it is judgmental, insensitive, and aggressive, which is nontherapeutic. Option 4 is incorrect because it indicates passivity on the nurse's part and uses rationalization to avoid the therapeutic nursing intervention.

Test-Taking Strategy: Use therapeutic communication techniques to answer the question. Option 2 is the statement that is nonjudgmental and direct.

7. 4

Rationale: Alcoholics Anonymous is a major self-help organization for the treatment of alcoholism. Option 1 is a group for families of alcoholics. Option 2 is for nicotine addicts. Option 3 is for parents of children who abuse substances.

Test-Taking Strategy: Focus on the subject, self-help groups for an alcoholic. If you are unfamiliar with these support groups, note the relation between *drinking* in the question and *Alcoholics* in the correct option.

8. 2

Rationale: The client receiving diagnostic tests is an appropriate roommate. The client with anorexia is most likely experiencing hematological complications, such as leukopenia. Having a roommate with pneumonia would place the client with anorexia nervosa at risk for infection. The client with anorexia nervosa would not be put in a situation in which he or she can focus on the nutritional needs of others or be managed by others, because this may contribute to sublimation and suppression of his or her own hunger.

Test-Taking Strategy: Note the subject, a state of starvation. Recalling the characteristics and complications associated with anorexia nervosa will direct you to the correct option.

9. 4

Rationale: Early signs of alcohol withdrawal develop within a few hours after cessation or reduction of alcohol and peak after 24 to 48 hours.

Test-Taking Strategy: Focus on the subject, when the first signs of alcohol withdrawal will be seen. This will assist in directing you to the correct option.

10. 1

Rationale: Al-Anon support groups are a protected, supportive opportunity for spouses and significant others to learn what to expect and to obtain suggestions about successful behavioral changes. Option 1 is the healthiest response because it exemplifies an understanding that the alcoholic partner is responsible for his behavior and cannot be allowed to blame family members for loss of control. The nonalcoholic partner should not feel responsible when the spouse loses control (option 2). Option 3 indicates that the group is being seen as an escape, not a place to work on issues. Option 4 indicates that the wife remains codependent.

Test-Taking Strategy: Focus on the subject of the question, benefiting from attending an Al-Anon group. This will direct you to the correct option.

11. 4

Rationale: Altered or distorted body image is a concern with clients with anorexia nervosa. Although the client may struggle with ambivalence and present with regressed behavior, the client's coping pattern relates to the basic issue of distorted body image. The client's behavior is not normal.

Test-Taking Strategy: Focus on the data in the question to determine that the subject relates to a distorted body image. This will direct you to the correct option.

12. 1

Rationale: The nurse can be charged with false imprisonment if a client is made to wrongfully believe that he or she cannot leave the hospital. Notifying the nurse supervisor is the correct option. Most health care facilities have documents that the client is asked to sign that relate to the client's responsibilities when he or she leaves against medical advice (AMA). The client would be asked to sign this document before leaving. The nurse would request that the client wait to speak to the PHCP before leaving, but if the client refuses to do so, the nurse cannot hold the client against his or her will. Restraining the client and calling security to block exits constitutes false imprisonment. Any client has a right to health care (option 3) and cannot be told otherwise.

Test-Taking Strategy: Keeping the concept of false imprisonment in mind, eliminate options 2 and 4 because they are comparable or alike. Eliminate option 3, knowing that any client has a right to health care.

13. 4

Rationale: Clients with bulimia nervosa may not initially appear to be physically or emotionally ill. They are often at or slightly below ideal body weight. During further inspection, the client demonstrates enlargement of the parotid glands with dental erosion and caries if he or she has been inducing vomiting. Electrolyte imbalances are present.

Test-Taking Strategy: Focus on the subject, bulimia nervosa. Note the strategic words, *need to further research*. These words indicate a negative event query and the need to select the incorrect characteristic of bulimia nervosa. Focusing on the client's diagnosis will direct you to option 4. Option 4 is a characteristic sign of anorexia nervosa, not bulimia nervosa.

14. 2

Rationale: Opioids are CNS depressants. Withdrawal effects include yawning, insomnia, irritability, rhinorrhea, diaphoresis, cramps, nausea and vomiting, muscle aches, chills, fever, lacrimation, and diarrhea. Withdrawal is treated by methadone tapering or medication detoxification. Option 2 identifies the clinical manifestations associated with withdrawal from opioids. Option 1 describes intoxication from hallucinogens. Option 3 describes withdrawal from alcohol. Option 4 describes withdrawal from cocaine.

Test-Taking Strategy: Focus on the subject of the question, the clinical manifestations associated with withdrawal from opioids. Recalling that opioids are CNS depressants will direct you to option 2.

15. 3

Rationale: Clients with anorexia nervosa have the desire to please others. Their need to be correct or perfect interferes with rational decision-making processes. These clients are moralistic. Rules and rituals help the clients manage their anxiety. Options 1, 2, and 4 are incorrect.

Test-Taking Strategy: Focus on the subject, managing anxiety. Eliminate options 2 and 4 because of the closed-ended word, *always*. Eliminate option 1 because it is not characteristic of the client with anorexia.

CHAPTER **64**

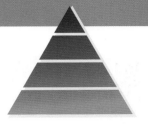

Crisis Theory and Intervention

PRIORITY CONCEPTS Coping; Interpersonal Violence

WHAT WOULD YOU DO?

A female victim of rape has just arrived at the emergency department. What would the nurse do?
Answer is located on p. 902.

I. Crisis Intervention

A. Description
1. Crisis is a temporary state of severe emotional disorganization caused by an event that presents a threat.
2. Everyone experiences crises; the outcome depends on coping mechanisms and support systems available at the time of the crisis.
3. The ability for decision making and problem solving is inadequate.
4. Treatment is aimed at assisting the client and the family through the stressful situation.

B. Phases of a crisis
1. Phase 1: External precipitating event (could be situational, developmental, cultural, or societal)
2. Phase 2
   a. Perception of the threat
   b. Increase in anxiety
   c. Client may cope or resolve the crisis.
3. Phase 3
   a. Failure of coping
   b. Increasing disorganization
   c. Emergence of physical symptoms
   d. Relationship problems
4. Phase 4
   a. Mobilization of internal and external resources
   b. Goal is to return the individual to at least a precrisis level of functioning.

C. Types of crises (Box 64.1)

D. Crisis intervention
1. Treatment is immediate, supportive, and directly responsive to the immediate current crisis.

2. The interprofessional team assists individuals in crisis to cope; interventions are goal directed.
3. Feelings of client are acknowledged.
4. Intervention provides opportunities for expression and validation of feelings.
5. Connections are made between the meaning of the event and the crisis.
6. Client explores alternative coping mechanisms and tries out new behaviors.

II. Grief

A. Grief is a natural emotional response to loss that individuals will experience as they attempt to accept it.

B. Grief usually involves moving through a series of stages or tasks to help with resolve (Box 64.2).

C. Depending on the type of loss, feelings associated with grief can include anger, frustration, loneliness, sadness, guilt, regret, or peace.

D. Healing can occur when the pain of the loss has lessened and the survivor has adapted to life without the deceased. The survivor will continue to experience memories of the deceased.

E. Types of grief
1. Normal grief: Physical, emotional, cognitive, or behavioral reactions can occur. The process of resolution can take months to years.
2. Anticipatory grief occurs before the loss and is associated with an acute, chronic, or terminal illness.
3. Disenfranchised grief occurs when a loss is experienced and cannot be acknowledged openly (societal norms do not define the loss as a loss within its traditional definition).
4. Dysfunctional grief occurs with prolonged emotional instability and a lack of progression to successful coping with the loss.
5. Children's grief is based on their developmental level (Box 64.3).

III. Loss

A. Loss is the absence of something desired or previously thought to be available.

BOX 64.1 Types of Crises

Maturational
Relates to developmental stages and associated role changes; examples include marriage, birth of a child, and retirement.

Situational
Arises from an external source, is often unanticipated, and is associated with a life event that upsets an individual or a group's psychological equilibrium; examples include loss of a job or a change in job, a change in financial status, death of a loved one, divorce, abortion, addition of new family members, and severe physical or mental illness.

Adventitious
Relates to a crisis of disaster or an event that is not a part of everyday life and is unplanned and accidental. This type of crisis may result from a natural disaster such as a flood, earthquake, hurricane, fire, or tornado; a national disaster such as war, riots, or acts of terrorism; or a crime of violence such as rape, assault, murder, or spousal or child abuse.

BOX 64.2 The Grief Response

Stage 1: Shock and Disbelief
The individual may have feelings of numbness, difficulties with decision making, emotional outbursts, denial, and isolation.

Stage 2: Experiencing the Loss
If the grief response is a result of a loss of a loved one, the individual may feel angry at the loved one who died or may feel guilty about the death.
Bargaining or depression may also occur in this stage.

Stage 3: Reintegration
The individual begins to reorganize his or her life and accepts the reality of the loss.

B. Actual loss can be identified by others and can arise in response to, or in anticipation of, a situation.
C. Perceived loss is experienced by one person and cannot be verified by others.
D. Anticipatory loss is experienced before the loss occurs.
E. Mourning
   1. The outward and social expression of loss
   2. May be dictated by cultural and religious beliefs
F. Bereavement
   1. Includes the inner feelings and the outward reactions of the individual experiencing the loss
   2. Includes grief and mourning

▲ IV. Nurse's Role: Grief and Loss (Box 64.4)
   A. Encourage client to express feelings within a trusting, supportive, and nonjudgmental environment.
   B. Allow ongoing opportunities for fully informed choices.

BOX 64.3 Children's Grief

Birth to 1 Year
The infant has no concept of death.
The infant reacts to the loss of their mother or caregiver.

1 to 2 Years
The child may see death as reversible.
Toddler may scream, withdraw, or become disinterested in the environment.
Grief response occurs only to the death of the significant person in the child's life.

2 to 5 Years
The child may see death as reversible.
The child has a sense of loss and is concerned about who will provide care.
Regression or aggressive behavior may occur.

5 to 9 Years
The child begins to see death as permanent.
The child may feel responsible for the occurrence.
The child has difficulty concentrating.

Preadolescent through Adolescence
The adolescent sees death as permanent.
The adolescent experiences a strong emotional reaction.
The adolescent may regress.

C. Facilitate the grief process; monitor the individual's grief and assist the individual to feel the loss and complete the tasks of the grief process.
D. Grief affects individuals physically, psychologically, socially, and spiritually; an interprofessional team approach, including a bereavement specialist, facilitates the grief process.

⚠ The nurse's role in the loss and grieving process includes communicating with the client, their family members, and significant other. The nurse needs to consider the individual's culture, spirituality, religion, family structure, individual life experiences, coping skills, and support systems.

V. COVID-19-Coping
   A. Description
      1. The unprecedented event of the COVID-19 pandemic and its emotional effect of acute traumatic stress has affected everyone and is in essence a direct threat to our lives.
      2. The normal way of life has changed and it is unknown if life will ever go back to normal or ever be the same.
      3. It is crucial that nurses recognize that the pandemic is a real threat to both physical and emotional well-being and that coping methods need to be in place to prevent prolonged psychological effects, such as depression or post-traumatic stress disorder or other types of emotional distress.

BOX 64.4	Communication During Grief and Loss

Determine how much the client and family want to know.

Determine whether there is a spokesperson for the family.

Be aware of cultural, spiritual, and religious beliefs and how they may affect the communication process. Consider personal space issues, eye contact, and touch.

Obtain an interpreter if necessary.

Allow opportunity for informed choices.

Assist with the decision-making process if asked. Use problem solving to assist with decision making, and avoid interjecting personal views or opinions.

Establish trust with the client and encourage expression of feelings, concerns, and fears within a trusting, supportive, and nonjudgmental environment.

Be honest and truthful, and let the client and family know that you will not abandon them.

Ask the client and family about their expectations and needs.

Be a sensitive listener. Sit in silence if necessary and appropriate.

Extend touch and hold the client or family member's hand if appropriate.

Encourage reminiscing.

If you do not know what to do in a particular situation, seek assistance.

If you do not know what to say to a client or family who is talking about death, listen attentively and use therapeutic communication techniques such as open-ended questions or reflection.

Acknowledge your own feelings. Let the client and family know that the topic of conversation is a difficult one and that you do not know what to say.

Realize that it is acceptable to cry with the client and family during the grieving process.

4. Supportive relations are key in promoting resilience and healing from trauma.

5. Moral injury is a concern particularly among health care workers who need to make difficult and even impossible choices during care and end up feeling responsible for the death of others.

6. Family members and friends may suffer from moral injury when witnessing upsetting situations such as when a loved one becomes ill and the impossibility to be with the loved one or help the loved one. (Refer to Chapter 62 for additional information on Moral Injury.)

7. Grief and loss is experienced; there may be a communal sense of grief because of the loss of how things were, and anticipatory grief because of the threat of loss of life. Many experience loss of jobs and financial loss. (Refer to Sections II and III for additional information on grief and loss.)

8. Each individual's personal experience with grief and loss differs and it is crucial for the nurse to understand this and accept the differences.

B. Data collection
1. Anxiety
2. Feelings of panic
3. Fear of the unknown and what the future will bring
4. Psychological stress of isolation and quarantine
5. Grief and loss: apathy, insomnia, change in appetite, weight changes, anxiety, anger, irritability, sadness, worries, numbness
6. Depression and other emotional effects including suicide
7. Survival guilt

C. Interventions for coping
1. Assess the client for signs of psychological stress and effects of grief and loss.
2. Assess for signs of depression and suicidal behaviors; intervene as necessary and appropriate.
3. Provide hope and foster resilience with the client and family.
4. Encourage the use of cognitive reappraisal approaches; assist the client to approach stressors with a positive view and emphasize that resources are available; encourage breathing techniques.
5. Encourage the client to think about and list what one can control.
6. Promote using safety behaviors such as physical distancing and handwashing and wearing masks; these decrease transmission of the virus and are a part of managing anxiety.
7. Limit COVID media exposure and avoid forwarding fearful media information to others.
8. Continue to seek connectedness and social support from family and friends via text, video methods, phone, email; it is comforting to know that others are doing well.
9. Encourage to care for self, eating well, activities and exercise, adequate sleep.
10. Encourage seeking out resources to assist in support and ways to cope with the traumatic stress, grief and loss.

VI. Suicidal Behavior

A. Description
1. Suicidal clients characteristically have feelings of worthlessness, guilt, and hopelessness that are so overwhelming they feel unable to go on with life and feel unfit to live.
2. The nurse caring for a depressed client always considers the possibility of suicide.

B. Individuals at risk
1. Clients with a history of previous suicide attempts
2. Family history of suicide attempts
3. Adolescents
4. Older clients

BOX 64.5   Suicidal Cues

Giving away personal, special, and prized possessions
Canceling social engagements
Making out or changing a will
Taking out or changing insurance policies
Positive or negative changes in behavior
Poor appetite
Sleeping difficulties
Feelings of hopelessness
Difficulty concentrating
Loss of interest in activities
Client statements that indicate intent to attempt suicide
Sudden calmness or improvement in a depressed client
Client questions about poisons, guns, or other lethal objects
Sudden deterioration in school/work performance

BOX 64.6   Suicidal Client: Data Collection

Plan
Does the client have a plan?
What is the plan, how lethal is the plan, and how likely is death to occur?
Does the client have the means to carry out the plan?

Client History of Attempts
What suicide attempts occurred in the past and what were the outcomes (i.e., physiological injuries)?
Was the client accidentally rescued?
Have the past attempts and methods been the same, or have methods increased in lethality?

Psychosocial Factors
Is the client alone or alienated from others?
Is hostility or depression present?
Do hallucinations exist? If yes, type of hallucination (audio/command, visual)?
Is substance abuse present?
Has the client had any recent losses or physical illnesses?
Has the client had any environmental or lifestyle changes?

5. Disabled or terminally ill clients
6. Clients with personality disorders
7. Clients with an organic brain syndrome or dementia
8. Depressed or psychotic clients
9. Substance abusers
10. Those who have been consistently bullied or rejected by peers or society
11. History of child maltreatment
12. Past psychiatric hospitalizations

C. Cues (Box 64.5)
D. Data collection (Box 64.6)
E. Interventions
1. Assess for suicidal intent or ideation and initiate suicide precautions.
2. The client's statements, behaviors, and mood are documented every 15 minutes.
3. Remove harmful objects.
4. Do not leave the client alone.
5. Provide a nonjudgmental, caring attitude.
6. Develop a contract (per psychiatrist prescription and agency procedures) that is written, dated, and signed and that indicates alternative behavior at times of suicidal thoughts.
7. Encourage the client to talk about feelings and identify positive aspects about self.
8. Encourage active participation in own care.
9. Keep the client active by assigning achievable tasks.
10. Check that visitors do not leave harmful objects in the client's room.
11. Identify support systems.
12. Do not allow the client to leave the unit unless accompanied by a staff member.
13. Continue to assess the client's suicide potential.

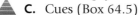 Provide one-to-one supervision at all times for the client at risk for suicide.

VII. Abusive Behaviors

A. Anger
1. A feeling of annoyance that may be displaced onto an object or person
2. Used to avoid anxiety and gives a feeling of power in situations in which the person feels out of control
B. Aggression can be harmful and destructive when not controlled.
C. Violence is the physical force that is threatening to the safety of self and others.
D. Data collection
1. History of violence or self-harm
2. Poor impulse control and low tolerance of frustration
3. Defiance and argumentativeness
4. Raising of voice
5. Making verbal threats
6. Pacing and agitation
7. Muscle rigidity
8. Flushed face
9. Glaring at others
E. Interventions
1. Ensure a safe and low-stimuli environment.
2. Use a calm approach and communicate with a calm, clear tone of voice. (Be assertive but not aggressive, and avoid verbal struggles.)
3. Maintain a large personal space, and use a nonaggressive posture (e.g., arms and hands at the side rather than folded across the chest or placed on the hips).
4. Listen actively and acknowledge the client's anger.
5. Determine what the client considers to be his or her need.

6. Provide the client with clear options that deal with the client's behavior, set limits on behavior, and make the client aware of the consequences of anger and violence.

7. Discuss the use of restraints (security devices) or seclusion if the client is unable to control angry behavior that may lead to violence.

8. Assist the client with problem solving and decision making regarding the options.

▲ **F.** Restraints (security devices) and seclusion

  1. Description

   a. Physical restraints: Any manual method or mechanical device, material, or equipment that inhibits free movement

   b. Seclusion: A process in which a client is placed alone in a specially designed room for protection and close supervision

   c. Chemical restraints: Medications given for the specific purpose of inhibiting a specific behavior or movement and that have an effect on the client's ability to relate to the environment

  2. Use of restraints and seclusion

   a. Restraints and seclusion would never be used as punishment or for the convenience of the health care staff.

   b. Restraints and seclusion are used when behavior is physically harmful to the client or others, and when alternative or less restrictive measures are insufficient in protecting the client or others from harm.

   c. The nurse needs to document the behavior leading to the use of restraints or seclusion.

   d. Restraints and seclusion are used when the health care team anticipates that a controlled environment would be helpful and requests seclusion.

   e. In an emergency, the qualified nurse may place a client in restraints or seclusion and obtain a written or verbal prescription as soon as possible thereafter.

   f. Per state guidelines, within 1 hour of the initiation of restraints or seclusion, the psychiatrist must make a face-to-face assessment and evaluation of the client and must continuously reevaluate the need for continued restraint or seclusion.

   g. While in restraints or seclusion, the client must be protected from all sources of harm by having one-to-one supervision with a staff member within an arm's length of the client.

   h. The client in restraints or seclusion needs constant one-to-one supervision. Physical, safety, and comfort needs must be assessed every 15 to 30 minutes, and these observations are also documented (such as food, fluids, bathroom needs, range-of-motion exercise, and ambulation).

   i. The nurse always follows agency procedures and policies regarding the use of restraints and must also be familiar with their use for the older client and juveniles.

   j. In most settings, a primary health care provider's prescription is required prior to the use of restraints.

VIII. Bullying

A. Bullying is the abuse of power by an individual on another through repeated aggressive acts.

B. It most often occurs in children and in high school or college environments but can also occur in the workplace or other environments.

C. The bully feels power from sources such as physical strength, maturity, a higher status within a peer group, from knowing the victim's weaknesses, or from support of others.

D. Bullying can occur in the form of physical harm, relational aggression, isolation and exclusion, and verbal harm such as slander, rumors, or threats; it is both intentionally cruel and unprovoked.

E. Cyberbullying is also a form of bullying and occurs in the form of internet messages on social media networks, text messages, e-mails, photos being posted, and rumors.

F. The bullied person is repeatedly experiencing negative actions from the bully(s).

G. These bully acts can lead to depression, low self-esteem, humiliation, isolation, and social withdrawal in the victim; it could result in self-harm such as cutting, suicide, and murder.

H. The nurse's responsibility is to observe for signs of bullying and to educate teachers, school administrators, and parents about bullying behaviors and signs that it may be occurring.

IX. Family Violence ▲

A. Description (Fig. 64.1)

  1. The violence begins with threats or verbal or physical minor assaults (tension building), and the victim attempts to comply with the requests of the abuser.

  2. The abuser loses control and becomes destructive and harmful (acute battering), while the victim attempts to protect himself or herself.

  3. After the battering, the abuser then becomes loving and attempts to make peace (calmness and a diffusion of tension); undoing behavior is characteristic of the abuser giving gifts and positive attention to the victim to undue the negative behavior.

  4. The abuser justifies that violence is normal and the victim is responsible for the abuse.

  5. Outsiders are usually not aware of what is happening in the family.

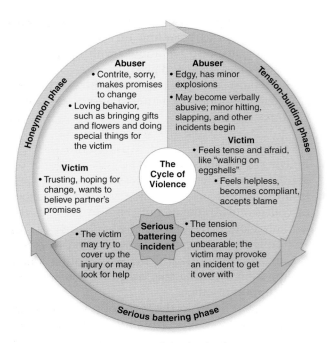

FIGURE 64.1 The cycle of violence.

6. Family members are isolated socially and lack autonomy and trust among one another. Caring and intimacy in the family are absent.
7. Family members expect other members of the family to meet their needs, but none are able to do so.
8. The abuser threatens to abandon the family.

B. Types of violence (Box 64.7)

C. The vulnerable person (victim)
1. The vulnerable person is the one in the family unit against whom violence is perpetrated.
2. Those most vulnerable are children and older adults.
3. The perpetrator of violence and the person targeted by the violence can be male or female.
4. Battering is a crime.

D. Characteristics of abusers
1. Impaired self-esteem
2. Strong dependency needs
3. Narcissistic and suspicious
4. History of abuse during childhood
5. Perceive victims as their property and believe that they are entitled to abuse them

E. Characteristics of victims
1. Some may have a dependent personality disorder.
2. Feel trapped, dependent, helpless, and powerless.
3. Victims of abuse may become depressed as they are trapped in the abuser's power and control cycle (see Fig. 64.1).
4. As the victim's self-esteem becomes diminished with chronic abuse, they may blame themselves for the violence and be unable to see a way out of the situation.

BOX 64.7 **Types of Violence**

Physical violence: Infliction of physical pain or bodily harm
Sexual violence: Any form of sexual contact without consent
Emotional violence: Infliction of mental anguish
Physical neglect: Failure to provide health care to prevent or treat physical or emotional illnesses
Developmental neglect: Failure to provide physical and cognitive stimulation needed to prevent developmental deficits
Educational neglect: Depriving a child of education
Economic exploitation: Illegal or improper exploitation of money, funds, or other resources for one's personal gain

F. Interventions
1. Report suspected or actual cases of child or adult abuse to appropriate authorities. (Follow state and agency guidelines.)
2. Assist to refer to appropriate Sexual Assault Domestic Violence (SADV) team or other appropriate agency team.
3. Check for evidence of physical injuries.
4. Ensure privacy and confidentiality during data collection, and provide a nonjudgmental and empathetic approach to foster trust. Reassure the victim that he or she has not done anything wrong. (See Box 64.8 for examples of data collection questions.)
5. Assist the victim with developing self-protective abilities and other problem-solving abilities.
6. Even if the victim is not ready to leave the situation, encourage the victim to develop a specific safety plan (a fast escape if the violence resumes) and the best place to obtain help (hotlines, safe houses, and shelters). An abused person is usually reluctant to call the police.
7. Assess the suicidal potential of the victim.
8. Assess the potential for homicide.
9. Check for the use of drugs and alcohol.
10. Determine family coping patterns and support systems.
11. Provide support and assistance with coping by contacting the legal system.
12. Assist in resolving family dysfunction with prescribed therapies.
13. Encourage individual therapy, as prescribed, for the victim that promotes coping with the trauma and prevents further psychological conflict.
14. Encourage individual therapy for the abuser that focuses on preventing violent behavior and repairing relationships.
15. Encourage psychotherapy, counseling, group therapy, and support groups as prescribed to assist family members with developing coping strategies.
16. Assist the family with accessing community and personal resources.
17. Maintain accurate and thorough medical health records.

> ### BOX 64.8 Data Collection Questions for Violence and Abuse
>
> "Has anyone ever touched you in a way that made you uncomfortable?"
>
> "Are these injuries a result of someone harming you?"
>
> "Is anyone hurting you now?"
>
> "How do you and your partner deal with anger (or disagreement)?"
>
> "Has your partner ever hit you?"
>
> "Have you ever been threatened by _____?"
>
> "Does your partner prevent you from seeing family or friends?"
>
> "Does your partner ever use the children to manipulate you?"
>
> "Did (or does) anyone in your family deal with anger by hitting?"

X. Child Abduction

A. Description

1. Child abduction is the kidnapping of a child (or infant) by an older person.

2. Occurrences

   a. A stranger may kidnap a child for criminal or mischievous purposes.

   b. A stranger may kidnap a child (or infant) to bring up him or her as that person's own child.

   c. A parent removes or retains a child from the other parent's care (often in the course of or after divorce proceedings).

 3. Because of the increased independence that occurs in the preschool-aged child, parents are less able to provide the constant protection they once did. When the child reaches this age, interventions that ensure protection (including teaching the child) are necessary.

 4. Questions that help to reveal the potential for abuse include: "Who do you play with the most often? Is there anyone you do not like playing with? Are there games you don't like playing?"

 B. Interventions

1. Instruct the parents to teach their child basic guidelines about personal safety that include the following:

   a. Do not go anywhere alone.

   b. Always tell an adult where he or she is going and when he or she will return.

   c. Say "no" if he or she feels uncomfortable with a situation.

   d. If any adult offers you anything without asking your parents first, step away, say "no", and tell someone.

   e. If any adult asks you for your help without asking your parent first, step away, say "no", and tell someone.

   f. If any adult asks you to keep a secret, step away, say "no", and tell someone.

   g. Do not help anyone look for a lost dog or cat and do not accept candy from a stranger.

   h. If lost in a store, do not wander around looking for the parent; go at once to a clerk or guard.

2. Children need to learn their full name, address, and parents' names and phone numbers.

3. Watch for posttraumatic stress disorder in any child who has experienced an abduction.

XI. Child Abuse

A. Description

1. Abuse is the nonaccidental physical injury or the nonaccidental act of omission of care by a parent or person responsible for a child; abuse comprises neglect and physical, sexual, and emotional maltreatment.

2. Neglect can be in the form of physical or emotional neglect and involves the deprivation of basic needs, supervision, medical care, or education and failure to meet a child's needs for attention and affection.

3. Sexual abuse can involve incest, molestation, exhibitionism, pornography, prostitution, or pedophilia; findings associated with sexual abuse may not be easily apparent in a child.

4. Shaken baby syndrome is caused by the violent shaking of an infant and results in intracranial (usually subdural hemorrhage) trauma; this can lead to cerebral edema and death.

B. Data Collection (Box 64.9)

C. Interventions

1. Support the child during a thorough physical assessment.

2. Check for injuries.

3. If shaken baby syndrome is suspected, monitor the infant for a decrease in level of consciousness, which can indicate increased intracranial pressure (ICP).

4. Report a case of suspected abuse; nurses are legally required to report all cases of suspected child abuse to the appropriate local or state agency.

5. Place the child in an environment that is safe, preventing further injury.

6. Document information related to the suspected abuse in an objective manner.

7. Assist with assessing the parents' strengths and weaknesses, normal coping mechanisms, and presence or absence of a support system.

8. Assist the family with identifying stressors, support systems, and resources.

9. Refer the family to appropriate support groups.

⚠ Nurses are legally required to report all cases of suspected child abuse or elder abuse to the appropriate local or state agency; state laws and procedures may vary and are always followed.

BOX 64.9 **Child Neglect and Abuse: Data Collection Findings**

Neglect
- Inadequate weight gain
- Poor hygiene
- Consistent hunger
- Inconsistent school attendance
- Constant fatigue
- Reports of lack of child supervision
- Delinquency

Physical Abuse
- Unexplained bruises, burns, or fractures
- Bald spots on the scalp
- Apprehensive child
- Extreme aggressiveness (typically boys) or withdrawal (typically girls)
- Fear of parents
- Lack of crying (older infant, toddler, or young preschool child) when approached by a stranger
- Spiral fractures without history of trauma from a sports injury
- Poor performance

Emotional Abuse
- Speech disorders
- Habit disorders such as sucking, biting, and rocking
- Psychoneurotic reactions
- Learning disorders
- Suicide attempts

Sexual Abuse
- Difficulty walking or sitting
- Torn, stained, or bloody underclothing
- Pain, swelling, or itching of genitals
- Deformities, bruises, bleeding, or lacerations in genital or anal area
- Unwillingness to change clothes or unwillingness to participate in gym activities
- Poor peer relations

Shaken Baby Syndrome
- External signs of trauma are usually absent
- Ophthalmoscopic examination reveals retinal hemorrhage
- Full bulging fontanels and head circumference greater than expected

---

XII. Latchkey Children

A. Description
1. Children who do not have adult supervision before or after school hours; they are left to care for themselves during these times.
2. Occurs when children are members of a single-parent family or when both parents work and need to leave the home before children are brought to school or arrive home after the children
3. This situation induces a stress-provoking environment for children and places them at risk for an unsafe situation, injury, and delinquent behavior.

B. Interventions
1. Identify the latchkey child.
2. Encourage the parent to teach the child about self-care and self-help skills.
3. Assist the parent with identifying possible alternatives to leaving the child alone.
4. Inform the parent about available community resources such as after-school programs for children.

XIII. Abuse of the Older Adult

A. Description
1. Abuse of an older adult involves physical, emotional, or sexual abuse; neglect; and economic exploitation.
2. Older adults at most risk include individuals who are dependent because of illness, immobility, or altered mental status.
3. Factors that contribute to abuse and neglect include long-standing family violence, caregiver stress, and the older adult's increasing dependence on others.
4. Victims may attempt to dismiss injuries as accidental, and abusers may prevent victims from receiving proper medical care to avoid discovery.
5. Victims are often socially isolated by their abusers.

B. Data Collection
1. Physical abuse
   a. Sprains, dislocations, or fractures
   b. Abrasions, bruises, or lacerations
   c. Pressure sores
   d. Puncture wounds
   e. Burns
   f. Skin tears
2. Sexual abuse
   a. Torn or stained underclothing
   b. Discomfort or bleeding in the genital area
   c. Difficulty in walking or sitting
   d. Unexplained genital infections or disease
3. Emotional abuse
   a. Confusion
   b. Fearful and agitated
   c. Change in appetite and weight
   d. Withdrawn and loss of interest in self and social activities
4. Neglect
   a. Disheveled appearance
   b. Dressed inadequately or inappropriately
   c. Dehydration and malnutrition
   d. Lacking physical needs, such as glasses, hearing aids, and dentures
5. Signs of medication overdose
6. Economic exploitation
   a. Inability to pay bills and fearful when discussing finances

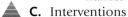

b. Confused, inaccurate, or no knowledge of finances

C. Interventions
1. Assist in assessing and treating physical injuries.
2. Ask if any injury is a result of someone harming them.
3. Report cases of suspected abuse to appropriate authorities (follow state and agency guidelines)
4. Separate the older adult from the abusive environment, if possible, and contact adult protective services for assistance in placement while the abuse is being investigated.
5. Explore alternative living arrangements that are least restrictive and disruptive of the victim.
6. The older adult who has been abused may need assistance for financial or legal matters.
7. Provide referrals to emergency community resources.
8. When working with caregivers, monitor the need for respite care or counseling to deal with caregiver stress. (see Priority Nursing Actions).

⚡ PRIORITY NURSING ACTIONS

Physical Abuse of an Older Client

1. Assess and treat the wounds.
2. Ensure that the victim is removed from the threatening environment.
3. Adhere to mandatory abuse reporting laws.
4. Notify the caseworker of the situation.
5. Document the occurrence, findings, actions taken, and the victim's response.

XIV. Rape and Sexual Assault

A. Description
1. Rape is engaging another person in a sexual act and/or sexual intercourse through the use of force and without the consent of the sexual partner.
2. The victim is not required by law to report the rape or assault.
3. Often, the victim is blamed by others and receives no support from significant others.
4. Acquaintance rape involves someone known to the victim.
5. Statutory rape is the act of sexual intercourse with a person under the age of legal consent, even if the minor consents.
6. Same sex rape
   a. Females: Involves sexual touching, oral sex, or penetration with a finger or some other object
   b. Males: Same as for females; often experiences stigma when seeking help

c. See https://www.cdc.gov/ViolencePrevention/index.html for more information.
7. Marital rape
   a. The belief that marriage bestows rights to sex whenever wanted and without consent of the partner contributes to the occurrence of marital rape.
   b. Victims of marital rape describe being forced to perform acts they did not wish to perform and being physically abused during sex.

B. Data collection
1. Female client
   a. Obtain the date of the last menstrual period.
   b. Determine the form of birth control used and the last act of intercourse before rape.
   c. Determine the duration of intercourse, orifices violated, and whether penile penetration occurred.
   d. Determine the use of a condom by the perpetrator.
2. Shame, embarrassment, and humiliation
3. Anger and revenge
4. Fear of telling others for fear of not being believed
5. Male client: It is important to note that males may be sexually abused both as children and as adults and are the usual targeted victim of pedophiles. Males may have more difficulty with disclosing their abuse.

C. Rape trauma syndrome
1. Sleep disturbances and nightmares
2. Loss of appetite
3. Fears, anxiety, phobias, and suspicion
4. Decrease in activities and motivation
5. Disruptions in relationships with partner, family, and friends
6. Self-blame, guilt, and shame
7. Lowered self-esteem and feelings of worthlessness
8. Somatic complaints
9. See Chapter 62 for information on posttraumatic stress disorder.

D. Interventions
1. Perform data collection in a quiet, private area.
2. Assist with referral to SADV nurse as appropriate.
3. Stay with the victim and provide client safety.
4. Monitor the client for physical injuries.
5. Assess the victim's stress level before performing treatments and procedures.
6. Victim would not shower, bathe, douche (female), or change clothing until an examination is performed.
7. Ensure that written consent is obtained for the examination, photographs, laboratory tests, release of information, and laboratory samples.
8. Assist with the female pelvic examination and obtain specimens to detect semen (the pelvic ex-

amination may trigger a flashback of the attack). A shower and fresh clothing would be made available to the client after the examination.

9. Preserve any evidence.
10. Treat physical injuries and provide client safety.
11. Assist to administer any prescribed medications.
12. Document all events in the care of the victim.
13. Reinforce to the victim that surviving the assault is most important. If the victim survived the rape, he or she did exactly what was necessary to stay alive.
14. Refer the victim to crisis intervention and support groups.

WHAT WOULD YOU DO?

Answer: The nurse would first take the victim to a quiet and private room and assess the victim's stress level before performing treatments and procedures. The nurse needs to stay with the victim. The victim must not shower, bathe, douche (female), or change clothing until an examination is performed. The nurse would obtain consent for an examination, photographs, laboratory tests, release of information, and laboratory samples. The nurse would assist with the female pelvic examination (the pelvic examination may trigger a flashback of the attack). A shower and fresh clothing would be made available to the client after the examination. Any evidence needs to be preserved, and physical injuries need to be treated. The nurse would provide for client safety, document all events in the care of the victim, and reinforce to the victim that surviving the assault is most important; if the victim survived the rape, he or she did exactly what was necessary to stay alive. When appropriate, the nurse would refer the victim to crisis intervention and support groups.

PRACTICE QUESTIONS

1. The nurse is caring for an older adult client who has recently lost her husband. The client says, "No one cares about me anymore. All the people I loved are dead." Which response by the nurse is therapeutic?
   1. "Right! Why not just 'pack it in'?"
   2. "That seems rather unlikely to me."
   3. "I don't believe that, and neither do you."
   4. "You must be feeling all alone at this point."

2. The nurse is planning care for a client who is being hospitalized because the client has been displaying violent behavior and is at risk for potential harm to others. The nurse would avoid which intervention in the plan of care?
   1. Facing the client when providing care
   2. Ensuring that a security officer is within the immediate area
   3. Keeping the door to the client's room open when with the client
   4. Assigning the client to a room at the end of the hall to prevent disturbing the other clients

3. Which behaviors observed by the nurse might lead to the suspicion that a depressed adolescent client could be suicidal?
   1. The client gives away a DVD and a cherished autographed picture of the performer.
   2. The client runs out of the therapy group swearing at the group leader and then runs to their room.
   3. The client gets angry with her roommate when the roommate borrows their clothes without asking.
   4. The client becomes angry while speaking on their cell phone and slams the phone down on her bed.

4. A client is admitted to the psychiatric unit after a serious suicidal attempt by hanging. What is the nurse's **most important** intervention to maintain client safety?
   1. Request that a peer remain with the client at all times.
   2. Remove the client's clothing and place the client in a hospital gown.
   3. Assign a staff member to the client who will remain with him or her at all times.
   4. Admit the client to a seclusion room where all potentially dangerous articles are removed.

5. The police arrive at the emergency department with a client who has seriously lacerated both wrists. Which is the **initial** nursing action?
   1. Administer an antianxiety agent.
   2. Examine and treat the wound sites.
   3. Secure and record a detailed history.
   4. Encourage and assist the client with venting their feelings.

6. The nurse is caring for a client with severe depression. Which activity is appropriate for this client?
   1. A puzzle
   2. Drawing
   3. Checkers
   4. Paint by number

7. A client experiencing a severe major depressive episode is unable to address activities of daily living. Which is the appropriate nursing intervention?
   1. Feed, bathe, and dress the client as needed until the client can perform these activities independently.
   2. Offer the client choices and consequences to the failure to comply with the expectation of maintaining activities of daily living.
   3. Structure the client's day so that adequate time can be devoted to the client's assuming responsibility for the activities of daily living.

4. Have the client's peers confront the client about how their noncompliance with addressing activities of daily living affects the milieu.

❖ 8. The nurse is preparing to care for a dying client and several family members are at the client's bedside. Which therapeutic techniques would the nurse use when communicating with the family? **Select all that apply.**
   ❏ **1.** Discourage reminiscing.
   ❏ **2.** Make the decisions for the family.
   ❏ **3.** Encourage expression of feelings, concerns, and fears.
   ❏ **4.** Explain everything that is happening to all family members.
   ❏ **5.** Extend touch, and hold the client or family member's hand if appropriate.
   ❏ **6.** Be honest and truthful, and let the client and family know that you will not abandon them.

9. The nurse is assisting with planning the care of a client being admitted to the nursing unit who has attempted suicide. Which **priority** nursing intervention would the nurse include in the plan of care?
   1. One-to-one suicide precautions
   2. Suicide precautions, with 30-minute checks
   3. Checking the whereabouts of the client every 15 minutes
   4. Asking the client to report suicidal thoughts immediately

10. The nurse is reviewing the health care record of a client admitted to the psychiatric unit. The nurse notes that the admission nurse has documented that the client is experiencing anxiety as a result of a situational crisis. The nurse would determine that this type of crisis could be caused by which event?
   1. Witnessing a murder
   2. The death of a loved one
   3. A fire that destroyed the client's home
   4. A recent rape episode experienced by the client

11. The nurse is gathering data from a client in crisis. When determining the client's perception of the precipitating event that led to the crisis, which is the **most appropriate** question to ask?
   1. "With whom do you live?"
   2. "Who is available to help you?"
   3. "What leads you to seek help now?"
   4. "What do you usually do to feel better?"

12. The nurse is assisting with creating a plan of care for the client in a crisis state. When developing the plan, the nurse would consider which about a crisis response?
   1. A crisis state indicates that the individual is suffering from a mental illness.
   2. A crisis state indicates that the individual is suffering from an emotional illness.
   3. Presenting symptoms in a crisis situation are similar for all individuals experiencing a crisis.
   4. A client's response to a crisis is individualized, and what constitutes a crisis for one person may not constitute a crisis for another person.

13. The nurse observes that a client with a potential for violence is agitated, pacing up and down in the hallway, and making aggressive and belligerent gestures at other clients. Which statement is appropriate to make to this client?
   1. "You need to stop that behavior now!"
   2. "You will need to be placed in seclusion!"
   3. "What is causing you to become agitated?"
   4. "You will need to be restrained if you do not change your behavior."

14. During a conversation with a depressed client on a psychiatric unit, the client says to the nurse, "My family would be better off without me." The nurse would make which therapeutic response to the client?
   1. "Have you talked to your family about this?"
   2. "Everyone feels this way when they are depressed."
   3. "You will feel better once your medication begins to work."
   4. "You sound very upset. Are you thinking of hurting yourself?"

15. An older client is a victim of elder abuse, and the client's family has been attending weekly counseling sessions. Which statement by the abusive family member indicates that he or she has learned positive coping skills?
   1. "I will be more careful to make sure that my father's needs are met."
   2. "Now that my father is moving into my home, I will need to change my ways."
   3. "I feel better able to care for my father now that I know where to obtain assistance."
   4. "I am so sorry and embarrassed that the abusive event occurred. It won't happen again."

ANSWERS

1. 4

Rationale: The client is experiencing loss and is feeling hopeless. The therapeutic response by the nurse is the one that attempts to translate words into feelings. In option 1, the nurse uses sarcasm, which gives advice and is nontherapeutic as a nursing response. In option 2, the nurse is voicing doubt, which is often used when a client verbalizes delusional ideas. In option 3, the nurse is disagreeing with the client, which implies that the nurse has passed judgment on the client's ideas or opinions.

Test-Taking Strategy: Use therapeutic communication techniques. Option 4 is the only option that focuses on the client's feelings.

2. 4

Rationale: The client needs to be placed in a room near the nurses' station and not at the end of a long, relatively unprotected corridor. The nurse would not isolate himself or herself with a potentially violent client. The door to the client's room would be kept open, and the nurse must never turn away from the client. A security officer or male aide needs to be within immediate call in case the possibility of violence is suspected.

Test-Taking Strategy: Focus on the subject, the intervention to avoid. This indicates the need to select the incorrect intervention. Keeping in mind that safety is the subject will direct you to the correct option.

3. 1

Rationale: A depressed, suicidal client often gives away that which is of value as a way of saying "goodbye" and wanting to be remembered. Options 2, 3, and 4 identify acting-out behaviors.

Test-Taking Strategy: Options 2, 3, and 4 are comparable or alike in that they deal with anger and "acting-out behaviors," which are often typical of some adolescents. Option 1 is different in nature and could indicate that the client may be saying goodbye.

4. 3

Rationale: Hanging is a serious suicide attempt. The plan of care must reflect action that will promote the client's safety. Constant observation status (one-on-one) with a staff member who is never less than an arm's length away is the safest intervention.

Test-Taking Strategy: Note the strategic words, *most important.* Also focus on the subject, suicide. Eliminate option 4 because seclusion would not be the initial intervention. Eliminate option 1 next because the responsibility to safeguard a client is not the peer's responsibility. Eliminate option 2 because removing one's clothing will not maximize all possible safety strategies.

5. 2

Rationale: The initial nursing action is to examine and treat the self-inflicted injuries. Injuries from lacerated wrists can lead to a life-threatening situation. Other interventions may follow after the client has been treated medically.

Test-Taking Strategy: Note the strategic word, *initial.* Use Maslow's Hierarchy of Needs Theory to prioritize. Physiological needs come first. Option 2 addresses the physiological need.

6. 2

Rationale: Concentration and memory are poor in a client with severe depression. When a client has a diagnosis of severe depression, the nurse needs to provide activities that require little concentration. Activities that have no right or wrong choices or decisions minimize opportunities for the client to put down himself or herself. The nurse can also process the client's feelings by sitting with the client and talking or encouraging the client to write in a journal.

Test-Taking Strategy: Note that options 1, 3, and 4 are comparable or alike, in that they all require concentration. It is important to remember that clients with depression have difficulty concentrating and need activities that require little concentration.

7. 1

Rationale: The client with depression may not have the energy or interest to complete activities of daily living. Often, severely depressed clients are unable to perform even the simplest activities of daily living. The nurse assumes this role and completes these tasks with the client. Options 2 and 3 are incorrect because the client lacks the energy and motivation to perform these tasks independently. Option 4 will increase the client's feelings of poor self-esteem and unworthiness.

Test-Taking Strategy: Note the subject, severe major depressive episode. Eliminate options 2 and 3 because the client lacks the energy and motivation to do these independently. In addition, option 2 may lead to increased feelings of worthlessness as the client fails to meet expectations. Option 4 will increase the client's feelings of poor self-esteem and unworthiness.

❖ 8. 3, 5, 6

Rationale: The nurse must determine whether there is a spokesperson for the family and how much the client and family want to know. The nurse needs to allow the family and client the opportunity for informed choices and assist with the decision-making process if asked. The nurse would encourage expression of feelings, concerns, and fears, as well as reminiscing. The nurse needs to be honest and truthful and let the client and family know that they will not be abandoned. It is important to extend touch and to hold the client or family member's hand if appropriate.

Test-Taking Strategy: Recalling therapeutic communication techniques and client and family rights will assist you in answering this question.

9. 1

Rationale: One-to-one suicide precautions are required for the client who has attempted suicide. Options 2 and 3 are not appropriate, considering the situation. Option 4 may be an appropriate nursing intervention, but the priority is stated in option 1. The best option is constant supervision so that the nurse may intervene as needed if the client attempts to cause harm to him or herself.

Test-Taking Strategy: Note the strategic word, *priority.* Recalling that one-to-one suicide precautions are the priority in caring for a suicidal client will direct you to the correct option.

10. 2

Rationale: A situational crisis is associated with a life event. External situations that could precipitate a situational crisis include loss or change of a job, the death of a loved one, abortion, change in financial status, divorce, and severe illness. Options 1, 3, and 4 identify adventitious crises. An adventitious crisis relates to a crisis, disaster, or event that is not a part of everyday life, is unplanned, and is accidental.

Test-Taking Strategy: Focus on the subject, situational crisis. This will assist in eliminating options 1, 3, and 4 because they are comparable or alike.

11. 3

Rationale: The nurse's initial task when gathering data from a client in crisis is to assess the individual or family and the problem. The more clearly the problem can be defined, the better the chance a solution can be found. Option 3 will assist with determining data related to the precipitating event that led to the crisis. Options 1 and 2 identify situational supports. Option 4 identifies personal coping skills.

Test-Taking Strategy: Note the strategic words, *most appropriate*, and focus on the subject, precipitating event. Eliminate options 1 and 2 because these data will determine support systems. Eliminate option 4 because this question would be asked when determining coping skills.

12. 4

Rationale: Although each crisis response can be described in similar terms as far as presenting symptoms are concerned, what constitutes a crisis for one person may not constitute a crisis for another person because each is a unique individual. Being in a crisis state does not mean that the client is suffering from an emotional or mental illness.

Test-Taking Strategy: Eliminate option 3 because of the closed-ended word, *all*. Next, eliminate options 1 and 2 because a crisis does not indicate "illness."

13. 3

Rationale: The best statement is to ask the client what is causing the agitation. This will assist the client with becoming aware of the behavior and will assist the nurse with planning appropriate interventions for the client. Option 1 is demanding behavior, which could cause increased agitation in the client. Options 2 and 4 are threats to the client and are inappropriate.

Test-Taking Strategy: Focus on the subject, an aggressive client. Eliminate option 1 because of the demand that it places on the client. Eliminate options 2 and 4 because they indicate threats to the client.

14. 4

Rationale: Clients who are depressed may be at risk for suicide. It is critical for the nurse to assess suicidal ideation and plan. The client needs to be directly asked if a plan for self-harm exists. Options 1, 2, and 3 are not therapeutic responses.

Test-Taking Strategy: Use therapeutic communication techniques. Option 4 is the only option that deals directly with the client's feelings. Additionally, clients at risk for suicide need to be directly assessed regarding the potential for self-harm.

15. 3

Rationale: Elder abuse sometimes occurs with family members who are being expected to care for their aging parents. This can cause family members to become overextended, frustrated, or financially depleted. Knowing where in the community to turn for assistance with caring for aging family members can bring much-needed relief. Taking advantage of these alternatives is a positive alternative coping strategy, which many families use.

Test-Taking Strategy: Focus on the subject, a coping strategy. Only option 3 identifies a means of coping with the subjects. The other options are statements of good faith or promises, which may or may not be kept in the future. Option 3 outlines a definitive plan for how to handle the pressure associated with the father's care.

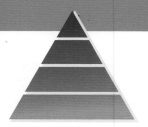

CHAPTER 65

Psychiatric Medications

PRIORITY CONCEPTS Anxiety; Mood and Affect

WHAT WOULD YOU DO?

A client has been taking alprazolam on a long-term basis for the treatment of anxiety. The primary health care provider (PHCP) has informed the nurse that the medication will be discontinued and the client needs instructions about tapering off of the medication. What would the nurse do?
Answer is located on p. 914.

I. Selective Serotonin Reuptake Inhibitors (SSRIs) (Box 65.1)

A. Description

1. Inhibit serotonin uptake and elicit an antidepressant response
2. Effective for depression with anxiety features as well as depression with psychomotor agitation
3. Relatively low side-effect profile compared with older antidepressants (tricyclics)
4. Do not cause anticholinergic effects, dry mouth, blurred vision, or urinary retention
5. May interact with other medications (e.g., digoxin, warfarin)
6. The potential for medication interactions is greatest when administered with a second serotonin-enhancing agent, such as a monoamine oxidase inhibitor (MAOI).
7. A complete medication assessment needs to be obtained and evaluated.
8. The nurse would inquire about the use of herbal therapies, especially St. John's wort.

B. Side and adverse effects

1. Dry mouth
2. Central nervous system (CNS) stimulation, including akathisia (restlessness, nervousness, agitation)
3. Blood pressure changes
4. Insomnia, somnolence (sleepy, drowsy), apathy
5. Weight loss or gain
6. Decreased libido
7. Apathy
8. Tremors

9. Seizure activity
10. Potential toxic effects (too high dose or interaction with other drugs)
    a. Abdominal pain, diarrhea
    b. Sweating, fever
    c. Tachycardia, elevated blood pressure
    d. Altered mental state (delirium)
    e. Myoclonus (muscle status), increased motor activity

C. Interventions

1. Monitor vital signs, because SSRIs can potentially lower or elevate blood pressure.
2. May cause sexual dysfunction or lack of sex drive. Inform primary health care provider if this occurs.
3. Initiate safety precautions and contact the PHCP if dizziness occurs.
4. Administer with a snack or meal to reduce the risk of dizziness and light-headedness.
5. The client is instructed to avoid alcohol.
6. Monitor the suicidal client, especially during improved mood and increased energy levels.
7. Instruct the client that taking ibuprofen with SSRIs increases the risk of an upper gastrointestinal (GI) bleed.
8. For the client on long-term therapy, monitor liver and renal function test results. Altered values may occur requiring dosage adjustments.
9. Monitor white blood cell and neutrophil counts. The medication may be discontinued if levels fall below normal.
10. Reinforce instructions to the client to change positions slowly to avoid a hypotensive effect.
11. Educate about the potential for discontinuation syndrome if medication is stopped abruptly rather than tapered. The syndrome is characterized by GI distress, behavioral or perceptual oddities, movement problems, and sleep disturbances.
12. Be aware of the potential for serotonin syndrome characterized by hyperactivity or restlessness, tachycardia, fever, elevated blood pressure, altered mental status (delirium), mood swings, seizures,

BOX 65.1 Reuptake Inhibitors

Selective Serotonin Reuptake Inhibitors
Citalopram
Escitalopram
Fluoxetine
Fluvoxamine
Paroxetine
Sertraline
Vilazodone

Serotonin-Norepinephrine Reuptake Inhibitors
Duloxetine
Desvenlafaxine
Levomilnacipran
Venlafaxine

Atypical Antidepressants
Brexanolone
Bupropion
Mirtazapine
Nefazodone
Trazodone
Venlafaxine

BOX 65.2 Tricyclic Antidepressants

Amitriptyline
Amoxapine
Clomipramine
Desipramine
Doxepin
Imipramine
Nortriptyline
Protriptyline
Trimipramine

---

muscle rigidity, and abdominal pain. This risk is greatly increased when SSRIs are given with monoamine oxidase inhibitors (MAOIs). Thus this medication combination needs to be avoided.

13. Reinforce instructions to the client that over-the-counter (OTC) cold medicines can increase the likelihood of serotonin syndrome.
14. During pregnancy, consultation with an obstetrician is recommended regarding taking these medications.
15. Monitor the medication response in children, adolescents, and the older client closely because the response may be different from in an adult client.
16. Encourage psychotherapy.
17. Serotonin-norepinephrine reuptake inhibitors (SNRIs) are similar to SSRIs, but they also work by blocking the effects of norepinephrine in addition to serotonin. Considerations are similar to those of SSRIs.

II. Tricyclic Antidepressants (Box 65.2)

A. Description
1. Block the reuptake of norepinephrine (and serotonin) at the presynaptic junction. They are used to treat depression.
2. Also affect other neurotransmitters, leading to a number of side effects
3. May reduce seizure threshold
4. May reduce effectiveness of antihypertensive agents
5. Concurrent use with alcohol or antihistamines can cause CNS depression.
6. Concurrent use with MAOIs can cause hypertensive crisis.
7. Cardiac toxicity can occur, and all clients need to undergo electrocardiographic (ECG) evaluation before treatment and periodically thereafter.

8. Overdose is life-threatening, necessitating immediate treatment (see **Priority Nursing Actions**).
9. The tricyclic antidepressant clomipramine may be used to treat obsessive-compulsive disorder.

⚡ PRIORITY NURSING ACTIONS

Tricyclic Antidepressant Overdose

1. Check airway and maintain a patent airway.
2. Administer oxygen and ventilation (as required).
3. Check vital signs and cardiac monitoring findings.
4. Assist with obtaining an electrocardiogram (ECG).
5. Prepare to assist with gastric lavage with activated charcoal if within 2 hours of ingestion.
6. Administer intravenous fluids as prescribed.
7. Prepare to assist with the administration of medications as prescribed to reverse the effects of the tricyclic antidepressant.
8. Document the event, actions taken, and the client's response.

B. Side and adverse effects
1. Anticholinergic effects: Dry mouth, difficulty voiding, dilated pupils and blurred vision, decreased gastrointestinal motility, constipation
2. Urinary retention
3. Cardiovascular disturbances such as tachycardia, dysrhythmia; orthostatic hypotension
4. Sedation
5. Seizure (with bupropion)
6. Weight gain or weight loss
7. Anxiety, restlessness, irritability, confusion
8. Decreased or increased libido with ejaculatory and erection disturbances
9. Symptoms of tricyclic antidepressant (TCA) toxicity (pseudo parkinsonism)
   a. Tardive dyskinesia: Involuntary movement of the face and jaw
   b. Akinesia: Loss of voluntary muscle movement
   c. Akathisia: State of agitation, distress, and restlessness
   d. Pseudoparkinsonism

C. Interventions
1. Monitor the suicidal client, especially during improved mood and increased energy levels.

Mental Health

2. Instruct client to change positions slowly to avoid hypotensive effect.
3. Monitor pattern of daily bowel activity.
4. Monitor for urinary retention.
5. For the client on long-term therapy, monitor liver and renal test results.
6. Administer with food or milk if gastrointestinal distress occurs.
7. Administer the entire daily oral dose at one time, preferably at bedtime because of the sedative effect. Do not split doses, such as taking half in the morning and half in the evening.
8. Instruct the client to avoid alcohol and nonprescription medications to prevent adverse medication interactions.
9. The client is instructed to avoid driving and other activities requiring alertness until the response is known. Sedation is expected during early therapy and may subside with time.
10. When the medication is discontinued by the PHCP, it would be tapered gradually.
11. The potential for medication interactions with OTC cold medications exists.
12. Good oral hygiene and the use of hard candies and mouth rinses to relieve dry mouth are encouraged.
13. Encourage psychotherapy.

⚠️ The client is informed that antidepressant medication may take several weeks to produce the desired effect. (The client response may not occur until 2–4 weeks after the first dose.)

III. **Monoamine Oxidase Inhibitors (MAOIs) (Box 65.3)**
A. Description
1. Inhibit the enzyme monoamine oxidase, which is present in the brain, blood platelets, liver, spleen, and kidneys
2. Monoamine oxidase metabolizes amines (dopamine, tyramine), norepinephrine, and serotonin, so the concentration of these amines increases with MAOIs.
3. Clients who have depression and have not responded to other antidepressant therapies, including electroconvulsive therapy, may be given MAOIs. These medications are not the first choice because of other available medications and the possible serious side and adverse effects that can occur.
4. Concurrent use with amphetamines, antidepressants, dopamine, epinephrine, levodopa/carbidopa, nasal decongestants, norepinephrine, tyramine-containing foods, or vasoconstrictors may cause hypertensive crisis.
5. Concurrent use with opioid analgesics may cause hypertension, hypotension, coma, or seizure.
B. Side and adverse effects
1. Orthostatic hypotension
2. Restlessness, insomnia
3. Dizziness and vertigo

| BOX 65.3 | Monoamine Oxidase Inhibitors |

Isocarboxazid
Phenelzine
Selegiline
Tranylcypromine

4. Weakness and lethargy
5. GI upset or constipation
6. Urinary hesitancy
7. Dry mouth
8. Weight gain
9. Peripheral edema
10. Anticholinergic effects
11. CNS stimulation (anxiety, agitation, mania)
12. Sexual dysfunction
13. Changes to cardiac rate and rhythm
C. Hypertensive crisis
1. Hypertension
2. Occipital headache radiating frontally
3. Neck stiffness and soreness
4. Nausea and vomiting
5. Sweating
6. Fever and chills
7. Clammy skin
8. Dilated pupils
9. Palpitations, tachycardia, or bradycardia
10. Constricting chest pain
11. Antidote for hypertensive crisis: Phentolamine by intravenous injection
D. Interventions
1. Monitor blood pressure frequently for hypertension.
2. Monitor for signs of hypertensive crisis.
3. If palpitations or frequent headaches occur, the medication is withheld and the PHCP is notified.
4. Administered with food if GI distress occurs.
5. The client is instructed that the medication effect may be noted during the first week of therapy, but maximum benefit may take up to 3 weeks.
6. The client is instructed to report headache, neck stiffness, or neck soreness immediately.
7. The client is instructed to change positions slowly to prevent orthostatic hypotension.
8. The client is instructed to avoid caffeine or OTC preparations such as weight-reducing pills or medications for hay fever and colds.
9. Monitor for client compliance with medication administration.
10. Instruct the client that they may take a missed dose within 3 hours of the scheduled time; otherwise, the client would skip the missed dose and take the next dose at the scheduled time.
11. The client is instructed to carry a Medic Alert card indicating that an MAOI medication is being taken.
12. Administering the medication in the evening is avoided because insomnia may result.
13. When the medication is discontinued by the PHCP, it would be discontinued gradually.

BOX 65.4	Foods to Avoid That Contain Tyramine

Avocados
Bananas
Beef or chicken liver
Brewer's yeast
Broad beans
Caffeine, such as in coffee, tea, or chocolate
Cheese, especially aged, except cottage cheese
Eggplant
Figs
Meat extracts and tenderizers
Overripe fruit
Papaya
Pickled herring
Raisins
Red wine, beer, sherry
Sauerkraut
Sausage, bologna, pepperoni, salami
Sour cream
Soy sauce
Yogurt

Note: These foods need to be avoided in the client taking a monoamine oxidase inhibitor (MAOI). Even a small amount of tyramine can increase the blood pressure and the force and/or rate of heart contractions.

14. Reinforce instructions to the client to avoid foods that require bacteria or molds for their preparation or preservation and those that contain tyramine (Box 65.4).

> ⚠ The client is taught about the foods that contain tyramine. Consuming tyramine-containing foods when taking an MAOI can cause hypertensive crisis.

IV. Mood Stabilizers (Box 65.5)

A. Description: Affect cellular transport mechanism and enhance serotonin and/or gamma-aminobutyric acid (GABA) function, which are associated with mood

B. Lithium

1. Concurrent use with diuretics, fluoxetine, or nonsteroidal anti-inflammatory drugs (NSAIDs) increases lithium reabsorption by the kidney or inhibits lithium excretion, either of which increases the risk of lithium toxicity.
2. Acetazolamide, theophylline, phenothiazines, or sodium bicarbonate may increase renal excretion of lithium, reducing its effectiveness.
3. The therapeutic dose is only slightly less than the amount producing toxicity.
4. The therapeutic drug serum level of lithium is 0.6 to 1.2 mEq/L. The actual dose at which the therapeutic effect is achieved and the levels at which toxicity occurs are highly variable among individuals.
5. The causes of an increase in the lithium level include decreased sodium intake; fluid and electrolyte loss associated with severe sweating, dehydration, diarrhea, or diuretic therapy; and illness or overdose.

BOX 65.5	Mood Stabilizers

Lithium Preparations
Lithium carbonate

Other Mood Stabilizers
Aripiprazole
Brexpiprazole
Carbamazepine
Clozapine
Fluoxetine
Gabapentin
Lamotrigine
Olanzapine
Olanzapine/fluoxetine
Oxcarbazepine
Paliperidone
Quetiapine
Risperidone
Valproate
Ziprasidone

6. Serum lithium levels would be checked frequently after initiation of therapy and then every 1 to 2 months or whenever any behavioral change suggests an altered serum level.
7. Blood samples to check serum lithium levels would be drawn in the morning, 12 hours after the last dose was taken.
8. Lithium has been associated with risks during pregnancy for both the mother and the unborn child; it crosses the placental barrier freely and has been associated with fetal toxicity and increased risk for congenital malformations.

C. Side and adverse effects
1. Polyuria
2. Polydipsia
3. Edema
4. Dysrhythmia
5. Anorexia, nausea
6. Dry mouth, mild thirst
7. Abdominal bloating
8. Soft stools or diarrhea
9. Fine hand tremors
10. Inability to concentrate
11. Muscle weakness
12. Headache
13. Hypothyroidism and goiter

D. Interventions
1. Monitor the suicidal client, especially during improved mood and increased energy levels.
2. The medication is administered with food to minimize GI irritation.
3. Reinforce instructions to the client to avoid excessive amounts of coffee, tea, or cola, which have a diuretic effect.
4. Diuretics are not administered while the client is taking lithium.

5. Reinforce instructions to the client to avoid alcohol.
6. Reinforce instructions to the client to avoid OTC medications.
7. Reinforce instructions to the client that he or she may take a missed dose within 2 hours of the scheduled time. Otherwise, the client would skip the missed dose and take the next dose at the scheduled time.
8. Reinforce instructions to the client not to adjust or stop the medication without consulting the PHCP because lithium needs to be tapered and not discontinued abruptly.
9. Reinforce instructions to the client regarding the signs/symptoms of lithium toxicity.
10. Reinforce instructions to the client to notify the PHCP if polyuria, prolonged vomiting, diarrhea, or fever occurs.
11. Reinforce instructions to the client that the therapeutic response to the medication will be noted in 1 to 3 weeks.
12. Monitor the electrocardiogram (ECG), renal function tests, and thyroid tests (ensure that these tests are performed before the start of therapy).
13. Monitor weight.

⚠️ The client taking lithium is instructed to maintain a fluid intake of six to eight glasses of water a day and an adequate salt intake to prevent lithium toxicity.

E. Lithium toxicity
1. Description
   a. Occurs when ingested lithium cannot be detoxified and excreted by the kidneys
   b. Symptoms of toxicity begin to appear when the serum lithium level is at 1.5 mEq/L.
2. Mild toxicity
   a. Serum lithium level of 1.5 mEq/L
   b. Apathy
   c. Lethargy
   d. Diminished concentration
   e. Mild ataxia
   f. Coarse hand tremors
   g. Slight muscle weakness
3. Moderate toxicity
   a. Serum lithium level of 1.5 to 2.0 mEq/L
   b. Nausea, vomiting
   c. Severe diarrhea
   d. Mild to moderate ataxia and incoordination
   e. Slurred speech
   f. Tinnitus
   g. Blurred vision
   h. Muscle twitching
   i. Irregular tremor
4. Severe toxicity:
   a. Serum lithium level greater than 2.0 mEq/L
   b. Nystagmus
   c. Muscle fasciculations
   d. Deep tendon hyperreflexia

BOX 65.6	Benzodiazepines

Alprazolam
Chlordiazepoxide
Clonazepam
Clorazepate
Diazepam
Lorazepam
Midazolam
Oxazepam
Temazepam
Triazolam

Nonbenzodiazepine Anxiolytics
Buspirone

---

   e. Visual or tactile hallucination
   f. Oliguria or anuria
   g. Impaired level of consciousness
   h. Tonic-clonic seizure or coma leading to death
5. Interventions for lithium toxicity
   a. Lithium is withheld and the PHCP is notified.
   b. Monitor vital signs and level of consciousness.
   c. Monitor cardiac status.
   d. Prepare to obtain samples to monitor lithium, electrolyte, blood urea nitrogen, and creatinine levels and perform a complete blood cell count.
   e. Monitor for suicidal tendencies and institute suicide precautions.

V. Antianxiety or Anxiolytic Medications
A. Description
   1. Antianxiety medications depress the CNS, thereby increasing the effects of GABA, which produces relaxation and may depress the limbic system.
   2. Benzodiazepines have anxiety-reducing (anxiolytic), sedative-hypnotic, muscle-relaxing, and anticonvulsant actions (Box 65.6).
   3. Benzodiazepines are contraindicated in clients with acute narrow-angle glaucoma and need to be used cautiously in children and older clients.
   4. Benzodiazepines interact with other CNS medications, producing an additive effect and therefore would only be considered for short-term use.
   5. Abrupt withdrawal of benzodiazepines can be potentially life-threatening, and withdrawal needs to occur only under medical supervision.
B. Side and adverse effects
   1. Daytime sedation
   2. Dizziness
   3. Headache
   4. Blurred or double vision
   5. Hypotension
   6. Tremor
   7. Amnesia
   8. Slurred speech
   9. Constipation or diarrhea

10. Lethargy

11. Behavioral change

C. Acute toxicity

    1. Somnolence

    2. Confusion

    3. Diminished reflexes and coma

    4. Flumazenil is a benzodiazepine antagonist that will reverse benzodiazepine intoxication in 5 minutes (it is administered intravenously).

    5. The client being treated for an overdose of a benzodiazepine may experience agitation, restlessness, discomfort, and anxiety.

D. Interventions

    1. Monitor liver and renal function test results and complete blood cell counts.

    2. Reduce the medication dose as prescribed for the older adult client and for the client with impaired liver function.

    3. Initiate safety precautions, because the older adult client is at risk for falling when taking the medication for sleep or anxiety.

    4. Assist with ambulation if drowsiness or light-headedness occurs.

    5. Inform the client that drowsiness usually disappears during continued therapy.

    6. Inform the client to avoid tasks that require alertness until the response to the medication is established.

    7. Inform the client to avoid alcohol.

    8. Reinforce instructions to not take other medications without consulting the PHCP.

    9. Reinforce instructions not to stop the medication abruptly (can result in seizure activity).

    10. Monitor for motor responses such as agitation, trembling, and tension.

    11. Monitor for autonomic responses such as cold, clammy hands and sweating.

    12. Monitor for paradoxical CNS excitement during early therapy, particularly in older adults and debilitated clients.

    13. Monitor for visual disturbances, because the medications can worsen glaucoma.

E. Withdrawal

    1. To lessen withdrawal symptoms, the dosage of a benzodiazepine needs to be tapered gradually over 2 to 6 weeks.

    2. Abrupt or too-rapid withdrawal results in the following:

        a. Restlessness

        b. Irritability

        c. Insomnia

        d. Hand tremors

        e. Abdominal or muscle cramps

        f. Sweating

        g. Vomiting

        h. Seizures

VI. Barbiturates and Sedative-Hypnotics (Box 65.7)

A. Description

> **BOX 65.7** **Barbiturates and Sedative-Hypnotics**
>
> **Barbiturates**
> Pentobarbital
> Phenobarbital
> Secobarbital
>
> **Sedative-Hypnotics**
> Chloral hydrate
> Eszopiclone
> Meprobamate
> Ramelteon
> Suvorexant
> Tasimelteon
> Zaleplon
> Zolpidem

    1. These medications depress the reticular activating system by promoting the inhibitory synaptic action of the neurotransmitter GABA.

    2. These medications are used for short-term treatment of insomnia or for sedation to relieve anxiety, tension, and apprehension.

B. Side and adverse effects

    1. Dizziness and drowsiness

    2. Confusion

    3. Irritability

    4. Allergic reactions

    5. Agranulocytosis

    6. Thrombocytopenic purpura

    7. Megaloblastic anemia

C. Overdose

    1. Tachycardia

    2. Hypotension

    3. Cold and clammy skin

    4. Dilated pupils

    5. Weak and rapid pulse

    6. Signs of shock

    7. Depressed respirations

    8. Absent reflexes

    9. Coma and death may result from respiratory and cardiovascular collapse.

D. Withdrawal

    1. Severe withdrawal symptoms begin within 24 hours after the medication is discontinued in an individual with severe medication dependence.

    2. Gradual withdrawal is used to detoxify a dependent client.

    3. Anxiety

    4. Behavioral changes

    5. Insomnia

    6. Nightmares

    7. Daytime agitation

    8. Tremors

    9. Delirium

    10. Seizure

E. Interventions

    1. Lower doses are administered as prescribed for the older client.

BOX 65.8 **Antipsychotic Medications**

Typical Antipsychotics
Chlorpromazine
Fluphenazine decanoate
Haloperidol
Loxapine
Perphenazine
Thiothixene
Thioridazine
Trifluoperazine

Atypical Antipsychotics
Aripiprazole
Asenapine
Brexpiprazole
Cariprazine
Clozapine
Iloperidone
Lurasidone
Olanzapine
Paliperidone
Pimavanserin
Quetiapine
Risperidone
Ziprasidone

BOX 65.9 **Side and Adverse Effects of Antipsychotic Medications**

Anticholinergic Effects
Dry mouth
Increased heart rate
Urinary retention
Constipation
Hypotension

Extrapyramidal Side and Adverse Effects
Parkinsonism
Tremors
Mask-like facies
Rigidity
Shuffling gait
Dysphagia
Drooling

Dystonias
Abnormal or involuntary eye movements, including oculogyric crisis
Facial grimacing
Twisting of the torso or other muscle groups

Akathisia
Restlessness
Constant moving about

Tardive Dyskinesia
Protrusion of the tongue
Chewing motion
Involuntary movements of the body and extremities

Other Side and Adverse Effects
Drowsiness
Blood dyscrasias
Pruritus
Photosensitivity
Elevated blood glucose level
Increased weight
Impaired body temperature regulation
Gynecomastia
Lactation

---

2. Medications need to be used with caution in the client who has suicidal tendencies or has a history of drug addiction.
3. Maintain safety by supervising ambulation and using side rails at night.
4. Reinforce instructions to take the medication as directed.
5. Reinforce instructions to avoid driving or operating hazardous equipment if drowsiness, dizziness, or unsteadiness occurs.
6. The client needs to avoid alcohol, because this allows an increase of medication to enter the brain, causing feelings of depression and drowsiness, dizziness, slow and difficult breathing, confusion, and coma.
7. For insomnia, the client would take the medication 30 minutes before bedtime; avoid taking with a large amount of food to help absorption.
8. Inform the client that a hangover effect may occur in the morning.
9. The client is not to discontinue the medication abruptly.
10. Inform the client taking chloral hydrate to take the medication with food and a full glass of water, fruit juice, or ginger ale to prevent gastric irritation.

VII. Antipsychotic Medications (Box 65.8)

A. Description
1. Improve the thought processes and the behavior of the client with psychotic symptoms, especially the client with schizophrenia

2. Affect dopamine receptors in the brain, thereby reducing the psychotic symptoms
3. Typical antipsychotics are more effective for positive symptoms of schizophrenia such as hallucinations, aggression, and delusions. Typical antipsychotic medications also block the chemoreceptor trigger zone and vomiting center in the brain, producing an antiemetic effect.
4. Atypical antipsychotics are more effective for the negative symptoms of schizophrenia, such as avolition, apathy, and alogia.
5. The effects of antipsychotic medications will be potentiated when given with other medications acting on the CNS.

B. Side and adverse effects (Box 65.9)
C. Extrapyramidal syndrome: Can cause parkinsonism, dystonia, akathisia, or tardive dyskinesia

D. Interventions
1. Monitor vital signs.
2. Monitor for symptoms of neuroleptic malignant syndrome (can occur with antipsychotic medications); refer to Section VIII.
3. Monitor urine output.
4. Monitor serum glucose level.
5. Administer the medication with food or milk to decrease gastric irritation.
6. For oral use, the liquid form might be preferred because some clients hide tablets to avoid taking them.
7. Note that the absorption rate is faster with the liquid form of oral medication.
8. Skin contact with the liquid concentrate is avoided to prevent contact dermatitis.
9. Protect the liquid concentrate from light.
10. Dilute the liquid concentrate with fruit juice.
11. Injectable form of risperidone is administered every 2 weeks for clients who have difficulty with medication adherence.
12. The client is informed that a full therapeutic effect of the medication may not be evident for 3 to 6 weeks after initiation of therapy. However, an observable therapeutic response may be apparent after 7 to 10 days.
13. The client is informed that some medications may cause a harmless change in urine color to pinkish to red-brown.
14. Reinforce instructions to use sunscreen, hats, and protective clothing when outdoors.
15. Inform the client to avoid alcohol or other CNS depressants because they may allow more of the medication to enter the brain, causing feelings of depression and drowsiness, dizziness, slow and difficult breathing, confusion, and coma.
16. Reinforce instructions to change positions slowly to avoid orthostatic hypotension.
17. Reinforce instructions to report signs of agranulocytosis, including sore throat, fever, and malaise.
18. Reinforce instructions to report signs of liver dysfunction, including jaundice, malaise, fever, and right upper abdominal pain.
19. When antipsychotics are discontinued, the medication dosage is reduced gradually to avoid sudden recurrence of psychotic symptoms.

⚠️ Monitor for extrapyramidal side and adverse effects in the client taking an antipsychotic medication.

VIII. Neuroleptic Malignant Syndrome

A. Description
1. A potentially fatal syndrome that may occur at any time during therapy with neuroleptic (antipsychotic) medications (typically with first-generation antipsychotics)
2. Although rare, neuroleptic malignant syndrome more commonly occurs at the initiation of therapy, after the client has changed from one medication to another, after a dosage increase, or when a combination of medications is used.

B. Data collection
1. Dyspnea or tachypnea
2. Tachycardia or irregular pulse rate
3. Autonomic dysfunction
   a. Hyperpyrexia
   b. Hypertension
   c. Tachycardia
   d. Tachypnea
   e. Diaphoresis
   f. Drooling
4. High or low blood pressure
5. Excessive weakness or fatigue
6. Altered level of consciousness
7. Seizure
8. Severe extrapyramidal side and adverse effects
9. Skeletal muscle rigidity
10. Difficulty swallowing
11. Oculogyric crisis
12. Elevated white blood cell count, liver function results, and creatinine phosphokinase level

C. Interventions
1. Notify the registered nurse, who will then notify the PHCP.
2. Monitor the vital signs.
3. Initiate safety and seizure precautions.
4. Prepare to discontinue the medication.
5. Monitor the level of consciousness.
6. Administer antipyretics as prescribed.
7. Use a cooling blanket to lower the body temperature.
8. Monitor electrolyte levels and assist with the intravenous administration of fluids, as prescribed.
9. Monitor for complications such as deep vein thrombosis (DVT) and rhabdomyolysis.

IX. Medications to Treat Attention-Deficit/Hyperactivity Disorder (Box 65.10)

A. Children with attention-deficit/hyperactivity disorder (ADHD) may require medication to reduce hyperactive behavior and lengthen attention span.

B. CNS stimulants are effective in controlling this disorder; these medications, which increase agitation and activity in adults, have a calming effect on children with ADHD and increase alertness and sensitivity to stimuli.

C. Side and adverse effects
1. Tachycardia

BOX 65.10 **Medications to Treat Attention-Deficit/Hyperactivity Disorder**

Amphetamine
Atomoxetine
Dexmethylphenidate
Dextroamphetamine
Dextroamphetamine and amphetamine
Guanfacine
Lisdexamfetamine
Methylphenidate

2. Anorexia and weight loss
3. Elevated blood pressure
4. Dizziness
5. Agitation
D. Interventions
1. Monitor for CNS side and adverse effects.
2. Obtain a baseline electrocardiogram (ECG).
3. Monitor the blood pressure.
4. The child and parents are instructed that OTC medications need to be avoided.
5. The child and parents are instructed that the last dose of the day would be taken at least 6 hours before bedtime (14 hours for extended-released forms) to prevent insomnia.
6. Monitor height and weight (particularly in children).
7. Reinforce that several weeks of therapy may be necessary before the therapeutic effect is noted.
8. Reinforce instructions to the child and parents that a drug-free period may be prescribed to demonstrate the continued need for the medication; a drug-free period temporarily removes side effects of the medication, which include sleep delay, appetite suppression, and tolerance to treatment.

X. **Medications to Treat Alzheimer's Disease (Box 65.11)**

A. Acetylcholinesterase inhibitors may be used to treat Alzheimer's disease to improve cognitive functions in the early stages.
B. Donepezil
1. An inhibitor of acetylcholinesterase used to treat mild to moderate dementia of Alzheimer's disease
2. Side and adverse effects include nausea and diarrhea.
3. Donepezil can slow the heart rate through its vagotonic effect.
C. Galantamine
1. An inhibitor of cholinesterase used to treat mild to moderate dementia of Alzheimer's disease
2. Side and adverse effects include nausea, vomiting, diarrhea, anorexia, and weight loss.
3. Can cause bronchoconstriction. Used with caution in clients with asthma and chronic obstructive pulmonary disease.
D. Memantine
1. An N-methyl-D-aspartate (NMDA) receptor antagonist is indicated for moderate to severe Alzheimer's disease.
2. Side and adverse effects include dizziness, headache, confusion, and gastrointestinal disturbances.

BOX 65.11	Medications to Treat Alzheimer's Disease

Donepezil
Galantamine
Memantine
Rivastigmine

3. Would not be used in combination with other NMDA antagonists such as amantadine or ketamine. Such combinations produce undesirable additive effects
4. Sodium bicarbonate and other medications that alkalinize the urine can decrease renal excretion of memantine. Accumulation to toxic levels can result.
5. Clearance is reduced with renal impairment, therefore used with caution.
E. Rivastigmine
1. Cholinesterase inhibitor used to treat mild to moderate dementia of Alzheimer's disease
2. Side and adverse effects include nausea, vomiting, diarrhea, abdominal pain, and anorexia.
3. Would be taken with food to reduce gastrointestinal side effects.
4. Used with caution in clients with peptic ulcer disease, bradycardia, sick sinus syndrome, urinary obstruction, and lung disease because it enhances cholinergic transmission, thus intensifying symptoms of these disorders.

WHAT WOULD YOU DO?

Answer: Alprazolam is a benzodiazepine and to prevent withdrawal or lessen withdrawal symptoms, the nurse would reinforce instructions to the client to taper the dose gradually over 2 to 6 weeks as specifically prescribed by the PHCP. The nurse needs to inform the client that abrupt or too rapid withdrawal can result in restlessness, irritability, insomnia, hand tremors, abdominal or muscle cramps, sweating, vomiting, and seizures. The nurse informs the client that if any of these manifestations occur during tapering, they need to be reported immediately to the PHCP.

PRACTICE QUESTIONS

1. A hospitalized client is taking clozapine for the treatment of a schizophrenic disorder. Which laboratory study prescribed for the client would the nurse specifically review to monitor for an adverse effect associated with the use of this medication?
1. Platelet count
2. Cholesterol level
3. White blood cell count
4. Blood urea nitrogen level

2. Disulfiram is prescribed for a client and the nurse is collecting data on the client and is reinforcing instructions regarding the use of this medication. Which is **most important** for the nurse to determine before administration of this medication?
1. A history of hyperthyroidism
2. A history of diabetes insipidus

3. When the last full meal was consumed
4. When the last alcoholic drink was consumed

3. The nurse is collecting data from a client, and the client's spouse reports that the client is taking donepezil hydrochloride. Which disorder would the nurse suspect that this client may have based on the use of this medication?
   1. Dementia
   2. Schizophrenia
   3. Seizure disorder
   4. Obsessive-compulsive disorder

4. Fluoxetine is prescribed, and the nurse reinforces instructions to the client regarding the administration of the medication. Which statement by the client indicates an understanding about the administration of this medication?
   1. "I should take the medication with my evening meal."
   2. "I should take the medication at noon with an antacid."
   3. "I should take the medication in the morning when I first arise."
   4. "I should take the medication right before bedtime with a snack."

5. A client receiving a tricyclic antidepressant arrives at the mental health clinic. Which observation indicates that the client is correctly following the medication plan?
   1. Reports not going to work for the past week
   2. Complains of not being able to "do anything" anymore
   3. Arrives at the clinic neat and appropriate in appearance
   4. Reports sleeping 12 hours per night and 3 to 4 hours during the day

❖ 6. A hospitalized client is prescribed phenelzine sulfate for the treatment of depression. The nurse reinforces instructions to the client and tells the client to avoid consuming which foods while taking this medication? **Select all that apply.**

❏ 1. Figs
❏ 2. Yogurt
❏ 3. Crackers
❏ 4. Aged cheese
❏ 5. Tossed salad
❏ 6. Oatmeal cookies

7. A client taking buspirone for 1 month returns to the clinic for a follow-up visit. Which would indicate medication **effectiveness?**
   1. No rapid heartbeats or anxiety
   2. No paranoid thought processes
   3. No thought broadcasting or delusions
   4. No reports of alcohol withdrawal symptoms

8. A client taking lithium carbonate reports vomiting, abdominal pain, diarrhea, blurred vision, tinnitus, and tremors. The lithium level is checked as a part of the routine follow-up, and the level is 3.0 mEq/L. The nurse knows that this is which level?
   1. Toxic
   2. Normal
   3. Slightly above normal
   4. Excessively below normal

9. A client arrives at the health care clinic and tells the nurse that they have been doubling their daily dosage of bupropion hydrochloride to help them get better faster. The nurse understands that the client is now at risk for which problem?
   1. Insomnia
   2. Weight gain
   3. Seizure activity
   4. Orthostatic hypotension

10. The nurse is performing a follow-up teaching session with a client discharged 1 month ago who is taking fluoxetine. Which information would be important for the nurse to gather regarding the adverse effects related to the medication?
    1. Cardiovascular symptoms
    2. Gastrointestinal dysfunctions
    3. Problems with mouth dryness
    4. Problems with excessive sweating

ANSWERS

1. 3
Rationale: Hematological reactions can occur in the client taking clozapine and include agranulocytosis and mild leukopenia. The white blood cell count would be checked before initiating treatment and would be monitored closely during the use of this medication. The client would also be monitored for signs indicating agranulocytosis, which may include sore throat, malaise, and fever. Options 1, 2, and 4 are unrelated to this medication.

Test-Taking Strategy: Focus on the subject, an adverse effect of clozapine. Remember, clozapine can cause agranulocytosis and mild leukopenia.

2. 4
Rationale: Disulfiram is used as an adjunct treatment for selected clients with chronic alcoholism who want to remain in a state of enforced sobriety. Clients need to abstain from alcohol intake for at least 12 hours before the initial dose of the medication is administered. The most important data are to determine when the last alcoholic drink was consumed. The

medication is used with caution in clients with diabetes mellitus, hypothyroidism, epilepsy, cerebral damage, nephritis, and hepatic disease. It is contraindicated in severe heart disease, psychosis, or hypersensitivity related to the medication.
Test-Taking Strategy: Note the strategic words, *most important*. Recall that the medication is used as an adjunct treatment for selected clients with chronic alcoholism. This will assist in directing you to the correct option.

3. 1
Rationale: Donepezil hydrochloride is a cholinergic agent used in the treatment of mild to moderate dementia of the Alzheimer type. It enhances cholinergic functions by increasing the concentration of acetylcholine. It slows the progression of Alzheimer's disease. This medication is not used to treat the disorders in options 2, 3, and 4.
Test-Taking Strategy: Focus on the subject, the use of donepezil hydrochloride. Remember, this medication is used to treat mild to moderate dementia.

4. 3
Rationale: Fluoxetine is a selective serotonin reuptake inhibitor (SSRI). It is administered in the early morning without consideration to meals. Options 1, 2, and 4 are incorrect.
Test-Taking Strategy: Focus on the subject, the administration of fluoxetine. Use medication guidelines to eliminate option 2. Next, eliminate options 1 and 4 because they are comparable or alike and indicate taking the medication with food.

5. 3
Rationale: Depressed individuals will sleep for long periods, are not able to go to work, and feel as if they cannot "do anything." Once they have had some therapeutic effect from their medication, they will report resolution of many of these complaints, as well as demonstrate an improvement in their appearance.
Test-Taking Strategy: Focus on the subject, the effects of tricyclic antidepressants. Observations identified in options 1, 2, and 4 are all symptoms of depression. The improvement in appearance indicates a therapeutic response to the medication, thus indicating compliance with the medication regimen.

❖ 6. 1, 2, 4
Rationale: Phenelzine sulfate is a monoamine oxidase inhibitor. The client would avoid consuming foods that are high in tyramine. Eating these foods could trigger a potentially fatal

hypertensive crisis. Some foods to avoid include yogurt, aged cheeses, smoked or processed meats, red wines, and fruits such as avocados, raisins, and figs.
Test-Taking Strategy: Focus on the subject, foods to avoid when taking a monoamine oxidase inhibitor. Recall that phenelzine sulfate is a monoamine oxidase inhibitor and foods high in tyramine need to be avoided. Next, from the food items listed in the question, identify the foods that contain tyramine.

7. 1
Rationale: Buspirone hydrochloride is not recommended for the treatment of drug or alcohol withdrawal, paranoid thought disorders, or schizophrenia (thought broadcasting or delusions). Buspirone hydrochloride is most often indicated for the treatment of anxiety and aggression.
Test-Taking Strategy: Focus on the subject, the use of buspirone hydrochloride. Recalling that this medication is an antianxiety medication will direct you to the correct option.

8. 1
Rationale: The therapeutic serum level of lithium is 0.6 to 1.2 mEq/L. A level of 3 mEq/L indicates toxicity.
Test-Taking Strategy: Focus on the subject, the therapeutic serum level of lithium. Remember the therapeutic level is 0.6 to 1.2 mEq/L.

9. 3
Rationale: Bupropion is an atypical antidepressant and does not cause significant orthostatic blood pressure changes. Seizure activity is common in dosages greater than 450 mg daily. Bupropion frequently causes a drop in body weight. Insomnia is a side effect, but seizure activity causes a greater client risk.
Test-Taking Strategy: Focus on the subject, the effects of doubling a dose of bupropion. Recalling that seizure activity can occur with higher-than-recommended doses will direct you to option 3.

10. 2
Rationale: The most common adverse effects related to fluoxetine include CNS and GI system dysfunction. This medication affects the GI system by causing nausea and vomiting, cramping, and diarrhea. Options 1, 3, and 4 are not adverse effects of this medication.
Test-Taking Strategy: Focus on the subject, adverse effects related to fluoxetine. It is necessary to recall that this medication causes CNS and GI system dysfunction.

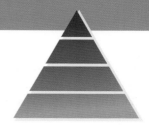

References

American Academy of Dermatology Association. (n.d.). *Isotretinoin: Treatment for acne*. Retrieved from https://www.aad.org/public/diseases/acne-and-rosacea/isotretinoin-treatment-for-severe-acne.

American Academy of Pediatrics (2020). *Car seats: Information for families*. Retrieved from https://www.healthychildren.org/English/safety-prevention/on-the-go/Pages/Car-Safety-Seats-Information-for-Families.aspx.

American Academy of Pediatrics. (n.d.). *Healthy foster care America*. Retrieved from https://www.aap.org/en-us/advocacy-and-policy/aap-health-initiatives/healthy-foster-care-america/Documents/HFCAJudgesToolkit.pdf.

American Academy of Pediatrics. (2014). *Policy statement: Screening for nonviral sexually transmitted infections in adolescents and young adults*. Retrieved from http://pediatrics.aappublications.org/content/early/2014/06/25/peds.2014-1024.

American Academy of Pediatrics. (2020). *Recommendations for preventive pediatric health care*. Retrieved from https://www.aap.org/en-us/Documents/periodicity_schedule.pdf.

American Cancer Society. (2014). *Signs and symptoms of cancer*. Retrieved from https://www.cancer.org/cancer/cancer-basics/signs-and-symptoms-of-cancer.html.

American Cancer Society. (2015). *Tools to help measure distress*. Retrieved from https://www.cancer.org/treatment/treatments-and-side-effects/emotional-side-effects/distress/tools-to-measure-distress.html.

American College of Rheumatology. (2017). *Juvenile arthritis: Fast facts*. Retrieved from https://www.rheumatology.org/I-Am-A/Patient-Caregiver/Diseases-Conditions/Juvenile-Arthritis.

American Heart Association. (2020). *Guidelines for Cardiopulmonary Resuscitation and Emergency Cardiovascular Care*. Retrieved from https://professional.heart.org/en/science-news/2020-aha-guidelines-for-cpr-and-ecc.

American Nurses Association. (2011). *ANAs Principles for social networking and the nurse*. Retrieved from https://www.nursingworld.org/~4af4f2/globalassets/docs/ana/ethics/social-networking.pdf

American Nurses Association. (n.d.). *Social networking privacy tool-kit*. Retrieved from https://www.nursingworld.org/practice-policy/nursing-excellence/social-networking-Principles/.

Ard, K. L. (n.d.). *Improving the health care of lesbian, gay, bisexual, and transgender people: Understanding and eliminating health disparities*. Retrieved from https://www.lgbthealtheducation.org/wp-content/uploads/Improving-the-Health-of-LGBT-People.pdf.

Arnett, D. et.al. (2019). ACC/AHA Guideline on the Primary Prevention of Cardiovascular Disease: Executive Summary: A Report of the American College of Cardiology/American Heart Association Task Force on Clinical Practice Guidelines. *Circulation*, 140:e563–e595. Retrieved from https://www.ahajournals.org/doi/10.1161/CIR.0000000000000677.

Benjamin, R. M. (2010). Multiple chronic conditions: A public health challenge. *Public Health Repository*, 125(5), 626–627.

Bohn, D. K., & Holz, K. A. (1996). Sequelae of abuse: Health effects of childhood sexual abuse, domestic battering, and rape. *Journal of Midwifery & Women's Health*, 41(6), 442–456.

Campinha-Bacote, C. (1999). A model and instrument for addressing cultural competence in health care. *Journal of Nursing Education*, 38(5), 203–207.

Centers for Disease Control and Prevention. (2018). *Interim guidance for environmental infection control in hospitals for Ebola virus*. Retrieved from https://www.cdc.gov/vhf/ebola/clinicians/cleaning/hospitals.html.

Centers for Disease Control and Prevention. (2018). *Guidance on personal protective equipment (PPE) to be used by healthcare workers during management of patients with confirmed Ebola or persons under investigation (PUIs) for Ebola who are clinically unstable or have bleeding, vomiting, or diarrhea in U.S. hospitals, including procedures for donning and doffing PPE*. Retrieved from https://www.cdc.gov/vhf/ebola/healthcare-us/ppe/guidance.html.

Centers for Disease Control and Prevention. (2018). *Hand hygiene in healthcare settings*. Retrieved from https://www.cdc.gov/handhygiene/.

Centers for Disease Control and Prevention. (2018). *Ebola (Ebola Virus Disease)*. Retrieved from https://www.cdc.gov/vhf/ebola/index.html.

Centers for Disease Control and Prevention. (2019). *Conjunctivitis (pink eye)*. Retrieved from https://www.cdc.gov/conjunctivitis/index.html.

Centers for Disease Control and Prevention. (2020). *Coronavirus (COVID-19)*. Retrieved from https://www.cdc.gov/coronavirus/2019-ncov/index.html.

Centers for Disease Control and Prevention. (2016). *Identify, isolate, inform: Emergency department evaluation and management for patients under investigation (PUIs) for Ebola Virus Disease (EVD)*. Retrieved from https://www.cdc.gov/vhf/ebola/clinicians/emergency-services/emergency-departments.html.

Cooper, K., & Gosnell, K. (2019). *Foundations and adult health nursing* (8th ed.). St. Louis, MO: Elsevier.

Crawford, L. & Yoost, B. (2020). *Fundamentals of nursing* (2nd ed.). St. Louis, MO: Elsevier.

deWit, D., Stromberg, H., & Dallard, C. (2017). *Medical-surgical nursing: Concepts & practice* (3rd ed.). St. Louis, MO: Saunders.

De Hert, M., Correll, C. U., Bobes, J., et al. (2011). Physical illness in patients with severe mental disorders. Prevalence, impact of medications and disparities in healthcare. *World Psychiatry*, 10(1), 52–77.

Dickison, P., Haerling, K. A., & Lasater, K. (2019). Integrating the National Council of State Boards of Nursing Clinical Judgment Model into nursing educational frameworks. *Journal of Nursing Education*, 58(2), 72–78.

Frich, L. M. (2003). Nursing interventions for patients with chronic conditions. *Journal of Advanced Nursing*, 44(2), 135–154.

Gahart, B., Nazareno, A., & Ortega, M. (2019). *Gahart's 2019 Intravenous medications* (35th ed.). St. Louis, MO: Mosby.

Global Citizen. (2018). *The 7 biggest challenges facing refugees and immigrants in the U.S.* Retrieved from https://www.globalcitizen.org/en/content/the-7-biggest-challenges-facing-refugees-and-immig/.

Guttmacher Institute. (2018). *Guttmacher Policy Review*. Retrieved from https://www.guttmacher.org/gpr?volume=21&language=en.

Harding, M. M., Kwong, J., Roberts, D., et al. (2020). *medical-surgical nursing: Assessment and management of clinical problems* (11th ed.). St. Louis, MO: Elsevier, p. 947.

Health Care for the Homeless Clinicians' Network. (2014). *Adapting your practice: Recommendations for the care of homeless patients with opioid use disorders.* Retrieved from https://nhchc.org/wp-content/uploads/2019/08/hch-opioid-use-disorders_adapting-your-practice-final-to-post.pdf.

Henry, J., & Kaiser Family Foundation. (2017). *Key facts about the uninsured population.* Retrieved from https://www.kff.org/uninsured/fact-sheet/key-facts-about-the-uninsured-population/.

Heuther, S., & McCance, K. (2017). *Understanding pathophysiology* (6th ed.). St. Louis, MO: Elsevier.

Hockenberry, M., Wilson, D., & Rodgers, C. (2017). *Wong's essentials of pediatric nursing* (10th ed.). St. Louis, MO: Mosby.

Hodgson, B., & Kizior, R. (2020). *Saunders nursing drug handbook 2020.* St. Louis, MO: Saunders.

Huber, D. (2018). *Leadership and nursing care management* (6th ed.). St. Louis, MO: Saunders.

Huber, D. (2010). *Leadership and nursing care management* (4th ed.). Philadelphia: Saunders.

iPLEDGE® program update. (2016). Retrieved from https://www.ipledgeprogram.com/iPledgeUI/home.u.

Issues in Science and Technology. (n.d.). *Correctional health is community health.* Retrieved from http://issues.org/32-1/correctional-health-is-community-health/.

Ignatavicius, D., Workman, M., & Rebar, C. (2018). *Concepts for interprofessional collaborative care* (9th ed.). St. Louis, MO: Saunders.

Ignatavicius, D., Workman, M., Rebar, C., Heimgartner, N. (2021). *Concepts for interprofessional collaborative care* (10th ed.). St. Louis, MO: Saunders.

Ignatavicius, D., Workman, ML. (2013). *Medical-surgical nursing: Patient centered collaborative care* (7th ed.). St. Louis, MO: Saunders.

International Council of Nurses. (2012). *The INC code of ethics for nurses.* Retrieved from https://www.icn.ch/sites/default/files/inline-files/2012_ICN_Codeofethicsfornurses_%20eng.pdf.

Jarvis, C. (2020). *Physical examination and health assessment* (8th ed.). St. Louis, MO: Saunders.

Joyful Heart Foundation. (2018). *Effects of domestic violence.* Retrieved from http://www.joyfulheartfoundation.org/learn/domestic-violence/effects-domestic-violence.

Keltner, N., Steele, D. (2019). *Psychiatric nursing* (8th ed.). St. Louis, MO: Mosby.

Lewis, S., Bucher, L., Heitkemper, M., et al. (2017). *Medical-surgical nursing: Assessment and management of clinical problems* (10th ed.). St. Louis, MO: Mosby.

Lewis, S., Dirksen, S., Heitkemper, M., Bucher, L., & Camera, I. (2014). *Medical-surgical nursing: assessment and management of clinical problems* (9th ed.). St. Louis, MO: Mosby.

Lilley, L., Rainforth Collins, S., & Snyder, J. (2020). *Pharmacology and the nursing process* (9th ed.). St. Louis, MO: Mosby.

Linton, A. (2016). *Introduction to medical-surgical nursing* (6th ed). St. Louis, MO: Saunders.

Maness, D. L., & Khan, M. (2014). Care of the homeless: An overview. *American Family Physician, 89*(8), 634–640.

May, M. E., & Kennedy, C. H. (2010). Health and problem behavior among people with intellectual disabilities. *Behavioral Annals of Practice, 3*(2), 4–12.

Mau, M., Blanchette, P., Carpenter, D-A., et al. (2010). *Health and health care of Native Hawaiian and other Pacific Islander Older Adults.* Retrieved from https://geriatrics.stanford.edu/ethnomed/hawaiian_pacific_islander.html.

McIntosh, J. (2015). *Single mothers at risk of poorer health later in life, study suggests.* Retrieved from https://www.medicalnewstoday.com/articles/293887.php.

McKinney, E., James, S., Murray, S., et al. (2018). *Maternal-child nursing* (4th ed.). St. Louis, MO: Elsevier.

Mehta, S. (2016). *The health toll of single motherhood.* Retrieved from https://www.healthify.us/healthify-insights/the-health-toll-of-single-motherhood.

Mosby's Medical Dictionary. (2017). 10th ed. St. Louis, MO: Elsevier.

National Academies of Sciences, Engineering, and Medicine. (2016). *Parenting matters: Supporting parents of children ages 0–8.* Washington, DC: The National Academies Press.

National Council of State Boards of Nursing: 2020 NCLEX-PN® detailed test plan, Chicago, 2019, National Council of State Boards of Nursing. Retrieved from http://www.ncsbn.org.

NCSBN. (Fall 2019). *Next Generation NCLEX News: Approved NGN Item Types.* Chicago: NCSBN.

National Health Care for the Homeless. (2018). *Federal issues and priorities.* Retrieved from https://www.nhchc.org/policy-advocacy/issue/.

National Institute of Neurological Disorders and Stroke (n.d.). *Know Stroke. Know the Signs. Act in Time* Retrieved from. http://www.stroke.nih.gov/.

Nix, S. (2017). *Williams' basic nutrition and diet therapy* (15th ed.). St. Louis, MO: Mosby.

Olenick, M., Flowers, M., & Diaz, V. J. (2015). US veterans and their unique issues: Enhancing health care professional awareness. *Advanced Medical Education Practice, 6,* 635–639.

Pagana, K., Pagana, T., & Pagana, T. N. (2019). *Mosby's diagnostic and laboratory tests reference* (14th ed.). St. Louis, MO: Mosby.

Pamper, F. C., Krueger, P. M., & Denney, J. T. (2010). Socioeconomic disparities in health behaviors. *Annual Review of Sociology, 36,* 349–370.

Perry, A., Potter, P., & Ostendorf, W. (2018). *Clinical nursing skills & techniques* (9th ed.). St. Louis, MO: Mosby.

Potter P, Perry AG, Stockert PA, Hall AM. (2013). *Fundamentals of nursing* (8th ed). St. Louis, MO: Mosby.

ProEdit. (2019). *Understanding Bloom's (and Anderson and Krathwohl's) Taxonomy.* Retrieved from http://www.proedit.com/understanding-blooms-and-anderson-and-krathwohls-taxonomy/.

Rapp, C. G., Mentes, J., & Titler, M. (2001). Acute confusion/delirium protocol. *Journal of Gerontological Nursing, 27*(4), 21–33.

Russell, L. (2010). *Fact sheet: Health disparities by race and ethnicity.* Retrieved from https://cdn.americanprogress.org/wp-content/uploads/issues/2010/12/pdf/disparities_factsheet.pdf.

Skidmore-Roth, L. (2017). *Mosby's nursing drug reference* (30th ed.). St. Louis, MO: Mosby.

Swain, G. R. (2017). How does economic and social disadvantage affect health? *Institute for Research on Poverty, 33*(1), 1–6.

Swearingen, P. (2016). *All-in-one care planning resource: Medical-surgical, pediatric, maternity, & psychiatric nursing care plans* (4th ed.). St. Louis, MO: Mosby.

Szilagyi, M. A., Rosin, D. S., Rubin, D., et al. (2015). Health care issues for children and adolescents in foster care and kinship care. *Pediatrics, 136*(4), e1142–e1146.

The Joint Commission. (2018). *Facts about the official "do not use" list of abbreviations.* Retrieved from https://www.jointcommission.org/facts_about_do_not_use_list/.

The Joint Commission. (2018). *Hospital national patient safety goals.* Retrieved from https://www.jointcommission.org/assets/1/6/2018_HAP_NPSG_goals_final.pdf.

The Joint Commission. (2018). *National patient safety goals.* Retrieved from https://www.jointcommission.org/assets/1/6/NPSG_Chapter_HAP_Jan2018.pdf.

Thomas, C., & Siela, D. (2011). The impaired nurse: Would you know what to do if you suspected substance abuse? *American Nurse Today, 6*(8). Retrieved from https://www.americannursetoday.com/the-impaired-nurse-would-you-know-what-to-do-if-you-suspected-substance-abuse/.

Touhy, T., & Jett, K. (2018). *Ebersole and Hess' gerontological nursing & healthy aging* (5th ed.). St. Louis, MO: Mosby.

Touhy, T., & Jett, K. (2012). *Ebersole and Hess' toward healthy aging* (8th ed.). St. Louis, MO: Mosby.

Traditional Chinese Medicine World Foundation. (n.d.). *TCM healing modalities.* Retrieved from https://www.tcmworld.org/what-is-tcm/healing-modalities/.

Trehearne, B., Fishman, P., & Lin, E. (2014). Role of the nurse in chronic illness management: Making the medical home more effective. *Nursing Economics, 32*(4), 178–184.

Urden, L., Stacy, K., & Lough, M. (2018). *Priorities in critical care nursing* (8th ed.). St. Louis, MO: Elsevier.

US National Library of Medicine. (2017). *Veterans and military health.* Retrieved from https://medlineplus.gov/veteransandmilitaryhealth.html.

US Department of Agriculture. *ChooseMyPlate* (n.d.). Retrieved from https://www.choosemyplate.gov/browse-by-audience/view-all-audiences/adults/moms-pregnancy-breastfeeding.

U.S. Department of Health and Human Services Office. (n.d.). *Health information privacy.* Retrieved from https://www.hhs.gov/hipaa/index.html.

Varcarolis, E. (2017). *Essentials of psychiatric mental health nursing: A communication approach to evidence-based care* (3rd ed.). St. Louis, MO: Saunders.

Wilson, A. F., & Giddens, J. F. (2013). *Health assessment for nursing practice* (5th ed.). St. Louis, MO: Mosby.

Wilson, A. F., & Giddens, J. F. (2009). *Health assessment for nursing practice* (4th ed.). St. Louis, MO: Mosby.

World Health Organization. (2018). *Migration and health: Key issues.* Retrieved from http://www.euro.who.int/en/health-topics/health-determinants/migration-and-health/migrant-health-in-the-european-region/migration-and-health-key-issues.

World Health Organization. (2005). Chronic diseases and their common risk factors. Retrieved from http://www.who.int/chp/chronic_disease_report/media/Factsheet1.pdf.

Zerwekh, J., & Zerwekh Garneau, A. (2018). *Nursing today: Transition and trends* (9th ed.). St. Louis, MO: Elsevier.

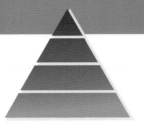

Glossary

ABO A type of antigen system. The ABO type of the donor should be compatible with the recipient's. Type A can match with type A or O; type B can match with type B or O; type O can match only with type O; type AB can match with type A, B, AB, or O.

Abuse When directed toward another, includes acts such as neglect, misuse, deceit, or exploitation. It is the wrongful or improper use or action toward another that results in willful infliction of pain, injury, maltreatment, mental anguish, or unreasonable confinement. Abuse can include verbal assaults, the demand to perform demeaning tasks, theft, or mismanagement of personal belongings (exploitation). Abuse inflicted can be physical, emotional, or sexual.

Accommodation Process whereby a clear visual image is maintained as the gaze is shifted from a distant to near point.

Accountability Moral concept that involves the acceptance of consequences of a decision or action by a professional nurse.

Acculturation Process of learning norms, beliefs, and behavioral expectations of a group other than one's own.

Active immunity A form of long-term acquired antibody protection that develops naturally after an initial infection or exposure to antigens, or artificially after a vaccination.

Acute kidney injury (AKI) The sudden loss of kidney function caused by renal cell damage from ischemia or toxic substances. It occurs abruptly and can be reversible. Acute kidney injury leads to hypoperfusion, cell death, and decompensation in renal function. The prognosis depends on the cause and condition of the client.

Addiction State of dependence or compulsive use. In relation to substance dependence, addiction incorporates the concepts of loss of control with respect to the use of a substance, consuming the substance despite related problems and complications, and a tendency to relapse.

Addisonian crisis A life-threatening disorder caused by adrenal hormone insufficiency. Crisis is precipitated by infection, trauma, stress, or surgery. Death can occur from shock, vascular collapse, or hyperkalemia.

Addison's disease Hyposecretion of adrenal cortex hormones (glucocorticoids and mineralocorticoids) from the adrenal gland, resulting in deficiency of the corticosteroid hormones. The condition is fatal if left untreated.

Adenocarcinoma A tumor that arises from glandular epithelial tissue.

Adrenalectomy The surgical removal of an adrenal gland. Lifelong replacement of glucocorticoids and mineralocorticoids is necessary with a bilateral adrenalectomy. Temporary replacement may be necessary for a unilateral adrenalectomy.

Advance directive Written document recognized by state law that provides directions concerning the provision of care when a client is unable to make his or her own treatment choices; the two basic types of advance directives include instructional directives, such as a living will, and durable power of attorney for health care.

Advocacy Acting on behalf of the client and protecting the client's right to make his or her own decisions.

Afterload The force against which the heart has to pump (peripheral resistance) to eject blood from the left ventricle. Factors and conditions that would impede blood flow increase left ventricular afterload.

Air embolism An obstruction caused by a bolus of air that enters the vein through an inadequately primed intravenous (IV) line, from a loose connection, during a tubing change, or during removal of an IV line.

Allen's test A test to assess for collateral circulation to the hand by evaluating the patency of the radial and ulnar arteries.

Amniotic fluid Pale, straw-colored fluid in which the fetus floats. It serves as a cushion against injury from sudden blows or movements and helps to maintain a constant body temperature for the fetus. The fetus modifies the amniotic fluid through the processes of swallowing, urinating, and movement through the respiratory tract.

Anuria Urine output of less than 100 mL/day.

Arterial pressure The pressure of the blood against the arterial walls. Pressure can be measured indirectly by sphygmomanometer or directly by arterial catheter. Readings are expressed as systolic over diastolic. Arterial pressure increases when the cardiac output, peripheral resistance, or blood volume increases.

Arterial steal syndrome A set of symptoms that can develop following the insertion of an arteriovenous fistula when too much blood is diverted to the vein and arterial perfusion to the hand is compromised.

Arteriovenous fistula Surgical creation by anastomosis of an opening between a large artery and a large vein to provide an access for hemodialysis. The flow of arterial blood into the venous system causes the vein to become engorged (maturity). Maturity is necessary so that the engorged vein can be punctured using a large-bore needle for hemodialysis.

Ascites The accumulation of fluid within the peritoneal cavity that results from venous congestion of the hepatic capillaries, which leads to plasma leaking directly from the liver surface and portal vein.

Asterixis A sign that occurs with liver disease. Causes a coarse tremor characterized by rapid, nonrhythmic extensions and flexions in the wrist and fingers; also termed liver flap.

Asthma (reactive airway disease) A chronic inflammatory disorder of the airways marked by airway hyperresponsiveness. Asthma causes recurrent episodes of wheezing, breathlessness, chest tightness, and coughing associated with airflow obstruction that is often reversible with treatment.

Astigmatism Visual distortion that results from an uneven curvature of the cornea or lens, in which light rays focus on two different points on the retina.

Atresia Congenital absence or closure of a body orifice.

Attenuated vaccines Vaccines derived from microorganisms or viruses; their virulence has been weakened as a result of passage through another host.

Auscultation The physical data collection technique that involves listening to sounds within the body. Special equipment such as a stethoscope may be needed to perform this technique.

Autonomic dysreflexia Syndrome characterized by hypertension, bradycardia, excessive sweating, facial flushing, nasal congestion, pilomotor responses, and headache. Occurs with spinal lesions above T6. Triggers include visceral stimulation from a distended bladder or impacted rectum. It is a neurological emergency and must be treated immediately to prevent a hypertensive stroke; also known as autonomic hyperreflexia.

Autonomy An ethical principle; respecting the client's right to make decisions about self and health care.

Babinski reflex Dorsiflexion of the big toe with extension; elicited by firmly stroking the lateral aspect of the sole of the foot.

Bacille Calmette-Guérin vaccine (BCG) A vaccine containing attenuated tubercle bacilli that may be given to persons in foreign countries or to those traveling to foreign countries to produce increased resistance to tuberculosis.

Ballottement Rebounding of the fetus against the examiner's finger on palpation. When the examiner taps the cervix, the fetus floats upward in the amniotic fluid. The examiner feels a rebound when the fetus falls back.

Bariatric surgery A surgical procedure used to treat severe obesity.

Baroreceptors Specialized nerve endings (also called pressoreceptors) located in the walls of the aortic arch and carotid sinuses. They are affected by changes in the arterial blood pressure (BP). An increase in arterial pressure stimulates baroreceptors and the heart rate, and arterial pressure decreases. A decrease in arterial pressure leads to a lessened stimulation of the baroreceptors, vasoconstriction occurs, and the heart rate increases.

Beneficence An ethical principle; the responsibility of the nurse to take positive actions to help the client.

Benign Usually refers to growths that are encapsulated, remain localized, and are slow growing.

Billroth I Partial gastrectomy with the remaining segment being anastomosed to the duodenum; also termed gastroduodenostomy.

Billroth II Partial gastrectomy with the remaining segment being anastomosed to the jejunum; also termed gastrojejunostomy.

Birth The expulsion or extraction of the neonate.

Blood The liquid pumped by the heart through the arteries, veins, and capillaries. Blood is composed of a clear yellow fluid (plasma), formed elements, and cell types with various functions.

Blood cell Any of the formed elements of the blood, including a red cell (erythrocyte), white cell (leukocyte), and platelet (thrombocyte).

Blood pressure (BP) The force exerted by the blood against the walls of the blood vessels. If the blood pressure falls too low, blood flow to the tissues, heart, brain, and other organs becomes inadequate. If the blood pressure becomes too high, the risk of vessel rupture and damage increases.

Body mechanics The coordinated efforts of the musculoskeletal and nervous systems to maintain balance, posture, and body alignment during lifting, bending, and moving to perform activities safely.

Brudzinski's sign Involuntary flexion of the hip and knee when the neck is passively flexed; indicates meningeal irritation.

Burn Cell destruction of the layers of the skin caused by heat, friction, electricity, radiation, or chemicals.

Calcium A mineral element needed for the process of bone formation, coagulation of blood, excitation of cardiac and skeletal muscle, maintenance of muscle tone, conduction of neuromuscular impulses, and the synthesis and regulation of the endocrine and exocrine glands. The normal adult reference range is 9 to 10.5 mg/dL.

Cancer A neoplastic disorder that can involve all body organs. Cells lose their normal growth-controlling mechanism, resulting in uncontrolled cell division.

Carbon monoxide poisoning Carbon monoxide is a colorless, odorless, and tasteless gas that has an affinity for hemoglobin 200 times greater than that of oxygen. Poisoning occurs from the inhalation of carbon monoxide. Oxygen molecules are displaced and carbon monoxide reversibly binds to hemoglobin to form carboxyhemoglobin. Tissue hypoxia results.

Carcinogen A physical, chemical, or biological stressor that causes neoplastic changes in normal cells.

Carcinoma A new growth or malignant tumor that originates from epithelial cells, the skin, gastrointestinal tract, lungs, uterus, breast, or other organ.

Carcinoma in situ A premalignant lesion with all of the histological characteristics of cancer except invasion of the basement membrane.

Cardiac output The total volume of blood pumped through the heart in 1 minute. The normal cardiac output is 4 to 7 L/minute. Cardiac output equals stroke volume multiplied by heart rate.

Cast A stiff dressing or casting made of plaster of Paris or synthetic material to stabilize a part or parts of the body until healing occurs.

Cataract An opacity of the lens that distorts the image projected onto the retina and that can progress to blindness.

Catheter embolism An obstruction caused by breakage of the catheter tip during intravenous line insertion or removal.

Chadwick's sign Violet coloration of the mucous membranes of the cervix, vagina, and vulva that is one of the early signs of pregnancy; caused by increased vascularity. This is considered a probable sign of pregnancy.

Chest tube Tube that returns negative pressure to the intrapleural space; used to remove abnormal accumulations of air and fluid from the pleural space.

Cholecystectomy Removal of the gallbladder.

Cholecystitis An inflammation of the gallbladder that may occur as an acute or chronic process. Acute inflammation is associated with gallstones (cholelithiasis). Chronic cholecystitis results when inefficient bile emptying and gallbladder muscle wall disease cause a fibrotic and contracted gallbladder.

Choledocholithotomy Incision into the common bile duct to remove a gallstone.

Chronic kidney disease (CKD) The progressive loss and ongoing deterioration in kidney function. It is characterized by a glomerular filtration rate of less than 60 mL/minute for a period of 3 months or longer. It is irreversible and eventually results in uremia or end-stage kidney disease. Chronic kidney disease requires dialysis or kidney transplantation to maintain life.

Chronic obstructive pulmonary disease A disease state characterized by pulmonary airflow obstruction that is usually progressive, not fully reversible, and sometimes accompanied by airway hyperreactivity. Airflow obstruction may be caused by chronic bronchitis and/or emphysema. In chronic hypercapnia, the stimulus to breathe is a low Pao_2 instead of an increased $Paco_2$.

Chronological age Age in years.

Chvostek's sign A sign of hypocalcemia. A spasm of the facial muscles elicited by tapping the facial nerve just anterior to the ear.

Circulatory overload A complication resulting from the infusion of blood or intravenous solutions at a rate too rapid for the size, age, physiological status, or clinical condition of the recipient.

Cirrhosis A chronic progressive disease of the liver characterized by diffuse degeneration and destruction of hepatocytes. Repeated destruction of hepatic cells causes the formation of scar tissue.

Client's (Patient's) Bill of Rights The rights and responsibilities of clients receiving care. These rights acknowledge the client's right to participate in her or his health care with an emphasis on autonomy.

Compartment syndrome Condition in which pressure increases in a confined anatomical space, leading to decreased blood flow, ischemia, and dysfunction of these tissues. Initial ischemia with pain, pallor, paresthesia, muscle weakness, and loss of pulses may progress to necrosis and permanent muscle cell dysfunction.

Compatibility Matching of blood from two persons by two different types of antigen systems, ABO and Rh, present on the membrane surface of the red blood cells, to prevent a transfusion reaction.

Compensation Refers to the body processes that occur to counterbalance a physiological disturbance such as an acid-base disturbance, or other disturbance such as that which occurs during heart failure.

Conductive hearing loss A mechanical dysfunction or blockage of sound waves to the inner ear fibers because of an external ear or middle ear disorder. Such disorders often can be corrected with no damage to hearing or minimal permanent hearing loss.

Conductivity The ability of the heart muscle fibers to propagate electrical impulses along and across cell membranes.

Confidentiality The nurse's responsibility of keeping a client's information private.

Confidentiality/information security In the health care system, refers to the protection of privacy of the client's personal health information.

Consent Voluntary act whereby a person agrees to allow someone else to do something.

Contractility The inherent ability of the myocardium to alter contractile force and velocity. Sympathetic stimulation increases myocardial contractility, so stroke volume increases. Conditions that decrease myocardial contractility reduce stroke volume.

Conversion The first step in the calculation of a medication problem. Conversion is necessary when a medication prescribed is written in one system but the medication label is stated in another.

Coping mechanism Method used to decrease anxiety.

Coronavirus The virus that causes the illness known as COVID-19. This virus can be transmitted from person to person primarily via respiratory droplets.

COVID COVID-19 means coronavirus disease 2019. In COVID-19, the 'CO' stands for 'corona,' the 'VI' for 'virus,' and the 'D' for disease. COVID is the illness caused by the coronavirus.

Crackles Audible high-pitched crackling or popping sounds heard during lung auscultation; result from fluid in the airways and are not cleared by coughing.

Crisis Temporary state of disequilibrium that can be physiological or psychological. An individual's usual compensatory or coping mechanisms and problem-solving methods fail. Crisis can result in further physiological disturbance, personality growth, or personality disorganization if left untreated.

Crohn's disease An inflammatory disease that can occur anywhere in the gastrointestinal tract but most often affects the terminal ileum; leads to thickening and scarring, a narrowed lumen, fistulas, ulcerations, and abscesses. The disease is characterized by remissions and exacerbations.

Crossmatching The testing of the donor's blood and the recipient's blood for compatibility.

Cullen's sign Bluish discoloration of the abdomen and periumbilical area seen in acute hemorrhagic pancreatitis.

Cultural assimilation Process in which individuals from a smaller group are absorbed by the larger cultural group and take on the characteristics of the larger culture.

Cultural awareness Learning about the cultures of clients being cared for; this includes a self-examination of one's own background, recognizing biases, prejudices, and assumptions about other people. The nurse is also responsible for asking clients about their health care practices and preferences.

Cultural competence Continued pursuit of acquisition of awareness, skill, and knowledge of a culture and its practices that facilitates provision of culturally appropriate health care.

Cultural diversity Differences that may exist among groups of people; differences may result from ethnic, racial, and cultural variables.

Cultural imposition Tendency to impose one's own beliefs, values, and patterns of behavior on individuals from another culture.

Culture The knowledge, beliefs, patterns of behavior, ideas, attitudes, values, and norms that are unique to a particular group of people.

Cushing's disease A metabolic disorder characterized by abnormally increased secretion (endogenous) of cortisol, caused by increased amounts of adrenocorticotropic hormone (ACTH) secreted by the pituitary gland.

Cushing's syndrome A metabolic disorder resulting from the chronic and excessive production of cortisol by the adrenal cortex or by the administration of glucocorticoids in large doses for several weeks or longer (exogenous or iatrogenic).

Cushing's triad A classic, late sign of increased intracranial pressure; the triad includes hypertension, bradycardia, and widened pulse pressure.

Cyanosis The bluish color that results in tissues, such as the nail beds and mucous membranes, when tissues are deprived of adequate amounts of oxygen.

Cycloplegia Paralysis of the ciliary muscles by medications that block muscarinic receptors. Cycloplegia causes blurred vision because the shape of the lens can no longer be adjusted for near vision.

Dawn phenomenon A nocturnal release of growth hormone, which may cause blood glucose level elevations before breakfast in the client with diabetes mellitus. Treatment includes administering an evening dose of intermediate-acting insulin at 10:00 p.m.

Decerebrate (extensor) posturing Stiff extension of one or both arms and possibly the legs; indicates a brainstem lesion.

Decorticate (flexor) posturing Flexure of one or both arms on the chest and possibly stiff extension of the legs; indicates damaged cortex.

Deep full-thickness burn Injury extends beyond the skin into underlying fascia and tissues, and muscle, bone, and tendons are damaged.

Deep partial-thickness burn Injury extends deep into the dermis and few healthy cells remain.

Defense mechanism Coping mechanism used in an effort to protect the individual from feelings of anxiety. As anxiety increases and becomes overwhelming, the individual copes by using defense mechanisms to protect the ego and decrease anxiety.

Delegation Process of transferring a selected nursing task in a situation to an individual who is competent to perform that specific task.

Delivery Actual event of birth; the expulsion or extraction of the neonate.

Dementia An organic syndrome identified by gradual and progressive deterioration in intellectual functioning. Long- and short-term memory losses occur with impairment in judgment, abstract thinking, problem-solving ability, and behavior, resulting in a self-care deficit. A common type of dementia is Alzheimer's disease.

Depression A mood disorder that can be identified by feelings of sadness, hopelessness, and worthlessness, and a decreased interest in activities.

Developmental age Age based on a child's maturational progress. It is determined by standardized resources such as body size, physical and psychological functioning, motor skills, and aptitude tests.

Diabetes insipidus The hyposecretion of antidiuretic hormone from the posterior pituitary gland, resulting in failure of tubular reabsorption of water in the kidneys and diuresis.

Diabetes mellitus A chronic disorder of glucose intolerance and impaired carbohydrate, protein, and lipid metabolism caused by a deficiency of insulin or resistance to the action of insulin. A deficiency of insulin results in hyperglycemia.

Diabetic ketoacidosis A life-threatening complication of diabetes mellitus that develops when a severe insulin deficiency occurs, resulting in hyperglycemia. Hyperglycemia progresses to ketoacidosis over a period of several hours to several days. Acidosis occurs in clients with type 1 diabetes mellitus, persons with undiagnosed diabetes, and persons who stop prescribed treatment for diabetes.

Dialysis A blood filtering procedure that is indicated when kidney function deteriorates and the accumulation of water and waste products interferes with life functions. Dialysis is performed via the bloodstream (hemodialysis) or through the peritoneal cavity (peritoneal dialysis).

Diastole The phase of the cardiac cycle in which the heart relaxes between contractions. Diastole represents the period of time when the two ventricles are dilated by the blood flowing into them.

Diastolic pressure The force of the blood exerted against the artery walls when the heart relaxes or fills.

Disaster Any human-made or natural event that causes destruction and devastation that cannot be alleviated without assistance; internal disasters are events that occur within a health care agency, whereas external disasters are events that occur outside the health care agency.

Diverticulitis Inflammation of one or more diverticula from penetration of fecal matter through the thin-walled diverticula, resulting in local abscess formation. A perforated diverticulum can progress to intraabdominal perforation with generalized peritonitis.

Diverticulosis Outpouching or herniations of the intestinal mucosa that can occur in any part of the intestine but are most common in the sigmoid colon.

Dumping syndrome Rapid emptying of the gastric contents into the small intestine, which occurs following gastric resection.

Embryo The earliest stage of fetal development beginning day 15 through approximately week 8 after conception. Then, the unborn baby is usually referred to as the fetus.

Emergency response plan A health care agency's preparedness and response plan in the event of a disaster.

Emphysema Abnormal permanent enlargement of air spaces distal to the terminal bronchioles in the lungs, with destruction of alveolar walls.

Endotracheal tube Tube used to maintain a patent airway; indicated when a client needs mechanical ventilation.

Enteral nutrition Administration of nutrition with liquefied foods into the gastrointestinal tract via a tube.

Ergonomic principles The anatomical, physiological, psychological, and mechanical principles used to ensure the efficient and safe use of an individual's energy.

Esophageal varices Dilated and tortuous veins in the submucosa of the esophagus caused by portal hypertension, often associated with liver cirrhosis; at high risk for rupture if portal circulation pressure rises.

Ethical principles Set of guidelines or codes that direct or govern actions for health care providers. The guidelines and codes identify the expectations of a profession and the standards of behavior for its members.

Ethics The ideals of right and wrong; guiding principles that individuals may use to make decisions.

Ethnic group People within a culture who share characteristics based on race, religion, color, national origin, or language.

Ethnicity An individual's identification of self as part of an ethnic group.

Evidence-based practice Approach to client care in which the nurse integrates the client's preferences, clinical expertise, and the best research evidence to deliver quality care.

External fixation Stabilization of a fracture by the use of an external frame, with multiple pins applied through the bone.

Fat embolism Sudden dislodgment of a fat globule that is freed into the circulation, where it can lodge in a blood vessel and obstruct blood flow to tissue distal to the obstruction.

Fat emulsion (lipids) A solution administered intravenously with parenteral nutrition therapy to prevent fatty acid deficiency.

Fertilization Uniting of the sperm and ovum, which occurs within 12 hours of ovulation and within 2 to 3 days of insemination, the average duration of viability for the ovum and sperm.

Fetor hepaticus The fruity, musty breath odor associated with severe chronic liver disease.

Fidelity An ethical principle; the nurse's responsibility to keep promises by following through with nursing actions and interventions.

Flaccid posturing No motor response display in any extremity.

Fluid volume deficit Dehydration, in which the fluid intake of the body is not sufficient to meet the fluid needs of the body.

Fluid volume excess Fluid intake or fluid retention that exceeds the fluid needs of the body. Also called overhydration or fluid overload.

Fowler's position The client is supine and the head of the bed is elevated to 45 to 90 degrees.

Fresh-frozen plasma A blood product administered to increase the level of clotting factors in clients with such a deficiency.

Full-thickness burn Involves injury and destruction of the entire epidermis and dermis; there are no skin cells to repopulate.

Functional age The age equivalent at which a child actually is able to perform specific self-care or related tasks.

Gastrectomy Removal of the stomach with attachment of the esophagus to the jejunum or duodenum; also termed esophagojejunostomy or esophagoduodenostomy.

Gastric resection Removal of the lower half of the stomach, usually including a vagotomy; also termed antrectomy.

Generic name Also known as the nonproprietary name of a medication, or the US adopted name; each medication has only one generic name. In most medication questions on the NCLEX®, the generic name will be the only name identified.

Glaucoma Increased intraocular pressure as a result of inadequate drainage of aqueous humor from the canal of Schlemm or from overproduction of aqueous humor. If untreated, the condition damages the optic nerve and can result in blindness.

Glomerulonephritis An immunological condition causing proliferative and inflammatory changes within the glomeruli of the kidneys that results in sclerosis (hardening) and loss of function.

Goodell's sign Softening of the cervix that occurs at the beginning of the second month of gestation. This is considered a probable sign of pregnancy.

Gravida A pregnant woman; called gravida I (primigravida) during the first pregnancy, gravida II during the second pregnancy, and so on.

Growth Measurable physical and physiological body changes that occur over time.

Grunting The sound made by forced expiration, which is the body's attempt to improve oxygenation when hypoxemia is present.

Health care–associated (nosocomial) infections Infections acquired in the hospital or other health care facility that were not present or incubating at the time of the client's admission; also referred to as hospital-acquired infections.

Health history The collection of subjective data when interviewing the client. It includes information such as the client's current state of health, the medications taken, previous illnesses and surgeries, family histories, and a review of systems.

Hegar's sign Compressibility and softening of the lower uterine segment that occurs at about week 6 of gestation. This is considered a probable sign of pregnancy.

Hemianopsia Blindness in half of the visual field.

Hemiparesis Weakness affecting one side of the body.

Hemiplegia Paralysis affecting one side of the body.

Hemoglobin A1c A blood test that measures the amount of glycosylated hemoglobin as a percentage of total hemoglobin. When glucose levels are elevated over time, a higher percentage of hemoglobin is glycosylated. When hemoglobin is glycosylated, the glucose remains attached for the life of the red blood cell, approximately 120 days. The hemoglobin A1c level is reflective of the degree of glycemic control over the previous 2 to 3 months. An estimated average daily glucose can be calculated from the hemoglobin A1c.

Hepatitis Inflammation of the liver caused by a virus, bacteria, or exposure to medications or hepatotoxins.

Hereditary Refers to the transmission of genetic characteristics from parent to offspring.

Herpes zoster (shingles) An acute viral infection of the nerve structure caused by varicella-zoster (chickenpox). Reactivation of the virus can occur in those who previously had chickenpox and is commonly seen in the older adult; a vaccine is available to prevent this occurrence. Herpes zoster can be contagious to individuals who have never had chickenpox and have not been vaccinated against the virus.

Hiatal hernia A portion of the stomach that herniates through the diaphragm and into the thorax. Herniation results from weakening of the muscles of the diaphragm and is aggravated by factors that increase abdominal pressure, such as pregnancy, ascites, obesity, tumors, and heavy lifting; also termed esophageal or diaphragmatic hernia.

High Fowler's position The client is supine and the head of the bed is elevated to 90 degrees.

Home safety Removing items from the home environment and avoiding situations or events that place the client at risk for accident or injury.

Homeostasis The tendency of a biological system to maintain relatively constant conditions in the internal environment while continuously interacting with and adjusting to changes originating within or outside the system.

Homonymous hemianopsia Loss of half of the field of view on the same side in both eyes.

Hyperglycemia Elevated blood glucose as a result of too little insulin or the inability of the body to use insulin properly.

Hyperopia Farsightedness; objects converge to a point behind the retina. Vision beyond 20 feet is normal, but near-vision is poor. The condition is corrected by a convex lens.

Hyperosmolar hyperglycemic syndrome (HHS) Extreme hyperglycemia without acidosis. A complication of type 2 diabetes mellitus, which may result in dehydration or vascular collapse but does not include the acidosis component of diabetic ketoacidosis. Onset is usually slow, taking from hours to days.

Hyperparathyroidism A condition resulting in the excess secretion of parathyroid hormone (PTH). Parathyroid hormone is responsible for calcium homeostasis in the body.

Hyperthyroidism A condition that occurs as a result of excessive thyroid hormone secretion.

Hypoglycemia Low blood glucose level that results from too much insulin, not enough food, or excess activity.

Hypothyroidism A hypothyroid state resulting from a hyposecretion of thyroid hormone.

Implantation Embedding of the fertilized ovum in the uterine mucosa 6 to 10 days after conception.

Inactivated vaccine A vaccine that contains killed microorganism(s).

Increased intracranial pressure Increased pressure within the skull caused by trauma, hemorrhage, growths or tumors, hydrocephalus, edema, or inflammation. Increased pressure can impede circulation to the brain and absorption of cerebrospinal fluid and can affect nerve cell functioning, leading to brainstem compression and death.

Infant A human born alive; also, a human from 28 days of age until the first birthday.

Infiltration Seepage of intravenous fluid out of the vein and into the surrounding interstitial spaces.

Informed consent A client's understanding of the reason for the proposed intervention, with its benefits and risks, and agreement with the treatment by signing a consent form.

Inspection The first physical data collection technique, which begins the moment the examiner meets the client. It involves a visual assessment of the client during the health history and making observations during the physical examination of specific body systems.

Internal fixation Stabilization of a fracture that involves the application of screws, plates, pins, a wire, or nails to hold the fragments in alignment.

Interprofessional collaboration Involves teamwork among health care professionals that promotes sharing of expertise to create a plan of care that will restore and maintain a client's health.

Irritable bowel syndrome (IBS) A functional gastrointestinal disorder characterized by chronic or recurrent diarrhea, constipation, and/or abdominal pain, and bloating.

Justice An ethical principle; refers to fairness when providing care to clients.

Kernig's sign Loss of the ability of a supine client to straighten the leg completely when it is fully flexed at the knee and hip; indicates meningeal irritation.

Labor Coordinated sequence of rhythmic involuntary uterine contractions resulting in effacement and dilation of the cervix, followed by expulsion of the products of conception.

Lateral (side-lying) position The client is lying on their side, head and shoulders aligned with the hips and spine, and parallel to the edge of the mattress. The head, neck, and upper arm are supported by a pillow. The lower shoulder is pulled forward slightly and, along with the elbow, flexed at 90 degrees. The legs are flexed or extended. A pillow is placed to support the back.

Leadership Interpersonal process that involves influencing others (followers) to achieve goals.

Lecithin-to-sphingomyelin (L/S) ratio Ratio of two components of amniotic fluid, used for predicting fetal lung maturity; normal L/S ratio in amniotic fluid is 2:1 or greater when the fetal lungs are mature.

Legally blind The best visual acuity with corrective lenses in the better eye of 20/200 or less, or the visual field is no greater than 20 degrees in its widest diameter in the better eye.

Leukemia Neoplasm involving abnormal overproduction of leukocytes, usually at an immature stage, in the bone marrow.

Lithotomy position The client is lying on the back with the hips and knees flexed at right angles and the feet in stirrups.

Lochia Discharge from the uterus that consists of blood from the vessels of the placental site and debris from the decidua; lasts for 2 to 6 weeks after delivery.

Lymphoma Neoplasm that originates from lymphoid tissue.

Macular degeneration Blurred central vision caused by progressive degeneration of the center of the retina. The condition may be atrophic or age related, or dry or exudative (wet).

Magnesium Concentrated in the bone, in the cartilage, and within the cell itself; required for the use of adenosine triphosphate as a source of energy. It is necessary for the action of numerous enzyme systems such as those involved in carbohydrate metabolism, protein synthesis, nucleic acid synthesis, and contraction of muscular tissue. It also regulates neuromuscular activity and the clotting mechanism. The normal adult level is 1.8 to 2.6 mEq/L.

Malignant Term for growths that are not encapsulated but grow and metastasize. These growths are cancerous lesions having the characteristics of disorderly, uncontrolled, and chaotically proliferating cells.

Malnutrition Deficiency of the nutrients required for development and maintenance of the human body.

Malpractice Type of negligence; failure to meet the standards of acceptable care, which results in harm to another person.

Management Accomplishment of tasks or goals by oneself or by directing others.

Mass casualty event Involves a number of casualties that exceeds the resource capabilities of the hospital; also known as a disaster.

Mechanical ventilation The use of a ventilator to move room air or oxygen-enriched air into and out of the lungs mechanically to maintain proper levels of oxygen and carbon dioxide in the blood. Types of ventilators include negative-pressure and positive-pressure ventilators. Various ventilator modes are adjusted to the client's individual needs.

Medication reconciliation An organized process to avoid medication errors by comparing the client's medication prescriptions when hospitalized with all medications that the client was previously taking.

Melena Black, tarry stools as a result of bleeding in the upper gastrointestinal tract.

Metabolic acidosis A total concentration of buffer base that is lower than normal, with a relative increase in the hydrogen ion concentration. This results from loss of buffer bases or retention of too many acids without sufficient bases and occurs in conditions such as kidney failure and diabetic ketoacidosis, from the production of lactic acid, and from the ingestion of toxins, such as acetylsalicylic acid.

Metabolic alkalosis A deficit or loss of hydrogen ions or acids or an excess of base (bicarbonate) that results from the accumulation of base or from a loss of acid without a comparable loss of base in the body fluids. This occurs in conditions resulting in hypovolemia, the loss of gastric fluid, excessive bicarbonate intake, the massive transfusion of whole blood, and hyperaldosteronism.

Metabolism Ongoing chemical process within the body that converts digested nutrients into energy for the functioning of cells.

Metastasis The transfer of disease from one organ or part to another not directly connected with it. Secondary malignant lesions, originating from the primary tumor, are located in anatomically distant places.

Milieu The safe physical and social environment in which an individual receives treatment.

Minority group Ethnic, cultural, racial, or religious group that constitutes less than a numerical majority of the population.

Miosis Constriction of the pupil, which occurs primarily by stimulation of the muscarinic receptors of the sphincter muscles. It is seen with the use of pilocarpine drops when treating glaucoma, when using opioids, or when there is brain damage of the pons.

Miotic A medication that causes constriction of the pupil.

Morality Behavior that is in accordance with customs or traditions and usually reflects personal or religious beliefs.

Multicasualty event Involves a limited number of victims or casualties and can be managed by a hospital with available resources.

Multidrug-resistant strain of tuberculosis (MDR-TB) A multidrug-resistant strain of tuberculosis can occur as a result of improper or noncompliant use of treatment programs and the development of mutations in the tubercle bacilli.

Murphy's sign A sign of gallbladder disease consisting of pain when taking a deep breath when the examiner's fingers are on the approximate location of the gallbladder.

Mydriasis A dilated pupil that occurs because of blockage of the muscarinic receptors of the sphincter muscles or by stimulation of the α-receptors of the dilator muscles. Enlarged pupils occur with stimulation of the sympathetic nervous system, use of dilating drops, acute glaucoma, or past or recent trauma.

Mydriatic A medication that causes dilation of the pupil.

Myeloma A malignant proliferation of plasma cells within the bone.

Myopia Nearsightedness; rays coming from an object are focused in front of the retina. Near vision is normal, but distant vision is defective. A biconcave lens is used for correction.

Myxedema coma A rare but serious disorder that results from persistently low thyroid production. Coma can be precipitated by acute illness, rapid withdrawal of thyroid medication, anesthesia and surgery, hypothermia, and the use of sedatives and opioid analgesics.

Nadir The period of time during which an antineoplastic medication has its most profound effects on the bone marrow.

Naegele's rule Determines the estimated date of birth based on the premise that the woman has a 28-day menstrual cycle. Subtract 3 months and add 7 days to the first day of the last menstrual period; then add 1 year if appropriate. Alternatively, add 7 days to the last menstrual period and count forward 9 months.

Nasal flaring A widening of the nares to enable an infant or child to take in more oxygen; a serious indicator of air hunger.

Neglect The failure to provide services necessary for physical or mental health; includes failure to prevent injury.

Negligence Conduct that falls below a standard of care; failure to meet a client's needs either willfully or by omission or failure to act.

Neoplasm An abnormal growth, which may be benign or malignant.

Nephrolithiasis The formation of kidney stones. Kidney stones are formed in the renal parenchyma.

Nephrotic syndrome A set of manifestations characterized by protein wasting and diffuse glomerular damage in which the client has severe diffuse edema.

Neurogenic shock Occurs most commonly in clients with injuries above T6 and is usually experienced soon after the injury. Massive vasodilation occurs, leading to pooling of blood in the blood vessels, tissue hypoperfusion, and impaired cellular metabolism.

Newborn; neonate A human from the time of birth to the 28th day of life.

Nonmaleficence An ethical principle; the obligation to do no harm or cause no harm to another.

Nuchal rigidity Stiff neck; flexion of the neck onto the chest causes intense pain.

Nutrients Carbohydrates, fats or lipids, proteins, vitamins, minerals, electrolytes, and water that must be supplied in adequate amounts to provide energy, growth, development, and maintenance of the human body.

Objective data Information about the client that is obtained by the examiner through the physical examination and the review of results obtained from laboratory, radiological, or other diagnostic studies.

Oliguria Urine output of less than 400 mL/day.

Packed red blood cells A blood product used to replace erythrocytes lost as a result of trauma or surgical interventions, or in clients with bone marrow suppression.

Palpation A physical data collection technique that involves using the hands to feel certain parts of the client's body, including some organs. The examiner uses this technique to assess texture, size, and consistency of the body part being examined.

Pancreatitis An acute or chronic inflammation of the pancreas, with associated escape of pancreatic enzymes into surrounding tissue. Acute pancreatitis can occur suddenly as one attack or can be recurrent with resolution. Chronic pancreatitis is a continual inflammation and destruction of the pancreas, with scar tissue replacing pancreatic tissue.

Para Number of pregnancies that have ended at 20 or more weeks, regardless of whether the infant was born alive or was stillborn.

Parenteral Given by injection, such as by the intravenous, intramuscular, subcutaneous, or intradermal route.

Parenteral nutrition (PN) A nutritional formula administered through a central or peripheral intravenous catheter. In the clinical setting, the term parenteral nutrition may be used interchangeably with the term hyperalimentation.

Partial parenteral nutrition A nutritional alternative to total parenteral nutrition that is usually administered through a peripheral intravenous access device or a peripherally inserted central catheter. It is used for clients who are still able to eat but are not able to take in enough nutrients to meet their needs.

Passive immunity A form of acquired immunity that occurs artificially through injection or is acquired naturally as the result of antibody transfer through the placenta to a fetus or through colostrum to an infant; is not permanent and does not last as long as active immunity.

Percussion A physical data collection technique that involves tapping the body to assess the size, borders, and consistency of some organs and to assess for the presence of fluid within body cavities. Direct percussion is performed by striking the fingers directly on the body surface. Indirect percussion is performed by striking a finger of one hand on a finger of the other hand as it is placed on the body surface, such as over an organ.

Perinatal nursing practice Perinatal nurses provide nursing care to women during pregnancy, childbirth, and postpartum. These nurses are sometimes referred to as obstetrical nurses or prenatal nurses and work in both inpatient and outpatient settings, including the private practices of midwives or obstetricians, hospitals, birth centers, or community health centers.

Perioperative nursing Nursing care given before (preoperative), during (intraoperative), and after (postoperative) surgery.

Peristalsis Wave-like rhythmic contractions that propel material through the gastrointestinal tract.

Phlebitis An inflammation of the vein that can occur from mechanical or chemical (medication) trauma or from a local infection.

Phosphorus (phosphate) Needed for generation of bony tissue. It functions in the metabolism of glucose and lipids, in the maintenance of acid-base balance, and in the storage and transfer of energy from one site in the body to another. Phosphorus levels are evaluated in relation to calcium levels because of their inverse relationship; when calcium levels are decreased, phosphorus levels are increased, and when phosphorus levels are decreased, calcium levels are increased. The normal adult level is 3.0 to 4.5 mg/dL.

Physical hazard Any situation or event that places the client at risk for accident, injury, or death.

Placenta Organ that provides for the exchange of nutrients and waste products between the fetus and the mother and produces hormones to maintain pregnancy. The placenta develops by the third month of gestation. Also called afterbirth.

Plasma The watery, straw-colored, fluid part of lymph and the blood in which the formed elements (blood cells) are suspended. Plasma is made up of water, electrolytes, protein, glucose, fats, bilirubin, and gases and is essential for carrying the cellular elements of the blood through the circulation.

Platelet transfusion A blood product administered to clients with a low platelet count and to thrombocytopenic clients who are bleeding actively or are scheduled for an invasive procedure.

Play An activity that is spontaneous or organized and provides entertainment or diversion. It is a part of childhood that is necessary for the development of a normal personality and social, physical, and intellectual skills.

Pneumothorax The accumulation of atmospheric air in the pleural space caused by a rupture in the visceral or parietal pleura. The loss of negative intrapleural pressure results in collapse of the lung. Diagnosis of pneumothorax is made by chest radiography.

Poison Any substance that impairs health or destroys life when ingested, inhaled, or otherwise absorbed by the body.

Polypharmacy Taking multiple prescription and/or over-the-counter medications together.

Portal hypertension A persistent increase in pressure within the portal vein that develops as a result of obstruction to flow.

Postural (orthostatic) hypotension A blood pressure decrease of more than 10 to 15 mm Hg of the systolic pressure or a decrease of more than 10 mm Hg of the diastolic pressure and a 10% to 20% increase in heart rate. Postural hypotension occurs when the client's blood pressure is not maintained adequately when moving from a lying to a sitting or standing position.

Potassium A principal electrolyte of intracellular fluid and the primary buffer within the cell itself. It is needed for nerve conduction, muscle function, acid-base balance, and osmotic pressure. Along with calcium and magnesium, potassium controls the rate and force of contraction of the heart and thus cardiac output. The normal adult level is 3.5 to 5.0 mEq/L.

Preload The volume of blood stretching the left ventricle at the end of diastole. Preload is determined by the total circulating blood volume and is increased by an increase in venous return to the heart.

Presbycusis Gradual nerve degeneration associated with aging; a common cause of sensorineural hearing loss.

Pressure injury Area of tissue damage that occurs as a result of skin and underlying soft tissue compression from pressure between a surface and a bony prominence.

Prioritizing Deciding which needs or problems require immediate action and which ones could tolerate a delay in action until a later time because they are not urgent.

Prodromal Pertaining to early symptoms that mark the onset of a disease.

Prone position The client is lying on the abdomen with the head turned to the side.

Puberty The period of time during which the adolescent experiences a growth spurt, develops secondary sex characteristics, and achieves reproductive maturity.

Pulse pressure The difference between the systolic and diastolic pressure. Normal pulse pressure is 30 to 40 mm Hg.

Pyelonephritis An inflammation of the renal pelvis and the parenchyma, commonly caused by bacterial invasion.

Pyloroplasty Enlarging the pylorus to prevent or decrease pyloric obstruction, thereby enhancing gastric emptying.

Quickening Maternal perception of fetal movement for the first time, occurring usually in the 16th to 20th week of pregnancy.

Race A grouping of people based on biological similarities; members of a racial group may have similar physical characteristics, such as blood group; facial features; and color of skin, hair, and eyes.

Racism Discrimination directed toward individuals or groups who are perceived to be inferior.

Reduction Correction or realignment of a bone fracture or joint dislocation.

Regurgitation An abnormal backward flow of body fluid.

Respiratory acidosis A total concentration of buffer base that is lower than normal, with a relative increase in hydrogen ion concentration; thus, a greater number of hydrogen ions is circulating in the blood than the buffer system can absorb. This is caused by primary defects in the function of the lungs or by changes in normal respiratory patterns as a result of secondary problems. Any condition that causes an obstruction of the airway or depresses respiratory status can cause respiratory acidosis.

Respiratory alkalosis A deficit of carbonic acid or a decrease in hydrogen ion concentration that results from the accumulation of base or from a loss of acid without a comparable loss of base in the body fluids. This occurs in conditions that cause overstimulation of the respiratory system.

Restraints (security/safety devices) Physical restraints include any manual method or mechanical device, material, or equipment that inhibits free movement. Chemical restraints include the administration of medications for the specific purpose of inhibiting a specific behavior or movement.

Retraction An abnormal movement of the chest wall during inspiration in which the skin appears to be drawn in between the ribs, and above and/or below the clavicle, and scapula; indicates respiratory difficulty.

Reverse Trendelenburg position The entire bed is tilted so that the client's foot of the bed is down. Position in which the lower extremities are low and the body and head are elevated on an inclined plane.

Rh factor Rh stands for rhesus factor. A person having the factor is Rh positive; a person lacking the factor is Rh negative. The presence or absence of Rh antigens on the surface of red blood cells determines the classification as Rh positive or Rh negative.

Safety measures Interventions that ensure protection of the client and the prevention of an accident or injury.

Sarcoma Neoplasm that originates from muscle, bone, fat, the lymph system, or connective tissue.

Seclusion Placing a client alone in a specially designed room that protects the client and allows for close supervision. Seclusion is the last selected measure in a process to maximize safety for the client and others.

Self-neglect The choice to avoid medical care or other services that could improve optimal function. Unless declared legally incompetent, an individual has the right to refuse care.

Semi-Fowler's position (low Fowler's) The client is supine and the head of the bed is elevated about 30 to 45 degrees.

Sensorineural hearing loss A pathological process of the inner ear or of the sensory fibers that lead to the cerebral cortex. Such hearing loss often is permanent and measures must be taken to reduce further damage or to attempt to amplify sound as a means of improving hearing to some degree.

Septicemia The presence of infective agents or their toxins in the bloodstream. Septicemia is a serious infection and must be treated promptly; otherwise, the infection leads to circulatory collapse, profound shock, and death.

Serum The clear and thin fluid part of blood that remains after coagulation. Serum contains no blood cells, platelets, or fibrinogen.

Shunt Movement of blood or body fluid through an abnormal anatomical or surgically created opening.

Sims' position The client is lying on the side with the body turned prone at 45 degrees. The lower leg is extended, with the upper leg flexed at the hip and knee to a 45- to 90-degree angle.

Skin cancer A malignant lesion of the skin that may or may not metastasize.

Smoke inhalation injury Respiratory injury that occurs as a result of inhalation of products of combustion during a fire.

Sodium An abundant electrolyte that maintains osmotic pressure and acid-base balance and transmits nerve impulses. The normal adult level is 135 to 145 mEq/L.

Somogyi phenomenon A rebound phenomenon that occurs in clients with type 1 diabetes mellitus. Normal or elevated blood glucose levels are present at bedtime; hypoglycemia occurs at about 2:00 a.m. to 3:00 a.m. Counterregulatory hormones, produced to prevent further hypoglycemia, result in hyperglycemia (evident in the prebreakfast blood glucose level). Treatment includes decreasing the evening (predinner or bedtime) dose of intermediate-acting insulin or increasing the bedtime snack.

Spinal shock Also known as spinal shock syndrome. It is a complete but temporary loss of motor, sensory, reflex, and autonomic function that occurs soon after the injury as the cord's response to the injury.

Spirituality A broad concept that may have different perspectives for individuals. It can relate to religious beliefs and values and to the soul or human spirit, rather than to material and physical things.

Staging A method of classifying malignancies on the basis of the presence and extent of the tumor within the body.

Standard precautions Guidelines used by all health care providers for all clients to reduce the risk of infection for clients and caregivers.

Stenosis The narrowing or constriction of an opening.

Stereotyping Expectation that all people within the same racial, ethnic, or cultural group act alike and share the same beliefs and attitudes.

Stretch receptors Nerve endings located in the vena cava and the right atrium that respond to pressure changes affecting circulatory blood volume. When the blood pressure decreases because of hypovolemia, a sympathetic response occurs, causing an increased heart rate and blood vessel constriction. When the blood pressure increases because of hypervolemia, an opposite effect occurs.

Stridor A shrill, harsh sound heard during inspiration, expiration, or both, produced by the flow of air through a narrowed segment of the respiratory tract.

Stroke volume The amount of blood ejected from the left ventricle with each contraction. The normal stroke volume is 70 to 130 mL/heartbeat. The stroke volume can be affected by preload, afterload, contractility, and the Frank-Starling law.

Subcultures Social group within a culture that has distinctive characteristics, such as patterns of behavior or beliefs.

Subjective data Information obtained from the client during the history-taking process. It is what the client says about himself or herself.

Suctioning A sterile procedure involving the removal of respiratory secretions that accumulate in the tracheobronchial airway when the client is unable to expectorate secretions; performed to maintain a patent airway.

Suicide The ultimate act of self-destruction in which an individual purposefully ends his or her own life.

Suicide attempt Any willful, self-inflicted, or life-threatening attempt by an individual that has not led to death.

Superficial partial-thickness burn Involves injury to the upper third of the dermis; an adequate blood supply remains.

Superficial-thickness burn Involves injury to the epidermis; cells and membranes needed for total regrowth remain.

Supine position The client is lying on her or his back. The head and shoulders are usually slightly elevated (depending on the client's condition) with a small pillow. The arms and legs are extended, and the legs are slightly abducted.

Surfactant Phospholipid that is necessary to keep the fetal lung alveoli from collapsing; amount is usually sufficient after 32 weeks' gestation.

Syndrome of inappropriate antidiuretic hormone The hypersecretion of antidiuretic hormone from the posterior pituitary gland resulting in increased intravascular volume, serum hypoosmolality, and dilutional hyponatremia.

Systole The phase of contraction of the heart, especially of the ventricles, during which blood is forced into the aorta and pulmonary artery.

Systolic pressure The maximum pressure of blood exerted against the artery walls when the heart contracts.

Thyroid storm An acute, potentially fatal exacerbation of hyperthyroidism that may result from manipulation of the thyroid gland during surgery, severe infection, or stress.

Thyroidectomy Surgical removal of the thyroid gland; may be done to treat persistent hyperthyroidism or thyroid tumors.

Total parenteral nutrition A nutritional solution administered through either a peripherally inserted central catheter or the subclavian or internal jugular veins via a central line. It is used when the client requires intensive nutritional support for an extended period of time.

Tracheostomy An opening made surgically directly into the trachea to establish an airway. A tracheostomy tube is inserted into the opening and the tube attaches to the mechanical ventilator or another type of oxygen delivery device.

Traction Exertion of a pulling force to a fractured bone or dislocated joint to establish and maintain correct alignment for healing and to decrease muscle spasms and pain.

Trade name Also known as the proprietary or brand name of a medication. The trade name is the name under which a medication is marketed. A medication can have many trade names; therefore, trade names must be approved by the US Food and Drug Administration (FDA) to ensure that no two trade names are alike. Trade names may be used in clinical practice settings but will not likely be identified in a medication question on the NCLEX®.

Transfusion reaction A hemolytic reaction caused by blood type or Rh incompatibility. An allergic transfusion reaction most often occurs in clients with a history of an allergy. A febrile transfusion reaction most commonly occurs in clients with antibodies directed against the transfused white blood cells. A bacterial transfusion reaction occurs after transfusion of contaminated blood products.

Transmission-based precautions Guidelines used in addition to standard precautions for specific syndromes that are highly suggestive of specific infections until a diagnosis is confirmed.

Trendelenburg position The entire bed frame is tilted so that the client's head of the bed is low and the body and legs are elevated. This position is contraindicated in clients with head injuries, increased intracranial pressure, spinal cord injuries, and certain respiratory and cardiac disorders.

Triage Classifying procedure that ranks clients according to their need for medical care.

Trousseau's sign A sign of hypocalcemia. Carpal spasm can be elicited by compressing the brachial artery with a blood pressure cuff for 3 minutes.

Tuberculin skin test (TST) Test used to determine infection with tuberculosis. The TST is performed by injecting 0.1 mL of tuberculin purified protein derivative (PPD) intradermally in the forearm. The skin test reaction is read between 48 and 72 hours later. The reaction is measured in millimeters of the induration (raised, hardened area).

Tuberculosis A highly communicable disease caused by *Mycobacterium tuberculosis,* an acid-fast rod bacterium. Tuberculosis is transmitted by the airborne route via droplet infection.

Tumor marker Substances that are produced by cancer or by normal cells of the body in response to cancer or certain benign (noncancerous) conditions.

Turner's sign A gray-blue discoloration of the flanks seen in acute hemorrhagic pancreatitis.

Ulcerative colitis Ulcerative and inflammatory disease of the bowel that results in poor absorption of nutrients. Acute ulcerative colitis results in vascular congestion, hemorrhage, edema, and ulceration of the bowel mucosa. Chronic ulcerative colitis causes muscular hypertrophy, fat deposits, and fibrous tissue with bowel thickening, shortening, and narrowing.

Unconscious client A state of depressed cerebral functioning with unresponsiveness to sensory and motor function. Causes include head trauma, cerebral toxins, shock, hemorrhage, tumor, or infection.

Undifferentiated cells Cells that have lost the capacity for specialized functions.

Unilateral neglect An inability to recognize a physical impairment on one side of the body. Also known as neglect syndrome.

Unit A measurement of a medication in terms of its action, not its physical weight.

Urolithiasis The formation of urinary stones or calculi. Urinary calculi are formed in the ureter.

Uterus Organ located behind the symphysis pubis, between the bladder and the rectum. It has 4 parts: fundus (upper part), corpus (body), isthmus (lower segment), and cervix.

Vaccine A suspension of attenuated or killed microorganisms administered to induce active immunity against an infectious disease.

Vagina Tubular structure located behind the bladder and in front of the rectum; it extends from the cervix to the vaginal opening in the perineum. It functions as the outflow tract for menstrual fluid and for vaginal and cervical secretions, as the birth canal, and as the organ for coitus.

Vagotomy Surgical division of the vagus nerve to eliminate the vagal impulses that stimulate hydrochloric acid secretion in the stomach.

Venipuncture Puncture into a vein to obtain a blood specimen for testing; the antecubital veins are the veins of choice because of ease of access.

Venous pressure The force exerted by the blood against the vein walls. Normal venous pressures are highest in the extremities (5–14 cm H_2O in the arm), and lowest closest to the heart (6–8 cm H_2O in the inferior vena cava).

Veracity An ethical principle; the responsibility and obligation to tell the truth.

Warfare agent Biological or chemical substance that can cause mass destruction or fatality.

Wheezing High-pitched musical whistle sounds heard with or without a stethoscope as air is compressed through narrowed or obstructed airways because of swelling, secretions, or tumors.

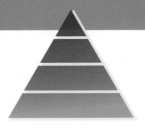

Index

Note: Page numbers followed by *b*, *t*, and *f* indicate boxes, tables, and figures, respectively.